Geriatric Medicine

Second Edition

Geriatric Medicine

Second Edition

Edited by
Christine K. Cassel
Donald E. Riesenberg
Leif B. Sorensen
John R. Walsh

With a Foreword by Robert N. Butler

With 150 Figures in 172 Parts, 28 in Full Color

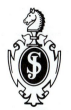

Springer-Verlag
New York Berlin Heidelberg
London Paris Tokyo Hong Kong

CHRISTINE K. CASSEL, M.D.
Chief, Section of General Internal Medicine
The University of Chicago Medical Center
Chicago, Illinois 60637, U.S.A.

DONALD E. RIESENBERG, M.D.
Senior Editor, Journal of the American
    Medical Association
Chicago, Illinois 60610, U.S.A.
and
Clinical Associate Professor of Medicine
Pritzker School of Medicine
University of Chicago
Chicago, Illinois 60637, U.S.A.

LEIF B. SORENSEN, M.D., PH.D.
Associate Chief, Department of Medicine
Pritzker School of Medicine
University of Chicago
Chicago, Illinois 60637, U.S.A.

JOHN R. WALSH, M.D.
Chief, Geriatric Medicine
Portland V.A. Medical Center
Portland, Oregon 97207, U.S.A.

Library of Congress Cataloging-in-Publication Data
Geriatric medicine / Christine K. Cassel . . . [et al.], editors. –
    2nd ed.
        p.   cm.
    Includes bibliographical references.
    ISBN 0-387-96977-2 (alk. paper)
    1. Geriatrics.   I. Cassel, Christine K.
    [DNLM: 1. Geriatrics.   WT 100 G36635]
    RC952.G393   1990
    618.97 – dc20
    DNLM/DLC
    for Library of Congress   89-21932

Printed on acid-free paper

© 1984, 1990 Springer-Verlag New York Inc.

Copyright is not claimed for Chapter 50 by Dr. Robert L. Kane.

Dr. Neil M. Resnick's chapter "Urinary Incontinence" is also appearing in Katzman and Rowe, eds., *Geriatric Neurology*, to be published by F.A. Davis.

Typeset by TCSystems, Shippensburg, Pennsylvania.
Printed and bound by Arcata Graphics/Halliday, West Hanover, Massachusetts.
Printed in the United States of America.

9 8 7 6 5 4 3 2 1

ISBN 0-387-96977-2 Springer-Verlag New York Berlin Heidelberg
ISBN 3-540-96977-2 Springer-Verlag Berlin Heidelberg New York

To our parents and grandparents

Foreword to Second Edition

The Second Edition of this outstanding textbook is further evidence that the field of geriatrics has made great strides; indeed, has come of age. The broad scope of this volume shapes a substantial answer to the question, "What is geriatrics and why should we be interested in it?" As I see it, there are at least five reasons.

First, the scientific or intellectual reason: gerontology is the study of aging from the biologic, psychological, and social perspectives. There is increasing interest in the fascinating insights into the biologic mechanisms of aging, free radical damage, failed cellular disposal, DNA repair mechanisms, alterations of the neuroendocrine system, changes in the immune system, genetic controls, and somatic mutations.

Second, the demographic reason: this is the century of old age. There has been a 26 year gain in the average life expectancy. This gain compares with that acquired from 3,000 years B.C. (the Bronze Age) to the year 1900, which was about 29 years. Therefore, in one century there has been a gain in the average life expectancy almost equal to 5,000 previous years of human history.

In 1830, one of three newborn infants survived beyond 60 years of age. Today 8 of 10 newborn babies are expected to live a full life. In 1870, only 44 of 100 women who did not die of scarlet fever, diphtheria, chicken pox, or other diseases, and who survived to 15 years of age, enjoyed what we take for granted as the natural course of human life today. In 1920, a 10-year-old child had about a 40 percent chance of having two of his or her four grandparents alive. At present, that probability is over 80 percent. From birth, women today will outlive men by nearly 8 years. This is a mixed blessing, because many of the problems of age are the special problems of women.

Third, the epidemiologic reason: the high incidence and prevalence of disease and disabilities with age is striking. There are "diseases of affluence," the consequence of life long exposure to unhealthy life styles, such as high fat diets and sedentary living. Certain diseases pose "silent epidemics," which rise with the aging population. One, senile dementia of the Alzheimer's type probably is the fourth leading cause of death; yet, it has received significant attention only recently. Another, osteoporosis, is unknown to 80 percent of the public according to one survey, but it is one of the main causes of disability. Along with senile dementia of the Alzheimer's type, osteoporosis is one of the true scourges of old age. These are only two examples of the kinds of medical disorders that affect great numbers of people advanced in age and that, nonetheless, have, until recently, attracted little research attention. These are frontiers of scientific knowledge that are now responding to inquiry and experimentation.

Fourth, the health costs: In 1988, about 11.2 percent of the gross national product, or some $500 billion, was spent on health care; some $90 billion on Medicare and Medicaid, largely but not exclusively for elderly persons. Of all health costs, 30 percent are associated with persons over 65 years of age; 40 percent of all Medicaid funds go to nursing homes. There are about 20,000 nursing homes in the United States, in which about 1.5 million people reside; 1.4 million are over 65 years of age. On any given day, there are more patients in nursing homes than there are in hospitals. Attempts to contain costs thus often focus on the elderly population. Considerations of health care policy are a critical part of effective, prudent, and humane geriatric practice.

Fifth, attitude: negativism toward old age. In my medical school days, I was offended by the use of the word "crock" and other insensitive epithets. These attitudes are deep, widespread, and undoubtedly part of the evident resistance to the development of geriatrics in our institutions of health care. Changing these negative attitudes requires more than exhortation. It requires developing a sense of competence in handling the clinical problems of elderly persons, a working knowledge of the social, economic, and institutional barriers to respectful treatment and how to change them, and the intellectual background to meet ethical issues with both analytic and humanistic skills.

Geriatrics clearly is a topic of great complexity and breadth. Some 40 to 50 percent of the time of most internists, family practitioners, and surgeons already is devoted to the diagnosis, treatment, and care of older persons. The field of geriatrics demands more than attention to biology. It requires a greater appreciation of the social and psychological forces that operate within us. In medical education, we emphasize the search for a single explanation in the diagnostic evaluation of a patient. We refer to a medieval philosopher, William Occam, and his "razor." He is said to have propounded the principle of searching for a single explanation to any complex group of symptoms. This has been a cardinal principle of differential diagnosis. Yet, the multiplicity of illnesses, their complexity, associated polypharmacy, the disguise of one disease by another, and the effect of the age of the host in altering the presentation and the course of diseases all must change our reasoning. Multiple interacting disorders are more likely than a single diagnosis to explain the problems of elderly persons. The same factors also may change the character of treatment response.

The future of medicine is coupled with the "graying of America" and "the triumph of survivorship." We will have 55 million people over 65 years of age in the range of the years 2020–2030. We see government and business engaged in increasing efforts at cost containment and regulation, as well as the growth of corporate medicine. It is possible that physicians will take a distant third place to business and government in the conduct of health delivery. Thus, understanding the social, political, and economic realities of health care systems is essential to a geriatrician as well as the physician in general.

In geriatrics, we stress the team, the collaboration of physicians, nurses, social workers, and other professionals. We stress the importance of assessing function and, even more importantly, maintaining and improving function. We can no longer depend on brief, mechanistic, overly economical, and, therefore, superficial forms of assessment. Older patients in contemporary hospitals deteriorate because they often are neglected after their acute episode has been treated. There frequently are no efforts toward continuing function, even ambulation. There should be signals that herald discharge planning at the very moment of admission. Hospitals and physicians should be prepared to respond on an urgent basis with rehabilitative and other restorative efforts when a high-risk older person is in a medical crisis. They should also be prepared to respond with common sense and compassion when there is nothing more that can be done realistically and death is at hand.

Charcot, the great French physician, one century ago said, "The importance of a special study of the diseases of old age would not be contested at the present time." However, it has taken time. An American physician, Ignatz Nascher, introduced the term "geriatrics" just after the turn of the century. In Great Britain in the late 1930s, a unique physician,

Marjorie Warren, took leadership in the development of geriatrics. In 1976, the National Institute of Aging inaugurated a Geriatric Medicine Academic Award. It also sponsored the Institute of Medicine, National Academy of Sciences, special task force under the leadership of Paul B. Beeson to study "aging and medical education." This report concurs with most leaders in geriatrics in not promoting a primary care practice specialty to which patients would be referred at some arbitrary age. However, most leaders in geriatrics do favor the creation of an academic specialty to ensure that there will be new ideas and innovations in diagnosis and treatment, as well as critical leadership in research and education. This specialty must represent a broad range of knowledge rather than a focused one, which is characteristic of other kinds of specialties. Both the American Board of Internal Medicine and the American Academy of Family Practice, fortunately, have established examinations for added qualification in geriatrics.

Not long ago, there were those who objected that geriatrics did not possess a distinct body of knowledge. This book demonstrates the falseness of that statement, containing work concerning the fundamentals of geriatric care, biomedicine, and psychiatry. It highlights the fact that geriatrics is distinct in the breadth of its concern rather than being a more narrow definition of a specialty. The goal of this unique book is to integrate biomedical and psychosocial information with the perspectives of ethics and social policy. This volume provides the basic information that most medical textbooks do not have, for example, on such topics as law and the role of rehabilitation medicine. All of these perspectives and data bases are necessary to achieve excellence in clinical practice and to foster the further evolution of this expanding field.

ROBERT N. BUTLER, M.D.

Preface to Second Edition

"The body immures the mind within a fortress; presently on all sides the fortress is besieged and in the end, inevitably, the mind has to surrender."*

Proust's poetic lament characterizes most people's attitudes towards aging—The "inevitable surrender of the mind." We now understand that not all the declines of aging are so inevitable, and just as importantly, we have better skills in caring for those declines we cannot prevent. Indeed, the siege of the body and surrender of the mind rank among modern medicine's greatest concerns. Because of the unprecedented growth, in developed countries, of the number and proportion of elderly persons, geriatrics now has taken its place among the distinct medical disciplines. Its purview goes even beyond mind and body, to include also society and to examine questions of values and meaning. We offer this second edition of *Geriatric Medicine* in response to continuing refinement of the art and science of medical care for older persons.

The years since publication of the first edition have seen unparalleled advances in geriatric medicine. Examples include the development of sophisticated diagnostic categories of urinary incontinence, resulting in better understanding of a condition that afflicts half of all people in nursing homes; clarification of the epidemiologic patterns of osteoporosis and falls, which, together, account for the excess burden (both morbidity and mortality) of fractures borne by elderly persons; the elucidation of discrete genetic patterns and neuropathological changes as they relate to certain forms of dementia; increasing visibility and importance of home care and of rehabilitation; and court decisions and institutional policies about end of life decisions that are prompting important and intense public discussion. Such progress foretells therapeutic and policy advances, some of which are nearing the horizon already.

Equally dramatic has been the academic maturation of geriatric medicine. Over three-fourths of all U.S. medical schools are now affiliated with long-term care institutions. One hundred twenty-five geriatrics fellowship programs were active as of 1987. Program directors can take pride in the fact that over 90 percent of their graduates who took the 1988 examination for certification of Added Qualifications in Geriatric Medicine passed, while other examinees did distinctly less well.

---

*Marcel Proust, *Remembrance of Things Past*.

That examination, itself a benchmark for the field of geriatric medicine, was administered jointly by The American Board of Internal Medicine and the American Board of Family Practice, bespeaking the primary-care nature of the field and codifying its distinct body of knowledge.

All of these events seemed to demand a second edition of this textbook, which we have focused into a single volume from the original two, a task that required doubling the number of editors. We have not eliminated topics by moving to one volume, but have focused better the rich tapestry of different disciplines that comprise the theoretical and clinical basis of geriatrics. This text combines traditional medical topics with the psychological, social, and ethical issues that are no less a part of the geriatrician's domain. In weaving this tapestry, it was inevitable that there be overlappings of one discipline into another. We believe that such duplication, rather than being redundant, is appropriate in a comprehensive resource. The areas of overlap provide differing perspectives on the same topic and will enrich the reader's understanding in the process. Extensive indexing and cross-referencing guide those seeking these different perspectives.

Medicine finds itself enmeshed in fierce debate about its very fabric. The cost and logic of ever increasing technological capabilities demand difficult choices. Nowhere are those choices confronted more frequently or more poignantly than in geriatrics, where a thorough understanding of technologies must go hand in hand with a discerning sense of judgement. The geriatrician is called upon to take seriously the role of patient advocate in all its meanings, no small act of courage. So the geriatric imperative is just that: growing numbers of older patients require competence, compassion, and judgement of their physicians.

For a project such as this, it is impossible to acknowledge adequately all those who helped. As with the first edition, the effort has resulted in a spirit of communal scholarship. During the three years of work, innumerable persons have contributed unqualified support. At Springer-Verlag, Shelley Reinhardt and Robin Brown ensured the soundness of the final product by their professionalism and encouragement. Juliann Lundell Tarsney and Kathleen Heller lent their considerable scholarship to the copyediting process. And Lois Danker and Joyce Eberhardt successfully managed the trafficking of manuscripts between busy universities throughout the country.

The contributors to this volume, who represent the very best that our discipline has to offer, have given freely of their time and expertise. We the editors thank them especially and proudly offer the second edition of *Geriatric Medicine* as a testimony to their excellence.

CHRISTINE K. CASSEL, M.D.
DONALD E. RIESENBERG, M.D.
LEIF B. SORENSEN, M.D., PH.D.
JOHN R. WALSH, M.D.

Preface to First Edition

"Old age ain't for sissies" *

In the last decade, two developments have changed the practice of medicine: the aging of the population and the dominance of medical technology. Both medical education and medical practice have responded to these events. Aging, chronic illness, and long-term care now are frequently written about in medical journals. Advances in diagnostic and therapeutic technologies have out-stripped our ability to evaluate or to pay for the new services. The field of geriatric medicine is a response to the first development and a reaction to the second.

The medical response to the demographic imperative of aging has been to codify a field of medical specialization that is relevant and useful to the increasing numbers of elderly persons. The reaction is to emphasize a broadly comprehensive, humane, and personal approach to patient care. There no longer is any doubt that there exists a body of scientific knowledge, which characterizes the field of geriatrics. In addition to a distinct body of knowledge, most geriatricians also will describe a special approach and philosophy that characterizes the practice of geriatrics. There is a growing awareness in academic medicine that special knowledge, skills, and attitudes are needed to deal effectively with elderly patients, particularly very old or frail patients. However, many physicians in primary care specialties such as internal medicine, family practice, and general surgery claim (and accurately so) that they function as geriatricians because many of their patients are elderly. In fact, in many instances, clinical practices of these generalists predominantly consist of elderly patients. Even with the advent of full-time geriatricians, the proportion of elderly persons in general practice populations will increase within the next 2 decades.

Both viewpoints are correct. Geriatrics is a specialty and also an essential component of almost any clinical practice. It is true that many physicians, especially those in primary care settings, will have a large proportion of elderly patients in their practice and (to a certain extent) will be practicing geriatrics. Until recently, most graduate training programs in medicine, family practice, or psychiatry did not include special consideration of geriatrics. Many physicians have learned some of the practical information on their own; however, the body of knowledge referred to in the recent Institute of Medicine report

---

*Moore, H: Sayings, in Alvarez J, Oldham P (eds): *Old Age Ain't For Sissies*.

and the theoretic and scientific progress in this field has not been generally accessible.†
It also is true that we have, in the last 5 years in the United States, codified a specialty of
geriatrics that includes training programs in geriatric medicine at the fellowship level.
Many of the graduates of these programs will assume academic roles and bring the content
of geriatrics to all relevant areas of health care education.

In these volumes, we have tried to assemble the material in a way that is useful for both
practicing clinicians and physicians-in-training, especially those who have selected training in geriatrics. In addition, this text is meant to be a comprehensive resource for a practitioner who needs information for the clinical demands of the moment. For a research
scientist or physician in advanced training, there is an introduction to the theoretical basis
of each subject and a substantial bibliography. We hope that, in this way, these volumes
also will provide access to the new areas of research and the new understandings that are
now emerging.

Because we attempt to bring together in one place the full content of geriatric medicine,
this work is deliberately compendious. Geriatrics has a broad basis; it includes clinical
medicine, humanities, and the social sciences. Also, *Geriatric Medicine* accordingly has
several sections organized into two volumes. The division into two volumes is primarily in
the interest of the reader's convenience and, thus, inevitably somewhat arbitrary. Nonetheless, our underlying concept is that the biological, the psychosocial, and the philosophical
are essential parts of a single whole. We have called on a large number of contributors, in
many different fields, to assure that the subject matter is treated authoritatively.

Aging is an important and exciting area of biomedical research, which is represented
largely in Volume I. The diseases that are the greatest scourges of old age are principally
the chronic and degenerative disorders such as osteoporosis, parkinsonism, stroke,
Alzheimer's disease, osteoarthritis, and peripheral vascular disease. Until recently, the
level of research activity into the causes and treatments of these disorders has been
markedly inadequate when measured against the numbers of people who are afflicted and
the costs—both financial and humanitarian—to our society. However, there are areas of
knowledge and research outside of biomedicine that also are critical to progress in geriatrics. These include disciplines that are based in social sciences and humanities, rather
than in biology and medicine. Health services research and bioethics are especially important to geriatrics. A geriatrician may need to emulate the Renaissance scholar. The body
of knowledge is broad and its relevance is undeniable.

Geriatrics is unique as a medical specialty, because it is broader, rather than narrower,
than the parent disciplines. An effective clinician must have some grasp of social gerontology, architectural design, law, psychology and psychiatry, spiritual counseling, health
policy and health care economics, interprofessional sociology, epidemiology, and philosophical ethics to claim a firm competence in the care of elderly persons. For this reason,
much of Volume II is devoted to chapters that are written by experts in these fields. These
authors provide information that is both practical and relevant to clinicians, and that also
may encourage a deeper exploration of this field.

The breadth of subjects covered in these two volumes is a demonstration of the need for
interdisciplinary practice in geriatrics and gerontology. No one person can be an expert in
each of these areas. Yet, each subject will be relevant to the needs of an elderly patient at
one time or another. It is important for a geriatrician to be able to work effectively with
other health care providers as well as with social scientists and policymakers, and to know
where his or her own limits have been surpassed and where consultation is necessary. For
appropriate and effective consultation, one must have a basic understanding of the sphere
of knowledge of consultants.

The theoretical and clinical basis of geriatrics is a rich tapestry of different disciplines.
In weaving this tapestry, it was inevitable that there would be overlappings and crossings
of one discipline into another. The reader occasionally may find material that is appar-

---

† Institute of Medicine: *Aging and Medical Education*. National Academy of Sciences, Washington,
DC, 1978.

ently redundant from one chapter to another. We feel that such duplication is appropriate in a comprehensive resource text such as this. In most cases, the areas of overlap will provide a different perspective on the same topic and will enrich the understanding of the reader in the process. We hope that the indexing and cross-referencing will provide guidance to those who are specifically seeking these different perspectives.

For a project of this magnitude, it is impossible to adequately acknowledge all those who helped. It has been a project of many rewards, both in the content and meaning of the work itself and in the expanding community of scholarship and advocacy. From inception to completion, this project has taken 3 years. During this time, innumerable persons have contributed significant support. The staff of Springer-Verlag has given us stimulating concepts and good ideas, in addition to steadfast sensible guidance. The details of organizing, phone-calling, letter-writing, library research, and manuscript preparation cannot be overemphasized in a work of this size and complexity. Special acknowledgment in these areas is due to Pamela Beere Briggs and Carol Saatzer. We also acknowledge the generous support of the Henry J. Kaiser Family Foundation.

We are aware that we have joined the beginning of a very important process. The profession of medicine is at a turning point; it is caught between the successes of scientific and technologic progress and concerns about the rising costs of care and the depersonalization of its delivery. Patients—disaffected, frustrated, and often in real need—are caught in between these unresolved issues. The moral center of the profession is at risk in the policy debates. An understanding of geriatrics requires competent familiarity with the capabilities of the latest in medical technology, a discerning sense of judgment about when and when not to use such interventions, and the courage and energy to take seriously the social role of advocate for a patient. The complexity, richness, and mystery of aging cannot be described better than it has been by T.S. Eliot in *East Coker:*

> Home is where one starts from. As we grow older
> The world becomes stranger, the pattern more complicated
> Of dead and living. Not the intense moment
> Isolated, with no before and after,
> But a lifetime burning in every moment
> And not the lifetime of one man only
> But of old stones that cannot be deciphered.

We choose to view the challenge posed by the geriatric imperative not as a burden, but as an opportunity for medicine to restructure its priorities and to respond to the real needs of modern society. Geriatrics can be a vehicle for returning the values of compassion, moderation, and moral judgment to both medicine and scientific progress. These volumes, in themselves, will not create the complete clinician, but they can provide the groundwork for the excellence that is possible in geriatrics. That excellence not only is possible, but it is a duty we owe to our patients, our profession, our society, and—in the final analysis—to ourselves.

CHRISTINE K. CASSEL, M.D.
JOHN R. WALSH, M.D.

Contents

NEUROLOGIC AND PSYCHIATRIC DISORDERS

COMMON PROBLEMS IN ELDERLY PERSONS

Contributors

Marilyn S. Albert, Ph.D.
Professor of Psychiatry and Neurology, Massachusetts General Hospital, Harvard Medical School, Boston, Massachusetts 02114, U.S.A.

Sharon Anderson, M.D.
Assistant Professor of Medicine, Department of Medicine, Harvard Medical School, Boston, Massachusetts 02114; Associate Physician, Renal Division, Brigham and Women's Hospital, Boston, Massachusetts 02115, U.S.A.

Jerry Avorn, M.D.
Associate Professor of Social Medicine, Harvard Medical School, Boston, Massachusetts 02114; Attending Physician, Gerontology Division, Beth Israel Hospital, Boston, Massachusetts 02115, U.S.A.

Dan G. Blazer II, M.D., Ph.D.
Professor of Psychiatry, Director, Affective Disorders Program, Duke University Medical Center, Durham, North Carolina 27706, U.S.A.

Jacob A. Brody, M.D.
Dean, School of Public Health, University of Illinois at Chicago, Chicago, Illinois 60680, U.S.A.

Robert A. Bruce, M.D.
Professor Emeritus, Department of Medicine, University of Washington; University Hospital, Seattle, Washington 98195, U.S.A.

Kenneth Brummel-Smith, M.D.
Associate Professor of Family Medicine, University of Southern California School of Medicine, Los Angeles, California 90007; Co-Chief, Clinical Gerontology Service, Rehabilitation Research and Training Center on Aging, Ranchos Los Amigos Medical Center, Downey, California 90242, U.S.A.

Edith A. Burns, M.D.
Assistant Professor, Department of Geriatrics, University of Wisconsin, School of Medicine, Milwaukee Clinical Campus, Milwaukee, Wisconsin 53211; Attending Physician, Sinai-Samaritan Geriatrics Institute, Milwaukee, Wisconsin 53233, U.S.A.

Robert N. Butler, M.D.
Chair, Department of Geriatrics and Adult Development, Mount Sinai Medical Center, New York, New York 10029, U.S.A.

Louis Caplan, M.D.
Professor and Chairman, Department of Neurology, Tufts University School of Medicine, Boston, Massachusetts, Neurologist-in-Chief, New England Medical Center, Boston, Massachusetts 02111, U.S.A.

Michael Carvell, M.D.
Assistant Professor, Division of Geriatric Psychiatry, Department of Psychiatry, Pennsylvania State University College of Medicine, Hershey, Pennsylvania, U.S.A.

Christine K. Cassel, M.D.
Chief, Section of General Internal Medicine, University of Chicago Medical Center, Chicago, Illinois 60637, U.S.A.

Donald O. Castell, M.D.
Professor of Medicine and Chief of Gastroenterology, Bowman Gray School of Medicine; North Carolina Baptist Hospital, Winston-Salem, North Carolina 27103, U.S.A.

Gerald W. Chodak, M.D.
Associate Professor of Urology, Department of Surgery, University of Chicago; Division of Urologic-Oncology, University of Chicago Medical Center, Chicago, Illinois 60637, U.S.A.

Thomas G. Cooney, M.D.
Professor of Medicine and Residency Program Director, Oregon Health Sciences University, Portland, Oregon 97201; Staff Physician, Section of General Medicine, Department of Veterans Affairs Medical Center, Portland, Oregon 97207, U.S.A.

David S. Cooper, M.D.
Associate Professor of Medicine, The Johns Hopkins University School of Medicine, Baltimore, Maryland 21218; Division of Endocrinology, Sinai Hospital of Baltimore, Baltimore, Maryland 21215, U.S.A.

Jeffrey L. Cummings, M.D.
Associate Professor of Neurology and Psychiatry and Biobehavioral Sciences, and Director, Dementia Research Program, University of California at Los Angeles School of Medicine, Los Angeles, California 90024, U.S.A.

Charles N. Ellis, M.D.
Associate Professor of Dermatology, Director, Dermatopharmacology Unit, University of Michigan Medical Center, Ann Arbor, Michigan 48109, U.S.A.

Robert S. Felder, D.D.S., M.P.H.
Assistant Professor, Public Health Dentistry, Oregon Health Sciences University, Portland, Oregon 97201; Director, Geriatric Dental Services, Department of Veterans Affairs Medical Center, Portland, Oregon 97207, U.S.A.

John R. Feussner, M.D.
Associate Professor and Chief, Division of General Internal Medicine, Department of Medicine, Durham, North Carolina 27706; Health Services Research and Development, Field Program, Department of Veterans Affairs Medical Center, Durham, North Carolina 27705, U.S.A.

Edward D. Frohlich, M.D.
Vice President, Academic Affairs, Alton Ochsner Distinguished Scientist, Alton Ochsner Medical Foundation, New Orleans, Louisiana 70121, U.S.A.

Michael T. Goldfarb M.D.
Lecturer, Department of Dermatology, University of Michigan Medical Center; University of Michigan Hospital, Ann Arbor, Michigan 48109, U.S.A.

James S. Goodwin, M.D.
Professor and Head of Geriatrics, Department of Medicine, University of Wisconsin, School of Medicine, Milwaukee Clinical Campus, Milwaukee, Wisconsin 53211; Sinai-Samaritan Geriatrics Institute, Milwaukee, Wisconsin 53213, U.S.A.

Jerry Gurwitz, M.D.
Merck Fellow in Geriatric Clinical Pharmacology, Instructor in Medicine, Harvard Medical School, Boston, Massachusetts 02114; Department of Medicine, Gerontology Division, Beth Israel Hospital, Boston, Massachusetts 02115, U.S.A.

Cynthia T. Henderson, M.D., M.P.H.
Associate Chairperson, Consultant in Gastroenterology and Clinical Nutrition, Department of Geriatric Medicine and Chronic Diseases, Oak Forest Hospital, Oak Forest, Illinois; Department of Medicine, Geriatrics Program, University of Chicago Medical Center, Chicago, Illinois 60637, U.S.A.

Patrick W. Irvine, M.D.
Assistant Professor, Department of Medicine, University of Minnesota, Minneapolis, Minnesota 55455; Director, Geriatric Medicine and Extended Care, Hennepin County Medical Center, Minneapolis, Minnesota 55415, U.S.A.

Lissy F. Jarvik, M.D., Ph.D.
Distinguished Physician, Department of Veterans Affairs Medical Center, Los Angeles, California; Professor, Department of Psychiatry and Biobehavioral Sciences, University of California at Los Angeles School of Medicine, Los Angeles 90024; Neuropsychiatric Hospital, Los Angeles, California, U.S.A.

L. E. Johnson, M.D., Ph.D.
Geriatric Fellow, University of California at Los Angeles Multicampus Division of Geriatric Medicine, San Fernando Valley Program, Department of Veterans Affairs Medical Center, Sepulveda, California 91343, U.S.A.

Fran E. Kaiser, M.D.
Assistant Professor of Medicine, University of California School of Medicine, Los Angeles, California 90024; Chief, Division of Geriatrics, Olive View Medical Center, Sylmar, California; Hospital-Based Home Care, Department of Veterans Affairs Medical Center, Sepulveda, California 91343, U.S.A.

Anthony Kales, M.D.
Professor and Chairman, Department of Psychiatry, Pennsylvania State University College of Medicine, Hershey, Pennsylvania, U.S.A.

Joyce D. Kales, M.D.
Professor and Director, Division of Community Psychiatry, Department of Psychiatry, Central Pennsylvania Psychiatric Institute, Pennsylvania State University College of Medicine, Hershey, Pennsylvania, U.S.A.

Rosalie A. Kane, D.S.W.
Professor, School of Social Work and School of Public Health, University of Minnesota, Minneapolis, Minnesota 55455, U.S.A.

Robert L. Kane, M.D.
Dean, School of Public Health, University of Minnesota, Minneapolis 55455, U.S.A.

Marshall B. Kapp, J.D., M.P.H.
Professor, Department of Medicine in Society, Wright State University School of Medicine, Dayton, Ohio 45435, U.S.A.

Harold G. Koenig, M.D.
Geriatric Medicine Fellow, Center for the Study of Aging and Human Development, Duke University Medical Center, Durham, North Carolina 27705, U.S.A.

Diana Koin, M.D.
Assistant Clinical Professor, Department of Medicine, Stanford University, Palo Alto, California 94305; Director, Hospital Based Home Care Program, Department of Veterans Affairs Medical Center, Palo Alto, California, U.S.A.

Eric B. Larson, M.D., M.P.H.
Professor of Medicine, University of Washington, Attending Physician, University Hospital, Seattle, Washington 98122, U.S.A.

Melinda A. Lee, M.D.
Assistant Professor of Medicine, Oregon Health Sciences University, Portland, Oregon 97201; Staff Physician, Geriatric Medicine Section, Department of Veteran Affairs Medical Center, Portland, Oregon 97207, U.S.A.

Joanne Lynn, M.D.
Associate Professor and Acting Director, Center for Aging Studies and Services, Department of Health Care Sciences, George Washington University, Washington, D.C. 20052; Medical Director, The Washington Home and Hospice of Washington, Washington, D.C., U.S.A.

Diane Meier, M.D.
Assistant Professor, Geriatrics and Adult Development, Chief, Geriatric Clinic, Co-Director, Osteoporosis and Metabolic Bone Disease Program, Mount Sinai Medical Center, New York, New York 10029, U.S.A.

Lane J. Mercer, M.D.
Associate Professor, Department of Ob/Gyn, Out-Patient Clinics, Director, Out-Patient Clinics, Obstetrics and Gynecology, University of Chicago Medical Center, Chicago, Illinois 60637, U.S.A.

Ernest Mhoon, M.D.
Associate Professor, Department of Surgery/Otolaryngology—Head and Neck Surgery, University of Chicago Pritzker School of Medicine; Director, Medical Student Education in Otolaryngology—Head and Neck Surgery, University of Chicago Medical Center, Chicago, Illinois 60637, U.S.A.

John E. Morley, M.B., B.Ch.
Professor of Medicine, Director, Division of Geriatrics, St. Louis University Medical School, St. Louis, Missouri; Department of Veterans Affairs Medical Center, St. Louis, Missouri 91343, U.S.A.

James F. Morris, M.D.
Professor of Medicine, Oregon Health Sciences University, Portland, Oregon 97201; Pulmonary Disease Section, Department of Veterans Affairs Medical Center, Portland, Oregon 97207, U.S.A.

Donald J. Murphy, M.D.
Assistant Professor, Department of Health Care Sciences, George Washington University, Washington, D.C. 20052; Thomas House, Washington, D.C., U.S.A.

James B. Nelson, M.D.
Senior Fellow, Gastroenterology Section, Bowman Gray School of Medicine, Winston-Salem, North Carolina 27103, U.S.A.

Bernice L. Neugarten, Ph.D., D.Sc.
Rothschild Distinguished Scholar, Center on Aging, Health and Society, Department of Medicine, University of Chicago, Chicago, Illinois 60637, U.S.A.

Thomas H. Norwood, M.D.
Professor of Pathology, Co-Director, Cytogenetics Laboratory, University of Washington, School of Medicine, Seattle, Washington 98195, U.S.A.

John G. Nutt, M.D.
Professor of Neurology, Oregon Health Sciences University, Portland, Oregon 97201, U.S.A.

Eugene Z. Oddone, M.D.
Associate in Medicine, Department of Medicine, Division of General Internal Medicine, Duke University Medical Center, Durham, North Carolina 27706; Research Associate, Health Services Research and Development Field Program, Ambulatory Care Service, Department of Veterans Affairs Medical Center, Durham, North Carolina 27705, U.S.A.

Gavril W. Pasternak, M.D., Ph.D.
Member, Department of Neurology, Memorial Sloan-Kettering Cancer Center, New York; Attending Neurologist, Memorial Hospital, New York, New York, 10021, U.S.A.

Richard Payne, M.D.
Associate Professor of Neurology, Attending Physician, University of Cincinnati Medical Center, Cincinnati, Ohio 45221, U.S.A.

Peter Pompei, M.D.
Assistant Professor, Department of Medicine, University of Chicago; Director, Windermere Senior Health Center, University of Chicago Medical Center, Chicago, Illinois 60637, U.S.A.

Lawrence A. Pottenger, M.D., Ph.D.
Associate Professor, Orthopaedic Surgery, Department of Surgery, University of Chicago; Director, Surgical Arthritis Clinic, University of Chicago Medical Center, Chicago, Illinois 60637, U.S.A.

Ruth B. Purtilo, Ph.D., P.T.
Professor and Program Director, Ethicist-in-Residence, Program in Ethics, Massachusetts General Hospital Institute of Health Professions, Boston, Massachusetts 02114; Lecturer, Orthopaedic Service, Harvard Medical School, Boston, Massachusetts 02115, U.S.A.

Neil M. Resnick, M.D.
Professor of Medicine, Harvard Medical School; Chief, Geriatrics and Director of the Continence Center, Brigham and Women's Hospital, Boston, Massachusetts 02115, U.S.A.

James B. Reuler, M.D.
Professor of Medicine, Oregon Health Sciences University, Portland, Oregon 97201; Chief, Section of General Medicine, Department of Veterans Affairs Medical Center, Portland, Oregon 97207, U.S.A.

L. F. Rich, M.S., M.D.
Associate Professor Ophthamology, Cornea and External Disease Service, Director, Adult Eye Clinic, Department of Ophthamology, Oregon Health Sciences University, Portland, Oregon 97201, U.S.A.

Don Riesenberg, M.D.
Senior Editor, *Journal of the American Medical Association*, Chicago, Illinois 60610; Department of Medicine, University of Chicago Pritzker School of Medicine, Chicago, Illinois 60637, U.S.A.

Greg A. Sachs, M.D.
Fellow in Geriatrics, Department of Medicine, University of Chicago Hospitals, Chicago, Illinois 60637, U.S.A.

Mary Shepard, M.D.
Assistant Professor of Medicine, Oregon Health Sciences University, Portland, Oregon 97201; Active Staff, Good Samaritan Hospital and Medical Center, Portland, Oregon, U.S.A.

Leif B. Sorensen, M.D., Ph.D.
Associate Chief, Department of Medicine, University of Chicago Pritzker School of Medicine, Chicago, Illinois 60637, U.S.A.

David O. Staats, M.D.
Assistant Professor, Department of Medicine, University of Illinois at Chicago, Chicago, Illinois 60637; Chief, Section of Geriatric Medicine, Assistant Chief, Medical Services, West Side Department of Veterans Affairs Medical Center, Chicago, Illinois, U.S.A.

Mary E. Tinetti, M.D.
Assistant Professor, Medicine, Yale University School of Medicine 06520; Associate Director, Continuing Care Unit, Yale-New Haven Hospital, New Haven, Connecticut, U.S.A.

Ruth Ann Tsukuda, M.P.H.
Director, Interdisciplinary Team Training in Geriatrics Program, Department of Veterans Affairs Medical Center, Portland, Oregon 97207, U.S.A.

Richard C. U'Ren, M.D.
Associate Professor of Psychiatry, Oregon Health Sciences University, Portland, Oregon 97201, U.S.A.

John J. Voorhees, M.D.
Professor and Chairman, Department of Dermatology, University of Michigan Medical Center, Ann Arbor, Michigan 48109, U.S.A.

John R. Walsh, M.D.
Chief, Geriatric Medicine, Department of Veterans Affairs Medical Center, Portland, Oregon 97207, U.S.A.

Nanette K. Wenger, M.D.
Professor of Medicine, Emory University School of Medicine, Atlanta, Georgia 30303; Director, Cardiac Clinics, Grady Memorial Hospital, Atlanta, Georgia, U.S.A.

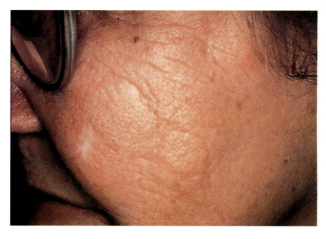

Fig. 29.1. Typical changes of solar elastosis, with deep wrinkling in the periorbital area.

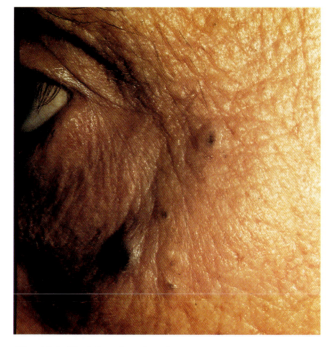

Fig. 29.2. Nodular elastoidosis with cysts and comedones.

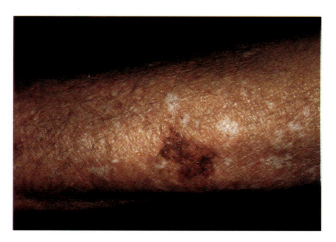

Fig. 29.3. Senile or Bateman's purpura on the dorsal forearm.

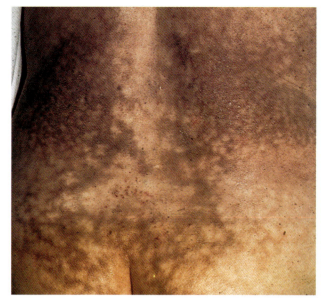

Fig. 29.4. Erythema ab igne on the lower part of the back. Note the reticulated brown pigmentation.

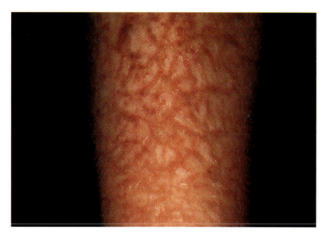

Fig. 29.5. Eczema craquelé of the pretibial area. Crisscrossing linear fissures and inflamed skin are the characteristic features.

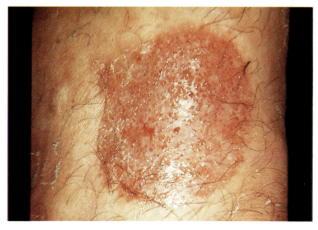

Fig. 29.6. Nummular eczema of the leg with erythema and vesiculations.

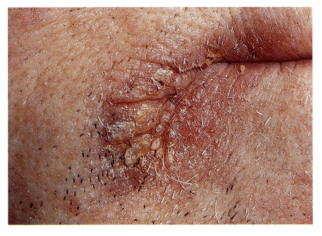

Fig. 29.7. Angular cheilitis with erythema, scaling, and crusting at the corner of the mouth.

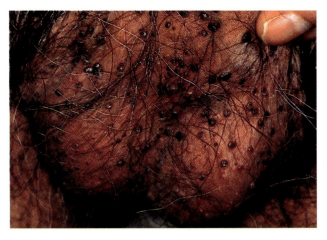

Fig. 29.10. Angiokeratomas of Fordyce, with numerous, red-purple papules located on the scrotum.

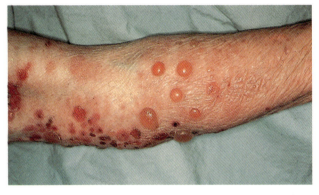

Fig. 29.8. Bullous pemphigoid characterized by tense bullae with clear serum on the flexural aspect of the arm.

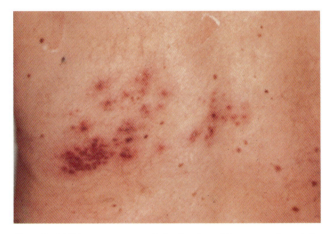

Fig. 29.11 Herpes zoster of the back, with grouped vesicles on an erythematous base in a dermatomal distribution.

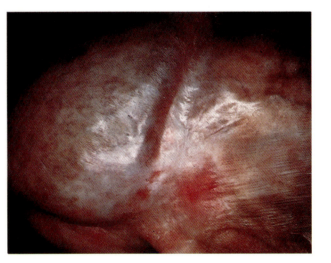

Fig. 29.9. Balanitis xerotica obliterans on the ventral aspect of the penis, appearing as a white, atrophic plaque.

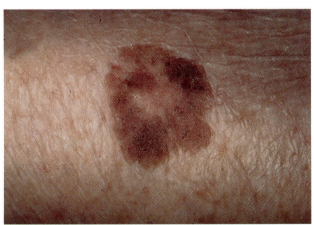

Fig. 29.12. Seborrheic keratosis with the classic appearance of a tan, sharply marginated lesion with a rough surface.

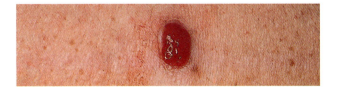

Fig. 29.13. (Left) Cherry angioma on the torso.

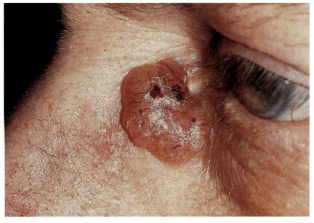

Fig. 29.14. *(Right)* Nodular basal cell carcinoma appearing as a pearly, translucent nodule on the side of the nose.

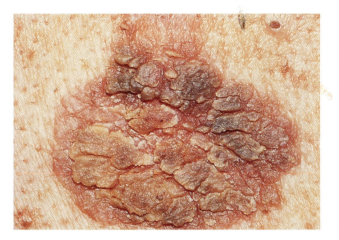

Fig. 29.15. Bowen's disease appears as a slightly elevated erythematous plaque with scales.

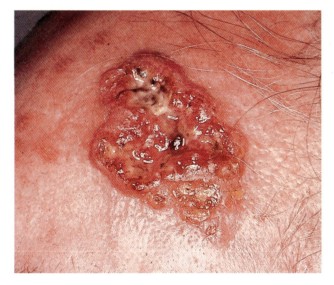

Fig. 29.16. Squamous cell carcinoma of the forehead, appearing as a large, firm lesion with ulcerations.

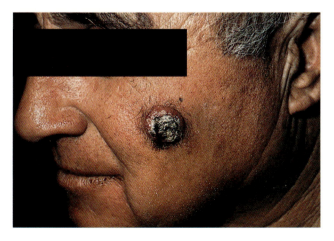

Fig. 29.17. Keratoacanthoma, a dome-shaped nodule with a central keratotic plug, located on sun-exposed skin.

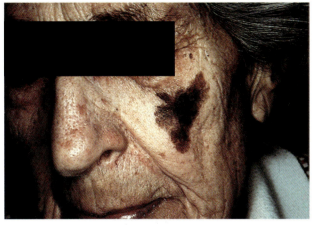

Fig. 29.18. Lentigo maligna melanoma appears as a large darkly pigmented lesion with nodules on a flat base.

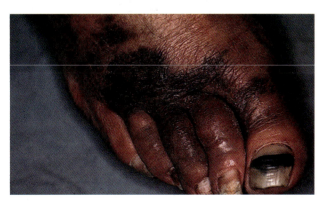

Fig. 29.19. Kaposi's sarcoma with multiple plaques located on the dorsum of the foot.

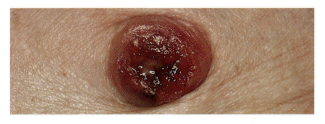

Fig. 29.20. Umbilical metastasis from a gastrointestinal tract malignancy presents as a firm, pink nodule.

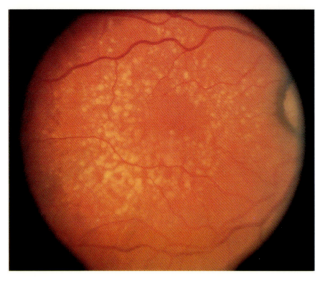

Fig. 30.3. Ocular fundus of patient with drusen.

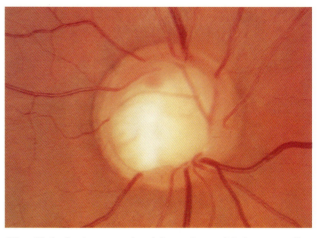

Fig. 30.6. Optic nerve head in patient with long-standing, uncontrolled glaucoma. Note large central cup with only thin rim of neural tissue remaining, indicating extensive damage to optic nerve. Compare Figures 30.4 and 30.5.

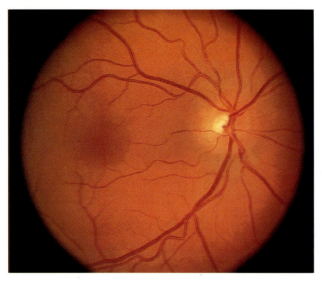

Fig. 30.4. Normal ocular fundus in young adult.

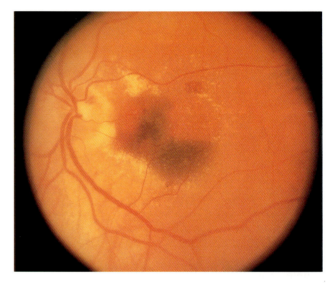

Fig. 30.7. Ocular fundus in patient with macular degeneration.

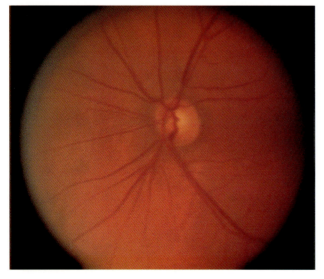

Fig. 30.5. Normal fundus in elderly person.

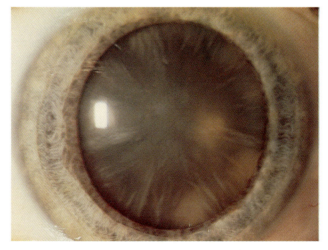

Fig. 30.8. Senile cataract as seen with diffuse light and patient's pupil dilated.

1

Cellular Aging

Thomas H. Norwood

The level of investigative activity into the mechanisms of aging at the cellular and molecular level has increased dramatically during the past two to three decades. While these efforts certainly have yielded a wealth of descriptive information and some fundamental changes in our perception of the aging process, definitive knowledge of the cause or causes of aging remains elusive. Investigative efforts in the area of cellular aging address a number of questions, the answers to which are only beginning to emerge. For example, it is not known if all cell populations in the body are vulnerable to aging, or if the nature of the aging process is similar in all cell populations in the body. Some scientists have suggested that the rate of aging is determined by one or a few critical cell populations; an alternative notion is that the manifestations of aging are the summation of subtle decrements of function in most or all of the cell populations in the body. Also, the role of aging at the cellular level in the pathogenesis of age-associated diseases, such as arteriosclerotic vascular disease and many carcinomas, remain, for the most part, speculative. While definitive answers to the questions posed above are not forthcoming at the present time, there is enough information to permit some speculation about future directions that may be pursued in the area of cellular aging. In this chapter, the current status of cellular aging will be discussed at a level that will provide geriatricians with a foundation of knowledge to assist them in following future developments in the field of basic gerontology.

A classification system based on cellular prolifera-

tive behavior provides a useful, if oversimplified, organizational infrastructure for a discussion of problems of cellular aging. In this system, the following three major populations of cells in the body can be recognized: (1) *postreplicative cells,* (2) *quiescent cells,* and (3) *continuously proliferating cells.* The group of postreplicative cells includes differentiated cell types that no longer respond to any known physiologic stimulus for cell division, with the prototype cell being the neuron. Other cell types in this group include the polymorphonuclear leukocyte, skeletal muscle cells, and cardiac muscle cells. The group of quiescent cells includes types that usually are nonproliferating but are capable of cell division in response to specific mitogenic stimuli. Most commonly, these proliferative stimuli are part of the response to tissue injury. Hepatocytes, renal tubular epithelial cells, connective tissue fibroblasts, and endothelial cells are some of the many cell types in this category. Continuously proliferating cells are the stem cells of those populations that undergo terminal differentiation and cell death and thus must be constantly renewed. Hematopoietic cells and many epithelial cell types, such as those of the epidermis and the gastrointestinal epithelium, are examples of this cell type. The continued capacity of these cells to proliferate is essential to the immediate survival of the organism.

Clearly one of the problems, even in the greatly simplified classification system outlined above, is to identify biologic marker(s) that will provide an operational definition of senescent cells within the population. An ideal biomarker of aging should (1) be universal, that is, provide a reliable assessment of biological aging in all cell types in a wide variety of species, (2) provide a reliable estimate of subsequent survival or longevity, (3) change significantly with age, and (4) be reproducible within an individual or population of cells.[1] Unfortunately, there are no markers of aging at either the cellular or the organismal level that satisfy all of these criteria. An important emphasis in this chapter will be to analyze how senescent populations are defined by biomarkers that are available and how these markers are used as experimental end points in studies designed to probe the basic mechanism of aging. In the case of postmitotic cells, there are no universal markers of aging, although some age-associated changes are widely distributed. On the other hand, the loss of proliferative capacity has provided an operational definition of aging in all cell populations capable of sustained cell division. This phenomenon and its application to the study of basic aging processes at the organismal level will be the major focus of the section below, dealing with aging in cell types capable of sustained proliferative activity.

Aging in Proliferating Cell Populations

It is not surprising that, after general acceptance of the concept that the cell is the basic living unit of all organisms, early cytologists began to speculate about the life span of somatic cells. With the development of cell culture systems that support sustained proliferative activity, the capacity of cells to sustain this basic function very quickly became a subject of scientific inquiry. However, the answer to this question has been remarkably elusive. It is now accepted by most, but not all, biologists that normal diploid cells from mammalian and probably all avian species have a finite growth potential. However, there remain many questions about the causal relationship between changes of proliferative activity and aging at the organismal level. This fundamental issue in aging has been studied both in cell culture systems (in vitro) and in experimental animal models (in vivo). These two experimental approaches are quite different and, therefore, will be discussed separately.

Studies of Proliferative Life Span in Vitro

As indicated above, in the first decades of the 20th century, scientists quickly perceived that cell cultures could provide an experimental approach to the question of the proliferative life span of somatic cells. The most influential studies that addressed the question were carried out with cultured cells derived from the

chick heart muscle by a well-known experimental biologist, Alexis Carrel.[2] He published a number of studies that described the prolonged growth capacity of these cells and finally concluded in a publication in the mid-1930s that somatic cells are, in fact, immortal.[2] This conclusion was supported by contemporary tissue culturists who were, for the most part, working with cultured cells derived from murine tissues.

The results of these studies strongly influenced the perception of gerontologists regarding the role of the somatic cell in the aging process; the prevailing notion was that aging does not occur at the cellular level and that the causes of aging should be sought at the level of organ dysfunction, possibly mediated by changes in extracellular substances, with emphasis on the decline of function due to some form of "wear and tear" analogous to that occurring in inanimate machines. It should be emphasized that these are not totally spurious or naive perceptions. Certainly, many age-associated decrements of form and function occur in all organs, and many changes in the extracellular matrix have been documented at the morphologic and biochemical level and are believed by most gerontologists to be responsible for some of the cosmetic and functional changes associated with aging.

In the 1960s, the notion of the proliferative immortality of somatic cell populations was first seriously challenged. Findings from initial reports that cultured human fibroblasts do not proliferate indefinitely were dismissed as manifestations of the technical limitations of cell culture techniques available to scientists at that time. Given the artificial environment present in tissue culture systems, this interpretation was very difficult to exclude. Despite these difficulties, Drs Leonard Hayflick and Paul Moorehead[3] were the first investigators to carry out extensive studies, with a series of fibroblast cultures derived from fetal lung tissue, to rule out trivial explanations for cessation of growth, such as nutritional depletion of the culture medium or the presence of biologic agents, such as viruses or mycoplasma. Hayflick[4] also observed that cell cultures derived from adult tissues consistently displayed a lower growth potential than those derived from fetal tissue. Based on the results of these studies, he concluded that the limited growth potential of human diploid fibroblasts was a manifestation of an intrinsic property of these cells and that this cell culture system might be a model for the study of cell aging. These conclusions ignited a scientific debate that continues to this day. Hayflick's basic observations regarding the limited growth potential of human diploid fibroblasts have been confirmed in many laboratories throughout the world and now are generally accepted as biologic fact. However, the notion that the cultured fibroblast is a model for some aspects of cellular aging continues to be debated.

This scientific debate has stimulated many studies designed to establish biologic correlates between the proliferative potential of cultivated cells, on the one hand, and aging in vivo, on the other. The most compelling observations that support the cultured diploid fibroblast as a model of cellular aging are as follows: (1) an inverse relationship between the age of the donor and the proliferative capacity of these cultures;[5,6] (2) a diminished growth potential in culture derived from individuals with certain genetic syndromes that display features of accelerated aging[7]; and (3) an apparent positive correlation between the growth potential of a culture and the maximum life span of the species from which it is derived.[8]

Proliferative Potential and Donor Age

The inverse relationship between donor age and the growth potential of cultured human diploid fibroblasts has been reported in a number of studies and is generally accepted. In the study shown in Fig. 1.1, a decline of the mean growth capacity of approximately 30% is evident from the third to the 10th decade. Note that there is considerable scatter in the data and that cultures derived from even the oldest individuals display a significant growth capacity. These observations serve to emphasize that the loss of proliferative capacity of fibroblasts and almost certainly of any other proliferating cell populations in the body is not a primary determinant of longevity, nor is the observed growth potential predictive of longevity.

It has been suggested that the decline of growth potential in cultures from aged donors reflects the extent of proliferation that has occurred in vivo. A number of morphologic and functional changes that are associated with serial subcultivation in vitro, such as the increased length of the cell cycle, increased cell size, and decreased number of cells when the cultures are permitted to achieve confluency, are more apparent in early-passage cultures from elderly donors, (age, >65 years) than in cultures of a comparable passage level derived from young donors (age, <35 years).[9] These changes, although not as extensive as those that occur with in vitro aging, suggest that similar physiologic changes may be occurring with age in vitro and in vivo.

Proliferative Potential and Donor Genotype

The observation that cultures derived from subjects with certain genetic disorders that are associated with accelerated aging display an attenuated growth capacity has stimulated increased interest in cell culture systems as models for the study of cellular aging. There are a number of genetic disorders that show, to a variable extent, features of premature aging and decreased life expectancy. This group of disorders has been collectively referred to as *progeroid syndromes*.[10] The Hutchinson-Gilford syndrome, sometimes called *true progeria,* and Werner's syndrome, sometimes called *adult progeria,* are clinically the most dramatic examples of this group of genetic disorders (Table 1.1.). Fibroblast cultures derived from patients with Werner's syndrome show the most dramatic attenuation of growth potential (Fig. 1.2.). Fibroblast cultures derived from donors with Hutchinson-Gilford syndrome display a greater variability of growth potential, but the extent of proliferation is consistently lower than that observed in cultures derived from normal donors.

Aside from the diminished growth capacity, comparatively few observations that distinguish the phenotype of Werner's and Hutchison-Gilford fibroblast cultures from each other or from fibroblast cultures derived from normal donors have been reported. One finding of considerable interest is the demonstration of multiple clonal chromosome aberrations in fibroblast cultures derived from donors with Werner's syndrome and not in cultures derived from donors with Hutchinson-Gilford syndrome or normal donors.[11] While the significance of these observations in relation to the primary defect in Werner's syndrome is unknown, the presence of chromosomal instability suggests that defects of DNA replication, DNA repair, and/or chromatin structure may be a facet of this

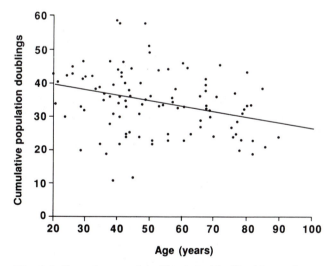

Fig. 1.1. Growth potential of human skin fibroblast cultures vs age of donor. Solid regression line, calculated by method of least squares, indicates decline of 0.18 cell doublings per year (P< .001). Cell cultures were initiated from skin biopsy specimens obtained ante mortem and post mortem from mesial aspect of arm (from Martin et al.[6] Effects of age on cell division capacity, in Danon D, Shock NW, Marois M [eds]: *Aging: A Challenge to Science and Society.* Oxford, Oxford University Press, 1981, Vol 1, p 128. Used by permission).

4 Thomas H. Norwood

Table 1.1. Comparison of selected features of three progeroid syndromes and normal aging in humans.

	Werner's syndrome	Hutchinson-Gilford syndrome	Down's syndrome (trisomy 21)	Normal aging
Inheritance	Autosomal recessive	Autosomal dominant (?)	Sporadic*	Polygenic (universal)
Growth failure	Primary	Primary	Primary	Secondary
Neoplasia	Meningiomas, possibly increased sarcoma	No increased incidence of neoplasia	Leukemia	Carcinoma
Presence of atherosclerotic vascular disease	Severe	Severe	Probably not more than expected for age	Variable (almost universal)
Neurodegenerative changes	Not present	Not present	Severe (almost universal by 5th decade)	Very frequent but not universal

* In most instances, the occurrence of Down's syndrome is sporadic. The phenotype is the result of unbalance (presence of extra copies) of multiple genes.

syndrome. However, no abnormalities have been observed in the metabolism of DNA or in the integrity of chromatin structure at this time.

The growth behavior of cultured fibroblasts derived from donors with other premature-aging syndromes has been less extensively studied. In general, the deviation from normal proliferative potential has been shown to be relatively subtle, certainly less dramatic than that observed in cultures derived from donors with Werner's and Hutchinson-Gilford syndromes.[7] In some cases, the growth capacity is within the normal range. This is certainly not surprising given the variable extent to which the individual progeroid syndromes show features of premature aging. Even in the case of Werner's and Hutchinson-Gilford syndromes, there are a number of facets of these phenotypes that are discordant with normal aging (Table 1.1.). For example, neurodegenerative changes, a common finding in normal elderly populations, have not been observed in association with these syndromes. It has been suggested that Down's syndrome, trisomy 21, may display the greatest number of features of premature aging, a conclusion of some interest in that Down's syndrome, like normal aging, is the result of the action of multiple genes.[10] Despite the fact that these progeroid syndromes are, as some authors have suggested, "caricatures" of the normal aging process, their value for the study of certain aspects of aging cannot be questioned.[12]

Growth Potential and Species Life Span

The most extensive study addressing this question has shown a positive relationship between growth potential in vitro and longevity of the species.[8] However, some caution must be exercised in the interpretation of findings from these studies. A relatively small number of mammalian species have been examined. Also, the origin of the so-called fibroblast in culture from the skin explants is uncertain and could be derived from one or several cell types that are normally resident in this tissue. Therefore, it is not clear if the same cell type is present in cultures derived from donors from different species. Another potential problem is that precise knowledge of the maximum life span of most mammalian species is lacking; thus, the values assigned to independent variables in these studies are, at best, estimates. Finally, the propensity of cultures initiated from certain species to undergo spontaneous neoplastic transformation to a cell type of apparently unlimited growth potential can obscure the senescent phase in the culture. This is a phenomenon of fundamental biologic significance and is discussed in depth below.

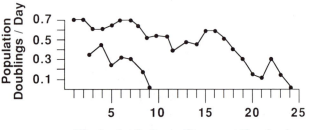

Fig. 1.2. Growth in vitro of fibroblasts derived from clinically normal individual (upper curve) and from individual with Werner's syndrome (lower curve). Normal culture ceased measurable proliferative activity at 80.7 population doublings (PDs), and culture with Werner's syndrome ceased at 20.1 PDs. These cultures are unusually long lived, both in cases of normal donors (usually 50 to 60 PDs) and of donors with Werner's syndrome (usually <15 PDs) (from Norwood TH, Hoehn H, Salk D, et al. Cellular aging in Werner's syndrome: a unique phenotype? *J Invest Dermatol* 1979;73:92-96. © by Williams & Wilkins, 1979.)

Neoplastic Transformation In Vitro

With the demonstration that some cell types have an intrinsic capacity for limited growth in vitro, a number of authors suggested that two fundamentally different cell types can be identified in culture.[3,13] Some of the distinguishing characteristics of the two broad classifications are listed in Table 1.2. The cell types with a finite life span can be viewed as the in vitro counterpart of reactive hyperplasia of normal somatic cells, and the apparently immortal cell types are an in vitro model of neoplasia. Many names for these two basic cell types have been proposed by various authors. In the current literature, they frequently are referred to as *normal diploid* or *nontransformed* and *transformed* or *immortalized,* respectively. It is important to emphasize that there is, in many of the individual cell lines, a significant overlap of the characteristics that distinguish these basic cell types. For example, some immortal cell lines exhibit a high-serum requirement but have a highly abnormal karyotype (eg, mouse 3T3 cell lines).

Cultured cells from many species transform spontaneously. The frequency of this event may, to a certain extent, be inversely related to the maximum life span of the species from which the culture was derived. Murine cells will almost invariably transform in culture. This occurs after the cell population has doubled 12 to 15 times and is associated with a "crisis" of growth when proliferation almost ceases but then begins to increase as the transformed cells emerge.[14] The failure of the early tissue culturists to appreciate these events in murine cultures is certainly an important reason for the widely held belief that normal somatic cells in culture possess an indefinite proliferative potential. In contrast, most human cell types in culture are remarkably stable with respect to tranformation; there are no confirmed reports of spontaneous transformation in a human fibroblast culture.

Transformation can be reproducibly induced by biologic, physical, and chemical agents that are oncogenic or carcinogenic in vivo. However, physical and chemical agents transform human fibroblasts in culture at a very low frequency. Cultured human fibroblasts can be transformed with high efficiency by a DNA virus called simian virus 40. This virus will, on infection, produce malignant tumors in certain rodent species but not in humans. In contrast to cultured human diploid cells, rodent cells in culture are quite susceptible to transformation by a variety of chemical and physical agents and following infection by a variety of oncogenic viruses. More recently, transformation has been induced by the introduction directly into the cells (transfection) of individual or combinations of genes known to be causally associated with cancer, ie, so-called oncogenes.

One of the concepts to arise from these in vitro transformation studies with cloned genes is that transformation and immortalization (acquisition of unlimited growth potential) may be distinct and independent events. For example, infection of a human fibroblast culture with SV40 will invariably result in morphologic transformation and dramatic changes in the growth behavior of the culture, but the establishment of an immortal cell line is a rare event. Most of the transformed cultures cease growing and die, an event that may or may not be identical to senescence in a normal (uninfected) culture. In contrast, the immortal murine 3T3 cell lines initiated from fetal tissues under rigidly controlled conditions require high concentrations of serum, are anchorage dependent, and are not tumorigenic in vivo (Table 1.2.). Certain strains of 3T3 cells are used in an assay system to screen for transformation activity in genomic or cloned DNA. This assay has been used to isolate genes with transforming activity from some human neoplasms.[15] These kinds of studies are of fundamental importance in cell and molecular biology and represent

Table 1.2. Selected characteristics of two major types of mammalian cells in culture.*

	Hyperplastoid, cell strain	Neoplastoid, cell line
Prototype cell	Human diploid fibroblast	HeLa cells†
In vivo counterpart	Reactive hyperplasia	Neoplasia
Growth potential	Finite	Unlimited
Karyotype	Remains diploid (or same as donor)	Generally abnormal (structural and numeric aberrations)
Serum requirement for growth	Generally high (≥10%)	Frequently low (growth at 1%-3%)
Growth substrate requirement	Attachment to solid surface obligate requirement for growth	Frequently able to grow in suspension
Tumorigenicity	Never tumorigenic following injection into recipient host	Some cell lines exhibit tumorigenicity in recipient host

* Modified from Martin and Sprague.[13]

† A human tumor cell line derived from an endocervical adenocarcinoma of the cervix.

the interface of gerontologic and cancer research. The mechanisms of cell transformation have been extensively reviewed elsewhere.[16,17]

Studies of Proliferative Life Span In Vivo

An implicit criticism of in vitro models to study cell function is that the observations may be a reflection of the technical limitations of the experimental system. Therefore, it is important to carry out parallel studies in vivo whenever feasible. The first attempts to quantitate the extent of age-associated change in proliferative activity in vivo were carried out by enumeration of tritium-labeled interphase and mitotic cells in autoradiographic preparations of tissue from laboratory animals that had previously been pulsed with labeled thymidine. This technology permits quantitation of the following phases of the cell cycle: pre-DNA synthesis (G_1), DNA synthesis, post-DNA synthesis (G_2), and mitosis (M). In general, these experiments have demonstrated a reduced fraction of dividing cells and an increased length of the duration of the cell cycle time primarily due to lengthening of the G_1 phase of the cycle.[18] While these observations certainly suggest that decrements of proliferative function occur with advancing age, they do not distinguish between intrinsic alterations in the cells and extracellular changes in the aging tissues as the primary cause of the functional decline.

The transplantation of cells or tissues provides an experimental approach that can potentially distinguish between intracellular and extracellular factors modulating proliferative function in aged individuals.[19] Serial transplantation studies, designed to determine if normal (nonneoplastic) proliferative tissues have a finite cell division potential, have been carried out in inbred strains of laboratory mice with a variety of tissues, including immunocytes (antibody-producing cells), skin, hematopoietic cells, and breast tissue (mammary epithelium). In the majority of these studies, it has been observed that these tissues can be transplanted a limited number of times, but that the extent of proliferation observed far exceeds that required for the life span of the animal. The general controls for these studies are numerous tumor cell lines that can be serially transplanted indefinitely, which are the in vivo equivalent of transformed cell lines in culture.

The interpretation of these studies' findings is not straightforward. The limited transplantability of normal (nonneoplastic) proliferating populations could reflect the finite growth potential of these cells or, alternatively, these tissues could be uniquely sensitive to the trauma of transplantation. Which of these interpretations is correct has yet to be determined

through experimental studies. However, transplantation studies with mammary epithelium suggest that the limited transplantability, at least in this tissue, is due to a limited cell division potential.[19] Breast epithelium is unique in that the extent of cell proliferation can be estimated: the extension through the fat pad of the developing breast is achieved by means of cell division. Thus, if the number of transplant generations is positively related to the proliferative potential of the ductal epithelium, one would expect that serial transplants of ductal tissue obtained in each generation from a location in the fat pad distant from the site of the previous transplantation could be carried through fewer transplant generations than ductal tissue obtained in each generation from near the site of the preceding implantation. Indeed, this was observed in studies carried out in the early 1970s.[19] The results of these experiments support the conclusion that, at least in the case of mammary epithelium, there is an intrinsically limited cell division capacity in vivo. However, it should be noted that other transplantation studies of hematopoietic tissue and immunocytes have shown that tissues from old and young donors display no significant differences in functional capacity or growth potential. Moreover, tissues from both youthful and old donors transplanted to old recipients display diminished functional and proliferative activity. These observations have led some authors to conclude that certain stem cell populations may not age.[20] However, a reasonable conclusion at the present time is that normal proliferative tissues have a finite growth potential, but the growth potential of any cell population is not a direct determinant of life span. These studies also have shown that extracellular factors exert a significant influence on the proliferative capacity of cells. Clearly, more precise knowledge about the changes in cell-to-cell and cell-to-matrix interactions with aging is essential before a definitive interpretation of these transplantation studies can be made.

Phenotype of Senescent Proliferative Cell

In the discussion above, the loss of proliferative activity has been the biomarker that defines the operational definition of cell senescence. An obvious objective of investigations of near-terminal or postmitotic populations is to establish more precise, independent markers for aging studies. Many descriptive studies have been published, and a variety of changes have been clearly demonstrated in senescent fibroblast cultures.[21-23] Morphologic studies have revealed a variety of consistent changes, including an increase in cell volume by threefold to fourfold and an increased frequency of binucleation and micronucleation (a small satellite nuclear structure that contains one or a few chromosomes). Structural studies via electron microscopy have demonstrated an increase in certain classes of filamentous proteins (primarily intermediate filaments) and a striking increase in lysosomes and dense bodies. Cytogenetic analyses reveal an increase in tetraploidy but no other consistent structural or numeric changes in the chromosomes. Significantly, no evidence of unstable aberrations, such as chromosome breaks and gaps, has been reported, suggesting that significant damage to chromatin structure does not occur before the loss of proliferative activity. Biochemical studies of macromolecular synthesis and turnover have been carried out in many laboratories. There is a complete cessation of DNA synthesis as proliferative activity declines. Total RNA synthesis declines in late-passage cultures, but the total RNA content increases as the cultures approach senescence. Protein content increases significantly in the enlarged senescent cells, which may be a result of the decreased activity in some of the protein degradation pathways known to exist in mammalian cells.

While the dramatic morphologic changes that have been observed with cell aging in vitro are not readily apparent in the tissues of elderly individuals, there is some evidence that similar changes occur with aging in vivo. Probably the best-documented example is the increased binucleation and tetraploidy in hepatocytes with age. There also is some evidence that cell size increases with age in some quiescent cell populations. The apparent absence of senescent cells in vivo may be due to the fact that only a small fraction of cells reach senescence and/or there are mechanisms to remove selectively senescent somatic cells. As will be discussed below, the failure to observe obviously senescent cells in aged tissue does not exclude the possibility that a decline of proliferative capacity plays a significant role in organismal aging.

Other Cultured-Cell-Type Models of Aging

So far, this discussion has been confined largely to the cultured fibroblast, a spindle-shaped cell type that has yet to be defined precisely. With advances in the technology of cell cultures, a variety of precisely defined cell types have been maintained successfully in vitro. A finite growth potential has now been demonstrated in these human cell types in culture (Table 1.3.). These other cell types have not been as extensively characterized as the cultured fibroblast; however, these specialized cells will almost certainly play an increasingly important role in in vitro studies of cellular aging. For example, it has recently been demonstrated that the expression of the gene for steriod 17α-hydroxylase is lost with senescence of bovine adrenocortical cells in culture.[24] The significance of the finding with respect to the aging process is as yet unclear. Elucidation of the mechanisms of the functional loss will provide an important marker for future studies, both in the cell biology and endocrinology of aging. In a more general sense, the availablity of well-defined cell culture models will provide new experimental approaches to study the role of cell aging in age-associated disease processes.

Proliferative Changes in Age-Associated Diseases

Whether changes in proliferative activity are causally related to decrements of function of specific systems and/or specific age-related diseases is an area of active investigation. Many of the age-associated pathologic processes are associated with inappropriate proliferation rather than diminished cell growth, an apparent paradox that has been emphasized by Martin.[25] Examples of age-associated hyperproliferative lesions include benign prostatic hyperplasia (glandular epithelium, smooth-muscle cells, and fibroblasts), degenerative joint disease (fibroblasts), benign lentigines (melanocytes), the early lesions of atherosclerosis (intimal smooth-muscle cells), and the ultimate hyperproliferative disease, carcinoma (most epithelial cell populations). This paradox may be due in part to the difficulty of detecting the consequences of a decline of

Table 1.3. Some human cell types for which there is evidence for limited growth in vitro and the appearance of aging-related markers.

Source, y	Cell type	Differentiating markers
Hayflick and Moorhead,[3] 1961, Martin et al,[5] 1970, and Martin et al,[6] 1981	Fibroblast (from multiple tissues)	No defining markers*
Bierman,[51] 1978	Vascular smooth-muscle cell	Morphology, growth characteristic in vitro
Glassberg et al,[52] 1982	Endothelial cell	Factor VIII, angiotensin converting enzyme
Rheinwald and Green,[53] 1975	Epidermal keratinocyte	Spectrum of cytokeratins
Walford et al,[54] 1981	T lymphocytes from peripheral blood	Growth characteristic, morphology, cell-surface antigens

* The fibroblast culture is undefined and may be a heterogeneous population of cell types depending on the tissue from which the culture is derived.[21]

proliferative activity in the tissues. The presence of these hyperproliferative lesions suggests that aging may be associated with an increasing frequency of inappropriate responses to mitogenic and antimitogenic stimuli. Thus, just as an aged call may fail to respond to an external signal to proliferate, it is also possible that cells approaching senescence may lose the capacity to respond to signals that normally would be antiproliferative. This notion has recently gained greater currency with the experimental observations that some growth factors, under certain conditions, exhibit antiproliferative activity.[26]

There is no direct evidence that associates the loss of proliferative activity with a specific condition or disease entity associated with aging. There are a number of disease states and decrements of physiologic functions that may be causally related to a decline of proliferative activity by one or more cell populations. For example, the duration of wound healing is known to increase with age.[27] In the case of cutaneous wounds, migration and proliferation of a variety of cell types, including epithelial cells (epidermis) and dermal fibroblasts, are important components of the wound-healing process. It is tempting to postulate that a decline in the proliferative capacity of these cells accounts for an increased wound-healing time. However, the process of wound healing is a complex phenomenon that involves an inflammatory response, as well as the immune system, and is influenced by integrity of the vascular system. In humans, vascular disease could play a role in retarding the rate of wound healing in elderly persons. In addition, there is an age-associated decline in immune function,[28] which almost certainly influences the quality and rate of repair of injured tissues. Thus, it is very likely that the decline in the rate of wound healing is caused by multiple factors, one of which very likely is decreased proliferative capacity of the various cell types involved in the reparative process.

The decline of immune function with age also is associated with decreased proliferative capacity. Most of the changes in immune responsiveness are related to T-cell functions, such as delayed hypersensitivity and T-cell–mediated cytotoxicity.[28] A number of laboratories have demonstrated a diminished response to the T-cell mitogen phytohemagglutinin with age (Fig. 1.3.).[29,30] The pattern of decline in responsiveness to specific mitogens is similar to that observed in late-passage fibroblast cultures, and these studies are believed to reflect changes that occur in vivo. Thus, the T-lymphocyte cultures will be a valuable model for the study of the relationship between proliferative competence and aging.

Of the age-associated diseases, cancer is most clearly associated with an alteration of proliferative

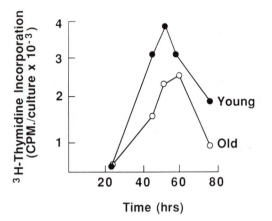

Fig. 1.3. Proliferation of peripheral blood lymphocytes from young (age, <32 years) and old (age, >65 years) donors as assessed by tritiated thymidine incorporation into DNA in culture stimulated by phytohemagglutinin (PHA). Addition of colchicine permits examination of first round of DNA synthesis only, because this drug prevents progression of cells through mitosis. cpm indicates counts per minute (from Hefton JM, et al: Immunologic studies of aging. V. Impaired proliferation of PHA responsive human lymphocytes in culture. *J Immunol* 124:1007, 1980. © by Amer. Assoc. of Immunologists).

behavior. Some experimental evidence indicates that the increased incidence of carcinomas reflects increased vulnerability to neoplastic transformation due to intrinsic, age-associated changes in certain epithelial cell populations. In murine studies, in which skin from old and young donors is transplanted to young donors, a threefold higher incidence of cancers in the old skin has been observed following exposure to carcinogens.[31] Although such observations are highly suggestive of an age-related susceptibility to transformation, more studies are required to determine the extent to which intrinsic and/or extracellular factors are involved.

The relationship of aging at the cellular level to the pathogenesis of atherosclerotic vascular disease, another very important age-associated disease, has been relatively unexplored. This disease process is associated with altered proliferative behavior; one of the earliest lesions that is anatomically evident is the proliferation of intimal smooth-muscle cells. Numerous theories predicting the cause(s) and the mechanisms of the pathogenesis of this disease have been proposed.[32] The so-called response-to-injury hypothesis has been the most extensively tested and can explain many, but not all, of the observed characteristics of this disease.[33] The proponents of this theory hold that a primary event is an injury to the endothelial lining of the luminal surface of the artery wall, with or without a loss of continuity of that cell layer. These injurious events in the intima lead to changes in the proliferative behavior of the subjacent intimal smooth-muscle cells. In the case of intimal injuries that result in the loss of continuity of the endothelium, the intimal smooth-muscle cells are exposed to a variety of constituents of the blood, some of which contain mitogens for the cells. Platelets, which rapidly adhere to the area of injury that is denuded of the protective endothelial barrier, contain a number of biologically active compounds, including platelet-derived growth factor—a potent mitogen for arterial smooth-muscle cells. This growth factor could be a mediator of the sustained proliferation of subjacent smooth-muscle cells and formation of the atherosclerotic plaque.

It should be emphasized that the precise mechanism(s) leading to the initial proliferative lesion is unknown at the present time.[33] However, one of the predisposing conditions to the loss of continuity of the endothelium in the cell population could be regional senescence. This suggestion is based primarily on the following properties of endothelial cells: (1) a finite growth potential in culture (Table 1.3.) and (2) repair of disruptions of the monolayer by migration of proliferating cells in the immediate vicinity of the "wound." Thus, repeated injury in a specific location of the intima could lead to a very localized area of proliferative exhaustion and, therefore, a permanent defect in the endothelium.[32] Alternatively, aging in endothelial cells and/or smooth-muscle cells could be associated with the loss of efficient secretion of growth regulatory factors that are involved in the maintenance of the quiescent state of other cell types in the region. This could lead to smooth-muscle proliferation without a loss of the continuity of the endothelium, a mechanism suggested by Martin and Sprague.[13] There are other hypotheses to explain the pathogenesis of atherosclerosis that place less emphasis on the loss of integrity of the endothelium. But it is clear that the cultured endothelial cell, because of its central role in the pathogenesis of degenerative vascular disease and the remarkable similarity of its growth behavior in vitro and in vivo, is becoming an important experimental system for the study of cellular aging.

Although the discussion above is in large part speculative, it is likely that relatively subtle decrements of proliferative function play a significant role in the pathogenesis of many age-associated diseases. The discovery of the mechanisms of the loss of proliferative competence remains an important objective. As Hayflick[34] has emphasized, attainment of this experimental objective may provide insight into the primary mechanism(s) of aging at the cellular and molecular level. Moreover, to be discussed in the next section, no such universal marker has been identified for postreplicative cells.

Aging in Postreplicative Cells

There are a large number of terminally differentiated (postreplicative) cell types that can be identified at the cytologic or molecular levels. For the purposes of this discussion, the following two broad groups of cells are identified: (1) cells with a short postreplicative life span (hours to days) and rapid replacement from stem cell precursors, such as red blood cells (RBCs) and polymorphonuclear leukocytes; and (2) cells with a long postreplicative life span and minimal or absent capacity for renewal from stem cell populations. This latter class includes neurons, skeletal muscle cells, myocardial cells, and oocytes.

While a universal marker that would define senescent cells in all postreplicative populations has not been identified, recent studies with RBCs indicate that changes occur in the plasma membrane that identify senescent cells and are involved in the mechanism for the removal of these senescent cells. These studies may provide a model for experimental approaches to the identification of biomarkers of senescence in other cell types and are described in some detail below.

Short-Lived Postreplicative Cells—The RBC

The kinetics of mature RBC turnover has been extensively studied in humans and in a number of experimental animal models. As every student of medicine learns early in training, the half-life of this cell in the circulation in humans is approximately 120 days. It is probably less well known that a reasonably close correlation between the survival time of RBCs and the maximum life span of the species has been reported.[8] The precision of RBC turnover suggested to a number of investigators that recognition and elimination of senescent RBCs may be initiated by specific changes in the cell. It is now known that phagocytosis of the senescent RBC is initiated by the binding of an IgG autoantibody to the modified cell-surface glycoprotein.[35] Antibodies raised to purified preparations of the "senescence protein" cross-react with a major transmembrane polypeptide. This peptide, constituting about 25% of the RBC membrane proteins, mediates anion exchange across the plasma membrane and may be involved in other fundamental biologic activities, such as glucose transport and attachment of the cytoskeleton to the plasma membrane. Modification of this antigen to the susceptibility of binding by the autoantibody can be brought about by storage of the RBC, exposure to detergent, and proteolytic cleavage.

These antigens have now been demonstrated to be present in a much lower concentration in the plasma membranes of a variety of other nucleated somatic cells, including neutrophils and squamous epithelial cells and in a variety of neoplastic cells but not hepatocytes.[34] The wide distribution of an antigenically similar membrane protein is not surprising given the basic biologic function of this peptide. Of interest for cellular aging is that these observations suggest the possibility of a generalized mechanism for the identification and elimination of senescent cells. Clearly, the exact mechanism would vary, depending on the anatomic location of the cells, eg, extravascular vs intravascular.

Long-Lived Postreplicative Cells

One of the problems in critically evaluating the results of descriptive studies of age-associated changes in long-lived postreplicative cells is that many of the observed changes are secondary or tertiary phenomena. For example, it has been pointed out that many of the changes in skeletal muscle may be related to disuse atrophy.[36] In this overview of cellular aging, only a few observations that may reflect direct manifestations of a primary mechanism will be examined.

The ultimate end point of cell aging is cell death. The estimate of age-associated loss of nonrenewable cells in an organ does not provide direct insights into the mechanism of cellular aging. However, such studies do provide data regarding the relative vulnerability of cells to aging and some information that correlates with changes of physiologic functions. The question of cell loss has been most extensively studied in the central nervous system of humans. This is in part due to the belief that this organ may be an important determinant in the rate of aging and, therefore, longevity of the organism. These studies are technically demanding, involving the application of quantitative morphometric techniques in conjunction with an accurate estimation of the volume of the anatomic region that is being analyzed.[37] Such studies have shown that the extent of neuronal loss varies from one anatomic region to another in the central nervous system. In some regions of the brain, no age-associated neuronal loss is apparent with the techniques for enumeration presently available. On the other hand, significant loss of Purkinje's cells in the cerebellum, neurons in the locus caeruleus, and dopamine-containing neurons in the midbrain has been documented. The precise physiologic consequences of neuronal loss in these regions are unknown at the present time. It has been suggested that neuronal loss in the locus caeruleus may be causally related to sleep disturbances that are frequently observed in elderly persons and that the decrease in the number of dopamine-containing neurons could be related to age-associated parkinsonism.[36]

Of particular interest in human studies has been the investigation of neuronal loss in the cerebral cortex. The earliest reports indicated that significant neuronal loss occurs with age in this region of the brain.[38] However, more recent investigations that have utilized sophisticated image analysis techniques have revealed a somewhat more modest neuronal loss in the cerebral cortex. Interestingly, a decrease in the proportion of large neurons (90-μm cross-sectional area) associated with a concomitant increase in a subpopulation of smaller neurons has been reported.[36] The authors interpreted this observation as shrinkage of the larger cells. While the biologic significance of this observation is unclear, it raises the possibility that neuronal size could be a useful marker of aging in these cell populations. In this study, as in earlier ones, the number of glial cells was observed to increase with age, yet another example of age-related hyperproliferation.

The extent of neuronal loss has not been as extensively studied in other animal species. One group of investigators found a decline in the number of large neurons in sonicated brain preparations that paralleled the age-specific mortality in one inbred strain of laboratory mice.[39] Certainly, the development of a well-characterized animal model will be essential for the exploration of the mechanism(s) of cell loss in the central nervous system and for a more precise knowledge of the physiologic consequences of this phenomenon.

The mechanism of cell death in long-lived postreplicative cell populations is unknown. However, given the variable extent to which cell loss occurs, it is possible that specific mechanisms of cell death are operant or, alternatively, certain critical cell types have evolved mechanisms that render them less vulnerable to the aging process. The identification of specific markers that would unambiguously identify aged cells in these populations, such as have been characterized in the erythrocyte, would greatly facilitate the study of age-related cell death.

To be sure, many studies have revealed a host of biochemical and anatomic changes in specific cell populations. For example, studies designed to evaluate qualitative and quantitative changes of receptors for neurotransmitters have been carried out, and the emerging picture is complex. Decreases in the number of one class of dopamine receptors (D-2) and the major classes of serotonin receptors have been demonstrated. However, another class of dopamine receptors (D-1) increases in number in aging humans, while in rodents, the levels of this receptor remain constant.[40] The authors suggest that these alterations may be causally related to age-associated neurodegenerative disorders, such as parkinsonism. However, the fact that interspecies variation is apparent serves to emphasize that the manifestations of aging at the cellular level are modulated by the genetic endowment of the species.

Anatomic changes that may have relevance to important functional change with age have also been described. For example, dramatic morphologic changes have been observed in the mitochondria of myocardial cells following prolonged hypoxia.[41] Biochemical studies by other investigators have revealed functional impairment of the mitochondria.[42] These studies obviously deal with a very important area of geriatric research, ie, the causes of age-associated decline of myocardial function. However, two other aspects of the design of these studies should be emphasized. The first important general experimental strategy in aging research is the application of stress (such as hypoxia in the example above) to the experimental system, which frequently increases the magnitude of change in the parameter under study in the aged subjects. The second aspect is the importance of a combined anatomic and biochemical approach to the study of cellular function in vivo, a point that has been emphasized by other gerontologists.[36] It is obvious that changes in the relative abundance of cell populations within tissues with age could profoundly influence the interpretation of observed alterations.

Many age-associated changes, such as those described above, are confined to a single tissue or narrow range of cell types and may reflect the highly specialized nature of these tissues. There is, however, one age-associated change that is almost universal in multicellular organisms—the intracellular accumulation of lipofuscin, ie, so-called age pigments. This insoluble yellow-brown material accumulates in a perinuclear location and is most prominent in the long-lived postreplicative cells, such as neurons and myocardial cells. Despite extensive analytic studies, the composition of lipofuscin is not known; it is thought to be composed of auto-oxidation products of various cellular macromolecules, including proteins but primarily unsaturated lipids.[43] However, the accumulation of lipofuscin with age has been well documented (Fig. 1.4.). It has been pointed out that a relationship to a maximum life span is apparent in comparisons of the rate of intracellular accumulation of this pigment in beagle dogs and humans.[36] Clearly, further studies comparing the rate of accumulation of lipofuscin in closely related species of differing longevities will be of interest.

The role of lipofuscin per se as direct cause of cellular dysfunction is uncertain. It has been suggested by some investigators that the accumulation of this pigment is an immediate cause of functional decline and death in many cell populations. This appears to be unlikely in light of observations that the neurons of the inferior olivary nucleus contain some of the largest

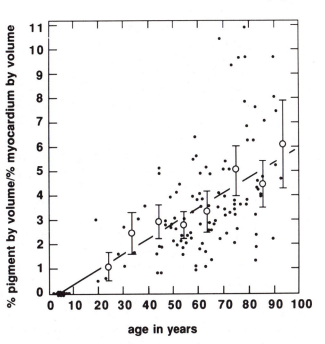

Fig. 1.4. Accumulation of lipofuscin in human myocardium plotted as function of age. (from Strehler BL, Mark DD, Mildvan AS, et al. Rate and magnitude of age pigment accumulation in the human myocardium. *J Gerontol* 1959;14:430-439. Used by permission).

accumulations of lipofuscin, despite the fact that this is one of the regions of the brain stem that does not show neuronal loss.[36] This does not, however, diminish the importance of this pigment as a useful biomarker. As will be discussed in the next section, the accumulation of products of auto-oxidation is predicted by a theory that postulates free-radical damage as a primary cause of aging.

Theories of Aging and Future Prospects

The fundamental importance of biomarkers is that they will provide end points for studies designed to test the theories of aging that attempt to explain primary causes of this process at the molecular level. Historically, theories of aging have fallen into two broad categories as follows: (1) those predicting that the quality and quantity of aging are primarily regulated by genetic mechanisms, referred to as the *programmed* theories of aging; and (2) those that propose that randomly occurring, injurious events are the primary causes of the aging process, sometimes referred to as *stochastic* theories. The most compelling evidence for the programmed hypotheses is the striking variation in the maximum achievable life span among mammalian species. If one assumes a conservative 100-year maximum life span for humans, the longest-lived mammalian species, and approximately 2 years or slightly less for the shortest-lived species, the shrew, then a 40- to 50-fold variation in life span is present in mammals alone. Also, there is an overall positive correlation between the time span from birth to sexual maturity and maximum life span, suggesting that longevity is related to the developmental process. As indicated above, even the growth potential of mammalian diploid cells appears to be positively related to life span. These observations indicate that the genotype of any species is a primary determinant of longevity.

There have been many stochastic theories put forward during the past century, with many being little more than refinements of ones previously proposed.[44] The following three injury theories have received the most attention during the last two decades: (1) *the protein error catastrophe theory,* which predicts that errors in transcription and/or translation result in production of abnormal proteins, a few of which will be involved in the synthesis of more abnormal species; this sequence ultimately will lead to an exponential increase of abnormal proteins (and other macromolecules) to functionally significant levels; (2) *the free-radical theory,* which proposes that aging primarily is the result of damage to macromolecules, particularly unsaturated lipids, but also to proteins and DNA, mediated by the action of free radicals derived from oxidative metabolism in the organism; and (3) *the somatic mutation theory,* which proposes that age is the result of the accumulation of mutations at the gene and/or chromosome levels in somatic cells. It is evident that these theories have extensive overlap and are not mutually exclusive. For example, somatic mutations could be caused by the action of free radicals or by the decreased replicative fidelity of an abnormal DNA polymerase, resulting from an erroneous protein synthesis. There is now a very extensive literature that describes in vitro and in vivo studies designed to test these various hypotheses.[44] At this time, there is no definitive experimental evidence that excludes any of the theories of aging that have been proposed. During the past decade, however, there has been a resurgence of interest in the free-radical theory with advancing knowledge of the biologic significance of these very reactive chemical entities.[45]

It would seem at first glance that the genetic or programmed theory of aging and the stochastic theories are mutually exclusive. However, given that the longevity has a strong genetic component, as evidenced by the interspecies differences in maximum life spans, the rate of aging must likewise be, at least in part, regulated by the genetic endowment of the species. It is possible that relatively few genes are directly involved in the determination of longevity.

Martin[46] has speculated that possibly as few as 7% of unique genes are of direct relevance to aging. This speculation is based on the fraction of known mendelian genetic disorders that are associated with a premature onset of one or more features of "normal" aging.

Assuming that there are relatively few genes that determine the nature and rate of aging in mammalian species, the obvious next question is regarding the nature of the genetic loci that may be direct determinants of longevity. While the answer to this question is unknown at the present time, several experimental observations suggest that genes involved in DNA repair, scavenging abnormal molecules, and possibly other "janitorial" activities are potential candidates. A study by Hart and Setlow[47] demonstrated a positive correlation between the magnitude of the DNA repair response in cultured fibroblasts following exposure to UV light and the maximum life span of the species from which the cells were derived, an observation that has been confirmed in other laboratories. In addition to DNA repair, there are enzyme systems that specifically metabolize abnormal proteins and free radicals (Table 1.4.). Indeed, there is at least one study that has shown a positive correlation between the activity of certain antioxidants and longevity.[48] While these observations must be considered preliminary, they provide a strong rationale for the vigorous exploration of the role of this class of genes as modulators of the aging process. The answer to these questions will certainly emerge, as the methods for detection of mutational events, free-radical damage, and the levels of abnormal proteins become more sensitive.

The role of changes of gene regulation in the aging process will be vigorously explored. There are now a number of observations that suggest that changes in gene action may be a factor in aging. For example, the levels of methylation of DNA have been shown to decrease with age in murine tissue and in human fibroblasts in vitro.[49,50] Methylation is, at the present time, the only molecular modification known to occur in DNA and clearly is involved in the regulation of gene activity. These observations may be relevant to the relationship between aging and the increased incidence of carcinomas; the extent of DNA methylation in many cancers is reduced relative to that observed in the normal tissue.[50]

The model systems that have been used for the study of aging at the cellular level have limited the types of questions that can be asked. This limitation has precluded the exploration of some very important areas of cell biology that may be very relevant to aging. For example, it is well known that many metabolic interactions occur between and within cell populations. In addition, cell function is influenced by

Table 1.4. Selected stochastic theories of aging, corresponding types of damage, and repair mechanisms.

Source, y	Name of theory	Molecular substrate	Mechanism of primary change	Responding repair or scavenger system
Rothstein,[55] 1987	Protein error catastrophe	Primary: proteins; secondary: errors of DNA synthesis	Random errors of transcription and translation	Extralysosomal degradation pathway, ubiquitin conjugation
Setlow,[56] 1987	Somatic mutation	Primary: DNA; secondary: production of abnormal proteins	Random errors during replication and repair, damage by physical and chemical mutagens	DNA repair, specific metabolic pathways for different types of damage
Katz and Robison,[43] 1986; Harman,[45] 1986	Free-radical	All macromolecules, lipids most frequently	Free-radical damage to macromolecules, eg, lipid peroxidation	Antioxidants and metabolic enzymes, eg, glutathione, superoxide dismutase, peroxidase

the extracellular matrix that is known to undergo qualitative and quantitative changes with age. The importance of age-associated changes in cell-to-cell and cell-to-matrix interactions has remained relatively unexplored. More sophisticated cell culture systems, in which these cell-to-cell and cell-to-matrix interactions can be more precisely defined certainly will be developed in the near future. Such systems will help to define the relative importance of intrinsic factors, such as the level of DNA methylation, and extrinsic events, such as the change in the quality or quantity of a component of the extracellular matrix, to cellular aging.

There are many potential experimental approaches to the study of the basic mechanism of aging at the cellular and molecular level. These surely will lead to significant advances in this field during the next several decades. However, it should be emphasized that the ultimate goal of basic biogerontologic research is identical to that of clinical geriatrics: to develop a rational basis for the treatment and, more importantly, the prevention of the age-associated decline of basic physiologic functions that is so destructive to the quality of life for many elderly persons.

References

1. Harrison DE. Experience with developing assays of physiological age. In: Reff ME, Schneider EL, eds. *Biomarkers of Aging.* Bethesda, MD:; 1981:2-12. National Institutes of Heatlh publication NIH 82-2221.
2. Carrel A. *Man, the Unknown.* New York, NY: Halycyon House; 1935:173.
3. Hayflick L, Moorhead PS. The serial cultivation of human diploid cell strains. *Exp Cell Res* 1961;25:585-621.
4. Hayflick L. The limited in vitro lifetime of human diploid cell strains. *Exp Cell Res* 1965;37:614-636.
5. Martin GM, Sprague CA, Epstein CJ. Replicative lifespan of cultivated human cells. effects of donor's age, tissue, and genotype. *Lab Invest* 1970;23:86-92.
6. Martin GM, Ogburn CE, Sprague CA. Effects of age on cell division capacity. In: Danon D, Shock NW, Marois M, eds. *Aging: A Challenge to Science and Society.* New York, NY: Oxford University Press Inc; 1981; 1:124-135.
7. Goldstein S. Human genetic disorders that feature premature onset and accelerated progression of biological aging. In: Schneider EL, ed: *The Genetics of Aging.* New York, NY: Plenum Publishing Corp; 1978:171-224.
8. Rohme D. Evidence for a relationship between longevity of mammalian species and life-spans of normal fibroblasts in vitro and erythrocytes in vitro. *Proc Natl Acad Sci USA* 1980;78:5009-5013.
9. Schneider EL, Mitsui Y. The relationship between in vitro cellular aging and in vivo human age. *Proc Natl Acad Sci USA* 1972;73:3584-3588.
10. Martin GM. Genetic syndromes in man with potential relevance to the pathobiology of aging. *Birth Defects* 1978;14:5-39.
11. Hoehn H, Bryant EM, Au K, et al. Variegated translocation mosaicism in human fibroblast cultures. *Cytogenet Cell Genet* 1975;15:282-298.
12. Epstein CJ, Martin GM, Schultz AL, et al. Werner's syndrome: a review of its symptomology, natural history, pathology features, genetics and relationship to the natural aging process. *Medicine* 1966;45:177-221.
13. Martin GM, Sprague CA. Life histories of hyperplastoid cell lines from aorta and skin. *Exp Mol Pathol* 1973;18:125-141.
14. Rothfels FH, Kupelweiser EB, Parker RC. Effects of X-irradiated feeder layers on mitotic activity and development of aneuploidy in mouse embryo cells in vitro. *Can Cancer Conf* 1963;5:191-223.
15. Weinberg RA. A molecular basis of cancer. *Sci Am* 1983;249:126-143.
16. Varmus HE. The molecular genetics of cellular oncogenes. *Annu Rev Genet* 1984;18:553-612.

17. Bister K, Jensen HW. Oncogenes in retroviruses and cells: biochemistry and molecular genetics. *Adv Cancer Res* 1986;47:99-188.

18. Thrasher JD, Greulich RC. The duodenal progenitor population, I: age related increase in the duration of the cryptal progenitor cycle. *J Exp Zool* 1965;159:39-46.

19. Daniel CW. Cell longevity in vivo. In: Finch CE, Hayflick L, eds. *Handbook of the Biology of Aging*. 1st ed. New York, NY: Van Nostrand Reinhold Co; 1977:122-158.

20. Harrison DE. Cell and tissue transplantation: a means of studying the aging process. In: Finch CE, Schneider EL, eds. *Handbook of the Biology of Aging*. 2nd ed. New York, NY: Van Nostrand Reinhold Co; 1985:322-356.

21. Norwood TH, Smith JR. The cultured fibroblast-like cell as a model for the study of aging. In: Finch CE, Schneider EL, eds. *Handbook of the Biology of Aging*. 2nd ed. New York, NY: Van Nostrand Reinhold Co; 1985:291-321.

22. Cristofalo, VJ, Stanulis-Praeger BM. Cellular senescence in vitro. In: Maramotosch K, ed. *Advances in Tissue Culture*. Orlando, Fla: Academic Press Inc; 1982;2:1-68.

23. Martin GM. Cellular aging—clonal senescence. *Am J Pathol* 1977;89:484-510.

24. Hornsby PJ, Hancock JP, Vo TP, et al. Loss of expression of a differentiated function give steroid 17α-hydroxylase, as adrenocortical cells senesce in culture. *Proc Natl Acad Sci USA* 1987;84:1580-1584.

25. Martin GM. Proliferative homeostasis and its age-related aberrations. *Mech Ageing Dev* 1979;9:385-391.

26. Takehara K, LeRoy EC, Grotendorst GR. TGF-β inhibition of endothelial cell proliferation: alteration of EGF binding and EGF-induced growth-regulatory (competence) gene expression. *Cell* 1987;49:415-422.

27. Eaglstein WH. Wound healing and aging. *Dermatol Clin* 1986;4:481-484.

28. Siskind GW. Aging and the immune system. In: Warner HR, Butler RN, Sprott RL, et al, eds. *Modern Biological Theories of Aging*. New York, NY: Raven Press; 1987:235-242.

29. Hefton JM, Darlington GJ, Casazza BA, et al. Immunologic studies of aging, V: impaired proliferation of PHA responsive human lymphocytes in culture. *J Immunol* 1980;125:1007-1010.

30. Tice RR, Schneider EL, Kram D, et al. Cytokinetic analysis of the impaired proliferative response of peripheral lymphocytes from aged humans to phytohemagglutinin. *J Exp Med* 1979;149:1029-1041.

31. Ebbesen P. Aging increases susceptibility of mouse skin to DMBA carcinogenesis independent of general immune status. *Science* 1974;183:217-218.

32. Gown AM, Norwood TH. Atherosclerosis and cellular aging. In: Blumenthal HT, ed. *Handbook of Disease of Aging*. New York, NY: Van Nostrand Reinhold Co; 1983:149-180.

33. Ross R. The pathogenesis of atherosclerosis—an update. *N Engl J Med* 1986;314:488-500.

34. Hayflick L. The cellular basis for biological aging. In: Hayflick L, Finch CE, eds. *The Handbook of the Biology of Aging*. 1st ed. New York, NY: Van Nostrand Reinhold Co; 1977:159-186.

35. Kay MMB. Aging of cell membrane molecules leads to appearance of an aging antigen and removal of senescent cells. *Gerontology* 1985;31:215-235.

36. Martin GM. Cellular aging—postreplicative cells. *Am J Pathol* 1977;89:513-530.

37. Terry RD, Hansen LA. Some morphometric aspects of Alzheimer disease and of normal aging. In Terry RD, ed. *Aging and the Brain*. New York, NY: Raven Press; 1988:109-114.

38. Brody H. Organization of the cerebral cortex, III: a study of aging in the human cerebral cortex. *J Comp Neurol* 1955;102:551-556.

39. Johnson HA, Erner S. Neuron survival in the aging mouse. *Exp Gerontol* 1972;7:111-117.

40. Morgan DG, May PC, Finch CE. Dopamine and serotonin systems in human and rodent brain: effects of age and neurodegenerative disease. *J Am Geriatr Soc* 1987;35:334-345.

41. Sulkin NM, Sulkin DF. Age differences in response to chronic hypoxia in the fine structure of cardiac muscle and autonomic ganglion cells. *J Gerontol* 1967;22:485-501.

42. Chen JC, Warshaw JB, Sanadi DR. Regulations of mitochondrial respiration in senescence. *J Cell Physiol* 1972;80:141-148.

43. Katz ML, Robison WG Jr. Nutritional influences on auto-oxidation, lipofuscin accumulation, and aging. In: Johnson JE Jr, Walford R, Harman D, et al, eds. *Free Radicals, Aging, and Degenerative Diseases*. New York, NY: Alan R Liss Inc; 1986:221-259.

44. Schneider EL. Theories of aging: a perspective. In: Warner HL, Butler RN, Sprott RL, et al, eds. *Modern Biological Theories of Aging*. New York, NY: Raven Press; 1987:1-4.

45. Harman D. Free radical theory of aging: role of free radicals in the origination and evolution of life, aging, and disease processes. In: Johnson JE, Walford R, Harman D, et al, eds. *Free Radicals, Aging, and Degenerative Diseases*. New York, NY: Alan R Liss Inc; 1986:3-49.

46. Martin GM. Genetic and evolutionary aspects of aging. *FASEB J* 1979;38:1962-1967.

47. Hart RW, Setlow RB. Correlation between deoxyribonucleic acid excision repair and lifespan in a number of mammalian species. *Proc Natl Acad Sci USA* 1974;71:2169-2173.

48. Cutler RG. Peroxide-producing potential of tissues: inverse correlation with longevity of mammalian species. *Proc Natl Acad Sci USA* 1985;82:4798-4802.

49. Wilson VL, Jones PA. DNA methylation decreases in aging but not in immortal cells. *Science* 1983;220:1055-1057.

50. Mays-Loope L, Chao W, Butcher HC, et al. Decreased methylation of the major mouse interspersed repeated DNA during and in myeloma cells. *Dev Genet* 1986;7:65-73.

51. Bierman EL. The effect of donor age in the in vitro lifespan of cultured human arterial smooth-muscle cells. *In Vitro* 1978;14:951-955.

52. Glassberg MK, Bern MM, Coughlin SR, et al. Cultured endothelial cells derived from the human iliac arteries. *In Vitro* 1982;18:859-866.

53. Rheinwald JO, Green H. Serial cultivation of strains of human epidermal keratinocytes: the formation of keratinizing colonies from single cells. *Cell* 1975;6:331-344.

54. Walford RL, Jawaid SQ, Nalim F. Evidence for in vitro senescence of T lymphocytes cultured from normal human peripheral blood. *Age* 1981;4:67-70.

55. Rothstein M. Evidence for and against the error catastrophe hypothesis. In: Warner HR, Butler RN, Sprott RL, et al, eds. *Modern Biological Theories of Aging.* New York, NY: Raven Press; 1987:139-154.

56. Setlow RB. Theory presentation and background summary. In: Warner HR, Butler RN, Sprott RL, et al, eds. *Modern Biological Theories of Aging.* New York, NY: Raven Press; 1987:177-182.

2

Demography, Epidemiology, and Aging

Christine K. Cassel and Jacob A. Brody

Demography

Demography is the study of populations—viewed regionally, nationally, or globally—describing the numbers of people and the dynamics of population change. Demographic studies reveal the phenomenon of increasing numbers and increasing proportion of older people in the United States and in other developed countries. This phenomenon is so predictable that it has become a measure of improved economic and health status of nations in the 20th Century. Aging populations are the result of three major factors: fertility, mortality, and immigration. This discussion concerns the United States, where in the last half century immigration has not been a major influence on mortality patterns, and thus will not discuss immigration in any detail.

Both increased longevity and decreased fertility contribute to the "squaring" of the population pyramid. The most influential factor in the shift in population profile to a greater proportion of elderly people is the decline in fertility rates. The fewer people in the younger generations and the more people surviving to old age, the less "pyramidal" the figure becomes (Fig 2.1). Historically and in most developing countries, women bear many children and high infant and early-life mortality rates cause the percentage of elderly persons in the population to be small. For example, Japan in 1950 had 7.7% of its population over the age of 60 years, and by the year 2000 it will have doubled that amount to between 15% and 16%, because of low birth rates and control of infant mortality. Similarly,

China's dramatic decrease in fertility rates, coincident with its "one child per family" policy begun in the 1970's sets the stage for very rapid population aging, with forecasts of the current 5% elderly population growing to more than 30% in the next 50 years.[1] Thus, in the modern world, a population can age simply because of decreasing birth rates, without necessarily any changes in the longevity of those who do survive into adulthood and early old age.

While more males than females are conceived and born, after birth the male death rate exceeds that of females at all ages. The ratio of women to men in the population increases with age because of what is seen as premature death among men. The female survival advantage is not well understood and is the subject of a number of new studies supported by the National Institute on Aging. The sex discrepancy has definite social importance, since old age in industrial countries is associated with widowhood—and thus poverty and institutionalization—for women who have no independent income separate from their deceased husbands and for whom family support is not available (Fig 2.2).

Mortality

Reductions in both infant mortality and adult deaths from acute diseases have resulted in increasing numbers of individuals surviving to later life. Infant mortality in developed countries has fallen from 150 or more per 1,000 population in the 19th century to approximately 10 per 1,000 today. The larger numbers

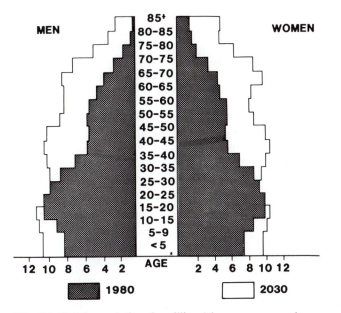

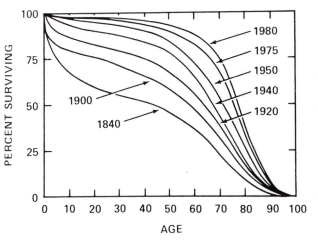

Fig. 2.3. Specific mortality survival curve.

Fig. 2.1. Total population (in millions) by age group and sex.

of survivors would produce a considerable increase in the elderly population even if mortality rates at older ages had not changed. These mortality rates, however, have declined dramatically, and life expectancy in the United States has increased at all ages. Between 1954 and 1982, the life expectancy of men at age 65 years increased by about 1.5 years, from 13.1 to 14.5 years, and that of women increased by about 3 years, from 15.7 to 18.9 years.[2]

Life expectancy from birth in the United States for 1984 was forecast to be approaching 75 years for men and 79 years for women.[3] These forecasts, made by the Office of the Actuary of the Census Bureau, have underestimated life expectancy in the past.[4] Experts in epidemiology, demography, and statistics are seeking greater accuracy by using models that incorporate hypotheses about trends in the treatment and prevention of chronic degenerative diseases.

Specific mortality can be shown in a survival curve, as illustrated in Figure 2.3, which shows survival

curves for Americans from 1840 to 1980. Note the initial drop due to decreased infant mortality at the beginning of the century and the fact that more than half of people died before middle age at that time. In 1900, life expectancy at birth was between 45 and 50 years, compared with 74 years for those born in 1980. Age-adjusted mortality rates throughout the whole population are decreasing, with the greatest declines occurring in the population over the age of 80 years.

Thus, not only are populations getting older, but elderly individuals are living longer and mortality rates even at higher ages are falling. In many countries, including the United States, those over the age of 80 years make up the fastest growing segment of the population, a segment expected to double in size by the end of the century (Fig 2.4). Changes in death rates at advanced ages have little effect on the age structure of the population as a whole, because the size of this age group is relatively small, but these changes do have a major impact on medical and social resources. Of the group over the age of 65 years, it is those over 85 years who are at greatest risk to suffer from impaired function and disability related to chronic illness. In 1986, almost 75% of all deaths occurred in

Year	At birth			At age 65		
	Male	Female	Difference	Male	Female	Difference
1990	71.6	79.2	7.6	15.0	19.5	4.5
2000	72.9	80.5	7.6	15.7	20.5	4.8
2010	73.8	81.5	7.7	16.1	21.2	5.1
2020	74.2	82.0	7.8	16.5	21.7	5.2
2030	74.6	82.5	7.9	16.8	22.1	5.3
2040	75.0	83.1	8.1	17.1	22.6	5.5
2050	75.5	83.6	8.1	17.4	23.1	5.7

Fig. 2.2. Projected life expectancy at birth and age 65 by sex: 1990-2050 (from Spencer, G, *Projections of the Population of the United States, by age, sex, and race: 1983-2080,* Current Population Reports, Series P-25, No. 952, May 1984).

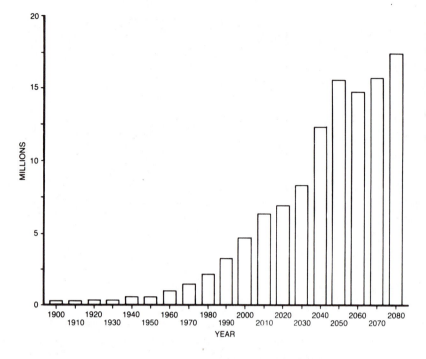

Fig. 2.4. Actual and projected increase in population 85 years and older: 1900-2080 (from Taeuber CM, *America in Transition: An Aging Society,* Current Population Reports, Series P-23, No. 128, September 1983, and Spenecer G, *Projections of the population of the United States, by age, sex, and race: 1983-2080,* Current Population Reports, Series P-25, No. 952, May 1984).

people aged 65 years and over. Thirty percent of deaths were in those aged 80 years and over, and 20% in those older than 85 years.[5]

Epidemiologists have questioned the degree to which the decline in mortality in developed countries in this century is related to modern medical care. While the mortality decline parallels the development of modern medical practices and institutions, it appears to be related more directly to factors of social progress, such as better sanitation, nutrition, and working conditions, than to any specific medical interventions.[6]

The primary lethal diseases in the year 1900 were infectious (Fig 2.5). Thus, not only has the age at which people die changed, but what they die of has also changed. The primary causes of death in 1980 were cardiovascular diseases, cancer, and stroke. It is possible to view these as diseases of older adults, since in the early part of the century—when few people lived long enough to manifest these disorders—they were not prominent causes of death.

These diseases, which account for more than 75% of deaths in our society, are the areas where the greatest resources have been invested in research on treatment and prevention, with substantial success in many areas. While there is no cure for any of the major three causes of death, both risk factor modification and treatment have improved, so that the onset of disease is delayed, and survival, even with disease, is prolonged. It is conceivable, then, that the surprising decreases in mortality in the very old age groups, especially those over 75 or 85 years, are in some way

related to these modern health care interventions. Where people previously would have died of pneumonia, heart attack, stroke, or malignancy, we are now able to prevent deaths from one of these causes or at least to delay them.

The concept of postponement is important to an understanding of the contemporary demographic debate. The public health and preventive medicine approach to chronic degenerative diseases of old age

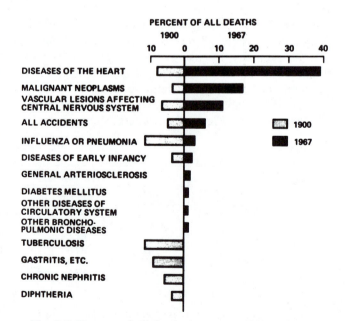

Fig. 2.5. Percent of all deaths by cause: 1900 and 1967.

uses the language of "prevention." Behavioral and medical risk factor alteration has become a fundamental part of medical practice, as reflected in the widespread pharmacologic treatment of hypertension (to "prevent" stroke or renal failure) and the recommendation of exercise and dietary changes (to "prevent" heart disease). In fact, it is very rare that diseases such as stroke and myocardial infarction are entirely prevented by risk factor intervention. Rather, much more commonly, their onset is delayed.[7] Early in the 1950s and 1960s, when cardiovascular mortality was reaching its peak, it was common for men to suffer a first heart attack in their 40s or 50s. Now, because of changes in life-style and (to some undetermined degree) invasive therapeutic methods, that first heart attack often does not occur until age 70 or 75 years, or even later. Heart disease has not been eradicated, however, or even decreased in incidence. The most common reported cause of death, even among the very elderly, is still cardiovascular disease.

The prevention of lung cancer by avoidance of cigarette smoking is one example of a disease that truly can be prevented by risk factor modification. The relations of other cancers (eg, bowel and breast cancer, leukemia, and lymphoma) to risk factor interventions are much less direct.

Epidemiology

Epidemiology is the study of patterns of disease in populations. Morbidity is a technical term referring to the presence of disease. Measures are made of both morbidity and mortality rates. As we delay the occurrence of death, we increase the duration of time during which people are susceptible to the degenerative and chronic diseases of senescence.

The nonlethal chronic illnesses of old age that have the greatest impact on function include degenerative neurologic disorders (such as Alzheimer's disease, Parkinson's disease, and stroke) and chronic musculoskeletal disorders (most prominently osteoarthritis and osteoporosis with resultant fractures). We can ameliorate the symptoms of chronic degenerative diseases, but in most cases we do not understand enough about their etiology or pathogenesis to delay or prevent them. While much research is going on in all of these areas, currently there is very little understanding of preventive measures. Thus, we delay the onset of lethal illnesses such as myocardial infarction, stroke, and certain malignancies and thereby expose people to an increased risk of suffering from a nonlethal but severely disabling degenerative disorder. This fact is illustrated by the huge and growing prevalence of Alzheimer's disease and related disorders. While only

5% of people over the age of 65 years have dementia, 20% or more of those over the age of 80 years are so afflicted, and the incidence increases more than linearly with age. At present, 2.5 million Americans have a dementing disorder.

Interestingly, the lethal disorders—cardiovascular disease, stroke, and cancer—have in many respects also become chronic illnesses. People are more likely to survive an initial heart attack, stroke, or malignancy and go on to receive treatment. If these disorders are not lethal within a short period of time, they may move into a chronic phase requiring "medical management." The patient enters into a relationship with the health care system, but the disease does not cause the person's death, or at least not until many years later.

Causes of Death

What do elderly people die of? In population studies, causes of death are usually determined from death certificates. As any experienced clinician knows, it is often difficult to establish a single cause of death when an older person dies. There have been proposals for a category called senescence or old age on the death certificate.

In a recent French study of people over the age of 65 years, "senility" was listed as an underlying cause of death in 2% to 3% of death certificates for those aged 70 to 74 years, compared with 25% for those aged 90 years and over.[8] In a Scandinavian study, up to one third of individuals over the age of 70 years died of "old age" rather than a single organ failure, in the view of certifying physicians.[9]

In the United States, however, death certificates most commonly point to cardiovascular diseases as being the final cause of death. While ischemic heart disease and stroke continue to be the major causes of death, even at very advanced ages (Table 2.1), these older groups also shared in the decrease in ischemic heart disease and stroke mortality that followed the 1960s. For white men, heart disease mortality rates increased dramatically until 1965, and since that time there has been a reversal, with each successive cohort showing a decrease. The US statistics for deaths from heart disease in white women have shown a continuous decline for successive birth cohorts from 1886 onward.

Mortality in old age from neoplastic diseases, however, is on the increase in about half of industrialized countries and falling in the other half. In the United States, breast cancer and lung cancer are the only categories in which there has been an increase in mortality.

Table 2.1. Leading chronic conditions in those 65 and over, by sex.

Men 65–74	Women 65–74
1. Arthritis	Arthritis
2. High blood pressure	High blood pressure
3. Hearing impairment	Hearing impairment
4. Ischemic heart disease	Cataracts
5. Tinnitus	Ischemic heart disease
6. Diabetes	Varicose Veins
7. Hardening of the arteries	Tinnitus
8. Cataracts	Diabetes
9. Cerebrovascular disease	Visual impairment
10. Varicose Veins	Hardening of the arteries

Men 75–84	Women 75–84
1. Arthritis	Arthritis
2. Hearing impairment	High blood pressure
3. High blood pressure	Hearing impairment
4. Cataracts	Cataracts
5. Ischemic heart disease	Ischemic heart disease
6. Other visual impairment	Other visual impairment
7. Tinnitus	Hardening of the arteries
8. Hardening of the arteries	Tinnitus
9. Malignant neoplasms	Varicose veins
10. Diabetes	Diabetes

Men 85+	Women 85+
1. Hearing impairment	Arthritis
2. Arthritis	High blood pressure
3. High blood pressure	Hearing impairment
4. Cataracts	Cataracts
5. Visual impairment	Visual impairment
6. Hardening of the arteries	Hardening of the arteries
7. Ischemic heart disease	Ischemic heart disease
8. Deaf both ears	Lower extremity orthopedic impairment
9. Lower extremity orthopedic impairment	Tinnitus
10. Malignant neoplasms	Varicose veins

Source: National Health Interview Surveys, 1984; S.O.A. Reference 16.

Demographic Transitions

The rate of decline in mortality with advances of civilization has not been a smooth slope (Fig 2.6). There have been periods in history when there were dramatic changes in mortality rates, known as demographic transitions.[10] Generally, the consequence of a transition was a redistribution of deaths from the young to the old. The epidemiologic transition theory, as it was originally set forth, described the three stages of the transition as the age of pestilence and famine (lasting until about 1850), the age of receding pandemics (lasting from 1850 to 1920), and the age of degenerative and manmade diseases (lasting from 1920

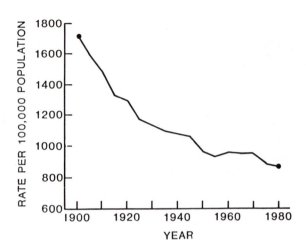

Fig. 2.6. Mortality rates for years 1900-1980 (all ages).

on). Gains on longevity in the United States since the middle of the 19th century reflect these epidemiologic transitions, in which deaths from infectious and parasitic diseases were replaced by deaths from degenerative diseases. The third transition was the early 20th century, when the mortality rate for all ages fell from 1,720 per 100,000 in 1900 to approximately 1,100 per 100,000 by 1920. The major reason for this decrease was not medical care but rather improved living environments and better sanitation and nutrition.[11] In Figure 2.7, the decline in mortality rate from tuberculosis from 1900 to 1980 is shown. Clearly, there has been a consistent and dramatic decline in tuberculosis deaths, independent of the introduction of specific antimicrobial chemotherapy. This observation led to a more sophisticated examination of the factors related to mortality reduction.

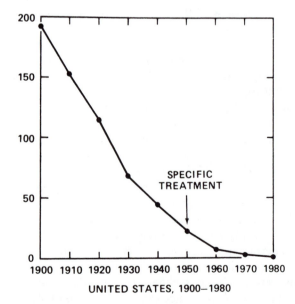

Fig. 2.7. Mortality rate from tuberculosis: 1900-1980.

By about 1945, half of the decline in mortality observed in this century for those over 65 years had been achieved. This decline was also probably related to social rather than medical influences, because it is hard to identify any special medical interventions that would have delayed death in older age groups before 1945.

After the third demographic transition, there was a plateau. In the population aged 65 years and over, mortality did not decline rapidly. From 1945 to the late 1960s, when the development of specific medical treatments was booming (eg, antibiotics, cardiac treatments, hormone replacements, and intensive care units), mortality actually increased among those age 65 years and over. This phenomenon could be interpreted as more people surviving to age 65 years and then dying within the next decade of age-associated diseases.

Policymakers have assumed a constant or even increasing mortality in the elderly, as more people survived to old age, and they have based public policies such as Social Security on these projections. Since 1970, however, mortality rates among the elderly population have consistently and dramatically declined, particularly among the very oldest. Figure 2.8 shows life expectancy in 1984 at selected ages by race and sex.

Recent trends in cause-specific mortality indicate that since the mid-1960s in the United States there have been rapid declines in the rate of deaths from major degenerative diseases, primarily among the population reaching advanced ages. This has resulted in unexpected increases in life expectancy at birth and at older ages that go beyond the general characteristics of what is described as the third stage of the epidemiologic transition. The timing and magnitude of this latest mortality transition is significant and distinct enough from the previous stages to qualify as the fourth stage of the epidemiologic transition—a stage characterized by the postponement of death from degenerative diseases.[12]

Can this recent decline be ascribed to modern medical or social developments? Since cardiovascular diseases have been the most common cause of death, this area is the obvious place to look for the impact of change. Deaths due to cardiac disease have not declined so much in number, but the age of occurrence has been dramatically delayed. This delay could be related in part to behavioral changes among Americans, such as cessation of cigarette smoking, increased exercise, and better diet. It may also be related to new medical and surgical treatments for cardiac disease. Attempts have been made[13] to sort out these factors, but without a controlled experiment the relative roles of social and medical advances will remain speculative.[14] Some studies had indicated that the hypothetical elimination of a single major cause of death would lead to only relatively small gains in life expectancy.[15] This phenomenon can be explained by the clinical observation that with advancing age, people are likely

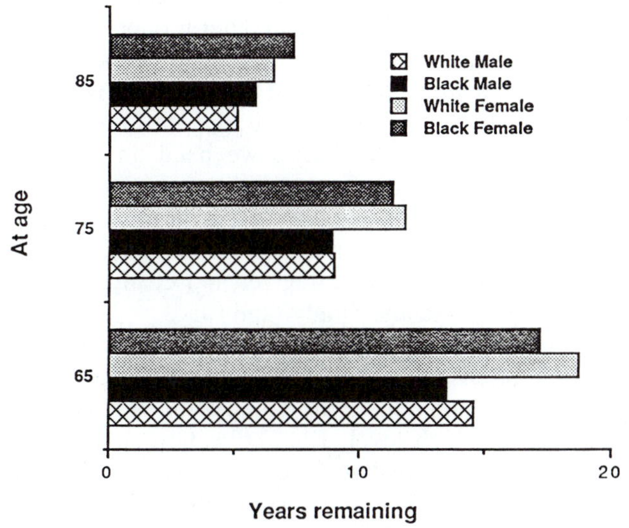

Fig. 2.8. Life expectancy of the elderly in 1984 from Havlik RG, Liu MG, Kovar MG, Health Statistics on Older Persons, United States 1986, Vital and Health Statistics series 3, No. 25. DHHS Pub. No. (PHS) 87-1409. Washington, DC: Government Printing Office, 1987.

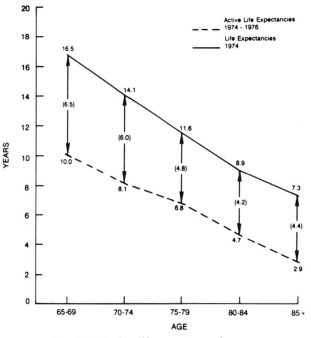

Fig. 2.9. Active life expectancy by age.

to have more than one chronic illness. If death from one cause, such as cancer, is avoided or postponed, the person may die relatively soon from another cause, such as heart attack. Most degenerative diseases of modern civilization share some common risk factors, and simultaneous multiple-cause elimination models have been shown to reflect general mortality trends from 1960 to the present more accurately than single-cause models.[16]

Active Life Expectancy

The epidemiology of chronic nonlethal disease in the elderly population is of great concern to health care planners and indeed to everyone as we face this optimistic future of increased longevity. Ideally, one would like to minimize the duration of disability while still extending life expectancy as far as possible. This has been called the "compression of morbidity."[17] The theory of compression of morbidity relies on the two assumptions that the biologic life span itself will not increase and that chronic disabling disorders can be prevented. Life expectancy, a measure of the probability of reaching that genetically determined life span, can thus increase only up to age 85 to 90 years, with very few people surviving past 100 years. If chronic disease is effectively delayed but death is not postponed, the period of predeath morbidity is decreased. This theory is considered by most analysts to be an unrealistic prediction within the foreseeable future. The major unresolved problems of chronic nonlethal disease and disability still remain.[18] Some analysts are even arguing that life span is not fixed and is increasing, albeit at a slower pace than life expectancy.[19] A recent report of the Census Bureau predicts that the number of centenarians in the United States will increase from 25,000 in 1985 to 110,000 by the year 2000, a huge increase for a 15-year period.[20]

While it is clear that people are living longer, the quality of that life has come under scrutiny. Since many diseases and disabilities are associated with old age, it seems logical that as people live longer they are more susceptible to these chronic illnesses and infirmities. Diseases in which there has been a substantial delay or mitigation are the ones that have caused the greatest number of deaths; heart disease, stroke, and cancer still account for 75% of all deaths. If one does not die (or dies later) from one of these diseases, one is more likely to develop one of the nonlethal disabling diseases of old age. The most disabling of these are primarily in three categories: the degenerative neurologic diseases, such as Alzheimer's disease and parkinsonism; degenerative musculoskeletal diseases, such as osteoporosis and osteoarthritis; and sensory loss, including deafness and blindness. Among these, only in osteoporosis is there enough etiologic understanding to believe that prevention or amelioration can be achieved through life-style changes, and even this is not proved. With all of the other diseases in these categories, we have at best a limited basis for assuming that they could be prevented or delayed.

Forecasts of Morbidity

In planning for our future medical and long-term care needs, the relationship between mortality and morbidity and the relationship between morbidity and functional impairment are critically important. For predeath dependency and disability to be forecast accurately, morbidity—defined as the occurrence of disease—must be linked with realistic clinical assessments of disease-related disability and with the interaction of multiple illnesses in causing disability. In addition, geriatric medicine has taught clinicians that psychological and social factors interact with disease to either enhance or diminish functional status. These factors should also be included in a model to predict measurements of functional independence in senescence, or what has been termed "active life expectancy."[21] Early studies have suggested that for each year of life gained in old age, 60% of the time will be spent in a disabled or dependent condition (Fig 2.9). Women have longer life expectancies at all ages, but in this study they showed only a modest advantage in active life expectancy over men in the 65- to 69-year age group, and no advantage in older groups.[21] If men eventually close some of the gap in life expectancy, then they too may look forward to longer survival with disability. In order to increase the usefulness and precisions of these forecasts, we need an array of information concerning comorbidities, codisabilities, loss of autonomy and ability to perform basic daily functions, and alterations in social situations, such as the loss of a spouse or caregiver and changes in the availability of friends, family, and funds.[22]

Despite the physiologic losses and the psychosocial stresses often associated with advanced age, most elderly individuals have the vitality and resilience to function at a high level. Data collection should take into account the positive aspects of aging rather than focusing solely on functional decline, disease, and mortality. Similarly, there needs to be more recognition of the capacity of function in some individuals to improve over time; thus, data sets should be conceptualized with a view to measuring some kinds of functional improvement, particularly in social parameters, rather than with the assumption that a progressive loss of function always leads to disability and ultimate mortality.

Increased longevity is a central fact of modern life and will be an important social reality in the 21st century. An appropriate goal of medical research is to improve the quality and productivity of those many years of advanced life. Projections of health care needs, however, must include an assumption that a substantial number of older people will suffer from chronic and disabling diseases and will need long-term care. According to projections by the National Center for Health Statistics, the number of nursing home beds, currently at 1.5 million, will need to rise to more than 5 million by the year 2040.[23] Nursing home occupancy is only one proxy measurement for extensive long-term care needs. Continuing care for most people occurs in the community and at home.

Epidemiology of Chronic Illness

Table 2.1 shows the most common chronic illnesses reported by persons over age 65 years living in the community. Women and men name the same major chronic conditions: arthritis, hypertension, chronic sinusitis, diabetes, heart disease, and visual and hearing impairments. Arthritis is the most prevalent of all chronic disorders and causes the greatest reported limitation of activity. For most nonfatal chronic diseases, older women have higher prevalence rates than do older men. The key exceptions are heart disease, some digestive diseases, and visual and hearing impairments. At older ages, prevalence rates for chronic diseases and impairments increase, but there is little change in leading problems for either sex: arthritis, hearing impairments, hypertension, heart disease, and

chronic sinusitis, in that order.[24] Looked at in another way, these figures mean 50% of those over age 65 years have arthritis, 40% have hypertension, 30% have hearing impairments, and 10% have visual impairments. Five percent have cognitive impairment from Alzheimer's disease or other dementing illnesses, but this percentage rises steeply with advancing age, to approximately 20% of those over the age of 80 years.

These disabling diseases generally are not life threatening, but they have an enormous impact on the quality of an individual's life. The statistical linking of morbidity or disease categories with disability or impaired function is just beginning to be explored systematically by physicians, demographers, statisticians, and epidemiologists (Fig 2.10). The first area between the morbidity and disability survival curves, labeled B, defines the number of person-years that can be expected to be lived by an individual from the cohort in a morbid, but disability-free, state. This portion of the figure has implications for acute or short-term health services but relatively little direct impact on long-term care services. The second area defined by the disability curve lies between it and the mortality curve and is labeled C. This area represents the person-years that can be expected to be lived by a person from this cohort in a chronically morbid and disabled state. Currently, in the age group from 65 to 74 years, 41% report some limitations of activity due to chronic diseases, compared with 51% of those aged 75 to 84 years and 60% of those aged 85 years or older. Among the population 65 to 74 years old, about 5% have limitations in the basic activities of daily living (see Chapter 50). Among people aged 85 years and over, more than a third are unable to carry out all the activities of daily living. A Bureau of the Census Study of people over the age of 100 years, found that they did

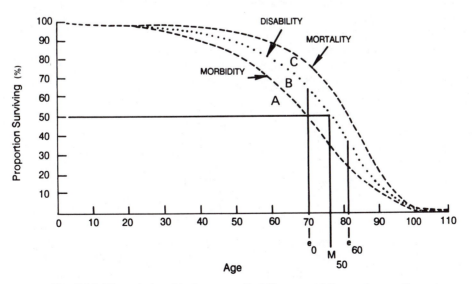

Fig. 2.10. The relationship between disability, morbidity, and mortality.

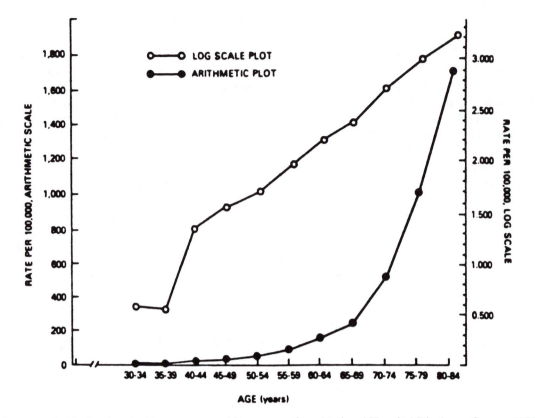

Fig. 2.11. Age-specific hip fracture incidence among white women (from National Hospital Discharge Survey 1975 to 1979).

not differ dramatically in dependency measures from those over the age of 85 years.[7] Only 40% of community-dwelling centenarians required help with daily activities.

Two specific examples illustrate the realities of chronic illness facing an aging population and the implications for health policy: hip fracture and Alzheimer's disease. National data indicate that the frequency of hip fractures starts to rise in the early 40s and thereafter increases exponentially, doubling every 6 years. The projected annual number of hip fractures will increase from 200,000 in 1980 to more than 650,000 by 2050. According to some estimates, this number will exceed 1 million per year. As indicated in Figure 2.11, if hip fractures can be delayed by only 6 years, or one cycle of doubling, the incidence will be decreased by 50%, because of the multiple-disease observation and the related assumption that many older people will die of something else without ever suffering hip fracture. Research on bone metabolism could provide a mechanism for delaying osteoporosis so as to postpone uniformly the onset of the exponential rise in hip fracture, and thus decrease the incidence of this condition by 50%. Research directed at the precursors of disability is the most effective means of postponing and hence preventing chronic diseases and attendant disabilities.

Figure 2.12 shows that in 1980 more than 2 million people had Alzheimer's disease or related disorders, and that their mean age was about 80 years. By the year 2000, that number will increase to approximately 4 million, and by 2050 to more than 8 to 10 million, of whom almost 5 million will be over the age of 85 years. Currently, no specific preventive or ameliorative interventions are known.

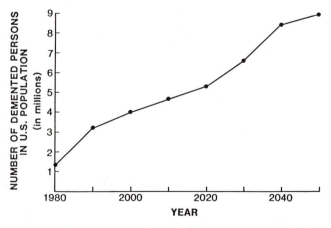

Fig. 2.12. Projected number of demented persons in the United States by age: 1980-2050 (from NIA prevalence estimates and U.S. Bureau of Census projections).

Aggressive research on dementing illness has only just begun, as with a number of other disabling conditions of old age, such as osteoarthritis, deafness, and macular degeneration. The effect on quality of life that awaits progress in these areas is enormous, and appropriate research must be pushed. Meanwhile, demographic and epidemiologic projections show that our aging society faces a major challenge of long-term care, because as longevity increases the chronic disabling disorders associated with age will take their toll in limitations of activity and in pain and suffering and will command the resources required to provide humane and effective care.

Global Trends and Comparisons

The numbers and proportions of older people are increasing in almost every country in the world. In the United States, the impact of this shift actually will be less than that occurring in other developed countries for the next 20 to 30 years (Fig 2.13). In most industrialized nations, approximately 15% of the population is currently at least 65 years old, while in the United States, the figure is about 11.5%. This is because our post–World War II baby boom comprises such a large percentage of the total population and is still relatively young. In effect, the baby boom provides our elderly population with a cushion of available children and other caretakers, which will persist until about 2010 to 2020. The situation will then reverse between 2020 and 2040, when the baby boom generation will be old, with relatively few offspring.

In Japan, the elderly population will have an enormous impact in the near future. Life expectancy in Japan is now the longest in the world, but Japan is in a unique position of currently having only 10% of the population over age 65 years, with the prospect of this population growing to almost 25% by the first decade of the next century. In Northern European countries, about 15% of the populations are over 65 years old, and this figure will slowly increase to 20% over the next 30 to 50 years.

A puzzling and poorly understood discrepancy in major causes of death exists among developed countries. Perhaps most noteworthy is the fact that only Canada, Australia, New Zealand, and the United States experienced the enormous declines in deaths from heart disease and cerebral vascular disease in the past 20 years. Thus, many countries with longer life expectancies at birth than the United States have achieved this status without the benefit of a sudden decline in the leading causes of death. Whether they will experience this decline with its population implications is a subject of conjecture.

In many of the Eastern Bloc countries, most notably in the Soviet Union, death rates have actually been increasing. This increase is probably a temporary phenomenon and could change rapidly. It is accompanied by very low birth rates, resulting in such problems as the inadequate size of the currently available labor force.

The rapid expansion of elderly populations in developing countries confronts their limited abilities to plan for and structure a rapidly aging society. They cannot divert their resources from basic food needs and preventive and curative medicine in their younger populations. A remarkable observation in the United States, Japan, and developing nations is that life

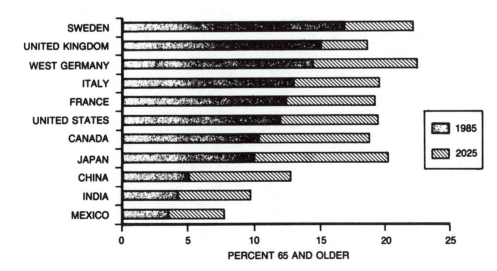

Fig. 2.13. Percent of population 65 and older in selected countries: 1985 (estimated) and 2025 (projected) (from Torey BB, Kinsella KG, and Taueber CM. *An Aging World.* US Bureau of the Census, in press).

expectancy has increased by an extraordinary amount in only one or two generations. When acute diarrheal diseases cease to be the leading cause of death in a developing society, the leading cause of death almost invariably becomes heart disease. From a public health point of view, it is relatively easy to eliminate acute diarrheal diseases as the primary cause of death, and this has occurred in almost every country in the world, with the exception of many African nations. Once heart disease becomes the primary cause of death, life expectancy increases by 20 to 30 years and this can occur within one or two generations.

The rapidity with which the population is aging in the developing world promises policy problems much more difficult than those in the US and is looked on with trepidation. China, a country that is developing rapidly, is currently facing a population of unmanageable size. This caused the Chinese government to take the extraordinary measure of attempting to limit families to one child. This approach has had some success, but the implications for future demographic profiles are sobering. The more successful the population control program is, the higher will be the percentage of the population over age 65 years, and within 20 to 50 years—with much less support from younger generations and greater longevity—social and health care needs will grow dramatically.

An analysis of data submitted to the United Nations from the 17 most developed countries in the world from 1950 to 1985 reveals that the United States is doing relatively well with regard to its older population.[22] This is of considerable interest, since most of the other countries have more formal national health services. Since 1950, the United States has been consistently ranked relatively low in life expectancy at birth, primarily because of its higher infant mortality rates. But for life expectancy at age 65 years, the United States has ranked in the upper half of the 17 countries over the entire period, and our life expectancy at age 75 years has been and continues to be among the longest in the world.

Policymakers in the United States are currently debating options for health policy, which must take the growing elderly population into account. It obviously will be difficult to evaluate the efficacy of policies by measuring longevity, since the specific age groups in which we expect improvement are already among the most long-lived in the world. New initiatives will have to consider the goals of health care in an aging society as an intergenerational network (see Chapter 47). The success of new policies will have to be determined according to social benefits and quality of life, as well as more conventional measures of health and economic productivity.

References

1. Grigsby JS, Olshansky SJ. The demographic components of population aging in china. *Population Dev Rev.* In press.
2. Brody J, Brock DB, Williams TF. Trends in the health of the elderly population. *Ann Rev Public Health* 1987;8:211-234.
3. *Health Statistics on Older Persons.* Washington, DC: 1986.
4. Olshansky SJ. On forecasting mortality. *Milbank Q* 1988;66:482-530.
5. *Annual Summary of Births, Marriages, Divorces, and Deaths: Vital Statistics.* Washington, DC: 1986.
6. Brody JA. Prospects for an aging population. *Nature* 1985;315:463-466.
7. Olshansky SJ. Pursuing longevity: delay vs. elimination of degenerative diseases. *Am J Pub Health* 1985;75:754-756.
8. Preston SH, Keyfitz N, Schoen R. *Causes of Death: Life Tables for National Populations.* New York, NY: Seminar Press; 1972.
9. Jonsson A, Hallgrimsson J: Comparative disease patterns in the elderly and the very old: A retrospective autopsy study. *Age Aging,* 1983;12:111-117.
10. Omran AR. The epidemiologic transition: a theory of the epidemiology of population change. *Milbank Q* 1971;49:508-538.
11. McKeown T. *The Role of Medicine.* Princeton, NJ: Princeton University Press; 1979.
12. Olshansky SJ. The fourth stage of the epidemiologic transition: the age of delayed degenerative diseases. *Milbank Q* 1987.
13. Stallones RA. The rise and fall of ischemic disease. *Sci Am* 1982;243:53-59.
14. Brody JA, Brock DB, and Williams TF. Trends in the health of the elderly population. *Ann. Rev. Public Health* 1987;8:211-234.
15. Keyfitz N. What difference would it make if cancer were eradicated: an examination of the Taeuber paradox. *Demography* 1977;14:411-418.
16. Olshansky SJ. Pursuing longevity: delay vs. elimination of degenerative diseases. *Am J Pub Health* 1985;75: 754-6.
17. Fries JF. Aging, death and the compression of morbidity. *N Engl J Med* 1980;303:130-135.
18. Schneider E, Brody J. Aging, natural death and the compression of morbidity: another view, *N Engl J Med* 1983;309:854.
19. Manton K, Woodburg M, Stallard E. Forecasting the limits for life expectancy: modeling mortality from epidemiological and medical data. In: Johansson SR, ed. *Aging and Dying: The Biological Foundations of Human Longevity.* Berkeley, Calif: University of California Press. In press.
20. National Institute of Aging and the U.S. Bureau of the Census, *America's Centenarians.* Washington, DC: Government Printing Office, 1987.
21. Katz S, Branch LG, Branson MH, et al. Active live expectancy. *N Engl J Med,* 1983;309:1218-1224.

22. Brody J. *Aging in the Twentieth and Twenty-first Centuries*. Washington, DC: National Center for Health Statistics; 1987.
23. Rice DP. Demographic realities and projections of an aging population. In: Andreopoulos S, Hogness JR, eds. *Health Care for an Aging Society*. New York, NY: Churchill Livingstone Inc.; 1989:15–46.
24. Verbrugge LM. Longer live but worsening health? trends in health and mortality of middle aged and older persons. *Milbank Q* 1984;62:475–517.

3

Social and Psychological Characteristics of Older Persons

Bernice L. Neugarten

The Aging Society

Long life is a major achievement of the 20th century in all developed countries of the world. The average life expectancy at birth in United States has now reached 75 years, and it is expected to keep rising (Table 3.1.). It is not only that people are living longer. Primarily because of lower birth rates, the proportions of older to younger people are increasing, producing a shift in the overall age distribution of the society that is expressed by the term, the aging society.

That the older population itself is growing older is reflected in the fact that during the next 20 years, the fastest growth rates will be, as now, in the group aged 85 years and older. The trend is dramatized even further by the fact that centenarians, while they are rare, are expected to quadruple in number and to reach nearly 110,000 by the year 2000.[1]

The older population is growing older because the newest gains in life expectancy are different from those of earlier decades. In the past, because they were due mainly to the conquest of infectious diseases, the gains were spread relatively evenly across the population, with the result that more people reached old age. But because, for the past two decades, mortality rates have been so low for persons younger than age 50 that they could not be much improved, the new gains have been those that affect older persons: gains that have come from new treatments of chronic diseases and from the amelioration of those conditions internal and external to the individual that are especially lethal to older people. While the effects of new infectious diseases, such as the acquired

immunodeficiency syndrome (AIDS), cannot be foreseen, it is nevertheless likely that future gains in longevity will continue to be those that lengthen the period of old age.

Health Status

The future health status of older people as a group is not altogether predictable. The evidence is clear that the vigorous and active part of the life span has been lengthening, and, in that sense, we have been producing a 20th century version of the Fountain of Youth. But advanced old age may continue to mean, for individuals, failure in one body organ after another.[2] Science and medicine may continue to develop palliative means that delay death, but that prolong rather than shorten the duration of terminal illnesses.[3]

At present, more and more people are surviving into the oldest age group where the need for supportive services is greatest, especially the need for long-term care. For the immediate future, this group will remain a small proportion of persons older than age 65 (Table 3.2.); however, as their numbers multiply, it is the population older than 85 that will dominate health planning for the foreseeable future.[4]

Economic and Social Health of Older People

Patterns of aging, and the quality of life once people grow old, are closely related to the economic and social health of the society at large. A strong case can

Table 3.1. Life expectancy at selected ages.*

| | Average remaining years of life at | | | |
	Birth	65 y	75 y†	85 y†
White women				
1960	74.1	15.9	9.3	4.7
1985	78.7	18.7	11.8	6.5
White Men				
1960	67.4	12.9	7.9	4.3
1985	71.8	14.6	9.0	5.2
Black women				
1960	65.9	15.1	10.1	5.4
1985	73.7	17.2	11.5	7.4
Black men				
1960	60.7	12.7	8.9	5.1
1985	65.3	13.4	9.0	6.0
Sex ratio, 1986				
(Men/100 Women)	105	83	64	40

* Data from references 5 and 14.
† Entries for the ages of 75 and 85 years are for 1983.

be made that the economic well-being of older persons and the social well-being that is so closely related to it reflect the society's economic level more than its political ideology or its cultural characteristics.

In the decades after World War II, but especially since the late 1960s, the economic condition of older people as a group has dramatically improved. Like other developed countries, the United States has a multitiered system that rests on public pensions, private pensions, and savings. The system supports people for as long as 30 or more years after retirement, a reflection of the fact that people are retiring earlier but living longer.

Economic Indicators

Most older persons are not poor, although the range of economic differences is very wide.[5] About as many older men have very high incomes as the number who live in poverty. The distribution is different for women, of whom a much larger proportion have incomes near or under the poverty level. This is related to the fact that the majority of women over 65 are widowed; they were in the labor force only intermittently, and as a consequence, they have meager or no Social Security benefits of their own, and few have private pensions. Very old widowed and never-married women are particularly disadvantaged groups.

Minority-group older people, especially blacks, also are very poorly off. In these groups, the social and economic disadvantages that have accumulated throughout their lives are accentuated in old age.

Older persons, on average, have substantially lower cash incomes than younger people. At the same time, they have certain economic advantages because of special income tax benefits provided to persons older than 65, government in-kind transfers that are not available to younger persons (primarily health care costs covered by Medicare), and lifetime accumulations of wealth (primarily the equity in their own homes). Some analysts contend that when these factors are taken into account, the average older person has economic resources roughly equivalent to an average person of working age. Still, there are sizable subgroups of older people who have very limited economic resources, especially very old women and members of minority groups.

Social Indicators

A few additional facts are helpful in rounding out the picture: The vast majority of persons retire before the age of 65 years and begin to draw Social Security benefits at the age of 62 or 63 years. At present, only 16% of men and only 7% of women are in the labor force after the age of 65, and most of them work only part-time.

Most men older than 65 years are married and living with their wives. Not only are most women widowed by the time they reach 65 years of age, but by the time they reach 75, more than half live alone.

Most older persons "grow old in place"; that is, they remain in the same communities, often in the same houses that they have occupied for most of their adult lives. Of the small proportion who move, most go to the Sunbelt states of the South and West.

About 75% of older people own their own homes, and about 80% of these homes are mortgage free. For the first time in 1980, more older people lived in suburbs than in the central cities.

The major point to be drawn from the kinds of data shown in Table 3.2. is that old age itself does not define a problem group in today's society. Some older people are economically and socially needy; others are not. On most socioeconomic measures, it is a small minority who are severely disadvantaged. These are mainly very old persons who, compared with persons born later, have been disadvantaged earlier in their lives with regard to education, occupational skills, medical care, and pension systems.

This picture will change rapidly as new cohorts of persons reach old age, a point to be elaborated in a later section of this chapter.

Social Participation and Attitudes

Measures of the social participation and social integration of older people reveal considerable heterogeneity.

Table 3.2. Selected characteristics of older people by age group.*

	65-74	75-84	85+	All 65+	All 75+
Numbers (millions), (1986)					
Men	7.2	3.3	0.7	11.2	4.0
Women	9.4	5.5	1.8	16.7	7.3
Projected total population (millions)					
2000	17.7	12.3	4.9	34.9	. . .
2020	29.9	14.5	7.1	51.4	. . .
Median income, (1985) (thousands)					
Families	20.4	16.4	15.1	. . .	. . .
Unrelated individuals	8.2	7.2	6.4	. . .	. . .
Percent below poverty level (1986)					
Men	7.0	10.7	13.3	8.5	. . .
Women	13.0	18.1	19.7	15.2	. . .
Percent in labor force (1986)					
Men	25.0†	. . .	. . .	16.0	10.4‡
Women	14.3†	. . .	. . .	7.4	4.1‡
Marital status (percents)§					
Men					
Married with spouse present	79	68	. . .	75	. . .
Widowed	9	23	. . .	14	. . .
Women					
Married with spouse present	49	23	. . .	38	. . .
Widowed	39	67	. . .	51	. . .
Living alone					
Men	13	. . .	. . .	15	19
Women	35	. . .	. . .	41	51
Living in nursing homes (1985)‖					
Men and Women	1	6	22	. . .	. . .
Median years of schooling (1986)					
Men	12.1	. . .	. . .	11.7	9.6
Women	12.1	. . .	. . .	11.9	10.4
Percent who are homeowners (1985)	. . .	. . .	. . .	75	. . .
(Percent of homes that are mortgage free)¶	. . .	. . .	. . .	80	. . .
Changed residence (from March 1983–March 1984)#					
Same county	. . .	. . .	. . .	3.8	. . .
Different county	. . .	. . .	. . .	1.0	. . .

* Data from references 5 and 15.

† Data are for those 65-69.

‡ Data are for those 70+.

§ Percent of the never married, married with spouse absent, and divorced are not shown in this Table.

‖ Of nursing home residents, over two-thirds are women.

¶ In 1980 for the first time a greater number of older persons lived in suburbs (over 10 million) than in central (8 million).

Fewer than 5% of persons 65+ moved in this one-year period, compared to 17% of persons of all ages and 34 persons aged 20-24. Of the small proportion of older persons who move, most migrate to the sunbelt states.

As Table 3.3. shows, however, the majority report that they have active family ties and close friends whom they see frequently. About the same proportion of younger people attend a church or synagogue, and sizable numbers, up through their 80s, report that they belong to organizations and are engaged in volunteer work.

Moreover, as shown in Table 3.4., a majority report their health to be excellent or good; and most report high levels of life satisfaction. Compared with younger adults, about the same proportion feel that life is better than they expected, and high proportions have positive self-images. Only a small fraction report that insufficient income is a serious problem, or loneliness; a somewhat larger fraction report that fear of crime or poor health poses a serious problem.

Overall, the picture that emerges is that persons over 65, as a group, exhibit relatively high levels of economic and social health.

The data in Tables 3.2. through 3.4. have, at the same time, been broken down to show some of the differences between younger and older subgroups.

Table 3.3. Indicators of social participation (self-reports) by age group.*

	Age, y			
	18-59	60-69	70-79	80+
Of those with children, %				
Saw child in last day or so	65	53	46	51
Give help to child or grandchild, %				
When someone is ill	74	73	75	78
By helping with money	26	21	23	25
Have close friends, %	97	95	94	90
Saw friend in last day or so, %	63	63	59	58
Spend "lot of time" in organizations, %	14	15	17	16

	Age, y		
	18-64	55-64	All 65+
Attended church/ synagogue in last week or two, %			
Year 1974	34	. . .	40
Year 1981	27	. . .	35
Attended senior center or golden age club in last week or two, %			
Year 1974	. . .	2	6
Year 1981	. . .	3	9
In past year 1984†	. . .	. . .	15
Used congregate meal services in past year			
Year 1984†	. . .	. . .	8
Spend "lot of time"			
in recreation and hobbies, %			
Year 1974	34	. . .	26
Year 1981	36	. . .	26
socializing with friends, %			
Year 1974	55	. . .	47
Year 1981	45	. . .	38
caring for younger/older family members, %			
Year 1974	53	. . .	27
Year 1981	50	. . .	20

	Age, y			
	65-69	70-79	80+	All 65+
Do volunteer work, %				
Year 1974	28	20	12	22
Year 1981	28	23	12	23

	Age, y			
	35-54	55-64	65-74	75+
Voted, %				
Year 1980‡	66	71	69	58
Year 1984‡	66	72	72	61

* Data from references 19 and 20.
† Data from reference 21.
‡ Data from reference 5 (pp 9,10,12,44,45,47,85,137,139,142).

The Life Cycle Perspective

It is important to recognize that aging processes are gradual and continuous, a progression of changes, some orderly and predictable, and others unpredictable. Social, as well as biological, timetables govern the sequence of change.

The life cycle perspective has important implications for health planners and providers. First, except for retirement, old age is not a separable period of life, neither abrupt in its onset nor, for most persons, marked by dramatic changes in interest patterns, personal commitments, or, until a major change in health occurs, in life style. The individual's social and health characteristics in old age are, in large part, the outcomes of earlier life-styles and earlier health histories.

Second, people grow old in very different ways, and they become increasingly different from one another with the passage of time, at least until the very terminal stage of life when biological losses may level out individual differences. Women age differently from men, and there are differences among racial, ethnic, and, particularly, socioeconomic groups. Add to this the idiosyncratic sequence of events that accumulate over a lifetime to create individual variation. The result is that older people are a very diverse group.

Although the incidence of illness and disability increases with age in the second half of life, the association between age and health is far from perfect. In probabilistic terms, age is a good predictor of health status, but for any given individual, it is a poor predictor of physical, mental, or social competence.

Third, some of the major variations in aging are due to cohort differences: each group of people who reach old age has certain unique characteristics. This is because of the changing historical and societal conditions that have influenced their lives. One example is the rising educational level of older persons: by 1990 about half of the population over age 65 will have had some education beyond high school. Another example relates to the increasing number of women in the labor force: now, for the first time, large groups of women are experiencing formal retirement. To plan health services for the next 20 years, health professionals will thus do well to study the characteristics of people who are presently middle aged.

Finally, social, psychological, and biological changes are not synchronous. Many older people suffer from ill health but consider themselves well; they go about their daily lives without taking on "the sick role." Others, when they retire or become great-

Table 3.4. Attitudes of older people by age group.*

	Age, y (1974)					Age, y (1981)
	18-59	60-69	70-79	80+	All 65+	All 65+
Health is excellent or good (self-report, 1981), %	. . .	64†	52	51	56	. . .
Life satisfaction, %‡						
Year 1974	. . .	27†	26	24	26	. . .
Year 1981	. . .	26†	24	24	25	. . .
"My life now compared with what I expected it would be," %						
Better than expected	38	30	33	27	. . .	. . .
Worse than expected	11	10	10	13	. . .	. . .
Self-image: "very useful member of my community," %	28	38	39	28	. . .	. . .
"People over 65 get too little respect," %	73	46	44	45	. . .	. . .
"Very serious problem for me," %						
Not enough money to live on	18	19	15	12	15	17
Fear of crime	14	21	26	19	23	25
Poor health	9	23	22	28	21	21
Loneliness	7	12	13	17	12	13
Transportation to stores, physicians, recreation (1981)	10§	. . .	. . .	. . .	. . .	14

* Data from references 19 and 20.
† For group aged 65 to 69 years.
‡ Median score on the Life Satisfaction Index Z, on scale ranging from 0 to 36.
§ For group aged 18 to 64 years.

grandparents, think of themselves as old even though their health may be excellent.

Expectations and Adaptations

Despite the diversities in patterns of aging, most older people become more preoccupied with their health than when they were young. This produces a greater readiness, not only to seek health services, but to learn about health maintenance. Older people of today are an eminently teachable group for the health educator.

Older men and women, like younger people, make continual adaptations to the changes that occur inside and outside the body. Most older people adapt successfully. As they accumulate life experience, they become practiced in making psychological adaptations. They look ahead with a certain sense of èquanimity and with an expectation that, given certain supports, they will succeed in coping with new transitions just as they have coped with earlier ones.

A significant factor in adapting to change is the nature of the individual's expectations. Most people develop a concept of the "normal, expectable life cycle," a set of anticipations that certain life events will occur at certain times, and an internalized social clock telling them whether they are on time or off time.[6]

Being on or off time is a compelling basis for self-assessment. Men and women compare themselves with their friends or siblings or parents in deciding whether they are doing well or poorly, always with a time line in mind. It is not the fact that one reaches 60 or 70 that is important, but rather, "How well am I doing for my age?" This probably poses special changes in self-image for those who reach 90, for they have few peers with whom to compare themselves. In coming years, there will be more people who survive to ages 90 and 100. We may then learn more about the psychology of that age group.

Expectable Life Events

For most people, the normal and expectable life events are not life crises. Marriage, parenthood, occupational achievements, children growing up and leaving home, the climacteric, grandparenthood, retirement, and great-grandparenthood are the normal turning points, the punctuation marks along the lifeline. They call forth changes in self-concept and identity, but whether or not they become critical events usually depends on their timing. For the majority, the departure of children from the home is not a crisis, nor is retirement. Even the death of one's spouse, if it occurs on time, does not usually create a mental health crisis.

The onset of chronic illness is another expectable event. This is one of the reasons why most older people describe their health as being good even when they have one or more chronic diseases (Table 3.4.). They mean that their health is as good or better than they had anticipated.

This is not to deny that illness precipitates crisis reactions in many older persons, nor to deny that some, but by no means all, of the major life events that occur in the second half of life are losses to the individual, accompanied by anxiety or grief. But most such events have been anticipated and rehearsed. Given the appropriate social supports, the psychological adjustment is made without shattering the sense of continuity of the life cycle or the individual's coping strategies.

Young-Old and Old-Old

Across the great range of differences among older people, the most useful distinction for the health planner is between young-old and old-old, a distinction based not on age itself, but on social and health characteristics.[7] The young-old are the large majority of older persons. They are vigorous and competent men and women who have retired or otherwise reduced their time investments in working or homemaking. They are relatively comfortable financially, relatively well-educated, and well-integrated members of their families and their communities.

Old-old persons, by contrast, are those who suffer major physical, mental, or social losses and who require a range of supportive and restorative health and social services. Essentially, these are persons who are in need of special care. While this group probably will remain a minority over the next few decades, their absolute numbers are growing rapidly as medical and social advances help to extend their lives.

It is estimated, based on recent health and social surveys, that, at any one moment, young-old men and women constitute about 80% or 85% of the whole population aged older than 65 years, and old-old persons, about 15% to 20%. These are gross estimates, and the proportions are different in successive age subgroups.

Young-old persons seek meaningful ways to use their time. Some stay at work, some move to part-time jobs, and some undertake second careers. Others seek self-fulfillment through education or various forms of leisure. Some serve as volunteers in health services, social services, or civic affairs. A large number are teaching, counseling, or tutoring in schools, social agencies, churches, or corporations. Young-old men and women are beginning to be recognized as a major resource to the society.[8]

Young-old men and women are also active politically, more so than younger adults, and are becoming more articulate about their political, economic, and social claims on both governmental and private agencies. Old-age advocacy groups are a manifestation of this new political consciousness; the proliferation of government agencies that serve the needs of older people is another. Young-old people are likely to make increasing demands on the health services system and, in doing so, to speak not only for themselves but for old-old persons, whom they see themselves becoming.

Oldest-Old

Recently, a new group has been delineated called the *oldest-old*. It refers to persons over 85, who presently constitute about 1% of the population, a percentage that is expected to grow to more than 2% by the year 2010 and to almost 3% by the year 2030 (by which time it will have reached nearly 9 million in number). This group holds special interest for gerontologists who are interested in studying the biological and social factors associated with survivorship, in the hope that to do so will add important new insights into the processes of aging.

From preliminary studies of this group, it already is clear that it is very heterogeneous: blacks and whites, rich and poor, and extremely high proportions of widowed women and extremely low-income persons. It includes competent, vigorous individuals who report no limitations of everyday activities due to health, and individuals who are in extreme states of disability and deterioration.[9] These preliminary facts seem to support the findings mentioned earlier, that the longer people live, the more different from one another they become, and accordingly, that age becomes an increasingly poor predictor of an individual's level of health or social competency.

Psychological Issues

Whatever the variations among individuals, and whatever the personality differences, there is a certain directionality of change and a certain ordering of psychological tasks and preoccupations across the long periods of adulthood and old age.[10]

Young Adulthood

We are accustomed to thinking that in adolescence, the major psychological task is identity formation, and in youth, it is finding a niche in society and preparing a script for one's life. In young adulthood, the issues are related to intimacy, to investing oneself in the lives of a few significant others, and to taking on responsibilities for those others, usually a spouse and children. New tasks also arise in meeting expectations in the world of work, developing competency and job mastery, and creating a balance between work and family.

A frequent preoccupation of the young adult is how to follow one's planned life script while accepting the reality that the script is being continually altered in ways that could not have been predicted and that can only partially be controlled.

Psychology of Middle Age

In middle age, the psychological issues are new. Some are related to family roles: the reworking of relationships between husbands and wives, with changing expectations of what it means to be male or female; and the realization that one's victories and defeats are reckoned by how well one's children are turning out. The appearance of a son-in-law or daughter-in-law often means establishing a quick but intimate relationship with a stranger, and for increasing numbers of middle-aged persons today, the need to adjust to the divorce of a child. The appearance of a grandchild brings a new awareness of aging, but also, for most men and women, a new source of pleasure.

Some of the psychological readjustments of middle age relate not to the creation of biological heirs, but to the creation of social heirs; the need to nurture and to act as a model or mentor to the young; and the concern not to overstep the delicate boundaries of one's authority either in the family or in the workplace. For women, there is often a sense of new freedom, increased time for oneself when children are gone, freedom from fear of unwanted pregnancy, and for many, a new pleasure in sexual relations that accompanies menopause.

At the same time, there are also the responsibilities that can be called *parent-caring*. Recent studies indicate that, with the increase of multigenerational families, the concern over providing care for aging parents is the major source of stress in the area of family life.[11]

Other issues relate to the occupational life: the concerns about moving up or moving down or reaching a plateau. With large proportions of middle-aged women now in the work force, there is often, for both women and men, increasing investment in work. For some, there are unwelcome job pressures; for others, the restlessness that comes with job boredom, or burnout. But for most middle-aged workers, there is a heightened competence and also a sense of being in the prime of life with regard to the value of one's experience and expertise.

Middle age is also the period of increased stocktaking: introspection and reflection become characteristic of the mental life. The assessment of where one has been and where one is going manifests itself in a number of ways: acceptance of limits and a moderation of ambition; dramatic new questions of identity; for some persons, depression in the face of unrealized hopes or unavoidable life events; and for others, a moving away from conventional patterns that leads to new careers, geographic moves, and new leisure activities.

Concerns Over Health

A psychological change that is probably of special interest to physicians as they interact with middle-aged patients is the heightened concern over health that usually comes as a person moves through the 40s and 50s.

For men, the most dramatic signs that they are entering middle age are often biological. Attention is increasingly centered on the decreasing efficiency of the body. It is not only one's performance on the golf course or one's sexual performance, but it is the heart attack in a friend that prompts many men to describe bodily changes as the most important feature of the transition from young adulthood to middle age.

Health changes are more salient markers for men than for women. The menopause and other manifestations of the climacteric are events to which middle-aged women seldom attach great psychological significance; despite the concerns over cancer, women refer less often than men to health or biological changes. It is, for instance, a false stereotype that the menopause leads to depression in most women.

Body monitoring nevertheless takes on new importance to both men and women as they develop a large variety of protective strategies for maintaining the body at given levels of performance and appearance. While these issues reflect a new sense of physical vulnerability in men, they often take a different form in women, ie, the mental "rehearsal for widowhood." Women often are more concerned over the body monitoring of their husbands than of themselves.

Changing Time Perspectives

A second set of psychological issues also is likely to be of special interest to physicians: namely, that both men and women are aware of a new way in which they think about their lifetimes. Life is restructured in terms of time-left-to-live rather than time-since-birth. Not only the reversal in direction, but also the awareness that time is finite is a conspicuous feature of middle age, especially for men. Death takes on a new reality; it becomes personalized, ie, it could now happen to oneself. There is at the same time a new awareness of increased longevity in the population at large and, for most people, the expectation that they will live much longer than their parents.

Many middle-aged persons think of time as a two-edged sword that acts in some ways as a brake on their activities, but in other ways, as a prod, in seeing how many more good years one can plan for and how many new activities one can undertake.

The sense of a long life still ahead has different implications for middle-aged men compared with middle-aged women. In at least some men, it is accompanied by a readiness to marry for a second time and to start a new family. Many women, sensitive to the reality that middle-aged or older women seldom remarry, worry that there may be many years of widowhood ahead and perhaps of living alone. Middle age, then, as is true of other periods of life, has a different set of psychological meanings for the two sexes.

Psychology of Old Age

Many of the concerns of middle age continue to preoccupy older persons, but new themes also arise.

Some of the new psychological issues are related to renunciation: adapting to losses of work, friends, and spouse, and yielding up positions of authority. The resolution of grief over the death of others becomes a repeated psychological task, and grief occurs over one's own approaching death. The sense of integrity is reformulated in terms of what one has been rather than what one is, and the concerns over legacy arise, as how to leave traces of oneself and a proper record of one's life.

There are also the triumphs of survivorship, for instance, the recognition that one has savored a wide range of experiences and therefore "knows about life" in ways no younger person can know. There is, in most old people, the knowledge that, in having lived through physical and psychological pain in the past, one recovers and can cope also with the contingencies that lie ahead. There is also a sense that one is now the possessor and conservator of some of the basic values of one's society and perhaps some of the eternal truths about living and dying.

These are only some of the themes and the preoccupations that give meaning to the long years of adulthood, and that call forth a changing sense of self and a changing set of adaptations. With the passage of time, lives become more, not less, complex, and for most persons, lives become enriched, not impoverished.

Psychology of Illness in Old Age

Older people have been described here as a very diverse group, most of whom, despite their differences, remain young-old for long periods of time and relatively well in terms of social, physical, and mental health. Older persons deal with illness in many different ways, just as is true of young people. This is not to say, however, that older people as a group are the same as younger people in the ways that they think about their health, their illnesses, and their medical care.

The important factor in the psychology of illness in late life is that young-old people become, whether for a very short or a very long period before their deaths, old-old people. Recognizing that this change will come, most men and women become particularly sensitive not only to the quality of the physical care that they are receiving from health professionals, but also the quality of psychological care, and to what kinds of care they can anticipate when they become frail.

The sensitivity to psychological care has many components. One is that older persons have ongoing, not only intermittent, concerns about their health and health care. Given the increased attention to health maintenance and preventive medicine by newspaper columnists, television commentators, and other educators, there is a wider understanding among older people today that many of their illnesses are treatable, and that some are reversible. As a consequence, many old men and women have higher expectations of being benefited by medical treatment than was true only a decade ago.

At the same time, old men and women recognize their biological vulnerability and the fact that the aging body becomes less able to cope with stress, internal or external. As mentioned earlier, illness and disability have different meanings if they occur "on time" or "off time" in the life cycle. To the old person, illness comes "on time," and understandably enough is usually accompanied by premonitions of death.

Most old people talk about death with their spouses or children or friends and are relatively willing to talk about it even with an interviewer who is a stranger. They usually express most concerns not about the fact that death will come, but about how long a period of dependency and deterioration will precede it, and about the manner in which it will come. With the recent advances in high-technology medicine and life-prolonging procedures, there is a new worry that one might die "on the machines." An increasing number of persons are signing a "living will," a directive that, should they be suddenly stricken and unable to make known their wishes, instructs their physicians in advance to forego the use of extreme forms of life-extending treatment.

Another factor is the difficulty for most older persons of acknowledging dependency, especially for women who have been for long periods of their lives the givers of physical and emotional care, rather than the receivers.

Some older persons, after experiencing a catastrophic medical event, such as a major stroke, express the fear of dependency by stating their willingness, even their eagerness, to die. The physician, in attempting to facilitate recovery, may be thwarted by such a patient's desires and may experience a sense of helplessness and frustration.

Other patients react differently to a personal medical catastrophe. They become preoccupied with "buying time"; they may challenge the competence of the physician by continually seeking additional opinions or by insisting on all the newest treatment procedures.

Whatever form the fear of dependency may take, or the fear of pain, or other motivations, older people usually want not the latest possible death that high technology can provide, but what they regard as the "best death," one that provides as much dignity and autonomy as possible.

Some old persons want to discuss this problem with their physicians; others are hesitant about broaching it. Physicians, for their part, have their own sensitivities to issues of death and dying that may, in some instances, create new opportunities for intimate communication with patients who are approaching death, but, in other instances, new difficulties of communication.

In a medical system that has been geared more to cure than to care, it is understandable that the psychological needs of old sick patients sometimes go unmet by otherwise competent physicians whose training has been focused more on scientific and technological than on humanistic aspects of medical practice.[12] The same problems of communication may occur in the interactions between physicians and young patients, but the problems become accentuated in the case of old patients whose remaining lifetimes are short, whose well-being often depends directly on the nature of the patient-physician relationship, and who are therefore especially in need of emotional support and understanding that only the physician can provide. This is especially true because most old-old people suffer from chronic illness, where the relationship with the physician becomes a long-lasting and increasingly complex one.

Although the patient-physician relationship and patient-physician communication are by no means new concerns among physicians or patients, new attention is presently being given to these issues by medical educators, in particular to the cultivation of empathy, caring, and compassion on the part of the physician.[13] It is not clear whether or not the appearance of the aging society plays a major role in bringing these concerns to the forefront. But because more physicians now and in the future will be dealing with increasing numbers of old patients, it is likely that the

psychology of illness in old age will command increasing attention, and that communication between physicians and old patients will be a central issue in medical training and in medical practice.

References

1. National Institute on Aging and the US Bureau of the Census. *America's Centenarians*. Washington, DC: US Dept of Health and Human Services, 1987.
2. Avorn JL. Medicine: The life and death of Oliver Shay. In: Pifer A, Bronte L, eds. *Our Aging Society*. New York, NY: WW Norton & Co Inc; 1986:283–297.
3. Brody JA, Brock DB, Williams TF. Trends in the health of the elderly population. *Annu Rev Public Health* 1987;8:211–34.
4. Katz S, Greer DS, Beck JC, et al. Active life expectancy: societal implications. In: Committee on an Aging Society, Institute of Medicine and National Research Council, eds. *America's Aging: Health in an Older Society*. Washington, DC: National Academy Press; 1985:57–72.
5. Special Committee on Aging, (US Congress, Senate) 1987. *Aging America: Trends and Projections*. US Dept of Health and Human Services publication, 1988:38–77.
6. Neugarten BN, Neugarten DA. Changing meanings of age in the aging society. In: Pifer A, Bronte L, eds. *Our Aging Society*. New York, NY: WW Norton & Co Inc; 1986:33–52.
7. Neugarten BN. Age groups in American society and the rise of the young-old. *Ann Am Acad Political Soc Sci* 1974;415:187–198.
8. Committee on an Aging Society, Institute of Medicine and National Research Council. *America's Aging: Productive Roles in an Older Society*. Washington, DC: National Academy Press; 1986.
9. Rosenwaike I. A demographic portrait of the oldest old. *Milbank Q* 1985;63:187–205.
10. Neugarten BN. Time, age, and the life cycle. *Am J Psychiatry* 1979;136:887–893.
11. Brody EM. Parent care as a normative family stress. *Gerontologist* 1985;25:19–29.
12. Odegaard CE. *Dear Doctor—A Personal Letter to a Physician*. Menlo Park, Calif: The Henry J. Kaiser Family Foundation; 1986.
13. White KL. *The Task of Medicine*. Menlo Park, Calif: The Henry J. Kaiser Family Foundation; 1988.
14. US Bureau of the Census, *Statistical Abstract of the United States: 1987* (107th edition), No. 82, Births and Birth Rates: 1960 to 1984. Washington, D.C.: Government Printing Office; 1986.
15. US Bureau of the Census, Current Population Reports, Series P-20, No. 418, *Marital Status and Living Arrangements: March 1986*, Washington, D.C.: Government Printing Office; 1986.
16. US Bureau of the Census, Current Population Reports, Series P-20, No. 407, *Geographical Mobility: March 1983 to March 1984*, Washington, D.C.: Government Printing Office; 1986.

17. Sherman SR. Assets of new retired-worker beneficiaries: findings from the New Beneficiary Survey. *Social Security Bulletin,* July 1985, vol 48, No. 7, pp 27–43.

18. US Bureau of the Census, Current Population Reports, Series P-25, No. 952, *Projections of the Population of the United States, by Age, Sex, and Race: 1983 to 2080,* Washington, D.C.: Government Printing Office; 1984.

19. Louis Harris & Associates, Inc. *The Myth and Reality of Aging in America: A Study for the National Council on the Aging, Inc.* Washington, DC: National Congress on the Aging, Inc.; 1975.

20. Louis Harris & Associates, Inc. *Aging in the Eighties: A Study for the National Council on the Aging, Inc.* Washington, DC: National Council on the Aging, Inc.; 1981.

21. National Center for Health Statistics. *Aging in the Eighties, Age 65 Years and Older: Use of Community Services.* Rockville, Md: National Center for Health Services; 1986 (advance data No. 124, September 1986).

4

Ethical Problems in Geriatric Medicine

Christine K. Cassel

Principles of Clinical Medical Ethics

The complexity of modern medical care produces dilemmas and conflicts in which an ability to understand and explicitly address issues of moral choice and value differences is essential to the practicing physician. Ethical dilemmas are not rare or esoteric events. It is impractical and unnecessary to take every ethical problem to court, and every health care institution does not have a consultant ethicist or an ethics committee. Day-to-day decisions must be made as they arise. Therefore, in addition to technical competence in medicine, the geriatrician also must attain a certain level of ethical competence.

A systematic approach to problems in clinical ethics begins with a few basic principles, which undergird public attitudes and the personal values of physicians and help to define relationships with patients, with other professionals, and with society.[1] The principles of ethical action are shaped by the context of Western culture. Traditions of Judaism and Christianity and secular, political, and social philosophies all contribute somewhat different perspectives. However, there are many areas of commonality among them, and respect for every individual value system is encompassed within the US constitutional provisions for the right to privacy and self-determination.

The description of principles that follows is widely used in the deliberations of modern biomedical ethics, including beneficence, respect for persons, fidelity, and justice. While this is not an exhaustive list of values related to medicine, most such values are included within one or another of these categories.

Beneficence

Beneficence combines the obligation to do what's best for the patient with the obligation to no harm: this is the most ancient and central principle of medical ethics. It encompasses the caring, empathic aspect of the physician's role. It also demands adequate knowledge and technical competence of the physician and, in current times, includes the science of prognosis.

It is important in understanding the principle of beneficence to distinguish doing what is best for the patient from paternalistic action. Paternalism is a stance in which one makes decisions on behalf of another, as a parent would for a child, either when that person cannot decide for himself or herself or when it is believed that he or she is making the wrong decision. The history of medicine largely is one of paternalistic attitudes toward patients. It is only recently that health professionals have begun a serious attempt to share medical information with their patients. The image of stoic family physicians who take all the troubles of the patient on their shoulders, make all the hard decisions alone, and simply tell the patient not to worry or that "I did everything I could" is fading from view. However, we should not reject all the qualities of that era, for there is a great deal of caring concern that emerges from such an image. In the new model of collaborative decision making, it is possible to lose the caring and beneficent aspect of health care practice in a colder and more impersonal negotiated contract. This risk is increased by physicians' fear of litigation.

Beneficence has a corollary that is an often-quoted Hippocratic statement: "Do no harm." The two aspects of this principle may come into conflict with each other. The most obvious example of this is when a very risky or painful therapy has a chance of benefiting a patient: one wants to do good but wonders if the decision to follow the more conservative route of doing no harm is not, in fact, the most ethical. In these dilemmas it is, whenever possible, the patient's own decision to make. In the case of an incommunicative, comatose, or severely demented person, one is helped enormously by prior knowledge of the patient, his or her life's values and plans, and contributing information from family and friends.

Beneficence includes the need to make decisions about letting a patient die to put an end to needless suffering that cannot be relieved. Merciful and compassionate treatment of dying patients is a very important part of any medical practice (see Chapter 46). The skills and knowledge in this area include courage and sensitivity needed to make the ethical decisions involved, and these should be a part of the training of every health care professional.[2]

Respect for Persons

Respect is an attitude that a physician should have toward any patient. This is not the kind of respect that grows from personal knowledge of another person's accomplishments or abilities, but rather a more basic respect for persons that derives from respect for human life itself. One aspect of respect for persons includes an understanding of autonomy. Autonomy is a trait or attribute of individuals. Our society supports the moral right to choose one's own plan of life as long as it does not interfere with the autonomy of others. Our legal system most highly prizes this principle of respect for autonomy in its emphasis on self-determination, as stated in a landmark court decision of 1914: "Every adult of sound mind has the right to decide what shall be done with his or her body."[3] Thus, respect for the patient's right of self-determination is essential to competent clinical care.

In medical care, respect for persons has major implications for disclosure of information and informed consent.[4] One should, in most cases, be frank with patients about their diagnosis and about what is known and not known about that diagnosis and enlist them as partners when decision making of any ambiguous nature needs to be done. The exceptions to this are the few cases when it seems truly medically or psychiatrically dangerous to give the information to patients or when patients request not to be told and ask that physicians make all decisions for them.[5] Physicians' attitudes about telling patients bad news have changed dramatically in the past 20 years in the United States,[6]

with wide acceptance of a patient's right to full disclosure.

Full disclosure about relevant medical information becomes difficult in cases of cognitive disorder, or, in aphasia, in which it is difficult to know how much the patient is understanding. Still, the effort must be made, and it is often surprising how much is understood in either case, especially if simple and clear language is used. With people who have memory deficits, one must be prepared to repeat patiently the information sometimes many times over. Informed consent, discussed in greater detail later in this chapter, often has to be an ongoing process of communication rather than a single encounter focused on the signing of a piece of paper.

Another aspect of respect for people is constituted by respectful action. If patients are not aware enough to engage in meaningful dialogue about the nature and prognosis of their disease, clinicians must take special care to treat those patients respectfully, because many of the usual components of human interaction that normally elicit respect are absent. This includes a whole range of concerns having to do with how patients are addressed, handled, clothed, and treated during the course of an office visit or hospitalization. Our actions toward those patients who are most vulnerable not only reflect our attitudes toward ourselves as members of the human community but also may strengthen or instill those attitudes in others.

Physicians also show respect for people in their ambulatory practice by doing what is possible to ensure that patients do not have a long wait in an uncomfortable situation, that they have ample time with the health care provider, that there is acoustic as well as visual privacy for the interaction, and finally that, whenever possible, the patient and the physician can openly discuss the patient's concerns and wishes about his or her death and aggressiveness of therapy in the event of severe incapacity.

Fidelity or Trust

The fiduciary relationship of the physician and patient is a balance between the beneficent, compassionate role and the respect for a patient's autonomous self-determination. Fiduciary means a relationship based on trust. The patient is in a position inherently more vulnerable, and the physician therefore has the greater responsibility to deserve and respect the patient's confidence.

Confidentiality is one important aspect of this trust. The physician's duty to maintain information about the patient in confidence takes special attention and effort in a world of computerized data systems and larger, impersonal institutions.[7] Even multidisciplinary teams can pose a threat to confidentiality. The only times when a breach of confidentiality is justified are when the public welfare, as established by statute, demands it, eg, reporting of seizure disorders to the bureau of motor vehicles or reporting of certain kinds of infectious diseases. Most states have regulations that require reporting of infectious diseases, such as acquired immunodeficiency syndrome, typhoid, tuberculosis, and hepatitis in food handlers and in hospital personnel.

In the law, a fiduciary relationship between two equal parties is a "contract" with rights and responsibilities stipulated for each party. In medicine, a "covenant" model is more appropriate, where because of the unequal status of the parties involved, a greater responsibility is on the physician to understand and communicate with the patient.[8] Communication thus becomes an essential skill for physicians and is a major theme of research in clinical medical ethics. Communication requires psychologic, logistic, and institutional, as well as moral, commitments by the physician to this aspect of patient care. Without adequate communication, critical ethical decisions are much more difficult.

Justice

Justice refers, in a general way, to fairness or equitable treatment. In a situation of limited resources, it is the basic principle that we seek for the allocation of those resources. In situations of truly dire scarcity, such as wartime or when hospital beds are unavailable for patients who truly need them, principles of "triage" must operate. Dire scarcity is rare in our social arrangements for medical care, however, except where natural resources are limited by availability, eg, organs for transplantation or blood for transfusion.

Relative scarcity is the more common and more troubling reality—it is troubling because the moral role of the physician is much less clear than in dire scarcity. In the current situation of extensive and expensive possibilities in medical care, the containment of medical spending has taken a prominent place in the attention of physicians and health care administrators. Some interventions are dramatically effective or even lifesaving, and others have only questionable efficacy and significant iatrogenic risks. This is "relative" scarcity because its limits are set by policy decisions rather than by the natural limits of biologic availability. The constraints on the use of resources, then, are determined on a "macro" level by the political process (national, local, and institutional) and on the "mirco" level by decisions of physicians in the care of each patient.

Physicians cannot avoid being involved in the issues of cost containment and rationing of health care services.[9] The traditional role of the physician, acting in the patient's best interests (beneficence) and with communication and consent from the patient (respect), does not include a cost-containment perspective. Until recently, ethicists, both philosophers and physicians, have asserted the primacy of patient care in the morality of the physician, leaving allocation of resources to representation by a broader social voice: "Society must decide." The further fragmentation of health care, and irrational incentives created by "society" through financing structures that overemphasize acute care and high technology interventions, have led many physicians to think that clinical knowledge is an essential component in decisions about the allocation of health care resources. This impression is strengthened in geriatrics, where chronic illness demands treatment that often is outside of the acute care model, where acute care costs themselves are greater than for any other group, and where the "productivity" of patients who are successfully treated cannot be measured in conventional economic terms.[10] Thus, physicians are becoming more involved in medical economics and health policy. Furthermore, most health care systems have dealt with financial constraints by making physicians the "gatekeepers," which has the logical advantage that physicians can better decide which resources have the greatest clinical utility.[11] This is a new role for physicians, however, that carries a risk of conflict of interest and that is not well defined by traditional ethics, by the law, or by health care regulation.

The appropriate ethical basis for physicians withholding clearly efficacious services on any basis other than the patient's refusal is highly questionable, and it has never been tested in courts of law. The following statements can be derived from the principles of beneficence, respect, and justice: (1) Physicians should never use or advocate the use of health care services that are known not to be efficacious. (2) Decisions about patient care should not be influenced by the physician's own profit from those decisions. (3) Physicians should learn the most cost-efficient method of diagnosis and treatment and keep themselves and their patients informed about new information in this area. (4) If functioning in a primary care "gatekeeper" role, the physician is first the advocate for the patient and only second the advocate for the hospital or health plan administration. (5) Whenever possible, physicians should participate actively in allocation decisions at the policy level to inform policy decisions with clinical knowledge.

Role of the Law, Government, and Institutional Policies

Most of the law relevant to medical ethics is not statutory law, but rather case law. This means it is the result of decisions passed by courts, mostly in civil suits, as they cumulatively develop into a body of precedents that judges will look to as each similar or related case comes up for decision.

The higher the courts, the more influential, but even the state supreme courts can be seen as relevant directly only to that state in which the judgment was passed. Thus, in the evolving precedents that deal with new medical technologies and difficult ethical issues, there are few absolute legal "rules" that govern. For this reason, the informed physician must keep up to date on the basics of key court cases in medical ethics and should freely consult legal experts, such as hospital attorneys, in uncertain situations. This does not mean, however, that all ethical dilemmas must be decided in courts. In fact, most courts have asserted the primary role of the physician, working in respect of the patient's wishes, to make clinical decisions.

The role of government in regulating clinical ethics is quite circumscribed. "Living will" statutes are examples of enabling legislation at the state level, which have been used in many courts as important evidence of a patient's wish to limit heroic treatments at the end of life, but which have not been tested in court as "binding." The federal government's role in decisions to forego life-sustaining treatments in critically ill infants ("Baby Doe") was overruled by the Supreme Court in 1984, leaving these decisions again at the individual level. No federal regulations have been enacted about such decisions in elderly patients. State governments are discussing regulations that require hospitals to establish policies about certain kinds of ethical issues, such as decisions not to resuscitate, obtaining consent for organ donation, and how to manage human immunodeficiency virus antibody testing.

Even aside from government regulations, institutional policies are being developed by many hospitals to establish both standards and procedures for decision making. The most widely reported of these, to date, are policies for "do not resuscitate" decisions, specifying the information relevant to such decisions and the process for their documentation. The Joint Commission for the Accreditation of Health Care Organizations now requires all facilities that it accredits to have explicit written policies about "do not resuscitate" orders. Similar requirements for institutional protocols that cover other kinds of clinical decisions to forego or withdraw life-sustaining treat-ment soon may be added to the "do not resuscitate" regulations.[12] Some hospitals and nursing homes have established ethics committees to assist in developing policies to foster education of staff and, in some cases, to assist in the decision-making process in especially difficult situations.[13]

Communication, Disclosure, and Informed Consent

Informed consent represents the basic tenets of the physician-patient relationship: communication and respect. Its necessary components are (1) full information, (2) free and uncoerced decision making, and (3) competence of the patient.

Full Information

The information given to a patient is judged to be adequate by two different standards: (1) information that is usually given by competent physicians in that community, ie, "community standards," and (2) information that a "reasonable person" would want or need (see Chapter 48). The second standard, while more subjective, leans more on the principle of respect for patient self-determination and, therefore, is probably the best standard to use.

Many studies have shown that patients desire substantial disclosure of information about their medical conditions, even if it is disturbing information. Except in very unusual situations, patients should be told (1) their medical status, including the likely course without treatment, and (2) interventions that might help, including a description of procedures and medications and their common adverse effects. Physicians in the beneficent and educator roles should do more than just describe alternatives; they also should be willing to make recommendations based on their own professional opinions, to continue to care for a patient if the patient makes another choice, and to convey this information in a genuine and caring way to the patient.

"Informed consent" is too often equated with a "consent form." Ethically and legally, consent does not refer only to a signature on a piece of paper, but rather also to a real communication, often over a period of time, and an agreement about the course of medical care and understanding of the valued outcomes.[14] It is an integral part of the physician-patient relationship. Communication experts have studied areas of misunderstanding or conflict in this process. Conflicts most frequently occur about the definition of the problem, the goals for treatment, and the conditions of treatment. Conflicts can be implicit or explicit and major or minor. Major conflicts threaten the fiduciary basis of the relationship and its therapeutic effectiveness. They should be identified and dealt with openly.

Conflict sometimes will occur when the patient or family wants or demands a certain kind of test or treatment that the physician does not think is necessary, eg, long-term use of sedative-hypnotics or laxatives. Studies of negotiation have shown that it is more effective to find mutual interests than to argue from preestablished positions, eg, both physician and patient may agree that relief of pain is important and thereby avoid a struggle over the hazards of addicting medication. Negotiation and compromise differ from capitulation by the physician, which often is due to a lack of interest, caring, or skill. Patients who are demanding of a physician's time, but without discernible medical problems, also need the physician's communication skills. A compromise on the definition of the problem, which includes the patient's psychologic needs, can establish a relationship of regular visits that is less stressful to both parties. By acknowledging the importance of the patient's position (to the patient) and by having a variety of options available, the physician can make concessions and still meet the goals of treatment.

Lack of Coercion

The second component of valid informed consent, lack of coercion, refers in most circumstances to the absence of psychologic pressures from the physician. Patients may fear that physicians will disapprove of a certain choice, treat them with less respect, or may abandon their care altogether and may then feel reluctant to express their preferences or to ask questions about things that are not understood. It is part of the physician's duty in communication to transmit an open and positive regard and willingness to respect the patient's choices.

Decision theory analysts have demonstrated that patients often have value systems that are very different from those held by physicians. In two important studies of cancer, patients overwhelmingly chose therapies that had less chance of cure but less potential for functional impairment from the treatment, eg, radiotherapy vs radical surgery for lung cancer and for laryngeal cancer.[15,16] In both cases, hypothetically, the physicians would make the opposite choice of "the long shot" for cure even if it held greater risk of immediate morbidity. These studies are just one example of ways in which patients may make decisions very differently from what physicians would expect.

The physician may disagree with the patient about the best course of evaluation or treatment, but if the physician understands communication and negotiation techniques, an effective interaction can usually be achieved. Only rarely should the conflict be irresolvable. In geriatric medicine, this situation may occur when a patient prefers to forego life-sustaining treatment, or a family, acting as proxy decision makers, make that choice on the incompetent patient's behalf. If the physician has a morally based disagreement with this strategy in a particular case, the physician may decide that he or she is unable to be effective in the care of this patient and may, with the patient's agreement, transfer care to another physician. In the case of a patient who wants unorthodox or ineffective therapy, such as amygdalin (Laetrile) and benzoic acid (Gerovital), the physician will do more good by not abandoning the patient but remaining available for other kinds of help and discussion of alternatives at any point in the illness.

Capacity to Decide

The third component of valid informed consent, competence, is the attribute of a patient who has the mental capacity to understand and communicate information, to reason and deliberate about choices, and to make choices in the light of specific goals and values. If a person is unable to meet any of these criteria, eg, is comatose, delirious, demented, or aphasic, then different decision-making processes are necessary. Sometimes, especially in emergencies, the physician must take a more paternalistic role, but in every case, the goal of decision making should be to respect the values and preferences of that particular person.

Determination of the capacity to decide is a clinical assessment. The physician should assume that most adult patients have the capacity to make their own decisions, but in the initial interview and other interactions with the patient, the physician should be assessing the components of adequate capacity to decide. A standardized mental status examination is useful in the case of questionable cognitive status, or in distinguishing delirium from depression, but there is no single quantitative score that indicates decisional capacity. An elderly person with mild or even moderate dementia, for example, may be able to understand enough about the issue at hand to deliberate and make a choice that is consistent with his or her lifelong values. If such a person refuses recommended surgery, the assessment of decision-making capacity benefits enormously from a sound and continuing physician, patient, and family relationship. A psychiatric consultation may be helpful, especially in cases where the patient's belief system appears to be delusional or other clues of underlying emotional instability or conflict are identified.

"Capacity to decide" is to be distinguished from "competence," a legal term with very specific meanings, usually without an explicit relation to health care decisions (see Chapter 48). A person must be adjudicated as incompetent by a judge (de jure incompetence), and a guardian must be appointed. Adjudicated incompetence may be very narrow, eg, incompetent to manage finances and requiring a guardian of the estate, or very broad, eg, globally incompetent and requiring a guardian of the person.

When a patient lacks the capacity to decide, other people are appropriately brought into the process. Unless a legal guardian has been appointed, however, no other person has the absolute right to make medical decisions on behalf of another adult. An elderly person is not automatically subject to the decisions of family members, in contrast to health care decisions for children where parents automatically have the legal authority. Family members and others who are close to the patient, of course, should be consulted about what the patient's own wishes would have been. The most closely connected people should be kept informed and involved in the ongoing process of decision making.

When the patient's own capacity for decision making fluctuates, the physician should examine every possible medical, pharmacologic, and environmental variable that might improve the patient's ability to make decisions. When a conflict between physician and family cannot be resolved, a court-appointed guardian *ad litem,* which can be obtained very quickly, may resolve the issue. Emergency treatment always may be instituted without formal consent.

Advance Directives

Because of the high value that society places on self-determination, every attempt is made to make medical decisions consistent with the patient's own values. If the patient cannot decide, or cannot express a decision, it is very helpful to the physician to have evidence of "prior expressed wishes" or "advance directives." State laws are being developed to allow specific instruments for this purpose. The most widespread are the "living will" statutes, currently extant in 36 states, which designate a legally valid statement to the effect that, in the event of critical or terminal illness where recovery is extremely unlikely, the patient does not wish to be kept alive by extraordinary measures.[17] These statements inevitably are imprecise but do provide evidence of the patient's own values. While living wills are not considered to be legally binding, they have been admitted as important evidence in a number of cases about decisions to forego life-sustaining treatment.

A second, more recently developed form of an advance directive is the "durable power of attorney for health care," which is statutory law currently in only a few states, wherein a specific person is designated as the patient's proxy decision maker if the need arises. This format is more comprehensive and flexible because it does not require every clinical situation to be anticipated and specified, but it does identify a person whom the patient trusts to make decisions on his or her behalf. The primary care physician should be especially aware of the responsibility, whenever possible, to talk with patients about their own values concerning death, disability, and medical care at the end of life. These conversations should be documented in the medical record.

While some people will not have thought about these issues, there are many who have and who are eager to discuss their views with an interested physician. As people age, most will have experienced the critical illness or death of someone close to them. Such people are more likely to have considered the implications for themselves of modern medical advances, especially life-sustaining technology. When possible, it is always better to have the patient's own views rather than those of a family member or surrogate. Even in very close families, proxy decision makers commonly make incorrect assumptions or misinterpreted judgments about what the patient would have wanted.[18] Especially in situations of critical illness, knowing the patient's own expressed wishes about extraordinary measures should be a major contribution of the primary care geriatrician.

Decisions to Forego Life-Sustaining Treatment

Brain Death

Irreversible loss of total brain function, (ie, function of the neocortex and brain stem) is increasingly accepted in statutory and case law as a sufficient basis for declaring death. The President's Commission for the Study of Ethical Problems in Medicine and Biomedical and Behavioral Research proposed the following model statute: "An individual who has sustained either 1) irreversible cessation of circulatory and respiratory function, or 2) irreversible cessation of all functions of the entire brain, including the brain stem, is [brain] dead. A determination of death must be made in accordance with accepted medical standards."[19] Patients who are brain dead are in a deep coma, lack all movement except for spinal segmental reflexes, lack brain-stem reflexes, and are totally dependent on a respirator. They usually, but not always, have flat electroencephalographic tracings. Cardiopulmonary "survival" rarely exceeds 4 to 6 weeks among such patients. When a diagnosis of brain death is established, no further treatment is required. A physician has no moral obligation to perform futile actions.

Persistent Vegetative State

Brain death must be distinguished from cortical or cerebral death, which is more precisely called "the persistent vegetative state (PVS)." In PVS, the neocortex is largely and irreversibly destroyed; brainstem function, however, may persist. Patients in this state may appear to be awake but without the ability consciously to interact with the environment. They may make spontaneous movements, and often are not dependent on a respirator. Courts have accepted that recovery is hopeless after 3 to 6 months in this condition, but many clinicians believe an accurate prognosis can be established much sooner.[20] Patients in this state can survive for many years, but for many people, such an existence is meaningless or, worse, abhorrent. In the past decade, ethical and legal standards for the care of PVS patients have been established by a number of important court cases in which the patient's right to have life-sustaining treatment withdrawn or withheld has been confirmed in every case, as long as there was reasonable evidence that such a decision is consistent with the patient's own values and preferences. It should not be necessary to take such cases to court, since the judgment in past precedents have been so consistent. Extraordinary measures usually are not indicated if this is in accordance with the patient's wishes and decisions are reached in consultation with relevant family members.

Quality of Life

In ethical dilemmas that concern elderly patients, one often encounters the issue of quality of life. Decisions made on the basis of quality-of-life considerations must be examined scrupulously, because there is a significant risk of generalizing one's own values in such an assessment. There is now ample empiric evidence that patients often have very different standards of an "acceptable" quality of life. Even physicians who had a long-standing relationship with the patient were frequently mistaken in their assessment of what a particular patient's quality-of-life decision would be.[21] This is a time when the golden rule must be viewed in the complexity added by the concept of respect for the views of others. This caveat is clearly exemplified by consideration of a patient with dementia. One often hears it said that a person who is demented, particularly one who is in a nursing home, has such a poor quality of life that it is not worth living. Clinical decisions may be made on this basis. Medical treatment in many such cases is limited, eg, fevers are not evaluated or treated. Although we may not explicitly acknowledge this, there is often an assumption that such people should be mercifully allowed to die.

Before such decisions are made and acted on, it is useful to examine the following issues.[22] First, decisions that are made to relieve the suffering of the patient must initially establish whether or not that patient is actually suffering. One of the most disconcerting aspects of dementing syndromes is that patients lose insight about their own conditions. If they are well cared for, patients with dementia often do not appear to suffer.

The caregivers, however, may suffer, seeing a potential future self-reflected in the patients. Physicians find the prospect of developing a dementing illness to be fearful and abhorrent. Physicians sometimes seem to value intelligence more highly than almost any other human characteristic. But not everyone shares this value. There may be a significance to life that goes beyond one's cognitive ability. For example, we do not generally limit medical treatment for retarded children, even though their cognitive function may not be any greater than that of a moderately demented elderly person.

Second, part of our concern for the suffering of demented patients is justified by the realities of poor treatment and inadequate resources in short- and long-term care facilities. If we must place patients in institutions where they are given poor care, are neglected, or even are mistreated, then concern for suffering is certainly warranted. But how can we justify a decision to allow a patient to die that is based on the miserable quality of life in the nursing home if, in fact, that condition is amenable to change? The moral obligation here is to take socially responsible action toward changing these conditions rather than to let the patient die because the conditions are so poor.

Life-Sustaining Nutrition and Fluid

There has been a growing acceptance that certain life-sustaining technologies are sometimes no longer indicated in a dying patient. Case law and medical practice have established that mechanical ventilation, cardiopulmonary resuscitation, intensive care units, and major surgical procedures ethically may be omitted if the patient refuses the treatment or if there is no reasonable chance that it will help. Life-sustaining food and fluid have not been seen in this category until the past few years. While there remains a considerable controversy about this issue, several state supreme court decisions have established precedents that, in permanently comatose or severely impaired patients expected to survive less than a year, nutritional support can be viewed as "extraordinary" treatment, and thus withheld, but only if there is evidence that the patient would have wished such support removed.[23]

The health care team should be considered in the analysis of consequences, in any difficult ethical decision. The inclusion of the feelings and ideas of several relevant caregivers in the decision process is not always simple but has the advantage of requiring clarification of ethical reasoning. Tube feeding is a common example of a practice in which the feelings of others are too easily overlooked.[24] A physician may decide not to institute tube feeding in an elderly mentally disabled patient in a long-term care facility because of the potential discomfort to the patient and because the physician feels some uneasiness with the level of aggressiveness that even tube feeding represents. Instead, in a patient who is not taking nourishment, the physician will write an order to the nursing staff to feed the patient aggressively. The people who actually have to carry out this order are generally nurses' aides who may spend most of their day trying to feed patients who do not want to eat or who cannot eat. Often, it seems to hurt the patient or causes choking. The patient may become combative, distressed, or frightened when a bolus of food is placed inside an unwilling mouth. For nurses' aides who must go through this with several patients day after day, distancing and dehumanization are probably the defenses that make it endurable. These psychologic consequences of the decision may therefore contribute to poor care of other and future patients.

In any ethical decision, as in any medical decision, the physician must be clear and direct. If it is not clear whether the patient may recover, a therapeutic trial, which includes adequate (if possible, optimal) nutrition, is necessary if any accurate conclusions are to be drawn about the patient's rehabilitation potential. Intravenous hyperalimentation for a defined period may be more acceptable to patient and staff. Feeding gastrostomy or jejunostomy also should be considered. It is up to the physician to provide leadership in finding solutions to the problem of how to manage this feeding. Such leadership may, for example, involve exerting administrative pressure to allow nurses, dietitians, psychologists, and rehabilitation therapists to perform their work in a humane context, and to allow frustrations and moral concerns to be expressed and discussed.

If a decision is then made that feeding is not of benefit to the patient, active and supportive involvement of the physician will help caregivers deal with inevitably difficult and painful feelings about the futility of treatment and the death of the patient. Once a decision is made, in particular, a decision to withdraw or not to institute an aggressive therapy, the ethical context includes the enactment of the decision. These actions take extraordinary sensitivity and extreme responsibility. The less dramatic, more intimate details of caring for a patient can and should continue and perhaps even intensify in that situation.

In such weighty matters, one must always consider the consequences to society. In fact, those who argue against the legalization of active euthanasia, even for terminal patients in extreme suffering, assert that it would erode the moral fiber of the profession and of society to allow physicians actually to administer a lethal dose of a drug to a patient.[25] This is the same argument that is used against having physicians involved in capital punishment even though the form of death thereby may be more merciful. One may counter this argument with the claim that compassionate care of dying patients may have to include instances of assisted voluntary suicide, but the influence on society could be positive because responsible caring for dying patients deepens our sense of humanity. This debate continues,[26] but there is no legal basis in the United States for mercy killing or euthanasia.

Nursing Homes

The same principles of ethics apply to patients in nursing homes as to those in acute care centers, hospitals, or ambulatory care settings. There are, however, certain special characteristics of the kinds of ethical dilemmas that arise in nursing homes and the ways in which they can be dealth with that deserve the attention of the geriatrician.[27]

First and very importantly, there is almost always more time to discuss the issues and explore the options when an ethical dilemma arises in the care of a nursing home patient. For example, in the case of a demented but otherwise healthy man who wanders, the staff is confronted with the dilemma of whether to limit his autonomy by the use of restraints or to take the risk that he may hurt himself. The nursing home setting provides a chance for exploration at length with all of the staff involved, administrators, various advocates for the patient, and family members. The longer time frame allows some kinds of decisions to be made on a trial basis for a period of time and then reevaluated and further discussed (eg, forego restraints for a week or two, then reconsider). This offers a chance for much deeper reflection and consideration of more complex concerns than is often the case in the acute care setting.

Second, it is always important, particularly in decisions about life-sustaining treatment, such as do not resuscitate or do not transfer orders, to distinguish clearly terminal illness from chronic progressive disease. The geriatrician should not make the mistake of assuming that all older people with chronic, progressive disease are suffering from terminal illness and therefore should not be treated for reversible conditions.

Third, there is a well-documented high prevalence of cognitive impairment in nursing home populations, precisely because patients with dementia, particularly advanced dementia, are very difficult to care for at home. One could all too easily assume—incorrectly—that all nursing home residents are incapable of making their own decisions. Even with borderline or mild dementia, often there is some ability of the person to take part in decision making. Therefore, cognitive function needs very careful testing, evaluation, and documentation.

Fourth, the staff in nursing homes often have very close relationships with the patients and can function as surrogate family members, particularly for those nursing home residents who do not have other family or friends. When the need for a decision arises and a patient is unable to voice his or her own decision, the physician will be looking for evidence of what that patient's wishes would have been. Staff who have had a chance to talk with the patient throughout weeks, months, or even years may be able to provide that information. An additional aspect of this role of staff as family is that deep feelings may have developed for the patient and those feelings need to be taken into account if any care plan is to be effective.

Fifth, there often is a lack of a dominant physician role in nursing homes; therefore, when ethical dilemmas arise, it may be more appropriate for another health professional to take the lead in discussions seeking a resolution. The role of the interdisciplinary team in an ethics committee may be more essential in long-term care than in the short-term care setting.

Finally, the nursing home, as with any health care institution, has institutional interests that it must protect.[28] Those interests are, to some extent, different from those of the acute care hospital. Nursing home administrators are responsible for making possible the highest quality of care in an institution that is incessantly beleaguered by severe shortages of financial resources. Nursing homes also are subject to strict government regulations that often limit their ability to individualize clinical decision making. Such regulations may, for example, require nursing homes to provide certain kinds of care to incompetent patients even if there is evidence that the patient would have refused it, or to transfer the patient to a hospital emergency room for treatment of an acute illness.

Conclusions

While significant factors may vary among the acute care hospital, the nursing home, and home care, the general principles apply in each case. As with any aspect of clinical care, certain general guidelines apply as follows: an emphasis on continuity of care and consistency of a care plan regardless of the site of care; adequate communication between the team of health care providers, and between the health care providers and the patient and family; good faith and technical competence in the delivery of care; respect and compassion for the patient; an ability to identify and analyze ethical problems; and a willingness to seek consultation if the resolution to a dilemma is not clear.

Ethics has always been a discipline central to the sound practice of medicine, but it has probably never been more important than now. The many advances of modern medicine carry both a promise of improved quality of life and increased longevity. These same advances may represent threats to the quality of life or autonomy of a patient, if prudence and thoughtfulness are not included in clinical decision making. In addition, the pressures of cost containment and shifting reimbursement incentives pose threats of both underutilization and overutilization of health care services with elderly people. Physicians can maintain the integrity of their relationship with patients and also deal with their social responsibilities by developing an ethically based framework for decision making.

References

1. Beauchamp TL, Childers JF. *Principles of Biomedical Ethics.* 2nd ed. New York, NY: Oxford University Press Inc; 1985.
2. The Hastings Center. *Guidelines on the Termination of Life-Sustaining Treatment and the Care of the Dying.* New York, NY: The Hastings Center; 1987.
3. *Schloendorff v Society of New York Hospitals,* 211 NY 125, 105 NE 92 (1914).
4. Katz J. *The Silent World of Physician and Patient.* New York, NY: Free Press; 1985.
5. Strull W, Lo B, Charles G. Do patients want to participate in medical decision making? *JAMA* 1984;252:2990–2995.
6. Novack D, Plumer R, Smith R, et al. Changes in physicians' attitudes toward telling the cancer patient. *JAMA* 1979;241:897–899.
7. Siegler M. Confidentiality in medicine: a decrepit concept. *N Engl J Med* 1982;247:2695.
8. May WF. Code, covenant, contract or philanthropy. *Hastings Cent Rep* 1975;5:29–38.
9. Evans R. Health care technology and the inevitability

of resource allocation and rationing decisions. *JAMA* 1983;249:2047, 2208.

10. Avorn J. Benefit and cost analysis in geriatric care: turning age discrimination into health policy. *N Engl J Med* 1984;310:1294–1298.

11. Eisenberg J. The internist as gatekeeper: preparing the general internist for a new role. *Ann Intern Med* 1985;102:537.

12. Miles SH, Cassel CK, Siegler MS, et al. *Institutional Policies About the Use of Life-Sustaining Treatments. Institutional Protocols for Decisions about Life-Sustaining Treatments, Special Report.* OTA-BA-389, Washington, DC: Government Printing Office, July 1988.

13. Glasser G, Zweibel NR, Cassel CK. The ethics committee in the nursing home: results of a national survey. *J Am Geriatr Soc* 1988;36:150–156.

14. President's Commission for the Study of Ethical Problems in Medicine and Biomedical and Behavioral Research *Making Health Care Decisions.* Washington, DC: LC 82-600637; 1984.

15. McNeil B, Weichselbaum R, Pauker S. Fallacy of the five-year survival in lung cancer. *N Engl J Med* 1978;299:1397.

16. McNeil B, Weichselbaum R, Pauker S. Speech and survival: tradeoffs between quality and quantity of life in laryngeal cancer. *N Engl J Med* 1979;301:444.

17. Society for the Right to Die: *Handbook of Living Will Laws.* New York, NY: Society for the Right to Die; 1987.

18. Steinbrook R, Lo B. Decision making for incompetent patients by designated proxy. *N Engl J Med* 1984;310:1598–1601.

19. President's Commission for the Study of Ethical Problems in Medicine and Biomedical and Behavioral Research *Defining Death.* Washington, DC: 1981, publisher LC 81-600150.

20. Levy DE, Bates D, Coronna JJ, et al. Prognosis in nontraumatic coma. *Ann Intern Med* 1981;94:293–301.

21. Pearlman R, Jonsen A. Use of quality of life considerations in medical decision making. *J Am Geriatr Soc* 1985;33:344.

22. Cassel CK, Jameton AL. Dementia in the elderly: an analysis of medical responsibility. *Ann Intern Med* 1981;94:802–807.

23. Lynn J, ed. *By No Extraordinary Means.* Bloomington, Ind: Indiana University Press; 1986.

24. Watts D, Cassel CK, Hickam D. Nurses' and physicians' attitudes toward tube-feeding decisions in long-term care. *J Am Geriatr Soc* 1986;34:607–611.

25. Meier D, Cassel CK. Euthanasia in old age: a case study and ethical analysis. *J Am Geriatr Soc* 1983;31:294–298.

26. Wanzer S, et al. Care of the hopelessly ill patient: a second look. *N Engl J Med* 1989;320:844–849.

27. Zweibel N, Cassel CK, eds. *Clinical and Policy Issues in the Care of the Nursing Home Patient: Clinics in Geriatric Medicine.* Philadelphia, Pa: WB Saunders Co; 1988.

28. Miles SH, Ryden M. Limited-treatment policies in long-term care facilities. *J Am Geriatr Soc* 1985;33:707.

5

Neuropsychological Testing

Marilyn S. Albert

A variety of cognitive disorders occur with increasing frequency as people age; these include progressive dementing disorders, acute confusional states, and cognitive disorders secondary to psychiatric syndromes. Epidemiological studies indicate that approximately 15% of the population older than 65 years of age suffers from some form of dementia.[1,2] However, the probability of having a dementing disorder increases dramatically with age. Recent data concerning the prevalence of dementia in a community-dwelling population indicate that between the ages of 65 and 74 years, the prevalence of probable and highly probable dementia ranges from 2% to 3%; this increases to 22% and 23% among those persons 75 to 84 years and to 47% and 48% among those persons aged 85 years and older.[3] Similarly striking figures pertain to the incidence and prevalence of acute confusion in hospitalized elderly patients. Several studies have reported that 25% to 35% of hospitalized geriatric patients on a general medical service who are cognitively intact at admission develop acute confusion.[4–6] The incidence of acute confusion in subjects younger than the age of 70 years in comparison with those older than the age of 70 years is 3.6% vs 30%, respectively.[4] There are few systematic studies of the prevalence of cognitive disorders secondary to psychiatric syndromes, but numerous clinical reports state that their prevalence is greater among the elderly patients than young patients.[7]

These cognitive disorders produce considerable morbidity and mortality, and although only some of them can be completely reversed with treatment, appropriate management can substantially improve the quality of life and reduce the development of secondary conditions. Thus, it is in the best interests of the patient for one to become increasingly attuned to the possible presence of cognitive dysfunction in older patients and to the appropriate procedures for workup and referral. The present chapter will focus on the role of neuropsychological testing in the assessment of cognitive dysfunction in elderly patients, particularly as it applies to the geriatrician, since there is much that a geriatrician can do to identify the presence of cognitive dysfunction and see that it is properly assessed.

Interview with Patient

There are two sources of information concerning the cognitive status of patients: (1) patients themselves and (2) patients' families. Unless a family member has approached the physician with concerns about the patient's cognitive function, it is not likely a family member will be routinely involved in a geriatric assessment. Therefore, the physician is initially limited to information that is obtainable from the patient. This information can be most easily gathered in two ways: (1) from an interview of the patient in the course of conducting a medical evaluation and (2) from brief mental status testing.

Observation During the Medical Examination

In the course of a routine medical examination, there is ample opportunity to converse with patients and gather information about their cognitive status. Since the most common causes of cognitive decline in elderly patients produce a memory disorder (specifically a difficulty with learning and retaining new information), the greatest emphasis should be placed on ascertaining information about the memory function of the patient. This may be accomplished by a discussion of current events. Appropriate subjects will differ according to the educational and socioeconomic background of the patient. For one patient, this may be politics, for another, sports, and for another, the stage of the planting season. If there is a particularly dramatic event in the news that most people are likely to have heard of (eg, a presidential election, a plane crash, etc), this may be useful for persons of diverse backgrounds. In any case, the task is to determine whether the person is familiar with the event in question and, if so, if it is a familiarity that is more than general. Many patients in the early stages of a dementing disorder can make general all-purpose remarks that appear to be appropriate while obscuring the fact that they do not have any substantive knowledge of the subject at hand.

In the course of conversing, one can also listen to the nature of the patient's linguistic output. Language problems are important to assess because they are common in both cerebrovascular disorders (eg, stroke) and dementing disorders. The patient's comprehension ability can be evaluated during a medical examination with relative ease because the patient is generally asked to perform tasks (eg, open your mouth, lift up an arm, etc), and the ability to comprehend these simple directions can be ascertained. Speech fluency also is relatively easy to observe. Patients who are nonfluent have an effortful and halting quality to their speech. Substantive words, such as nouns and verbs, are present, but small connective words (eg., "if's," "and's," "but's") are generally missing. Disturbances in fluency, like problems with comprehension, often are indicative of a stroke.[8,9] Naming ability also can be assessed in the course of conversation. A person with naming problems frequently hesitates over names of objects or persons and may attempt to circumvent the difficulty in a variety of ways (eg, giving a lengthy description of the object or person, substituting associated words, etc). If naming problems are suspected, a further evaluation can be carried out by using common objects at hand. Very familiar objects, such as a watch or a door, are easy to name. Thus, only a person with a relatively severe naming problem will have difficulty with them. In general, however, parts of objects are harder to name (eg, the stem of a watch, the knob on a door, etc). The use of both common objects and parts of objects as stimuli will assess a range of naming ability.

Thus, with little additional expenditure of time,

memory and language, ie, the two aspects of cognitive function most frequently affected by cerebrovascular disease and common dementing disorders, can be briefly assessed. The goal is not to undertake a detailed or thorough evaluation, but to determine whether any problems are present that suggest an underlying abnormality.

Mental Status Testing

It should, however, be pointed out that it takes a considerable amount of experience to become skilled in drawing sound clinical conclusions from a conversational approach to the assessment of cognitive function. Therefore, it is ideal if this can be supplemented by a brief test of mental status. The most widely used tests are listed below.

- Mini-Mental State Examination[10] (Chapter 33)
- Short Portable Mental Status Questionnaire[11]
- Mental Status Questionnaire[12]
- Blessed Dementia Scale[13]
- East Boston Memory Test[14]

These tests vary in length of administration from about 3 to 10 minutes. The shorter tests tend to evaluate only one major area of cognitive function, such as memory (eg, the East Boston Memory Test), while the longer ones assess a broader range of cognitive abilities, such as memory, calculations, language, and spatial ability (eg, the Mini-Mental State Examination). However, all screening mental status tests have a number of aspects in common. First, all are particularly prone to the confounding effects of education. Individuals with a high premorbid ability can score in the unimpaired range and still have experienced a substantial amount of cognitive decline. Similarly, individuals with low educational achievement are frequently misidentified as impaired.[15] One must therefore be extremely cautious in interpreting the poor screening test results of an elderly individual with little or no education or in ignoring the good test results of a highly educated person who is complaining of cognitive dysfunction. In addition, the cutoff points on many of the existing screening tests are generally designed to identify moderately to severely impaired individuals, to minimize falsely identifying persons who are well (ie, false positives). Thus, individuals' conditions can, by a lengthier examination, be diagnosed as the early stages of a dementing disorder, such as Alzheimer's disease, and these individuals may still perform above the standard cutoff scores on a short screening test. It is also important to note that such tests, by their very nature, were not designed to measure subtle aspects of behavior. Thus, the scores may show little or no decline over time in patients whose conditions can be shown, by other measures, to have declined substantially.

Despite these shortcomings, mental status screening tests are extremely useful tools. In a brief period of time, one can administer a standardized series of questions that have proved to be helpful in identifying persons with cognitive dysfunction. Most of the tests are effective in screening memory ability. Thus, they are useful in identifying persons with dementing disorders, such as Alzheimer's disease, or acute confusion, conditions that are particularly difficult to diagnose. If used repeatedly over time, they are helpful in establishing a numerical baseline against which future performance can be compared. And if clinicians use the same test with frequency, they will begin to learn how to use test results to formulate referral questions. It is, for example, much more useful for a patient to be referred for further neuropsychological testing with a statement, such as "the patient has declined four points on the Mini-Mental State Exam over the last year and appears to have particular difficulty with memory testing" rather than "referral for question of dementia."

Interview with Family

If cognitive dysfunction is suspected, it is extremely important to obtain a good history of the cognitive changes that have recently occurred. Since the patient's self-report may be unreliable, it is important to obtain a cognitive history from one or more family members.

Obtaining a good cognitive history is one of the most difficult and yet important aspects of an evaluation for cognitive dysfunction. A comprehensive history should include information concerning the onset, nature, and progression of behavioral change. Cognitive histories are difficult to obtain because most patients and family members are not attuned to subtle behavioral symptoms. They do not know how to isolate important aspects of the medical history or how to focus on individual cognitive functions in isolation from one another. For example, the family may state that the first symptom of disease was the patient's anxiety and depression about work and, only when asked, remember several episodes that preceded the onset of work-related anxiety in which the patient could not remember how to deal with a complex situation or how to use new equipment in the workplace.

Family members also may have difficulty in understanding why certain subtle distinctions are important for diagnosis. For example, a family member may say that the patient's first symptom was forgetfulness, but when asked to provide instances of forgetfulness, the family member may explain that the patient had trouble installing a new drawer pull in the kitchen or had trouble knowing how to find a familiar location, both of which would suggest spatial difficulty more than memory difficulty. In addition, an unwillingness to admit that certain impairments exist can prevent family members from providing accurate information.

Finally, family members can sometimes misinterpret even fairly direct questions. For example, a history of a gradually progressive disorder is essential to the diagnosis of Alzheimer's disease. Yet, frequently family members say that a disorder came on suddenly when it did not. The realization that the patient is having cognitive problems often coincides with an unusual external event, such as a trip to an unfamiliar place. An unfamiliar environment generally prevents persons from employing overlearned habits and routines and, thus, exposes their cognitive problems. Since family members notice these difficulties suddenly, they may conclude that the disease onset is sudden. If this misconception appears to be the case, it is then necessary to determine whether any symptoms of cognitive change preceded the external event. Most commonly, family members then recall episodes of an earlier change in cognitive function.

As mentioned earlier, a good cognitive history must first establish the time at which cognitive changes became apparent. This will provide important clues regarding the nature of the disorder, because some diseases are well known for their particularly rapid rate of decline (eg, Creutzfeldt-Jakob disease). It will also enable the clinician to give the family some tentative feedback regarding the course of the illness. If the point at which the disorder began is known, the rate of decline can be determined by seeing how long it has taken the patient to reach the present level of function. While estimates of the rate of progression can be only roughly approximated, it is extremely helpful for the family to have an estimate in making plans for the future. Repeated cognitive testing can provide further help in establishing the course of disease.

Second, it is important to determine the nature of the behavioral changes that were evident when the disease began. This also will provide essential information regarding the diagnosis. For example, an early symptom of Pick's disease is generally thought to be a change in personality (eg, inappropriate behavior), while the most common early symptom of Alzheimer's disease is a gradually progressive decline in the ability to learn new information. Several years after the disease has begun, which is when most patients' conditions are actually diagnosed, the cognitive symptoms of the two disorders may be very similar, so that information regarding the initial symptoms may be critical.

Third, it is important to determine whether the initial symptoms came on suddenly or gradually. If the onset of illness is gradual and insidious, as in Alzheimer's disease, it is often only in retrospect that the family realizes that a decline has occurred. In contrast, a series of small strokes, even if not evident on computed tomographic or magnetic resonance imaging scans, produce a history of sudden onset and stepwise progression. There is generally an incident (eg, a fall or a period of confusion) that marks the beginning of the disorder. Acute confusional states generally have an acute onset as well, although if they are the result of a condition such as drug toxicity, this may not be the case.

The manner in which the symptoms have progressed over time also provides important diagnostic information. A stepwise deterioration, characterized by sudden exacerbations of symptoms, is most typical of multi-infarct dementia. However, a physical illness in a patient with Alzheimer's disease (eg, pneumonia, a hip fracture, etc) can cause a rapid decline in cognitive function. The sudden worsening of symptoms in a psychiatric patient (eg, depression) also can produce an abrupt decrease in mental status. Careful questioning is therefore necessary to determine the underlying cause of a stepwise decline in function.

It is also important to determine the patient's current functional status. A substantial discrepancy between the functional and cognitive status of the patient suggests the presence of a psychiatric illness.

Detailed Neuropsychological Testing

If one suspects the presence of cognitive deficits and is going to refer a patient for neuropsychological testing, it is important to know that there are at least two basic approaches to the selection of a neuropsychological test protocol. Some neuropsychologists use a predetermined test battery, such as the Halstead Reitan Battery[16] or the Luria Nebraska Battery.[17] Other neuropsychologists select from a group of tests that seem to be particularly relevant to the diagnostic question. Even in the latter case, however, there tends to be a core group of tests that are relied on more heavily than others. However, regardless of the approach of the neuropsychologist, it is reasonable to expect that the neuropsychological report be formed in terms of the following major areas of cognitive ability: attention, language, memory, spatial ability, conceptualization, and general information.

Attention is important to consider because simple attentional abilities must be preserved for any other task to be performed adequately. If the subject has difficulty in keeping his or her mind on a task for 1 to 3 minutes at a time, it will not be possible to assess other areas of function. Commonly used tests of attention are as follows:

• Letter Cancellation[18]
• Digit Span[19]
• Continuous Performance Task[20]

A complete language evaluation can include an assessment of naming, fluency, grammar, comprehension, repetition, vocabulary, reading, and writing. However, if an aphasia is not suspected, the language evaluation is likely to be limited to an assessment of confrontation naming, since decreases in naming ability are a prominent symptom of a number of cognitive disorders common in elderly patients (eg, Alzheimer's disease). Tests of language function include the following:

• Boston Diagnostic Aphasia Examination[21]
• Western Aphasia Battery[22]
• Token Test[23]
• Boston Naming Test[24]

A careful evaluation of memory is perhaps most essential to the cognitive workup of an elderly person. Memory dysfunction occurs in almost all of the cognitive disorders common in elderly patients, and the nature and severity of the memory impairment can serve as one of the major guidelines to the diagnosis. The neuropsychological assessment of memory should at least distinguish between the patient's immediate and delayed memory function, since the difference between immediate and delayed recall is very striking in early Alzheimer's disease and, if present, can be diagnostic, whereas loss of information during a brief delay is less severe in patients with other dementing and psychiatric disorders.[25] Some of the most commonly used tests of memory are listed below.

• Wechsler Memory Scale[26]
• Rey Auditory Verbal Learning Test[27]
• Selective Reminding Test[28]
• Delayed Recognition Span Test[29]
• California Verbal Learning Test[30]
• Randt Memory Test[31]
• Fuld Object Memory Test[32]

The assessment of visuospatial ability should, if at all possible, include figure copying. Figures can be chosen to span a great range of difficulty and, if the patient has visuosensory deficits, visual stimuli can be adapted accordingly (by using photographic enlargements of drawings or making the figures with felt-tipped pens). There are other tests of spatial ability that use blocks, sticks, or design recognition as follows:

- Benton Visual Retention Test[33]
- Block Design subtest of Wechsler Adult Intelligence Test–revised (WAIS-R)[19]

Tasks that examine conceptualization include tests of concept formation, abstraction, set shifting, and set maintenance. These abilities are often affected in both depression and most of the major dementing disorders[34] and therefore should be assessed separately from tests of general intelligence. Below are listed examples of some of the tests that can be used.

- Similarities subtest of WAIS-R[19]
- Proverbs Test[35]
- Trail Making Test[36]
- Modified Card Sorting Test[37]
- Visual-Verbal Test[38]

Tests of general intelligence are also useful to administer, if time permits. This will allow one to determine whether the individual has access to previously acquired knowledge. For example, early in the course of Alzheimer's disease, some patients have a normal IQ although they have a striking memory deficit and difficulty with conceptualization. A relatively preserved IQ in a patient with Alzheimer's disease often relates to higher levels of functioning at home and tends to be a good prognostic sign.

Full-scale IQ tests are, however, very lengthy. One should therefore consider administering a brief test that provides a good estimate of general intelligence. Once such test is a reduced version of the WAIS or WAIS-R.[39]

The referring physician should encourage the neuropsychologist to formulate his or her clinical report in terms of the six broad areas of cognitive function described above. A neuropsychological report organized in this fashion will make it easier for an individual with less neuropsychological expertise to interpret the results. It will also be easier to determine whether the patient has spared areas of cognitive function. This is important, since knowing the patient's pattern of spared and impaired abilities can provide an important guide to diagnosis. For example, patients with Alzheimer's disease have an approximately equal impairment in both verbal and nonverbal memory. Therefore, a patient whose verbal memory skills are disproportionately deficient relative to nonverbal testing is unlikely to have Alzheimer's disease.

The description of a patient's major cognitive impairments and major cognitive strengths also can be used to maximize function. For example, early in the course of Alzheimer's disease, most patients have striking difficulty in retaining new information during a brief delay and have problems with conceptualization that make it hard for them to integrate a number of individual tasks into a complex whole or to plan activities in the future. However, mildly impaired patients with Alzheimer's disease frequently have spared spatial abilities and a preservation of well-learned skills; therefore, they can be encouraged to carry out a wide variety of sports and leisure activities with the knowledge that they will be successful. Table 5.1 provides a summary of the major strengths and weaknesses in mild and moderately impaired patients who have typical symptoms of Alzheimer's disease.

The number and nature of the patient's impairments will also enable the skilled clinician to formulate a reasonable prognosis. For example, even though a patient with Pick's disease might have only a mild memory deficit, early evidence of severe conceptuali-

Table 5.1. Strengths and weaknesses in mild and moderately impaired patients with Alzheimer's disease.

Disease

Mild
  Memory—very defective new learning, relatively preserved recall of remote events
  Conceptualization—defective ability to plan and execute complex activity, problems switching from 1 task to another, impaired ability to form conceptual generalities, and preserved ability to understand concrete ideas
  Language—word-finding deficits, preserved conversational abilities
  Visuospatial skills—difficulty with complex spatial tasks, relatively preserved figure copying and spatial skills needed for activities of daily living (dressing, bathing, sports, etc)
  Personality—less interest in usual activities, occasional irritability, preserved general personality profile
Moderate
  Memory—severely defective new learning, moderately affected remote memory, preserved recall of most distant remote events
  Conceptualization—difficulty with anything requiring abstract thinking, can understand only simplest concrete ideas
  Language—increased word-finding deficits, difficulty with comprehension of complex language, relatively fluent speech
  Visuospatial skills—difficulty in copying simple drawings; problems with spatial skills needed for activities of daily living (dressing, bathing, sports, etc); can engage in physical activity, such as walks and simple exercise
  Personality—increased likelihood of behavioral disturbances, such as hallucinations, delusions, and agitation; can enjoy simplified and restructured activities.

zation difficulties and inappropriate behavior suggests that the patient will need to be in a supervised environment relatively soon and the family needs to plan for that eventuality. On the other hand, a patient with Alzheimer's disease with a striking memory deficit who has some preservation of conceptualization skills and shows good judgment by, for example, not cooking when food has been repeatedly burned, or not going for a long walk if this has previously led to being lost, is likely to be able to remain in a relatively unsupervised environment for a long period of time.

The assessment of cognitive function in an older person can thus serve many useful purposes if it is well focused and integrated into the general evaluation of the patient. A geriatrician who understands the potential utility of neuropsychological testing can substantially contribute to its appropriate application.

References

1. Katzman R. The prevalence and malignancy of Alzheimer's disease. *Arch Neurol* 1976;33:217–218.
2. Mortimer JA, Schuman LM, French LR. Epidemiology of dementing illness. In: Mortimer JA, Schuman LM, eds. *The Epidemiology of Dementia.* New York, NY: Oxford University Press Inc; 1981:3–23.
3. Evans D, Funkenstein H, Albert M, et al. Prevalence of Alzheimer's disease in a community-based population of older persons: marked increase beyond age 85 years. *JAMA* (in press).
4. Gillick MR, Serrell NA, Gillick LS. Adverse consequences of hospitalization in the elderly. *Soc Sci Med* 1982;16:1033–1038.
5. Hodkinson HM. Mental impairment in the elderly. *J R Coll Physicians Lond* 1973;7:305–307.
6. Hodkinson HM. Organic impairment in the elderly. *J R Coll Physicians Lond* 1981;15:141–167.
7. Reifler BV, Larson E, Hanley R. Coexistence of cognitive impairment and depression in geriatric outpatients. *Am J Psychiatry* 1982;139:623–626.
8. Albert ML, Helm-Estabrooks N. Diagnosis and treatment of aphasia, I:*JAMA* 1988;259:1043–1047.
9. Albert ML, Helm-Estabrooks N. Diagnosis and treatment of aphasia, II: *JAMA* 1988;259:1205–1210.
10. Folstein MF, Folstein SE, McHugh PR. 'Mini-Mental State': a practical method for grading cognitive state of patients for the clinician. *J Psychiatr Res* 1975;12:189–198.
11. Pfeiffer E. SPMSQ: Short Portable Mental Status Questionnaire. *J Am Geriatr Soc* 1975;23:433–441.
12. Kahn RL, Goldfarb AL, Pollack M, et al. Brief objective measures for the determination of mental status in the aged. *Am J Psychiatry* 1960;111:326–328.
13. Blessed G, Tomlinson BE, Roth M. The association between quantitative measure of dementia and of senile changes in the cerebral gray matter of elderly subjects. *Br J Psychiatry* 1968;114:797–811.
14. Scheer PA, Albert MS, Funkenstein H, et al. Correlates of cognitive function in an elderly community population. *Amer J Epidemiol* 1988;128:1084–1101.
15. Anthony JC, LeResche L, Niaz U, et al. Limits of the Mini-Mental State as a screening test for dementia and delirium among hospital patients. *Psychol Med* 1982;12:397–408.
16. Halstead WC. *Brain and Intelligence.* Chicago, Ill: University of Chicago Press; 1947.
17. Golden CJA, Hammeke TA, Purisch AD. Manual for the Luria-Nebraska Neuropsychological Battery. Los Angeles, CA: Western Psychological Services, 1980.
18. Talland G. *Deranged Memory.* Orlando, Fla: Academic Press Inc; 1965.
19. Wechsler D. *WAIS-R Manual.* New York, NY: Psychological Corp; 1981.
20. Mirsky A. Attention: a neuropsychological perspective. In Chall J, Mirsky A, eds: *Education and the Brain.* Chicago, Ill: Univ Chicago Press; 1978.
21. Goodglass H, Kaplan E. *Assessment of Aphasia and Related Disorders.* Philadelphia, Pa: Lea & Febiger; 1972.
22. Kertesz A. *Aphasia and Associated Disorders.* New York, NY: Grune & Stratton; 1979.
23. DeRenzi E, Vignolo LA. The Token Test: a sensitive test to detect disturbances in aphasics. *Brain* 1962;85:665–678.
24. Kaplan E, Goodglass H, Weintraub S. *Boston Naming Test.* Philadelphia, Pa: Lea & Febiger; 1983.
25. Moss M, Albert MS. Alzheimer's disease and other dementing disorders. In: Albert MS, Moss M, eds. *Geriatric Neuropsychology.* New York, NY: Guilford Press; 1988:145–178.
26. Wechsler D. A standardized memory scale for clinical use. *J Psychol* 1945;19:87–95.
27. Rey A. *L'examen clinique in psychologie.* Paris, France: Presses Universitaires de France; 1964.
28. Buschke H, Fuld PA. Evaluating storage, retention, and retrieval in disordered memory and learning. *Neurology* 1974;11:1019–1025.
29. Moss M, Albert M, Butters N, et al. Differential patterns of memory loss among patients with Alzheimer's disease, Huntington's disease and alcoholic Korsakoff's syndrome. *Arch Neurol* 1986;43:239–246.
30. Delis DC, Kramer JH, Kaplan E, et al. *California Verbal Learning Test.* New York, NY: Psychological Corp; 1987.
31. Randt CT, Brown ER, Osbourne DJ. A memory test for longitudinal measurement of mild to moderate deficits. *Clin Neuropsychol* 1980;2:184–194.
32. Fuld PA. Guaranteed stimulus-processing in the evaluation of memory and learning. *Cortex* 1980;16:255–272.
33. Benton AL. *The Revised Visual Retention Test.* New York, NY: Psychological Corp; 1974.
34. Caine ED. The neuropsychology of depression: the pseudodementia syndrome. In: Grant I, Adams KM, eds. *Neuropsychological Assessment of Neuropsychiatric Disorders.* New York, NY: Oxford University Press Inc; 1986:221–243.
35. Gorham DR. A proverbs test for clinical and experimental use. *Psychol Rep* 1956;1:1–12.

36. Reitan RM. Validity of the Trail Making Test as an indication of organic brain damage. *Percept Mot Skills* 1958;8:271–276.
37. Nelson HE. A modified card sorting test sensitive to frontal lobe defects. *Cortex* 1976;12:313–324.
38. Feldman MJ, Drasgow JA. A visual-verbal test for schizophrenia. *Psychiatr Q* 1951;25(suppl):55–64.
39. Satz P, Mogel S. An abbreviation of the WAIS for clinical use. *J Clin Psychol* 1962;18:77–79.

6

Instruments to Assess Functional Status

Rosalie A. Kane

The essence of geriatric practice is the expert management of a patient's needs. To accomplish this goal, a geriatric team must translate its knowledge about a patient's functional abilities and limitations, psychologic state, social support, and personal preferences into recommendations that often have far-reaching effects on the patient's life-style. This requires a physician to become involved in collecting, synthesizing, interpreting, and weighting a formidable amount of patient-specific information. Much of this information differs, in kind, from the laboratory values, physical signs and symptoms, radiology results, and other data that are combined to reach a medical diagnosis. In 1987, a Consensus Panel convened by the National Institute on Aging agreed that functional assessment, ie, assessment of the patient's "ability to function in the arena of everyday living," is integral to medical decision making.[1-2]

The gerontologic and geriatric disciplines have spawned a large family of diverse and unruly assessment tools to measure various aspects of the physical, mental, and social functioning of old people.[3-4] These instruments range from brief screening tools to comprehensive multidimensional batteries that yield multiple scores. Some of the latter instruments have become enshrined as multipurpose instruments that are used, without adaptation, to identify persons at risk, to develop the information base for care planning, to monitor care, and to generate outcome measures for evaluating the care programs. Unfortunately, the effective all-purpose geriatric assessment tool is as illusory as the proverbial free lunch. Instead of seeking the universal instrument,

those persons working with elderly patients should tailor the instruments to the purposes at hand.

This chapter discusses considerations for the physician in choosing assessment tools to incorporate into clinical practice. The choice of instruments depends on the purpose of the measurement (eg, screening, initial care planning, monitoring, or program evaluation) and the expected characteristics of the population that is being assessed. Beyond the choice of instruments, a geriatric team needs to consider its general assessment strategy, which includes criteria for deciding who collects the information, when, where, using which informants, and with what level of detail.

What Is Measured?

Physical, mental, and social factors seem to be almost inextricably intertwined in the etiology of functional impairment in elderly persons. A clinician needs both a measure of the extent and nature of the functional impairment itself (eg, what the patient can do, what does the patient do) and measures of the separate components that might account for the functional results (eg, physical health, pain or discomfort levels, depression, and social circumstances). The latter determinations offer clues to the cause of functional impairments; therefore, they suggest appropriate strategies to address functional impairments identified in the more general measure.

A general functional measure takes into account the capabilities of the patient, the social environment in which a patient is located, and the resources (financial and otherwise) at a patient's disposal to minimize the functional effects of physical or mental impairments. For convenience, the characteristics to be measured can be separated into several domains.

Physical Functioning

General physical health can be measured through combinations of symptoms, diagnoses, physical handicaps, categories of drugs that are taken, and reports of disruptions due to illnesses (eg, hospital days per year, bed days per year, or days unable to perform usual activities) to produce a summary statement of a person's health status.[5] Self-ratings and professional ratings of health may also be incorporated into such measures. This approach offers an overview of morbidity levels (actual and self-perceived) that can be incorporated into self-completed questionnaires, which are supplemented by checklists completed by a physician or other caregivers. Pain and discomfort also merit measurement (both alone and to contribute to a summary score); however, at present, our ability to gauge this characteristic systematically is rudimentary.

Self-care Abilities/Independent Living Skills

Geriatricians concur in the importance of measuring abilities that are linked to self-care. Conventionally, a distinction has been made between (1) activities of daily living (ADLs) that involve basic self care, such as eating, dressing, toileting and bathing, and (2) more complex, so-called instrumental activities of daily living (IADLs) that may be necessary for independent living. The IADLs include cooking, cleaning, laundry, using the telephone, using public or private transportation, managing money, or taking medicines. Measurement of ADLs and IADLs has been refined in the last decade, as described by Branch and Meyers[6] in a comprehensive review of a wide range of unidimensional and multidimensional measures that vary in their source of information, their level of detail, and the time period used as a frame of reference.

The performance of ADL and IADL functions depends on a happy combination of physical abilities, mental acuity, motivation, and social circumstances. Social factors, in particular, must not be overlooked. For example, it is easier to use public transportation if the bus stop is nearby. Some men who cannot prepare meals may simply not know how to cook. Labor-saving equipment may change laundry from an impossibility to a manageable task. Self-medication may become possible through a combined strategy of simplifying the regimens, making containers more readily

distinguishable, and eliminating childproof caps. The care team can exercise ingenuity in its efforts to improve IADL scores, which (in turn) are related to independent community living.

Mental Functioning

Although general measures of mental functioning are available, it is a disservice to elderly patients to combine information about cognitive and affective status into a summary statement. As it is, cognitive and affective states interact, and it is worthwhile to measure the dimensions separately. Cognition can be further divided to include (for example) memory, perception, judgment, calculation, and social intactness. Some persons can participate lucidly and appropriately in a wide range of social experiences and make judgments about an immediate situation, despite considerable memory loss. Cognitive measures[7] should be sensitive enough to pick up these distinctions, which have practical implications for care planning.

Affective status measures[8] must include a measure of depression that differentiates the saddened mood states that are prevalent in the whole population from a sustained and severe depressive state that puts the individual at risk for deteriorating functioning, self-destructive behavior, and high mortality rates. Anxiety is a second affective component worthy of attention, especially because it may propel patients into hasty decisions about their futures.

Social Functioning

Social functioning includes social contacts and relationships, social roles, resources, and activities.[9] These characteristics have an objective and a subjective component. The frequency and range of social contacts and activities can be enumerated; however, only the patient can indicate whether the observable social circumstances are perceived as satisfactory. A geriatric team is interested in the extent and nature of the available social support from the following two perspectives: (1) its potential for providing care and assistance to a patient, and (2) its potential for meeting a patient's needs for human affiliation (eg, companionship and the giving and receiving of confidences). The geriatric field also has developed summary measures of perceived social well-being that measures abstractions, such as morale, life satisfaction, or contentment.[10–12] Finally, a new and promising area of instrumentation is evolving to measure "person-environment fit." This requires that information about a person's functional abilities and value preferences be combined with objective information about a given social environment. The resultant score measures the desirability of the environment for that person.

Need for Care

The geriatric team increasingly is being asked to determine how much care is needed, of what type, and for how long. This requires not only assessment of a patient's functional capabilities, but also assessment of unmet needs, ie, needs not currently filled by the patient's family or through care that is being purchased for the patient. Some tools have been developed to help a care planner decide what is needed on the basis of observed functioning, the likelihood of ameliorating that functioning, and measured levels of help already available.

Of course, the formulas used to move from assessment to prescription of health care and services require assumptions that are based on value judgments. How much risk should people be permitted to take? How protective should care be? How great are our expectations that relatives will provide care? It is crucial that a physician examine and consider the assumptions embedded in the tools used to establish program eligibility in his or her state, locality, or organization.

Family Burden

Sometimes, the geriatric team recommends community services for a patient, not because a patient's needs are currently unmet, but because family members who are supplying the necessary care are being unreasonably, or even harmfully, burdened. To make such a judgment, one must consider the amount of help that the family members are giving, the family members' own health, the competing responsibilities of the family caregiver (eg, for minor children, for other functionally impaired adults, and for participation in the labor force), and the perception of burden or stress associated with giving care. Since the first edition of this volume was published, measurement of family burden has developed considerably.[13–15]

Providing care to a family member can have far-reaching effects on other family relationships, social activities, leisure time, mobility, career development, and income. But research suggests that burden also is a subjective phenomenon. Some family caregivers are stressed to the point that their own mental health is in jeopardy by situations that others take in stride. In these latter situations, not only can outside help be marshaled, but also the family caregiver may benefit by direct supportive mental health services. Scales to measure family burden, thus, tend to have both objective and subjective components.

Why Measurement?

Measurements are distinguished from nonstandardized clinical judgment by the specificity and uniformity that they bring to the assessment process. The implication of measurements is that standardized techniques will be used to gather and record information. Clinicians sometimes argue that such standardization dehumanizes and oversimplifies the complex phenomena being observed, hampers the artistry of the intuitive caregiver, and interferes with the physician-patient relationship.

This argument creates a spurious dichotomy between measurement and clinical assessment. The instruments used to measure functional status gauge the limitations of capability or performance, but they do not explain the etiology of the observed phenomena. A full medical history and physical examination, with its accompanying tests, are still needed to determine what is wrong. Clinical judgments often can become incorporated into measures. None of the assessment tools discussed in this chapter can be used to reach a diagnosis. Conversely, a diagnosis alone gives little information about the capacity for independence. Once a patient's condition is diagnosed as arthritis, diabetes, heart disease, or dementing illness, little has been explained about that patient's capabilities and prognosis for independent living.

Measurements are needed to evaluate the effects of treatment on functional status, or simply to monitor changes in the functional areas that are so important to the patient. Without systematically looking for changes in the psychologic and social functioning associated with medical treatment, a physician will find such changes only in a haphazard fashion. Also, without implementing a measurement strategy that is applied consistently, physicians are hampered in interpreting their observations. A precipitous change in any measurement may be more important than the measurement itself. For example, we may note two patients whose weekly social contact is limited to one face-to-face encounter and one daily telephone call. However, for one patient, this may represent a continuation of a stable pattern, whereas for the other patient, it may be an ominous change in a previously gregarious person.

Measurements are also needed to identify cases from a target population and to determine both their need and eligibility for publicly funded services. The eligibility is a quasi-legal matter, with equity demanding consistency in assessment approaches. Measurements also can be organizing tools for a geriatric team and even for the patients and their families. They provide a systematic way of considering all the circumstances and factors relevant to developing a plan to maximize a patient's independence. Optimal care plans flow from good assessment.

Measurements also serve a community function beyond planning and evaluating one's individual care. For want of a nail, the nursery rhyme tells us, the battle was eventually lost. Perhaps, for want of sensible and inexpensive services (eg, hearing aids or home modifications), patients experience undue functional impairments and ultimately end up receiving more disruptive and expensive services (eg, nursing home care or daily in-home service). However, we only can document such situations through an aggregation of cases that have been assessed in a uniform manner. Similarly, this systematic assessment forms the basis for program evaluation and for many quality assurance techniques that use patient-specific outcome measures.

Finally, systematic measurement has strategic significance for training in the health professions, for resocializing previously trained practitioners, and for demonstrating the importance of geriatric programs. Appropriate assessment tools that can demonstrate positive changes can combat the pervasive prejudice that geriatric care makes no difference. For instruments to have this power, they must be able to capture increments of improvement or deterioration at the lower end of the functional spectrum. Some measures perpetrated on an older patient are akin to measuring nail growth in yards—there is little likelihood that the nail's growth so measured will ever occur! Armed with suitable assessment tools, one also can teach paraprofessionals (eg, nurses' aides, or home health providers), family members, or even patients themselves to monitor important changes and to take appropriate actions to intervene or summon other assistance. Even when assessment tools have been designed for an older population, many still are insensitive to meaningful functional levels in frail elderly nursing home residents.

Types of Measures and Scores

Available measurements differ in their scope and detail. Some are designed as screening tools, whereas others are designed for thorough evaluations. Both screening tools and detailed instruments may be unidimensional (ie, measuring a single dimension of functioning) or multidimensional (ie, measuring more than one domain or aspect of functioning).

Instruments also differ in the extent to which they summarize information through one or more scores. Some instruments used in geriatric assessment are, in actuality, standardized recording formats. An early example is the Patient Appraisal and Care Evaluation methodology developed for multidisciplinary assessment and care planning for nursing home residents.[16–17] This technique involves applying decision rules to making a large number of observations, but no effort is made to summarize the information through scoring. Similarly, many of the tools used to measure social functioning are purely descriptive, with no effort to weigh the information to summarize the adequacy of that functioning.

Standardized recording formats are an important step to permit comparisons among patients and across settings. They also serve as checklists to remind caregivers of multiple dimensions of the patient's well-being. In late 1987, by congressional mandate, the Secretary of Health and Human Services appointed a commission to recommend a minimal data set to assess the needs of older people at discharge from hospitals. This work may incorporate some brief scales, but is expected to be largely an organized recording format.[18] Similarly, in 1988, the Health Care Financing Administration commissioned a study to develop a standardized assessment tool for nursing home care.[19] Both these efforts are designed to improve care through systematic assessment and to encourage comparable information that can be used by regulators and perhaps even by payers.

In contrast to recording formats, other multidimensional tools do provide scores. There are screening instruments, for example, that score cognitive functioning, complete with cutoff scores to suggest when a patient is an unreliable informant because of cognitive confusion.[20,21] There are multidimensional assessment tools that yield a single score, such as the Sickness Impact Profile,[22–24] or that yield a score for each domain, such as the Older Americans Resources and Services (OARS) instrument,[25–27] the Multilevel Assessment Instrument (MAI) developed at the Philadelphia Geriatric Center,[28] and the Comprehensive Assessment and Referral Evaluation (CARE) instrument developed at Columbia University, New York, NY.[29–31] Since the first edition of this book, substantial work has been done on the OARS instrument, the MAI, and the CARE instrument to create and test scales contained within the batteries and to develop shortened versions.

The development and interpretation of scores on assessment batteries involve several considerations.

Norms

Before drawing conclusions that certain patterns are pathologic, one needs information about their normal distribution. There is danger that we will focus on observed problems and functional impairments in the patients who are being assessed and then undertake protective interventions without realizing that the phenomenon is prevalent in the population at large. Similarly, without population-based norms, a program may be held responsible for poor outcomes that exist independently of that program (eg, a nursing home held responsible for depression when its prevalence mirrors that of the general population).

Thresholds

For the voluminous descriptive information to have clinical significance, one must define thresholds below which the observations connote a problem. The geriatrician should not be as interested in developing the perfect scale to capture the range of social behavior as in developing mechanisms for determining when a person has reached a level of social isolation, depression, or fragile social support that requires professional attention. An example of this is found in the efforts of Gurland and colleagues[32] to identify clinically significant thresholds for dementia in the community. Another example is the Index of Vulnerability developed by Morris and colleagues.[33]

Cultural Differences

Interpretations must take into account differences based on ethnicity or social class. The interpretations also must consider age-cohort characteristics, which may involve behavior patterns and preferences that differ from those of the care providers and the assessors.

Selecting an Instrument

Reliability and Validity

Reliability and validity, of course, are general considerations for choosing an instrument. Reliability—the property of producing the same result in repeated applications in the absence of real change—is poorly established for many instruments now in use. Interrater reliability most often is established through asking several interviewers to complete the form on the basis of a standardized stimulus, such as a videotaped interview. When multiple interviewers gather information independently, it is much more likely that interviewer styles and sensitivities or extraneous circumstances or a particular interview introduce unreliable results. (However, this mirrors the way information is collected in the real world and, thus, produces a more appropriate test than the simulated interview or group interview, although the latter is useful for training new interviewers to a standard of reliability.) Professional

ratings have a better chance of being reliable, but even so they are not necessarily valid. For example, consider when floor nurses rate the ADL capacity of their patients based on widely shared beliefs but without empiric verification.

Validity—the property of measuring what one intends to measure—is difficult to achieve confidently when given the abstractions that we examine in geriatrics. There is an ever-present danger that scales purporting to measure complex qualities (eg, cognitive ability, social support, family burden, or morale) become too trusted. Sometimes, we act as though the measurement were a concrete manifestation of the property measured (like height and weight) instead of an approximation of an elusive concept. Because action based on such measures can set in motion a self-fulfilling prophecy, it is important that the geriatrician examine the items in the scales used and understand the arguments made for their validity.

Information Source

Information may be gathered from the patient, a family member, or a professional caregiver. The choice of informant can influence the results rather markedly.[34] In general, there is too much reluctance to get information directly from an elderly patient and too great a propensity to trust family members as a source of information. Of course, some patients will be unreliable informants by dint of cognitive or communicative incapacity, and someone else will need to supply information as their proxy. In such cases, it is better to leave information on subjective matters, such as satisfaction and mood, blank than to presume to guess what the patient thinks.

Type of Information

Related to the choice of informant is the decision about the type of information that will be used. Functioning may be rated based on general knowledge of a patient, based on specific observations, or based on demonstrations of abilities. Finally, patients may report and rate their own performance.

Capacity vs Performance

Functional abilities may be measured according to the capacity to perform a function or according to the actual behavior in performing that function. For example, we can measure the extent to which patients *can* bathe themselves or the extent to which they *do* bathe themselves. Capability can be assessed through self-report (eg, "can you walk 10 ft?" or "in the last few weeks, have you walked at least 10 ft?"), through observer reports (eg, "in the past few weeks, has the patient walked 10 ft or more?"), or through demonstration (eg, "show me how you would walk 10 feet."). The first method is subject to distortions due to an exaggeration or underestimation of abilities; the second is limited by the observer's ability to know; and the third method can be cumbersome. However, it is possible to apply assessment techniques by using demonstrations for a wide variety of functions, such as making change, using the telephone, dressing, taking medicine, reading, or writing. The Performance ADL Test[35] is a good example of a measure that requires patients to demonstrate their abilities. This approach was adapted and used successfully in a large-scale study in nursing homes,[36] where too often patient limitations are assumed rather than tested.

Sometimes, it is appropriate to assess actual performance rather than the capacity to perform. For example, a physician may seek a patient-specific assessment to determine whether the quality of life is adequate in a particular long-term care facility. In that case, it is much more important to know whether the patient does go out than whether he or she can go out, or whether he or she does bathe by himself or herself than whether he or she can do so. If the question were posed in terms of capacity, real restrictions in independence might slip by unnoticed.

Time Frames

Available instruments vary in the time frames established for measurement. They may probe a patient's behavior or feelings right now, during a recent short period (eg, 1 day, 1 week, or 1 month), during a longer period (eg, 1 year), or even during an entire lifetime (eg, "have you *ever* felt short of breath?"). The more recent the time period in question, the more likely that accurate information can be recalled. However, if the object is to assess a particular patient rather than describe a whole population, a short time frame is inappropriate to tap relatively rare but important social events. For example, "in the last week" would be an injudicious time period on which to base an understanding of a patient's contact with out-of-town relatives.

Place and Time of Measurement

Too often, elderly persons are at a disadvantage when they are assessed. In an acute care hospital, for example, they experience the unfamiliarity and dependency-engendering nature of the surroundings. Furthermore, they still may be recovering from an acute episode. Inevitably, some assessment must occur in an acute care hospital, but the assessor should

regard that information as a likely understatement of a patient's capabilities. When in doubt, it may be worthwhile to send a patient home and assess what occurs under those circumstances, even if a patient falls into the large group of hospital dischargees who technically are eligible for nursing home care because of their functional impairments.

Amount of Detail

Assessment tools vary considerably in the amount of detail that they offer. For example, let us consider the measurement of ADLs. The most commonly included items are bathing, dressing, getting to the toilet, transferring, and feeding. A parsimonious way of measuring these items is used in the Activities of Daily Living (ADL) described by Katz et al,[37] where each function is dichotomously rated as either independent or dependent (Table 6.1). A three-point version of Katz and colleagues'[37] scale has been developed and used in a number of demonstration projects.[38] Other ADL scales introduce wider response choices that differentiate between complete independence, independence with equipment, dependence on help from others, or complete dependence, yielding four-point or greater scales. Detail is also increased by the number of items and the subdivision of tasks. For example, the Self-Care Rating Scales described by Mahoney and Barthel[39] have expanded the response categories and also increased the items. Accordingly, eating is divided into drinking from a cup or eating from a plate. (See Table 6.2 for a portion of Barthel Self-Care Rating Scales.) In another modification of ADL measurement, originally designed for an arthritis program, separate ratings are made of the speed of performance and the pain or discomfort that accompany the performance.[40] In rehabilitation settings, extremely detailed approaches to ADL measurement that divide each task into numerous subcomponents are available.[41–44]

Purpose of Measurement

The purpose of the measurement should influence the choice of the assessment tool and the general assessment strategy.

Screening

If the instrument is to be used for screening and case finding, then brevity is important. The items included on a brief instrument should be selected to achieve the desired sensitivity and specificity. To screen for depression in a recently bereaved person, one seeks a tool that specifically picks up severe depression. Ask-

Table 6.1. Katz index of ADL*

Index of Independence in Activities of Daily Living

The Index of Independence in Activities of Daily Living is based on an evaluation of the functional independence or dependence of patients in bathing, dressing, going to the toilet, transferring, continence, and feeding. Specific definitions of functional independence appear below the index.

A   Independent in feeding, continence, transferring, going to the toilet, dressing, and bathing.
B   Independent in all but one of these functions.
C   Independent in all but bathing and one additional function.
D   Independent in all but bathing, dressing, and one additional function.
E   Independent in all but bathing, dressing, going to toilet, and one additional function.
F   Independent in all but bathing, dressing, going to toilet, transferring, and one additional function.
G   Dependent in all six functions.
Other   Dependent in at least two functions, but not classifiable as C, D, E, or F.

Independence means without supervision, direction, or active personal assistance, except as specifically noted below. This is based on actual status and not on ability. A patient who refuses to perform a function is considered as not performing the function, even though he or she is deemed able.

BATHING (Sponge, shower or tub)
Independent: assistance only in bathing a single part (as back or disabled extremity) or bathes self completely
Dependent: assistance in bathing more than one part of body; assistance in getting in or out of tub or does not bathe self

DRESSING
Independent: gets clothes from closets and drawers; puts on clothes, outer garments, braces; manages fasteners; act of tying shoes is excluded
Dependent: does not dress self or remains partly undressed

GOING TO TOILET
Independent: gets to toilet, gets on and off toilet; arranges clothes, cleans organs of excretion (may manage own bedpan used at night only and may or may not be using mechanical supports)
Dependent: uses bedpan or commode or receives assistance in getting to and using toilet

TRANSFER
Independent: moves in and out of bed independently and moves in and out of chair independently (may or may not be using mechanical supports)
Dependent: assistance in moving in or out of bed and/or chair; does not perform one or more transfers

CONTINENCE
Independent: urination and defecation entirely self-controlled
Dependent: partial or total incontinence in urination or defecation partial or total control by enemas, catheters, or regulated use of urinals and/or bedpans

FEEDING
Independent: gets food from plate or its equivalent into mouth (precutting of meat and preparation of food, as buttering bread, are excluded from evaluation)
Dependent: assistance in act of feeding (see above); does not eat at all or parenteral feeding

Evaluation Form

Name _____ Date of Evaluation _____

For each area of functioning listed below, check description that applies. (The word "assistance" means supervision, direction, or personal assistance.)

BATHING—either sponge bath, tub bath, or shower

☐
Receives no assistance (gets in and out of tub by self if tub is usual means of bathing)

☐
Receives assistance in bathing only one part of body (such as back or a leg)

☐
Receives assistance in bathing more than one part of body (or not bathed)

DRESSING—gets clothes from closets and drawers—including underclothes, outer garments, and using fasteners (including braces, if worn)

☐
Gets clothes and gets completely dressed without assistance

☐
Gets clothes and gets dressed without assistance except for assistance in tying shoes

☐
Receives assistance in getting clothes or in getting dressed, or stays partly or completely undressed

TOILETING—going to the "toilet room" for bowel and urine elimination; cleaning self after elimination and arranging clothes

☐
Goes to "toilet room," cleans self, and arranges clothes without assistance (may use object for support such as cane, walker, or wheelchair and may manage night bedpan or commode, emptying same in morning)

☐
Receives assistance in going to "toilet room" or in cleansing self or in arranging clothes after elimination or in use of night bedpan or commode

☐
Does not go to room termed "toilet" for the elimination process

(Continued)

Table 6.1. Continued

TRANSFER		
☐	☐	☐
Moves in and out of bed as well as in and out of chair without assistance (may be using object for support such as cane or walker)	Moves in or out of bed or chair with assistance	Does not get out of bed
CONTINENCE		
☐	☐	☐
Controls urination and bowel movement completely by self	Has occasional "accidents"	Supervision helps keep urine or bowel control; catheter is used or is incontinent
FEEDING		
☐	☐	☐
Feeds self without assistance	Feeds self except for getting assistance in cutting meat or buttering bread	Receives assistance in feeding or is fed partly or completely by using tubes or intravenous fluids

* Katz S, Ford AB, Moskowitz RW, et al: Studies of illness in the aged. The index of ADL: A standardized measure of biological and psychosocial function. *JAMA* 185:914–919. 1963. Copyright 1963 American Medical Association.

Table 6.2. Examples of items from Barthel Self-Care Rating Scales.

	Score	Items
		Transfer/chair
0	Intact	Able to approach, sit down, or get up from a regular chair safely; if in wheelchair, able to approach a bed or another chair, lock brakes, lift foot rest, and safely perform either a standing pivot or sliding transfer; able to return safely, changing the position of the wheelchair if necessary; able to remove and replace arm rest if necessary.
1	Limited	As above but requires adaptive or assisting devices such as a sliding board or a lift, or takes more than a reasonable time, but does not require assistance.
2	Helper	Minimal assistance or lifting is required.
		Dress upper body
0	Intact	Able to dress and undress upper body, including obtaining clothes from their customary places such as drawers and closets; able to handle bra, slip, pullover garment and front-opening garment, as well as manage zippers, button, and snaps.
1	Limited	Requires prior retrieval or arrangement of clothes, or able to dress presentably in spite of omission of some of above or through use of special closures, or takes more than a reasonable time.
2	Helper	Patient performs at least one-half the effort him- or herself.
		Bladder continence
0	Intact	Complete voluntary and elective control of bladder (never incontinent).
1	Limited	Has catheter, urinary-collecting device or urinary diversion; able to clean, sterilize, and set up the equipment for irrigation without assistance; able to assemble and apply condom drainage or an ileal appliance without assistance; able to empty, put on, remove and clean leg bag or empty and clean ileal appliance bag; no accidents. May have bladder urgency.
2	Helper	Needs assistance with external device, or has occasional accidents, or cannot wait to get bedpan or to the toilet in time.
3	Null	Incontinent despite aids or assistance.
		Bowel continence
0	Intact	Complete voluntary and elective control of the bowels (never incontinent).
1	Limited	Regularly requires stool softeners, digital stimulation, suppository, laxative, or enema, but does not require assistance; has colostomy but does not require assistance; no accidents. May have bowel urgency.
2	Helper	Needs assistance using suppository or taking an enema or has occasional accidents.
3	Null	Incontinent despite aids or assistance

Source: Sherwood SJ, Morris J, Mor V, et al: *Compendium of Measures for Describing and Assessing Long Term Care Populations.* Boston, Hebrew Rehabilitation Center for Aged, 1977, mimeographed.

ing "how often have you thought of killing yourself?" is more useful than asking "how often do you feel sad and blue?" The latter question would pick up so many false positives that another layer of screening would be needed to identify those persons at greatest risk. When a condition frequently occurs in the population and ranges in its severity, the specific approach seems to be indicated even if some real cases are missed. In contrast, when screening for a relatively rare condition and/or one with life-threatening implications (eg, elder abuse), a more sensitive screening tool is desirable, The false positives can later be eliminated without enormous expense.

We may appropriately question whether the tools that are currently being used to screen for dementia[20,21,45] are too sensitive, especially given the frequency of at least some memory loss, the heavy use of prescription drugs, and the lack of social milestones (particularly for those in institutions) to prompt one's memory for date and place. They may be useful when used routinely to alert a clinician to memory loss and to set in motion a process of ruling out alternative causes. Such screening tools should never form the basis for a diagnosis of dementia (Chapter 5).

Sometimes, screening measures are combined with longer assessment tools so that those who fall out of an initial screening receive a more in-depth assessment. However, such strategies reduce a major advantage of screening, ie, doing a preliminary sorting inexpensively. For the convenience of both patients and professionals, screening tools should be refined so that they can be administered by telephone or by receptionists. There is also considerable untapped potential for self-report screening tools that can be used by patients and their families before encounters with a physician.

Comprehensive Assessment

Comprehensive assessment tools need to be conducive to the needs, pace, and constraints of clinical encounters. They should contain branching questions, so that patients need not be offended, inconvenienced, or made anxious by questions that are either too easy or too difficult. They should be keyed to thresholds with clinical significance. They should be capable of measuring functioning in increments that reflect improvements or deteriorations that are meaningful to the patient. The comprehensive assessment tool should provide the basis for care decisions and, thus, should provide information about capacity, as well as performance; it also should provide for notation of information relevant to the etiology of a functional limitation. Assessments should be easily incorporated into office routines. Here, a physician might consider

assigning a nurse or a social worker to administer comprehensive assessments. The least rigorous approach is one in which the physician rates the patient's functioning in a variety of areas. Good reliability has been reported for the Rapid Disability Rating Scale[46]; yet, the typical primary care physician would be unlikely to have the information necessary to make accurate global judgments on the dimensions included.

Monitoring

One monitors for the following two general reasons: (1) to observe any change in problems that have been noted and, perhaps, treated, and (2) to rescreen in areas where no problems were found. The frequency and detail of the monitoring should depend on the type of problem, the type of regimen introduced, and the expected frequency of change. Although medical providers generally appreciate the importance of developing a monitoring strategy for the use of potent drugs, they are less conscious of the need to monitor the effects of socially oriented decisions (eg, nursing home placements or decisions to send a patient home under the care of a frail relative). The effects of such interventions can be monitored with the help of specially designed tools. It also is feasible to involve paraprofessional personnel, relatives, and patients themselves in this monitoring.

Role of Value Judgments

Assessment instruments have a veneer of science. One easily forgets that they embody value judgments at every step. Values are reflected in the choice of items to be measured and the way results are scored (ie, the way items are weighted in an overall score). Most of all, value judgments are reflected in the decision rules by which the information generated by the assessment is translated into an action plan.

Half Empty or Half Full?

No matter how detailed an assessment, eventually a judgment is required about what the information means. Does a describable set of social conditions add up to an adequate or inadequate environment for self-care? Does a 5 on a scale of 1 through 10 in physical functioning mean that a patient can or cannot live alone? Such questions are interpreted according to the optimism or pessimism of the beholder.

A physician may not be fully aware of the implications of a recommendation that a patient receive substantial amounts of assistance. Such a prescription can set in motion a chain of events whereby care at the intervals and intensity suggested is deemed too expensive to deliver in the community. Thus, a benevolently protective interpretation of assessment data may lead to iatrogenic dependency and social disruption. This is particularly true if a concerned and risk-averse family is acting on a physician's advice. The interpretations are further tempered by philosophic beliefs about whether it is better to err by offering too much or too little care.

The very act of assessment entails taking inventory of a person's limitations, which then may add up to a heavy weight of problems. A more optimistic stance requires considerations of the strengths that a person brings to the situation. Sometimes, the instrument itself seeks out evidence of strength; an example is the inclusion of "positive cognition" in the criteria for identifying dementia.

Setting Goals

Assessment should lead to care plans that will improve or help maintain functional status. However, this chapter has argued for a far-ranging assessment of physical, emotional, cognitive, and social domains of functioning; each of these categories can be further divided into numerous dimensions. For clinicians to establish goals for care, they must determine which outcomes are to be maximized. Value preferences are at the heart of that determination. If activity comes at the expense of physical comfort, if mental alertness comes at the expense of pain, and if social participation comes at the expense of considerable risk to safety, what goals should a health care team adopt? Should the preferences of the patient be consulted? Those of the family? Should professional caregivers themselves be consulted? Or, perhaps, should the preferences of the party that pays the bill be consulted? These decisions require thoughtful attention. An assessment will not, in itself, provide the answer, but it will provide the basis for predicting a variety of likely outcomes of various care strategies.

References

1. Consensus Development Panel, Solomon D, chairman: National Institutes of Health Consensus Development Conference Statement. Geriatric assessment methods for clinical decision-making. *J Am Geriatr Soc* 1988;36:342–347.
2. Solomon D. Geriatric assessment: methods for clinical decision making. *JAMA* 1988;259:2450–2452.
3. Kane RA, Kane RL. *Assessing the Elderly: A Practical Guide to Measurement.* Lexington, Mass: DC Heath & Co; 1981.
4. Israel L, Kozerevic D, Sartorius N. *Source Book of Geriatric Assessment.* New York, NY: S Karger AG; 1984.
5. Rosencranz HA, Philbad CT. Measuring the health of the elderly. *J Gerontol* 1970;25:129–133.
6. Branch L, Meyers AR. Assessing physical function in the elderly. *Clin Geriatr Med* 1987;3:29–51.
7. Gurland BJ, Cote LJ, Cross PS, et al. The assessment of cognitive function in the elderly. *Clin Geriatr Med* 1987;3:53–63.
8. Gallagher D. Assessing affect in the elderly. *Clin Geriatr Med* 1987;3:65–85.
9. Kane RA. Assessing social function in the elderly. *Clin Geriatr Med* 1987;3:87–98.
10. Lawton MP. The Philadelphia Geriatric Morale Scale: a revision. *J Gerontol* 1975;30:85–89.
11. Havighurst R, Neugarten B, Tobin S. The measure of life satisfaction. *J Gerontol* 1961;16:134–143.
12. Bloom M, Blenker M. Assessing functioning of older persons living in the community. *The Gerontologist* 1970;10:331–337.
13. Zarit SH, Reever KE, Bach-Peterson JM. Relatives of the impaired elderly: correlates of feelings of burden. *The Gerontologist* 1980;20:649–655.
14. Robinson B. Validation of a caregiver strain index. *J Gerontol* 1983;38:344–348.
15. Montgomery RJ, Stull DE, Borgatta EF. Measurement and the analysis of burden. *Res Aging* 1985;7:137–152.
16. US Dept of Health, Education, and Welfare. *Working Document on Patient Care Management.* Washington, DC: Government Printing Office; 1978.
17. US Dept of Health, Education, and Welfare. *Long-term Care Minimum Data Set: Preliminary Report of the Technical Consultant Panel on Long-term Care Data Set.* Washington, DC: US National Committee on Vital and Health Statistics, 1978.
18. *Omnibus Budget Reconciliation Act,* §9305, 1986.
19. Health Care Financing Administration. *Development of a Resident Assessment System and Data Base for Nursing Home Care.* RFP-HCFA-88-039/EE, 1988 mimeo.
20. Pfeiffer E. A short portable mental status questionnaire for the assessment of organic brain deficiencies in elderly patients. *J Am Geriatr Soc* 1975;23:433–441.
21. Kahn RL, Goldfarb AI, Pollack M, et al. Brief objective measures for the determination of mental status in the aged. *Am J Psychiatry* 1960;117:326–328.
22. Bergner M, Bobbitt RA, Kressel S, et al. The Sickness Impack Profile: conceptual formulation and methodology for the development of a health status measure. *Int J Health Serv* 1976;6:393–415.
23. Bergner M, Bobbitt RA, Pollard WE, et al. Sickness Impact Profile: validation of a health status measure. *Med Care* 1976;14:57–67.
24. Gilson BS, Gilson JS, Bergner M, et al. The Sickness Impact Profile: development of an outcome measure of health care. *Am J Public Health* 1975;65:1304–1310.
25. Duke University Center for the Study of Aging and Human Development. *Multidimensional Functional Assessment: The OARS Methodology.* Durham, NC: Duke University Press; 1978.
26. George LK, Fillenbaum GG. OARS methodology: a

decade of experience in geriatric assessment. *J Am Geriatr Soc* 1985;33:607–615.

27. Fillenbaum GG. Screening the elderly: a brief instrumental activities of daily living measure. *J Am Geriatri Soc* 1985;33:698–706.

28. Lawton MP. A research and service-oriented Multilevel Assessment Instrument. *J Gerontol* 1982;37:91–99.

29. Gurland BJ, Wilder DE. The CARE interview revisited: development of an efficient, systematic clinical assessment. *J Gerontol* 1984;39:129–137.

30. Golden RR, Teresi JA, Gurland BJ. Development of indicator scales for the comprehensive assessment and referral evaluation (CARE) interview schedule. *J Gerontol* 1984;39:138–146.

31. Gurland BJ, Golden RR, Teresi JA, et al. The SHORT-CARE: an efficient instrument for the assessment of depression, dementia, and disability. *J Gerontol* 1984;39:166–169.

32. Gurland BJ, Dean LL, Copeland J, et al. Criteria for the diagnosis of dementia in the community elderly. *The Gerontologist* 1982;22:180–186.

33. Morris JN, Sherwood S, Mor V. An assessment tool for use in identifying functionally vulnerable persons in the community. *The Gerontologist* 1984;24:373–379.

34. Rubenstein LZ, Schairer C, Wieland GD, et al. Systematic biases in functional assessment of the elderly adults: effects of different data sources. *J Gerontol* 1984;39:686–691.

35. Kuriansky JB, Gurland BJ. Performance test of activities of daily living. *Int J Aging Hum Dev.* 1976;7:343–352.

36. Kane RL, Bell R, Riegler S, et al. Assessing the outcomes of nursing-home patients. *J Gerontol* 1983;38:385–393.

37. Katz S, Ford AB, Moskowitz RW, et al. Studies of illness in the aged: the Index of ADL: a standard measure of biologic and psychosocial function. *JAMA* 1963;185:914–919.

38. Mathematica Research Incorporated and Temple University. *National Long-term Care Demonstration: Clinical Baseline Assessment Instrument: Community Version, June 22, 1983, and Institutional Version, July 8, 1983.* 1983. US Dept of Health and Human Services contract HHS 100-80-0157. Princeton, NJ: Mathematica.

39. Mahoney FI, Barthel DW. Functional evaluation: the Barthel Index. *Maryland State Med J.* 1965;14:61–65.

40. Jette AM, Denniston OL. Inter-observer reliability of a functional status instrument. *J Chronic Dis* 1978;31:537–580.

41. Schoening HA, Iversen IA. Numerical sorting of self-care status: a study of the Kenny Self-Care Evaluation. *Arch Phys Med Rehab* 1968;49:221–229.

42. MacKenzie R, Charlson ME, DiGioia D, et al. A patient-specific measure of change in maximal function. *Arch Intern Med* 1986;146:1325–1329.

43. Carey RG, Seibert MA, Posavic EJ. Who makes the most progress in inpatient rehabilitation? *Arch Phys Med Rehabil* 1988;69:337–343.

44. Carey RG, Posavic EJ. Rehabilitation program evaluation using the revised Level of Rehabilitation Scale (LORS-II). *Arch Phys Med Rehabil* 1986;67:367–370.

45. Folstein MF, Folstein SE, McHugh PR. Mini-Mental State: a practical method for grading the cognitive state of patients for the clinician. *J Psychiatr Res.* 1975;12:189–198.

46. Linn MW, Linn BS. The Rapid Disability Rating Scale-2. *J Am Geriatr Soc* 1982;30:378–382.

7

Principles of Pharmacology

Jerry Avorn and Jerry Gurwitz

The proper use of medications represents one of the most important ways in which the practice of geriatric medicine differs importantly from conventional medical care. Pharmacotherapy is perhaps the single most important medical intervention in the care of elderly patients, and its proper performance requires a special understanding of the unique physiologic properties of drugs in this group, as well as a grasp of the sociocultural and epidemiologic aspects of medication use in aging. The advent of Medicare coverage of some prescription medications taken by elderly persons has focused attention on the special problems and opportunities offered by pharmacotherapy in geriatrics at a time of growing public awareness of the benefits, risks, and costs of prescription drugs. Thus, physicians have both an opportunity and a responsibility to examine this topic in all its aspects, from those as "micro" as receptor physiology and the molecular biology of aging, to those as "macro" as the study of adverse drug effects in large populations and the questions raised by governmental coverage of medication costs.

Pharmacodynamics

At its most basic level, a pharmacologic effect, whether therapeutic or toxic, occurs with the action between a drug and a receptor on (or in) a specific target cell. While the study of receptor physiology is much more recent than the older, more traditional aspects of pharmacology (see below), important progress has been made in recent years in understanding the nature of drug-receptor interactions and the effect of the aging process on this interplay. For reasons that are not well understood, the aging process appears to be associated with an increase in the sensitivity of the receptors for many commonly used medications. The study of this phenomenon is complicated by the fact that for many drugs, pharmacologic effect is magnified in elderly persons because of reduced clearance of the drug (see below), resulting in higher serum levels. Therefore, in studying the effects of aging on receptor sensitivity, one must control for the concentration of drug made available to the receptor. This has been accomplished in a small but growing number of ingeniously conducted studies that are helping to clarify the unique contribution of receptor sensitivity to the overall picture of drug response in aging.

One of the first studies describing changes in receptor sensitivity with age involved patients between the ages of 30 and 90 years undergoing elective cardioversion.[1] The clinical end point used was the patient's inability to respond to vocal stimuli, with preservation of response to a painful stimulus. It was found that the serum level of diazepam at which this effect occurred was significantly lower in elderly patients than in younger ones. Analogous findings emerged from a study of the performance of patients given a single dose of another benzodiazepine, nitrazepam.[2] Serum levels of the drug were similar in both young and old patients, but elderly patients showed a deterioration in their performance on psychomotor testing after administration of a single dose of the drug, while comparable deterioration was not seen in younger patients. Similar results have come from a study of the efficacy of metoclopramide in reducing the vomiting caused by cancer chemotherapy.[3] Although patients over age 65 years had serum levels that were virtually identical to those of younger patients, the older patients experienced greater symptomatic relief, as reflected in a significant reduction in episodes of emesis.

Thus, the apparent increase in receptor sensitivity in older patients can result in greater therapeutic effect as well as an increased potential for toxicity. Such enhanced receptor sensitivity probably underlies the common clinical observation that elderly patients may experience toxic effects from medications such as digoxin or aminophylline even when their serum drug levels are within the so-called "normal" therapeutic range. Increases in medication sensitivity with age have also been suggested for a number of other medications, including warfarin[4,5] and the opiates[6–8] (Figs 7.1, 7.2).

By contrast, β-adrenergic receptors seem to behave in precisely the opposite way: they appear to become

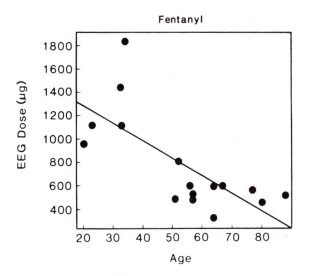

Fentanyl

Fig. 7.2. The relationship between age and response to the opiate fetanyl. The "EEG dose" represents the amount of drug required to produce a threshold cerebral effect, as indicated by electroencephalographic changes ($r = -.72$; $p < .01$). No age-related changes in the *pharmacokinetics* of fentanyl were found. Reprinted from JC Scott & DR Stanski. Decreased fentanyl and alfentanil dose requirements with age. A simultaneous pharmacokinetic and pharmacodynamic evaluation. Journal of Pharmacology and Experimental Therapeutics. 1977;240:159–66, © by American Society for Pharmacology and Experimental Therapeutics.

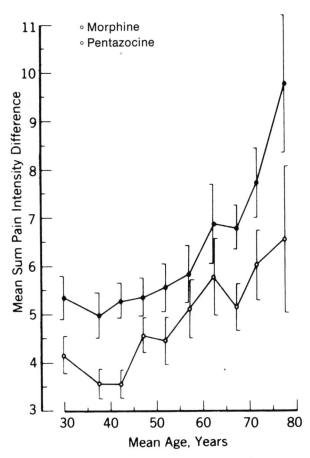

Fig. 7.1. The relationship between age and analgesic efficacy of two drugs. All patients received 10 mg of morphine sulfate or 20 mg of pentazocine for acute postoperative pain; older patients reported more pain relief with an equivalent dose. Reprinted from Bellville et al. JAMA 1971;217:1835–41, Copyright 1971. American Medical Association.

less sensitive with the advancing age. This phenomenon has clinical ramifications for β-adrenergic agonists, such as isoproterenol, as well as antagonists, such as the β-blockers. In studies that used as their end point an increase in resting heart rate of 25 beats per minute, elderly subjects were shown to require higher doses of isoproterenol to accelerate heart rate, as well as higher doses of propranolol to reduce heart rate to a similar degree.[9] Interestingly, a similar decrease in sensitivity to β-blockers has been observed in epidemiologic studies of β-blocker–induced depression, in which younger patients appeared to be much more sensitive to this side effect than those over age 65 years.[10]

Controversy remains as to the mechanism underlying changes in receptor sensitivity; it is unclear whether the predominant cause is a change in the affinity of receptors for drug, the number of receptors, or postreceptor events within the cell. Nonetheless, the changes in receptor sensitivity that have been observed (primarily increases, with the notable exception of the β-adrenergic system) must be considered in making therapeutic decisions for the aging patient, as these effects will interact importantly with the better-understood pharmacokinetic changes described below.

Changes in Drug Distribution

Of the four traditional components of pharmacokinetics—absorption, distribution, metabolism, and excretion—only the last three are meaningfully affected by age. In the absence of malabsorptive syndromes, most medications are absorbed as well in old age as in youth. Of course, the same concerns apply in elderly patients as in those of any age concerning the possible adsorption of medications by antacids and the relation between the ingestion of meals and the taking of medications. However, the well-reported changes in gastric motility and blood flow to the gut do not appear to alter meaningfully the efficiency with which medications move from the alimentary tract into the circulation.[11]

Another aspect of drug distribution that is not affected by normal aging is the binding of drugs to carrier proteins, such as serum albumin. In large populations, clinically meaningful decreases in serum albumin have not been found, although there is a very modest (albeit statistically significant) downward drift with advancing age.[12] Previous studies that purported to show an age-related decline in serum albumin levels were probably marred by the problem of confounding illness with aging. Nonetheless, they served to bring attention to the fact that serum albumin levels may be markedly decreased in older patients suffering from malnutrition or advanced disease.[13]

One of the more important risks of diminished binding proteins is an iatrogenic one, resulting from misinterpretation of serum drug levels. Most assays measure the total amount of drug that is present in serum, bound and unbound combined. For a patient with hypoalbuminemia or another deficiency in binding protein, any given serum drug "level" will reflect a much higher proportion of unbound drug than the same level would signify in a patient with a normal binding capacity. Because it is the unbound component of the drug level (the "free fraction") that accounts for drug effects, a hypoalbuminemic patient with a normal-appearing total serum drug level actually may have a free fraction concentration that is unacceptably high. For extensively protein-bound drugs whose binding is reduced due to hypoproteinemia, clinicians should expect both therapeutic and toxic events at lower total serum concentrations.[14]

One aspect of drug distribution that does vary importantly with age is the volume of distribution. This is the theoretical space in a given patient that is available for a particular drug to occupy. The volume of distribution is importantly affected by the relative contribution of lean body mass versus fat. Lipid-soluble drugs will have a greater volume of distribution in a patient with increased body fat, and water-soluble drugs will have a greater volume of distribution in patients with proportionately greater muscle mass and less fat. The aging process has been associated with an increase in fat at the expense of muscle.[15] Thus, drugs that are highly lipid soluble (such as the benzodiazepines and some β-blockers) will have a greater volume of distribution in older than in younger patients. Conversely, drugs that are predominantly distributed in lean body mass (eg, lithium) will have a smaller volume of distribution in older than in younger patients (Fig 7.3). Combined with changes in clearance, discussed below, these alterations in body composition will have important implications for both the half-life and the steady-state concentration of many medications, as presented in the following section.

Drug Clearance and Aging

The liver represents the major site of metabolism for many medications. Hepatic biotransformations of drugs are categorized into phase I (preparative) and phase II (synthetic) reactions. Phase I reactions include oxidations (hydroxylation, N-dealkylation, and sulfoxidation), reductions, and hydrolyses. Phase II reactions involve conjugations of the drug molecule to glucuronides, sulfates, or acetates.

Studies employing animal models have suggested reduced activity of liver microsomal drug-metabolizing enzymes and alterations in liver microsomal enzyme induction with normal aging. However, data on hepatic drug metabolism in aging human subjects are much more limited. Therefore, the evidence for altered hepatic metabolism in humans largely is indirect and frequently has been inconsistent. The consensus at present is that phase I oxidative metabolism may be impaired with advancing age but that aging has little impact on phase II metabolic pathways.[11]

Other factors may be expected to reduce hepatic metabolism in elderly persons. Autopsy studies have demonstrated a progressive decrease in liver mass after the age of 50 years. Regional blood flow to the liver at age 65 years is reduced by 40% to 45% relative to that of an individual at age 25 years, although this observation may partially reflect a fall in cardiac output with advancing age. Such changes may result in reduced clearance rates for drugs exhibiting flow-dependent clearance characteristics ("first pass effects"), although results of studies concerning two such drugs in this regard, propranolol and lidocaine, have been ambiguous.[16]

Antipyrine frequently is used as a marker compound to evaluate hepatic drug metabolizing capacity. Although many studies have reported reduced metabolic

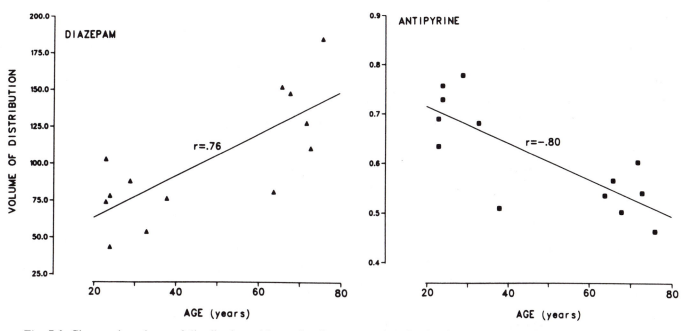

Fig. 7.3. Changes in volume of distribution with age for diazepam and antipyrine in healthy male volunteers. Because of an age-related increase in body fat, lipid-soluble drugs such as diazepam are more extensively distributed in elderly patients. By contrast, the volume of distribution of water-soluble agents such as antipyrine decreases with advancing age. Reprinted with permission from *The New England Journal of Medicine,* 306: 1084, 1982.

clearance of antipyrine in older subjects, as with many age-related differences, interindividual variation exceeded the variance in clearance related to advancing age.[17] This important finding suggests that genetic, environmental, and other patient-specific factors may have a far greater impact on liver drug metabolism than the aging process itself. Pharmacotherapeutic concerns about drug metabolism in elderly patients therefore should be based on individual patient characteristics as well as physiologic changes due to aging.

Renal Excretion

Early cross-sectional studies of renal function in aging suggested that there is a linear decrease in renal function between young adulthood and old age, amounting on average to a reduction in glomerular filtration rate by nearly a third.[18] While this is true in the aggregate, more recent longitudinal studies show that a third of subjects studied showed constant creatinine clearance with advancing age. One subgroup did show a linear decrease with age, while still others actually showed improvement in renal function as they got older.[19] Thus, although the aggregate findings have been enshrined in conventional gerontologic wisdom and in nomograms used to calculate drug dosing with

age, the key facts emerging from these more recent longitudinal studies are that the effect of age on renal function (and therefore on the excretion of many drugs) is quite variable and that differences among patients often will be more impressive than the changes attributed to the aging process itself. Thus, little comfort can be taken in formulas or general principles, and the clinician must maintain a high index of suspicion concerning the possibility of excessive or inadequate dosing of drugs excreted by the kidneys in older patients (see also Chapter 24).

Similarly, little comfort can be taken from standard laboratory tests of renal function. While blood urea nitrogen (BUN) and serum creatinine levels are useful markers of glomerular filtration rate, it must be remembered that each is susceptible in its own way to perturbations that may be seen in aging but have nothing to do with renal function directly. For example, the BUN reflects the concentration of urea in the blood. However, the origin of much of this urea is ingested protein, so that a malnourished older patient may not consume enough nitrogen to produce a rise in BUN, even in the face of renal impairment. Similarly, serum creatinine is produced by muscle, and if a patient has a markedly diminished muscle mass, whether because of chronic illness or any other cause, he or she may not produce enough creatinine to reflect a change in the ability of the kidney to excrete this substance.

Half-life and Steady-State Concentration

Drug Elimination Half-life

The elimination half-life of a medication ($t\frac{1}{2}$) is determined by the volume of distribution (Vd) for that medication in a given individual, divided by its clearance (Cl) in that subject, generally through metabolism in the liver and/or renal excretion. This can be expressed as an equation:

$$t\tfrac{1}{2} \approx \text{Vd/Cl}.$$

From this equation, it can be seen that the half-life of a medication will increase as the clearance (Cl) decreases if the volume of distribution (Vd) remains constant. If the volume of distribution also increases (as with a lipophilic drug), the half-life will be prolonged further.

The clinical implications of these pharmacokinetic relationships are illustrated by the benzodiazepine hypnotic flurazepam. In a study comparing the kinetics of flurazepam in young and elderly subjects, the drug was found to have an elimination half-life of 160 hours in elderly men, as compared with 74 hours in young men.[20] This difference probably is accounted for by an age-related reduction in the clearance of

flurazepam by the oxidative pathways in the liver and an increase in the volume of distribution for this highly lipid-soluble drug, associated with the changes in body composition that occur with advancing age. These findings concerning the drug's very prolonged elimination half-life likely contribute to the increased frequency of adverse effects attributed to flurazepam in elderly patients[21] (Fig. 7.4).

Steady-State Drug Concentration

Often a major goal of long-term pharmacotherapy is to achieve and maintain a therapeutic steady-state serum concentration. This concentration frequently is an important determinant of clinical outcome. The steady-state drug concentration (Css) is proportional to the medication dosing rate (dose/dosing interval) and inversely proportional to drug clearance. It can be expressed as follows:

$$\text{Css} \approx \text{(Dose/Dosing Interval)/Clearance}.$$

This has a number of important clinical ramifications for the prescriber. Although drug clearance is a biologically determined variable in each individual patient, over which the provider has no control, medication dose and dosing interval are variables that can be modified. To prevent the excessive accumulation of a

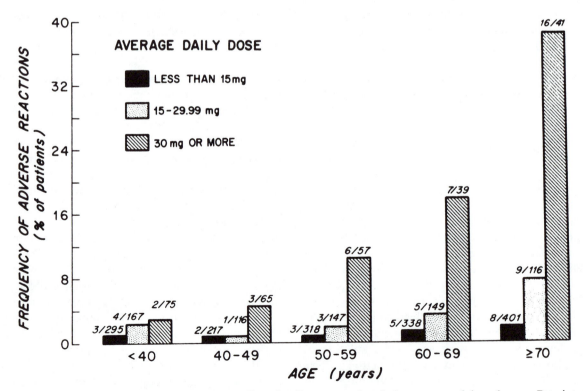

Fig. 7.4. Frequency of adverse reactions to the benzodiazepine flurazepam, in relation to age and drug dosage. Reprinted from DJ Greenblatt et.al. Toxicity of high-dose flurazepam in the elderly. Clinical Pharmacology and Therapeutics. 1977; 21:259.

drug when its clearance is reduced (as may be the case in an elderly patient), one can reduce the medication dose, increase the interval between doses, or both, depending on the particular situation.

Recognizing and Preventing Adverse Drug Effects in Elderly Patients

Adverse drug effects can mimic almost any clinical syndrome in geriatrics. Clinicians are most familiar with mental status changes as adverse effects of psychoactive drugs in the elderly; indeed, one study of reversible dementia found that drug-induced cognitive impairment was among the most common and treatable causes of syndromes that might be mistaken for senile dementia.[22] It is less commonly recognized that "nonpsychoactive" medications also can cause profound central nervous system toxicity in elderly patients. The toxic effects include cognitive impairment, which can be caused by β-blockers, histamine antagonists, and digoxin, to name only a few.

Equally important are the somatic side effects that can be caused by any drug, including psychoactive medications. Anticholinergic toxicity can be responsible for numerous symptoms apparently unrelated to the indication for which the drug was prescribed, and drugs with strong anticholinergic properties run the gamut from antiarrhythmics to antipsychotics (Table 7.1). Because acetylcholine serves as a neurotransmitter in numerous key roles in both the parasympathetic and central nervous systems, its blockade by medications with strong anticholinergic properties can yield a host of problems. As with all drug side effects, this effect is far more likely to occur in elderly patients because of the decreased drug clearance noted above and a diminished physiologic reserve to compensate for drug-induced perturbations in normal homeostatis.

The diagnosis of drug-induced illness in elderly patients is further complicated by ignorance of the physiology of normal aging and the tendency by patients, families, and even physicians to mislabel many symptoms as signs of "just growing old." As a result, drug-induced incontinence, confusion, fatigue, depression, and many other needless sufferings are attributed to the human condition, when they may well be amenable to appropriate diagnosis and therapeutic action. A useful antidote to these problems is a very high index of suspicion for drug-induced illness in elderly patients. An overstatement that is of great clinical use and forms a fine starting point for the evaluation of an older person may be stated as follows: "Any symptom in an elderly patient may be a drug side effect until proved otherwise." Or, as stated by

Table 7.1 Anticholinergic toxicity in elderly patients.*

Mechanism	Symptom	Possible misinterpretation or adverse consequences
Reduction in salivation	Dry mouth	Loss of appetite, trouble swallowing food, ill-fitting dentures
Reduction in gastrointestinal motility	Constipation	Gastrointestinal tract workup, over-use of laxatives
Disordered acetylcholine transmission in central nervous system	Confusion	Unnecessary dementia workup, mislabeling as "senility," treatment of symptoms with another drug
Reduction of impulses needed to contract detrusor muscle of bladder	Urinary retention with or without overflow	Diagnosis of "prostatic obstruction" or urinary incontinence, unnecessary treatment with prostatectomy or drug therapy, continuation of urinary symptoms

* Drugs with anticholinergic potential include disopyramide; antipsychotic medications, particularly low-potency drugs such as chlorpromazine and thioridazine; and belladonna-type drugs (eg, atropine).

Paracelsus (1493–1541), "All substances are poisons; there is none which is not a poison. The right dose differentiates a poison from a remedy."

Clinical Strategies

One maneuver with very useful diagnostic as well as therapeutic potential is the "therapeutic untrial" of a medication of dubious value that is currently in a patient's regimen. Older patients are at risk of accumulating layers and layers of drug therapy as they move through time, and often from physician to physician, forming the pharmacologic equivalent of a reef with accumulating layers of coral. Medications used for symptomatic relief (eg, of insomnia) are fairly easy to "prune," as their removal does not put the patient at any significant medical risk. However, even this must be done carefully, as chronic benzodiazepine users may be at high risk of the serious withdrawal symptoms that can occur after discontinuation of the drug.[23,24]

More challenging is the reassessment of medications that may be vital to the patient's regimen or may be presenting the risk of toxicity with no therapeutic benefit; examples include digoxin, quinidine, thiazides, antihypertensives, and anticonvulsants. Very often, these agents will have been prescribed many years previously, for reasons that were either poorly documented or transitory (eg, digoxin for mild transient congestive heart failure following a myocardial infarction or phenytoin for a poorly described seizure occuring immediately after a stroke or in the setting of alcohol withdrawal). Some clinicians argue that if a patient is stable and in no overt distress, it is too risky to change the regimen by removing drugs that may not be needed. However, it is often not appreciated that any medication that has the potential for toxicity with no continuing indication can represent a "time bomb" to a patient. Progressive diminution of renal or hepatic clearance, an acute hypovolemic state accompanying a transient respiratory or gastrointestinal illness, confusion on the part of the patient or caregiver regarding dosing—each of these can result in unexpected toxicity from a medication that is not currently producing symptoms. Another form of risk is the mild subclinical diminution in function that may result from the use of a medication with no clear purpose: slight postural instability from excessive antihypertensive therapy, mild blunting of affect or cognitive function with psychoactive drug use, subclinical depression from β-blockers, and so forth. Often, the presence of these symptoms is clear only in retrospect, when they have disappeared after withdrawal of the offending drug. The patient then may notice how much better he or she feels without a customary state of mild disability. To address these questions, a number of investigators have engaged in careful withdrawal of several medications from patients in whom no clear ongoing indication was evident.

In a study of the feasibility of discontinuing potentially unnecessary antihypertensive medications in elderly persons, 105 patients who were normotensive on therapy were withdrawn from their medication. Eleven months later, 41% of them remained normotensive without treatment.[25] A number of studies have suggested that many patients with compensated heart failure in sinus rhythm can be withdrawn from digoxin with no adverse clinical or hemodynamic effects. This may be particularly true of patients receiving concurrent diuretic and vasodilator therapy.[26,27] Another study found that withdrawal of anticonvulsant medication in patients free of seizures for 2 years was both practical and safe.[28] Although this study did not specifically address the geriatric population, it does suggest clinical guidelines under which such a maneuver might be undertaken.

"Pruning" of the drug regimen, however, can be accomplished only if the physician is aware of precisely what medications the patient is taking. This is best accomplished by a rigorous periodic review (at least every 6 months in a stable patient) of *all* medications taken by each elderly patient. Careful drug regimen review has been said to be one of the most useful interventions available to modern geriatric medicine, yet it fails to receive the attention it merits. Particular attention should be paid to eliciting information about medications that are (1) prescribed by another physician, (2) used only sporadically, (3) obtained over the counter, or (4) taken by some route other than by mouth (and hence often not thought of by patients as "drugs," eg, eyedrops for glaucoma, estrogen or steroid cream, medications applied via transdermal patch). A wise clinician once observed, "What you don't take can't hurt you." Periodic drug regimen review makes it possible to identify those medications that are truly enhancing a patient's clinical status and those that have become accidents of history and pose nothing but an ongoing risk.

Compliance

The failure of a patient to adhere to a thoughtfully prescribed therapeutic regimen is discouraging to every physician. The effects of noncompliance may be obvious, but often they are not fully appreciated. The worsening of a chronic condition that results from failure to take a prescribed medication may lead to the prescription of a larger dose or a more potent agent. This in turn can lead to serious toxicity should the patient begin taking the medication as prescribed. When noncompliance leads to unnecessary morbidity and mortality, the physician is left to consider what factors contributed to these adverse consequences and what strategies might have prevented their occurrence.

The problem of noncompliance with prescribed medical therapies is certainly not restricted to elderly patients. Across various patient age groups, compliance with long-term medication regimens has been found to be approximately 50%.[29] However, for a number of reasons, including increased use of both prescription and nonprescription medications, impaired homeostasis related to age-related decrements in many physiologic parameters, an increased prevalence of multiple coexisting chronic disease states, and the financial burden of substantial out-of-pocket costs in the face of fixed incomes, the compliance issue demands special attention in the geriatric population.

There are many types of noncompliant behavior associated with prescribed pharmacotherapy.[30] The most common type of noncompliance is simply the failure of the patient to take a medication. Other categories of noncompliance include the premature discontinuation of a medication, the taking of a medication at the wrong time, the excessive consumption of a medication ("if one pill is good, then two must be better"), and the use of medications not currently prescribed for the patient. This last category includes the inappropriate use of over-the-counter medications and the use of medications shared by family members and friends.[31,32]

Although problems with visual impairment, functional disability, and cognitive dysfunction have been frequently assumed as the prime contributors to therapeutic noncompliance in elderly patients, the results of a number of studies have confirmed that the major factor predicting compliance with a medication regimen is the total number of concurrently prescribed medications: the more prescriptions, the lower the compliance[33-35] (Fig. 7.5). Other factors contributing to noncompliance in the elderly include poor labeling instructions, difficulty in opening childproof containers, and misunderstanding of verbal instructions.[35]

In addition, confusion may lead to noncompliance when multiple drugs of similar appearance are prescribed for the same patient.[36]

A variety of strategies have been proposed for improving patient compliance with medication regimens.[29,30] Since the prescription of multiple concurrent medications reduces compliance, a primary strategy in improving compliance is to limit prescribing to the smallest possible number of medications and to make dosing instructions as simple as possible. Tailoring the regimen to the patient's schedule, such as mealtimes or other regularly scheduled activities, can be helpful. Compliance aids, such as commercially prepared or homemade pill boxes and medication calenders, also may be helpful. Family members and friends can be enlisted as informal social support networks to supervise and encourage compliance, and this support can be crucial to maintaining compliance with both long and short-term therapies. A regular reminder telephone call by a family member may be all that is required to complete an important course of therapy.

Medication Use in the Nursing Home

Since the advent of Medicaid and Medicare, nursing homes have taken on an increasingly prominent role in the medical care of many disabled elderly persons.[37]

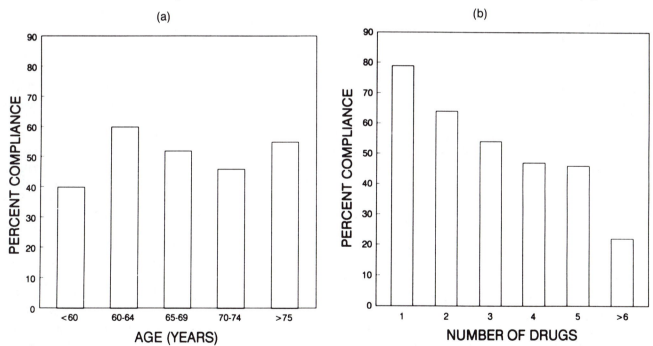

Fig. 7.5. (a)Compliance with medication regimens by age. No clear age-related differences are seen. (b), Compliance with medication regimens according to the number of prescribed drugs. Compliance is inversely related to the number of drugs prescribed. Reprinted with permission from the American Geriatrics Society, Medication use by ambulatory elderly by JC Darnell, et al., (*J Am Geriatr Soc,* 1986;34:1–4, pg. 33).

Nursing home patients are often heavily medicated[38]; polypharmacy is the rule rather than the exception in the nursing home. A 1976 study by the Office of Long Term Care reported an average of 6.1 drugs per patient, with a range in the number of prescriptions from zero to 23.[39]

There is compelling evidence to suggest misuse of medications in the nursing home. A 1980 study of Medicaid patients residing in Tennessee nursing homes reported that 43% received antipsychotic drugs.[40] Of even greater concern were observations that as the size of their nursing home practices increased, physicians prescribed more antipsychotic medication per patient, and that more antipsychotic medication was prescribed in larger nursing homes, implying that these drugs were being used excessively as a behavioral management strategy. Similar high levels of psychoactive drug use in nursing homes have been reported in other studies.[39,41–43] An Institute of Medicine report on improving the quality of care in nursing homes recently concluded that excessive use of tranquilizers and antipsychotic drugs suggested poor quality of care in nursing homes.[44]

Problems with inappropriate prescribing also have been found for a number of other drug classes. A survey of 3,032 nursing home patients found that the use of cimetidine appeared unjustified in 90% of patients receiving this drug.[45] In the case of another widely prescribed medication, the medical literature has suggested that many patients are receiving maintenance digoxin therapy unnecessarily and may have it withdrawn without detriment.[46–49] (The Office of Long Term Care study of physicians' drug prescribing patterns in skilled nursing facilities reported that nearly a quarter of sampled nursing home patients had a prescription for digoxin.[39])

An ominous consequence of excessive antibiotic use is the development of increasingly virulent bacterial strains in nursing homes, forcing reliance on potentially more toxic and expensive antibiotic regimens.[50] Systemic antibiotics are used in 8% to 16% of nursing home patients at any one time.[39,50–52] In one survey, documented evidence of the need for an antibiotic was inadequate in 38% of cases.[53]

The occurrence of preventable adverse drug reactions is the most important consequence of inappropriate drug prescribing in nursing homes. It has been consistently demonstrated that the incidence of adverse drug reactions increases substantially with the number of medications taken.[54] An increase in the incidence of adverse drug reactions with increasing age also has been suggested.[55] These two factors make the nursing home patient particularly vulnerable. Supporting this conclusion are a variety of studies that have suggested an association of medication use with a number of disorders prevalent in the institutionalized elderly population. These include cognitive impairment,[22] falls,[56–61] hip fractures,[62,63] depression,[64,65] and incontinence.[66] Many of these adverse reactions may be unavoidable consequences of the use of powerful and effective therapeutic agents in the elderly ill, yet the numerous studies documenting the extent of inappropriate drug prescribing in nursing homes suggest that a sizable proportion of them may be due to poor pharmacotherapeutic decision making.

Many factors contribute to inappropriate drug use in the nursing home. Training programs for physicians in internal medicine generally do not include formal training or experience in long-term care.[67] In general, physician visits to nursing home patients tend to be infrequent and brief and are precipitated more often by regulations rather by than any specific medical event involving the patient.[68] The general lack of organized medical staffs further impairs the ability of nursing homes to institute educational programs or to enforce standards of drug usage in this setting.

Since approximately 50% of all medication orders for nursing home patients are written by a physician with directions for administration as needed,[38] the nursing staff, by default, takes responsibility for a substantial proportion of pharmacotherapeutic decisions, including the frequency of dosing and the specific dosage of many medications. In addition, the bulk of direct care for nursing home patients is provided by nurses' aides, who often have little experience or formal training.[69] Current federal regulations allow nurses' aides to deliver all resident care in intermediate care facilities without the supervision of a registered, licensed, or vocational nurse from 3 PM to 7 AM every day.[44] Important pharmacotherapeutic decisions by physicians are by necessity often based on clinical information provided by nurses' aides.

Superimposed on this tenuous health care delivery system for the institutionalized elderly population are a number of additional factors contributing to suboptimal medication use. These include a reliance on advertising in therapeutic decision making, a failure to review medication orders frequently and critically, a lack of knowledge regarding the principles of geriatric pharmacology, an insulation from cost considerations in drug prescribing owing to third-party coverage, and poor communication with the nursing staff and the pharmacist. As the number of elderly patients in nursing homes continues to outstrip the number in acute care hospitals on any given day, increasing attention will need to be paid to improving the accuracy of medication use in this important setting.

Development and Testing of New Therapeutic Agents

Even though many drugs are likeliest to be used by the geriatric population, progress has been slow toward systematic inclusion of older patients in the drug evaluation and approval process. In the past, it has been advantageous for pharmaceutical manufacturers and clinical researchers to test new drugs prior to marketing primarily in healthy younger patients, because they are likeliest to yield "clean" results uncomplicated by concomitant therapy with other drugs, comorbidity, or pharmacokinetic complications. However, this leaves open the possibility that one of these "complicating factors" will prove to have a clinically meaningful effect on the new drug once it is marketed and taken by elderly persons in large numbers.

A particularly obvious example of this problem occurred with benoxaprofen, which was marketed as a nonsteroidal anti-inflammatory drug in the early 1980s without extensive premarketing testing on elderly patients.[70] A number of fatalities occurred after it was released for widespread use, particularly in elderly patients. As a result, the manufacturer was forced to withdraw the drug from the marketplace abruptly. The public outcry that resulted caused the Food and Drug Administration to float a series of discussion papers and proposed guidelines on the mandatory inclusion of older patients in premarketing testing of new drugs, particularly those with a geriatric target population.[71] This discussion began in 1982, but despite a number of congressional hearings, no such requirements have yet been put into place at this writing. The pharmaceutical industry has stated that companies are moving toward voluntary compliance within the spirit of these guidelines, but others question whether an issue so important should be left to voluntary compliance.

Research on Adverse Drug Reactions in Elderly Patients

Coupled with this lack of information regarding the effects of new drugs in the elderly, there is likewise a dearth of information on the unique properties in the aged patient of several commonly used medications, including both therapeutic and adverse effects. This represents an important and growing area of research in geriatric medicine. For example, while existing drug studies may or may not include elderly patients, they very rarely contain measurement of the end points of interest to geriatricians, which include cognitive impairment, functional status, and gait stability. Only recently has such research begun to appear, and the findings are of great consequence to clinicians. For example, there appears to be a greater degree of impairment in a variety of quality of life measures in patients taking β-blockers and methyldopa than in those taking other antihypertensives.[65]

The other major sector of medication research in geriatrics is in the domain of pharmacoepidemiology: the study of adverse drug effects in large populations. For example, one elegant study used Medicaid data to demonstrate the epidemiologic soundness of a clinical observation often made by clinicians, namely, that there is a marked increase in the risk of falls and fractures in elderly patients given long-acting benzodiazepine hypnotics, as compared with comparable patients given short-acting drugs or no hypnotics at all.[62] Using computer-assisted analysis of such large data sets, a number of studies are proceeding to determine the nature and magnitude of adverse drug effects in elderly patients. Current plans call for the new drug entitlement under Medicare to be implemented by means of a massive nationwide database that would keep track of every prescription filled by every American over age 65 years. Should this go forward as planned, it would provide an enormous reservoir of information concerning the medication taking behavior of older Americans. This could then be linked with other data from Medicare claims that deal with hospitalization and other forms of care, providing nearly limitless opportunities for the study of drug-disease interactions in this age group.

Conclusion

As the most prominent consumers of prescription medications, elderly patients benefit the most and are at greatest risk of toxicity from our increasingly complex, effective, and costly pharmacopoeia. The basic question (and often the most important one) is not, "Which drug should I prescribe?" but rather "Is a drug indicated at all?" For some common geriatric problems, nonpharmacologic treatment often is equally effective and considerably safer. When pharmacotherapy is indicated, choosing the right drug in the right dose for an elderly patient represents one of the most difficult challenges in all of medicine but also can yield the most gratifying outcomes. Likewise, few interventions in geriatric practice are as elegant in process, and as "heroic" in outcome, as diagnosing and treating adverse drug effects. Thorough knowledge of some of the overarching principles outlined above will enable the clinician to wield this powerful double-edged sword with the least possible risk and with the maximum benefit for patients.

References

1. Reidenberg MM, Levy M, Warner H, et al. Relationship between diazepam dose, plasma level, age, and central nervous system depression. *Clin Pharmacol Ther* 1978;23:371–374.
2. Casteden CM, George CF, Marcer D, et al. Increased sensitivity to nitrazepam in old age. *Br Med J* 1977;1:10–12.
3. Meyer BR, Lewin M, Dreyer DE, et al. Optimizing metoclopramide control of cisplatin-induced emesis. *Ann Intern Med* 1984;100:393–395.
4. O'Malley K, Stevenson IH, Ward CA, et al. Determinants of anticoagulant control in patients receiving warfarin. *Br J Clin Pharmacol* 1977;4:309–314.
5. Shephard AMM, Hewick DS, Moreland TA. Age as a determinant of sensitivity to warfarin. *Br J Clin Pharmacol* 1977;4:315–320.
6. Bellville JW, Forrest WH, Miller E, et al. Influence of age on pain relief from analgesics. *JAMA* 1971;217:1835–1841.
7. Kaiko RF. Age and morphine analgesia in cancer patients with postoperative pain. *Clin Pharmacol Ther* 1980;28:823–826.
8. Scott JC, Stanski DR. Decreased fetanyl and alfentanil dose requirements with age: a simultaneous pharmacokinetic and pharmacodynamic evaluation. *J Pharmacol Exp Ther* 1987;240:159–166.
9. Vestal RE, Wood AJJ, Shand DG. Reduced beta-adrenoreceptor sensitivity in the elderly. *Clin Pharmacol Ther* 1979;26:181–186.
10. Avorn J, Everitt DE, Weiss S, et al. Increased antidepressant use in patients prescribed beta-blockers. *JAMA* 1986;255:357–360.
11. Schmucker DL. Aging and drug disposition: an update. *Pharmacol Rev* 1985;37:133–148.
12. Campion EW, deLabry LO, Glynn RJ. The effect of age on serum albumin in healthy males: report from the Normative Aging Study. *J Gerontol* 1988;43:M18–M20.
13. MacLennan WJ, Martin P, Mason BJ. Protein intake and serum albumin levels in the elderly. *Gerontology* 1977;23:360–367.
14. Greenblatt DJ, Sellers EM, Koch-Weser J. Importance of protein binding for the interpretation of serum or plasma drug concentrations. *J Clin Pharmacol* 1982;22:259–263.
15. Buskirk ER. Health maintenance and longevity: exercise. In: *Handbook of the Biology of Aging,* 2nd ed. Finch CE, Schneider EL (eds.) New York: Van Nostrand Reinhold Company 1985;pp. 898–899.
16. Mooney H, Roberts R, Cooksley WGE, et al. Alterations in the liver with aging. *Clin Gastroenterol* 1985;14:757–771.
17. Vestal RE, Norris AH, Tobin JD, et al. Antipyrine metabolism in man: influence of age, alcohol, caffeine, and smoking. *Clin Pharmacol Ther* 1975;18:425–432.
18. Rowe JW, Andres R, Tobin JD, et al. The effect of age on creatinine clearance in man. *J Gerontol* 1976;31:155–163.
19. Lindeman RD, Tobin JD, Shock NW. Longitudinal studies on the rate of decline in renal function with age. *J Am Geriatr Soc* 1985;33:278–285.
20. Greenblatt DJ, Divoll M, Harmatz JS, et al. Kinetics and clinical effects of flurazepam in young and elderly insomniacs. *Clin Pharmacol Ther* 1981;30:475–486.
21. Greenblatt DJ, Allen MD, Shader RI. Toxicity of high-dose flurazepam in the elderly. *Clin Pharmacol Ther* 1977;21:355–361.
22. Larson EB, Kukull WA, Buchner D, et al. Adverse drug reactions associated with global cognitive impairment in elderly persons. *Ann Intern Med* 1987;107:169–173.
23. Greenblatt DJ, Harmatz JS, Zinny MA, et al. Effect of gradual withdrawal on the rebound sleep disorder after discontinuation of triazolam. *N Engl J Med* 1987;317:722–728.
24. Busto U, Sellers EM, Naranjo CA, et al. Withdrawal reaction after long-term therapeutic use of benzodiazepines. *N Engl J Med* 1986;315:854–859.
25. Danielson M, Lundback M. Withdrawal of antihypertensive drugs in mild hypertension. *Acta Med Scand* 1981;646(suppl 1):127–131.
26. Fleg JL, Gottlieb SH, Lakatta EG. Is digoxin really important in treatment of compensated heart failure? a placebo-controlled crossover study in patients with sinus rhythm. *Am J Med* 1982;73:244–250.
27. Gheorghiade M, Beller GA. Effect of discontinuing maintenance digoxin therapy in patients with ischemic heart disease and congestive heart failure in sinus rhythm. *Am J Cardiol* 1983;51:1243–1250.
28. Callaghan N, Garrett A, Goggin T. Withdrawal of anticonvulsant drugs in patients free of seizures for two years. *N Engl J Med* 1988;318:942–946.
29. Sackett DL, Snow JC. The magnitude of compliance and noncompliance. In: Haynes RB, Taylor DW, Sackett DL, eds. *Compliance in Health Care.* Baltimore, Md: The Johns Hopkins University Press; 1979, pp. 11–12.
30. Simonson W. *Medications and the Elderly: A Guide for Promoting Proper Use.* Rockville, Md: Aspen Systems Corp; 1984.
31. Ostrom JR, Hammarlund ER, Christensen DB, et al. Medication usage in the elderly population. *Med Care* 1985;23:157–164.
32. Hammarlund ER, Ostrom JR, Kethley AJ. The effects of drug counseling and other educational strategies on drug utilization of the elderly. *Med Care* 1985;23:165–170.
33. Darnell JC, Murray MD, Martz BL, et al. Medication use by ambulatory elderly: an in-home survey. *J Am Geriatr Soc* 1986;34:1–4.
34. German PS, Klein LE, McPhee SJ, et al. Knowledge of and compliance with drug regimens in the elderly. *J Am Geriatr Soc* 1982; 30:568–571.
35. Kendrick R, Bayne JRD. Compliance with prescribed medication by elderly patients. *Can Med Assoc J* 1982; 127:961–962.
36. Mazzullo J. The nonpharmacologic basis of therapeutics. *Clin Pharmacol Ther* 1972;13:157–158.

37. Trends in Nursing and Related Care Homes and Hospitals: United States, Selected Years 1969–80. National Center for Health Statistics; 1984. US Dept of Health and Human Services publication PHSS 84-1825.

38. Robers PA. Extent of medication use in U.S. long-term-care facilities. *Am J Hosp Pharm* 1988;45:93–100.

39. *Physicians' Drug Prescribing Patterns in Skilled Nursing Facilities*. Office of Long Term Care; 1976. US Dept of Health, Education, and Welfare publication OS 76-50050.

40. Ray WA, Federspiel CF, Schaffner W. A study of antipsychotic drug use in nursing homes: epidemiologic evidence suggesting misuse. *Am J Public Health* 1980;70:485–491.

41. Ingman SR, Lawson IR, Pierpaoli PG, et al. A survey of the prescribing and administration of drugs in a long-term care institution for the elderly. *J Am Geriatr Soc* 1975;23:309–316.

42. Beers M, Avorn J, Soumerai SB, et al. Psychoactive medication use in intermediate-care facility. *JAMA.* 1988;260:3016–3020.

43. Buck JA. Psychotropic drug practice in nursing homes. *J Am Geriatr Soc* 1988;36:409–418.

44. Institute of Medicine Committee on Nursing Home Regulation. *Improving the Quality of Care in Nursing Homes*. Washington, DC: National Academy Press; 1986:378–379.

45. Sherman DS, Avorn J, Campion EW. Cimetidine use in nursing homes: prolonged therapy and excessive doses. *J Am Geriatr Soc* 1987;35:1023–1027.

46. Dall JLC. Maintenance digoxin in elderly patients. *Br Med J* 1970;2:705–706.

47. Fonrose HA, Ahlbaum N, Bugatch E, et al. The efficacy of digitalis withdrawal in an institutionalized aged population. *J Am Geriatr Soc* 1974;2:208–211.

48. Hull SM, Mackintosh A. Discontinuation of maintenance digoxin therapy in general practice. *Lancet* 1977;2:1054–1055.

49. Wilkins CE, Khurana MS. Digitalis withdrawal in elderly nursing home patients. *J Am Geriatr Soc* 1985;33:850–851.

50. Garibaldi RA, Brodine S, Matsumiya. Infections among patients in nursing homes: policies, prevalence and problems. *N Engl J Med* 1981;305:731–735.

51. Zimmer JG, Bentley DW, Valenti WM. Systemic antibiotic use in nursing homes: A quality assessment. *J Am Geriatr Soc* 1986;34:703–710.

52. Crossley K, Henry K, Irvine P, et al. Antibiotic use in nursing homes: prevalence, cost, and utilization review. *Bull NY Acad Med* 1987;63:510–518.

53. Zimmer JG, Bentley DW, Valenti WM. Systemic antibiotic use in nursing homes: a quality assessment. *J Am Geriatr Soc* 1986;34:703–710.

54. Nolan L, O'Malley K. Prescribing for the elderly, I: sensitivity of the elderly to adverse drug reactions. 1988;36:142–149.

55. Seidl CG, Thornton GF, Smith JW, et al. Studies on the epidemiology of adverse drug reactions, III: reactions in patients on a general medical service. *Bull Johns Hopkins Hosp* 1966;119:299–315.

56. Granck E, Baker SP, Abbey H, et al. Medications and diagnoses in relation to falls in a long-term care facility. *J Am Geriatr Soc* 1987;35:503–511.

57. Lipsitz LA, Wei JY, Rowe JW. Syncope in an elderly, institutionalized population: prevalence, incidence, and associated risk. *Q J Med* 1985;55:45–54.

58. Prudham D, Evans JG. Factors associated with falls in the elderly: a community study. *Age Aging* 1981;10:141–146.

59. Sobel KG, McCart GM. Drug use and accidental falls in an intermediate care facility. *Drug Intell Clin Pharm* 1983;17:539–542.

60. Wells BG, Middleton B, Lawrence G, et al. Factors associated with the elderly falling in intermediate care facilities. *Drug Intell Clin Pharm* 1985;19:142–145.

61. Stephen PJ, Williamson J. Drug-induced parkinsonism in the elderly. *Lancet* 1984;2:1082–1083.

62. Ray WA, Griffin MR, Schaffner W. Psychotropic drug use and the risk of hip fracture. *N Engl J Med* 1987;316:363–369.

63. MacDonald JB, MacDonald ET. Nocturnal femoral fracture and continuing widespread use of barbiturate hypnotics. *Br Med J* 1977;2:483–485.

64. Avorn J, Everitt DE, Weiss S, et al. Increased antidepressant use in patients prescribed beta-blockers. *JAMA* 1986;255:357–360.

65. Croog SH, Levine S, Testa MA, et al. The effects of antihypertensive therapy on quality of life. *N Engl J Med* 1986;314:1657–1664.

66. Resnick NM. Urinary incontinence in the elderly. *Med Grand Rounds* 1984;3:281–290.

67. Katz PR. Training internists for a role in long-term care. *J Gen Intern Med* 1987;2:450–452.

68. Mitchell JB. Physician visits to nursing homes. *Gerontologist* 1982;22:45–48.

69. Waxman HM, Klein M, Carner EA. Drug misuse in nursing homes: an institutional addiction. *Hosp Community Psychiatry* 1985;36:886–887.

70. Taggart HM, Alderdice JM. Fatal cholestatic jaundice in elderly patients taking benoxaprofen. *Br Med J Clin Res* 1982;284:1372.

71. Temple R. *FDA Discussion Paper on Testing of Drugs in the Elderly*. Washington DC: Food and Drug Administration; 1983.

8

Screening for Disease in Elderly Persons

John R. Feussner and Eugene Z. Oddone

Decisions to Seek Early Diagnosis

Early detection of disease, or screening, is an attractive diagnostic strategy for physicians. Screening for disease facilitates detection of disease early in its clinical course, before many pathologic changes have occurred and while the disease may be more amenable to treatment. As attractive as early detection may seem, however, certain principles should be considered to assure the appropriateness of any decision to seek early diagnoses (Table 8.1).[1] Such considerations include the importance or seriousness of the target disease; the presence of an early presymptomatic period; the accuracy and acceptability of available diagnostic tests; the risk associated with invasive diagnostic testing; the efficacy, cost, and availability of treatment; and the risk of treatment, such as adverse drug effects or adverse outcomes of surgery. The absence of clear information about any one of these considerations may diminish the potential value of any screening strategy no matter how attractive it may seem.

The disease being considered as a potential target for early detection should be an important problem; that is, it should occur frequently, be more readily treated when detected early, or be readily treatable even though the prevalence is low. Sackett and colleagues state the principle succinctly: the disease should be so common or so awful as to justify the effort and expense of early detection.[2] An example of an important target disease in the elderly population is cancer of several organs. Age is an important risk factor for the development of cancer. The incidence

rates per 100,000 whites in the United States increase beyond age 65 years and peak between ages 90 and 94 years for digestive tract cancer, between 85 and 89 years for prostrate cancer, and between 85 and 90 years for breast cancer.

Interest in screening should imply an understanding of the natural history of the target disease. The physician should know that early detection of disease is likely to be useful because the disease has an early presymptomatic stage. If this were not true, the physician need only await the development of symptoms before pursuing diagnostic evaluation. Natural history data are equally important when considering treatment options. Knowledge of the clinical course of the target disease is necessary in judging whether available treatment is effective. Patient outcomes that should be considered when establishing efficacy include improved quality of life, reduced disability, and reduced mortality.

For a screening program to be feasible, diagnostic tests must be available that are accurate and acceptable to patients. The screening test should minimize false-positive results (healthy patients with positive test results) and false-negative results (patients with disease who have negative test results). The test should be acceptable; for example, in screening for colorectal cancer, flexible sigmoidoscopy may be a more acceptable screening test than rigid sigmoidoscopy. Because screening tests are frequently not definitive, it is important also that patients who agree to screening understand that additional definitive diagnostic procedures may be required. If patients are unwilling to proceed through the diagnostic process to

Table 8.1. Considerations in deciding to seek an early diagnosis.*

1. Is the target disease an important clinical problem?
   (*a*) Does the burden of disability warrant early action?
2. Is the natural history of the target disease understood?
   (*a*) Is there a latent or early presymptomatic period?
3. Is the screening diagnostic strategy effective?
   (*a*) Is the accuracy of testing established? The sensitivity and specificity?
   (*b*) Is the test acceptable to patients, with little discomfort and low risks?
   (*c*) If the screening test is positive, will patients accept subsequent diagnostic evaluation?
4. Is there a known treatment for the target disease?
   (*a*) Is the treatment effective and available?
   (*b*) Is the cost of testing balanced by the benefit of treatment?

* For more extensive discussion, see references 1 and 2.

some acceptable treatment, then screening will be of little value. Before embarking on a screening program, the physician should discuss with the patient the possible results of the tests and the available treatments to determine whether the patient values early disease recognition and will accept treatment.

The decision to screen for disease in elderly persons is problematic, as few studies evaluating the efficacy of screening programs have included elderly patients. Few data are available about the specific utility of diagnostic tests in elderly patients, the precise risks of testing, or the efficacy and risks of treatment. Even when studies have demonstrated the feasibility of a screening program, the definitive next step of demonstrating that a screening program actually improves patient outcomes is often lacking. Furthermore, bias sometimes works against elderly patients, in that they are assumed not to be candidates for screening programs because the risks of testing are thought to be higher or the benefits of treatment lower. As geriatricians already know, functional status and comorbid disease are more relevant considerations than chronologic age. Alternatively, screening strategies could be viewed as especially attractive in the elderly population. Unlike younger age cohorts, elderly persons often experience higher rates of multiple diseases. Screening tests perform better in situations where disease prevalence is high, because the number of false-positive tests is lower.

Diagnostic Tests: Accuracy and Predictive Value

Part of any decision to adopt a screening strategy must rest on the accuracy and safety of available screening tests. Screening tests are not usually definitive. For example, screening for breast cancer with breast self-examination or mammography does not establish a diagnosis. However, subsequent biopsy of a suspicious lesion will establish a diagnosis. The physician prefers a diagnostic test that accurately discriminates between patients with and without disease. In many screening situations, it is more important to avoid missing patients with disease, thereby minimizing false-negative test results. The tradeoff here is that the proportion of patients with false-positive test results increases, requiring additional definitive diagnostic testing to establish the presence or absence of disease. Stated differently, when a test's sensitivity is higher (low false-negative rate), its specificity is often lower (high false-positive rate).

In order to compare and interpret diagnostic test results, one must understand the operating characteristics—the sensitivity and specificity—of any given test (Table 8.2). Sensitivity is the characteristic of a test that describes how it performs in patients who have disease; it is the number of patients with a positive test and disease divided by the total number of patients with disease. Specificity is the characteristic of a test that describes how it performs in patients without disease; it is the number of patients with a negative test and no disease divided by the total number of patients without disease. The sensitivity and specificity of diagnostic tests are stable characteristics of the test and do not depend on the frequency of disease. In general, they should not change when applied to different populations.

As shown in Table 8.2, the prevalence of disease in a given population is expressed as the number of patients with disease divided by the total number of

Table 8.2. Operating characteristics of a diagnostic test.*

		Disease	
		Present	Absent
Test result	Positive	True positive (*A*)	False positive (*B*)
	Negative	False negative (*C*)	True negative (*D*)

* Sensitivity = $A/(A + C)$; specificity = $D/(D + B)$; accuracy = $(A + D)/(A + B + C + D)$; prevalence = $(A + C)/(A + B + C + D)$; positive predictive value = $A/(A + B)$ =

$$\frac{p(\text{Sensitivity})}{p(\text{Sensitivity}) + (1 - p)(1 - \text{Specificity})};$$

and negative predictive value = $D/(C + D)$ =

$$\frac{(1 - p)\text{Specificity}}{p(1 - \text{Sensitivity}) + (1 - p)(\text{Specificity})},$$

where p = probability that a patient has disease before a test result is known. (Positive predictive value is the probability that a patient has disease given a positive test result; negative predictive value, the probability that a patient does not have disease given a negative result.)

patients tested. Predictive values for diagnostic tests can be calculated to help predict the probability that a patient with a positive test will have the disease or that a patient with a negative test will not. Unlike sensitivity and specificity, the predictive value of a test is highly dependent on the prevalence of disease. When the prevalence of disease increases, as is frequently the case in the elderly population, the probability of disease in patients with positive test results (positive predictive value) also increases. For example, if a disease prevalence is only 2% and a test's sensitivity and specificity are 95%, the positive predictive value is only 28%. If the disease prevalence is raised to 20% with the same sensitivity and specificity, the positive predictive value is 83%. Thus, when accurate diagnostic tests are used in low-prevalence situations, the result is a high false-positive rate and a low positive predictive value. Screening in low-prevalence situations is inefficient and expensive, especially considering the additional diagnostic evaluation required for the patients with false-positive results.

Economic Issues: Cost-benefit and Cost-effectiveness Analysis

Decisions to screen for disease in the elderly population are complicated further by economic concerns. These decisions include the choice of a screening test, the frequency of testing, the size of the target population, and the cost and efficacy of treatment, and they are influenced by economic issues such as scarce resources, large copayments, and reduced reimbursement. Increasingly, the methods of health economics are being used to address decisions regarding early disease detection. Both cost-effectiveness analysis and cost-benefit analysis deal with the costs and consequences of clinical activities. While both methods may help physicians make decisions, they are somewhat different. Cost-effectiveness analysis usually deals with a single clinical effect (prolonged survival) that is common to two (or more) alternative diagnostic strategies but that may be achieved to differing degrees and at different costs. For example, the physician could use two different strategies to detect colon cancer: annual fecal occult blood testing or annual fecal occult blood testing plus annual sigmoidoscopy. While the diagnostic strategies are different, they both seek to identify disease early, thereby improving patient survival. However, the costs of the two strategies are clearly different. For this type of analysis, the data are presented in units relevant to the clinical outcome, increased survival; thus the data would be expressed as costs (dollars) per added survival (months). Were the efficacy of the two diagnostic strategies similar, one would simply choose the less expensive strategy. Eddy performed such economic analyses for several common tests used to detect cancer and estimated the influence on life expectancy of performing diagnostic tests at different intervals.[3] Concerning screening for colorectal cancer, one can show the difference in cost and efficacy when different diagnostic strategies are used (Fig. 8.1). Eddy's analysis suggested that life expectancy changed very little over a spectrum of testing intervals ranging from annual fecal occult blood testing and annual sigmoidoscopy to annual fecal occult blood testing and every-5-year sigmoidoscopy. The costs, however, are remarkably different, with the most frequent testing costing

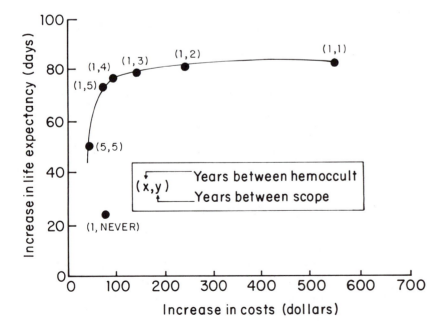

Fig. 8.1. Influence of varying the periodicity of fecal occult blood testing and rigid sigmoidoscopy on the cost of screening for colon cancer and on life expectancy. For a more complete discussion of the data, see reference 3. From ref. 3 with permission.

over five times more than the least frequent (annual fecal occult blood testing plus every 5-year sigmoidoscopy). Cost-effectiveness analysis assumes that the diagnostic strategy or treatment program is worthwhile and seeks to find which of several different strategies is most cost-effective.

Cardiovascular Disease Risk Factors

Hypertension

Hypertension has emerged as the major risk factor for stroke and a significant contributing factor for heart attacks in the United States.[4] The risk from hypertension is well documented for middle-aged people, and within the last 15 years several large trials have demonstrated that elevations of systolic and diastolic blood pressure also are associated with increased morbidity and mortality in elderly persons. Recent epidemiologic studies have shown that isolated systolic hypertension, which exists almost exclusively in older people, is also a significant risk factor for cerebrovascular and cardiovascular morbidity and mortality, independent of diastolic blood pressure.[5] The importance of hypertension in elderly persons is exemplified by its high prevalence. Even when conservative thresholds defining hypertension are used (blood pressure > 160/95 mm Hg), many people over age 65 years (45.1%) are classified as affected (Table 8.3). A smaller percentage of elderly people (7%) are estimated to have isolated systolic hypertension (systolic blood pressure greater > 160 and diastolic pressure < 90 mm Hg).[6]

Hypertension continues to be a risk factor for stroke and cardiovascular morbidity and mortality into the 9th decade.[7] The importance of screening for hypertension in the elderly population is supported by the well-documented efficacy of antihypertensive therapy, which significantly reduces cerebrovascular and cardiovascular morbidity and, in some studies, mortality. In the Hypertension Detection and Follow-up Program study, patients 60 to 69 years old who were randomized to stepped-care treatment experienced 16.4% lower total mortality than controls receiving usual care. This result was strikingly similar to the 16.9% mortality reduction in the 30- to 69-year old treatment group.[7] The Australian Therapeutic Trial in Mild Hypertension Study showed a 24% reduction in stroke and ischemic heart disease events in treated hypertensive patients over age 60 years.[8] The European Working Party on Hypertension in the Elderly, designed specifically to assess antihypertensive therapy in patients over age 60 years,[9] showed a 27% reduction in cardiovascular mortality, which was defined as fatal myocardial infarction, fatal congestive heart failure, and stroke. The results of these trials and others support the contention that treating hypertension in elderly patients affords benefits similar to those achieved in younger patients. The exact treatment threshold chosen in the several studies were as follows: the Hypertension Detection and Follow-up Program required a diastolic blood pressure of 90 mm Hg or higher, the Australian Study required a diastolic blood pressure of 95 to 109 mm Hg, and the European Working Party on Hypertension in the Elderly required a systolic blood pressure of 160 to 239 mm Hg.

Physicians should routinely screen for both systolic and diastolic hypertension in elderly patients, at least annually and on visits for other reasons (Table 8.4). The available evidence indicates that treatment for diastolic hypertension should be initiated at a blood pressure of 90 mm Hg. Specific recommendations for treatment of isolated systolic hypertension in elderly patients will have to await completion of the Systolic Hypertension in the Elderly Program study.

Hypercholesterolemia

Any approach to screening for hypercholesterolemia in elderly patients is complicated by two factors. First, people who survive to old age may have physiologic differences that distinguish them from their counterparts who died at a young age. Second, it may be difficult to detect a small reduction in mortality afforded by risk factor modification in elderly patients, given the high all cause mortality rates for older persons. These factors, among others, make it particularly important to establish that screening strategies and therapeutic initiatives aimed at reducing cholesterol levels in elderly persons result in lower cardiovascular morbidity and mortality. The two major interventional trials, the Lipid Research Clinics Coronary Primary Prevention Trial and the Helsinki Heart

Table 8.3. Prevalence of hypertension among noninstitutionalized men and women, aged 65 to 74 years.*

	% of Population	
	Blood pressure ≥160/95 mm Hg	Blood pressure ≥140/90 mm Hg
Black women	72.8	82.9
Black men	42.9	67.1
White women	48.3	66.2
White men	37.5	59.2
Total blacks	59.9	76.1
Total whites	43.7	63.1
Total (all races)	45.1	64.3

* Data modified from reference 4.

Table 8.4. Recommendations concerning frequently considered screening activities in elderly persons.

Disease	Test	Frequency	Recommendation
Hypertension	Sphygmomanometry	Annually, and on visits made for other reasons	Include in screening program
Hypercholesterolemia	Serum lipid profile	Uncertain	Not routine until treatment efficacy established
Cigarette smoking	History and counseling	Annually, and on visits made for other reasons	Include in screening program
Cerebrovascular disease	Physical examination	Uncertain	Not routine until treatment efficacy established
Tuberculosis in the nursing home	Purified protein derivative	Nursing home entry, annually thereafter	Include in screening program
Hearing impairment	Pure tone audiometry or Welch-Allen audioscope plus HHIE-S*	Annually	Include in screening program
Diminished Visual acuity	Snellen chart and ophthalmoscopy	Annually	Include in screening program
Open-angle glaucoma	Funduscopic examination, tonometry	Uncertain	Not routine until treatment efficacy established
Depression	Beck Depression Inventory, Geriatric Depression Scale, Brief Carroll Depression Rating Scale	Uncertain	Not routine until treatment efficacy established
Alcoholism	CAGE, VAST	Uncertain	Not routine until treatment efficacy established
Dental disease	Oral examination	Annually	Refer for dental evaluation
Injury prevention	History and physical examination	Uncertain	Not routine until screening strategy and effective treatment established
Osteoporosis	Dual-photon absorptiometry	Uncertain	Not recommended in elderly patients

* HHIE-S indicates Hearing Handicapped Inventory for the Elderly–Screening Version.

Study, limited their patient selection to middle-aged men (< 60 years). [10,11] Additionally, the best available epidemiologic data from the 30-year follow-up of the Framingham cohort suggested a lack of association between total serum cholesterol levels and mortality for patients over age 50 years. [12] The Framingham investigators proposed that a possible "harvest effect" may account for the lack of association, that is, deaths associated with high serum cholesterol levels tend to occur before age 50 years.

The recent National Heart, Lung, and Blood Institute expert panel report on cholesterol strongly advocates an aggressive cholesterol screening and treatment program. [13] Their recommendations include a screening program for all Americans beginning at age 20 years, with testing every 5 years as long as the total serum cholesterol level is less than 200 mg/dL. For those individuals whose total cholesterol level is above 200 mg/dL, they recommend measuring low-density lipoprotein, high-density lipoprotein, and triglyceride levels. The suggested therapeutic plan begins with a two-stage diet, followed by medication therapy if necessary. These recommendations are modified by

the presence or absence of other cardiovascular risk factors. The recommendations assume that routine screening continues into old age. However, the adoption of routine screening in elderly patients may lead to aggressive diet or drug therapy, with its attendant expense and adverse effects. Before routine screening is recommended for the elderly population, its efficacy should be established. Since we know of no studies to date that have demonstrated efficacy, we cannot support routine screening for hypercholesterolemia in elderly patients (Table 8.4).

Smoking

The causal association between cigarette smoking and multiple serious diseases, including cardiovascular and respiratory diseases and cancer, is well established. Less is known about smokers who survive to old age. Many physicians are reluctant to urge older patients to stop smoking, as the benefits of stopping may not significantly alter their functional status or survival. However, a few epidemiologic studies have reported improved health outcomes for older persons who do stop smoking. Jajich and colleagues, in a cohort study of people aged 65 to 74 years, showed a lower relative risk of cardiovascular mortality in elders who had quit smoking for as little as 1 to 5 years.[14] Hermanson et al recently reported 6-year survival data for an elderly cohort of men and women with angiographically proved coronary artery disease who were part of the Coronary Artery Surgery Study registry.[15] They demonstrated improved survival for patients over age 65 years who were able to stop smoking, compared with their counterparts who did not stop. The relative risk of death was 1.7 for patients over age 65 years who continued to smoke, compared with those who quit. In a cross-sectional study, Rogers et al measured cerebral blood flow in older smokers, nonsmokers, and smokers who had recently quit.[16] They showed significantly higher cerebral perfusion in nonsmokers, but more importantly, a small group of smokers who had recently quit showed significant and gradual improvement in their cerebral perfusion. We recommend that physicians continue to ask their patients about smoking at least annually and advise older patients to stop smoking (Table 8.4).

Cancer Screening

Breast Cancer

Breast cancer is the most commonly occurring malignancy in women and is the second leading cause of cancer-related deaths. The American Cancer Society estimates that one of every 10 women in the United States will develop breast cancer during her lifetime. The age-specific annual breast cancer incidence rates for all races, derived from the National Cancer Institutes Surveillance, Epidemiology and End Results Program, indicate a progressive rise in annual cancer incidence to age 85 years and beyond.

Several screening strategies have been recommended for the detection of breast cancer including breast self-examination, breast physical examination, and mammography. O'Malley and Fletcher, reporting for the US Preventive Services Task Force on screening with breast self-examination, indicate that breast self-examination has a low sensitivity, between 20% and 30%, that is even lower among older women. The task force did not advocate the use of breast self-examination as a screening test for breast cancer, especially among elderly women.[17] The American Cancer Society recommends clinical breast examination by a physician annually. Screening mammography is recommended annually after age 50 years.[18] Their recommendation suggests that screening for breast cancer is a lifetime requirement for women because

the incidence of disease continues to rise with age. The sensitivity for mammography alone is approximately 70%, but the sensitivity of combined mammography and clinical breast examination may be as high as 87%,[19] suggesting that the tests should be used together. For women over age 65 years, clinical breast examination and mammography are preferred screening tests (Table 8.5).

Several studies, beginning with the Health Insurance Plan of Greater New York study, have shown effectiveness of breast cancer screening in reducing mortality from breast cancer.[20] In this study, mammography was coupled with breast physical examination. The results for women over age 50 years were impressive in that screening decreased mortality by more than 50% at 5 years. However, this study has limited direct value for elderly patients, as women over 65 years at entry were not included in the study. A Swedish study, also a randomized clinical trial, used mammography alone to screen women between the ages of 40 and 74 years.[21] As in the Health Insurance Plan study, there was a clear decrease in mortality (40%) for women over age 50 years. Other studies confirm these positive results, without clearly distinguishing the respective contributions of breast physical examination and screening mammography.[19]

Despite the high incidence of breast cancer, the availability of screening tests, and the proved efficacy of early detection in improving survival, as many as 50% of women 65 years of age and older may not be adequately screened. An American Cancer Society survey of physicians showed that only 49% of physicians performed baseline or routine mammography in older patients. Ongoing efforts are required to educate physicians and elderly women about the benefits of routine breast cancer screening with clinical breast examination and mammography.

Table 8.5. Recommendations for cancer screening in elderly persons.

Disease	Test	Frequency
Breast	Breast physical examination	Annual
	Mammography	Every 1–2 years
Cervical	Pap test	At least once if underscreened
Skin	Physical examination	Annual
Colon	Fecal occult blood test	Annual
	Sigmoidoscopy	Every 3–5 years
Prostate	Digital rectal examination	Annual
Lung	Chest radiography	Not recommended
	Sputum cytology	Not recommended

Cervical Cancer

Cervical cancer continues to be a major health problem for women; approximately 20,000 new cases and 7,500 deaths occur annually. Surprisingly, elderly women account for a disproportionate amount of the case burden; 24% of new cases of cervical cancer and 41% of annual deaths from cervical cancer occur in women 65 years of age and older.[22] The age-specific incidence for invasive disease also increases with increasing age, from 17.5 cases per 100,000 for women aged 30 to 34 years to 30 cases per 100,000 for women aged 80 years and older.

The Papanicolaou (Pap) smear technique for detecting cervical cancer at a presymptomatic stage was developed in the 1940s. The sensitivity of a single routine cervical Pap smear is only 66% for the detection of cervical cancer.[23] The specificity of Pap testing is difficult to determine, since women with normal results are not subjected to the definitive diagnostic test, cone biopsy. There continues to be great variability concerning recommendations for the optimum frequency of screening. The American College of Obstetricians and Gynecologists recommends annual screening for all women. The American Cancer Society recommends less frequent Pap testing after a women has had at least three consecutive normal annual examinations. The National Institutes of Health consensus statement on cervical cancer screening recommends that screening be discontinued at age 60 years if two negative Pap smears have been obtained.[24] Finally, the Canadian Task Force on Cervical Cancer Screening recommends a stepped approach with annual screening for ages 18 to 35 years, then testing every 5 years until age 60 years at which time screening is stopped.[25]

A major premise of these policy statements is that older women have undergone screening throughout their lives. Several recent studies cast doubt on this assumption. Mandelblatt and colleagues offered cervical cancer screening to urban women aged 65 years and older.[22] Twenty-five percent of their patients had never had a Pap smear, and only 26% had undergone regular screening. A case-controlled study by Celentano et al found that 55% of women over age 65 years with a diagnosis of cervical cancer reported never having had a Pap smear, compared with only 15% for controls, for a relative risk of 14.1.[26] These and other studies indicate that older women may belong to a cohort who have not undergone routine cervical cancer screening. Because recent data suggest that elderly women are underscreened, it would seem prudent to obtain a Pap test at least once if functional status and medical conditions would permit therapy for any lesion discovered (Table 8.5).

Skin Cancer

Cutaneous cancers are among the most common malignancies, and their incidence increases markedly with age. Unlike other malignancies, they are readily visible, providing an opportunity for early detection and treatment. Surprisingly, there is little evidence substantiating the effectiveness of screening programs for this common cancer. The three most common types of skin cancer to be considered for screening programs are basal cell carcinoma, squamous cell carcinoma, and malignant melanoma.

Basal cell carcinoma compromises approximately 80% of the nonmelanoma skin cancers in the United States. This tumor occurs most often in the head and neck area, but it can also be found in sun-protected areas. Squamous cell carcinoma has a much greater proclivity for sun-exposed areas. Seventy-five percent of lesions are found on the face, 15% on the upper extremity, and 10% elsewhere.[27] Unlike basal cell carcinoma, squamous cell has a tendency to metastasize (in 3% to 11% of cases). Malignant melanoma carries a much graver prognosis due to its propensity for metastasis. The incidence of and death rate from melanoma are increasing significantly in the United States, having doubled in the last decade. The prognosis of melanoma is linked closely to the extent of disease at resection. Lesions limited to the epidermis (Clark I) have a 98% 5-year survival, compared with only 44% for those extending to subcutaneous tissue.[27]

There are no data from experimental studies to support the efficacy of a routine screening program. For example, we do not know if an intensive screening program uncovers more cancers at an earlier stage than a strategy that relies on patient recognition. However, we believe that the recommendations from the Canadian Task Force are prudent regarding screening for skin cancer. They recommend inspection by physical examination of sun-exposed skin.[28] The frequency of screening has not been determined, but the screening physical examination is simple and without risk (Table 8.5).

Colorectal Cancer

Colorectal cancer is the second most common malignancy in the United States, with approximately 145,000 new cases and 60,000 deaths occurring annually. Colorectal cancer is predominantly a disease of older people, with over 90% of cancers found in persons over age 50 years. The risk of colorectal cancer begins near age 40 years and doubles for each successive decade, with a maximum incidence at age 80 years. As with other cancers, long-term survival is related to stage at the time of diagnosis. For example, patients with in situ cancer (Duke's A) experience a 5-year survival of over 90% compared with less than 50% for patients with lymph node metastases (Duke's C).[29] The natural history of colon cancer is fairly well understood. The majority of carcinomas arise from premalignant adenomas, which pass through a stage of carcinoma in situ before invasion occurs. The time frame for this progression is probably 5 to 10 years, which defines the lead time for diagnosis.[29] Pathologic evidence also supports the suggestion that adenomatous polyps are precursors to cancer.

There are several screening tests available aimed at detecting the presymptomatic stage of colorectal cancer. The digital rectal examination and the fecal occult blood test (FOBT) are the most commonly used screening tests. Unfortunately, the sensitivity of these tests in the detection of precancerous lesions is low, ranging from 50% to 76%.[30,31] The specificity is not reliably known, as patients who have negative screening results do not systematically undergo definitive diagnostic evaluation. Several large trials have demonstrated a shift to earlier stage disease in patients tested with FOBT compared to controls.[30,32] Several characteristics of FOBT are evident from these trials. First, the overall positive rate in asymptomatic patients is between 2% and 4%. Second, the positive predictive value is only 8% to 10% for cancer and 24% to 29% for adenomas.[31] The predictive value increases with advancing age as the incidence of adenomas increases. However, as yet there is no evidence that screening with FOBT alone reduces mortality from colorectal cancer.

Sigmoidoscopy, either rigid or flexible, is another screening modality. A large trial from the Memorial Sloan-Kettering Cancer Center and Strang Clinic in New York compared screening with rigid sigmoidoscopy alone to screening with FOBT plus sigmoidoscopy. In patients over age 70 years, FOBT plus sigmoidoscopy increased the detection of cancers and benign adenomas,[31] with no increased morbidity from sigmoidoscopy.

We are unaware of any direct evidence showing that a screening program for colon cancer with any combination of screening tests in any age group reduces mortality from colon cancer. FOBT is a universally available test that is acceptable to patients and, when applied to large populations, results in a shift toward more local cancer and precancerous lesions. The test has a high false-positive rate, leading to unnecessary diagnostic evaluation for the majority of patients with positive test results. Sigmoidoscopy improves the detection of precancerous lesions more than FOBT alone, especially in an older population. Despite the lack of evidence to establish the efficacy of screening

for colorectal cancer, the American Cancer Society recommends digital rectal examination and FOBT annually (Table 8.5) for persons over age 50 years, with sigmoidoscopy every 3 to 5 years beginning at age 50 years.[18] This interim recommendation may require modification pending results from ongoing controlled trials.

Prostate Cancer

Prostate cancer is the second most common malignancy in men in the United States and the third most common cause of cancer deaths in men. The incidence and mortality rates for carcinoma of the prostate among black men in the United States are almost twice those for white men. As expected, age has a major effect on the incidence of prostate cancer. The disease is uncommon in men under 50 years of age, but the incidence rate increases rapidly to more than 1,000 per 100,000 man-years for men aged 85 years and older.

Early diagnosis would be attractive if prostate cancer could be identified at an early stage. However, screening tests to detect prostate cancer are disappointing. The digital rectal examination is the current test of choice for the early detection of prostate cancer (Table 8.5). Urologists, using the prostate biopsy as a reference standard, found that the rectal examination was the best screening test, with a sensitivity of 69% and a specificity of 89% when studied in a population with a 23% disease prevalence.[33] Digital rectal examination performed by internists to detect prostate cancer has not been examined. Transrectal ultrasonography of the prostate is a relatively recently developed screening test for prostate cancer. Unfortunately, the sensitivity and specificity of prostatic ultrasound are unsatisfactory for mass screening purposes.[34] Recent studies evaluating prostate ultrasound and digital rectal examination for screening show no benefit of ultrasonography over digital rectal examination alone.[34] Therefore, digital rectal examination remains the best available screening test; it is simple, safe, and performed routinely at physical examination. The American Cancer Society recommends annual digital rectal examinations for men over age 40 years (Table 8.5).[18] As with colorectal cancer screening, there are no data establishing efficacy of screening for prostate cancer.

Lung Cancer

Lung cancer is the leading cause of cancer deaths for both men and women in the United States. The risk of lung cancer is particularly high for male smokers and increases with increasing age. One half of all lung cancer cases occur in patients over age 64 years. The

5-year survival rate for lung cancer has increased very slightly over the past 15 years, remaining below 15%. In the 1970s, the National Cancer Institute Cooperative Early Lung Cancer Detection Program screened more than 30,000 male smokers over age 45 years for lung cancer. This study failed to demonstrate a benefit for the screening strategy.[35] The low incidence of lung cancer in screening studies and the failure to show a reduction in lung cancer mortality have resulted in pessimistic conclusions for the role of screening in lung cancer. The American Cancer Society does not recommend routine lung cancer screening (Table 8.5).[18]

While mass screening for lung cancer is not efficacious, it is less clear whether selective screening for lung cancer in elderly persons may be useful. Population-based epidemiologic data indicate that lung cancer incidence rates are two- to three-fold higher in older age groups. For example, the lung cancer incidence rate for men aged 65 years and older is 483 per 100,000 per year, compared with a rate of 151 per 100,000 per year for men aged 45 to 64 years.[36] In addition, several studies suggest that lung cancer is more likely to be diagnosed at a local stage in older age groups than in younger age groups.[37,38] Additional research is needed to study the efficacy of selective screening in high-risk target groups, such as elderly smokers, before any changes in the American Cancer Society recommendations can be considered.

Cerebrovascular Disease

Stroke is one of the most common causes of death in the United States, ranking third behind heart disease and cancer. Death rates from stroke for men and women increase progressively with age, for example, from 12 per 100,000 in men aged 40 to 44 years to 2,198 per 100,000 in men aged 85 years and older. These death rates are similar for women in all age groups. More than 400,000 new cases of stroke occur annually, and approximately 75% of strokes occur in the distribution of the carotid circulation. Atherosclerotic disease in the carotid artery contributes to cerebral ischemia or infarction by diminishing blood flow distal to a stenotic lesion or because of embolization of material from the site of stenosis or ulceration. Theoretically, if atherosclerotic disease in the carotid arteries could be identified before a stroke occurred, appropriate treatment might prevent some cases of stroke.

A marker for atherosclerotic disease in the extracranial carotid circulation is a neck bruit. The presence of a neck bruit identifies a high-risk patient population whose prevalence of hemodynamically significant disease exceeds 39%.[39] However, despite the high prevalence of hemodynamically significant disease, the incidence of stroke in the absence of premonitory symptoms is only 1%; in patients with the most severe (>75%) carotid artery stenosis, the incidence of stroke is as high as 3% per year.[40] The majority of patients with significant carotid artery disease experience transient neurologic symptoms before the occurrence of irreversible stroke.

The best available diagnostic test for evaluation of carotid artery disease, duplex ultrasonography, has a sensitivity of approximately 85% and a specificity of approximately 90%. Unfortunately, definitive diagnostic evaluation is invasive, requiring conventional carotid angiography, which carries a complication rate between 0.1% and 5%.[41] Screening for carotid artery disease represents a situation where the disease is common and reasonably accurate noninvasive diagnostic strategies are available, but the risk of invasive testing and the risk of carotid endarterectomy may outweigh any benefit from screening.

Feussner and Matchar have used the methods of decision analysis to evaluate the utility of screening for carotid artery disease.[41] The screening strategy used noninvasive diagnostic tests to establish the presence of significant carotid artery disease and invasive carotid angiography to establish the presence of an operable lesion. Because the clinical course of asymptomatic neck bruits is relatively benign, the critical issue is whether the risk of invasive diagnostic testing is offset by the benefit of surgery. Using their decision model, the relative benefit of carotid endarterectomy was plotted as a function of the annual risk of stroke (Fig 8.2). Even with an annual stroke rate of 3%, any benefit of surgery was offset by the risk of definitive diagnostic testing (carotid angiography). In their analysis, the authors assumed a low risk for endarterectomy—1% mortality and 4% stroke rate.[41] In a recent report concerning the appropriateness of carotid endarterectomy, Winslow and colleagues found a 30-day mortality rate exceeding 3% and a stroke rate exceeding 6%.[42] Thus, screening for asymptomatic carotid disease seems neither prudent nor justified (Table 8.4).

One other issue in this area concerns patients with asymptomatic bruits undergoing other major vascular surgery, either peripheral vascular reconstruction or coronary artery bypass grafting. The issue is whether these patients are at increased risk for stroke and whether prophylactic carotid endarterectomy would be efficacious. With regard to major vascular reconstructive surgery, there does not appear to be an increased perioperative stroke rate when neck bruits are present. Therefore, treatment with prophylactic

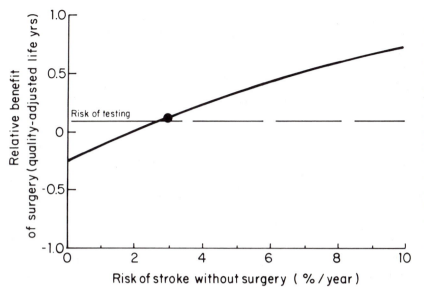

Fig. 8.2. Relative benefit of carotid endarterectomy as a function of the annual risk of stroke. The dashed horizontal line indicates the level of surgical benefit needed to offset the risk from invasive diagnostic testing (carotid angiography). The dot represents the relative benefit from carotid endarterectomy when the annual stroke rate for patients with asymptomatic neck bruits is as high as 3%. At this point any benefit of surgery is offset by the risk of invasive diagnostic testing. For a more complete discussion of the data, see reference 41. Reproduced with permission from: Feussner JR, Matcher DB, when and how to study the carotid arteries. Ann Intern Med. 1988;109:805–818.

endarterectomy is not necessary in those patients. The overall stroke rate is higher for patients with asymptomatic neck bruits undergoing coronary artery bypass grafting. However, the combined risk of diagnostic testing and prophylactic carotid endarterectomy is similar to the perioperative stroke rate for patients undergoing coronary bypass grafting alone. The combination of prophylactic carotid endarterectomy plus coronary artery bypass grafting cannot be justified here either, as the risk of stroke from the combined procedure exceeds the risk from the untreated carotid bruit.[41]

Tuberculosis Screening in the Nursing Home

Infection by *Mycobacterium tuberculosis* has declined with the advent of effective antituberculous therapy. However, the proportion of cases and deaths occurring in people over age 65 years is rising. Powell and Farer reported an increase in the percentage of persons with tuberculosis over the age of 65 years, from 13.8% in 1953 to 28.6% in 1973.[43] Stead and Lofgren's exhaustive cataloging of cases in Arkansas disclosed an even more drastic proportional increase in tuberculosis among the elderly population.[44] In Arkansas in 1961, 18.8% of people with tuberculosis were 65 years of age or older, compared with 50.7% in 1981. Stead and Lofgren reported further that nursing home residents are especially susceptible to tuberculosis; the risk of infection is five times greater for nursing home residents than for nonresidents.[44] No accurate information exists concerning increased death rates from tuberculosis infection in elderly

persons. A general figure of 8.1% for the case fatality rate can be derived from Centers for Disease Control data reported in 1985.

The tuberculin skin test remains the screening method of choice for the detection of tuberculosis among nursing home residents. Stead and To identified three major problems with the tuberculin test in elderly patients: (1) as many as 25% of persons who are clinically ill with tuberculosis may show no reaction to 5 units of tuberculin; (2) some people will show no reaction when tested a first time but will show a significant response when tested with the same dose 1 week later (booster effect); and (3) the great majority of persons who have a positive reaction to the test will show no evidence of clinical infection.[45] The same investigators monitored results of tuberculin skin tests and incidence of infection in 49,467 Arkansas nursing home residents.[45] Their protocol involved intradermal testing (with 5 TU) of all nursing home residents. If less than 10 mm of induration was noted, a second identical dose was given 10 to 21 days later. The test was considered positive when more than 10 mm of induration occurred. The prevalence of positive tests at entry to the nursing home was age dependent, with a peak prevalence of 30% for 60- to 69-year-olds and a low prevalence of 15% of 90- to 99-year-olds. There were 285 recorded cases of tuberculosis (0.6%) among nursing home residents during the study; 256 of these occurred in residents with positive tuberculin tests. The majority of recorded cases (61%) occurred in previous reactors, with 32% occurring in new converters.[46] The authors demonstrated that untreated new converters were 150 times more likely to develop tuberculosis than nonreactors (3% vs 0.02%). Thus, the Arkansas database indicates that the tuberculin test can identify a group of elders at higher risk for tuberculous infection.

Once elders at risk for tuberculosis have been identified, subsequent treatment depends upon the balance between the efficacy of isoniazid prophylaxis and the risk of serious adverse drug effects. Stead et al presented data on nearly 2,000 nursing home residents who were treated with isoniazid for the prevention of tuberculosis.[46] Among nursing home residents who were reactive to tuberculin testing at entry, isoniazid was 85% effective in preventing tuberculosis, but the prevalence of disease was low at 2.5%. Isoniazid was 99.6% effective in preventing tuberculosis among new converters, whose prevalence of disease was 9.7%.[46] Isoniazid was discontinued in 10% of treated patients due to hepatotoxic or other drug reactions; there were no reported deaths from hepatotoxicity.[46] The Public Health Service Surveillance Study reported eight cases of hepatotoxicity per 1,000 patients treated over age 65 years, and the case fatality rate among patients with isoniazid hepatitis was 4.6%.[47]

Based on available evidence, nursing home patients should be screened with a tuberculin skin test at admission and at 1 year if they still reside in the nursing home (Table 8.4). While the incidence of infection is low, treatment is known to be effective, and nursing homes, as closed communities, pose additional risks for epidemic infection.

Deficits in Special Senses

Screening for Hearing Impairment

Hearing loss is common in people over age 65 years, with 25% to 40% suffering some type of hearing impairment. Typically, these people are not deaf but have high-frequency sensorineural hearing loss that diminishes their understanding of conversational speech. Preliminary work by Mulrow and colleagues suggests that functional handicaps are associated with hearing loss in old age.[48] Elderly persons often accept this loss of function, believing that hearing loss is a concomitant of normal aging. Unfortunately, physicians often fail to initiate appropriate evaluation and treatment even when they recognize progressive hearing loss.

The reference standard for establishing hearing impairment is pure tone audiometry; however, initial screening may be possible in the physician's office, thus reducing the need for audiographic testing by audiology specialists. Lichtenstein and colleagues suggest that the combined use of two instruments, the Welch-Allen audioscope and the Hearing Handicapped Inventory for the Elderly–Screening version (HHIE-S), provides a reliable and inexpensive way to screen for hearing loss in the office.[49] Audioscopy alone had a good sensitivity in the detection of hearing impairment (94%) but a reduced specificity of 72%. Use of the two instruments together produced a test accuracy of 83%.[49]

In its 1984 update on the periodic health examination, the Canadian task force suggested that early detection of hearing impairment is efficacious and that screening for this condition should be included in a periodic health examination.[28] Simple strategies such as questioning the patient about hearing loss and assessing the patency of the auditory canal are part of the routine physical examination. Additional screening strategies like those suggested by Lichtenstein et al could be considered as an alternative to pure tone audiometry (Table 8.4).

Screening for Visual Acuity

Nearly 5% of people in the general population have some degree of visual impairment. Visual problems are even more prevalent in elderly persons. More than half of all blind people in the United States are over age 64 years. The leading causes of legal blindness in elderly persons include senile cataracts, glaucoma, diabetic retinopathy, and macular degeneration. Screening for loss of vision should include questioning the patient about visual loss, and if vision is changing visual acuity can be tested readily with a Snellen chart. Funduscopic examination also should be performed to screen for cataracts and diabetic retinopathy. Patients with abnormal or questionable findings should be referred to an ophthalmologist.

The literature suggests that screening for visual problems is efficacious. For example, for persons aged 65 to 74 years, the Framingham Eye Study showed an 18% prevalence of cataracts diminishing visual acuity to 20/30 or worse, increasing to 46% for those aged 75 to 84 years.[50] Straatsma and colleagues demonstrated that a visual acuity of 20/40 or better was achieved in 88% of patients undergoing cataract surgery with lens implantation.[51] Applegate and colleagues prospectively studied almost 300 elderly patients and similarly demonstrated sustained improvement in visual acuity (improved to 20/40) 1 year after cataract surgery and intraocular lens implantation.[52] Applegate et al also demonstrated marked improvement in postoperative physical functioning in elderly patients, including improvements in subjective measures of functional assessment, mental status, and timed manual performance at 1-year follow-up.[52] On the basis of this evidence, it seems prudent to screen elderly patients routinely for visual loss (Table 8.4).

Glaucoma Screening

The National Society to Prevent Blindness estimates that blindness in elderly persons is due to glaucoma in approximately 14% of cases. Open-angle glaucoma accounts for 50% to 80% of all cases of glaucoma.[53] The exact incidence of open-angle glaucoma in elderly persons is unknown. The best available evidence is derived from the Framingham study (Table 8.6), which indicates an increasing prevalence and increasing 5-year incidence with advancing age. The overall prevalence for people over age 55 years was 1.2%, with a peak prevalence of 4.4% in those aged 80 to 84 years.[50]

There are three screening tests available to detect open-angle glaucoma: tonometry, ophthalmoscopy, and perimetry. Tonometry measures the intraocular pressure by measuring the resistance of the eye to an applied force, either with direct contact (Schiotz) or with a noncontact device that shoots a puff of air onto the eye. Ophthalmoscopy is used to assess the surface appearance of the optic nerve, which becomes more cupped as glaucoma progresses, thus increasing the cup-to-disk ratio. Lastly, with perimetry dots of light are projected onto the patient's retina, and the patient's ability to detect the patterns is recorded. While this test can be used in screening, it is expensive, time consuming, and positive only in cases of actual visual loss.

Tonometry is the most common and most studied screening tool. The goal of tonometry is to identify people with ocular hypertension. However, not all people with ocular hypertension have or will develop glaucoma, and those with low-tension glaucoma will be missed by tonometry. Hollows and Graham demonstrated that the prevalence of ocular hypertension in 4,231 people aged 40 to 75 years was about 9%.[53] When people with elevated pressures were evaluated further, only seven (0.16%) were found to have open-angle glaucoma, 75% had persistent elevated pressure

without glaucoma, and 25% had normal pressures at follow-up. Stromberg screened 7,275 people over age 40 years and found that the prevalence of ocular hypertension was 4.5%. Again, on reexamination, only 11 (.15%) of those initially screened had open-angle glaucoma.[54] Other studies have attempted to establish the sensitivity and specificity of tonometry. A community-based study in New Orleans estimated the sensitivity of tonometry for glaucoma to be 72% and the specificity to be 30%, with a threshold level of 22 mm Hg.[55]

Ophthalmoscopy also has been advocated as a screening tool for glaucoma. Unfortunately, the test is limited by significant physician-observer variability as well as poor sensitivity and specificity. Ford and colleagues found the sensitivity of ophthalmoscopy to be 72%, with a specificity of 64%[56] for identifying open-angle glaucoma in a community-based screening program.

The high false-positive rate of both screening tests results in an extraordinarily large cost of further evaluation and potentially unnecessary treatment. Eddy et al performed a cost-effectiveness analysis estimating the results of screening 100,000 asymptomatic men and women over age 40 years.[57] Approximately 4,500-9,000 would have ocular hypertension. Further diagnostic evaluation would identify 160 patients (0.16%) with glaucoma. Of the remaining people with ocular hypertension, 75% would have confirmed ocular hypertension without glaucoma and 25% would have normal repeat pressures. An additional 160 patients with low-tension glaucoma (50% of all glaucoma patients) would not be identified by screening tonometry.

There is little evidence that available treatment modalities affect the clinical course of glaucoma. There are no randomized controlled trials establishing the effectiveness of therapy. Graham randomly assigned 201 patients with ocular hypertension to receive either pilocarpine and epinepherine or saline drops.[58] After 2 years the intraocular pressure decreased significantly in both groups, but there was no difference in the number of patients who progressed to glaucoma. Grant and Burke followed up a cohort of treated patients with early glaucoma and found that 25% were blind at 5 years, 38% at 10 years, and 75% at 20 years.[59]

As with many of the screening strategies that we have examined, the available information is incomplete and imprecise. Available screening tests for the early detection of glaucoma are not sufficiently accurate or reliable. Furthermore, the efficacy of treatment for glaucoma has yet to be established definitively. Until results are available from ongoing controlled

Table 8.6. Estimated prevalence and 5-year incidence of open-angle glaucoma, the Framingham study.*

Age, y	Prevalence, %	Incidence, %
55–59	0.5	0.2
60–64	0.7	0.3
65–69	0.9	0.5
70–74	1.7	0.7
75–79	2.0	1.1
80–84	4.4	. . .
Total	1.2	. . .

* Data modified from reference 50.

trials evaluating treatment efficacy, routine screening for glaucoma cannot be recommended.

Screening for Depression

Depression is a common illness. Blazer and Williams, surveying nearly 1,000 elderly persons, found that 4% had symptoms sufficient to establish the diagnosis of depression.[60] Studies of medically ill patients, whether outpatients or hospitalized, found higher rates of depression using *DSM-III* (Diagnostic & Statistical Manual for Mental Disorders, 3rd Edition) criteria. For example, the rate of major depression was as high as 12%, for elderly medical inpatients[61] and 29% for elderly medical outpatients.[62]

While there is little controversy concerning the high prevalence of depression among elderly medically ill patients, questions remain regarding the validity of screening instruments used to detect depression in such patients. Two recent studies have validated several screening instruments that can be used by physicians to screen for depression. Norris and colleagues studied geriatric medical outpatients and sought to validate the Beck Depression Inventory and the Geriatric Depression Scales.[62] Both screening instruments were compared with the *DSM-III* diagnosis of depression and the research diagnostic criteria for depression. At a threshold score of 10 for both screening instruments, the Beck Depression Inventory had a sensitivity of 89% and a specificity of 82%, and the Geriatric Depression Scale had a sensitivity of 89% and a specificity of 73%. Because of the relatively low specificities, the false-positive rate for either instrument is in the 20% to 30% range.[62] Other potential screening instruments have been validated in hospitalized elderly patients. Koenig and colleagues reported on the Geriatric Depression Scale and correlated results with a *DSM-III* diagnosis of depression.[61] At a cutoff score of 11, the Geriatric Depression Scale had a sensitivity of 92% and a specificity of 89%. With a 12% prevalence of major depression, the Geriatric Depression Scale had a positive predictive value of only 53%. In the same study, the Brief Carroll Depression Rating Scale, at a cutoff score of 6, had a sensitivity of 100%, a specificity of 93%, and a positive predictive value of 66%.[61]

The efficacy of treatment with antidepressant agents has been demonstrated in healthy elders over a short time frame. Low-dose tricyclic antidepressants have been shown also to be safe and effective when used to treat depressive symptoms in frail elderly patients.[63] What has yet to be established, however, is the efficacy and safety of antidepressant therapy in elderly patients whose depression is secondary to a serious medical illness.[64] Future research should seek to establish the value of coupling a systematic screening program for depression in elderly persons, whether medically ill or not, with antidepressant therapy. If the detection rate for screening is sufficiently high and the treatment sufficiently effective and safe, then routine screening for depression in elderly patients would be justified (Table 8.4—see also Chapter 36).

Alcoholism Screening

Alcoholism is the third most common mental health disorder among elderly men, following dementia and anxiety disorders. The 6-month prevalence of alcohol abuse or dependency in a community-based prevalence study was 3.0% to 3.7% for men over age 65 years and less than 1% for elderly women.[65] These prevalence figures were much lower than those for the younger age group. A retrospective review of inpatient treatment of elderly alcoholic patients from the Mayo Clinic reported a higher-than-expected frequency of serious medical disorders among elderly alcoholic patients.[66] While the prevalence of alcoholism generally declines with age, alcoholism remains a serious problem in the elderly population, especially for men, with considerable medical and psychiatric morbidity.

Several screening instruments have been used in an effort to detect alcoholism early. These include instruments like the CAGE questionnaire, the MAST (Michigan Alcoholism Screening Test), and the VAST (Veterans Alcohol Screening Test). The CAGE questionnaire has a sensitivity of 72% to 91%, and a specificity of 77% to 96%. It is easily understood and easy to administer. The CAGE questions are (1) Have you ever felt you should *C*ut down on your drinking? (2) Have people *A*nnoyed you by criticizing your drinking? (3) Have you ever felt bad or *G*uilty about your drinking? and (4) Have you ever had a drink first thing in the morning to steady your nerves or get rid of a hangover (*E*ye-opener)? Mayfield and colleagues, using a threshold of two or more positive responses on the CAGE, determined its sensitivity and specificity to be 81% and 89% respectively.[67] The prevalence of alcoholism in this hosptial-based study was 39%. Magruder-Habib and colleagues validated the VAST against the MAST in medical and surgical outpatients.[68] The VAST is a 24-question instrument and represents an improvement over the MAST; it uses the original MAST questions but also scores those questions on a time scale. The VAST can distinguish current and past alcoholics, making it especially useful in elderly persons. The reported sensitivity and specificity of the MAST are approximately 86% and 81%, respectively[69]; the VAST must be at least that good.

While screening instruments are available, it is unclear whether early detection, even when coupled with treatment, has a favorable influence on patient outcomes. Additional research on the influence of screening on the natural history of alcoholism is necessary before routine alcoholism screening can be recommended (Table 8.4).

Preventive Dentistry

Until recently little was known about the oral health status of elderly people in the United States. In 1985 and 1986, the National Institute of Dental Research conducted a descriptive epidemiologic survey of nearly 21,000 adults aged 18 to 103 years, which included oral examinations performed by dentists trained by the National Institute of Dental Research.[70] The goals of the survey were to assess the prevalence of toothlessness, dental caries, and periodontal disease. Results from the survey indicated a high prevalence of most dental diseases among elderly persons. Of people over 65 years of age, 42% were endentulous and only 2% had all 28 permanent teeth remaining.

Both coronal and root caries were evaluated in the survey. People over age 65 years had an average of 20 decayed or filled coronal surfaces, out of 128 possible surfaces. Young and old groups were similar in that 95% of coronal lesions were filled. This indicates a high level of dental care, at least for the population surveyed. Unlike coronal caries, root caries were three times more extensive in the elderly persons than in younger working adults. Fully 63% of the elderly patients surveyed had root caries, and only about half of these lesions were filled. Periodontal disease also was common in elderly persons. Gingival bleeding was present in 47% of those over age 65 years, and periodontal attachment loss was present in 95%.[70]

The survey also queried people about their past dental care. For elderly people who were dentate, 76% indicated that they had visited a dentist in the past 2 years. Half of those indicated that their main reason for visiting the dentist was a prevention checkup. For individuals who were endentulous, only 29% had visited the dentist within the past 2 years, 70% of those for prosthodontics.[70] The overall conclusions from the survey were that the oral health status of American adults has improved and that more people are keeping their teeth longer (see Chapter 32).

The preferred strategy for early detection of dental disease should focus on periodontal disease and root caries. Physicians should ask patients about their dental care methods during office visits for other reasons and encourage patients to use preventive dental services annually (Table 8.4).[71]

Injury Prevention

Injuries are the sixth leading cause of death in people over age 74 years. Falls account for the majority of these deaths. Even more striking are the statistics attesting to the significant morbidity from falls. For every fall that results in a death, there are approximately 20 that result in a hip fracture. The risk of falling and the risk of serious injury or mortality from falls increases exponentially after the age of 65 years (Fig 8.3). An estimated one third of all people over age 65 years fall each year. Additionally, over one half of those patients admitted to the hospital after a fall will be dead within a year. The cost in terms of morbidity and mortality is clearly significant. Holbrook et al estimated that the annual direct cost of hip fractures alone was approximately $7 billion in the United States.[72]

The incidence of falls in elderly persons and the morbidity from falls varies in different environmental situations. The lowest rates (0.2 to 0.6 falls per person per year) are found in free-living community-based elderly persons. These falls produce less major morbidity with fewer than five percent resulting in a fracture, most of which are in the upper extremity.[73] The highest rate of falls is found in long-term care

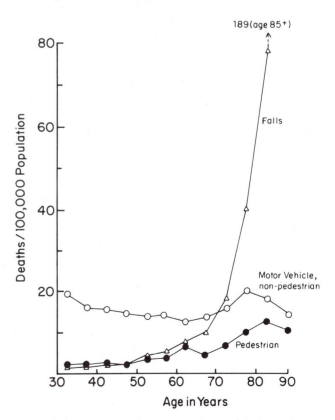

Fig. 8.3. Deaths from falls, pedestrian accidents, and non-pedestrian motor vehicle accidents in the United States in 1977 (data modified from ref. 81).

facilities (two falls per person per year) with up to six percent resulting in hip fractures.[73] Frail elders with multiple medical problems and multiple medications are at high risk for falls.

Despite the frequency of falls in elderly persons, there is surprisingly little information regarding screening for people at risk, and even less information about how to treat those who are indentified at high risk. Some investigators have attempted to correlate poor scores on standardized tests of balance with an increased risk of falls.[73,74] These tests add little predictive information beyond what is available on careful history and physical examination. Interventions in patients identified at high risk for falls have failed to show an impact on falls prevention. More research is needed to identify useful screening strategies and to establish the efficacy of preventive interventions (Table 8.4) (See also Chapter 4).

Osteoporosis Screening

Melton has estimated that at least 1.3 million fractures can be attributed to osteoporosis each year.[75] The burden of disease is almost exclusively borne by older women. Approximately one third of women over age 65 years will have vertebral fractures; for those who survive to age 90 years, one third will have hip fractures. The actual lifetime risk of developing a hip fracture is 15% for women and 5% for men.[75]

The majority of the fractures attributed to osteoporosis occur in the distal radius (Colles' fractures), vertebrae, and hip. The risk of these fractures rises exponentially for women beyond the 7th decade of life (Fig 8.4). Fractures due to osteoporosis are also associated with increased mortality. Hip fractures are associated with an approximate 12% to 20% reduction in 12-month survival.[76] The mortality is greatest for those who sustain fractures after age 75 years, with a tenfold reduction in expected 1-year survival compared with those with similar fractures who are less than age 65 years.[76] There is also a significant risk of prolonged institutionalization among patients who recover from hip fractures; approximately 8% of all nursing home admissions are related to hip fractures.[72]

A reduction in bone mineral content is an eventuality of the aging process. The physician must distinguish individuals with more rapid bone loss, who are at a higher risk of fractures. Women lose 10% to 15% of trabecular bone and a slightly lower percentage of cortical bone each decade after age 50 years. The important feature of this bone loss is that it occurs more rapidly in the 1st decade after menopause.[77] There is no current therapy that has been proved to reverse osteoporosis safely in women 10 years or more beyond the menopause. Unfortunately, if therapy is postponed to the 7th or 8th decade, the majority of bone mass that will be lost already has been lost.

There are three generally available noninvasive screening tests used to detect osteoporosis: single-photon absorptiometry, dual-photon absorptiometry, and quantitative computed tomographic scanning of vertebral bodies. The Health and Public Policy Committee of the American College of Physicians reviewed the performance of these tests and concluded that actual measurements of bone mineral content were more useful for following the course of the disease, monitoring drug complications, and assessing the effect of therapy for osteoporosis than for routine screening.[78] The dilemma in screening for osteoporosis in elderly persons is that a majority of experts, including the National Institutes of Health Consensus Conference on Osteoporosis, advocate estrogen replacement therapy for women after oopherectomy or natural menopause, independent of the results from any screening tests.[79,80] Osteoporosis screening questions are more relevant to younger women than to those over 65 years. Screening and treatment decisions need to be made in the menopausal period, or certainly within 10 years after menopause has occurred.

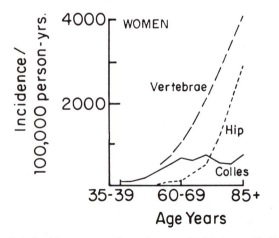

Fig. 8.4. Incidence rates for osteoporotic fractures (Colles, hip, and vertebral) in women, plotted as a function of age at the time of fracture. Reprinted with permission from *The New England Journal of Medicine*, 312, pp. 1677, 1986.

References

1. Wilson JMG, Jungner G. *Principles of Early Disease Detection.* Geneva, Switzerland: World Health Organization; 1968;34:27–39. Public Health Papers.
2. Sackett DL, Haynes RB, Tugwell PX. *Clinical Epidemiology: A Basic Science for Clinical Medicine.* Boston, Mass: Little Brown & Co Inc; 1985:139–155.

3. Eddy DM. The economics of cancer prevention and detection: getting more for less. *Cancer* 1981;47:1200–1209.

4. Working Group on Hypertension in the Elderly. Statement on hypertension in the elderly. *JAMA* 1986;256:70–74.

5. Siegel D, Kuller L, Lazarus NB, et al. Predictors of cardiovascular events and mortality in the Systolic Hypertension in the Elderly Program pilot project. *Am J Epidemiol* 1987;126:385–399.

6. Curb JD, Burhni NO, Entwiske G, et al. Isolated systolic hypertension in 14 communities. *Am J Epidemiol* 1985;121:362–370.

7. Hypertension Detection and Follow-up Cooperative Group. Five-year findings of the Hypertension Detection and Follow-up Program. *JAMA* 1979;242:2572–2577.

8. The Australian Therapeutic Trial in Mild Hypertension, the Management Committee. Treatment of mild hypertension in the elderly. *Med J Aust* 1981;2:398–402.

9. Amery A, Birkenhager W, Brixbe P, et al. Morbidity and mortality results from the European Working Party on Hypertension in the Elderly trial. *Lancet* 1985;293:1146–1151.

10. National Heart, Lung, and Blood Institute Lipid Research Clinics Coronary Primary Prevention Trial results, I. reduction in incidence of coronary heart disease. *JAMA* 1984;251:351–364.

11. Frick MH, Elo Q, Haapa K, et al. Helsinki Heart Study: primary prevention with gemfibrozil in middle age men with dyslipidemia. *N Engl J Med* 1987;317:1237–1245.

12. Anderson KM, Castelli WP, Levy D. Cholesterol and mortality. 30 years of follow-up from the Framingham study. *JAMA* 1987;257:2176–2180.

13. National Heart, Lung, and Blood Institute. Report of the National Cholesterol Education Program Expert Panel on Detection, Evaluation, and Treatment of High Blood Cholesterol in Adults. *Arch Intern Med* 1988;148:36–69.

14. Jajich CL, Ostfeld AM, Freeman DH. Smoking and coronary heart disease in the elderly. *JAMA* 1984;252:2831–2834.

15. Hermanson B, Omenn GS, Kronmal RA, et al. Beneficial six-year outcome of smoking cessation in older men and women with coronary artery disease: results from the CASS Registry. *N Engl J Med* 1988;319:1365–1369.

16. Rogers RL, Myer JS, Judd BW, et al. Abstention from cigarette smoking improves cerebral perfusion among elderly chronic smokers. *JAMA* 1985;253:2970–2974.

17. O'Malley MS, Fletcher SW. Screening for breast cancer with breast self-examination: a critical review. *JAMA* 1987;257:2196–2203.

18. American Cancer Society. Guidelines for the cancer-related checkup. *CA* 1980;30:194–240.

19. Baker LH. Breast Cancer Detection Demonstration Project: five year summary report. *CA* 1982;32:194–225.

20. Shapiro S, Venet W, Strax P, et al. Ten-to-14-year effect of screening on breast cancer mortality. *JNCI* 1982;69:349–355.

21. Tabar L, Gad A, Holmberg LH, et al. Reduction in mortality from breast cancer after mass screening with mammography: randomized trial from the Breast Cancer Screening Working Group of the Swedish National Board of Health and Welfare. *Lancet* 1985;1:829–832.

22. Mandelblatt J, Gobal I, Wisterick M. Gynecological care of elderly women. *JAMA* 1986;256:367–371.

23. Richart RM, Barron BA. Screening strategies for cervical cancer and cervical intraepithelial neoplasia. *CA* 1981;47:1176–1181.

24. National Institute of Health Consensus Statement: cervical cancer screening. *Br Med J* 1980;281:1264–1266.

25. Walton RJ, Blauchet M, Boyes DA. Cervical cancer screening programs. *Can Med Assoc J* 1976;114:1003–1033.

26. Celentano DD, Klassen AC, Weisman CS, et al. Cervical cancer screening practices among older women: results from the Maryland cervical cancer case-control study. *J Clin Epidemiol* 1988;41:531–541.

27. Pollack SV. Skin cancer in the elderly. *Clin Geriatr Med* 1987;3:715–729.

28. Canadian Task Force on the Periodic Health Examination. The periodic health examination, II. 1984 update. *Can Med Assoc J* 1984;130:1278–1285.

29. Winawer SJ, Millard D. Screening for colorectal cancer. *Bull WHO* 1987;65:105–111.

30. Hardcastle JD, Armitage NC, Chamberlain J, et al. Fecal occult blood screening for colorectal cancer in the general population. *Cancer* 1986;58:397–403.

31. Simon JB. Occult blood screening for colorectal cancer: a critical review. *Gastroenterology* 1985;88:820–837.

32. Gilbertsen VA, McHugh RB, Schuman L, et al. The earlier detection of colon cancers: a preliminary report of the results of the occult blood study. *Cancer* 1980;45:2899–2901.

33. Guinan P, Bush I, Ray V, et al. The accuracy of the rectal examination in the diagnosis of prostate carcinoma. *N Engl J Med* 1980;303:499–503.

34. Transrectal ultrasonography in prostate cancer: Diagnostic and Therapeutic Technology Assessment (DATTA). *JAMA* 1988;259:2757–2760.

35. Berlin NI, Buncher RC, Fontana RS, et al. The National Cancer Institute Cooperative Early Lung Cancer Detection Program: results of the initial screen (prevalence)—early lung cancer detection: introduction. *Am Rev Respir Dis* 1984;130:545–549.

36. Baranovsky A, Myers MH. Cancer incidence and survival in patients 65 years of age and older. *CA* 1986;36:27–41.

37. Goodwin JS, Samet JM, Key CR, et al. Stage at diagnosis of cancer varies with age of the patient. *J Am Geriatr Soc* 1986;34:20–26.

38. O'Rourke MA, Feussner JR, Feigel P, et al. Age trends of lung cancer stage at diagnosis: implications for lung cancer screening in the elderly. *JAMA* 1987;258:921–926.

39. Yatsu FM, Grotta JC, Pettigrew LC. Asymptomatic carotid bruit and stenosis. *Semin Neurol* 1986;6:262–266.

40. Chambers BR, Norris JW. Outcome in patients with asymptomatic neck bruits. *N Engl J Med* 1986;315:860–865.

41. Feussner JR, Matchar DB. When and how to study the carotid arteries. *Ann Intern Med* 1988;109:805–818.

42. Winslow CM, Solomon DH, Chassin MR, et al. The appropriateness of carotid endarterectomy. *N Engl J Med* 1988;318:721–727.

43. Powell KE, Farer LS. The rising age of the tuberculosis patient: a sign of success and failure. *J Infect Dis* 1980;142:946–948.

44. Stead WW, Lofgren JP. Does the risk of tuberculosis increase with old age? *J Infect Dis* 1983;147:951–55.

45. Stead WW, To T. The significance of the tuberculin test in elderly person. *Ann Intern Med* 1987;107:837–842.

46. Stead WW, To T, Harrison RW, et al. Benefit-risk reduction in preventive treatment for tuberculosis in elderly persons. *Ann Intern Med* 1987;107:843–845.

47. Kopanoff DE, Snider DE, Caros GJ. Isonazide related hepatitis: a U.S. Public Health Service Cooperative Surveillance Study. *Am Rev Respir Dis* 1978;117:991–1001.

48. Mulrow CD, Agular C, Hill J, et al. Functional handicaps in elderly individuals with hearing impairment. *Clin Res* 1988;36:91A.

49. Lichtenstein MJ, Bess FH, Logan SA. Validation of screening tools for identifying hearing-impaired elderly in primary care. *JAMA* 1988;259:2875–2878.

50. Kahn HA, Lieboritz HM, Ganley JP, et al. The Framingham Eye Study: outline and major prevalence findings. *Am J Epidemiol* 1977;106:17–32.

51. Straatsma BR, Meyer KJ, Bastek JV, et al. Posterior chamber intraocular lens implantation by ophthalmology residents. *Ophthalmology* 1983;90:327–335.

52. Applegate WB, Miller ST, Elam JT, et al. Impact of cataract surgery with lens implantation on vision and physical function in the elderly. *JAMA* 1987;257:1064–1066.

53. Hollows FL, Graham PA. Intraocular pressure, glaucoma, and glaucoma suspects in a defined population. *Br J Ophthalmol* 1966;50:570–586.

54. Stromberg V. Ocular hypertension: frequency, course, and relation to other disorders occurring in glaucoma. *Acta Ophthalmol* 1969;69(suppl):1962.

55. Power EJ, Wagner JL, Duffy BM, eds. *Screening for Open-Angle Glaucoma in the Elderly*. Office of Technology Assessment; 1988.

56. Ford VJ, Zimmerman TJ, Kooner K. A comparison of screening methods for the detection of glaucoma. *Invest Ophthalmol Vis Sci* 1982;22(suppl);257.

57. Eddy DM, Sanders LE, Eddy JF. The value of screening for glaucoma with tonometry. *Surv Ophthalmol* 1983;28:194–205.

58. Graham PA. The definition of preglaucoma: a prospective study. *Trans Ophthalmol Soc UK* 1968;88:153–165.

59. Grant WM, Burke JF. Why do some people go blind from glaucoma? *Ophthalmology* 1982;89:991–998.

60. Blazer D, Williams CD. Epidemiology of dysphoria and depression in an elderly population. *Am J Psychiatry* 1980;137:439–444.

61. Koenig HG, Meador KJ, Cohen HJ, et al. Self-rated depression scales and screening for major depression in the older hospitalized patient with medical illness. *J Am Geriatr Soc* 1988;36:699–706.

62. Norris JT, Gallager D, Wilson A, et al. Assessment of depression in geriatric medical outpatients: the validity of two screening measures. *J Am Geriatr Soc* 1987;35:985–995.

63. Harris RE, Mion LC, Patterson MB, et al. Severe illness in older patients: the association between depressive disorders and functional dependency during the recovery phase. *J Am Geriatr Soc* 1988;36:890–896.

64. Winokur G, Black DW, Nasrallah A. Depression secondary to psychiatric disorders and medical illness. *Am J Psychiatry* 1988;145:233–237.

65. Myers JK, Weissman MM, Tischler GL, et al. Six-month prevalence of psychiatric disorders in three communities. *Arch Gen Psychiatry* 1984;41:959–967.

66. Hurt RD, Finlayson RE, Morse RM, et al. Alcoholism in elderly persons: medical aspects and prognosis of 216 inpatients. *Mayo Clin Proc* 1988;63:753–760.

67. Mayfield D, McLeod G, Hall P. The CAGE questionnaire: validation of a new alcoholism screening instrument. *Am J Psychiatry* 1974;131:1121–1123.

68. Magruder-Habib K, Harris KE, Fraker GG. Validation of the Veterans Alcoholism Screening Test. *J Stud Alcohol* 1982;43:910–926.

69. Mayfield DG, Johnston RGM. Screening techniques and prevalence estimation in alcoholism. In Fann WE, ed. *Phenomenology and Treatment of Alcoholism*. New York, NY: Spectrum Press; 1981.

70. *Oral Health of United States Adults: The National Survey of Oral Health in U.S. Employed Adults and Seniors: 1985–1986—National Findings*. 1987. National Institutes of Health publication 87-2868. US Department of Health and Human Services Public Health Service Washington, D.C.

71. Canadian Task Force on the Periodic Health Examination. *Can Med Assoc J* 1979;121:1–45.

72. Holbrook TL, Grazier K, Kelsey JL, et al. *Frequency of Occurrence, Impact and Cost of Selected Musculoskeletal Conditions in the U.S.* Chicago, Illinois: American Academy of Orthopedic Surgery; 1984.

73. Rubenstein LZ, Robbins AS, Schulman GNP, Rosado J, Osterweil D, Josephson KR. Falls and instability in the elderly. *JAGS* 1988;36:266–78.

74. Nayak US, Gabell A, Simons MA, et al. Measurement of gait imbalance in the elderly. *J Am Geriatr Soc* 1982;30:516–520.

75. See Chapter 5 in this book.

76. Cummings SR, Kelsey JL, Nevitt MC, et al. Epidemiology of osteoporosis and osteoporotic fractures. *Epidemiol Rev* 1985;7:178–208.

77. Richelson LS, Wahner HW, Melton LJ, et al. Relative contributions of aging and estrogen deficiency to postmenopausal bone loss. *N Engl J Med* 1984;311:1273–1276.

78. Health and Public Policy Committee, American College of Physicians. Radiologic methods to evaluate bone mineral content. *Ann Intern Med* 1984;100:908–911.

79. NIH Consensus Conference. Osteoporosis. *JAMA* 1984;252:799–802.

80. Cummings SR, Black D. Should peri-menopausal women be screened for osteoporosis? *Ann Intern Med* 1986;104:817–823.

81. National Safety Council. *Accidents Facts*. Chicago, ILL. 1983.

82. Riggs BL, Melton LJ. Involutional osteoporosis. *N Engl J Med* 1986;314:1676–1686.

9

Patterns of Disease: The Challenge of Multiple Illnesses

Patrick W. Irvine

Much of the illness seen in elderly patients is predictable and may be preventable. Indeed, common patterns of disease recur often enough to provide clinicians with the opportunity to prevent major disabilities. Unfortunately, there is a common feeling that the care of elderly persons is more frustrating than it is rewarding. Many professionals, when overwhelmed by seemingly hopeless circumstances, fail to appreciate how small interventions can make a major impact on the quality of life. Sometimes, elderly patients are seen with one disorder after another as part of an inexorable downhill course, reinforcing beliefs that little can be accomplished for these patients. Most major illnesses, however, do not occur by accident, but result from preexistent conditions that contribute to a greater risk of developing further disease. By minimizing or eliminating antecedent risk factors, clinicians can prevent subsequent disease. Therefore, contrary to prevailing attitudes, a major goal of geriatric medicine is the anticipation of disease, and then accordingly, the prevention of disease.

Basic Clinical Principles of Geriatric Medicine

To understand fully the complex interactions that occur in the health of elderly persons, certain principles of geriatric medicine need emphasis (Table 9.1). These demonstrate the complexity of decision making in this population—perhaps a greater level of complexity than is present in almost any other patient group.

Multiple Diseases Commonly Coexist:

Care of elderly persons forces clinicians to coordinate the effects of multiple active problems. A single disease rarely links concurrent signs and symptoms together into a unified pathophysiologic process. Generally, the unitary disease hypothesis does not apply.[1(pp6–8)] Acute and chronic illnesses in older patients often involve multiple-organ systems that may be related by symptoms, physical findings, functional capacity, and treatment. Psychologic and social consequences of physical conditions also must be considered in the interrelationships.

The Spectrum of Illness Is Relatively Unique:

Certain medical problems tend to appear in old age. Prostate cancer, temporal arteritis, polymyalgia rheumatica, osteopenia, and osteoarthritis represent a few such conditions.[2] Functional disturbances and disabilities associated with illness are more likely to develop. Problems with mobility, cognition, incontinence, and metabolic homeostasis occur frequently.[3] Iatrogenic disorders also are more prominent than among younger patients.[4] Since most conditions known to occur among young adults also occur in elderly persons, the differential diagnosis is broader for each condition. Such a wide spectrum of possibilities available to explain a given condition places greater importance on understanding the relative risk of diseases, and on developing an organized approach to clinical decision making.

Table 9.1 Basic clinical principles of geriatric medicine.

Principle
Multiple diseases commonly coexist
The spectrum of illness is relatively unique
Illness may present in unusual ways
The aging process plays a relatively minor clinical role
Health problems are frequently underreported
Goals of health care become more function based

Illness May Present in Unusual Ways:

The nonspecific presentation of illness is relatively common in advanced age. Classic symptoms frequently are absent. The physiologic response to illness may be tempered in old age either by the physiology of aging or by another pathologic process. Nonspecific symptoms, such as delirium, falls, and incontinence, often herald a serious underlying disorder, although the symptom itself may bear little direct relationship to the diseased organ.[1(pp27-28)] Sepsis without fever is not unusual.[5] Up to 40% of older people with a myocardial infarction may not experience chest pain.[6] Pnuemonia may occur without cough or fever.[5] Onset of an acute abdomen may be marked by delirium or anorexia. Given such unusual presentations, clinicians must be exceedingly vigilant and perceptive.

The Aging Process Plays a Minor Clinical Role:

It is a major challenge to differentiate the effects of "normal" aging from manifestations of treatable disease. Many geriatricians believe that patients, families, and professionals have been too willing to implicate the aging process as the chief cause of maladies in old age. This bias causes treatable conditions to go undiagnosed and untreated. Since humans possess considerable reserve capacity beyond what is necessary for ordinary functional needs, it is unlikely that aging, per se, causes serious symptoms in the absence of associated disease, except in very old individuals. The physiology of aging, although heterogeneous among individuals, generally portends about a 1% decrement in function each year after the age of 35 years. Considering that functional capacity in youth is often fourfold to 10-fold in excess of average needs, most functions will not be seriously compromised in old age unless adverse effects of disease also are present.[7]

Health Problems Are Frequently Underreported:

According to popular stereotypes, older patients are thought of as chronic complainers who say, "every-

thing is always wrong." On average, however, they probably complain no more than other adults when considering the relative number of actual problems that they have to report. In fact, Williamson and colleagues[8] found that older persons complained less often than they should have about their health problems. Recognized in Great Britain as the iceberg of illness, unreported health concerns represent a major problem with some elderly people. Although undoubtedly due to a variety of factors, one plausible explanation rests with prevalent opinions that confuse disease with problems attributed to normal aging. If a problem is considered as normal for age, it is unlikely to be reported. Because of such misconceptions, it is unacceptable in modern medical practice to tell a patient: "it's just old age."

Goals for Health Care Become More Function Based:

In younger patients, health care providers concentrate primarily on curing disease and preventing premature death, while in elderly patients, efforts naturally shift toward maximizing functional independence.[9] This makes the approach toward elderly patients more complex by introducing limited treatment concepts into the care process (see Chapter 4). Difficult decisions regarding prolongation of life, quality of life, and cost of care enter the decision-making equations. Adding "life to years" is a most difficult challenge that requires meticulous attention to functional aspects of medical care.[10]

Important Factors Contributing to Complexity of Illness

To understand fully the nature of illness in elderly persons, important dimensions beyond the physical domain must be appreciated. Within each individual, as illustrated by Fig. 9.1., aging is a process with which chronic and acute conditions interact. In a young individual, aging plays a minor role; yet, as one approaches maximal life span, aging becomes a force of greater and greater importance. The overall health status of each individual represents a synthesis of these three effects.

Three primary domains influence comprehensive function as illustrated in Fig. 9.2. Physical, psychologic, and social function become more interdependent with advancing age; no single area is more important than the other two. Young healthy individuals may demonstrate some independence among these three domains, whereas older persons characteristically develop a tightly linked dependency. That these domains

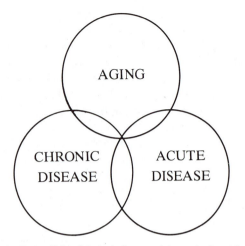

Fig. 9.1. Overall health is influenced by relationships that exist among aging, chronic disease, and acute disease. Modified from Kane RL. Essentials of Geriatrics, pg. 36. McGraw-Hill: 1984.

are so interdependent in elderly persons emphasizes that, in a truly geriatric patient, a physician cannot meet all the needs alone and that an interdisciplinary team approach is imperative for effective comprehensive care.

Interrelationships of Illnesses

Several chronic diseases often coexist in advanced age. When this occurs, acute and chronic conditions interact with one another, influencing their clinical expression, detection, and treatment. Some of the important clinical effects of disease-disease interactions are described in Table 9.2.

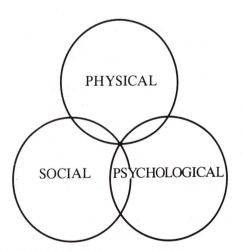

Fig. 9.2. Social, psychological, and physical domains become more interdependent with advancing age. Modified from Kane, RL. Essentials of Geriatrics, pg. 36. McGraw-Hill: 1984.

Table 9.2 Interrelationships of disease.

Relationship	Example
Masks expression	Disease X prevents expression of disease Y
Alters presentation	Disease X presents unusually secondary to disease Y
Alters therapy	Treatment of disease X is modified by disease Y
Enhances pathologic condition	Disease X intensifies disease Y
Simulates disease	Disease X appears identical to disease Y
Cascades of disease	Disease X leads to disease Y, which leads to disease Z, and so on
Cycles of disease	Disease X contributes to disease Y, which contributes to disease X, and so on

Disease Expression May Be Masked:

Masking occurs when one disease prevents the expression of a coexistent disease. Rheumatoid arthritis, for example, may mask coronary artery disease and angina pectoris. Since a patient with rheumatoid arthritis may be unable to exercise sufficiently to exceed myocardial oxygen demand and thus to experience anginal pain, angina may not occur until coronary artery disease becomes very advanced. A myocardial infarction or angina at rest might be the first symptom.

Similar masking may occur in patients with coexistent chronic obstructive pulmonary disease (COPD) and peripheral arterial vascular disease. Early ischemic symptoms in the lower extremities or claudication may not be experienced because exercise tolerance is limited primarily by COPD.

When masking occurs, symptoms and signs of disease may be absent or subtle before the onset of advanced disease states. This places additional importance on careful histories and physical examinations for patients with multiple illnesses.

Disease Presentation May Be Altered:

Diseases also may influence the manner in which another pathologic process presents itself. For example, hyperthyroidism may be more likely to present as supraventricular tachycardia in an individual with preexistent cardiac conduction disease.[11] In this circumstance, the cardiac conduction system would represent the "weakest link in the chain" of organ systems; its threshold for dysfunction may be lower because of preexistent disease. Similarly, when an individual with Alzheimer's disease develops a urinary tract infection, deterioration in cognition may be the only clinical clue; cognitive impairment leaves the individual unable to recognize and express urinary symptoms. Aging-related alterations in physiology, reduced ability to report disease, and the presence of coexistent diseases modify the presentation of illness among elderly persons.

Disease Treatment May Need to Be Altered:

When diseases coexist, the treatment of one condition may require consideration of another pathologic condition that is present. This common clinical problem is illustrated by certain drug therapy for hypertension in the presence of coexistent COPD. Whereas a β-blocking agent, such as propranolol, might be an excellent choice as the second-step antihypertensive in the absence of COPD, it is an extremely poor choice with COPD present. Similarly, an ophthalmic β-blocking agent, such as timolol maleate (Timoptic), might be a less desirable choice for the treatment of glaucoma for that same patient. Treatment incompatibilities are not unfamiliar to physicians; but, in elderly patients with greater numbers of coexistent chronic illnesses and increased use of medications, careful consideration of such disease-therapy interactions is very important.

Diseases May Enhance Pathologic Conditions of Other Diseases:

Illnesses may aggravate other diseases. For example, when an individual with osteoarthritis of the left hip and knee sprains the right ankle, greater stress will be transferred to the arthritic left hip and knee in ambulation. The patient may return 1 or 2 weeks later with increased pain in the uninjured hip or knee. Consider an individual with symptomatic ischemic heart disease and hypothyroidism: unless thyroid replacement is initiated in extremely small doses and advanced very slowly, life-threatening ischemia or arrhythmias may occur.

Diseases May Simulate Other Diseases:

Diseases commonly appear to be like other conditions. That several individual diagnoses might cause the same clinical constellation demonstrates this point. Often, symptoms of acid-peptic disease simulate ischemia of coronary artery disease. By history, intermittent claudication may sound exactly like bursitis, osteoarthritis, or lumbar spinal stenosis. Depression may be misdiagnosed as dementia or coexist with dementia in an elderly patient. Sorting out the differential diagnosis, therefore, becomes a major challenge as the history, physical examination, and laboratory data are influenced by the presence of other illnesses.

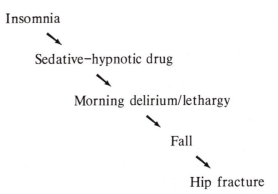

Fig. 9.3. Cascade of drug-induced illness.

Diseases May Contribute to a Cascade of Problems:

In this clinical scenario, an initial problem leads to a new condition that contributes to the development of a third problem, and so on. Such a cascade develops when the stepwise effects of several interdependent problems lead successively to other difficulties. Whereas cascades may be simple, they also may be complex, involving multiple-organ systems and several complications.

One simple example points out how the administration of a sedative-hypnotic medication can contribute to an untoward event, such as a hip fracture, as one of several possible adverse consequences (Fig 9.3.). Particularly if the sedative-hypnotic agent accumulates in an elderly person, such as may occur with flurazepam, the medication may impair cognitive performance.[12] If not properly evaluated, the patient might lose control of personal care or even be placed in a nursing home. If the sleeping medication had never been prescribed, the hip fracture or concerns over cognition might never have resulted.

Consider a second example whereby an elderly person receives phenytoin to prevent seizures (Fig. 9.4.). The drug is prescribed at a dose that produces

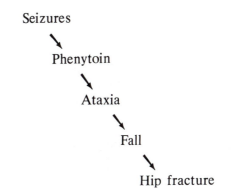

Fig. 9.4. Cascade of drug-induced illness.

therapeutic serum levels, and the individual does not experience impairment of balance under normal conditions. Under stressed conditions, however, such as a slip requiring optimum gait and balance performance, the patient may fall due in part to subclinical effects of phenytoin. When the fall occurs and results in a fractured hip, the fracture might be considered as the endpoint of a cascade of events that began with the onset of seizures.

In a third example, consider an older individual who has become constipated by inactivity; the constipation causes bloating, anorexia, and vomiting; adequate fluids no longer are ingested, and mild dehydration ensues; and dehydration leads to symptomatic orthostatic hypotension that contributes to a serious fall (Fig. 9.5.). Through mechanisms illustrated by this cascade, benign conditions, such as constipation, lead to serious disorders. Being aware of such common cascade effects permits prevention of adverse outcomes.

Diseases May Become Self-Nurturing and Cyclical:

When several related problems become self-nurturing, a cycle or "vicious circle" may result.[13] Cycles rarely stand alone; they are usually associated with cascade effects. Figure 9.6. illustrates how delirium and dehydration often relate in a cyclical manner. In the initial stages, when delirium and dehydration are subclinical, attempts of the kidneys to conserve salt and water may be mildly impaired by the effects of aging.[14] The degree of dehydration may enhance the stress placed on compromised homeostatic mechanisms, creating a progressive cycle that eventually leads to clinical dehydration and delirium. The development of clinical dehydration and delirium is even more probable when other illnesses coexist. For example, diuretic therapy

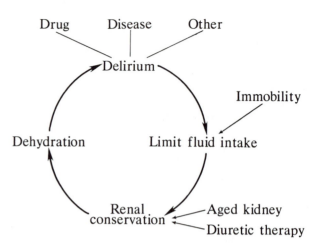

Fig. 9.6. Cycle of delirium and dehydration.

for hypertension would intensify salt and water loss, and immobility would limit access to additional fluids.

A second example illustrates how a febrile person may enter a self-perpetrating cycle (Fig. 9.7.). As the patient becomes dehydrated, delirium ensues, and

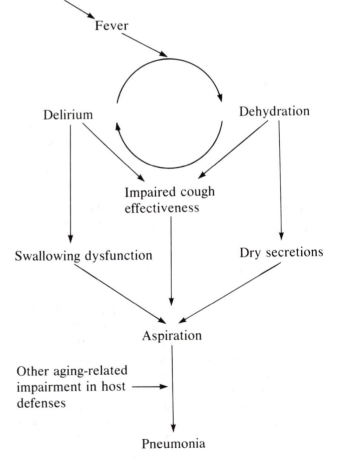

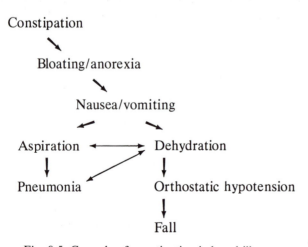

Fig. 9.5. Cascade of constipation-induced illness.

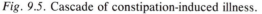

Fig. 9.7. Cycle and cascades leading to pneumonia.

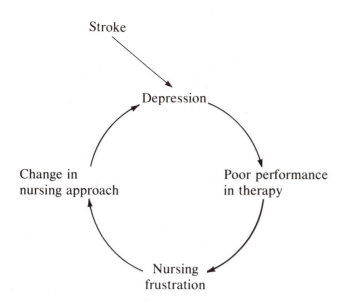

Stroke

Depression

Change in
nursing approach

Poor performance
in therapy

Nursing
frustration

Fig. 9.8. Cycle of depression and staff response.

secretions dry out. These conditions promote increased microaspiration, decreased cough reflex and force, and immobility. All of these factors contribute to the eventual development of pneumonia. The initiating event in this scenario was the dehydration-delirium cycle, which emphasizes the critical importance of preventing dehydration in acute illness.

In a third example, consider an older patient who suffers a stroke and becomes depressed (Fig. 9.8.) One manifestation of the depressive illness—poor performance in self-care activities on a hospital ward—is noted by the professional staff, and coordinated efforts to improve self-care activities are undertaken. Perhaps because of their lack of success with rehabiliation, the nursing staff confront the patient with failure; this strategy causes counterproductive patient frustration, anger, and further depression.

This cycle illustrates how members of the health care team play key roles in clinical care. Negative communications about patient performance in a clinical nursing conference may be passed on from shift to shift and even amplified if the team is not interactive and introspective. In other words, members of the professional team participate in these patterns of care. In some cases, they participate as productive professionals, while in other cases, they contribute to deterioration in patient status.

Despite these potential problems, clinical care is approached most effectively through professional teams because of the complexity of disease patterns that occur among elderly patients. Interdisciplinary teams dissect out the components of disease and dysfunction more successfully than physicians who work alone. When teams are orchestrated well, true integration of the social, psychological, and physical aspects of care is accomplished.

References

1. Hodkinson HM. How elderly patients are different. In: Harrison RJ, Asscher AW, eds. *An Outline of Geriatrics.* Orlando, Fla: Academic Press Inc; 1975.
2. Besdine RW. Geriatric medicine: an overview. In: Eisdorfer C, ed. *Annual Review of Gerontology and Geriatrics.* New York, NY: Springer-Verlag NY Inc; 1980;1:140–145.
3. Cape R. *Aging: Its Complex Management.* New York, NY: Harper & Row Publishers Inc; 1978:81–82.
4. Steel K, Gertman PM, Crescenzi C, et al. Iatrogenic illness on a general medical service at a university hospital. *N Engl J Med.* 1981;304:638–666.
5. Smith IM. Infections in the elderly. *Hosp Pract Off.* 1982;17:69–85.
6. Tinker GM. Clinical presentation of myocardial infarction in the elderly. *Age Aging.* 1981;10:237–240.
7. Fries JF. Aging, natural death, and the compression of morbidity. *N Engl J Med.* 1980;202:130–135.
8. Williamson J, Stokoe IH, Gray S, et al. Old people at home: their unreported needs. *Lancet.* 1964;1:1117–1120.
9. Kane RL, Solomon DH, Beck JC, et al. *Geriatrics in the United States: Manpower Projections and Training Considerations.* Santa Monica, Calif: Rand Corp; 1980.
10. Cluff LE. Chronic disease function and quality of care. *J Chronic Dis.* 1981;34:299–304.
11. Blum M. Thyroid function and disease in the elderly. *Hosp Pract Off.* 1981;16:105–116.
12. Conrad KA, Bressler R. Drug therapy for the elderly. St Louis, Mo: CV Mosby Co; 1982;73.
13. Exton-Smith AN, Overstall PW. *Geriatrics.* Lancaster, England: MTP Press Ltd;1979;1984.
14. Epstein M. Effects of aging on the kidney. *FASEB J.* 1979;38:168–171.
15. Kane RL, Ouslander JG, Abrass IB, eds. Essentials of clinical geriatrics. New York: McGraw-Hill Book Company; 1984.

10

Clinical Evaluation of the Patient

Christine K. Cassel, John R. Walsh, Mary Shepard, and Don Riesenberg

Much of what transpires between physician and patient in the examination room is not measurable, but nonetheless, a major effort has been expended recently to understand and teach clinical evaluation.[1,2] The objectives of this effort are to encourage physicians to appreciate patients in the context of their life histories, to enhance humanism and ethical conduct, and to enable physicians to communicate more effectively, especially to listen well.

Such goals are commensurate with the geriatrician's focus on the whole patient. Nowhere is the need greater to incorporate social and functional findings into the more traditional medical evaluation than in the assessment of an elderly patient. Here clinician involvement often occurs at critical life junctures, such as the time of nursing home placement, loss of independence due to a stroke, loss of family support due to the death of a significant other, or during the throes of a terminal illness. In such settings, information gathering and problem management require considerable skill, time, and effort to achieve an optimal outcome for the patient.

This chapter discusses the general aspects of an interview and physical examination that are peculiar to the older population; more detailed descriptions of specialized areas will be found in other chapters. An attitude contaminated with untrue biases interferes with an appropriate assessment of elderly persons. Therapeutic nihilism predictably leads to a superficial evaluation. Similarly, in situations that are dominated by psychiatric or psychosocial problems, a thorough medical examination should not be neglected. Thoroughness is, in fact, the guiding principle that pro-duces useful data that will contribute to appropriate diagnostic and therapeutic decision making. However, a clinician should pace the evaluation according to the urgency of the clinical presentation and a patient's stamina. The complete history and physical examination, which we physicians consider so necessary, may be too tiring to finish in a single session. In the absence of emergent conditions, and even then with regard to other parts of a complete evaluation, it is far better to break the complete assessment up throughout several days or several clinic visits.

Special Considerations

Evaluation of Common Disorders

The problem of underreporting and underinvestigation is well known in geriatrics. An example of a condition that is found more commonly in the older population, but often is underinvestigated and untreated, is falling. A history of falling may not be volunteered by an older person: many consider such an event too embarrassing to discuss or an inevitable part of old age. The interviewer specifically must inquire about falls, especially in persons aged more than 75 years, for whom the incidence of falls increases, parallel to that of intellectual, neurologic, and physical impairment. The evaluation of falls is the subject of Chapter 40; our intent here is to emphasize that uncovering such problems may require active pursuit by the interviewer. The patient's not volunteering information on such matters cannot be considered negative evidence;

too often physicians control the interview in a way that discourages full disclosure.[3] Aggressively seeking and evaluating all of the information available, such as in the case of falls, may be time consuming, but often prevents serious morbidity.

Atypical Presentation of Disease

Disease presentation is not always straightforward in an elderly person for a variety of reasons.[4] Persons with impaired cognitive abilities are unable to relate symptoms and may manifest illness through behavioral changes that are noted by attentive care-givers. Pneumonia, sepsis, pyelonephritis, stroke, and congestive heart failure may present with minimal symptoms other than cognitive or behavioral changes. Even in previously health elderly persons, myocardial infarction and other major organ system diseases may initially produce such nonspecific changes as confusion and anorexia.

Barriers to Communication

Many elderly persons suffer from auditory and visual impairments. An examiner should optimize a patient's sight and hearing to enhance information gathering. If a patient has eyeglasses and a hearing aid, they should be used during the interview. For a hearing impairment, the examiner should sit directly in front of the patient at eye level in a well-lighted room and speak slowly and distinctly. Refrain from putting a hand near the mouth when speaking; not only does this decrease the volume of the voice, but many people compensate for a hearing loss by lipreading. Shouting often is inappropriate (see below).

Functional Assessment

The American College of Physicians,[5] as well as other national organizations involved in geriatric medicine,[6] recognize comprehensive functional assessment as an important tool in geriatric practice. The complex interaction of cognitive, medical, and functional decline in frail elderly persons, as well as their high risk of iatrogenesis, institutionalization, and social and economic deprivation, mandates inclusion of functional assessment skills in undergraduate and graduate medical curricula.

Unlike younger individuals whose functional limitations are resolved completely during hospitalization (eg, a broken femur after a skiing accident), an older person is at greater risk for long-term impairment. Hence, functional assessment is necessary to determine the effect of physical and mental impairment on his or her ability to perform activities of daily living.

An accurate sense of the range of possible functional outcomes in a given patient will provide for more effective disposition planning and more appropriate rehabilitation prescribing. Chapter 6 covers the details of functional assessment, including examples of specific instruments and their use.

Home Living Assessment

It is not always practical for an older individual to visit a physician every time his or her condition changes. Some system for home evaluation is useful, especially for patients with major functional limitations that compromise mobility. The evaluation of any person with a functional impairment is not complete without a home visit by a physician, visiting nurse, social worker, or rehabilitation team. The objective of such a visit is to evaluate the adequacy of the living arrangements to meet an elderly person's functional needs. Particular importance is placed on safety, hygiene, physical comfort, social supports, nutrition, and medication compliance.

Social Network

Social networks are invaluable sources of help for the activities of daily living and in times of crisis. The people who make up such networks may include family, neighbors, friends, and church or club members. It is good planning to record names and telephone numbers in the event that an urgent need arises. The decision to involve others in a patient's care is, of course, made in consultation with the patient.

Financial Assessment

Physicians should be aware of a patient's financial situation and may need to tailor the evaluation and management more carefully for a person with limited financial resources. This does not mean, however, that needed tests or procedures should be foregone because of their costs. Social work assistance is crucial to sort through and uncover sources of reimbursement and special programs. Insurance policies may have been forgotten and should be scrutinized for benefits that Medicare excludes. In addition, special community programs may provide assistance.

Nutritional Assessment

Multiple factors contribute to the nutritional state of an older person, and a thorough nutritional assessment may suggest modifications that could improve well-being (see Chapter 41). Nutritional deficiencies stem from various sources. Some may be medical; others may involve inadequate funds to purchase food, an inability to shop, or an omission of meals due to forgetfulness. Some people on fixed incomes feed their pets rather than themselves. A disinterest in food may be a manifestation of depression or may be due to cancer, congestive heart failure, infection, or gastrointestinal disease. Visual and hearing impairments can produce difficulty in negotiating the marketplace, while a diminished sense of taste and smell, common in elderly persons, limits interest in food. Physical problems such as stroke, arthritis, or Parkinson's disease, can interfere with preparing food, to say nothing of getting it from the plate to the mouth. Finally, some medications affect appetite and eating, eg, the dry mouth caused by anticholinergic drugs.

Preventive Measures

Health maintenance and preventive medicine are legitimate areas of interest in elderly age groups as in younger age groups.[7] Evaluating and advising an elderly person on good nutrition is just one of many areas. The cessation of smoking and moderation in the use of alcohol should be advocated. Women should be encouraged to learn breast self-examination.

Patients should be asked about pneumococcal, influenza, and tetanus immunizations, and the dates should be recorded in the problem list or another conspicuous place in a patient's record. The prevention of falls, removal of causes of incontinence, and avoidance of iatrogenesis also are preventive components of geriatrics. Chapter 8 deals with the complex issue of periodic screening for disease in elderly persons.

Medication

A notorious cause of illness and disability in an elderly person is medication side effects. Any medication (but especially those recently added or changed in dosage) should be suspect when new symptoms arise. Elderly persons not only take multiple medications, but they are subject to more errors because of poor vision, memory impairment, and limited dexterity. A review of all medications taken, including over-the-counter drugs, as well as medications found in the medicine chest on a home visit, is indicated. Inquiry may reveal that a patient is taking medicine that has been prescribed for a spouse or a neighbor. Often, it is helpful to ask a patient or spouse to bring all medicines, including over-the-counter preparations, to a subsequent clinic visit. If there are suspected problems of drug compliance, a home visit by a physician or nurse may reveal the cause.

The Value History

The technologic accoutrements of modern medicine have created the need, fully discussed in Chapter 4, for the physician and patient to have an understanding about the vigor with which life-prolonging measures will be pursued, in the event of a critical or terminal illness. Part of such an understanding comes from knowledge about the patient as a person and his or her past values and beliefs—the so-called value history.[8] It is never too early for the geriatrician to begin such a dialogue, building to a full understanding with subsequent sessions with the patient and, where appropriate, the family.

History Taking in Elderly Patients

Source and Reliability

Unless patients are unable to give an adequate history because of obtundation or severe dementia, they should be interviewed alone. Patients with diminished cognitive function often can provide useful information, and a clinician may even be unaware of the cognitive defect until a mental status examination is done. Subsequent discussions with friends and family may reveal behavioral problems, incontinence, apathy, weight loss, sleep disturbances, and other problems that have not been mentioned by a patient. Initially, it is best for a physician to interview the person privately to allow discussion of concerns, fears, and symptoms that he or she may be reluctant to share with spouse, children, or friends. However, each case must be individualized, and some patients may prefer to be interviewed with a care-giver in attendance.

Old medical records are an invaluable source of information about past illnesses and surgeries. Even mentally intact individuals often have gross misunderstandings about their medical history and past treatments.

Chief Complaint(s)

Multiple problems are typical with older persons, and the clinician should seek multiple areas of concern rather than a single chief complaint. One must be patient in eliciting problems—the major source of a patient's distress may be hidden in a rather rambling story. Sometimes, while ascertaining the reason for a visit to a physician, other problems with more significant health consequences are uncovered. Thus, incontinence, falls, weight loss, and anorexia often are discovered only by direct questioning. A patient may consider these to be a consequence of aging or be fearful because he or she perceives them as very serious. The major problem may not be of concern to the patient, but rather one that is observed by the care-giver. A patient and physician each may be concerned with different problems; the problems perceived by both must be addressed. A patient's complaint should never be ignored.

Present Illness

A present illness provides the opportunity to explore the chief complaints, which may be various combinations of physical, mental, and social problems. The possibility that changes in the environment may intensify confusion or even bring on incontinence in a minimally demented indivual should be explored. Similarly, a patient with well-compensated heart failure may have an exacerbation after moving to a new living situation, if inadequate attention is given to the amount of salt used in meal preparation.

Medical History

A list of surgeries, the subsequent course, and complications is useful in predicting the future risk of anesthesia and surgery. Facts about a tumor type, extent, and nodal involvement that are obtained from surgical and pathology reports should be noted in the case of cancer surgery.

Major medical illnesses and complications, both self-limited, eg, pneumonia, and chronic, eg, diabetes, should be outlined, and all treatments and hospitalizations should be reviewed. A wallet-sized card with a list of diagnoses and medications, as well as a copy of an electrocardiogram, can be very useful to an unfamiliar physician in emergency situations.

Drug Allergies

Persons with serious allergies, regardless of age, should be encouraged to wear a medi-alert bracelet or necklace. In the event a patient becomes unconscious, it is to be hoped that the physician will have had the foresight to note any and all drug allergies in the problem list of the permanent medical record.

Habits

Alcohol, tobacco, tea, coffee, and other drug use (licit or illicit) should be quantitated. Terms, such as *alcohol* (or) *tobacco abuser,* do not accurately portray these problems late in life. Special attention needs to

be focused on a patient for whom this is a new pattern; older people sometimes begin to use alcohol in an attempt to cope with losses and loneliness during a period of uncertainty. They deny or minimize the use of alcohol in medical interviews. Relatives and friends may first bring the problem to a physician's attention. Occult alcoholism may provide an explanation for enigmatic falling episodes, confusional periods, or nutritional deficiencies.

Family History

Most familial diseases have manifestations in earlier adulthood and do not pertain to elderly individuals. It is valuable to inquire about contact with tuberculosis in family members. Alzheimer's disease and some malignant diseases may have a genetic predisposition that is manifested in later years. The family history also can provide information relevant to physician-patient rapport. For example, a person's attitude about certain diseases or about the medical profession may stem from earlier experiences: if a family member has had complications of an illness, this knowledge may instill fear in a patient.

Review of Systems

This inventory is designed to survey the problems that are known to be occult, but nevertheless common, in the elderly population. The goal is to uncover these symptoms early enough to plan an intervention for the patient's benefit. A thorough review of systems requires time and patience, especially with a slowly responsive or partially deaf patient, but it is well worth the effort if treatable or modifiable conditions are uncovered.

Instead of the usual typical set of symptoms, the only evidence of physical or mental health impairment may be an insidious, slowly progressive decline in function. A disinterest in life, weight loss, and agitated or reclusive behavior all may be subtle manifestations of thyroid disease, chronic infection, malignancy, uremia, dementia, an adverse drug effect, congestive heart failure, or depression. These vague symptoms may be noted initially by a neighbor or relative rather than by the patient, who may be unaware, or unwilling to admit, that anything is wrong. A careful review of the duration of decline and the temporal relationship to the death of a loved one, a move to a new residence, or a change in drug dosage may provide an answer. As mentioned previously, the symptoms of depression, anorexia, vague and poorly characterized pain, or confusion should not be attributed to old age alone, until a careful investigation has been carried out to exclude other diagnoses.

The *skin* of an elderly person is notably thin, and increased capillary fragility results in a history of easy bruisability (senile purpura). However, bruising also may reflect a vitamin deficiency, coagulopathy, or elderly abuse. Pruritus, with or without a rash, should arouse suspicion of liver disease or environmental factors, eg, new soap or clothing.

Diminished *hearing* may be noticed by an elderly person's family or friends before the patient is aware of it. Some persons purposely ignore it, because they wish to avoid a hearing aid and the negative stigma of aging that is associated with such devices. Hearing loss may invoke paranoia in older persons who hear sounds indistinctly and incorrectly assume that a conversation is about them, which generates feelings of resentment and hostility. Hearing loss restricts daily activities by preventing telephone conversations, listening to the radio, and social interactions.

Presbycusis is a gradual bilateral loss of hearing in an older person that sometimes is accompanied by a ringing in the ears. There is difficulty in understanding speech, especially with simultaneous background noise and other conversations. The presence of disruptive background noise at social gatherings, stores, and restaurants sometimes makes communication so taxing that one retreats from social interactions. High-frequency sounds are difficult for an elderly person to hear, and certain loud sounds are uncomfortable. A person may hear only parts of words, not the consonants (which are of a higher frequency), but only the lower frequency vowels. Speaking loudly or shouting often causes distortion by increasing the higher frequency sounds. Not all older adults are hard of hearing, and those who are not resent being shouted at.

Dyspnea is a commonly elicited symptom that may indicate cardiac or pulmonary disease. Dyspnea alone may be an anginal equivalent, with the shortness of breath overshadowing or replacing chest pain as the marker of coronary insufficiency.[9] Weakness and confusion alone may be the initial symptoms of congestive heart failure. Similarly, the first manifestation of a myocardial infarction is variable. An older person may feel weak and faint or experience syncope in the absence of any chest pain. Classic chest pain occurs in only 25% of older patients, although some form of chest discomfort is reported by about 60%.[9]

Weakness, faintness, vertigo, and syncope are common complaints that lead to falls. Postural hypotension is just one of the many possible causes. The worsening of a chronic stable anginal pattern or of congestive heart failure should alert a physician to consider thyrotoxicosis, a change in dietary habits, or

medication noncompliance. *Pedal edema* often is not cardiac in origin; chronic venous insufficiency, hypoproteinemia, liver disease, and sedentary habits are among the causes of this common complaint.

Anorexia may occur with infection, depression, dementia, or medication side effects, and it need not imply the presence of a gastrointestinal pathologic condition, which may, however, be of an insidious onset with minimal symptoms of early satiety or weight loss. *Dysphagia* is a common problem that may be due to motility disorders, mass lesions, strictures, or pseudobulbar palsy. Classically, liquids are more troublesome with a neuromuscular or motility disorder, while solids are more difficult for those with intraluminal obstructions.

Constipation can be particularly troublesome in a sedentary person, especially with a diet that contains new bulk foods, poor fluid intake, and medications with anticholinergic side effects. Diarrhea may have various causes, but if it alternates with constipation, than one should be suspicious of a fecal inpaction or overuse of laxatives.

Rectal bleeding has multiple causes that include hemorrhoids, vascular lesions, inflammatory bowel disease, neoplasms (benign and malignant), and diverticula. This should be investigated as in any other age group. Fecal incontinence always should be thoroughly evaluated.

Frequency of urination (especially nocturia) and *urinary incontinence* lead to major disabilities. Thorough questioning is indicated to evaluate possible diabetes, bladder infection, prostrate obstruction, and the many other causes of incontinence, so that studies can be obtained for treatment or referral to a urologist (see Chapters 21 and 38). *Nocturia* not only is a nuisance, but it may subject an individual to injuries from accidental falls at night; dysuria and frequency may point to an infection. The patient should be questioned about evening fluid intake or the administration of an afternoon diuretic as possible modifiable causes. Nevertheless, elderly persons are known to excrete a larger proportion of the 24-hour urine volume overnight, in the absence of a urinary pathologic condition.

Concerns about *sexuality* are common among medical outpatients, and neither age nor sex influence the prevalence of sexual problems.[10] Physicians should try to be tactfully candid on the topic of sexuality. Open-ended questions, such as "Is your sexual life as fulfilling as you would like it?" indicate a willingness to discuss these problems.

Geriatricians should be alert to clues about mental health problems while they are taking the history. Because of the reluctance of some older persons to discuss emotional difficulties, and because of the lack of familiarity with such illnesses among many non-psychiatrists, a short questionnaire can improve recognition and management of mental health problems.[11]

Physical Examination

The physical examination begins by observing a patient before the interview. As he or she enters the room, sits, stands, and answers questions, hearing, visual, and neurologic disabilities may be obvious immediately.

Vital Signs

Blood pressure should be taken in both arms, although differential readings that indicate a possible subclavian steal syndrome are uncommon. More importantly, determinations should be made with a patient lying, standing, and sitting. Normal asymptomatic elderly patients are unlikely to demonstrate significant orthostatic hypotension, which is defined as a drop of 20 mm Hg or more in systolic pressure on standing.[12] When such a drop is observed, it may or may not be symptomatic. If it is accompanied by tachycardia, the cause may be volume depletion due to dehydration or blood loss. When there is no increase in heart rate, an autonomic nervous system disturbance and the ingestion of β-blocking medication should be considered as possible causes.

The *temperature* should be routinely measured. Poor thermoregulatory control that is manifested by cold and heat intolerance is a consequence of autonomic nervous system dysfunction. The conservation of heat (via cutaneous vasconstriction) and increase in heat production (via shivering) are impaired in elderly persons. Conversely, older individuals have a diminished capacity for sweating, which impairs the lowering of body temperature in an overheated environment. Physicians should have available low-reading rectal thermometers to detect hypothermia (see Chapter 44).

Weight is a useful measurement; unfortunately, it often is not recorded. It may be used both to monitor a patient's nutritional status and to judge the efficacy of diuretic therapy for congestive heart failure. Several recordings over periods of time provide reference information when patients complain of weight loss. Weight is a vital sign that home health staff can follow in homebound elderly patients.

Skin

As mentioned above, the skin is fragile in older persons. This frequently results in senile purpura. Because of decreased elasticity, the evaluation of dehydration of the skin is less reliable than in younger age groups. In patients who are confined to bed or wheelchair, a diligent search should be conducted for early pressure sores, which have a predilection for bony prominences, eg, heels, occiput, sacrum, and scapulae.

Eyes

Wrinkling and loosening of the skin around the eyelids produce an eversion or ectropion of the eyelids with exposure of the conjunctiva, often accompanied by inflammation or excess tears. Entropion, or incurving of the eyelids, may produce an irritation of the eyelids by the eyelashes. Tear production usually is diminished in elderly persons.

Visual acuity should be checked with and without eyeglasses, using Snellen's chart or, in its absence, convenient printed material, such as a magazine. Visual fields can be screened quickly in a cooperative patient by the confrontation method.

A careful ophthalmologic examination is mandatory, noting cataracts (many of which can be seen readily with the ophthalmoscope) and retinal findings. The optic disc should be scrutinized for pressure atrophy due to glaucoma; the macula should be checked for evidence of macular degeneration; and the retinal field should be evaluated for diabetic or hypertensive angiopathy. Many older patients have had cataracts extracted, in which case the ophthalmoscope should be used with a +-diopter lens. Measurement of intraocular tension is done easily in either the office or home, and it may alert the physician to an early case of glaucoma, but its value is uncertain (see Chapter 8).

Oral Cavity

The gums, teeth, tongue, and buccal mucosa should be checked for infection, caries, and intraoral lesions. If a person wears dentures, he or she should be evaluated for the fit and state of repair. Mucosal lesions should be sought, especially in smokers.

Hearing

Profound hearing problems will be obvious during an interview. Mild losses, however, may be missed unless testing is included in the examination. The external canal always should be checked for wax buildup. Assessment of the patient's ability to hear a ticking watch provides gross information, and relatively inexpensive, handheld instruments now are available that combine an otoscope with three-level audiometer capability. For refined testing of frequencies, the patient should be referred to an audiologist.

Pulmonary Examination

Older individuals may have subtle but significant pulmonary pathologic conditions, particulaly if there is a long history of smoking or occupational exposure to lung toxins. Obstructive disease, pneumonia, pulmonary embolism, tuberculosis, congestive heart failure, and cancer are prominent considerations in elderly persons. An examination should determine the ability to generate a cough, the pattern of respiration, expansion of the chest, and auscultation of the lung fields. In a cooperative patient, an estimate of the forced expiratory volume can be made after a patient takes a deep breath and subsequently counts while exhaling forcefully. Bibasilar crackles may be heard in an otherwise apparently healthy elderly person.

Breast Examination

Atrophic breasts, being under less cyclic hormonal influence, often are easier to examine than those of younger women. The breast examination provides an opportunity for teaching self-examination and for arranging mammography, probably the most important tool in breast cancer screening.

Cardiovascular Examination

Carotid and femoral pulses should be auscultated for bruits. An asymptomatic carotid bruit serves to arouse suspicion of generalized atherosclerosis, especially in the coronary tree, rather than to predict the presence of a specific carotid lesion. The character of the carotid pulse may be an indicator of aortic valvular disease if it is significantly slow in the upstroke (stenosis) or rapidly collapsing (insufficiency). However, this sign may be obscured by the vessel stiffening seen in some elderly persons.

An S_3 gallop in old age generally indicates left ventricular dilatation and failure. A chronic fourth heart sound is heard frequently enough to be considered almost the norm; this probably reflects a decreased compliance of the left ventricle, but not failure. However, an S_4 gallop that develops suddenly in a person with angina pectoris may indicate an acute change, such as a silent myodardial infarction.

Systolic murmurs are common in elderly persons, and determination of their exact origin may be difficult.[13,14] Those that originate from the aortic area often are due to dilatation of the aortic annulus and ascending aorta, which is associated with sclerosis or calcification of the aortic ring. This murmur is shorter in duration and less intense (grades 1/6 to 2/6) than that of aortic valvular stenosis. Weight loss and anemia in a patient with a new murmur that is sug-

gestive of aortic insufficiency or mitral regurgitation should make a physician suspicious of bacterial endocarditis, especially in an individual who has undergone recent urologic or dental manipulation.

Atrial fibrillation is common, but may indicate a systemic disease, such as thyrotoxicosis or pulmonary emboli. Tachycardia can be due to thyrotoxicosis or occult blood loss and may be the only significant abnormal finding on examination.

Abdomen

A palpable abdominal aortic aneurysm should be carefully distinguished from a simple tortuous aorta, which is less than 3 cm wide and seldom has an associated bruit. An intra-abdominal pathologic condition, eg, appendicitis, gallbladder disease, and bowel obstruction, may present atypically with poorly localized pain.

Rectal Examination

This examination provides invaluable information about the prostrate gland in men and the cervix, uterus, rectal wall, and contents of the lower abdominal cavity in women. A digital rectal examination still is considered the best screening examination for prostatic carcinoma. Fecal impactions and rectal masses can be detected, and the stool can be tested for occult blood.

Genitourinary Examination

Men should have an inguinal examination for hernias. Women should have a periodic pelvic examination, done cautiously and without trauma. The vaginal mucosa may be friable, in which case it can tear easily. A thorough examination must be done on symptomatic patients, or if estrogens are used. Some authorities recommend no further Papanicolaou smears be performed in women older than 65 years of age who have had regular screening in earlier years. However, members of lower socioeconomic groups may not have had regular (or any) screening when younger. Other experts suggest that, after three negative annual smears, a woman should have the test every 3 years for life. A history of a hysterectomy must be confirmed by examination, because of the practice in earlier times of excluding the uterine cervix from a simple hysterectomy. Endometrial carcinoma is more frequent in elderly women who are taking estrogen; most cases are discovered after symptoms occur, rather than on a routine examination. Potential benefits of the pelvic examination must be weighed against discomfort in a very old, infirm woman who has no pelvic or vaginal symptoms.

Neurologic Assessment

Neurologic disease is a major cause of disability in old age and often produces significant functional impairment. Special consideration must be given to an examination of the nervous system because of age-related changes of posture and balance, and of disease entities related to stroke, parkinsonism, and dementia that cause a loss of functional capability and (frequently) falls.

Studies of volunteers without known neurologic disease has shown a sharp increase with age in the prevalence of "abnormal" neurologic signs.[15] For example, the palmomental and glabellar reflexes are found in some normal old persons, but are observed more frequently in persons with dementia.[16] Absent ankle jerks and a diminished vibratory perception in the ankle and foot are characteristic findings in elderly persons. An age-related peripheral neuropathy itself is not functionally significant, but it may be meaningful when associated with visual, muscular, or postural abnormalities. Moreover, when neuropathy is discovered, a careful search should be conducted for such commonly associated conditions as diabetes, alcoholism, and malignancy.

A systematic mental status examination is important in the examination of every elderly person. The physician can rapidly administer one of several validated screening examinations (eg, the Mini-Mental State—see Chapter 15) to evaluate certain critical functions in every patient. These should include the level of consciousness, orientation, attention, expressive and receptive language, memory of immediate, recent, and past events, contructional ability, abstract verbal reasoning, proverbs, and statements that require judgment. Such a systematic examination will occasionally uncover obvious deficits in garrulous, older patients who have good social skills and have learned to cope with an intellectual impairment in a gradually constricting environment.

A very old person stands with feet apart, flexed at the knees and hips, bent over, and looking upward (although women may adopt a narrow-based, waddling gait). Short shuffling steps with very little flexion at the ankles cause older persons to trip and stumble more frequently. The flexion at the knees causes increased work and fatigue of the thigh muscles. There is a loss of arm motion on walking, and turning around is done en bloc. In some cases, this senile gait appears to be a subtle form of parkinsonism, although it lacks many other features, such as tremor and the cogwheel phenomenon. The bent-over posture is attributed to degenerative changes in the intervertebral disks. In addition to describing the gait, the functional abilities in sitting, standing, and walking should be noted.

Basic Laboratory Tests

Laboratory tests usually are guided by a patient's particular problems, ability to cooperate, and limitations of intended therapy. For example, in the long-term care setting, a short, relatively inexpensive battery of tests will detect almost all conditions on which the physician is likely to act.[17] It is of little value to test for problems in which there is no intent of resolution due to a far-advanced or terminal disease. In most geriatric practices, however, this is not often the case. In almost all patients, there are conditions, such as anemia, electrolyte disturbances, and infections, that, if discovered, can be treated in a way that will substantially improve even seriously impaired patients. For a routine evaluation, a complete blood cell count, serum creatinine level, electrolyte panel, and urinalysis suffice. Thyroid function and glucose level should be assessed in any older person with a cognitive, cardiac, or neurologic disorder and probably performed at some point in asymptomatic patients. A stool guaiac test should be a part of every initial physical examination and the evaluation of anemia.

Chest x-ray films should be ordered for symptomatic patients or for those who are at risk for pulmonary disease, eg, smokers. Electrocardiograms should be initially obtained in all elderly patients and repeated at appropriate intervals in patients with pacemakers, conduction disturbances, and symptoms of severe angina.

Although physicians always should be cautious not to squander wastefully health care resources and although laboratory tests should never be done "routinely" without good reason, it also is essential not to err on the opposite side. Failing to investigate a protean symptom may lead to a cascade of illnesses that could significantly impair and possibly shorten a person's life.

Conclusion

The essence of geriatric practice is deciding what information to obtain, knowing how best to obtain it, and synthesizing the data into a set of diagnoses and a plan of action. The patient or caregivers have to be involved in these decisions, in order for evaluation and management to reflect individual values.

Appropriate and meticulous medical evaluation and treatment can improve the quality and, sometimes, duration of life for elderly patients, each of whom is different and must be assessed as an individual, not as a representative of a certain chronologic age group. As with all medical practice, time devoted to interacting with the patient is well spent.

References

1. Stillman PL, Swanson DB, Smee S, et al. Assessing clinical skills of residents with standardized patients. *Ann Intern Med.* 1986;105:762–771.
2. Lipkin M Jr, Quill TE, Napodano RJ. The medical interview: a core curriculum for residencies in internal medicine. *Ann Intern Med.* 1984;100:277–284.
3. Beckman HB, Frankel RM. The effect of physician behavior on the collection of data. *Ann Intern Med.* 1984;101:692–696.
4. Levkoff SE, Cleary PD, Wetle T, et al. Illness behavior in the aged: implications for clinicians. *J Am Geriatr Soc.* 1988;36:622–629.
5. Health and Public Policy Committee, American College of Physicians. Comprehensive functional asessment for elderly patients. *Ann Intern Med.* 1988;109:70–72.
6. Consensus Development Panel. National Institutes of Health Consensus Development Conference statement: Geriatric assessment methods for clinical decision-making. *J Am Geriatr Soc.* 1988;36:342–347.
7. Council on Scientific Affairs. Medical evaluations of healthy persons. *JAMA.* 1983;249:1626–1633.
8. McCullough LB. Medical care for elderly patients with diminished competence: an ethical analysis. *J Am Geriatr Soc.* 1984;32:150–153.
9. Tinker GM. Clinical presentation of myocardial infarction in the elderly. *Age Ageing.* 1981;20:237–240.
10. Ende J, Rockwell S, Glasgow M. The sexual history in general medicine practice. *Arch Intern Med.* 1984;144:558–561.
11. German PS, Shapiro S, Skinner EA, et al. Detection and management of mental health problems of older patients by primary care providers. *JAMA.* 1987;257:489–493.
12. Mader SL, Josephson KR, Rubenstein LZ. Low prevalence of postural hypotension among community-dwelling elderly. *JAMA.* 1987;258:1511–1514.
13. Noble RJ, Rothbaum DA. History and physical examination. In: Noble RJ, Rothbaum DA, eds. *Geriatric Cardiology.* Philadelphia, Pa: FA Davis Co Publishers; 1981:55–64.
14. Lembo NJ, Dell'Italia LF, Crawford MH, et al. Bedside diagnosis of systolic murmurs. *N Engl J Med.* 1988;318:1572–1578.
15. Jenkyn LR, Reeves AG, Warren T, et al. Neurologic signs in senescence. *Arch Neurol.* 1985;42:1154–1157.
16. Jacobs L, Grossman M. Three primitive reflexes in normal adults. *Neurology.* 1980;30:184–188.
17. Levinstein MR, Ouslander JG, Rubenstein LZ, et al. Yield of routine annual laboratory tests in a skilled nursing home population. *JAMA.* 1987;258:1909–1915.

11

Preoperative Assessment and Perioperative Care

Peter Pompei

Epidemiology and Risks of Surgery in the Elderly

The ever-increasing number of elderly patients being operated on is due to the expanding elderly population and to important advances in surgical and anesthetic techniques in the second half of this century. As our population ages, there are increasing numbers of individuals who have accumulated chronic diseases requiring surgical intervention, such as cataracts, prostatic hypertrophy, colorectal cancer, and peripheral vascular disease.[1] Falls and osteoporosis predispose elderly persons to fractures of the femoral neck, which often require surgical repair. The introduction of neuroleptic anesthesia, effective prophylaxis against deep venous thrombosis, and sophisticated perioperative monitoring technology have contributed to lower surgical mortality for elderly patients.[2] In a retrospective study of over 17,000 operations, the surgical mortality rate declined from 3.6% in 1964 to 1.8% in 1974, while the mean age of patients and the percentage who were 70 years of age or older remained constant.[2] It has been estimated that about half the people who reach 60 or 70 years of age will require an operation before they die.[3] The lowered risk of operative mortality has encouraged physicians and patients to consider surgical therapy more readily.

Although the safety of operative therapy for elderly patients has improved considerably, significant risks of mortality and morbidity persist. In contrast to the 1.5% operative mortality reported for young and middle-aged patients,[4] a prospective study of complications in elderly surgical patients reported a mortality rate of 5.8%.[5] In this study, 65% of the 258 elderly patients suffered at least one complication. The most common medical complications were pulmonary complications (39.5%), congestive heart failure (10.1%), delirium (9.7%), and thromboembolism (3.2%). Factors associated with an increased risk for various complications were the following: age 75 years or older, emergency procedures, the anatomic site of the operation, and the preoperative activity level of the patient. The relative importance of these factors was not examined in a multivariate model, nor was the impact of preexisting medical conditions assessed. Other studies have shown an important correlation between comorbid disease and surgical mortality.[6–8] The age of the patient has been found to be less important than the severity of comorbid conditions and the physiologic status.

Role of the Medical Consultant in Perioperative Assessment and Management of the Elderly Patient

The relatively high risk elderly patients face when undergoing an operation is a major reason that surgeons and anesthesiologists request preoperative consultations from internists or geriatricians. Though the request is often for "preoperative clearance," both the unstated expectations of the requesting physician and the responsibility of the consultant are much more specific. The purpose of a preoperative assessment is to identify factors associated with increased risks of specific complications related to the anticipated procedure and to recommend a management plan that would minimize these risks. During the perioperative period, the consulting physician will often be called on to assist in the management of specific medical problems. The consultant must give careful attention to the extent and severity of comorbid conditions, the current and anticipated pharmacologic therapy, and the functional and psychological state of the patient. In addition, patient-related risk factors are only a part of the required assessment; the type and technical difficulty of the procedure, the skill of the surgeon, and the anesthetic management all contribute to the overall risk of complications.

The specific reasons surgeons requested consultations from a general medicine consultation service at a university hospital have been reported by Charlson and colleagues.[9] Of the 289 requests for consultation from surgeons, 73% were for preoperative assessments. The reasons for consultation were as follows: 56% for chronic medical problems, 18% for specific symptoms or signs (eg, chest pain, fever, symptoms of thyroid disease), 15% for electrocardiographic or laboratory abnormality, 6% for an acute illness, and 5% for specific management issues (eg, antibiotic prophylaxis for valvular heart disease, steroid coverage, management of anticoagulation). Requests during the postoperative consultations were for chronic illnesses (38%), specific symptoms and signs (31%), electrocardiographic and laboratory abnormalities (15%), acute illness (15%), and specific management (1%). It is obvious that the assessment and management of chronic diseases is a primary clinical task of the geriatrician providing perioperative consultations.

Quantitative Assessment of Operative Risk

Patients and physicians frequently seek a quantitative assessment of risk before selecting therapy. The average risks associated with various procedures are usually known; the consultant is often called on to estimate the patient-related risks. A committee of the American Society of Anesthesiologists (ASA) developed a taxonomy of grading physical status in 1941; the purpose of this taxonomy was not to estimate risk but rather to describe the preoperative condition of patients in a subjective but standardized way.[10] The classification system has been modified over the years and now consists of the five classes shown in Table 11.1 Several investigators have observed an important relationship between the ASA status and operative

Table 11.1. ASA classification system.

Class I	A normally healthy patient undergoing an elective operation
Class II	A patient with mild systemic disease
Class III	A patient with severe systemic disease that limits activity but is not incapacitating
Class IV	A patient with incapacitating systemic disease that is a constant threat to life
Class V	A moribund patient not expected to survive 24 hours with or without operation.

mortality.[11,12] The ASA status has evolved into a useful global index of operative risk, in spite of institutional differences in death rates and inconsistency in ratings between observers.

Other indexes have been developed specifically to predict operative mortality. A computerized system to define a fitness score has been developed in Great Britain.[13] This score takes into account age, signs and symptoms of acute and chronic diseases, measures of nutritional status, and results of common blood tests. The total score ranges from 0 (fit) to 10 (unlikely to survive) and has been shown to predict prognosis from major abdominal operations when tested prospectively in about 1,500 patients. The authors did not compare their index with the ASA status. Some authors have attempted to develop instruments to predict operative mortality specifically designed for elderly patients. Lewin and associates examined physiologic measures that might improve the predictive value of the ASA classification system.[14] They report that the combination of a measure of overall cardiac function (an index derived by examining the relation between left ventricular work and central venous pressure) and the alveolar-arterial oxygen gradient is useful in predicting the mortality of poor-risk patients (ASA class III, IV, or V). Another group combined a modified ASA classification with patient age and diagnosis to develop a prognostic index.[15] In predicting overall operative mortality, the benefit of using any of these more complicated indexes rather than the commonly used ASA classification has yet to be proved.

Since cardiac complications are among the most

common and most lethal postoperative problems, significant attention has been focused on estimating cardiac risk, especially in noncardiac surgical procedures. Goldman and associates examined the association of preoperative factors with the development of cardiac complications in patients over 40 years of age.[16] The nine independent predictors they identified and the predictive values of four risk categories are shown in Tables 11.2 and 11.3. This predictive index has been tested in other populations, where it has been shown to be useful in stratifying patients according to their risk of cardiac complications.[17-21]

The multifactorial index developed by Goldman et al of cardiac risk has become a standard assessment tool

Table 11.2. Determination of the *cardiac* risk index.*

Criteria†	Multivariate discriminant function coefficient	Points
History		
Age > 70 y	0.191	5
MI* in previous 6 mo	0.384	10
Physical examination		
S3 gallop or JVD	0.451	11
Important VAS	0.119	3
Electrocardiography		
Rhythm other than sinus or PACs on last preoperative ECG	0.283	7
> 5 PVCs/min documented at any time before operation	0.178	7
General status		
Po_2 < 60 or Pco_2 > 50 mm Hg, K < 3.0 or HCO_3 < 20 mEq/L BUN > 50 or Cr > 3.0 mg/dL, abnormal AST, signs of chronic liver disease, or patient bedridden for noncardiac causes	0.132	3
Operation		
Intraperitoneal, intrathoracic, or aortic operation	0.123	3
Emergency operation	0.167	4

*From Goldman et al. Reprinted by permission of N Engl J Med[16]
†MI denotes myocardial infarction; JVD, jugular vein distention; VAS, valvular aortic stenosis; PACs, premature atrial contractions; ECG, electrocardiogram; PVCs, premature ventricular contractions; PO_2, partial pressure of oxygen; Pco_2, partial pressure of carbon dioxide; K, potassium; HCO_3, bicarbonate; BUN, blood urea nitrogen; Cr, creatinine; and AST, aspartate aminotransferase.

Table 11.3. Predicting morbidity and mortality using the cardiac risk index.*

Class	Point	No or only minor complication, %	Life-threatening complication,† %	Cardiac deaths, %
I	0–5	99	0.7	0.2
II	6–12	93	5	2
III	13–25	86	11	2
IV	26	22	22	56

*From Goldman et al. Reprinted by permission of N Engl J Med.[16]
†Documented intraoperative or postoperative myocardial infarction, pulmonary edema, or ventricular tachycardia without progression to cardiac death.

in many institutions. A recent study has confirmed its usefulness in predicting cardiac complications in elderly patients undergoing noncardiac surgery.[19] These investigators also found that while the results of preoperative rest and exercise radionuclide ventriculography added little prognostic information to this index, the inability to exercise for 2 minutes on a stationary bicycle was the only independent predictor of complications. After exercise ability was taken into account, the index provided no additional information about risks of complications. Detsky and colleagues have attempted to improve the Goldman index by proposing specific modifications.[20] In addition, they suggest combining the score from this modified index with preoperative estimates of complication rates based on the local experience with a given procedure to calculate more precisely the risk of a cardiac complication in an individual patient.

Management of Selected Problems in the Elderly Surgical Patient

In addition to identifying and quantifying the risks elderly patients face when surgery is being planned, geriatricians are also called on to assist in minimizing the risks and managing specific medical problems. A comprehensive review of the management of all possible medical problems in surgical patients and of the specific problems related to particular operations is beyond the scope of this chapter. The reader is referred to recent publications that address many of these important issues.[22-24] The remainder of this chapter will focus on the management of selected perioperative medical problems commonly faced by medical consultants.

Hypertension

The prevalence of hypertension among elderly Americans has been estimated to be 40%.[25] Uncontrolled hypertension is a well-established risk factor for stroke, myocardial infarction, and renal dysfunction, and a diastolic blood pressure of 110 mm Hg or greater in the preoperative period is an indication for postponing elective operations.[26] An increased incidence of myocardial ischemia is seen not only in patients with preoperative hypertension but also in those who have major deviations in blood pressure during a surgical procedure.[26,27] This variability is more common in hypertensive patients; significant elevations in blood pressure were observed in 25% of hypertensive patients during the perioperative period, irrespective of the control of their blood pressure preoperatively.[26]

The causes of perioperative variability in blood pressure among elderly patients include anesthetic agents and other medications, age-related changes in the cardiovascular system, changes in intravascular volume, and pain or other stimuli to the nervous system. The work of Prys-Roberts et al[28] has demonstrated some of the expected changes in blood pressure during surgery. Induction of anesthesia usually reduces systemic vascular resistance. The normal compensatory responses of increased heart rate and increased stroke volume may be limited in elderly patients, and these decreased responses will result in a reduced cardiac output and a fall in blood pressure. Intubation generally causes significant stimulation of the sympathetic nervous system and a sharp rise in blood pressure. Changes in intravascular volume and depth of anesthesia contribute to fluctuations in blood pressure during the operation. While the anesthesiologist attends to the variability of blood pressure in the immediate perioperative period, the geriatric consultant is more likely to have a role in preoperative assessment and the management of patients after they have left the recovery room.

Hypertensive patients undergoing elective operations are probably at no increased risk as long as the diastolic pressure is stable and less than 110 mm Hg and as long as large fluctuations in the mean arterial pressure can be avoided intraoperatively.[26] For this reason, and because of the potential for untoward responses to newly introduced antihypertensive agents, it generally is not advisable to begin a new drug regimen for blood pressure control in the few days before surgery. When therapy needs to be initiated or adjusted, it is preferable to postpone the procedure until the patient's response to a new regimen can be observed and a steady state achieved. Oral medications used to control hypertension preoperatively should be taken on the day of surgery with a sip of water. They should be restarted as soon as possible postoperatively.

In the postoperative period, sudden and significant elevations in blood pressure should be treated. Hydralazine has commonly been used to treat postoperative hypertension. The advantage of this drug is that it acts quickly when given parenterally. However, it is a vasodilator and may cause a reflex increase in heart rate and left ventricular contractility, thereby increasing myocardial oxygen demand. Its use can be hazardous in the subset of patients with hypertensive hypertrophic cardiomyopathy who have a small left ventricular chamber and good contractile function; these patients depend heavily on adequate filling pressures, which can be compromised by rapid vasodilation. β-Blockers can be administered parenterally for a rapid response. There are concerns about using this class of drugs in patients predisposed to congestive heart failure because of negative inotropic effects. The negative chronotropic effects could blunt the patient's ability to respond to a sudden loss of intravascular volume, such as a major postoperative bleeding episode. Other relative contraindications to this class of drugs include a history of bronchospasm, claudication, and diabetes mellitus. In a small study of elderly patients, sublingual nifedipine was found to be effective, with a rapid onset and a relatively long duration of action.[29] There were no reports of drug-induced hypotension, angina, or myocardial ischemia. Sodium Nitroprusside can be used very effectively to control significant hypertension, but its use requires very careful monitoring of the patient, usually in an intensive care unit with an intraarterial catheter to monitor blood pressure.

Atherosclerotic Disease

Many elderly surgical patients have atherosclerotic disease. The identification and management of occlusive coronary disease in the surgical patient is especially important, because the mortality of perioperative myocardial infarction has been estimated to be between 50% and 80%.[25] Two facts about postoperative ischemia support the practice of ordering follow-up electrocardiograms in patients at risk: the incidence is highest on the 3rd postoperative day, and more than half the time the ischemia is silent.[25] While stable angina has not been found to be associated with an increased risk of postoperative cardiac complications,[16] patients with unstable angina should have elective procedures delayed until they have been fully evaluated and treated. Patients who have undergone coronary bypass grafting for the treatment of ischemic heart disease have a low risk of cardiac complications after noncardiac surgery.[30] In contrast, patients who recently have suffered an acute myocardial infarction have a significantly increased risk of operative mortality: 30% for patients operated on within 3 months of a myocardial infarction, 10% at 3 to 6 months, and 5%

after 6 months.[31] For this reason, elective procedures should be delayed for at least 6 months after a myocardial infarction.

Carotid occlusions and peripheral vascular disease are prevalent among elderly patients and raise important management questions. The presence of a carotid bruit has not been found to be associated with an increased incidence of postoperative stroke.[32] Patients with transient ischemic attacks who have an indication for endarterectomy should undergo this procedure prior to elective noncardiac surgery. Peripheral vascular disease is often associated with atherosclerotic coronary artery disease. If the vascular disease is significant enough to limit the patient's activity, exertional angina may never have been experienced. Symptoms or signs of arterial disease should prompt the consultant to evaluate the patient for the presence of ischemic heart disease.

Congestive Heart Failure

Congestive heart failure is an important complication of ischemic heart disease but can also be due to other cardiomyopathies or valvular heart disease. In the multifactorial index of cardiac risk developed by Goldman et al., the presence of an S_3 gallop or jugular venous distention, two signs of uncompensated congestive heart failure, is the most important single factor predictive of an adverse outcome. In managing surgical patients with congestive heart failure, it is important to optimize their medication regimen and to monitor carefully their volume status and cardiac function. The use of diuretics, positive inotropic agents, and vasodilators is the standard in the treatment of heart failure. Heart rate and rhythm contribute significantly to cardiac output and may require special interventions. Swan-Ganz catheters have significantly improved our ability to monitor accurately the volume status of patients and optimize ventricular filling pressures. Intraoperative transesophageal echocardiography has become popular in some centers.[33] The advantages of this technique over the Swan-Ganz catheter are that estimates of left ventricular end-diastolic volumes can be made, changes in regional wall motion can be observed, and the observed ejection fraction area can be used to assess contractility. The disadvantage is that the device is used intraoperatively only, and unless a right heart catheter is also placed, management of postoperative volume status must be based on imprecise clinical measures.

Valvular Heart Disease

The primary perioperative risks associated with valvular heart disease are congestive heart failure and bacterial endocarditis. It has been estimated that 20% of surgical patients who have significant valvular heart disease will develop new or worsening congestive heart failure perioperatively.[31] Critical aortic stenosis has been identified as the valvular lesion most commonly associated with complications. Preoperative identification of this lesion by noninvasive means may be difficult. Clinical findings include a harsh systolic murmur radiating to the neck, which occurs late in systole, is prolonged, and may obscure the second heart sound; diminished carotid pulses; left ventricular hypertrophy on the electrocardiogram; and radiographic evidence of aortic valvular calcification.[3] Chun and Dunn have suggested that the constellation of a history of syncope, a palpable lag time between the carotid and apical impulses, shudder waves on the upstroke of the percussion wave on carotid pulse tracing, and left ventricular hypertrophy on the electrocardiogram successfully predict the aortic valve area.[34] If significant aortic stenosis is suspected, an echocardiogram can confirm the diagnosis. It has been suggested that patients with angina, heart failure, or syncope who have significant aortic stenosis established by means of echocardiography should undergo cardiac catheterization to assess the need for valve replacement prior to elective operations.[35] Other types of valvular heart disease are not absolute contraindications to elective surgery. Nevertheless, patients with stenotic or incompetent valves require careful hemodynamic monitoring during perioperative fluid management.

Patients who have significant valvular heart disease or prosthetic valves and are undergoing operations associated with a substantial risk of transient bacteremia require antibiotic prophylaxis. The procedures for which prophylactic antibiotics are indicated are listed in Table 11.4[36]; the recommended antibiotic regimens are summarized in Table 11.5.[37]

Rhythm Disturbances and Heart Block

A cardiac rhythm other than sinus rhythm is associated with an increased risk of cardiac complications,[16] most commonly myocardial ischemia or congestive heart failure.[35] If a patient is receiving antiarrhythmic medication, this should be given on the day of surgery and restarted as soon as possible postoperatively. Parenteral forms of many of these drugs are available and can be used until the patient is able to tolerate oral medications. Patients at increased risk for developing postoperative supraventricular tachycardia include those with subcritical valvular heart disease or a history of a paroxysmal rhythm disturbance. Pulmonary operations, valvular heart procedures, and cardiac surgery in patients with electrocardiographic

Table 11.4. Procedures for which endocarditis prophylaxis is indicated.

All dental procedures likely to induce gingival bleeding (not simple adjustment of orthodontic appliances or shedding of deciduous teeth)
Tonsillectomy and/or adenoidectomy
Surgical procedures or biopsy involving respiratory mucosa
Bronchoscopy, especially with a rigid bronchoscope*
Incision and drainage of infected tissue
Genitourinary tract surgery and instrumentation
Cystoscopy, prostatic surgery, urethral catheterization (especially in the presence of infection), urinary tract surgery, vaginal hysterectomy
Gastrointestinal tract surgery and instrumentation
Gallbladder surgery, colonic surgery, esophageal dilation, sclerotherapy of esophageal varices, colonoscopy, upper gastrointestinal tract endoscopy with biopsy, proctosigmoidoscopy biopsy

*The risk with flexible bronchoscopy is low, but the necessity for prophylaxis is not yet defined. Reprinted from Shulman et al.[36] by permission of the American Heart Association, Inc.

Table 11.5. Drugs for prevention of bacterial endocarditis.* From ref. 37 with permission.

	Dosage for adults
Dental and upper respiratory procedures	
Oral treatment†	
Pencillin V potassium	2 g 1 h before procedure and 1 g 6 h later
Erythromycin base (penicillin allergy)	1 g 1 h before procedure and 500 mg 6 h later
Parenteral treatment†	
Ampicillin sodium	2 g IM or IV‡ 30 min before procedure
Plus gentamicin sulfate	1.5 mg/kg IM or IV 30 min before procedure
Vancomycin hydrochloride (penicillin allergy)	1 g IV infused slowly over 1 h beginning 1 h before procedure
Gastrointestinal and genitourinary tract procedures	
Oral treatment	
Amoxicillin trihydrate	3 g 1 h before procedure and 1.5 g 6 hours later
Parenteral treatment	
Ampicillin sodium	2 g IM or IV 30 min before procedure
Plus gentamicin sulfate	1.5 mg/kg IM or IV 30 min before procedure
Vancomycin hydrochloride (penicillin allergy)	1 g IV infused slowly over 1 h beginning 1 h before procedure
Plus gentamicin sulfate	1.5 mg/kg IM or IV 30 min before procedure

*For patients with valvular heart disease, prosthetic heart valves, most forms of congenital heart disease (but not uncomplicated secundum atrial septal defect), idiopathic hypertrophic subaortic stenosis, and mitral valve prolapse with regurgitation.
†Oral regimens are more convenient and safer. Parenteral regimens are more likely to be effective; they are recommended especially for patients with prosthetic heart valves, those who have had endocarditis previously, or those taking continuous oral penicillin for rheumatic fever prophylaxis. A single dose of the parenteral drugs is probably adequate, because bacteremias after most dental and diagnostic procedures are of short duration. However, one or two follow-up doses may be given at 8- to 12-hour intervals in selected patients, such as hospitalized patients judged to be at higher risk.
‡IM indicates intramuscularly; IV, intravenously.

evidence of myocardial infarction are all associated with postoperative supraventricular tachycardia.[38,39] Digitalis may be useful in preventing the arrhythmia and in controlling the ventricular response rate[38,39]; therefore, the prophylactic use of digitalis is recommended for patients at high risk for developing supraventricular tachycardia. The initiation of other antiarrhythmic regimens in the perioperative period should be reserved for patients with arrhythmias that are either symptomatic or associated with hemodynamic compromise or myocardial ischemia.

The indications for a pacemaker are not influenced by the fact that a patient may be facing an operative procedure. The presence of bifascicular block does not significantly increase the risk of developing complete heart block in the immediate perioperative period and is not considered an indication for the insertion of a temporary pacemaker.[40,41] Patients who have sick sinus syndrome should have a temporary pacemaker placed preoperatively only if it is anticipated that they will require a permanent pacemaker. When there is an indication for a pacemaker in a patient about to undergo an operation associated with significant bacteremia, a temporary pacemaker should be placed. Postoperatively, when the risk of infecting an implanted foreign body is reduced, the permanent pacemaker should be inserted.[35]

Pulmonary Disease

Pulmonary problems are among the most common postoperative complications. In a prospective study of elderly surgical patients, respiratory problems were the cause of postoperative morbidity in 39.5% of patients.[4] Elderly patients may be particularly prone to pulmonary complications because of age-related changes in the respiratory system and the accumulation of chronic respiratory diseases over time. The principle structural changes that occur with aging are a decrease in elasticity due to changes in collagen content and structure; increased chest wall stiffness due to calcification of cartilage, arthritic changes, and diminished intervertebral space; and insufficient respiratory muscle strength to match the added work load of breathing imposed by the increased chest wall stiffness.[42] These structural changes result in the important changes in respiratory function listed in Table 11.6.

There are also important non–age-dependent changes in respiratory function that occur as a result of anesthesia and operations. The combination of the supine position and the induction of anesthesia results in a significant decrease in functional residual capacity and an associated increase in airway resistance.[43] The fall in functional residual capacity is most severe on about the 4th postoperative day but can persist for more than a week.[44] Vital capacity can be decreased as much as 25% to 50%, especially after upper abdominal incisions.[44] Postoperative pain and analgesics both contribute to a reduction in tidal volume and impaired clearing of secretions through normal cough mechanisms. Gas exchange is impaired and postoperative hypoxemia is especially common in the elderly patient, in whom it may persist several days,[45] as shown in Figure 11.1.

Considerable attention has been focused on pulmonary function tests to identify patients at high risk for respiratory complications.[44,46] Tisi[44] recommends that preoperative pulmonary function tests should be considered for (1) patients scheduled for thoracic or upper abdominal surgery, (2) patients with a history of heavy smoking or pulmonary disease, (3) obese patients, and (4) patients over 70 years of age. He suggests that a maximal breathing capacity of less than 50% of the predicted value, a forced expiratory volume in 1 second of less than 2 L, and an arterial carbon

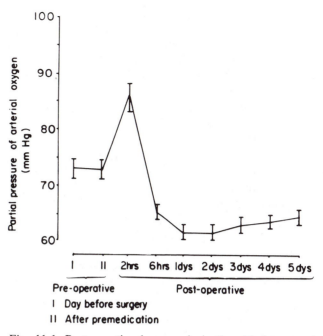

Fig. 11.1. Postoperative hypoxemia in the elderly general surgical patient. From ref. 45 with permission.

dioxide pressure of greater than 45 mm Hg indicate a high risk of morbidity and mortality. For patients undergoing pulmonary resections, quantitative ventilation-perfusion scans are useful in predicting the postoperative flow rates.[47] When the predicted postoperative forced expiratory volume in 1 second is 0.8 L or greater, the patient is a reasonable operative risk.[48]

After identifying the patient at risk for postoperative pulmonary complications, what can be done to help reduce the risk? Prospective studies in high-risk patients have identified specific interventions that reduce morbidity and mortality from respiratory problems. Stein and Cassara[49] found that "poor-risk" patients treated with a regimen of preoperative smoking cessation, antibiotics "when indicated," perioperative bronchodilator therapy, inhalation of humidified gas, postural drainage, and chest physiotherapy had fewer pulmonary complications, lower mortality, and shorter hospital stays than nontreated patients. Data on the impact of cigarette smoking suggest that as many as 6 weeks of abstinence may be required before there is improvement in small-airways disease, hypersecretion of mucus, tracheobronchial clearance, and immune function, although cardiovascular function can be enhanced through the elimination of carbon monoxide and nicotine for even 12 to 24 hours.[50]

A study of the effect of antibiotics, chest physiotherapy, bronchodilators, and postoperative analgesia on respiratory complications in men undergoing elective upper abdominal surgery found that only the use of antibiotics was significantly associated with reduced

Table 11.6. Changes in respiratory function with aging.

Increases:
    Functional residual capacity
    Residual volume
    Alveolar-arterial oxygen
       difference
No change:
    Total lung capacity
Decreases:
    Forced vital capacity
    Expiratory flow rates
    Diffusing capacity
    Arterial oxygen tension
    Respiratory muscle strength
    Ventilatory drive
    Respiratory sensation

* Reprinted from Mahler et. al.[42]

pulmonary morbidity.[51] Postoperative chest physiotherapy consisting of 15 minutes of breathing exercises with assisted coughing and vibration of the chest wall has been credited with a significant decrease in the frequency of chest infections.[52] Incentive spirometry may reduce the rate of postoperative complications.[53] A recent survey reports that this procedure is prescribed in 95% of American hospitals for the prevention of pulmonary atelectasis.[54] There is little consensus about the benefit of other treatments, such as instruction in respiratory maneuvers, bronchodilators, minimization of postoperative narcotic analgesics, and early mobilization of the elderly patient.[55] A pragmatic approach to the preoperative preparation of an elderly patient with chronic lung disease includes eradication of acute tracheobronchial infections, relief of bronchospasm, efforts to improve sputum clearance, and therapy for uncompensated right heart failure.

Thromboembolic Disease

Thromboembolic disease is prevalent in the perioperative period. It has been estimated that between 20% and 30% of patients undergoing general surgery develop deep venous thrombosis, and the incidence is as high as 40% in hip and knee surgery, gynecologic cancer operations, open prostatectomies, and major neurosurgical procedures.[56] Though fatal pulmonary embolism occurs in between 1% and 5% of all surgical patients, it accounts for a larger proportion of operative deaths in middle-aged and elderly individuals.[57] Since venous thrombosis and pulmonary emboli can be difficult to diagnose and treat, considerable effort has been focused on prophylactic therapy. Various treatment regimens, including heparin, warfarin, aspirin, dextran, and compressive devices, have been used. In a review of over 70 randomized trials,[58] it was found that the perioperative use of subcutaneous heparin can prevent about half of the pulmonary emboli and two thirds of the deep-vein thromboses. A significant reduction in the number of deaths attributed to pulmonary embolism also was observed. The beneficial effects were related to the type of operation, but it is notable that patients undergoing urologic and orthopedic surgery did benefit from the heparin therapy. There was an increased risk of bleeding after treatment with subcutaneous heparin, but the absolute increase of clinically important bleeding was small. These results provide strong evidence for the prophylactic use of subcutaneous heparin in surgical patients. Some surgeons may prefer other regimens based on the type of surgery they do and their own personal experience with thromboembolic disease and anticoagulation therapy. The geriatric consultant should discuss with the surgeon the advisability of prophylactic perioperative anticoagulation therapy in all patients.

Renal, Fluid, and Electrolyte Disorders

Renal function is of critical importance in the perioperative period, because of the critical role of the kidneys in drug metabolism and fluid and electrolyte balance. The age-related changes in kidney structure and function, combined with the effects of anesthesia and surgery, can have important consequences in the management of the elderly surgical patient. With aging there is a loss of renal mass, primarily in the cortex, which results in a 30% to 50% decrease in the number of glomeruli by the 7th decade.[59] This loss of filtering surface is associated with a fall in renal blood flow and reduction in glomerular filtration rate (GFR). The decrease in GFR is generally coincident with a decline in muscle mass, so that the serum creatinine level may remain normal. In the clinical setting, it may be difficult to measure GFRs accurately in elderly patients because of problems in obtaining complete urine collections. Estimates of GFR can be calculated from commonly available clinical information with use of the following equation, proposed by Cockcroft and Gault[60]:

$$C_{Cr} \text{ (mL/min)} = [140 - \text{Age (y)}] \times \text{Weight (kg)}/[72 \times \text{Serum Cr (mg/dl)}],$$

where C_{Cr} indicates creatinine clearance; and Cr, creatinine level. (This formula is for men; the result should be multiplied by 0.85 for women.) The estimates obtained from this formula have been shown to correlate with measured creatinine clearance in elderly patients.[61,62] This measure, while not precise, allows the clinician to initiate appropriate medication dosages, which should then be adjusted based on clinical response and measured drug levels when possible.

Diminished preoperative renal function increases the risk of postoperative acute renal failure. Renal blood flow can be compromised intraoperatively because of the decline in cardiac output secondary to the negative inotropic effects of inhalational anesthetic agents, the effects of positive pressure ventilation, and loss of intravascular volume. These factors and nephrotoxic medications can result in postoperative acute reversible intrinsic renal failure.[63] Oliguria, isosthenuria, and a rising serum creatinine level are early clinical signs. When acute renal failure is suspected, the urine sediment should be examined for epithelial cell casts, granular casts, and tubular epithelial cells. The urine sodium level is generally greater than 40 mEq/L, and the urine-plasma creatinine ratio is generally less than 10:1. In contrast, prerenal azotemia is associated with a urine sodium level of less than 40 mEq/L and a urine-plasma creatinine ratio of greater than 10:1. Management of acute intrinsic renal failure includes discontinuing potentially nephrotoxic drugs and carefully monitoring volume status. Dialysis is occasionally necessary to manage hypervolemia, hyperkalemia, metabolic acidosis, or uremic encephalopathy. Even with appropriate treatment, acute postoperative renal failure has a mortality rate of between 40% and 80%.[64] The efforts of the consultant, surgeon, and anesthesiologist should be focused on preventing this ominous complication.

The role of the kidneys in regulating body osmolality and fluid volume also can be compromised by both aging and surgery. With aging, the loss of functioning nephrons results in an increase in the solute load per nephron, and changes in the pattern of renal blood flow may adversely affect the normal counter current concentrating mechanism.[59] These changes can lead to volume depletion through a reduction in renal concentrating capacity and excessive losses of free water. Older individuals also have a diminished thirst perception, which compromises their ability to respond to significant free water loss and hyperosmolality.[65] This is particularly important postoperatively, when third-space losses of fluid and bleeding may cause severe intravascular volume depletion. On the other hand, volume overload sometimes results from the delayed response to sodium restriction and salt wasting observed in older individuals.[66] This can be exacerbated by the elevated levels of vasopressin seen in the postoperative state. Sodium and water retention after surgery may last for several days. These physiologic changes are compounded by the difficulties in the clinical assessment of volume status in elderly patients. Postural hypotension is an important sign of intravascular volume depletion but can be observed in euvolemic elderly patients and may be difficult to assess properly in the immediate postoperative period. When the assessment of volume status becomes critically important, it is often necessary to measure pulmonary capillary wedge pressure with a Swan-Ganz catheter.

Intravenous fluid management must be adjusted for the elderly surgical patient, because there is a decline in both total body water and intracellular water with advancing age. For men between 65 and 85 years of age and weighing between 40 and 80 kg, the intracellular volume represents 25% to 30% of body weight.[67] For women of the same age and weight ranges, the intracellular volume is estimated as 20% to 25% of body weight. In the absence of acute stress and conditions known to affect salt and water balance, the daily metabolic requirements per liter of intracellular fluid are as follows: water, 100 mL; energy, 100 kcal;

protein, 3 g; sodium, 3 mmol; and potassium, 2 mmol. For example, an 80-year-old woman weighing 40 kg, has an estimated intracellular volume of 10 L. Daily maintenance requirements would be 1 L of water, 1,000 kcal, 30 g of protein, 30 mmol of sodium, and 20 mmol of potassium. Fluid and electrolyte status must be closely monitored and adjusted according to the response of the patient and the development of other pathophysiologic conditions.

Endocrine and Metabolic Disorders

Diabetes mellitus, usually type II, is a common problem in elderly patients. It has been estimated that of the diabetic patients undergoing surgery, more than 75% are over the age of 50 years.[68] Diabetes not only complicates the management of surgical patients but also predisposes the patient to an increased risk of morbidity and mortality from cardiovascular and infectious complications.[69] Several predictable perioperative metabolic changes can exacerbate hyperglycemia. There is an increase in corticosteroids, corticotropin, and catecholamines associated with the stress and tissue injury of surgery. The hormonal changes stimulate gluconeogenesis, and the catecholamines can directly depress the release of insulin from the pancreas and blunt insulin activity at the cellular level.

In all diabetic patients undergoing surgery, it is important to monitor blood glucose levels frequently. Values should be obtained preoperatively, during the procedure, and in the recovery room. Afterwards, the frequency of monitoring will be determined by the management regimen and the patient's condition and glucose control. Frequent monitoring has been facilitated by the ready availability of capillary glucose monitoring devices that give accurate measurements within a few minutes. For patients whose blood glucose levels can be maintained in the normal range by diet and exercise therapy, no special preoperative preparation is required. Patients receiving oral hypoglycemic medications should have these discontinued 1 day before the operation unless they are receiving chlorpropamide, which has a half-life of about 36 hours and should be discontinued at least 3 days before surgery. For patients receiving insulin, several management regimens are possible. Commonly, the patient is given one third to one half of the usual dose of insulin on the morning of surgery and a glucose-containing intravenous solution is administered. Management is facilitated if a constant rate of the glucose solution is maintained while non–glucose-containing intravenous fluids are used to adjust for changes in intravascular volume. Additional doses of regular insulin should be administered to control blood glucose levels; an every-6-hour schedule is often used. Constant insulin infusions can be used successfully but require more careful monitoring because of the rapid changes in glucose and potassium levels. In addition to meticulous attention to blood glucose levels, it is important to monitor diabetic surgical patients for other complications. Infections and impaired wound healing are commonly seen in diabetic surgical patients. Cardiovascular complications are also common, since diabetes is an important risk factor for atherosclerosis. Myocardial ischemia can be silent and may be detected unexpectedly on postoperative electrocardiograms.

Thyroid disease is not as prevalent as diabetes in elderly patients, but if undetected, it can result in major complications perioperatively. The prevalence of hypothyroidism in hospitalized elderly patients has been reported to be 9.4%, and the prevalence of hyperthyroidism 0.8%.[70] It is well known that elderly patients may have nonspecific or atypical manifestations of thyroid illness, so it is important to maintain a high index of suspicion for thyroid illness in all elderly patients. The consequences of operating on a patient with unsuspected hypothyroidism can be significant. These patients metabolize medications more slowly and their increased sensitivity to central nervous system depressants can result in respiratory insufficiency. In addition, cardiac reserve is diminished, and the response to pressors may be blunted. While the potential for these complications should be suspected and preventive measures instituted, hypothyroidism should not be considered an absolute contraindication to necessary operative procedures.[71] Emergency surgery and trauma are indications for rapid replacement. When hypothyroidism is severe, an intravenous dose of 300 to 500 μg of levo-thyroxine sodium will significantly improve basal metabolic rate within 6 hours. Corticosteroids should also be given in the perioperative period, since the acute rise in basal metabolic rate can exhaust the adrenal reserves.

The increased perioperative risks associated with hyperthyroidism include hyperpyrexia, arrhythmias, and congestive heart failure. Elective operations should be delayed until treatment with thioamide medications render the patient euthyroid. When an emergency operation is necessary, the patient can be treated with 1,000 mg of propylthiouracil by mouth and a β-blocker to control the increased catecholamine effects. Sodium iodide is often given to inhibit the release of thyroid hormone and transiently inhibit organification. Iodide can be given either by mouth or intravenously; administration should be delayed until at least 1 hour after the propylthiouracil to allow time for the latter to block organification. Supplemental corticosteroids are also recommended for hyperthyroid patients undergoing emergency operations. These are given to protect against the possibility of adrenal insufficiency related to the chronic hypermetabolic state, and because corticosteroids may lower serum thyroxine and thyroid-stimulating hormone levels.

Management of Nutrition in the Perioperative Period

Surgery causes increased energy demands, and in a malnourished elderly patient when the body's carbohydrate stores are depleted, protein catabolism and a negative nitrogen balance can result. Malnutrition has been found to be associated with increased morbidity and mortality in patients without cancer undergoing elective operations.[72] Patients with poor nutritional status, as indicated by body weight, the percentage of weight loss, arm muscle circumference, and serum albumin levels, have significantly longer hospital stays and more complications than do well-nourished patients. As yet, there is no consensus on the best method for assessing a patient's nutritional status, especially in elderly patients.[73,74] (See Chapter 41 for a discussion of the factors contributing to nutritional deficiencies in old age.)

There have been conflicting results from studies examining the effectiveness of perioperative parenteral nutrition in reducing morbidity and mortality. A recent meta-analysis of 18 controlled trials concluded that, although statistical significance was not achieved there is a trend favoring the use of parenteral nutrition.[75] Additional studies are needed in the groups of patients most likely to benefit from perioperative parenteral nutrition: those who are severely malnourished before major surgery and those who undergo operations causing, or develop complications resulting in, prolonged periods of inadequate enteral intake.

Neuropsychiatric Disorders

Neuropsychiatric problems are common in elderly patients and can be associated with an increased risk of perioperative complications. The prevalence of dementia is about 3% among persons aged 65 years and older; it increases to about 25% in those 80 years of age and older. A study of elderly patients admitted for repair of hip fractures in Sweden reported a prevalence of dementia of 15%.[76] Depression also is prevalent in older persons and can be exacerbated by any acute illness or hospitalization. Anesthesia and surgery can have profound effects on mental functioning. The metabolic changes associated with surgery, along with the previously discussed effects on all the vital organ systems, can compromise cerebral function and exacerbate or precipitate neuropsychiatric disorders. These are important because they can result in prolonged hospital stays and an increased risk of complications. The physiologic and behavioral manifestations of these disorders can significantly complicate perioperative care.

The most common psychiatric problem in the postoperative period is delirium. The major manifestation of this condition is an alteration in consciousness, and it is, by definition, a transient disorder.[77] The *DSM-III* R criteria for establishing this diagnosis are listed in Table 11.7.[78] Prospective studies have been done to determine the patients at greatest risk for this complication and to define the common causes and consequences. One study reported an incidence of 44% among elderly patients undergoing repair of hip fractures.[79] The presence of depression, the use of anticholinergic medications, and the presence of hypoxemia were associated with delirium. Neither the

Table 11.7. Diagnostic criteria for delirium.[78]

1. Reduced ability to maintain attention to external stimuli (eg, questions must be repeated because attention wanders) and to shift attention appropriately to new external stimuli (eg, perseverates answer to a previous question)
2. Disorganized thinking, as indicated by rambling, irrelevant, or incoherent speech
3. At least two of the following:
   (a) Reduced level of consciousness (eg, difficulty keeping awake during examination)
   (b) Perceptual disturbances (misinterpretations, illusions, or hallucinations)
   (c) Disturbance of sleep-wake cycle with insomnia or daytime sleepiness
   (d) Increased or decreased psychomotor activity
   (e) Disorientation to time, place, or person
   (f) Memory impairment (eg, inability to learn new material, such as the names of several unrelated objects after 5 minutes, or to remember past events, such as history of current episode of illness)
4. Clinical features developing over a short period (usually hours to days) and tending to fluctuate over the course of a day
5. Either (a) or (b):
   (a) Evidence from history, physical examination, or laboratory tests of a specific organic factor (or factors) judged to be etiologically related to the disturbance
   (b) In the absence of such evidence, an etiologic organic factor can be presumed if the disturbance cannot be accounted for by any nonorganic mental disorder (eg, manic episode accounting for agitation and sleep disturbance)

*Reprinted with permission from the *Diagnostic and Statistical Manual of Mental Disorders, Third Edition, Revised.* Copyright 1987 American Psychiatric Association.

duration of the procedure nor the type of anesthetic used (halothane vs epidural) were predictors of an acute confusional state.

The differential diagnosis of delirium is very broad. A careful clinical assessment of the patient should focus on the possibility of infection, metabolic derangements, central nervous system events, myocardial ischemia, sensory deprivation, or drug intoxication. Lidocaine, cimetidine, atropine, aminophylline preparations, antihypertensives, steroids, and digoxin are medications commonly associated with delirium, but all drugs should be considered as possible causes. The best management strategy is prevention of delirium by meticulous attention to the factors known to precipitate it. When it cannot be prevented, it is important to recognize it early and identify and treat the underlying cause. Often, empirical treatment of the symptoms of delirium is indicated. This involves modifying the patient's environment to promote orientation and using the appropriate medications. If anticholinergic drugs are thought to be a contributing cause, 1 to 2 mg of physostigmine salicylate can be given parenterally, unless contraindicated by heart disease, asthma, or bowel or bladder obstruction. When sedation is required for agitated behavior, 0.5 to 2 mg of haloperidol lactate can be given parenterally and repeated every 30 minutes as necessary. The minimum dose sufficient to control symptoms is recommended, and dosages exceeding 20 mg over a 24-hour period are rarely indicated. Frequent assessment of patients suffering from delirium is mandatory to monitor both response to therapy and potential drug toxicity. It is important to ask patients about their hallucinations and illusions, to discuss and clarify these frightening experiences, and to reassure them if the underlying cause is reversible.

Alcoholism is a serious and common problem among the elderly; it has been estimated that there are at least 1.5 million alcoholics in this country who are 65 years of age or older.[80] Some of the sequelae of alcoholism require surgical intervention, and the associated postoperative complications can be devastating. The geriatric consultant should carefully explore current alcohol use with all patients, and a screening tool such as the Michigan Alcoholism Screening Test may be useful in establishing the diagnosis preoperatively.[81] When alcoholism is suspected, the patient should be questioned about symptoms or signs of physiologic dependence and organ damage. Chronic alcohol use can cause important metabolic derangements as well as cardiac, hepatic, hematologic, and neurologic dysfunction. Liver disease has a variable effect on drug metabolism. The rate of metabolism of many drugs is slowed, but microsomal enzyme induction may result in increased dose requirements of many anesthetic agents. The patients for whom a withdrawal syndrome seems likely should be treated with thiamine and short-acting benzodiazepines, and elective surgery should be delayed. The consultant is commonly called to assist in the management of delirium tremens or seizures occurring postoperatively. Seizures are effectively treated with benzodiazepines and often do not require long-term antiepileptics. Delirium tremens usually occurs 24 to 48 hours after the last drink but can occur after 7 to 10 days of abstinence. The classic signs are fever, tachycardia, confusion, and visual hallucinations.Oxazepam or lorazepam are given in sufficient doses to sedate the patient. The other principles of treating patients with delirium also apply.

References

1. Keating HJ III. Preoperative considerations in the geriatric patient. *Med Clin North Am* 1987;71:569–583.
2. Palmberg S, Hirsjarvi E. Mortality in geriatric surgery. *Gerontology* 1979;25:103–112.
3. Shipton EA. The peri-operative care of the geriatric patient. *S Afr Med J* 1983;63:855–860.
4. Santos AL, Gelperin A. Surgical mortality in the elderly. *J Am Geriatr Soc* 1975;23:42–46.
5. Seymour DG, Pringle R. Post-operative complications in the elderly surgical patient. *Gerontology* 1983;29:262–270.
6. Anderson B, Ostberg J. Survival rates in surgery of the aged: assessment of long-term prognosis according to coexisting disease. *Gerontol Clin* 1972;14:354–360.
7. Boyd JB, Bradford B, Watne AL. Operative risk factors of colon resection in the elderly. *Ann Surg* 1980;192:743–746.
8. Greenberg AG, Saik RP, Pridham D. Influence of age on mortality of colon surgery. *Am J Surg* 1985;150:65–69.
9. Charlson ME, Cohen RP, Sears CL. General medicine consultation: lessons from a clinical service. *Am J Med* 1983;75:121–128.
10. Saklad M. Grading of patients for surgical procedures. *Anesthesiology* 1941;2:281–284.
11. Vacanti CJ, Van Houten RJ, Hill RC. A statistical analysis of the relationship of physical status to postoperative mortality in 68,388 cases. *Anesth Analg* 1970;49:560–566.
12. Marx CF, Mateo CV, Orkin LR. Computer analysis of post-anesthetic death. *Anesthesiology* 1973;39:54–58.
13. Playforth MJ, Smith GMR, Evans M, et al. Preoperative assessment of fitness score. *Br J Surg* 1987;74:890–892.
14. Lewin I, Lerner AG, Green SH, et al. Physical class and physiologic status in the prediction of operative mortality in the aged sick. *Ann Surg* 1971;174:217–231.
15. Reiss, R, Haddad M, Deutsch A, et al. Prognostic index: Prediction of operative mortality in geriatric patients by use of stepwise logistic regression analysis. *World J Surg* 1987;11:248–251.
16. Goldman L, Caldera DL, Nussbaum SR, et al. Multifactorial index of cardiac risk in noncardiac surgical procedures. *N Engl J Med* 1977;297:845–850.
17. Zeldin RA, Math B. Assessing cardiac risk in patients who undergo noncardiac surgical procedures. *Can J Surg* 1984;27:402–404.
18. Jeffrey CC, Kunsman J, Cullen DJ, et al. A prospective validation of the cardiac risk index. *Anesthesiology* 1983;58:462–464.
19. Gerson MC, Hurst JM, Hertzberg VS, et al. Cardiac prognosis in noncardiac geriatric surgery. *Ann Intern Med* 1985;103:832–837.
20. Detsky AS, Abrams HB, McLaughlin JR, et al. Predicting cardiac complications in patients undergoing non-cardiac surgery. *J Gen Intern Med* 1986;1:211–219.
21. Charlson ME, Ales KL, Simon R, et al. Why predictive indexes perform less will in validation studies. *Arch Intern Med* 1987;147:2155–2161.
22. Goldmann DR, Brown FH, Levy WK, et al, eds. *Medical Care of the Surgical Patient*. Philadelphia, Pa: JB Lippincott; 1982.
23. Merli GJ, Weitz HH. Preoperative consultation. *Med Clin North Am* 1987;71:353–590.
24. Brindley GV Jr. Common surgical problems. *Geriatr Clin North Am* 1985;1:311–495.
25. Gibson JR Jr, Mendenhall MK, Axel NJ. Geriatric anesthesia: minimizing the risk. *Geriatr Clin North Am* 1985;1:313–321.
26. Goldman L, Caldera DL. Risks of general anesthesia and elective operation in the hypertensive patient. *Anesthesiology* 1979;50:285–292.
27. Prys-Roberts C, Meloche R, Foex P. Studies of anesthesia in relation to hypertension, I: cardiovascular responses of treated and untreated patients. *Br J Anaesth* 1971;43:122–137.
28. Prys-Roberts C, Greene LT, Meloche R, et al. Studies of anesthesia in relation to hypertension, II: haemodynamic consequences of induction and endotracheal intubation. *Br J Anaesth* 1971;43:531–546.
29. Adler, AG, Leahy JJ, Cressman MD. Management of perioperative hypertension using sublingual nifedipine: experience in elderly patients undergoing eye surgery. *Arch Intern Med* 1986;146:1927–1930.
30. Mahar LJ, Steen PA, Tinker JH, et al. Perioperative myocardial infarction in patients with coronary artery disease with and without aorto-coronary bypass grafts. *J Thorac Cardiovasc Surg* 1978;76:533–537.
31. Goldman L, Caldera DL, Southwick FS, et al. Cardiac risk factors and complications in non-cardiac surgery. *Medicine* 1978;47:357–370.
32. Ropper AH, Wechsler LR, Wilson LS. Carotid bruit and the risk of stroke in elective surgery. *N Engl J Med* 1982;307:1388–1390.
33. Cahalan MK, Litt L, Botvinick EH, et al. Advances in noninvasive cardiovascular imaging: implications for the anesthesiologist. *Anesthesiology* 1987;66:356–372.
34. Chun PKC, Dunn BE. Clinical clue of severe aortic stenosis: simultaneous palpation of the carotid and apical impulses. *Arch Intern Med* 1982;142:2284–2288.
35. Goldman L. Cardiac risks and complications of noncardiac surgery. *Ann Intern Med* 1983;98:504–513.
36. Shulman ST, Amren DP, Bisno AL, et al. Prevention of bacterial endocarditis. *Circulation* 1984;70:1123A–1127A.

37. Medical Letter Consultants. Prevention of bacterial endocarditis. *Med Letter* 1987;29:109.

38. Goldman L. Supraventricular tachyarrhythmias in hospitalized adults after surgery: clinical correlates in patients over 40 years of age after major noncardiac surgery. *Chest* 1978;73:450–454.

39. Chee TP, Prakash NS, Desser KB, et al. Postoperative supraventricular arrhythmias and the role of prophylactic digoxin in cardiac surgery. *Am Heart J* 1982;194:974–977.

40. Pastore JO, Yurchak PM, Janis KM, et al. The risk of advanced heart block in surgical patients with right bundle branch block and left axis deviation. *Circulation* 1978;57:677–680.

41. Bellocci F, Santarelli P, DiGennaro M, et al. The risk of cardiac complications in surgical patients with bifascicular block. *Chest* 1980;77:343–348.

42. Mahler DA, Rosiello RA, Loke J. The aging lung. *Geriatr Clin North Am* 1986;2:215–225.

43. Wahba WM. Influence of aging on lung function: clinical significance of changes from age 20. *Anesth Analg* 1983;62:764–776.

44. Tisi GM. Preoperative evaluation of pulmonary function: validity, indications, and benîfts. *Am Rev Respir Dis* 1979;119:293–310.

45. Helms U, Weihrauch H, Jacobitz K, et al. Die postoperativen veranderungen der blutgase mach unkemplizierten oberbaucheingriffen bei hochbetagten menchen. *Prakt Anasth* 1978;13:275–283.

46. Gass GD, Olsen GN. Preoperative pulmonary function testing to predict postoperative morbidity and mortality. *Chest* 1986;89:127–135.

47. Wernly JA, DeMeester TR, Kirchner PT, et al. Clinical value of quantitative ventilation-perfusion scans in the surgical management of bronchogenic carcinoma. *J Thorac Cardiovasc Surg* 1980;80:835–843.

48. Boysen PG, Block AJ, Olsen GN, et al. Prospective evaluation for pneumonectomy using the technitium lung scan. *Chest* 1977;72:422–425.

49. Stein M, Cassara EL. Preoperative pulmonary evaluation and therapy for surgery patients. *JAMA* 1970;211:787–790.

50. Jones RM. Smoking before surgery: the case for stopping. *Br Med J* 1985;290:1763–1764.

51. Collins CD, Darke CS, Knowelden J. Chest complications after upper abdominal surgery: their anticipation and prevention. *Br Med J* 1968;1:401–406.

52. Morran CG, Finlay IG, Mathieson M, et al. Randomized controlled trial of physiotherapy for postoperative pulmonary complications. *Br J Anaesth* 1983;55:1113–1117.

53. Bartlett RH, Gazzaniga AB, Geraghty T. The yawn maneuver: prevention and treatment of postoperative pulmonary complications. *Surg Forum* 1971;22:196–198.

54. O'Donohue WJ Jr. National survey of the usage of lung expansion modalities for the prevention and treatment of postoperative atelectasis following abdominal and thoracic surgery. *Chest* 1985;87:76–80.

55. Mohr DN, Jett Jr. Preoperative evaluation of pulmonary risk factors. *J Gen Intern Med* 1988;3:277–287.

56. National Institutes of Health Consensus Conference. Prevention of venous thrombosis and pulmonary embolism. *JAMA* 1986;256:744–749.

57. Dalen JE, Paraskos JA, Ockene IS, et al. Venous thromboembolism: scope of the problem. *Chest* 1986;89 (suppl):370S–373S.

58. Collins R, Scrimgeour A, Yusuf S, et al. Reduction in fatal pulmonary embolism and venous thrombosis by perioperative administration of subcutaneous heparin: overview of results of randomized trials in general, orthopedic and urologic surgery. *N Engl J Med* 1988;318:1162–1173.

59. Frocht A, Fillit H. Renal disease in the geriatric patient. *J Am Geriatr Soc* 1984;32:28–39.

60. Cockroft DW, Gault MH. Prediction of creatinine clearance from serum creatinine. *Nephron* 1976;16:31–41.

61. Gral T, Young M. Measured versus estimated creatinine clearance in the elderly as an index of renal function. *J Am Geriatr Soc* 1980;28:492–496.

62. Goldberg TH, Finkelstein MS. Difficulties in estimating glomerular filtration rate in the elderly. *Arch Intern Med* 1987;147:1430–1433.

63. Griffith GL, Maull KI, Coleman C, et al. Acute reversible intrinsic renal failure. *Surg Gynecol Obstet* 1978;146:631–640.

64. Beck LH. Postoperative acute renal failure. In: Goldmann DR, Brown FH, Levy WK, et al, eds. *Medical Care of the Surgical Patient*. Philadelphia, Pa: JB Lippincott; 1982:201–217.

65. Phillips PA, Rolls BJ, Ledingham JGC, et al. Reduced thirst after water deprivation in healthy elderly men. *N Engl J Med* 1984;311:753–759.

66. Epstein M, Hollenberg NK. Age as a determinant of renal sodium conservation in normal man. *J Lab Clin Med* 1976;87:411–417.

67. Miller RD. Anesthesia for the elderly. In: Miller RD, ed. *Anesthesia*. New York, NY: Churchill Livingstone Inc; 1986:1801–1818.

68. Galloway JA, Shuman CR. Diabetes and surgery: a study of 667 cases. *Am J Med* 1963;34:177–191.

69. Scarlett JA. The surgical patient with diabetes. In: Goldmann DR, Brown FH, Levy WK, et al, eds. *Medical Care of the Surgical Patient*. Philadelphia, Pa: JB Lippincott; 1982:144–152.

70. Livingston, EH, Hershman JM, Sawin CT, et al. Prevalence of thyroid disease and abnormal thyroid tests in older hospitalized and ambulatory persons. *J Am Geriatr Soc* 1987;35:109–114.

71. Ladenson PW, Levin AA, Ridgway EC, et al. Complications of surgery in hypothyroid patients. *Am J Med* 1984;77:261–266.

72. Warnold, I, Lundholm K. Clinical significance of preoperative nutritional status in 215 noncancer patients. *Ann Surg* 1984;199:299–305.

73. Mullen JL, Buzby GP, Matthews DC, et al. Reduction of operative morbidity and mortality by combined preoperative and postoperative nutritional support. *Ann Surg* 1980;192:604–613.

74. Baker JP, Detsky AS, Wesson DE, et al. Nutritional assessment: a comparison of clinical judgment and objective measurements. *N Engl J Med* 1982;306:969–972.

75. Detsky AS, Baker JP, O'Rourke K, et al. Perioperative parenteral nutrition: a meta-analysis. *Ann Intern Med* 1987;107:195–203.
76. Gustafson Y, Berggren D, Brannstrom B, et al. Acute confusional states in elderly patients treated for femoral neck fracture. *J Am Geriatr Soc* 1988;36:525–530.
77. Tune L, Folstein F. Post-operative delirium. *Adv Psychosom Med* 1986;15:51–68.
78. American Psychiatric Association. *Diagnostic and Statistical Manual of Mental Disorders*. 3rd ed, revised. Washington, DC. American Psychiatric Association; 1987:103.
79. Berggren D, Gustafson Y, Eriksson B, et al. Postoperative confusion after anesthesia in elderly patients with femoral neck fractures. *Anesth Analg* 1987;66:497–504.
80. Solomon DH. Alcoholism and aging. *Ann Intern Med* 1984;100:411–412.
81. Willenbring ML, Christensen KJ, Spring WD Jr, et al. Alcoholism screening in the elderly. *J Am Geriatr Soc* 1987;35:864–869.

12

Rehabilitation

Kenneth Brummel-Smith

Rehabilitation assists disabled persons in recovering from and adapting to the loss of physical, psychological, or social skills so that they may be more independent, live in personally satisfying environments, and maintain meaningful social relationships. This type of care can be provided in any health care setting, including the home, office, acute or rehabilitation hospital, and long-term care institution. An interdisciplinary team approach is required due to the complex nature of the various interventions. Patients and their families must be involved in decisions regarding rehabilitation treatment. Indeed, rehabilitation is a philosophical approach to the patient that recognizes that diagnoses are poor predictors of functional abilities,[1] that having a disability does not diminish one's social worth, and that the psychosocial aspects of care are at least as important as the medical aspects of care.

The rate of disability in the population increases markedly with age. Almost all problems that lead to disability are more frequently seen in the older population. Clinical geriatrics emphasizes the "functional approach" in the care of the patient. By enhancing the person's functional abilities, the impact of a disability can be lessened. For these reasons, rehabilitation is a basic foundation of geriatric care. The geriatrician can provide a rehabilitation focus in all aspects of patient care.

Definitions of Disability

Some basic concepts and definitions are needed when discussing geriatric rehabilitation. "Impairment" refers to alterations of function at the organ level. Older persons may have many impairments. Some physiologic decline in organ function is seen in almost all systems. These declinations, however, may not affect the person's ability to carry on with daily activities. An impairment severe enough to affect the person's daily functioning is a "disability." When persons with a disability have received appropriate rehabilitation training and have adapted to the change in functional status, they often can be fully independent. However, if subjected to policies that limit rehabilitation interventions because of age or to public buildings accessible only to those who are able bodied, these persons become "handicapped." Therefore, there are no handicapped persons, there are only handicapping societies. Although this chapter will be devoted to the problems of aged persons with a disability, the sociopolitical implications of rehabilitation must not be forgotten (Table 12.1).

Demographics of Disability

A large percentage of persons with a disability are elderly. Forty percent of disabled persons are over age 65 years, and 63% are over 75 years.[2] Conditions for which rehabilitation interventions are beneficial disproportionately affect the elderly population. Seventy-five percent of strokes occur after age 65 years.[3,4] The peak incidence of hip fractures is in the 8th decade.[5] Most amputations are performed in the geriatric age group. Even without such catastrophic diagnoses, the prevalence of limited activities due to chronic conditions is very high, particularly in those over age 75 years.[6]

Table 12.1. Definitions of disability.

Impairment: Organ level
Disability: Person Level
Handicap: Societal level

The type of disability also is important in the way it affects the care-giving system. A decreased ability to walk, feed, or toilet more strongly predicts dependency and increases the burden on caregivers.[7] The decision to institutionalize an older family member is very much related to the level of disability, in that a greater burden of illness creates greater needs for care. Interventions designed to enhance functional abilities and support caregivers have been shown to be cost-effective and lead to fewer hospitalizations, greater levels of independence, and lower mortality.[8,9]

Rehabilitation Principles

Components of Rehabilitation

Rehabilitation comprises a number of components of care. These are summarized in Table 12.2. Each of these components will require special attention in geriatric patients. With older persons, it is not always possible to stabilize the primary problem completely, in that there often is more than one "primary problem." An 80-year-old man with a recent amputation may have underlying cardiac disease, diabetes, and mild renal failure necessitating close supervision by the geriatrician during an inpatient rehabilitation stay. He also may be more prone to secondary complications than a younger person. Preventing such complications is crucial in geriatric populations due to the remarkable ease with which such events develop and the great risks involved. Secondary complications frequently seen in older patients are summarized in Table 12.3.

These complications also disproportionately affect older patients. Decreased subcutaneous fat, poor capillary function, and low blood volumes increase the risk of developing pressure sores. Besides adding great costs to the care of the patient, a sacral pressure sore may delay wheelchair training after a stroke. The enforced lack of exercise may then increase the risk

Table 12.2. Components of rehabilitation.

Stabilization of primary problem(s)
Prevention of secondary complications
Restoration of lost functional abilities
Adaptation of persons to environments
Adaption of environments to person
Promotion of family adaptation and accommodation

Table 12.3. Common secondary complications in geriatric patients.

Psychological dependency	Deconditioning
Confusion	Contractures
Depression	Pneumonia
Anorexia	Pressure sores
Incontinence	Venous thrombosis

of other secondary complications, such as deconditioning or psychological dependence. The development of a number of secondary complications can lead to a "cascade of disasters" (see Chapter 9). Contractures, muscle shortening causing a decrease in the functional range of motion, begin to develop within 24 hours of the cessation of activity.[10] Some contractures may lead to permanent disability, while others may require months of intense physical therapy and serial casting to recover the full range of motion. Muscle strength rapidly declines with immobilization or just decreased physical activity. In younger persons who are immobilized, muscle strength is lost at the rate of 5% per day. Recovery of lost strength occurs at a rate of only 2% per day. The loss of strength in immobilized older persons has not been studied, but it is reasonable that the rate of loss would at least equal that in younger persons, and recovery probably would be slower. Lastly, the quality of "help" given may contribute to the development of secondary complications. Patients encouraged to maintain activities of daily living may lose abilities less rapidly than those who are helped with all activities.[11] A conscious effort by all members of the team, including the patient, is required to prevent the development of secondary disabilities

The foundation of rehabilitation is the restoration of lost functional abilities. By using directed exercises, with the assistance of physical, occupational, and often communication therapists, the patient can "relearn" how to carry out daily activities. Various adaptive equipment, such as rocker knives, sock-donners, and dressing sticks may enable a person to function independently (Figs. 12.1, 12.2).

Another key component in geriatric rehabilitation is adaptation of the environment to the disabled person. The older person may be less able than a younger person to maintain an activity that is extremely demanding physiologically. For instance, a 20-year-old paraplegic may be able to walk using canes and braces. An 80-year-old with spinal stenosis and diminished cardiac reserve most often will need to learn wheelchair mobility skills. Similarly, the evaluation of the home environment plays a large role in geriatrics. Opportunities for obtaining new housing or for modifying the home may be limited by financial concerns and personal preferences.

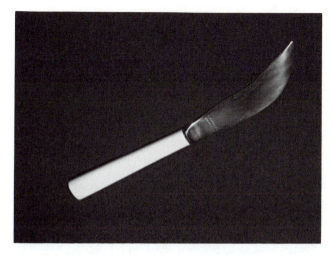

Fig. 12.1. A rocker knife allows the patient to cut with one hand.

Finally, the family must be assisted in the adaptation and support of the older person with a disability. Eighty-five percent of all health care for dependent elders is provided by the family.[12] Often the caregivers themselves are elderly (spouses and older children). The approach to the training of family caregivers is similar to that used with other students. Their knowledge regarding the disabilities and care-giving needs must be assessed and enhanced, their skills in providing care should be evaluated, and their attitudes toward the care-giving role should be elicited.

In summary, each component of rehabilitation must receive attention from a team of clinicians to ensure that the greatest level of functional independence is achieved.

Rehabilitation Teams

Both multidisciplinary and interdisciplinary teams are used in rehabilitation (see also Chapter 52). Geriat-

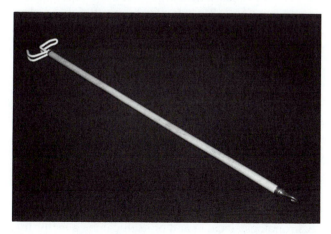

Fig. 12.2. A dressing stick is used to assist with donning coats or sweaters, unhooking velcro closures on shoes, pulling off socks, and so on.

ricians and physiatrists (specialists in physical medicine and rehabilitation) are often involved in interdisciplinary teams, while most primary care physicians function in a multidisciplinary setting. A multidisciplinary team works in a consulting relationship, each person seeing the patient individually and communicating with other team members by written notes or telephone calls. The decision to involve other team members usually is made by the physician. An interdisciplinary team functions in a setting where all team members can meet periodically to discuss the patient's problems and progress. Although each team member has a specific area of expertise, often there is considerable overlap in roles. With more complex cases, such as those seen in inpatient or long-term care rehabilitation, an interdisciplinary team is usually required.

Specific areas of functioning are addressed by different team members. Speech therapists, or communication disorders specialists, do much more than help people talk. In addition to training patients in a wide variety of communication techniques and helping the family adapt to the patient's communication needs, they assess cognitive skills. Occupational therapists are primarily concerned with assessment and treatment of the patient's deficits in basic and instrumental activities of daily living. Cognitive retraining programs as well as perceptual and sensory evaluations are also provided by occupational therapists. An occupational therapist can assist the geriatrician by providing driver training and by making recommendations for automobile modifications.

Physical therapists assess strength, range of motion, coordination, balance, and gait, but these are only a few of the services they provide. Some also assess bulbar function and provide swallowing training programs. The use of electrical stimulation for functional activities and pain control often is managed by physical therapists. Retraining in ambulation, the use of walking aids (canes and walkers), general strengthening, and wheelchair mobility are within the province of physical therapists. As there are hundreds of types of wheelchairs, these are best prescribed by physical therapists.

Recreation therapists serve an important role in geriatric rehabilitation. The ability to resume one's favorite leisure activity can be a powerful force encouraging participation in the rehabilitation program. The quality of life can be greatly enhanced by the resumption or learning anew of hobbies and enjoyable activities.

Each of these specialists have specific requirements for certification or registration. Most have certified aides, assistants, or technicians who provide some portion of the therapeutic program under the supervision of the registered therapist. Physical therapists and, in some states, occupational therapists have ventured into the private practice arena and are available for outpatient consultation and referral. When this is not the case, consultation can be obtained by referral to the appropriate hospital department.

Rehabilitation nurses play a crucial role in promoting the gains made by all the other therapists. They, besides attending to the patient's nursing needs, help the patient practice activities of daily living, make transfers in and out of bed or to the toilet, and learn new medication regimens. They also train family members in care-giving skills and serve as the usual avenue whereby patients and their families bring up questions, discuss concerns and fears, and learn to cope with disability.[13]

Vocational counselors have a role in geriatric rehabilitation as well. Many older persons are capable of work. Rehabilitation counselors are beginning to shift their focus from a purely vocational model to an independent living model when working with older clients.[14]

Ideally, team members should meet periodically to discuss their assessments, establish goals, provide updates on progress toward those goals, and estimate the length of the program needed to meet the goals. Patients should attend these meetings when possible. If they are unable to attend, their input and response to the team's treatment plan should be elicited. A written summary of the meeting is placed in the patient's record. Some teams also provide a copy to the patient and the family.

The role of the physician on the team is to provide medical expertise and often to serve as facilitator of the team process. Physicians must be extremely careful in this dual role as both the "expert" and the "facilitator." Hierarchical relationships are common in medical settings, and the physician-expert may inhibit the functioning of other team members. If that happens, the flow of information necessary to make critical decisions may be impeded. Although the final responsibility of the clinical decision rests with physicians, they must always promote the reasoned deliberation of other team members. Group communication skills and knowledge of team dynamics, attributes often ignored in medical school training, are important for efficient and mutually satisfying team work.

Special Aspects of Rehabilitation and the Older Patient

One of the most important aspects of geriatric care is that treatment of older persons differs in many fundamental ways from treatment of younger persons. This also is true in rehabilitation. The differences can be divided into categories, including those that are patient specific, provider specific, environment specific, and goal specific.

Patient-Specific Differences

A difference that is specific to the patient could be due to age or could be due to disease. Only those changes that may affect the patient's rehabilitation program will be discussed.

Age-Related Changes: Biologic

There is controversy over the degree of physiologic change that is expressly age related. Most investigators agree that some change in cardiac and pulmonary function and muscle strength is inevitable. Because rehabilitation involves fairly intense exercise, these changes are likely to affect the older person more significantly. Aerobic capacity (Vo_2 max) declines with advancing age.[15] The "typical" hospital patient, who may be deconditioned or may have had poor exercise habits before becoming disabled, is likely to have an even lower aerobic capacity. Decreases in vital capacity and minute volume also may affect exercise tolerance.[16] Lean muscle mass and strength decrease with age.[17] Orthostatic changes are common, particularly in those recently bed bound. Finally, the risk of hypertensive episodes with new exercise programs rises with increases in peripheral vascular resistance.

Age-Related Changes: Psychological

Functionally significant changes in cognitive function are not normal. Certain normal changes may nonetheless alter the older persons method of participation in a rehabilitation program. Older adults tend to have a slower pace of learning and require more repetitions to ensure learning.[18] Patients may have rather fixed ideas regarding the role of exercise in their lives. Values have been shown to remain rather stable throughout age,[19] and if the person believes is that one cannot recover from major losses, this belief may impede the learning process. Older persons are less likely to believe that they will be able to recover from a disabling condition and more likely to feel that they do not have enough time left to adjust.[20]

Age-Related Changes: Social

The existence of ageism is perhaps the greatest age-related change in the social realm. As Abdellah notes, "Chronological age in and of itself can be a factor that causes a person not to meet criteria of eligibility for rehabilitation services."[21] Older patients may not be referred for rehabilitation services due to fear of their failing or being harmed. Fewer than 5% of the caseloads of rehabilitation counseling departments are persons over the age of 65 years. Some older persons may share the view implicit in these facts and may feel that they do not deserve rehabilitation services or that the money should be spent on younger persons.

Disease-Related Changes: Biologic

Multiple diseases, rather than a single disabling condition, are the rule in geriatrics. In a study of community-dwelling elderly Hispanic patients, 40% had more than four medical problems.[23] Usually, inpatient rehabilitation programs treat patients from acute hospitals, who may have been bed bound for many days. Contractures, deconditioning, and loss of strength are common. With 20° knee flexion contracture, the energy costs of walking are increased by 35%.[24] In the person with subclinical coronary insufficiency, this increased demand may be enough to provoke angina. When upper-extremity walking aids or wheelchairs are used, oxygen consumption increases. In the person with underlying pulmonary insufficiency, this increased consumption may limit exercise capability. A poststroke patient, even with training, will have approximately twice the normal energy expenditures when walking with a hemiparetic gait.[24] Upper extremity osteoarthritis may limit the use of a walker in rehabilitation after a hip fracture. Thus geriatric rehabilitation patients may have multiple disabling diseases with which to contend.

Disease-Related Changes: Psychological

Underlying cognitive and affective problems often are unrecognized in medical and rehabilitation settings.[25,26] In the acute hospital, patients are not taxed intellectually and their cognitive deficits may go unnoticed. Depression is a common problem among patients being evaluated for or provided with rehabilitation services. Depression may present as not wanting to be bothered, feelings of hopelessness, (more subtly) decreased energy, lack of interest in activities, or decreased participation in therapeutic exercises. Depression may occur in as many as half of patients experiencing a stroke.[27] In another study, 28% of all patients undergoing rehabilitation were clinically depressed and half of these had depressive histories that antedated their disability.[28] It is appropriate to assess each geriatric patient for underlying cognitive or affective disorders at the beginning of the rehabilitation program.

The difficulties in motivating geriatric patients are a frequent topic of discussion in rehabilitation settings. This complaint usually means that the provider is unable to get patients to do what the provider would like them to do. Motivation can be assessed more completely by looking at the components of decision making that influence a person's choices.[20] These components can be illustrated by the following equation:

$$Motivation = (W \times E \times R)/C.$$

To determine a person's motivation to do something, one must know what that person wants (W), what he or she expects (E) will occur if the plan is accomplished, and what reinforcements or rewards (R) are likely to be encountered. These elements are affected by the costs (C): physical, economical, emotional, and social. Thus, persons are very motivated when they strongly desire the intervention, expect that it will benefit them, receive a modicum of positive rewards (the sooner the better), and incur low costs. Persons with "low motivation" may not want the goal, may not expect or believe they can achieve it, or may find the results to be not very satisfying or the costs to be too high.

There are some changes in motivation related to age. When faced with a choice, older persons tend toward the status quo. Moreover, they tend to take fewer risks in new situations and need more time to make decisions. Older persons try to avoid failure.[20] Because of these changes, older patients may appear less motivated in clinical situations. Practitioners can minimize the effect of the changes by explaining the reasons for a particular activity, by projecting a nonjudgmental attitude, and by allowing more time to practice.

Disease-Related Changes: Social

As noted above, society handicaps disabled persons to the extent that they are prevented from functioning at their highest possible level. Indeed, the major impact of a disability is in the social realm.[29] Many disabled people feel that the most difficult area of adjustment is relating to society. Unlike the physical and psychological adaptation to a disability, which usually is accomplished within the first 2 years after the disabling problem begins, the social adaptation continues for the rest of a person's life. Access to public buildings and reimbursement guidelines that do not limit access to rehabilitation on the basis of age or residency (eg, a nursing home) need to be promoted. Handicapping of disabled people can be minimized by legal protection of the rights of the disabled, adequate financing of rehabilitative interventions, and public education directed toward enhancing the standing of disabled persons in the community.

Provider-Specific Differences

In geriatric settings, the roles of various providers often overlap. The most obvious circumstance is when both a geriatrician and a physiatrist are working with the same person. Often geriatricians coordinate rehabilitation interventions in outpatient settings or in facilities where there are no physiatrists. However, even when physiatrists are available, the geriatrician may have to intervene for the patient to receive services. Ideally, the geriatrician helps manage the complex, multiple medical problems while the physiatrist coordinates the rehabilitation team.

There are other roles that overlap. Often nurses provide family support and counseling, psychologists may recommend psychotropic medications, and occupational or speech therapists may diagnose cognitive problems. A rehabilitation team is effective only insofar as it allows individual team members to express their full potential. In geriatric rehabilitation, where the patients have multiple problems and psychosocial issues predominate, it is crucial that each team member's viewpoint be considered.

Even small gains in function can mean a significant difference in independence. One must be careful to not miss opportunities to promote such small gains. With advanced age, loss of family members, or preexisting medical problems, the adjustment to a disability is made more difficult. A variety of simple but fun physical activities performed in a group setting may accomplish more in recovering range of motion or strength than a rigorous training program. During recreational therapy, a patient can pay less attention to performance but still accomplish worthwhile goals. A therapeutic pass, so that the patient can try out newly learned skills overnight, may help with depression and enable the patient to see more value in hospital-based therapies. Even when ambulation is not possible, a prosthesis for cosmetic purposes may allow the amputee to engage in community activities, thereby promoting self-respect.

Finally, it is important to be aware of our own ageist attitudes that influence decisions regarding rehabilitation. There is little evidence that age, alone, affects rehabilitation. Age has not been shown to be detrimental in stroke rehabilitation[30]; even persons over age 85 years can benefit.[31] Rehabilitation is also cost-effective.[32] In spite of these facts, providers of rehabilitation may have rather negative attitudes toward elderly persons.[33,34] Therefore, when decisions are made regarding cessation of therapy, one must consider the possibility that "therapeutic hopelessness" exists.

Environment-Specific Differences

Although all persons interact with their environment, this interaction becomes potentially more precarious as persons age. Physiologic reserves, underlying medical problems, affective states, and a host of other factors complicate the relationship between the person and his or her environment.

Often the response to this precarious relationship is to modify the environment to make it "safer." Assistive aids or home modifications may be recommended, but these interventions are subject to differences when dealing with older persons. Most of the commonly prescribed assistive aids are unattractive, and many are difficult to use. Unlike eyeglasses, in which case the "disabled" person now can choose a pair that looks appealing, walkers, chrome-plated grab bars, and wheelchairs project an image of illness. Furthermore, older persons are less likely to be able to install home modifications themselves. Some Retired Senior Volunteer Programs have carpenters available for this purpose, but many communities do not have such support services.

The reimbursement environment also may be different when one is dealing with elderly clients. Current Medicare guidelines stipulate that, when receiving acute rehabilitation services, the patient must receive physical, occupational, and/or speech therapy for at least 3 hours a day, 6 days a week. Such an aggressive program may be impossible for some geriatric patients, yet they could benefit from a less intensive schedule. The reason for this requirement is suspect; there is evidence that persons receiving 3-hour intervention do not improve significantly more than those receiving less intense and less costly therapy.[35] When a program provides a 2-week trial of rehabilitation in the hospital, it may not be reimbursed if the patient is discharged to a nursing home, in spite of the patient's improvement in functional status. It is more difficult with geriatric patients than with younger patients to obtain funding to equip a car with hand controls. Such problems may provoke a decision not to provide rehabilitation services, based on the likelihood of reimbursement rather than on the likelihood of functional improvement.

Goal-Specific Differences

With geriatric clients, there are differences in the goals of rehabilitation. For example physical therapists are often concerned with the patient's gait in terms of safety. Yet, older persons may prefer to walk "incorrectly" rather than not walk at all. These decisions are strongly related to values; the older person with a gait problem may prefer to risk a fall than be placed in a nursing home. Some older persons fear the loss of independence more than they fear death. The ultimate goal in rehabilitation is to promote independence, as defined by the patient.

Rehabilitation Techniques in Geriatric Care

Geriatrics has long promoted the functional approach in health care. Function is believed to encompass the physical, psychological, and social components of a person's life. In this regard, geriatrics and rehabilitation are synonymous. The enhancement of a person's ability to live independently must be addressed in all medical settings, not just in rehabilitation. Therefore, geriatricians must constantly assess the functional impact of the problem being treated and of the intervention being offered. (Instruments and techniques used to measure function, such as the various scales used to detect changes in cognitive, self-care, or social skills, are discussed in Chapters 5 and 6.) By attending to such matters not directly related to rehabilitation (such as in treating hypertension), the geriatrician practices rehabilitation interventions. Geriatricians also can benefit their patients by identifying needs for consultation with allied health practitioners. For instance, an adjunct to the primary treatment of the depressed patient may be a gait-retraining program that addresses the state of deconditioning.

Rehabilitation in Different Care Sites

Rehabilitation interventions can be provided in a variety of continuing-care sites. Medicare may cover some of these services, but Medicaid's reimbursement policies vary from state to state.

An ideal site for providing rehabilitation is the patient's home. The problem of transportation is relieved, and services can be rendered at lower costs than in hospitals.[36] Medicare may reimburse for some in-home services provided by nurses, as well as physical and occupational therapists. The patient's ability to function with available equipment can be assessed, the family is usually supportive, and carryover of techniques taught during therapy can be monitored. In one study, patients cared for at home obtained the greatest degree of functional improvement from home modifications, the next best improvement from instruction in the proper use of assistive-aid devices, and the least from exercises.[37] For the patient thought to be able to benefit from rehabilitation in outpatient settings but unable to attend clinics because of transportation difficulties, limited endurance, psychological reasons, or personal choice, home care is a valuable option.

Outpatient centers provide a large proportion of rehabilitation services. These centers may be found in physicians' offices, private physical (and occupational) therapy practices, Certified Outpatient Rehabilitation Facilities, day health centers, and hospital-affiliated facilities. Their advantages are (1) their access to a wider variety of practitioners and technology, (2) the stimulation for patients of being around other people (a disadvantage to some patients), and (3) their ability to serve more patients with fewer practitioners. Transportation to the clinic often is a major problem with the very old.

Perhaps the greatest unmet need for rehabilitation is in the acute hospital. The potential negative effects of acute hospitalization have been well documented.[38] In acute hospitals, functional disability often goes undetected.[39] Over half of these patients have difficulties with activities of daily living, and the hospital environment itself may interfere with functional recovery. With the advent of diagnosis-related groups and prospective payment, it is essential to obtain early allied health consultation as well as discharge planning so that the patient in need of rehabilitation receives preventive measures while awaiting more intensive interventions. When possible, patients should be kept out of their beds, walked to the bathroom or diagnostic studies, and encouraged to dress and feed themselves.

The classic site for providing rehabilitation is the specialized rehabilitation hospital. Such institutions may be freestanding or affiliated with an acute hospital. A full complement of rehabilitation specialists is on site. Usually, a physiatrist or, (in the case of geriatric rehabilitation units), a geriatrician coordinates the team. In order to receive Medicare reimbursement, patients must undergo 3 hours per day of physical, occupational, or speech therapy and must make regular progress toward specific goals. Periodic team meetings are held at least biweekly, and progress must be documented in the chart. A number of hospitals are developing specialized centers with the creation of geriatric units, geriatric-orthopedic units,[40] stroke units,[41] and assessment units.[42] Geriatric rehabilitation has been shown to be effective,[43,44,45] and age need not be a deterrent to providing rehabilitation.[30,31,50]

The nursing home is another important site for providing rehabilitation. For patients requiring physical or occupational therapy, Medicare funding can be obtained. In selected patients, the cost is less than acute care or intensive rehabilitation and the results are satisfactory.[46] About one fifth of patients treated in a rehabilitation-oriented skilled nursing facility are able to return home.[47] Some community- dwelling elderly persons may be able to use the nursing home as a primary site of rehabilitation. However, current Medicare regulations require a 3-day stay in an acute hospital before allowing reimbursement. Adelman et al

Table 12.4.

Physical health and impairments	
Cardiopulmonary:	Response to exercise, presence of coronary insufficiency or chronic obstructive pulmonary disease
Musculoskeletal:	Limitations of functional range of motion, pain deformities, foot problems
Neurologic:	Sensory deficits, presence of neglect, apraxia, agnosia, perseveration
Functional status:	Activities of daily living, continence, nutritional needs
Mobility:	Gait, balance, history of using walking aids, skin integrity
Cognitive and psychological functioning	
Mental status	
Affective state	
Motivation and desire to participate in program	
Goals and wishes for the future	
Social and support environment	
Family and friends (neighbors, church associates, etc)	willing to provide support
Home environment:	Accessibility, safety, modifications needed, feelings regarding potential need for relocation
Prior experiences in "learning situations":	Education, hobbies, work
Community Programs:	Availability of nutrition, transportation, and case management programs
Economic resources	
Health insurance coverage for rehabilitation	
Disposable income	
Assets	
Support from family	
Personal values regarding expending resources	

reported that 57% of community-dwelling elderly persons undergoing rehabilitation in a nursing home were able to return home.[48] It is obvious from this discussion that rehabilitation is a process that depends more on the type of intervention than on the site where the care is provided.

Assessment for Rehabilitation Potential

The first step in the assessment for rehabilitation potential is the geriatrician's awareness that rehabilitation interventions may be of benefit. Once that idea is entertained, a number of features must be considered. Factors associated with a better prognosis include recent (rather than long-term) health changes, less severe deficits, an assertive personality, a supportive family system, and adequate economic resources. A poorer prognosis exists for patients with low motivation, more severe health problems (especially if associated with cognitive impairments), and inadequate economic resources or support systems. On the other hand, no single factor should automatically exclude a person from a trial of rehabilitation interventions.

When there is doubt, the patient should undergo a multidisciplinary assessment before a final determination is made. The assessment should identify what demands the patient will encounter in the expected living environment and whether he or she has the ability to meet those demands. A complete assessment includes evaluations of the patient's physical impairments, cognitive and psychological functioning, the social environment, and economic resources.[49] The patient's prior level of functioning and present capabilities should both be determined, and the factors to be considered are outlined in Table 12.4.

In addition to these general considerations, factors specific to each disabling condition play a role in determining the appropriateness of rehabilitation. These are discussed in the specific problem areas below. The evaluation often is performed by a physiatrist, a nurse practitioner trained in rehabilitation, or a rehabilitation team. The consultant also must decide which site would be best for providing rehabilitation. In some cases, the geriatrician may be called on to advocate more intensive interventions on the patient's behalf.

Rehabilitation of Common Geriatric Conditions

Stroke

Stroke is a prototypic illness insofar as rehabilitation is concerned. Risks, prevention, and early treatment of stroke are covered in Chapter 34. Rehabilitation interventions begin on the same day as the stroke. Initially, the goals of rehabilitation primarily are preventive. In the immobilized patient, pressure sores can develop within 2 hours, and early contractures can be seen within 24 hours.

Functional return is to some degree dependent on chance. Rehabilitation interventions are designed (1) to prevent the occurence of secondary disabilities, (2) to train the patient in alternate methods for performing functional activities, (3) to promote adaptation to persistent deficits, and (4) to help the patient and family adapt to their new roles.

Most of the return of function will be seen in the 1st month. In some cases, however, motor function may return as late as 6 months after the stroke. Sensory deficits or swallowing problems may improve later. In spite of these endogenous improvements, rehabilitation efforts following stroke are cost-effective and lead to higher functional levels.[8] Age, by itself, does not affect rehabilitation outcome.[30] Patients and their families need accurate prognostic information soon after the stroke in order to make informed decisions about care. The highest mortality is in the 1st week. About 10% of survivors recover completely, 40% have minimal residual of disability, 40% have significant levels of dysfunction, and 10% need total care. Therefore, rehabilitation can benefit about 80% to 90% of stroke survivors.

Acute Phase

In the acute phase, rehabilitation efforts are geared toward preventing secondary disabilities and identifying patients who need more intensive rehabilitation. Prevention of secondary disabilities should begin soon after admission. The patient must be turned regularly to prevent the development of pressure sores. Daily ranging of the extremities and exercise of the uninvolved limbs to prevent deconditioning should be provided. Attention to bowel and bladder function also is important.

Immediately after the stroke, the patient usually has flail limbs. The arm needs to be properly placed to prevent subluxation of the shoulder, so that when motor function returns the arm will be more functional. Reflex sympathetic dystrophy (the "hand-shoulder syndrome") also can be prevented by regular ranging, close attention to proper bed positioning, and protecting the shoulder when moving the patient.[50] Proper body positioning usually will prevent nerve palsies from developing. The use of a footboard to prevent plantar flexion contractures is controversial and should not take the place of active ranging.

Although temporary urinary incontinence is common, other causes (eg, infections) should be ruled out.

Because the patient's cognitive state usually is clear after a single stroke, the presence of confusion should lead to investigation of possible treatable causes. During the acute phase the patient must be medically stabilized, blood pressure and other confounding medical problems must be controlled, and unnecessary drugs must be discontinued.

In the initial phase it is possible to make some prognostication of outcome. Factors associated with a poor prognosis[51] include flaccid hemiplegia of greater than 2 months' duration, dementia, persistent bowel or bladder incontinence, severe neglect or sensory deficits, and global aphasia. Patients who exhibit none of these features should be evaluated for intensive rehabilitation.

Rehabilitation Phase

Once the patient's condition is reasonably stable, intensive rehabilitation can begin. Total stability is elusive in the older person, and risks of an intervention must be weighed against risks of continued bed rest. Motor return follows a fairly predictable pattern. Initially, the limbs are flaccid with hyperactive reflexes. The next stage is mass flexor synergism, ie, the limb will flex at multiple joints when movement is attempted. A mass extensor synergism usually will occur next. Once the patient has an extensor synergy pattern, even with poor control, ambulation may be possible with a brace and adequate physical training. If the motor return progresses, selective flexion of individual joints usually follows, and finally selective extension with decreased flexor tone returns. Unfortunately, the return of sensory function is much less predictable. The return of motor function tends to be more important to ambulation (a value held highly by patients), while sensory return relates more to upper extremity function and activities of daily living.

It is in this phase that allied health specialists play crucial roles. Physical therapists work with patients to develop strength, evaluate transfer abilities, enhance balance abilities (sitting, then standing), and increase endurance. When being tested for strength, patients should attempt to stand (with assistance if necessary), because supine testing may give falsely weak results. When the lower extremities have "good strength" (4/5) and the patient can balance on the uninvolved side, gait training can be initiated.

When the patient has difficulties advancing the limb, a brace, hemicane, or walker may be required (Figs 12.3, 12.4). Ankle-foot orthoses are most commonly used in the elderly stroke patient (Fig 12.5). Two types are commonly employed: the double adjustable upright, used to stabilize the ankle and provide some proprioceptive feedback to the knee, and the posterior

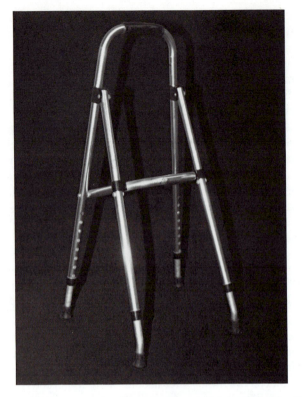

Fig. 12.3. A hemi-walker can be used by persons with hemiplegia.

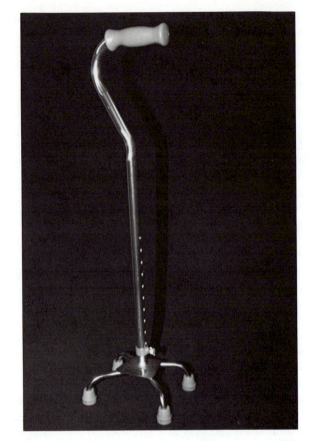

Fig. 12.4. A four-prong cane adds stability to the traditional cane.

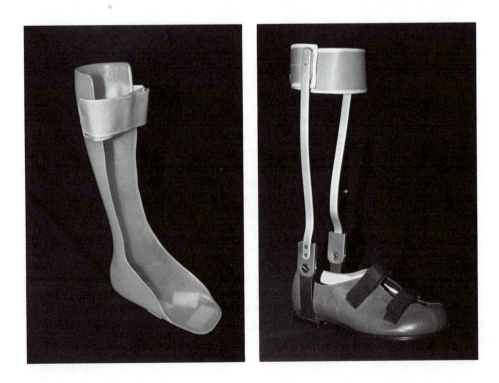

Fig. 12.5. Ankle-foot-orthoses: polyethlyene lower leg brace (left) and double adjustable upright lower leg brace (right).

plastic splint, which prevents footdrop but requires a more stable ankle. Functional electrical stimulation is often used to supplement the patient's muscular activity as well as reeducate paralyzed muscles.

The occupational therapist works with the patient to provide training in daily self-care activities. Perceptual deficits are commonly seen, particularly in right-sided cerebrovascular accidents. These deficits may go undetected until the patient's ability to organize motor tasks in sequence is evaluated. Simple remedies may provide great self-care benefits. For instance, spasticity sometimes can be controlled with the use of weighted utensils. Other types of special utensils—such as rocker knives, plate guards, and reachers—enable persons with hemiplegia to function more independently. A cognitive retraining program also may be provided by occupational therapists, or sometimes by speech therapists. Early assessment for aphasia is critical to providing other team members with recommendations regarding communication needs.

Special attention must be given to two common, and often related, problems. Poststroke depression is very common, especially with left hemisphere damage.[52] Treatment of depression facilitates the gains made in rehabilitation. Psychotherapy and the judicious use of antidepressant medication are usually needed. The second problem seen too often in rehabilitation is malnutrition. A swallowing evaluation, dietary consultation and, in some cases, short-term use of enteral feedings may be required.

Attention to premorbid problems must be especially vigilant in geriatric patients. Having access to one's dentures, eyeglasses, and clothing promotes self-esteem and may enhance the ability to participate in the rehabilitation program. The patient's family should be involved in the treatment program through training in care-giving skills. A bedside graph to document progress made by the patient and a chart that specifies goals to be achieved also can be helpful.

Chronic Phase

The chronic phase begins when the person who has suffered a stroke returns to society as a person with a disability. The home will usually need modifications, especially the bathroom. Installation of raised toilet seats with arm frames, grab bars, and a bathtub bench with a hand-held shower hose will be required. Kitchen modification also may be necessary. Prior to discharge, the home should be assessed for door widths, the presence of stairs, the need for ramps, the adequacy of lighting, safety features, and needed modifications.

Because the adjustment process to a major disability may take up to 2 years, ongoing psychological support

often is necessary. The patient may benefit from individual or group psychotherapy, a day health center, or a stroke recovery group. Frank information should be provided regarding the safety of sexual activities following a stroke.

Social activities should be strongly encouraged. A vocational rehabilitation counselor can assess and help with the return to employment if desired. Arrangements for transportation are particularly important, as many geriatric patients will stop driving after a stroke. For patients with right hemisphere lesions and neglect, driving is inadvisable unless the neglect remits.

Hip Fractures

Hip fractures are commonly encountered in geriatrics. Many of these patients can benefit from a rehabilitative intervention. The geriatrician also plays an important role in advocating the surgical procedure that will promote maximum independence and early ambulation. A general rule is to use techniques that allow the greatest amount of weight bearing soon after surgery. It is very difficult for older persons to "toe-touch" weight bear during ambulation, owing to general deconditioning and weak upper extremities.

Two types of hip fractures, subcapital and trochanteric, are most common. The distinguishing feature is the high rate of avascular necrosis of the femoral head seen in subcapital fractures. In elderly patients, most subcapital fractures are treated with installation of an Austin-Moore (or similar) prosthesis. Weight bearing to tolerance is allowed by the 2nd or 3rd day, an important consideration in light of the negative consequences of immobilization in this age group. Aggressive treatment of trochanteric fractures by internal fixation with a compression screw also is indicated in most cases. With this procedure, the patient usually can bear weight as tolerated by the 2nd day.[53] In the patient with a trochanteric fracture who has preexisting joint disease, a prosthesis also may be indicated.[54]

Non–weight-bearing status for up to 8 weeks has often been recommended in those patients treated with pins or nails. Such a period of inactivity is much too long for the geriatric patient. Weight bearing can be attempted as soon as 1 week after such procedures and, in the absence of pain, it appears to be safe and well tolerated by most patients. It is best to reserve conservative treatment with closed reduction for those patients who are unable to tolerate a surgical procedure and those who were bed bound before the fracture.

Rehabilitation efforts should begin as soon as the patient is admitted to the hospital. Stabilization of life-threatening medical problems should occur before surgical repair. If the patient is alert, preoperative evaluation by physical and occupational therapy and training in the exercises to be performed in bed can begin immediately. The patient can begin quadriceps contractions and, on the 1st postoperative day, can sit up and perform isometric exercises as well as gentle flexion-extension at the hip. Adduction, excessive flexion, and abduction at the hip should be avoided.

The patient can begin supervised ambulation with parallel bars by the 2nd or 3rd postoperative day, advancing to the use of a walker or cane. A properly fitted cane should have a one inch (or 2–3 cm) rubber tip and be long enough to allow 20° to 30° of flexion at the elbow when held at the side (Fig 12.6). The patient should support no more than 20% to 25% of total body weight on the cane. The hand opposite the injured hip should use the cane. By the 6th or 7th postoperative day, the patient can begin proning exercises to strengthen the hip extensors. Stair training begins during the 2nd week and consists of going up stairs with the uninvolved leg first and coming down with the involved leg first ("up with the good, down with the bad").

If the patient lacks upper body strength or is unstable with a cane, a walker should be prescribed (Fig. 12.7). Patients need to practice advancing the walker

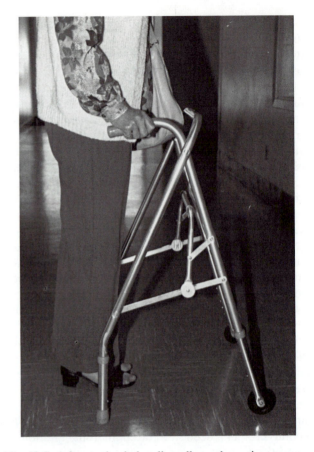

Fig. 12.7. A front-wheeled walker allows the patient to move more smoothly and decreases the risk of falling backwards.

about 20 to 30 cm, then advancing the weak leg, and then the good leg. Some older persons may find it easier to advance the good leg first, but this practice increases the risk of falls. Crutches are very difficult for most older persons to use. It must be remembered that special walkers are needed for going up stairs, and it is very difficult to carry objects while using a walker.

Depending on the preexisting health and social support status of the patient, the site for rehabilitation after hip fracture will vary. The patient's general medical condition is the most important factor affecting recovery.[55] Dementia and neurologic diseases are the greatest threats. Early discharge and home rehabilitation should be considered for those with (1) good health (the absence of significant medical problems), (2) strong social supports (someone who can provide assistance), and (3) adequate performance of ambulation and activities of daily living within 2 weeks of surgery. The remainder may require more intensive therapy than can be provided in the home.

Amputation

Three quarters of all amputations occur in people over age 65 years. Below-the-knee (BK) amputations are

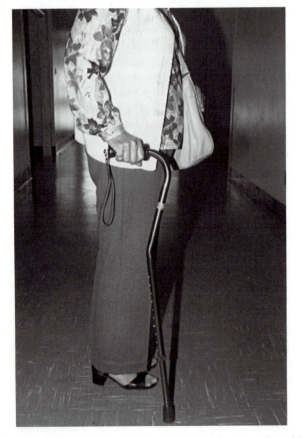

Fig. 12.6. Note elbow flexion at 20-30° in the adjustable cane.

the norm. The predominant cause is peripheral vascular disease. The older person's care is more complex after amputation due to weak upper extremities, underlying cardiovascular problems, skin that is prone to breakdown, and poor balance mechanisms. Older persons are more likely to have subsequent amputations on the contralateral side.[56] The geriatrician plays a crucial role in managing these problems and in helping to determine the most appropriate surgical intervention.

If at all possible, a BK amputation should be performed rather than an above-the-knee (AK) procedure. With a BK procedure, there is a lower postoperative mortality rate, the energy costs of using a prosthesis are less, and the chance of walking without the use of canes or walkers is better. Indeed, the energy cost of walking with bilateral BK amputations is lower than that of walking with a single AK amputation.[57] In a younger person such energy costs may be insignificant, but in the older patient they may precipitate angina where there is underlying coronary insufficiency.

Patients with poor cognition, preexisting joint disease of the affected knee, and contralateral sensory deficits may have difficulties learning to use a BK prosthesis. If the patient has contralateral vascular disease a prosthesis may be contraindicated. However, this is a very individual decision, and the motivated patient still may benefit from a prosthesis trial.

Even if a prothesis is not going to be used, patients can benefit from rehabilitation. Training in the use of a special amputation-style wheelchair should be provided. Bed, chair and toilet transfers also must be learned. Home modifications will need to be made. Because the energy costs of using a wheel chair are higher than those of walking, patients with chronic obstructive pulmonary disease and cardiovascular insufficiency will need to be stabilized.

All geriatric patients should be considered for the fitting of a prosthesis. Age should not be a determinative factor in this consideration. The decision should be based on the patient's medical state, motivation, and mobility needs. As in the case of hip fractures, rehabilitation should begin before the surgical procedure. Exercise training, including strengthening of the upper body, quadriceps, and hip extensors and practice lying prone, should begin as soon as the amputation is considered. Contractures of the hip and knee are the most common complications of amputations. They must be prevented by active and passive ranging daily. The bed should be kept flat, and pillows should not be placed under the knees.

Following the operation the patient must be trained in care of the stump. Massage techniques, wrapping with an elastic bandage or stump shrinker, inspection for skin integrity, and hygiene should receive attention. The patient should begin transfers with and without the prosthesis immediately postoperatively. Many geriatric patients will use a wheelchair for longer distances, so they also must receive training in its use. Sitting and single-limb balance training also is important.

A prosthesis is usually fitted 6 to 8 weeks postoperatively to allow for stump shrinkage and wound healing. A temporary pylon prosthesis is often employed in the meantime. Some surgeons have used casts placed at the time of the operation to promote early ambulation. The experience of using cast/prostheses in older persons is limited. A physiatrist or orthotist usually prescribes and fits a prosthesis. A patella-tendon-supracondylar socket with a solid-ankle, cushioned-heel foot is often used in elderly patients, as it is lightweight and easy to use.

The outcome of prosthetic training in elderly persons is quite good, with about 75% of unilateral BK amputees achieving independent ambulation. Unfortunately, only 50% of bilateral BK amputees and less than 50% of unilateral AK amputees will walk with a prosthesis.[57] Although one third of amputees will have phantom limb sensation, less than 5% have severe pain. Massage and physical therapy, along with small doses of antidepressant medication, usually suffice to treat such pain. The older person also may experience a change in the socket size with large weight changes (weight loss affects size more than weight gain), and neuroma formation and local skin problems can occur.

Parkinson's Disease

The peak incidence of Parkinson's disease is between the ages of 60 and 69 years, with as many as 40,000 to 50,000 new cases per year. Although drug treatment has led to significant improvements in the care of patients with Parkinson's disease, specific physical interventions also may be helpful. The physical treatment of Parkinson's disease can be considered an example of "preventive" geriatric rehabilitation.

The patient should be trained in techniques used to counter the effects of the disease. Strengthening and endurance training and proper use of assistive equipment also are important. Such training is best provided early in the course of the illness as an outpatient. Involvement in a support group may help to maintain newly learned skills.

Gait and balance training emphasizes a safe gait and improved balance. The patient should be taught to keep the head up, to counter the flexed posture consciously, and to lift the toes during the swing phase of the gait. It also may help to take longer steps and widen the base. The therapist often prescribes a home program of regular exercises to maintain or improve strength, range of motion, and flexibility. Some patients may benefit from speech therapy for articulation and breathing exercises. Other patients find singing to be helpful.

Canes should be avoided when walking aids become necessary. Due to the posture of Parkinson's disease, protraction and internal rotation of the shoulder may place the tip of the cane between the legs, causing a fall. When the walker is prescribed it should be fitted with front wheels, as pick-up walkers may induce a backward fall. In the home, shag or throw rugs should be removed, rails should be installed on all steps, and bathroom equipment (including raised toilet seats or arm frames and grab bars) should be prescribed.

Deconditioning and Immobility

Deconditioning, which usually can be traced to excessive bed rest in the home or institution, is a common geriatric phenomenon. With modern medical therapies there really are no diseases for which absolute bedrest is indicated. Conditioning reflexes can be maintained by simply sitting in a chair for 1 to 2 hours. Following hospitalization, some patients may be unable to return home because of deconditioning, in spite of having had their admitting diagnoses "successfully" treated. Therefore, the mainstay of treatment is prevention. In the acute hospital, patients should have orders for regular out-of-bed activities, be encouraged to walk to diagnostic studies if possible, and be taught bed and chair exercises if activities are limited. In some cases group exercise programs may be better tolerated and less costly.

If patients do not stress their cardiopulmonary or muscular systems, the presence of deconditioning may go unnoticed. This disorder can be recognized by an exaggerated heart rate or blood pressure response to exercise, decreased muscle power, and decreased endurance. Measurements of a person's "capacity" for exercise should be based on the expected demand in the anticipated living environment. For example, if the person is to be ambulatory in the community, it has been determined that he or she will need to be able to walk 332 meters at $\geq$ 50% normal velocity ($>$ 40 m/min), as well as negotiate three steps and a 3% ramp with rails and a curb.[58] One does not need to achieve total cardiovascular fitness to improve skills in independent living. Velocity and safety, not cardiovascular fitness, determine how well the person functions in community settings.

Rehabilitation is directed at enhancing strength, gait stability, and velocity in building endurance. In severely deconditioned patients, the time required to recover lost strength can be estimated to be three times as long as they were immobilized. Patients with premorbid cardiac or pulmonary disease may need inpatient rehabilitation to regain independence.

Other Conditions

A wide variety of other problems are amenable to rehabilitation interventions. A minority of patients with spinal cord injuries are elderly. One study showed that over 73% of persons suffering spinal injuries after age 60 years were able to return home with rehabilitation.[59] The most common chronic illness in the geriatric age group is arthritis. Rehabilitation techniques are used to maintain function of arthritic joints, enhance mobility, and prevent deterioration. Joint replacement surgery is being used increasingly in older populations, and rehabilitation is very important following these procedures. The cornerstones of arthritis rehabilitation are the use of adaptive equipment and training in joint protection and energy conservation techniques. Rehabilitation has even been used in Alzheimer's disease.[60] Caregivers can be trained in techniques that will allow the patient with Alzheimer's disease to maintain activities of daily living and thereby reduce care-giving stress.[61]

Conclusion

Rehabilitation, as both a philosophical approach and a technical intervention, is a treatment that should be considered in all geriatric patients with functional losses. Every intervention provided to older persons has the potential for enhancing or limiting functional abilities. If we are to be truly successful in treating the conditions associated with aging, patients should leave our care with higher functional capabilities than when they began treatment.

References

1. Williams TF. Keynote speech. Presented at the Aging and Rehabilitation Conference; December 2, 1984; Philadelphia, Pa.
2. Wedgewood J. The place of rehabilitation in geriatric medicine: an overview. *Int Rehabil Med* 1985;7:107–108.
3. *National Survey of Stroke*. Bethesda, Md: National Institute of Health publication 80-2064.
4. Clark G, Blue B, Bearer J. Rehabilitation of the elderly amputee. *J Am Geriatr Soc* 1983;31:439–448.
5. Kumar VN, Redford JB. Rehabilitation of hip fractures in the elderly. *Am Fam Physician* 1984;29:173–180.
6. *A Chartbook of the Federal Council on Aging*. 1981:29–31. Department of Health and Human Services publication, Washington DC; (OHDS) 81-2070.

7. Enright RB, Friss L. *Employed Care-givers of Brain-Damaged Adults: An Assessment of the Dual Role*. San Francisco, Calif: Family Survival Project, 1987.

8. Lehman JF, Wieland, GD. Stroke: does rehabilitation affect outcome? *Arch Phys Med Rehabil* 1975;56:375–382.

9. Rubenstein LZ, Josephson KR, et al. Effectiveness of a geriatric evaluation unit: a randomized trial. *N Engl J Med* 1984;311:1664–1670.

10. Sharpless JW. *Mossman's: A Problem Oriented Approach to Stroke Rehabilitation*. Springfield, Ill: Charles C. Thomas Publishers; 1982.

11. Avorn J. Induced disability in nursing home patients. *J Am Geriatr Soc* 1980;30:397–400.

12. Brody E. Informal support systems in the rehabilitation of the disabled elderly. In: Brody SJ, Ruff GE, eds. *Aging and Rehabilitation*. New York, NY: Springer Publishing Co Inc; 1986.

13. Hamberger SG, Tanner RD. Nursing interventions with families of geriatric patients. *Top Geriatr Rehabil* 1988;4:32–39.

14. Bozarth JD. The rehabilitation process and older people. *J Rehabil* 1981;47:28–32.

15. Shepard RJ. World standards of cardiorespiratory performance. *Arch Environ Health* 1966;13:664–672.

16. Kohn R. *Principles of Mammalian Aging*. Englewood Cliffs, NJ: Prentice Hall International Inc; 1978.

17. Shock NW, Norris AH. Neuromuscular coordination as a factor in age changes in muscular exercise. In: Brunner D, Jokl E, eds. *Physical Activity and Aging*. New York, NY: S Karger AG; 1970.

18. Huyck MH, Hoyer WJ: *Adult Development and Aging*. Belmont, Calif: Wadsworth Inc; 1982: chap 5.

19. Troll LE. Personal development. In: *Continuations: Adult Development and Aging*. Monterey, Calif: Brooks/Cole Publishing Co; 1982: chap 5.

20. Kemp B. Psychosocial and mental health issues in rehabilitation of older persons. In: Brody S, Ruff G, eds. *Aging and Rehabilitation*. New York, NY: Springer Publishing Co; 1986:pp.122–158.

21. Abdellah FG. Public health aspects of rehabilitation of the aged. In: Brody S, Ruff G, eds. *Aging and Rehabilitation*. New York, NY: Springer Publishing Co Inc; 1986.

22. Benedict RC, Ganikos ML. Coming to terms with ageism in rehabilitation. *J Rehabil* 1981;47:19–27.

23. Lopez-Aqueres W, Kemp B, Plopper M, et al. Health needs of hispanic elderly. *J Am Geriatr Soc.* 1984; 32:191–198.

24. Lehmann JF. Gait analysis: diagnosis and management. In: Kotke FJ, ed. *Krusen's Handbook of Physical Medicine and Rehabilitation*. Philadelphia, Pa: WB Saunders Co; 1971: chap 30, pp 583–603.

25. Garcia CA, Tweedy JR, Blass JP. Underdiagnosis of cognitive impairment in a rehabilitation setting. *J Am Geriatr Soc* 1984;32:339–342.

26. McCartney JR, Palmateer LM. Assessment of cognitive deficit in geriatric patients. *J Am Geriatr Soc* 1985; 33:467–472.

27. Collin SJ, Lincoln NB. Depression after stroke. *Clin Rehabil* 1987;1:27–32.

28. Gans JS. Depression diagnosis in a rehabilitation hospital. *Arch Phys Med Rehabil* 1981;62:386–389.

29. Gill C. *Social Aspects of Disability: Geriatric Rehabilitation Grand Rounds Presentation*. Downey, CA: Rancho Los Amigos Medical Center, 1985.

30. Adler MK, Brown CC, Acton P. Stroke rehabilitation: is age a determinant? *J Am Geriatr Soc* 1980;28:499–503.

31. Parry F: Physical rehabilitation of the old, old patient. *J Am Geriatr Soc.* 1983;31:482–484.

32. Bennett AE. Cost-effectiveness of rehabilitation for the elderly: preliminary results from the community hospital research program, *Gerontologist* 1980;20:284–287.

33. Burdman GDM. Student and trainee attitudes on aging. *Gerontologist* 1974;14:65–68.

34. Rasch JD, Crystal RM, Thomas KR. The perception of the older adult: a study of trainee attitudes. *J Appl Rehabil Counseling* 1977;8:121–127.

35. Johnston MV, Miller LS. Cost-effectiveness of the Medicare three hour regulation. *Arch Phys Med Rehabil* 1986;67:581–585.

36. Jarnlo GB, Ceder L, Thorngren KG. Early rehabilitation at home of elderly patients with hip fractures and consumption of resources in primary care. *Scand J Prim Health Care* 1984;2:105–112.

37. Liang MH, et al. Evaluation of comprehensive rehabilitation services for elderly homebound patients with arthritis and orthopedic disability. *Arthritis Rheum* 1984;27:258–266.

38. Steel K, Gertmon PM, Crescenzi C, et al. Iatrogenic illness on a general medical service at a University hospital. *N Engl J Med* 1981;304:638–642.

39. Warshaw G, Moore JT, Friedman W, et al. Functional disability in the hospitalized elderly. *JAMA* 1982; 248:847–850.

40. Sainsbury R, et al. An orthopedic geriatric rehabilitation unit: the first two years experience. *NZ Med J* 1986;99:583–585.

41. Feigenson JS, Gitlow HS, Greenberg SD. The disability oriented rehabilitation unit: a major factor influencing stroke outcome. *Stroke* 1979:10:5–8.

42. Applegate WB, Akins DA, Elam J, et al. A geriatric rehabilitation and assessment unit in a community hospital. *J Am Geriatr Soc* 1983;31:206–210.

43. Strax TE, Ledebur J. Rehabilitating the geriatric patient: potential and limitations. *Geriatrics* September 1979; 34:99–101.

44. Keith RA, Breckenridge K, O'Neil WA. Rehabilitation hospital patient characteristics from the hospital utilization project system. *Arch Phys Med Rehabil* 1977; 58:260–263.

45. Liem PH, Chernoff R, Carter WJ. Geriatric rehabilitation unit: a 3-year outcome. *J Gerontol* 1986;41:44–50.

46. Sutton MA. 'Homeward bound': a minimal care rehabilitation unit. *Br Med J* 1986;293:319–320.

47. Reed JW, Gessner JE. Rehabilitation in the extended care facility. *J Am Geriatr Soc* 1979;27:325–329.

48. Adelman RD, et al. A community-oriented geriatric rehabilitation unit in a nursing home. *Gerontologist* 1987;27:143–146.

49. Klingbeil G. The assessment of rehabilitation potential in the elderly. *Wis Med J* 1982;81:25–27.

50. Kozin F, et al. The reflex sympathetic dystrophy syndrome, *Am J Med* 1976;60:321–338.
51. McDowell FH. Rehabilitating patients with stroke. *Postgrad Med* 1976;59:145–149.
52. Collin SJ, et al. Depression after stroke. *Clin Rehabil* 1987;1:27–32.
53. Kumar VN, Redford JB. Rehabilitation of hip fractures in the elderly. *Am Fam Physician* 1984;29:173–180.
54. Sim FH, Sigmond ER. Acute fractures of the femoral neck managed by total hip replacement. *Orthopedics* 1986;9:35–38.
55. Ceder LF, Thorgren KG, Wallden B. Prognostic indicators and early home rehabilitation in elderly patients with hip fractures, *Clin Orthop* 1980;152:173–184.
56. Mazet R. The geriatric amputee. *Artif Limbs* 1967;11:33.
57. Clark GS, Blue B, Bearer JB. Rehabilitation of the elderly amputee. *J Am Geriatr Soc* 1983;31:439–448.
58. Cohen JJ, Sven JD, Walker JM, et al. Establishing criteria for community ambulation. *Top Geriatr Rehabil* 1987;3:71–77.
59. Watson N. Pattern of spinal cord injury in the elderly, *Paraplegia* 1976;14:36–40.
60. Reifler BV, Teri L. Rehabilitation and Alzheimer's disease. In: Brody S, Ruff G. *Aging and Rehabilitation* New York, NY: Springer Publishing Co Inc; 1986.
61. Levy LL. A practical guide to the care of the Alzeheimer's disease victim: the cognitive disability perspective. *Top Geriatr Rehabil* 1986;1:16–26.

13

Hypertension

Edward D. Frohlich

Hypertension is persistent elevation of the systolic and/or diastolic arterial pressure on either a primary (essential) or secondary basis. Uncontrolled, such pressure elevations lead to functional impairment of target organs—heart, brain, and kidneys—and accompanying morbidity and mortality.

Epidemiology

When individuals with borderline hypertension are included, half of all persons older than the age of 65 years in the United States have an abnormally elevated systolic and/or diastolic pressure.[1] According to the Joint National Committee,[2] systolic hypertension is termed *borderline* in the range of 140 to 159 mm Hg; above 159 mm Hg, when accompanied by a normal diastolic pressure, it is called *isolated systolic pressure.* Elevation of diastolic pressure, usually referred to as *systemic arterial hypertension,* has been labeled mild from 90 to 104 mm Hg, moderate from 105 to 114 mm Hg, and severe at 115 mm Hg and beyond.

Despite this high prevalence of elevated blood pressure in elderly persons, it must not be inferred that hypertension in this age group is an innocuous accompaniment of the aging process itself.[3-5] The pharmacologic control of diastolic hypertension in elderly persons has resulted in a favorable change in total and cardiovascular morbidity and mortality.[6-8] Interestingly, data from the United States[9-12] and other coun-

tries[13,14] suggest that the degree of elevation of *systolic* pressure is a better predictor of cardiovascular hypertensive morbidity and mortality than diastolic pressure elevation. In fact, isolated systolic hypertension increases the risk of cardiovascular death by a factor of 2 and of stroke by $2\frac{1}{2}$ compared with normotensive persons.[15]

The risk of developing serious complications of hypertension, such as stroke, congestive heart failure, dissecting aneurysm stroke, intermittent claudication, and progressive renal functional impairment, is reduced significantly when effective antihypertensive therapy is maintained, although prevention of myocardial infarction remains unresolved.[6-8] In Europe, fatal myocardial infarction in elderly persons has decreased by 60% in the face of effective antihypertensive therapy.[16,17] It is clear that reductions in the incidence of fatal stroke (by 50%) and myocardial infarction (by 35%) in the United States during the past decade[18] are related to the increased awareness and treatment of patients with elevated arterial pressure.

Insurance data, prospectively designed epidemiologic studies, and several national health surveys have confirmed that both systolic and diastolic pressures rise progressively with aging (at least until 60 years of age).[12,19,20] Later, diastolic pressure may decline, even though the systolic pressure continues to rise.[21] By contrast, in certain less acculturated societies, there is no rise in systolic or diastolic pressure with age. This has been attributed to a sodium intake of less than 60 mEq/d.

Pathophysiology

There are no qualitative differences between causes of hypertension in elderly and younger persons. However, some differences do exist with respect to prevalence of the various causes of pressure elevation. For example, renal arterial abnormalities are more common in older patients with hypertension (Table 13.1).[21]

Approximately 85%, possibly more, of the 60 million people in the United States with hypertension have no identifiable cause for their pressure elevations and are said to have "essential hypertension." The remaining patients have a specific abnormality that causes the elevated arterial pressure (i.e., "secondary hypertension.") Because of the greater prevalence of occlusive (ie, atherosclerotic) renal arterial disease, elderly persons are more likely to have secondary hypertension.

Which of these elderly patients are more likely to have an occlusive renal arterial lesion? Clues include a negative history for hypertension in earlier life, no family history of hypertension, abrupt escape from control after a sustained period of adequate blood pressure control with antihypertensive therapy, and spontaneous hypokalemia. The Joint National Committee's fourth report[2] recommends that such patients undergo at least a basic laboratory evaluation (see "Laboratory Data" subsection below).

Pressor Mechanisms

In recent years, we have learned that arterial pressure is maintained at normal levels by a wide variety of mechanisms.[22] It therefore follows that in the development and maintenance of essential hypertension any or all of these mechanisms, gone awry, may participate. Most authorities now consider essential hypertension to be multifactorial in causation, involving: (1) increased activity of the adrenergic nervous system (including the synthesis, release, and reuptake of catecholamines); (2) the renopressor system (including the extrarenal autocrine/paracrine renin-angiotensin systems in brain, heart, and blood vessels)[23,24]; (3) altered regulation of fluid and electrolyte metabolism (owing to subclinical renal parenchymal disease or humoral factors that affect this balance); and (4) reduced distensibility of, or obstructions in, the large arteries, which decreases vessel compliance and left ventricular impedance. Recently, various vasodepressor systems (kallikrein-kinin, prostaglandins, etc), circulating polypeptides (including atrial natriuretic hormone), and the renal medullary phospholipid substance have been shown to participate in control of arterial pressure (Table 13.2).

In most elderly patients with essential hypertension,

Table 13.1. Systemic arterial hypertensions in elderly patients.[21]

Primary essential hypertension: hypertension of undetermined cause
  Borderline (labile) essential hypertension: at times, diastolic pressures are normal (ie, <90 mm Hg), but on at least 3 occasions, diastolic pressures exceed 90 mm Hg
  Established essential hypertension
    Mild (diastolic pressures, 90–104 mm Hg)
    Moderate (diastolic pressures, 105–114 mm Hg)
    Severe (diastolic pressure, ≥115 mm Hg)
Secondary hypertension: hypertension of attributable cause
  Renovascular hypertension
    Atherosclerotic renal arterial disease
    Nonatherosclerotic (fibrosing) renal arterial diseases
    Renal arterial aneurysms
    Extravascular occlusion of renal arteries (eg, tumors, fibrosis)
    Embolic renal arterial disease
  Renal parenchymal diseases
    Chronic pyelonephritis
    Chronic glomerulonephritis
    Polycystic disease
    Diabetic glomerulosclerosis
    Radiation fibrosis
    Others (amyloid, excretory obstructive disease, etc)
  Hormonal diseases
    Thyroid diseases
      Hyperthyroidism
      Hypothyroidism
    Adrenal diseases
      Cushing's disease or syndrome
      Primary hyperaldosteronism
        Adenoma(s)
        Bilateral hyperplasia
      Adrenal enzyme abnormalities
    Pheochromocytoma
    Others (eg, ectopic production of pressor hormones in metastatic tumors, growth hormone, hypercalcemic diseases, hyperparathyroidism)
  Coarctation of aorta
  Drugs, chemicals, and foods[32]
    Excessive alcohol ingestion
    Excessive dietary sodium intake
    Steroidal compounds (eg, steroids for treating malignancies, oral estrogens, etc)
    Over-the-counter cold preparations (eg, nasal decongestants, phenylpropanolamine)
    Milk-alkali syndrome, hypervitaminosis D
    Cyclosporine
    Others (licorice, snuff, etc)
  Secondary to specific therapies for elderly patients
    Antidepressant therapy (eg, tricyclics, monoamine oxidase inhibitors)
    Long-term steroid administration
    β-Adrenergic receptor agonists
    Steroids for treating malignancies, asthma, etc
    Estrogens for treating malignancies, osteoporosis

*Adapted from Reference 21.

Table 13.2. Factors affecting vascular resistance.

Factor
Vasoconstriction
Passive
Increased blood viscosity
Cold
Vessel wall waterlogging
Edema: extravascular compression
Obstruction: thrombosis, embolus
Active
Adrenergic stimulation
Renopressor: angiotensin II
Cations: increased Ca^{++}, K^+
Other humoral factors, eg, vasopressin, some
prostaglandins, serotonin
Vasodilation
Passive
Decreased blood viscosity
Heat
Active
Dopamine
Some prostaglandins
Kinins: bradykinin, kallidin
Histamine
Renal medullary phospholipid substance
Peptides, eg, atrial natriuretic factor, vasoactive
intestinal polypeptide, endorphins

* Adapted from Reference 21

the plasma volume progressively contracts as arterial pressure and total peripheral resistance rise. Nevertheless, the renopressor system seems to be suppressed (in comparison with younger patients), thus attenuating the relationship between intravascular volume and renopressor mechanisms. This may account for the enhanced responsiveness, reported in some elderly hypertensive patients (especially those with isolated sytolic hypertension), to the administration of diuretics.[25]

However, an occasional elderly patient will have hyperthyroidism as the basis for systolic hypertension, and aortic insufficiency, malnutrition (ie, beriberi), arteriovenous fistula, and even fever also may be associated with elevation of systolic pressure.[25]

Hemodynamics

Arterial pressure is the product of cardiac output and the total peripheral resistance. Total peripheral resistance means the resistance to the forward flow of blood through the systemic circulation, which may be affected by the adrenergic nervous system, the renopressor system, and a variety of circulating factors[22] (Table 13.2).

Cardiac output, in turn, is the product of heart rate and stroke volume. The latter may be increased by extrinsic and intrinsic factors that enhance myocardial contractility. Additionally, because of the frequency of atherosclerotic vascular disease in elderly persons, diminished large artery distensibility occurs, favoring development of systolic pressure elevation in an attempt, by the left ventricle, to eject its stroke volume through the more rigid, less compliant aorta. Thus, isolated systolic hypertension is related to reduced distensibility of the aorta and other large arteries and increased left ventricular outflow impedance.[23,24]

Ventricular Hypertrophy

Increased vascular resistance progressively increases the afterload imposed on the left ventricle. The heart adapts to this by the development of concentric left ventricular hypertrophy.[26] However, the elderly normotensive person also may develop cardiac enlargement,[27] which, in part, may be due to ventricular hypertrophy, but also may be caused by fibrosis and deposition of collagen associated with coexisting ischemic heart disease.[28] A recent analysis of Framingham data confirmed that obesity, valvular disease, and age itself also are associated with the development of left ventricular hypertrophy.[29]

The Pascal relationship is an important hemodynamic consideration in the elderly hypertensive patient. Here, myocardial oxygen consumption is directly related to left ventricular wall tension. This physical factor is the product of the left ventricular diameter and the systolic pressure generated within this chamber during contraction. In hypertension—and in normotensive elderly persons–both left ventricular diameter and systolic pressure are increased. The increased tension increases the demand of the left ventricle for oxygen (a relationship that holds in both diastolic and isolated hypertension). This is of primary importance in the development of coronary insufficiency and angina pectoris and speaks to the need to reduce arterial pressure even in patients with only mildly elevated pressures. The hypertensive elderly individual demonstrates left ventricular enlargement, which may represent structural adaptation by the left ventricle to increasing arterial pressure and ventricular afterload, but also may be due to other factors mentioned above. When myocardial ischemia coexists with pressure overload, there may be associated insufficiency of blood supply to the myocardium—even if the arterial pressure is not dramatically elevated.[28] This represents the increased demand of the myocardium for oxygen owing to the elevated systolic pressure and chamber diameter that enhance ventricular chamber tension. Thus, numerous other age-associated conditions may contribute to cardiac enlargement and eventual cardiac failure in the elderly individual, eg, a decreased number of β-adrenergic receptors, amyloid, collagen, or fat deposition, and increased tension that mandates greater arterial oxygen demand.

Obesity

Hypertension also may be exacerbated by exogenous obesity, a separate but closely related entity, frequently observed in patients with essential hypertension,[29] which is associated with expanded intravascular volume, venous return to the heart, and cardiac output.[30] Both problems, hypertension and exogenous obesity, are closely associated with non–insulin-dependent diabetes mellitus,[31] but the mechanisms underlying this relationship remain to be elucidated (see also Chapter 18).

Endogenous and Exogenous Chemical Agents

It is important to consider the possibility of underlying endocrine diseases when the physician is confronted with an elderly patient who has recently developed hypertension. Other endocrinopathies also must be kept in mind, including hyperparathyroidism, hyperaldosteronism, pheochromocytoma, and tumor-associated humoral factors (Table 13.1). Elderly persons often have multiple diseases. But, in addition, the physician should consider the possibility of the myriad medications that may be prescribed (including over-the-counter preparations) for coexisting and intercurrent diseases. Some of the following medications predispose the hypertensive patient to certain complications: laxative abuse, corticosteroids, and the combination of digitalis and a diuretic all increase the risk of hypokalemia and attendant cardiac dysrhythmias. Cyclosporine-A, monoamine oxidase inhibitors (especially accompanied by ingestion of tyramine-containing foods), and over-the-counter cold preparations, including nose drops that contain phenylpropanolamine, all may elevate arterial pressure. Chemicals, toxins, and certain foods can account for the development or aggravation of hypertension (Table 13.1).[32]

Clinical Presentation and Diagnosis

The term *silent disease* is never more fitting than when applied to uncomplicated hypertension. However, elevated arterial pressure may be associated with symptoms in certain patients, even in those without target organ involvement. Patients may experience cardiac awareness (eg, palpitations, rapid heart action, skipped beats, etc) that accompanies a hyperdynamic

circulation. Some authors have suggested an increased frequency of headaches, epistaxis, and tinnitus in hypertensive patients, but to depend on such complaints is unwise, since these symptoms are just as frequent in normotensive persons.[33] An exception may be the severe headache that should alert the clinician to the possibility of certain forms of secondary hypertension (eg, pheochromocytoma, brain tumor) or the rupture of a berry aneurysm in the circle of Willis producing a subarachnoid hemorrhage. Moreover, the occurrence of symptomatic complaints in patients with either essential or secondary hypertension suggests target organ involvement.

Blood Pressure Measurement

It is appropriate to underscore the proper technique of blood pressure measurement, especially in the elderly individual. Pressure must be measured in both arms. Not infrequently, occlusive atherosclerotic disease of the subclavian or brachial arteries will reduce systolic pressure in one upper extremity. This should be considered if, on subsequent examinations, the systolic pressure is inexplicably and abruptly reduced. Furthermore, blood pressures should be obtained in all elderly hypertensive patients in the supine, sitting, and standing positions, since postural hypotension is not uncommon, especially in patients who are receiving antihypertensive medication and even in untreated and normotensive individuals shortly after a meal.

If office blood pressures are persistently and strikingly elevated, but cardiac size is normal as demonstrated by a chest roentgenogram and electrocardiogram (ECG), the physician should suspect "pseudohypertension" or "white coat hypertension." In some of these patients, this may be explained by the failure of the occluding cuff to compress sclerotic brachial arteries. This type of pseudohypertension may be detected by "Osler's maneuver," which is the ability to palpate the pulseless radial or brachial artery distal to a point of occlusion (manually or by cuff pressure).[34]

Cardiac and Coronary Artery Involvement

The earliest complaints in patients with cardiac involvement are easy fatigability, palpitations, and ectopic (atrial and/or ventricular) beats. Chest pain in the patient without occlusive coronary arterial disease may suggest increased myocardial oxygen demand, which is related to a persistently elevated arterial pressure associated with an increased left ventricular diameter (ie, greater wall tension). With more advanced stages of cardiac involvement come the classic symptoms and signs of left ventricular decompensation: exertional dyspnea, nocturia, orthopnea, peripheral edema, and increased ventricular irritability. Development of a fourth heart sound (ie, the atrial gallop rhythm) suggests reduced distensibility and compliance of the hypertrophied left ventricle. Sudden onset of back pain in the patient with hypertension should alert the physician to the possibility of aortic dissection.[21]

The chest roentgenogram and the ECG have served as the classic clinical tests for detection of cardiac involvement in hypertension. The chest roentgenogram is less sensitive for cardiac enlargement than the ECG; even before left ventricular hypertrophy can be detected by the usual ECG criteria of increased QRS complex voltage, delayed intrinsicoid deflection of the QRS complex, or left ventricular "strain" pattern, there may be still earlier ECG evidence of left ventricular hypertrophy in the form of left atrial enlargement.[21,35,36]

The enlarged left atrium does not reflect atrial disease, but rather reduced left ventricular distensibility, resulting from the developing left ventricular hypertrophy. The echocardiogram is an even more sensitive means of detecting the early stages of left ventricular hypertrophy. This is clearly demonstrable echocardiographically in patients with only ECG evidence of a left atrial abnormality.[36] Before systolic functional changes occur in patients with left ventricular hypertrophy, alterations in diastolic function are revealed by a reduced left atrial filling index on echocardiographic[37] or radionuclide studies.[38]

Renal Involvement

The earliest symptom of renal involvement is nocturia; later symptoms are those of functional impairment, ie, frequency, proteinuria, anemia, and edema. Elevation of the creatinine level (or blood urea nitrogen level) and diminished creatinine clearance (ie, glomerular filtration rate) occurs when approximately 60% of renal function is already lost. Both the aging process and essential hypertension are associated with histologically demonstrable nephrosclerosis. The renal blood flow and glomerular filtration rate decrease in proportion to the reduction of cardiac output in response to both hypertension and to advancing years (see Chapter 24).

In the untreated patient with essential hypertension, the lower the renal blood flow, the higher the serum uric acid concentration.[39] This may explain the great frequency of hyperuricemia in untreated young and elderly patients with hypertension. Usually, echocardiographic evidence of left ventricular hypertrophy precedes this expression of impaired renal hemodynamic function in hypertension; this is detected physi-

ologically by measurement of a reduced renal blood flow or clinically by an elevated uric acid concentration.[40]

Proteinuria is infrequent in patients with uncomplicated essential hypertension. If daily urinary protein excretion exceeds 400 mg, it is unlikely to be related to nephrosclerosis alone, and the possibility of coexisting parenchymal disease of the kidney should be considered. Fresh urine with an alkaline pH suggests primary hyperaldosteronism, but this should be accompanied by unexplained hypokalemia before more extensive studies are conducted.[21] The presence of anemia in hypertension usually is indicative of parenchymal disease of the kidney (if hemoglobinopathy is excluded), but another extremely important consideration in the elderly patient is the coexistence of an occult neoplasm.

Retinal Involvement

The physician should diligently determine the presence and severity of hypertensive retinopathy. In elderly patients, hypertensive retinal vascular changes should not be confused with sclerotic changes of increased arteriolar light-striping, nicking, and tortuosity. By contrast, arteriolar and venular constriction and appearance of hemorrhages, exudates, and papilledema suggest advancing and more severe degrees of hypertensive vascular disease.

Vascular Involvement

A search for renal (see "Secondary Hypertension" subsection below), carotid, brachial, and femoral bruits should be undertaken.[20] The presence, for example, of a carotid bruit and symptoms compatible with transient cerebral ischemia suggests embolic phenomena. Other vascular bruits may signal diffuse atherosclerotic disease.

Secondary Hypertension

Certain signs and symptoms increase the probability of secondary forms of hypertension. The patient with pheochromocytoma may complain of headache, flushing, and lability of blood pressure. Occlusive renal arterial disease, the most common of the secondary hypertensions in elderly persons, may present as a sudden onset or worsening of blood pressure elevation accompanied by headaches and renal artery bruits that are systolic and (more significantly) diastolic in timing.[2,20] Patients with thyroid disease will demonstrate the appropriate symptoms of thyroid hormone excess, as modified in elderly persons (see Chapter 19). Primary hyperaldosteronism causes symptoms related to hypokalemia (eg, muscle weakness, nocturia, isosthenuria, and altered carbohydrate metabolism) and to hypokalemic alkalosis. Cushing's syndrome also should be suspected in the presence of spontaneous hypokalemia, when accompanied by hirsutism, purplish striae, buffalo hump, or cushingoid facies.[21]

Laboratory Data

Which laboratory studies to obtain in the hypertensive patient should be based on the results of the physical examination and the medical history.[21] As a minimum, the following are indicated: complete blood cell count; urinalysis; ECG; fasting blood glucose, serum creatinine, uric acid, and potassium levels; and probably a lipid profile, including measurement of high-density cholesterol.[2] Because of lower costs, an automated battery of blood chemistry studies that contain these tests may be wiser.

Hyperuricemia suggests that the patient is taking a diuretic or that the patient already has a reduced renal blood flow as discussed above. Hypercalcemic states not infrequently are associated with hypertension; this should raise the suspicion of hyperparathyroidism or malignancy. Moreover, diuretic therapy also can elevate the serum calcium level.

Treatment

At present, there are no completely effective established means for the primary prevention of hypertensive cardiovascular disease. Nevertheless, it as appropriate to advise the patient against smoking, to control body weight, to reduce alcohol intake, and to take steps to correct elevated levels of blood glucose and lipids.[2] These so-called nonpharmacologic approaches[41] may not control arterial pressure completely, but may add to the overall therapeutic program in a way that allows for the administration of fewer antihypertensive drugs or lower doses.

Achievement of ideal body weight, moderation in alcohol (ie, ethanol) (<1 ounce/d), and reduced dietary sodium especially are important. Some patients with less severe hypertension who are successful with these life-style changes will be able to discontinue medications,[42] but whether they remain normotensive indefinitely is controversial.[21,43] Additionally, patients who take antihypertensive drugs and smoke develop more complications than those receiving treatment who do not smoke. For these reasons, therapy for hypertension, outlined in Fig. 13-1, should begin with nonpharmacologic approaches.

Mild Hypertension

Patients, who have diastolic pressures between 90 and 104 mm Hg, often respond to lower doses of a diuretic.

Baseline: Nonpharmacologic Approaches

Step 1: Select One agent from Diuretic (Thiazide or Chlorthalidone)
or
β-Adrenergic Receptor Blocker
or
Angiotensin Converting Enzyme Inhibitor
or
Calcium Antagonist

Response   No response

Proceed to   Switch to   Add a
Full Dose   an Alternative   Second
                  Agent   Agent

Step 2: Add a Second Agent from an Alternative of the Above Four

Step 3: Add a Third Agent

Fig. 13.1. Therapy for hypertension.

β-adrenergic receptor blocker, angiotensin converting enzyme (ACE) inhibitor, or calcium antagonist in submaximal doses.[2] If such doses are inadequate to control pressure, the selected agent may be increased to full dosage or a second agent may be added.[2] For example, addition of a β-blocker to hydrochlorothiazide, 12.5 or 25 mg daily, may control the blood pressure elevation and prevent development of hypokalemia, hyperuricemia, etc. Elderly patients generally have been said to be responsive to diuretics, but a β-blocker (eg, propranolol [80 mg], metoprolol [50 to 100 mg], or atenolol [50 to 100 mg] daily) may be equally effective monotherapy,[2] and patients with coronary artery disease may benefit from the cardioprotective action of a β-blocker.

Calcium antagonists should be considered, especially if the elderly patient also is black or has side effects from other drugs. These agents have considerable appeal in the geriatric population because of a relatively low incidence of adverse effects (Table 13.3). Angiotensin converting enzyme inhibitors also have been shown to be effective in mild hypertension at low dosages, alone or combined with a diuretic if necessary.[2,44]

Isolated Systolic Hypertension

Whether treating isolated systolic hypertension in elderly patients reduces complications has not yet been demonstrated by appropriate studies. However, as discussed above, these patients have increased myocardial oxygen demand. At the present time, a large multicenter study of Systolic Hypertension in the Elderly (Program)—SHEP–is being conducted by the

Table 13.3. More frequent and important adverse effects of antihypertensive agents.*

Drugs	Selected side effects†	Precautions and special considerations
Diuretics		
Thiazides and related sulfonamide diuretics	Hypokalemia, hyperuricemia, glucose intolerance, hypercholesteremia, hypertriglyceridemia, sexual dysfunction, weakness	May be ineffective in renal failure, hypokalemia increases digitalis toxicity, may precipitate acute gout, may cause an increase in blood levels of lithium
Loop diuretics		Effective in chronic renal failure, hypokalemia, and hyperuricemia as above
Potassium-sparing agents	Hyperkalemia	Danger of hyperkalemia or renal failure in patients treated with an ACE inhibitor or nonsteroidal anti-inflammatory drug, may increase blood levels of lithium
Spironolactone	Gynecomastia, mastodynia	Interferes with digoxin immunoassay
Triamterene		Danger of renal calculi
Amiloride		
Adrenergic inhibitors		
β-adrenergic blockers‡ (acebutolol, atenolol, metoprolol, nadolol, penbutolol sulfate, pindolol, propranolol hydrochloride, timolol)	Bronchospasm, peripheral arterial insufficiency, fatigue, insomnia, sexual dysfunction, exacerbation of congestive heart failure, masking of symptoms of hypoglycemia, hypertriglyceridemia, decreased HDL cholesterol (except for pindolol and acebutolol)	Should not be used in patients with asthma, COPD, congestive heart failure, heart block (>1st-degree), or sick sinus syndrome; use with caution in insulin-treated diabetics and patients with peripheral vascular disease; should not be discontinued abruptly in patients with ischemic heart disease
Centrally acting adrenergic inhibitors		
Clonidine	Drowsiness, sedation, dry mouth, fatigue, sexual dysfunction	Rebound hypertension may occur with abrupt discontinuance, particularly with prior administration of high doses or with continuation of concomitant β-blocker therapy
Guanabenz	Same as for clonidine	Same as for clonidine
Guanfacine hydrochloride	Same as for clonidine	Same as for clonidine
Methyldopa	Same as for clonidine	May cause liver damage and Coombs-positive hemolytic anemia, use cautiously in elderly patients because of orthostatic hypotension, interferes with measurements of urinary catecholamine levels
Clonidine TTS (patch)	Same as for clonidine, localized skin reaction to patch	
Peripheral-acting adrenergic inhibitors		
Guanadrel sulfate	Diarrhea, sexual dysfunction, orthostatic hypotension	Use cautiously because of orthostatic hypotension
Guanethidine monosulfate	Same as for guanadrel	Same as for guanadrel
Rauwolfia alkaloids	Lethargy, nasal congestion, depression	Contraindicated in patients with history of mental depression, use with caution in patients with history of peptic ulcer
Reserpine	Same as for *Rauwolfia* alkaloids	Same as for *Rauwolfia* alkaloids

Table 13.3. Continued

Drugs	Selected side effects†	Precautions and special considerations
α₁-Adrenergic blockers		
Prazosin hydrochloride	"First-dose" syncope, orthostatic hypotension, weakness, palpitations	Use cautiously in elderly patients because of orthostatic hypotension
Terazosin hydrochloride	Same as for prazosin hydrochloride	Same as for prazosin hydrochloride
Combined α- and β-adrenergic blockers		
Labetalol‡	Bronchospasm, peripheral vascular insufficiency, orthostatic hypotension	Should not be used in patients with asthma, COPD, congestive heart failure, heart block (>1st-degree), or sick sinus syndrome; use with caution in insulin-treated diabetics and patients with peripheral vascular disease
Vasodilators	Headache, tachycardia, fluid retention	May precipitate angina pectoris in patients with coronary artery disease
Hydralazine	Positive antinuclear antibody test	Lupus syndrome may occur (rare at recommended doses)
Minoxidil	Hypertrichosis	May cause or aggravate pleural and pericardial effusions, may precipitate angina pectoris in patients with coronary artery disease
ACE inhibitors	Rash, cough, angioneurotic edema, hyperkalemia, dysgeusia	Can cause reversible, acute renal failure in patients with bilateral renal arterial stenosis or unilateral stenosis in solitary kidney; proteinuria may occur (rare at recommended doses); hyperkalemia can develop, particularly in patients with renal insufficiency; rarely can induce neutropenia; hypotension has been observed with initiation of ACE inhibitors, especially in patients with high plasma renin activity or in those receiving diuretic therapy
Calcium antagonists	Edema, headache	Use with caution in patients with congestive heart failure, contraindicated in patients with 2nd- or 3rd-degree heart block
Verapamil	Constipation	May cause liver dysfunction
Diltiazem hydrochloride	Constipation	May cause liver dysfunction
Nifedipine	Tachycardia	
Nitrendipine	Tachycardia	

* ACE indicates angiotension converting enzyme; HDL, high-density lipoprotein; and COPD, chronic obstructive pulmonary disease.
† The listing of side effects is not all inclusive, and health practitioners are urged to refer to the package insert for a more detailed listing.
‡ Sudden withdrawal of these drugs may be hazardous in patients with heart disease.
§ Sexual dysfunction, particularly impotence in men, has been reported with the use of all antihypertensive agents.

National Heart, Lung and Blood Institute, The feasibility portion was conducted in only five centers, but those results suggested (without demonstrating statistical significance) that elevated systolic pressure should be controlled.[21] That study has shown that a diuretic (eg, chlorthalidone, first 25 mg, and later, if necessary, 50 mg daily) may be enough to control pressure. Alternatively, a β-adrenergic receptor–blocking drug or a calcium antagonist may be adequate. If any one of these agents does not control systolic pressure, a second may be added (eg, a diuretic and β-blocker).

More Severe Stages of Hypertension

Patients with moderate (diastolic pressure, 105 to 114 mm Hg) and severe (diastolic pressure, >115 mm Hg) hypertension may respond to any of the four classes of antihypertensive agents recommended in the most recent Joint National Committee report[2] (diuretics, β-blockers, ACE inhibitors, and calcium antagonists). As with milder hypertension, if pressure is not adequately controlled, an alternative agent may be substituted; a second or even a third agent may be necessary. These may be added in sequential fashion by using lower doses first and then increasing dosage or adding other agents (Fig. 13.1).

Recent evidence suggests that it is possible to provide a more rational individualized stepped care for patients by "tailoring" therapy.[2] The goal is to wed the mechanism of action of the pharmacologic agent to the involved pressor mechanism(s) of disease. Thus, the black or obese patient, who is more volume dependent and has lower plasma renin activity, may respond better to a diuretic or calcium antagonist. The patient with renal arterial disease (providing it is unilateral renal arterial disease or not present in a solitary kidney) or the patient with congestive heart failure and hypertension may benefit more from an ACE inhibitor.[2]

Patients with a history of myocardial infarction, angina pectoris, migraine headache, or glaucoma may initially receive a β-blocker if there are no other contraindications. (In patients with glaucoma, the oral β-blocker will not be adequate therapy for the eye disease, but knowing that these patients have tolerated β-blocker eye drops provides some degree of confidence that the oral preparation also will be tolerated.)

Hypertensive Urgencies and Emergencies

Patients who present with hypertensive encephalopathy, acute left ventricular failure, or dissecting aortic aneurysm, as well as those with extreme blood pressure elevation who require emergency surgery, require

rapid lowering of arterial pressure. Intravenous nitroprusside, diazoxide, ACE inhibitors, or labetalol may be used when immediate pressure reduction is required. Intravenous methyldopa, parenteral hydralazine, oral calcium antagonists, and intravenous furosemide have a less rapid onset of action, generally 20 to 30 minutes.[2,44] As with the prior discussion of therapy, one should be extremely careful in these situations to wed the mechanism of action of the pharmacologic agent to the pathophysiologic mechanisms that operate in the specific hypertensive emergency.[2,44] Extreme caution and constant monitoring are required in these situations.

Side Effects

As with any therapeutic agent, side effects, whether adverse or additional, should be anticipated. The more frequent and important of these are presented in Table 13.3. If the patient already is using digitalis, the use and follow-up of diuretic therapy should be done with extreme care. Close supervision of the serum potassium level is in order to obviate cardiac dysrhythmias associated with hypokalemia. On the other hand, potassium-sparing agents may produce hyperkalemia and, when combined with ACE inhibitors or nonsteroidal anti-inflammatory agents, renal failure may be precipitated.

All antihypertensive agents, but, in particular, diuretics and adrenergic inhibitors (including β-blockers) may produce sexual dysfunction and impotence. This is particularly important in elderly men, since sexual dysfunction may be inappropriately ascribed to aging by patient and physician alike. Sexual dysfunction also may be produced in women. The ACE inhibitors and calcium antagonists appear to cause fewer adverse effects in elderly patients. Moreover, these agents generally are not associated with alterations in lipid levels.

Findings from the Hypertension Detection and Follow-up Program[6] have shown that elderly patients with uncomplicated hypertension have no more side effects from prolonged treatment than younger individuals. Nevertheless, we should remember that orthostatic hypotension is more frequent in older persons; therefore, this should be considered in all elderly individuals who are taking antihypertensive drugs (particularly on arising in the morning and postprandially). It also should be borne in mind that agents with central effects are more likely to exacerbate complaints of depression, forgetfulness, vivid dreams or hallucinations, sleep problems, dry mouth, gait disturbances, and constipation.

Finally, the patient with chronic obstructive lung disease or asthma should not take β-blockers. Calcium antagonists may be more appropriate for such patients, as well as for those with slower heart rates. The frequency of comorbidity in elderly hypertensive patients makes therapy for hypertension complex. Clearly, more drug trials involving older subjects are needed.

References

1. Drizd T, Dannenberg A, Engel A. Blood pressure levels in persons 18–74 years of age in 1976–80, and trends in blood pressure from 1960–80 in the United States. *Vital Health Stat 11* 1986.

2. The Joint National Committee on the Detection, Evaluation and Treatment of High Blood Pressure: the 1988 report of the Joint National National Committee on Detection, Evaluation and Treatment of High Blood Pressure. *Arch Intern Med* 1988;148:1023–1038.

3. Genest J, Larochelle P, Kuchel O, et al. Hypertension in the elderly: atheroarteriosclerotic hypertension. In: Genest J, Kuchel O, Hamet P, et al, eds. *Hypertension: Physiopathology and Treatment.* 2nd ed. New York, NY: McGraw-Hill International Book Co; 1983:913–921.

4. Kannel WB, Doyle JT, Ostfeld AM, et al (Atherosclerosis Study Group). Optimal resources for primary prevention of atherosclerotic diseases. *Circulation* 1984;70(suppl):157A–205A.

5. Kannel WB. Implications of Framingham study data for treatment of hypertension: impact of other risk factors. In: Laragh HG, Buhler FR, Seldin DW, eds. *Frontiers of Hypertension Research.* New York, NY: Springer-Verlag NY Inc; 1981:17–21.

6. Hypertension Detection and Follow-up Program Cooperative Group. Five-year findings of the Hypertension Detection and Follow-Up Program, III: reduction in stroke incidence among persons with high blood pressure. *JAMA* 1982;247:633–638.

7. National Heart Foundation of Australia. Treatment of mild hypertension in the elderly: report by the Management Committee. *Med J Aust* 1981;2:398–402.

8. Amery A, Birkenhager W, Brixho P, et al. Mortality and morbidity results from the European Working Party on High Blood Pressure in the Elderly Trial. *Lancet* 1985;1:1349–1354.

9. Kannel WB. Prevalence and natural history of electrocardiographic left ventricular hypertrophy. *Am J Med* 1983;75(3A):4–11.

10. Kannel WB, Castelli WP, McNamara PM, et al. Role of blood pressure in the development of congestive heart failure: the Framingham Study. *N Engl J Med* 1972;207:781–787.

11. Kannel WB, Dawber TR, Sorkie P, et al. Components of blood pressure and risk of atherothrombotic brain infarction: the Framingham Study. *Stroke* 1976;7:327–331.

12. Kannel WB, Gordon T. Evaluation of the cardiovascular risk in the elderly: the Framingham Study. *Bull NY Acad Med* 1978;54:573–591.

13. Hughes G, Schnaper HW. The Isolated Systolic Hypertension in the Elderly Program. *Int J Ment Health* 1982;2:76–97.

14. WHO Expert Committee. Arterial Hypertension. *WHO Tech Rep Ser* 1978.

15. Shekelle RB, Ostfeld AM, Klawans HL Jr. Hypertension and risk of stroke in an elderly population. *Stroke* 1974;5:71–75.

16. European Working Party on High Blood Pressure in the Elderly: Antihypertensive therapy in patients above age 60 with systolic hypertension. *Clin Exp Hypertens A* 1982;4:1151–1176.

17. Amery A, Hansson L, Andren L, et al. Hypertension in the elderly. *Acta Med Scand* 1981;210:221–229.

18. Frohlich ED: Multicenter clinical trials: potential influence of consumer education. *Hypertension* 1987;9(suppl 3):75–79.

19. Health and Nutritional Examination Study (HANES). Blood pressure levels of persons 60–74. *Vital Health Stat 2* 1977.

20. Working Group on Hypertension in the Elderly. Statement on hypertension in the elderly. *JAMA* 1986;256:70–74.

21. Frohlich ED. Hypertension in the elderly. *Curr Probl Cardiol* 1988;13:313–367.

22. Frohlich ED. Mechanisms contributing to high blood pressure. *Ann Intern Med* 1983;98:709–714.

23. Dzau VJ, Gibbons GH. Autocrine paracrine mechanisms of vascular myocytes in systemic hypertension. *Am J Cardiol* 1987;60:99–103.

24. Re RN. Cellular mechanisms of growth in cardiovascular tissue. *Am J Cardiol* 1987;60:104–109.

25. Frohlich ED, ed. *Pathophysiology: Altered Regulatory Mechanisms in Disease.* 3rd ed. Philadelphia, Pa: JB Lippincott; 1984.

26. Frohlich ED, Tarazi RC, Dustan HP. Clinical-physiological correlations in the development of hypertensive heart disease. *Circulation* 1971;44:446–455.

27. Lakatta EG. Alterations in the cardiovascular system that occur in advanced age. *FASEB J* 1979;38:163–167.

28. Dunn FG, Frohlich ED. Hypertension and angina pectoris. In: Yu PN, Goodwin JF, eds. *Progress in Cardiology.* Philadelphia, Pa: Lea & Febiger, 1978:163–196.

29. Levy D, Anderson KM, Savage DD, et al. Echocardiographically detected left ventricular hypertrophy: prevalence and risk factors—the Framingham Study. *Ann Intern Med* 1988;108:7–13.

30. Frohlich ED, Messerli FH, Reisin E, et al. The problem of obesity and hypertension. *Hypertension* 1983;5(suppl 3):71–78.

31. Frohlich ED. Achievements in hypertension: a 25-year overview. *J Am Coll Cardiol* 1983;1:225–239.

32. Oren S, Grossman E, Messerli FH, et al. High blood pressure: side effects of drugs, poisons, and food. In: Ram CV, ed. *Cardiology Clinics of North America;* 1988; 6,2:467–474. Philadelphia, Pa: WB Saunders Co. In press.

33. Weiss NS. Relation of high blood pressure to headache, epistaxis, and selected other symptoms: the United States Health Examination Survey of Adults. *N Engl J Med* 1972;287:631.

34. Messerli FH, Ventura HO, Amodeo C. Osler's maneuver and pseudohypertension. *N Engl J Med* 1985;312:1548–1551.

35. Tarazi RC, Miller A, Frohlich ED, et al. Electrocardiographic changes reflecting left atrial abnormality in hypertension. *Circulation* 1966;34:818–822.

36. Dunn FG, Chandraratna PN, Basta LL, et al. Pathophysiologic assessment of hypertensive heart disease with echocardiography. *Am J Cardiol* 1977;39:789–795.

37. Dreslinsky GR, Frohlich ED, Dunn FG, et al. Echocardiographic diastolic ventricular abnormality in hypertensive heart disease: atrial emptying index. *Am J Cardiol* 1981;47:1087–1090.

38. Inouye I, Massie B, Loge D, et al. Abnormal left ventricular filling: an early finding in mild to moderate systemic hypertension. *Am J Cardiol* 1984;53:120–126.

39. Messerli FH, Frohlich ED, Dreslinski GR, et al. Serum uric acid in essential hypertension: an indicator of renal vascular involvement. *Ann Intern Med* 1980;93:817–821.

40. Kobrin I, Frohlich ED, Ventura HO, et al. Renal involvement follows cardiac enlargement in essential hypertension. *Arch Intern Med* 1986;146:272–276.

41. Frohlich ED, Gifford R Jr, Horan M, et al. Nonpharmacologic approaches to the control of high blood pressure: report of the Subcommittee on Nonpharmacologic Therapy of the Joint National Committee on Detection, Evaluation, and Treatment of High Blood Pressure, 1984. *Hypertension* 1986;8:444–467.

42. Stamler R, Stamler J, Grimm R: Nutritional therapy for high blood pressure: final report of a four-year randomized control trial—the hypertension control program. *JAMA* 1987;257:1484–1491.

43. Dustan HP, Page IH, Tarazi RC, et al. Arterial pressure responses to discontinuing antihypertensive drug treatment. *Circulation* 1968;37:370–379.

44. Frohlich ED. Hypertension. In: Rackel R, ed. *Conn's Current Therapy*. Philadelphia, Pa: WB Saunders Co. 1989, pp 225–241

14

Cardiovascular Disease

Nanette K. Wenger

Introduction

The World Health Organization's *World Health Statistical Annual 1987* identifies that aging of populations, common in the industrialized world, is rapidly becoming a characteristic of developing nations as well. Two thirds of the world's 600 million people aged 60 or older are projected to reside in developing nations by the year 2000. Not only is the elderly population increasing worldwide, but the aged population itself is becoming older as more people survive to higher ages. Cardiovascular disease increases dramatically with aging and is the major cause of death and disability in elderly persons. The problem facing all societies is how to pay for the care, rather than cure, that is characteristic of chronic illness. Elderly patients constitute a highly heterogeneous group, with widely differing functional status, severities of illness, expectations of medical therapy, and psychosocial needs, none of which relates substantially either to each other or to chronologic age. The challenge is to identify the characteristics of people who remain active and energetic into old age, to determine how life-style components, including nutrition, obesity, exercise, psychosocial features, work, retirement, and others, affect aging. This information can guide the preventive measures that may decrease disability in later life.

Cardiovascular Changes of Aging

Both the structural and the physiologic changes that occur in the cardiovascular system with aging decrease cardiac functional reserve capacity, limit exercise performance, and lessen the ability to tolerate a variety of stresses, including cardiovascular disease.

Maximal heart rate and maximal aerobic capacity decrease with age,[1] independent of habitual activity status, whereas the maximal oxygen uptake and maximal work capacity reflect the level of physical fitness, as well as as the effects of cardiovascular disease. Cardiac dilatation and an increased stroke volume compensate for the diminished heart rate response to maintain the increase in cardiac output required for exercise.[2,3] Vascular stiffness increases with aging, with a resultant increase in arterial systolic pressure. Progressive left ventricular hypertrophy parallels the rise in arterial systolic pressure.

Aging changes in the heart also include the following features: its altered geometric contour; a decrease in ventricular compliance, the diastolic dysfunction of aging; a prolonged duration of myocardial contraction and relaxation; and lessened chronotropic and inotropic responses to catecholamine stimulation.[4] Although consequences of postural hypotension, particularly falls, have been attributed to the sluggish baroreceptor reflex of aging, recent studies in community-dwelling elderly individuals show that they have preserved baroreceptor responsiveness.[5]

These changes constitute the substrate on which cardiovascular disease is superimposed, and the cardiovascular manifestations of aging must be differentiated from those of disease.

Limitations of History and Physical Examination in Diagnosis of Cardiovascular Disease in Elderly Persons

Over 70% of elderly US residents are healthy, alert, and functional, and they live independently at home well into their eighth and ninth decades. Although many of these elderly persons have serious illnesses and varying disabilities, only 10% to 15% of the US elderly population have dementia, and only 5% are in nursing homes or require other custodial care. However, some elderly individuals consider illness and disability inevitable consequences of aging; these negative attitudes often inappropriately lower their expectations of functional capabilities and recovery after illness.

Limitations in obtaining information from the clinical history include the potential altered mental acuity with aging, as well as cognitive disturbances related to illness, medications, or a combination of these features. The coexistence of multiple diseases also hinders the accurate evaluation of symptoms. Habitual activity levels differ substantially, but often decrease with progressive aging, so that many symptoms do not retain their activity-precipitated characteristics. Depression also may obscure or complicate the patient's clinical history, and confirmatory data often must be obtained from family members or medical records.

The increased vascular stiffness of aging causes the upstroke of the arterial pulse to appear more brisk than usual, potentially masking the slowly rising carotid pulse of aortic stenosis. Frequent findings in an elderly population include the early-peaking basal systolic murmur of aortic sclerosis, typically accompanied by a fourth heart sound at the cardiac apex as evidence of reduced ventricular compliance.

Importance of Noninvasive Diagnostic Tests and Their Limitations

Because of difficulties in obtaining a clinical history and in interpreting findings at physical examination, noninvasive diagnostic tests assume greater importance.[6] However, many of these have limitations unique to an elderly population.

Resting Electrocardiogram

About 50% of elderly individuals have abnormalities of the resting electrocardiogram,[7] most commonly intraventricular conduction abnormalities, reduction in QRS voltage, and a leftward shift of the frontal plane QRS axis. These occur in addition to the arrhythmias described below. Electrocardiographic evidence of myocardial infarction occurs far more frequently than would be suspected from the clinical history.

Long-term (24-Hour) Ambulatory Electrocardiography

The 24-hour ambulatory electrocardiogram is the most useful diagnostic technique to identify symptomatic arrhythmias, particularly when diary evidence is available to correlate symptoms with these spontaneously occurring arrhythmias. The limitation of utility of this study is the high prevalence of both supraventricular and ventricular arrhythmias in the absence of cardiac disease, even arrhythmias as potentially serious as nonsustained ventricular tachycardia.[8]

Echocardiography

The echocardiogram is more accurate than the chest roentgenogram in the assessment of cardiac chamber size, because the kyphoscoliotic chest deformity and sternal depression common in elderly persons may cause a factitious increase in heart size on the chest roentgenogram. The echocardiogram is also more accurate for the determination of left ventricular hypertrophy than is the electrocardiogram; in addition to identifying left ventricular wall thickness and mass, wall motion abnormalities can be detected as can pericardial effusion. However, a technically adequate echocardiogram cannot be recorded in some elderly patients because of the chest configuration.

Doppler echocardiography appears to be reliable for determining the aortic valve area and estimating the pressure gradient in elderly patients with significant aortic stenosis; there is a good correlation of the calculated echocardiographic valve area with cardiac catheterization data.[9]

Exercise Testing and Exercise Radionuclide Studies

Exercise testing can be undertaken with the same safety and efficacy in elderly patients as in younger patients, ie, among elderly patients who are able to perform an exercise test. A normal response to exercise testing has the same favorable prognosis as in a younger population, and an abnormal response to exercise imparts comparable risk as in younger individuals. An unmet need is the ability to assess activity-induced ischemia in elderly patients who are unable to perform a standard treadmill or bicycle exercise test or arm ergometry adequately, often because of arthritis, claudication, or cerebrovascular or musculoskeletal disorders. Thallium-201 myocardial imaging after coronary vasodilatation with intravenous dipyridamole appears to be well tolerated by elderly patients, with a lesser tachycardia and a delayed decrease in systolic blood pressure compared with younger individuals; however, correlation with coronary arteriography has not been described for elderly patients, nor has the prognostic value of dipyridamole-thallium imaging been defined.[10]

Careful explanation of the test procedure, a practice session on the bicycle or treadmill before the actual test, meticulous skin preparation and electrode placement, and selection of an appropriately low-intensity exercise protocol increase the likelihood of a satisfactory exercise test. The Naughton protocol or a modification of the standard Bruce protocol are preferable. The exercise test can help to determine if the chest discomfort represents myocardial ischemia, to characterize risk status in the elderly patient with angina or following myocardial infarction, to guide recommendations for a physical activity regimen, and to assess the suitability for return to work when appropriate.

The presence and extent of exercise-induced thallium-201 scintigraphic abnormalities are described to permit effective risk stratification in elderly patients, including determination of risk status among elderly patients who had nondiagnostic exercise test electrocardiograms.[11]

Ventricular function is best assessed by radionuclide ventriculography; although it is more expensive than echocardiography, it is more readily applicable to larger numbers of elderly patients.

Perfusion Lung Scanning

Because there is progressive nonuniformity of lung function with aging, perfusion defects may occur in the absence of pulmonary embolism, rendering this test less reliable in an elderly population.

Manifestations of Cardiovascular Disease

Congestive Heart Failure

Although the prevalence of heart failure increases with increasing age, this problem tends to be both under-diagnosed and overdiagnosed in elderly patients.

Echocardiography, in particular, but also other non-invasive techniques for evaluating cardiac function, such as radionuclide ventriculography, have substantially improved the recognition of heart failure in elderly patients and helped to differentiate between predominant systolic and diastolic ventricular dysfunction. Coronary atherosclerotic heart disease, hypertensive cardiovascular disease, and calcific aortic stenosis are the most prevalent causes, and the occurrence of heart failure is more common in men. Heart failure is more frequently precipitated or exacerbated by associated medical problems than in younger patients. The occurrence of congestive heart failure adversely affects the prognosis of most cardiovascular disorders.

Although ventricular systolic dysfunction with cardiac enlargement is the most frequent finding in elderly patients with heart failure, diastolic dysfunction is a prominent cause of heart failure in elderly patients, particularly among those with problems characterized by left ventricular hypertrophy and with normal- or near-normal–sized hearts.[12] Even with normal ventricular systolic function, the decreased ventricular compliance of aging increases the likelihood that even exercise of low to moderate intensity may induce dyspnea. Differentiation from predominant systolic dysfunction is important in that therapies differ markedly.[13]

Manifestations of heart failure may be masked by the sedentary life-style of many elderly patients, whereas exertional dyspnea may reflect another common problem, chronic pulmonary disease, rather than cardiac failure.

The responsiveness of heart failure to vasodilator therapy with nitrate drugs and hydralazine[14] may be especially prominent in an aging population, as the characteristic abnormalities are often superimposed on the increased arterial stiffness of aging. Because of the importance of the atrial contribution to ventricular filling in the poorly compliant aged ventricle, reversion of atrial fibrillation or atrial flutter to sinus rhythm can substantially augment the cardiac output and improve heart failure.

Arrhythmias and Conduction Abnormalities

Both arrhythmias and conduction abnormalities are encountered with increased frequency in an aged population, due to the age-related changes in specialized conducting tissue (Table 14.1).

Syncope may result from either tachyarrhythmias or bradyarrhythmias. Owing to the decrease in cerebral blood flow with aging, a lesser severity of bradyarrhythmia or tachyarrhythmia than required in younger patients may cause an alteration of conscious-

Table 14.1. Ambulatory ECG findings in elderly subjects with no clinical heart disease.*

Variable	Finding
Heart rate, beats/min	34-180
Longest sinus pauses, s	1.8-2
Supraventricular premature complexes (>20/h), %	66
Paroxysmal supraventricular tachycardia, %	13-28
Ventricular premature complexes (>10/h), %	32
Ventricular couplets, %	8-11
Ventricular tachycardia, %	2-4

* Modified from Marcus et al. ECG indicates electrocardiographic. Reprinted with permission from American College of Cardiology (*J Am Coll Cardiol* 1987; 10:68A).

ness or true syncope. Because syncope of a cardiovascular origin carries an enormous 1-year mortality rate, 24%, identification of its mechanism is urgent to enable appropriate therapy; elderly patients with syncope of a noncardiac cause have a more favorable outlook, with their annual mortality approximating 3%.[15,16]

The incidence of supraventricular premature beats increases with aging and is present in virtually all individuals older than 80 years of age, even in the absence of heart disease. Atrial fibrillation also increases in prevalence with increasing age and is a major contributor to stroke in elderly patients, even in the absence of valvular disease.[17] Anticoagulation is advisable, particularly when atrial fibrillation is associated with mitral valve disease or left ventricular dysfunction, despite the greater prevalence of bleeding complications than at a young age.

Ambulatory electrocardiography in elderly individuals who are presumably free of cardiac disease shows that ventricular premature complexes (PVCs) are pervasive, with frequent paired and multiform PVCs and occasional short runs of ventricular tachycardia. Although these arrhythmias do not appear to impart a significant risk in healthy elderly patients, those with congestive cardiac failure or evidence of myocardial ischemia are placed at an increased risk of sudden cardiac death by these findings. Very frequent ventricular premature beats are thought to signify a poor prognosis in very old people with ischemic heart disease.[8] At least 75% suppression of an arrhythmia should be observed to consider that pharmacologic therapy is beneficial. Adverse antiarrhythmic drug reactions are more common in elderly patients due to their altered metabolic function and drug elimination, as well as to the frequent polypharmacy; plasma drug levels should be monitored to maintain therapeutic values and minimize adverse effects. Refractory symptomatic ventricular tachyarrhythmias in elderly

persons may respond well to cardiac surgery (left ventricular endocardial resection or aneurysmectomy), as well as to automatic defibrillator implantation.[18]

Bradyarrhythmias, both the sick sinus syndrome and complete atrioventricular block, occur frequently in an elderly population, and symptomatic bradyarrhythmias are the major indications for pacemaker implantation. Digitalis and calcium- and β-blocking drugs may accentuate the bradycardia of the sick sinus syndrome; in elderly patients with this problem, pacemaker implantation may be required to permit treatment of the tachyarrhythmias with digitalis, β-blocking drugs, or calcium-blocking drugs. Pacemaker implantation in this setting has dramatically improved both survival and life quality. Increasingly, dual-chamber pacemakers are used for reasonably active elderly patients because maintenance of the atrial contribution to ventricular filling improves the cardiac output and activity tolerance in these patients with impaired ventricular compliance of aging.

Coronary Atherosclerotic Heart Disease

Morbidity and mortality from coronary atherosclerotic heart disease increase progressively with age, and coronary disease is responsible for over two thirds of all cardiac deaths among the US elderly population. In the United States, most patients with coronary disease, with new episodes of acute myocardial infarction, and with chronic congestive heart failure secondary to ischemic heart disease are older than 65 years of age.[19] Nevertheless, there is a wide variation in the severity of coronary illness and in the functional status of elderly coronary patients. Furthermore, the characteristic male preponderance among younger coronary patients virtually disappears by the eighth decade.

Angina Pectoris

The presentation of angina pectoris, both as an isolated event and following myocardial infarction, is more likely to be atypical, owing to a combination of a habitually decreased activity level, associated diseases, and possibly an altered sensitivity to pain in elderly persons; furthermore, angina is more likely to be precipitated by a concurrent medical or surgical problem. Severe unstable angina is more common in elderly persons.[20] When unresponsive to intravenous nitroglycerin, with calcium- and β-blocking drugs added as tolerated, urgent coronary arteriography is indicated to evaluate for myocardial revascularization.

As in younger patients, intravenous heparin or oral aspirin therapy appears to be prudent for treating unstable angina.

Myocardial Infarction

Acute myocardial infarction, because of its atypical presentation, is more often unrecognized in aged patients, despite the fact that infarction in elderly persons characteristically is of an increased severity, has a greater occurrence of complications, entails a longer hospital stay, and results in a higher mortality than in a younger age group. Based on Framingham data, unrecognized myocardial infarction is more common in elderly women than in elderly men.

Elderly patients frequently have atypical manifestations for acute myocardial infarction (Table 14.2): chest pain is far less common as the presenting symptom, the electrocardiographic diagnosis is limited by the increased occurrence of non–Q-wave infarction, and elevated MB fractions of creatine kinase (CK) are common in the presence of a normal total CK level, due to a decreased lean-body mass with aging.[21] Although the myocardial infarction may be painless, the clinical presentation is often not asymptomatic and may include acute dyspnea, exacerbation of heart failure, syncope, stroke, vertigo, acute confusion, palpitations, peripheral arterial emboli, or acute renal failure; more subtle changes involve altered mentation, excessive fatigue, and changes in eating pattern or in other usual behaviors. As is the case with angina pectoris, acute myocardial infarction in elderly patients is more often precipitated by a medical or surgical problem associated with hypovolemia, blood loss, infection, hypotension, and the like.

Although a number of small, often noncontrolled studies of thrombolytic therapy in patients with myocardial infarction older than 65 years of age have shown comparable reperfusion and no excess of mortality or bleeding complications than in younger patients, the large Gruppo Italiano per lo Studio della Streptochinasi nell'Infarto Miocardico trial[22] that included more than 1,000 patients older than 75 years of age showed no statistically significant benefit in the patients older than 65 years of age. However, there was no apparent increase in adverse events in elderly patients, and the survival trend was in the direction of benefit,[22] suggesting that the decision to use thrombolytic therapy must be made on an individual basis, with consideration of potential benefit and harm. Also to be considered is that coronary arteriography is often undertaken following successful thrombolysis to determine the need for myocardial revascularization procedures.

In-hospital mortality is greater in patients older than 70 years of age, in that complications, including hypotension, atrioventricular block, atrial arrhythmias, congestive cardiac failure, and cardiac rupture, occur more commonly in elderly patients. Posthospital mortality is also increased following myocardial infarction.

Except as noted above, the management of acute myocardial infarction is comparable with that of a younger population, save for the increased risk and lesser benefit of prophylactic lidocaine used for ventricular arrhythmias in acute infarction; the baseline prevalence of ventricular arrhythmias, even in the absence of myocardial ischemia, coupled with the greater risk of complications of lidocaine therapy with aging, renders this a less desirable prophylactic intervention. β-Blockade with timolol following myocardial infarction conferred comparable benefit in elderly patients to that observed in younger patients.[23]

Exercise testing, typically performed for risk stratification following myocardial infarction to select the subset of patients requiring more intensive diagnostic and therapeutic interventions,[24] can also be used to recommend the intensity of physical activity that can be performed with safety following discharge from the hospital. Many elderly patients can exercise safely without supervision; the predischarge exercise test can also identify the subset of patients for whom initially supervised exercise is most appropriate. Exercise, in addition to improving physical work capacity,[25] is reported to enhance psychologic and cognitive

Table 14.2. Atypical manifestations: acute myocardial infarction in elderly patients.

Presentation
  Painless infarction more common
  Acute symptoms
    Dyspnea
    Exacerbation of heart failure
    Syncope
    Stroke
    Vertigo
    Acute confusion
    Palpitations
    Peripheral arterial emboli
    Acute renal failure
  Subtle manifestations
    Altered mentation
    Excessive fatigue
    Changes in eating pattern
    Changes in other usual behaviors
Common precipitating factors
  Hypovolemia
  Blood loss
  Infection
  Hypotension

functioning (see Chapter 42).[26] Exercise test results can also guide recommendations for return to preinfarction physical activities, including resumption of remunerative work when appropriate.

Myocardial Revascularization

Elderly patients with chronic symptomatic angina, unresponsive or poorly responsive to medical management, or with persisting chest pain following myocardial infarction, are candidates for coronary arteriography to assess their suitability for myocardial revascularization. Older patients with evidence of myocardial ischemia at low work loads also constitute a high-risk group for early recurrent coronary events and should be evaluated for myocardial revascularization.

Older age patients now constitute an increasing proportion of the population undergoing cardiac catheterization, coronary angioplasty,[27] and coronary bypass surgery.[28] Although the risk of angioplasty is slightly increased in very elderly patients, high success rates with low mortality have been described, with striking 1- to 2-year persistence of symptomatic improvement.[29]

Although patients older than 70 years of age sustain a higher operative mortality from elective coronary artery bypass surgery than do younger individuals, as well as an increased incidence of stroke and a low cardiac output state requiring intra-aortic balloon pump support, the symptomatic improvement and late outcome among elderly survivors of coronary bypass surgery suggest that an optimistic approach to the management of symptomatic elderly patients with advanced obstructive coronary disease is reasonable.[30] Emergency coronary bypass surgery in elderly patients entails a substantially increased mortality risk. Elderly patients can be anticipated to have a longer hospital stay following coronary bypass surgery, with an increased period of time spent in an intensive care setting. In elderly patients with preserved ventricular function and without major associated medical problems, 5-year survival following successful coronary bypass surgery approximates 90%.

Hypertension

Even in normotensive elderly persons, blood pressure should be measured annually. Hypertension contributes importantly to accelerated coronary atherosclerotic heart disease, congestive heart failure, cerebrovascular accident, renal failure, and aortic aneurysm rupture in elderly persons, as well as in younger populations. Although only 20% of patients in the

Veterans Administration Cooperative Study on Antihypertensive Agents were older than 60 years of age, half of all the morbidity, heart failure, and stroke occurred in this age group.[31] Control of hypertension decreases the risk of complications: cardiovascular death, congestive heart failure, and stroke in elderly patients;[32,33] particularly in elderly patients with mild hypertension, nonpharmacologic approaches should be initially considered because of potential problems of drug treatment. Hypertension is discussed in more detail in Chapter 13.

Valvular Heart Disease, Congenital Heart Disease, and Infective Endocarditis

Aortic Stenosis

Hemodynamically significant symptomatic calcific aortic stenosis is the most frequent form of valvular heart disease that requires surgical correction in elderly patients.

Symptomatic severe aortic valvular stenosis is characterized by the same presentations in elderly persons as in a younger population: angina pectoris, exertional dizziness or syncope, and dyspnea or congestive cardiac failure; however, these symptoms are often misinterpreted as being due to other cardiac problems, such as coronary artery disease or neurologic disease when the presentation is with syncope.[34] Symptoms are less often effort related than in younger patients, due to a more frequent sedentary life-style with aging. Dyspnea is often associated with the hemodynamic abnormalities of left ventricular failure. Differentiation is required from the benign, but pervasive, early-peaking basal systolic murmur of aortic sclerosis. The classic slow-rising arterial (carotid) pulse of a younger patient may be masked by vascular stiffness in an elderly patient; this may also mask the usual narrow pulse pressure. Systemic arterial hypertension, rarely seen in younger individuals with severe aortic stenosis, is not uncommon in elderly persons. Hyperexpansion of the lungs may limit the palpatory evidence of the sustained apex impulse of left ventricular hypertrophy and, at times, the systolic thrill; the harsh basal systolic murmur may become softer as cardiac output lessens. Lack of commissural fusion with calcific aortic stenosis in elderly persons further mutes the harsh characteristics of the murmur and also explains the absence of an ejection sound. Atrial fibrillation rarely occurs in younger patients with aortic stenosis, but often precipitates congestive heart failure in elderly ones, due to a loss of the atrial contribution to ventricular filling in combination with the lessened ventricular filling due to the rapid heart rate. There is frequently a coexisting murmur of aortic regurgitation, but aortic regurgitation of hemodynamic significance is unusual.

Echocardiographic evidence of aortic valve calcification is virtually universal, with an increased left ventricular wall thickness evident in most patients. Doppler echocardiography can reasonably assess the severity of aortic valvular obstruction. There is characteristic electrocardiographic evidence of left ventricular hypertrophy as well, with a normal electrocardiogram suggested by some as excluding the presence of critical aortic stenosis. Cardiac catheterization and coronary arteriography are warranted, nonetheless, because coexistent coronary disease is frequent.[35]

Aortic valve replacement can be performed at an acceptable risk, even in patients with left ventricular dysfunction, and dramatically improves both survival and the patient's quality of life.[36,37]

The role of balloon valvuloplasty remains to be defined,[38] but it may provide palliation in symptomatic elderly patients who are poor candidates for general anesthesia and surgical valve replacement.[39]

Aortic Regurgitation

Aortic regurgitation, due to myxomatous valvular degeneration, congenital valvular abnormalities, rheumatic heart disease, infective endocarditis, systemic arterial hypertension, and a number of other disorders, can usually be diagnosed by clinical examination. Echocardiography and Doppler studies can help to assess the hemodynamic severity. The results of aortic valve replacement for aortic regurgitation are less satisfactory than for aortic stenosis, at least in part because of the significant depression of ventricular function. Vasodilator therapy and digitalis help to control congestive heart failure.

Mitral Regurgitation

Mitral valve prolapse may be asymptomatic in some elderly patients, and be diagnosed only by the classic auscultatory findings. In others, however,[40] disabling chest pain occurs; because of frequently associated nonspecific repolarization abnormalities on the electrocardiogram, an erroneous diagnosis of angina pectoris may be made. Palpitations should suggest an associated arrhythmia. In contrast to younger patients, mitral valve prolapse in elderly patients may result in severe mitral regurgitation and symptomatic congestive heart failure. There may be complicating infective endocarditis or ruptured chordae tendineae; again, in contrast to the female predominance in the

younger population, congestive heart failure secondary to mitral valve prolapse predominates in elderly men.

Other common causes of mitral regurgitation in elderly patients include mitral annular calcification and papillary muscle dysfunction, secondary to coronary disease. The diagnosis of mitral regurgitation usually can be made by clinical examination, but echocardiographic examination often suggests the cause. Doppler echocardiography may help to quantify the severity of the mitral regurgitation, and assessment of exercise capacity and noninvasive documentation of left ventricular systolic function can identify patients for whom cardiac catheterization is appropriate to assess suitability for operative intervention.

The mortality rate of combined mitral valve replacement and coronary bypass surgery or of mitral and aortic valve replacement and coronary bypass surgery is over 50% in patients in the eighth and ninth decades, presumably because of the significant antecedent left ventricular dysfunction.[41]

Mitral Stenosis

Mitral stenosis, usually rheumatic in origin, rarely assumes hemodynamic significance in the elderly age group.

Congenital Heart Disease

Congenital cardiac lesions rarely cause de novo hemodynamic problems in an elderly population. Atrial septal defect and persistent ductus arteriosus are the more commonly encountered lesions that may have associated hemodynamic significance, and surgical correction in symptomatic elderly patients entails only a modestly greater risk than in a younger age group. Most congenital cardiac lesions of hemodynamic significance have been corrected in childhood or young adult life.[42] Too few patients with corrected congenital heart disease have yet reached elderly age for determination to be made regarding their risks of arrhythmia, ventricular dysfunction, and other abnormalities.

Infective Endocarditis

Although one third of all cases of infective endocarditis occur in elderly patients, its recognition is often delayed or missed in this age group because of fewer symptoms and an absent or minimal febrile response. Elderly persons constitute an increasing percentage of patients with infective endocarditis, and the problem is likely to increase further in prevalence as more elderly persons are hospitalized and undergo complex invasive procedures. Endocarditis is associated with a higher mortality than in younger patients,[43] in part due to the delay in diagnosis and in the initiation of appropriate therapy. Invasive vascular procedures are the most common sources of infection. In addition to the organisms usually encountered in a younger population, enterococci, *Streptococcus bovis,* and coagulase-negative staphylococci occur with excessive frequency in elderly patients.

Cardiomyopathy

Hypertrophic cardiomyopathy is commonly under-diagnosed in elderly patients,[44] and may be incorrectly labeled as aortic valvular disease, mitral regurgitation, or coronary atherosclerotic heart disease. An incorrect diagnosis, with resultant inappropriate drug therapy (eg, digitalis, excessive diuretic use), may exacerbate the outflow obstruction and result in serious complications. Hypertrophic cardiomyopathy is more often symmetric, and the prognosis appears to be better than in a younger population, as serious arrhythmias or sudden cardiac death are unusual. Echocardiography aids in diagnosis; prophylaxis against infective endocarditis is appropriate. Calcium- or β-blocking drug therapy is advisable.

Dilated cardiomyopathy is infrequent in an elderly population, as the majority of patients with this problem do not survive to an elderly age. The management is as for systolic ventricular dysfunction, and includes digitalis, diuretics, and vasodilator therapy; anticoagulation is recommended, particularly when there is associated atrial fibrillation, despite the increased risk of bleeding when elderly patients receive anticoagulant drugs.

Restrictive cardiomyopathy is unusual in elderly patients. Although senile cardiac amyloidosis has a high prevalence among the oldest old patients, atrial fibrillation, rather than restrictive cardiomyopathy seems to be the more frequent manifestation. However, as more patients who have had coronary artery bypass surgery reach the elderly age group, postoperative restrictive pericarditis may be anticipated to occur with increased frequency.

Pulmonary Heart Disease

Pulmonary embolism is a frequent and often unrecognized complication of many systemic illnesses in elderly patients. The combination of prolonged bed rest, a sedentary life-style, and cardiopulmonary disease are the major predisposing factors, as is atrial fibrillation. Furthermore, anticoagulation, the management of choice, carries a greater risk of bleeding than in younger patients.

Pulmonary heart disease is superimposed on the decreased elastic properties of the aged lung, as well as the loss of pulmonary vascular reserve and the decrease in ventilatory function with aging. The most common form of chronic pulmonary heart disease that causes cor pulmonale and right ventricular failure is chronic obstructive pulmonary disease. The predominant mortality from this problem is among elderly patients, related, at least in part, to their coexisting cardiovascular disease. Therapeutic problems are accentuated with concomitant cardiac and pulmonary disease, in that the nonselective β-blocking drugs used to treat coronary disease or hypotension may induce bronchospasm; conversely, theophylline and β-agonist drugs used to manage chronic obstructive pulmonary disease may adversely affect cardiac function and induce arrhythmias. Elderly patients have a favorable response, comparable with that of a younger population, to continuous low-flow oxygen therapy, when significant hypoxemia is present.

Cardiovascular Drug Therapy: Problems that Predominate with Aging

Drug therapy in elderly patients is discussed in detail in Chapter 7. Both drug toxicity and adverse drug reactions are considerably more frequent in patients older than 65 years of age. Contributing factors include noncompliance or errors in medication-taking, often related to visual or cognitive impairment; drug interaction with age-related physiologic changes; differences in drug metabolism, excretion, bioavailability, and in receptor activity or affinity; and the multiple drug treatments and concomitant multisystem chronic diseases that are characteristic of many elderly patients.[45] Limited income may pose an added problem in adherence to drug therapy.

On the other hand, data from the Hypertension Detection and Follow-up Study suggest that elderly patients may comply better with medication-taking than younger age groups. In other studies, including the Systolic Hypertension in the Elderly Pilot Study,[47] elderly patients also appear to be both willing and able to adhere to medication regimens.

General principles that may limit problems with pharmacotherapy in elderly patients include the initiation of drug therapy at a low dosage, gradual dosage increases, simplification of the drug regimen as much as possible, avoidance of unnecessary drugs, and periodic reassessment of drug therapy. Clearly written directions can enable family members and friends to help the elderly patient with medication-taking.

Digitalis toxicity is accentuated in the elderly because of the limited volume of distribution of the drug, the lesser lean-body mass, and diminished renal excretion of the drug (even with a normal serum creatinine concentration).

Although reduction in drug dosage is often indicated in elderly patients, this is not universally so, as aged patients are relatively resistant to some categories of compounds, particularly β-blocking agents.[48]

Noncardiac Surgery in Elderly Patients with Cardiovascular Disease

Because there is far more heterogeneity in an elderly population than within any other age group, chronologic age per se poorly predicts either a patient's physiologic age or functional capabilities. Furthermore, negative stereotypes of elderly persons as being seriously ill and disabled often inappropriately bias recommendations and decisions about medical care and particularly suitable surgical interventions for elderly cardiac patients.

Age alone should not constitute a contraindication to surgical therapy; the increased complications in elderly patients relate predominantly to their associated diseases, and these should prominently influence clinical decisions. Mental status, cognitive ability, and expectations from medical care are other attributes to be considered. Both overt and occult cardiovascular disease, but particularly coronary disease, contribute to the increased risk of perioperative cardiovascular complications. General nutritional status[49] is also an important determinant of the ability to tolerate the stress of an operation and the postoperative period (See also Chapter 11).

Preventive and Rehabilitative Approaches to Care

As increased numbers of reasonably healthy and active individuals enter the elderly age group, more precise assessment of their functional capabilities will be required to determine suitable vocational, as well as recreational and leisure, activities. This less impaired elderly population can be anticipated to have greater interest in and requirements for preventive cardiovascular care.

At the same time, an overriding concern among elderly persons is maintenance of a self-sufficient and independent life-style; loss or deterioration of functional capability is viewed as a threat to that valued feature.

Preventive strategies are increasingly being applied to the elderly population. The fact that elderly persons are health conscious is shown by their disproportionate representation in most health screening programs. Most of the traditional risk factors for cardiovascular disease, ie, hypertension, hyperlipidemia, diabetes, obesity, physical inactivity, and smoking, are prevalent among elderly patients. Although their relative importance decreases somewhat with age, they continue to impart substantial risk due to the high incidence and prevalence of coronary disease in elderly patients. Coronary risk factors continue to predict morbidity and mortality even in very elderly patients (Table 14.3).

The lesser risk relationship of cholesterol in older adults is offset by the far greater occurrence of coronary heart disease in elderly persons.[50] Whereas total serum cholesterol levels are poor predictors of coronary risk in elderly persons, the high- and low-density lipoprotein fractions remain good indicators of future coronary risk. Vegetarians, who have lower cholesterol levels than nonvegetarians, also show lower coronary heart disease rates even in the 75- to 84-year-old age category.[51] Women constitute a greater proportion of the elderly population, and the occurrence of myocardial infarction is comparable in elderly men and women, so that detection and management of coronary disease must significantly involve elderly women. Although mean blood cholesterol levels are higher in men before the fifth decade, women subsequently have higher mean total cholesterol levels.

The Adult Treatment Panel of the National Cholesterol Education Program recommends that all adults with total blood cholesterol values above 200 mg/dL be evaluated and that those with elevated low-density lipoprotein cholesterol levels be treated.[52] Recommendations for cholesterol lowering in the elderly population are based predominantly on extrapolation of data derived from younger populations. Dietary therapy is recommended for the older adult; this consists of a diet restricted in saturated fat and cholesterol and high in fruits, vegetables, and grains; additional dietary components include lean meats, fish, and low-fat dairy products. A trained nutritionist or dietitian can often help elderly individuals initiate appropriate dietary management, while assuring adequate nutrition. This diet may confer other health benefits as well. Drug therapy to lower cholesterol levels is currently rarely indicated in the elderly population.

Increasingly, recommendations are made for a physically active life-style for elderly patients, incorporating a planned exercise regimen designed to improve functional status and thereby minimize or delay

Table 14.3. Impact of risk factors on cardiovascular disease incidence* by age in men and women at 30-year follow-up: Framingham Study.

| Risk factor | Multivariate logistic regression coefficients† at | | | |
| | Age, 35-64 y‡ | | Age, 65-94 y‡ | |
	Men	Women	Men	Women
Systolic pressure	341§	0.361§	0.410§	0.207§
Diastolic pressure	0.302§	0.288 ‖	0.259§	0.089¶
Serum cholesterol level	0.230§	0.202§	0.091#	0.040¶
Blood glucose level	0.087 ‖	0.176§	0.146§	0.173§
Relative weight	0.080#	0.134 ‖	0.044¶	0.052¶
Vital capacity	−0.089#	−0.252§	−0.109¶	−0.216§
Cigarettes	0.333§	0.183§	0.045¶	0.083¶
ECG-LVH**	0.121§	0.112§	0.142§	0.229§
Intraventricular block	0.049¶	0.075#	0.096#	0.096#
NSA-ST-T**	0.052¶	0.130§	0.187§	0.147§

* Modified from Kannel et al. Coronary events, stroke, cardiac failure, and peripheral arterial disease. Reprinted with permission from American College of Cardiology (*J Am Coll Cardiol* 1987;10:25A-28A).
† Covariates for each variable cited in "Risk Factor" column: blood pressure, cholesterol, cigarettes, and electrocardiographic evidence of left ventricular hypertrophy.
‡ Age at biennial examination.
§ $P < .001$.
‖ $P < .01$.
¶ Not significant.
# $P < .05$.
** ECG-LVH indicates electrocardiographic evidence of left ventricular hypertrophy; NSA-ST-T, nonspecific ST segment and T-wave abnormalities.

subsequent disability and dependence (see Chapter 42). Exercise recommendations must be individualized, avoiding excessive fatigue or exhaustion and limiting musculoskeletal injuries by restriction of running, jumping, and other high-impact activities. Brisk walking is generally recommended.

Hypertension, both elevation of the systolic and the diastolic blood pressures, continues to impart risk in elderly persons. Electrocardiographic evidence of left ventricular hypertrophy, intraventricular conduction disturbances, and nonspecific repolarization abnormalities all independently predict future cardiovascular events. The decline in coronary mortality in the United States from 1963 to 1981 affected all ages, but less prominently the elderly population; since most cardiovascular risk factors can be modified in elderly persons, attention to this aspect seems to be appropriate. Because the average life expectancy for a 65-year-old woman in the United States is about 19.5 years and that for a 65-year-old man 15.1 years, preventive approaches are indicated and have the potential to affect survival favorably. Based on the Framingham data,[19] the 10% of individuals aged 65 to 74 years with the highest multivariate coronary risk scores had a two-times greater occurrence of coronary events for men and four-times greater occurrence among women. Benefits of risk reduction, however,

must be extrapolated from intervention trials in younger aged patients; however, conventional risk modification may favorably affect other health aspects as well.

Risk status can be ascertained by standard clinical examinations and simple laboratory tests. Most preventive measures that are appropriate for older individuals are reasonable and relatively simple modifications of existing habits; unfavorable life-style behaviors can be modified to affect favorably cardiovascular risk.

References

1. Higginbotham MB, Morris KG, Williams RS, et al. Physiologic basis for the age-related decline in aerobic work capacity. *Am J Cardiol* 1986;57:1374–1379.
2. Rodeheffer RJ, Gerstenblith G, Becker LC, et al. Exercise cardiac output is maintained with advancing age in healthy human subjects: cardiac dilatation and increased stroke volume compensate for a diminished heart rate. *Circulation* 1984;69:203–213.
3. Hitzhusen JC, Hickler RB, Alpert JS, et al. Exercise testing and hemodynamic performance in healthy elderly persons. *Am J Cardiol* 1984;54:1082–1086.
4. Lakatta EG, Gerstenblith G, Angell CS, et al. Diminished inotropic response of aged myocardium to catecholamines. *Circ Res* 1975;36:262–269.

5. Mader SL, Josephson KR, Rubenstein LZ. Low prevalence of postural hypotension among community-dwelling elderly. *JAMA* 1987;258:1511–1514.

6. Gerstenblith G. Noninvasive assessment of cardiac function in the elderly. In: Weisfeldt M, ed. *The Aging Heart: Its Function and Response to Stress.* New York, NY: Raven Press; 1984:247–267.

7. Campbell A, Caird FI, Jackson TF. Prevalence of abnormalities of electrocardiogram in old people. *Br Heart J* 1974;36:1005–1011.

8. Ingerslev J, Bjerregaard P. Prevalence and prognostic significance of cardiac arrhythmias detected by ambulatory electrocardiography in subjects 85 years of age. *Eur Heart J* 1986;7:570–575.

9. Come PC, Riley MF, McKay RG, et al. Echocardiographic assessment of aortic valve area in elderly patients with aortic stenosis and of changes in valve area after percutaneous balloon valvuloplasty. *J Am Coll Cardiol* 1987;10:115–124.

10. Gerson MC, Moore EN, Ellis K. Systemic effects and safety of intravenous dipyridamole in elderly patients with suspected coronary artery disease. *Am J Cardiol* 1987;60:1399–1401.

11. Iskandrian AS, Heo J, Decoskey D, et al. Use of exercise thallium-201 imaging for risk stratification of elderly patients with coronary artery disease. *Am J Cardiol* 1988;61:269–272.

12. Dougherty AH, Naccarelli GV, Gray EL, et al. Congestive heart failure with normal systolic function. *Am J Cardiol* 1984;54:778–782.

13. Topol EJ, Traill TA, Fortuin NJ. Hypertensive hypertrophic cardiomyopathy of the elderly. *N Engl J Med* 1985;312:277–283.

14. Cohn JN, Archibald DG, Ziesche S, et al. Effect of vasodilator therapy on mortality in chronic congestive heart failure: results of a Veterans Administration Cooperative Study. *N Engl J Med* 1986;314:1547–1552.

15. Lipsitz LA, Wei JY, Rowe JW. Syncope in an elderly institutionalized population: prevalence, incidence, and associated risk. *Q J Med* 1985;55:45–54.

16. Gordon M, Huang M, Gryfe CI. An evaluation of falls, syncope and dizziness by prolonged ambulatory cardiographic monitoring in a geriatric institutional setting. *J Am Geriatr Soc* 1982;30:6–12.

17. Wolf PA, Abbott RD, Kannel WB. Atrial fibrillation: a major contributor to stroke in the elderly. *Arch Intern Med* 1987;147:1561–1564.

18. Tresch DD, Platia EV, Guarnieri T, et al. Refractory symptomatic ventricular tachycardia and ventricular fibrillation in elderly patients. *Am J Med* 1987;83:399–404.

19. Wenger NK, Furberg CD, Pitt E. *Coronary Heart Disease in the Elderly: Working Conference on the Recognition and Management of Coronary Heart Disease in the Elderly, National Institute of Health, Bethesda 1985.* New York, NY: Elsevier Science Publishing Co Inc; 1986.

20. Mock MD, Fisher LD, Gersh BJ, et al. Prognosis of coronary heart disease in the elderly patient: the CASS experience. In: Coodley EL, ed. *Geriatric Heart Disease.* Littleton, Mass: PSG Publishing Co Inc; 1985:358–363.

21. Hong RA, Licht JD, Wei JY, et al. Elevated CK-MB with normal total creatine kinase in suspected myocardial infarction: associated clinical findings and early prognosis. *Am Heart J* 1986;111:1041–1047.

22. Gruppo Italiano per lo Studio della Streptochinasi nell'Infarto Miocardico (GISSI). Effectiveness of intravenous thrombolytic treatment in acute myocardial infarction. *Lancet* 1986;1:397–401.

23. Gundersen T, Abrahamsen Am, Kjekshus J, et al, for the Norwegian Multicentre Study Group. Timolol-related reduction in mortality and reinfarction in patients ages 65–75 years surviving acute myocardial infarction. *Circulation* 1982;66:1179–1184.

24. Saunamaki KI. Early post-myocardial infarction exercise testing in subjects 70 years or more of age: functional and prognostic evaluation. *Eur Heart J* 1984;5(suppl E):93–96.

25. Williams MA, Maresh CM, Esterbrooks DJ, et al. Early exercise training in patients older than age 65 years compared with that in younger patients after acute myocardial infarction or coronary artery bypass grafting. *Am J Cardiol* 1985;55:263–266.

26. Dustman RE, Ruhling RO, Russell EM, et al. Aerobic exercise training and improved neuropsychological function of older individuals. *Neurobiol Aging* 1984;5:35–42.

27. Mock M, Holmes D Jr, Vlietstra R, et al. Percutaneous transluminal coronary angioplasty (PTCA) in patient >60 years of age registered in the NHLBI Registry. *Circulation* 1982;66(suppl II):II–329. Abstract.

28. Kern MJ, Deligonul U, Galan K, et al. Percutaneous transluminal coronary angioplasty in octogenarians. *Am J Cardiol* 1988;61:457–458.

29. Dorros G, Janke L. Percutaneous transluminal coronary angioplasty in patients over the age of 70 years. *Cathet Cardiovasc Diagn* 1986;12:223–229.

30. Gersh BJ, Kronmal RA, Schaff HV, et al, and participants in the CASS Study. Comparison of coronary artery surgery and medical therapy in patients 65 years of age or older: a nonrandomized study from the Coronary Artery Surgery Study (CASS) Registry. *N Engl J Med* 1985;313:217–224.

31. Veterans Administration Cooperative Study Group on Antihypertensive Agents. Effects of treatment on morbidity in hypertension, III: influence of age, diastolic pressure, and prior cardiovascular disease: further analysis of side effects. *Circulation* 1972;45:991–1004.

32. The Working Group on Hypertension in the Elderly. Statement on hypertension in the elderly. *JAMA* 1986;256:70–74.

33. Amery A, Birkenhager W, Brixko P, et al. Mortality and morbidity results from the European Working Party on High Blood Pressure in the Elderly Trial. *Lancet* 1985;1:1349–1354.

34. Nylander E, Ekman I, Marklund T, et al. Severe aortic stenosis in elderly patients. *Br Heart J* 1986;55:480–487.

35. Lombard JT, Selzer A. Valvular aortic stenosis: a clinical and hemodynamic profile of patients. *Ann Intern Med* 1987;106:292–298.

36. Murphy ES, Lawson RM, Starr A, et al. Severe aortic stenosis in patients 60 years of age or older: left ven-

tricular function and 10-year survival after valve replacement. *Circulation* 1981;64(suppl II):II–184–188.

37. Teply JF, Grunkemeier GL, Starr A. Cardiac valve replacement in patients over 75 years of age. *Thorac Cardiovasc Surg* 1981;29:47–50.

38. Rahimtoola SH. Catheter balloon valvuloplasty for aortic and mitral stenosis in adults. *Circulation* 1987;75:885–901.

39. Schneider JF, Wilson M, Gallant TE. Percutaneous balloon aortic valvuloplasty for aortic stenosis in elderly patients at high risk for surgery. *Ann Intern Med* 1987;106:696–699.

40. Kolibash AJ, Bush CA, Fontana MB, et al. Mitral valve prolapse syndrome: analysis of 62 patients aged 60 years and older. *Am J Cardiol* 1983;52:534–539.

41. Tsai TP, Matloff JM, Chaux A, et al. Combined valve and coronary artery bypass procedures in septuagenarians and octogenarians: results in 120 patients. *Ann Thorac Surg* 1986;42:681–684.

42. Cheitlin MD. Congenital heart disease in the adult. *Mod Conc Cardiovasc Dis* 1986;55:20–24.

43. Terpenning MS, Buggy BP, Kauffman CA. Infective endocarditis: clinical features in young and elderly patients. *Am J Med* 1987;83:626–634.

44. Krasnow N, Stein RA. Hypertrophic cardiomyopathy in the aged. *Am Heart J* 1978;96:326–336.

45. Lowenthal DT, Affrime MB. Cardiovascular drugs for the geriatric patient. *Geriatrics* 1981;36:65–74.

46. Hypertension detection and follow-up program cooperative group. Five-year findings of the hypertension detection and follow-up program: II. Mortality by race-sex and age. *JAMA* 1979;242:2572–2577.

47. Black DM, Brand RJ, Greenlick M, et al. Compliance to treatment for hypertension in elderly patients: the SHEP Pilot Study. *J Gerontol* 1987;42:552–557.

48. Vestal RE, Wood AJ, Shand DG. Reduced beta-adrenoreceptor sensitivity in the elderly. *Clin Pharmacol Ther* 1979;26:181–186.

49. Schneider EL, Vining EM, Hadley EC, et al. Recommended dietary allowances and the health of the elderly. *N Engl J Med* 1986;314:157–160.

50. Kannel WB, Doyle JT, Shephard RJ, et al. Prevention of cardiovascular disease in the elderly. *J Am Coll Cardiol* 1987;10:25A–28A.

51. Snowdon DA, Phillips RL, Fraser GE. Meat consumption and fatal ischemic heart disease. *Prev Med* 1984;13:490–500.

52. The Expert Panel. Report of the National Cholesterol Education Program Expert Panel on Detection, Evaluation, and Treatment of High Blood Cholesterol in Adults. *Arch Intern Med* 1988;138:36–69.

53. Marcus FI, Ruskin JN, Surawicz B. Arrhythmias. *J Am Coll Cardiol* 1987;10:66A–72A.

15

Disorders of Skeletal Aging

Diane Meier

Skeletal pathology is a leading cause of serious morbidity and functional loss in old age. However, it is difficult to distinguish between disease and normal age changes in the clinical approach to bone disorders, and this has lead to substantial controversy over the diagnosis and treatment of the most common metabolic bone disease, osteoporosis. For example, loss of skeletal calcium is a nearly universal concomitant of aging, independent of body size, race, or gender, but the process does not become pathologic until it is of sufficient magnitude to lead to osteoporotic fracture, with associated adverse consequences such as pain, immobility, deformity, and (in the case of hip fracture) premature death. Defining the point at which these age-related skeletal changes require intervention presents a major challenge to researchers and clinicians alike. Reasons for these difficulties include the fact that there is a long latent period of bone loss before the onset of clinically apparent disease, that current diagnostic procedures are unable to separate those at risk of fracture from those not at risk, that available treatment modalities have not been subject to randomized long-term study, and in particular, that studies of treatments for older adults are almost completely lacking. Research efforts directed at these issues have increased dramatically as a result of demographic changes leading to a large aging female population at high risk for osteoporosis and because of rapidly developing technologies in the measurement of bone mineral content.

Physiology of Skeletal Aging

The skeleton is composed of two distinct types of bone: cortical (or compact) and trabecular (or cancellous) bone. Cortical bone comprises the outer layer of the long bones and the cortex of the remainder of the skeleton, accounting for roughly 75% of total bone mass. Trabecular bone is a honeycomblike lattice of intersecting bone plates (or trabeculae) that form the central portion of bone. Trabecular bone has a much higher surface-to-volume ratio than cortical bone and is therefore more subject to blood-borne metabolic influences. The parts of the skeleton most susceptible to fracture are proportionately highest in trabecular bone volume (vertebrae, 66%; distal forearm, 25%; and femoral head, 50%).

Skeletal calcium losses are a nearly universal concomitant of aging and reflect an imbalance of bone remodeling, with osteoclastic bone resorption exceeding osteoblastic formation of new bone. This continuous process of bone remodeling is highly responsive to local and systemic metabolic influences and therapeutic interventions directed at altering the balance of resorption and formation. During childhood and young adulthood, new bone formation exceeds bone resorption, leading to net increases in bone mass. After about age 30 years, when peak skeletal bone mass has been achieved, resorption begins to exceed formation, with subsequent skeletal calcium losses and a decline in bone density. While other factors (for example, bone geometry and quality, presence of microfractures) also contribute, bone density is a major determinant of fracture risk. If this skeletal calcium loss is of sufficient magnitude, an increased vulnerability to fracture ensues.

Bone loss rates vary depending on the type of bone measured (cortical or trabecular), the technique of densitometry used, the part of skeleton evaluated, and the type of population studied. In white women, slow bone loss (at a rate of 0.5% to 1% per year) occurs between the ages of 25 and 50 years, followed by an acceleration during the menopausal and immediate postmenopausal years (2% to 4% per year), corresponding to the hormonal alterations of menopause. Bone loss rates slow down again after age 55 to 60 years, to approximately 0.5% to 1% per year through old age. In men, cortical bone loss may begin later (at age 50 to 60 years) and is slower (0.3% to .5% per year). No accelerated phase of bone loss comparable to that seen at the female menopause is observed in men. In both sexes, trabecular bone loss may begin earlier and progress more quickly than that observed in the cortical skeletal compartment. Thus, age-related bone loss is not a linear or homogeneous process and may have quite different etiologies at various ages.

Adult skeletal mass is the net result of two factors: the maximum or peak bone mass achieved at skeletal maturity and the subsequent rate and duration of bone loss. Influences on achievement of maximal peak bone mass are not well understood but probably include genetic factors, activity levels, nutritional status, and body habitus of children, adolescents, and young adults. Factors influencing the rate and duration of bone loss after skeletal maturity include gonadal hormone status, calcium intake and bioavailability, vitamin D status, physical activity, and other endocrine influences (parathyroid hormone, glucocorticoids, thyroid hormone, growth hormone, and calcitonin). The complex interaction of these variables in both normal age-related and pathologic bone loss remains poorly understood.[1]

Known age changes in factors influencing bone homeostasis occur in calcium, vitamin D, and gonadal hormone status. Dietary intake of calcium, gastrointestinal absorption of calcium, and 1,25-dihyroxyvitamin D synthesis are all decreased with age. Similarly, decreased dietary intake of ergocalciferol (vitamin D_2) and decreased skin absorption of vitamin D_3 due to inadequate sunlight exposure also may contribute to vitamin D deficiency with age.[2] The influence of menopause-induced hypogonadism on bone loss of women is clear, and although no accelerated decline in bone mass has been observed in men, a linear fall in free testosterone levels with age has been observed

and may contribute to age-related bone loss in men as well.

Osteoporosis

Of all metabolic bone disorders, osteoporosis is the most common, particularly among older adults. Osteoporosis is defined as a state of inappropriately low bone volume for age, gender, and race in association with normal mineralization processes and a normal ratio of unmineralized osteoid matrix to mineralized bone on bone histomorphometry. As such, it must be differentiated from osteomalacia, another disorder of low bone mineral content, which is characterized by normal bone volume and a decrease in mineralization processes. This low bone mass increases susceptibility to fracture. Osteoporosis may result from a variety of processes, which must be appropriately differentiated in the clinical approach to diagnosis and treatment.

Epidemiology

Osteoporosis affects over 20 million North Americans and is associated with a fracture incidence of 1.3 million in persons over age 45 years. These include approximately 210,000 hip fractures, 600,000 vertebral fractures, and over 400,000 radial and other limb fractures per year. The total cost of osteoporosis and osteoporotic fractures was estimated in 1983 to exceed $6 billion annually. The human costs of disability, dependency, and premature death associated with these fractures are enormous and are increasing rapidly as the population ages.[3]

Vertebral deformities (greater than 15% reduction in anterior vertebral height), occurring eight times as frequently in women as in men, affect at least 40% of women by age 80 years. If radiographic evidence of spinal osteopenia is taken as the diagnostic criterion, 65% of women over age 60 years and virtually 100% of women over age 90 years are affected. True vertebral crush fractures are less common, affecting about 5% of white women by age 70 years.[4] Vertebral fractures may be asymptomatic but can be associated with substantial short-and long-term disability due to pain and skeletal deformity ("dowager's hump").

Colles' fractures of the distal radius are the most common fractures occurring in white women under age 75 years. One study estimated[5] that a 50-year-old white woman has a 15% lifetime risk of a distal radial fracture. These fractures are associated with short-term pain and disability and seldom require hospitalization or extensive rehabilitation.

Hip fractures primarily afflict adults over age 75 years and occur in 32% of women and 17% of men by age 90.[6] The total number of hip fractures has been increasing with the growth in the elderly population, but age-adjusted incidence rates do not appear to be increasing in the United States,[7] although they are clearly on the rise in Europe.[8] Hip fracture affects twice as many women as men, and the rate in women quadruples with every decade past age 50 years. One study estimated that a white woman with an average life expectancy of 80 years has a 15% risk of a hip fracture during her lifetime. By age 80 years, a white woman has a 1% to 2% annual risk of hip fracture. These fractures are associated with severe consequences, including hospitalization, surgery, and a mortality rate 15% to 20% higher than that of age-and sex-matched controls in the first 4 months after fracture.[3] Whether this increased mortality is due to the hip fracture per se or to the fact that persons with greater illness and disability are more likely to sustain a hip fracture is unclear from available data. More than 25% of the survivors of hip fracture are discharged to nursing homes, and approximately 35% never resume independent walking. Predictors of nursing home placement and poor functional capacity after a hip fracture include preexisting cognitive or functional impairments and comorbidities.[3]

Age, Gender, and Racial Dimorphism

The primary demographic factors associated with osteoporosis are increasing age, female sex, and white race. Riggs and Melton have reported two major classes of osteoporosis, distinguished by age at onset.[9] Type 1 (or postmenopausal) osteoporosis is seen primarily in women (6:1 female-male ratio) in the peri- and immediate postmenopausal period and results in trabecular bone loss leading to increased vulnerability to vertebral crush fractures. The proposed etiology involves a primary loss of estrogen with subsequent decreased synthesis of 1,25-dihydroxyvitamin D, diminished gastrointestinal calcium absorption, and secondary hyperparathyroidism. In contrast, type II (or senile) osteoporosis is seen in both women and men (2:1 female to male ratio) usually over age 75, and is characterized by both cortical and trabecular bone loss leading to hip and vertebral fractures. Bone mineral density and bone loss rate measurements in type II fracture patients are not distinguishable from those observed in healthy age-matched controls. The mechanism is a postulated primary defect in renal 1α-hydroxylation of 25-hydroxyvitamin D with subsequent decrease in gastrointestinal calcium absorption and secondary hyperparathyroidism (Table 15.1). Thus age-related bone loss appears to encompass at least two distinct syndromes, affecting men and women differently. The clear gender difference in

Table 15.1. Characteristics of type I and type II osteoporosis

Characteristic	Type I	Type II
Age, y	50–65	75
Female-male ratio	6:1	2:1
Skeletal compartment lost	Trabecular	Trabecular and cortical
Site of fracture	Spine and wrist	Spine and hip
Primary cause	Estrogen deficiency	1,25-dihydroxy-vitamin D deficiency
Parathyroid hormone levels	Decreased	Increased
Calcium absorption	Decreased	Decreased
Abnormal vitamin D synthesis	Secondary	Primary

osteoporosis risk, most marked in the postmenopausal decade, has been attributed to both lower peak bone mass at skeletal maturity and more rapid bone loss (associated with menopause) in women than in men. Many investigators have reported higher bone mass and lower fracture rate in blacks (and recently in Hispanics), but the reasons for these racial differences in risk are unclear.[3] Possibilities include racial differences in attainment of higher peak bone mass, slower rates of bone loss, or other factors such as body habitus, activity, and diet. Comparison studies of multiple racial groups are needed to clarify the influence of heritable factors on osteoporosis risk.

Pathogenesis

Primary osteoporosis of unclear etiology is the cause of metabolic bone disease in the majority of individuals afflicted. Only 5% of cases are secondary to drugs or to other disease processes, including gastrointestinal disorders, nutritional deficiencies, neoplasms, and various endocrinopathies (Table 15.2). As noted above, the fundamental abnormality in all types of osteoporosis is a disturbance in bone remodeling leading to net bone loss, usually excess resorption, although a primary decrease in bone formation may also occur. Many hormonal agents affect bone remodeling but the most critical in the pathogenesis of osteoporosis in women is estrogen deficiency. Recent research has discovered estrogen receptors on bone osteoblasts.[10,11] Other indirect skeletal effects of estrogen deficiency include increased osteoclast responsiveness to the resorptive effects of parathyroid hormone and decreased renal synthesis of 1,25-dihydroxyvitamin D. However, not all postmenopausal women develop osteoporosis; therefore, other pathogenetic factors must play an important part.

Table 15.2. Secondary causes of osteoporosis

Immobilization
Nutritional deficiency
Lactase deficiency
Alcoholism
Chronic illness
   Rheumatoid arthritis
   Renal failure
   Chronic lung disease
Neoplasia
   Multiple myeloma
   Lymphoma
   Leukemia
   Metastatic disease
Endocrinopathy
   Hyperparathyroidism
   Hypercortisolism
   Hyperthyroidism
   Hypogonadism
   Diabetes mellitus
Gastrointestinal disease
   Malabsorption
   Gastrectomy
   Small-bowel resection
   Hepatic failure
Drugs
   Glucocorticoids
   Thyroid hormone
   Heparin
   Methotrexate
   Aluminum-containing antacids
   Diuretics (furosemide)
   Vitamin A excess
   Vitamin D excess
   Anticonvulsants

Aging is associated with a number of disorders of vitamin D metabolism, including decreased conversion of 25-hydroxyvitamin D to the active metabolite and decreases in basal and stimulated 1,25-dihydroxyvitamin D_3 levels. The efficiency of intestinal calcium absorption diminishes with age, more so in osteoporotic persons. Dietary intake of calcium also decreases with age, further exacerbating this calcium-deficient state. However, the contribution of vitamin D deficiency to bone loss remains unclear, and therapeutic trials have not defined a clear role for replacement vitamin D in the treatment of osteoporosis.

Other hormonal parameters (such as calcitonin availability and response, parathyroid hormone status, and end-organ sensitivity) also may have a pathogenetic role in osteoporosis. The observed associations of age, gender, and race to risk of osteoporotic fracture are due to their influence on more proximate variables (such as gonadal hormone levels and calcium and vitamin D status) affecting maximal bone mass and subsequent bone loss. Multiple etiologic factors are likely involved in the pathogenesis of osteoporosis.

Risk Factors

While the presence of risk factors associated with osteoporosis is of clinical utility in the detection of individuals at risk, clear public health evidence of etiologic risk factors is lacking. The proportion of all fractures actually attributable to a known risk factor is small, in part owing to the difficulty of assessing the impact of increments in relative risk without careful study of extremely large numbers of subjects.[12] It is clear that age, female sex, white race, estrogen deficiency, and low body weight are risk factors for the development of osteoporosis. Cigarette smoking is the most common potential risk behavior associated with osteoporotic fractures, and this habit has become substantially more widespread among women during this century. Since cigarette smoking is estimated to increase the relative risk of hip fracture by 1.5 to 2.0,[13] the incidence of hip fracture may increase by as much as 15% over the next several decades. Low calcium intake (below the recommended daily allowance of 800 mg) has been observed in about 75% of American women.[14] Even if the increased relative risk of hip fracture due to this factor were small, the very large numbers of women affected could ultimately lead to a high percentage of fractures due to low calcium intake.[12] Other risk factors associated with osteoporotic fracture are listed in Table 15.3.

Table 15.3. Risk factors associated with osteoporotic fracture

Age
Female sex
White race
Gonadal hormone deficiency
Early natural or surgical menopause
Heredity
Inactivity
Smoking
Low body weight
Rheumatoid arthritis
Falls
Psychotropic drugs
Previous hip fracture
Inadequate calcium intake
Lactose intolerance
Alcoholism
Excessive intake of protein
Excessive intake of coffee
Scoliosis

Clinical Presentation

Vertebral fractures often are asymptomatic and detected on routine chest radiographs. The most common sites for fractures are the lower thoracic and upper lumbar spine. Fractures occuring in the cervical and upper thoracic (above T-6) vertebrae should suggest a secondary or pathologic cause (such as a tumor or infection). An acute vertebral compression fracture may present with sudden onset of pain at the site of the fracture and associated radiation of pain laterally, paravertebral muscle spasm, and constipation and/or urinary retention. Bed rest and use of a brace may be helpful but should be minimized because of the potential for worsening bone loss due to disuse. Analgesics and muscle relaxants are often needed until the acute pain syndrome resolves. The pain usually resolves within several months; persistence of pain beyond 6 months mandates reevaluation for pathologic causes of fracture or other sources of pain. Vertebral fractures may occur in clusters of five or six over short periods. In elderly persons special attention must be paid to prevention of constipation, urinary retention, falls, and confusion as a consequence of the fracture and its treatment. In the absence of radiographic evidence of fracture or bone scan evidence of microfracture, back pain should not be attributed to osteoporosis. Sufficient numbers of wedge or crush fractures may lead to height loss, kyphosis, and dowager's hump with—in some but not all patients—attendant back pain and impaired functional capacity. Associated abdominal distention, discomfort, and pulmonary restriction may also occur in severe cases of thoracic kyphosis.

Distal radial fractures usually occur in middle-aged women who attempt to break a fall with outstretched arms and hands ("parachute reflex"). Presentation with pain and deformity usually is straightforward, as are treatment and the healing phase. Rehabilitation exercises of the hand and forearm may be necessary.

Hip fractures are associated with substantial morbidity and mortality and occur primarily in persons over age 75 years. They are almost always associated with a fall, but whether the fracture precedes or follows the fall is not always clear. Occasionally a patient with an impacted hip fracture retains the ability to walk, but most persons with a fractured hip are unable to stand. The involved limb may appear shorter and externally rotated. Prompt surgical stabilization and fixation of the fracture are critical to preventing complications of immobility in elderly persons: altered mental status, pneumonia, fat embolism, venous thrombosis, and pulmonary embolism. Current recommendations for prophylaxis of venous thromboembolism suggest that warfarin anticoagulation should be started preoperatively, with maintenance of the prothrombin time at less than 1.5 times the control level. Other alternatives include intravenous dextran, adjusted-dose subcutaneous heparin, or intravenous dextran with intermittent pneumatic compression.[15] Displaced femoral head and neck fractures within the joint capsule (intracapsular fractures) may be complicated by aseptic necrosis and poor healing due to fracture-related disruption of the blood supply. Intertrochanteric (extracapsular) fractures usually are unstable and may be associated in elderly patients with substantial blood loss and hemodynamic compromise. Depending on the type of fracture, the surgical approach may require internal fixation with nail and plate, placement of a prosthetic femoral head and neck, or total hip replacement. Active rehabilitation with physical therapy and gait training is required. Patients incapable of walking prior to a hip fracture may be considered for surgery if necessary to prevent bleeding, fat embolism, or flexion contractures.

Diagnosis

Primary osteoporosis accounts for 95% of nontraumatic fractures in postmenopausal women and 60% of those in older men. In contrast, premenopausal women and middle-aged or younger men rarely suffer fractures due to primary osteoporosis, and secondary or pathologic causes of fracture are likely in younger persons. It follows that the diagnostic evaluation must be appropriate to the age and sex of the individual in question. Osteoporosis is asymptomatic until the late stages when a fracture occurs; therefore, early detection is critical to prevention. Once a fracture has occurred, however, other causes of metabolic bone disease (such as malignancy, osteomalacia, and other secondary osteoporoses [Table 15.2]) must be excluded, a process usually requiring a thorough history, physical examination, and selected laboratory studies.

Because of the uncertain value of individual risk factors in predicting the likelihood of osteoporotic fracture, there is increasing interest in bone mass measurements as a means of determining fracture risk. An ideal technique would be highly accurate and reproducible (to permit reliable assessment of bone loss rates) and sufficiently specific to distinguish normal from at-risk individuals. Such a technique does not exist, and decisions to use densitometry for diagnostic purposes must take into account the limitations of currently available methods. Potential uses for bone densitometry include screening of asymptomatic persons to assess their risk of future fracture, diagnostic density measurements in persons with known risk factors for osteopenia, and repeated measurements to detect changes in bone mass over time in response to disease or treatments.[16]

Screening

The criteria for utility of a screening test require that (1) the disorder cause sufficient morbidity, mortality, and cost to warrant screening; (2) the screening test is safe and affordable; (3) treatment in an asymptomatic phase would reduce fractures; (4) screening would affect a patient's decision to accept treatment; and (5) the screening test can accurately predict the risk of fracture.[17] It is clear that osteoporosis (particularly hip fracture) causes substantial mortality, morbidity, and cost. Densitometry has been generally acceptable to patients, involves relatively low radiation doses, and costs from $50 to $400, depending on the method used. Menopausal estrogen replacement therapy has been shown to decrease risk of hip and vertebral fractures by 50%,[18] and many patients would be substantially influenced in their decision to take estrogen by a low bone mass measurement. The major issue affecting bone mass measurement as a screening tool is its uncertain accuracy in predicting fracture risk. Substantial overlap in bone mineral content has been observed between patients with fractures and age-matched controls, making accurate prediction of fracture risk difficult. This problem is encountered with all currently available techniques and suggests not only that technical error is occurring but also that fractures are probably a result of many factors, and not just low bone mineral content. For example, several studies have shown that women with hip fractures have hip bone densities in the normal range for age.[19] In contrast, women with vertebral fractures tend to have lower vertebral bone densities than age-matched controls, suggesting that a lower vertebral bone mass may be predictive of vertebral fracture risk.[20] However, at present, prospective data adequate to determine the capability of bone mass measures in predicting hip and spine fractures are not available, suggesting that mass screening of asymptomatic women is not appropriate.[21]

Patients with known risk factors for osteopenia may benefit from bone mass measurements if the results of the test will influence a treatment decision. A white or Asian postmenopausal woman with or without additional risk factors (see Table 15.3), may wish to receive preventive estrogen replacement therapy if there are no contraindications to this mode of therapy. If, however, uncertainty exists regarding such treatment, a bone mass measurement may be of great value in helping patient and physician balance the risks and benefits of estrogen replacement. Similarly, a low bone mass value in a patient receiving corticosteroids or anticonvulsants may prompt efforts to decrease or discontinue these drugs or to initiate specific treatments. Clearly, patients with multiple risk factors who are hesitant to begin recommended treatment may benefit from the additional information provided by a bone density measurement.[16]

Serial Measurements to Assess Bone Loss Rates:

Serial densitometry is helpful in determining the need for treatment in patients who have a normal baseline bone mass but are at risk for rapid loss (for example, during the immediate postmenopausal period or during corticosteroid therapy). Similarly, in persons undergoing treatment with variable (sodium fluoride) or dose-related (calcitonin) efficacy, information on bone mass changes over time may help in assessing the effectiveness of therapy. The measurement of rates of change in bone mass is dependent on the actual in vivo change in bone density, the reproducibility of the densitometric technique used, and the number of measurements taken. Presently available methods are not sufficiently precise for measurement of bone mass changes unless multiple measurements are taken (increasing cost) or expected changes in bone mass are very large. The precision of currently available techniques is not sufficient to permit actual determination of bone loss rates with a reasonable number of measurements.[17,21] Precision is a measure of the degree of variation in a result on repeated measures, defined as 100 (SD repeated measures/mean of repeated measures). The short-term precision of commonly used densitometric techniques varies from 1% to 5% even in research settings with stringent quality control requirements. Long-term precision and precision in nonresearch settings is worse. Since bone loss rates in humans generally do not exceed 1% per year, except during the immediate postmenopausal years or in pathologic states, the potential for error in bone loss rate assessment in individuals is obvious. Increasing the number of measurements will improve the accuracy of the estimate but at the expense of increased cost to the patient and lost treatment time.[17,21]

When patients undergo treatments expected to produce large (>10%) losses or gains of bone mineral (substantially in excess of the precision limits of the technique), serial measurements may help identify nonresponders or patients requiring a change in therapy. Serial measurements are not useful in assessing bone mass response to preventive measures such as estrogen replacement or calcium supplements, since expected rates of change are small by comparison with the precision variability of the technique. There are no prospective data supporting the ability of serial measures of bone loss rates to predict fracture risk.

Single-Photon Absorptiometry:

Photon absorptiometry uses a beam of photons passing through the bone region of interest; the amount of beam passing through the bone and detected by the scintillation counter is inversely proportional to the bone mass. This technique measures the sum of cortical and trabecular bone at the middle (95% cortical), distal (75% cortical), or ultradistal (where radius and ulna are 5 mm apart)—(75% trabecular) radius, with a precision of approximately 2%.[22] Radiation exposure is low (2 to 5 mrem), the cost is low (around $50), and patient acceptability is high. A major drawback of this technique is its poor correlation with bone mass measurements at predominately trabecular spinal sites of clinical interest. Second, while the relatively good precision of single-photon absorptiometry compared with other techniques suggest its utility for serial measurements, the slow turnover of cortical as compared with trabecular bone in most metabolic bone disorders limits its application. However, in disorders with preferential cortical bone loss, such as primary hyperparathyroidism,[23] the single-photon technique is probably superior, both for baseline measures as well as for assessment of bone loss rates. Finally, a substantial overlap in bone mass has been observed between patients with known vertebral fracture and age-matched controls, greatly limiting the utility of single-photon absorptiometry in diagnosing spinal osteopenia.[24,25]

In summary, low bone density as shown by single-photon absorptiometry is a reliable and specific indicator of severe generalized skeletal osteopenia. However, the converse is not true: a normal single-photon value may be seen in patients with spinal osteopenia and multiple vertebral fractures (poor sensitivity).

Dual-Photon Absorptiometry

Dual-photon absorptiometry is used to measure bone mass of the lumbar spine, hip, and whole skeleton. The dual (two-energy) photon beam permits computer adjustment for soft-tissue variations surrounding the bone region of interest. Bone mineral content is calculated by measuring the photon beam reaching the scintillation counter, and, as in single-photon absorptiometry, represents the sum of cortical and trabecular bone in the spine. The radiation dose is low (15 to 30 mrem), the cost is moderate (around $250), and patient acceptibility is high. Precision in vivo ranges from 2% to 4% in research centers.[24,25] The overlap between values for patients with osteoporotic fracture and values for age-matched controls is less than that observed with single-photon absorptiometry, which may permit improved prediction of vertebral fracture risk. By contrast, hip bone mass as measured by dual-photon absorptiometry does not appear to differ between patients with hip fracture and age-matched controls in most studies; thus, the technique has not yet proved useful in the prediction of hip fracture risk.

Drawbacks to the dual-photon method include its inability to distinguish betwen nonbone calcium—such as degenerative calcific changes or vascular calcifications—and bone calcium, yielding falsely high values in elderly patients with athersclerosis or osteophytic degenerative joint disease. Similarly, lumbar vertebral compression fractures also can give artifactually high readings. These risks of artifact mandate predensitometry spine films in elderly patients (with concomitant increase in radiation exposure and cost). In the presence of severe degenerative joint disease, vascular calcification, or lumbar compression fractures, dual-photon absorptiometry of the spine is probably useless.

The primary virtues of dual-photon absorptiometry are its comparatively good separation of patients with vertebral fracture from age-matched controls and its ability to measure a skeletal site of largely trabecular bone with high vulnerability to fracture. Again, a low value is a reliable indicator of spinal osteopenia, but a normal value may be seen in a patient with vertebral fractures. The reproducibility of the technique is too poor to permit accurate assessment of bone loss rates without a prohibitively high number of measurements, and technical difficulties limit application to the elderly population.

Quantitative Computed Tomography (CT)

Because of the wide availability of CT scanners, vertebral bone densitometry performed with quantitative CT is an attractive alternative to dual-photon absorptiometry. The technique is the only available method that is able to separately quantitate cortical and trabecular bone, potentially demonstrating signs of bone loss occurring earliest in the trabecular skeletal compartment. Short-term precision in vivo ranges from 1.5% to 5% in research settings,[26] limiting its applicability to serial determinations of bone loss rates. The radiation dose per scan is substantial (300 mrem), the cost is high (around $350), and patient acceptability is accordingly limited. The overlap between bone mass values for patients with fracture and those for matched normals is less than that observed with dual-photon absorptiometry and may permit better prediction of the future risk of vertebral fracture. Technical problems similar to those affecting dual-photon absorptiometry (vascular calcifications, degenerative changes, crush fractures) also affect the accuracy of quantitative CT in elderly patients.

The virtues of vertebral quantitative CT densiometry are its wide availability, its ability to separately quantitate trabecular and cortical bone compartments, and its superior separation of osteoporotic patients from controls. Its poor precision, high radiation dose, and cost greatly limit its utility for serial measurements.

Prevention and Treatment

Currently available studies of modalities for the prevention and treatment of osteoporosis are limited by not being blinded, randomized, and controlled; by follow-up periods too short to detect the long-term impact on fractures, side effects, and toxicities; and by an almost complete lack of data on effective treatments for elderly persons.

Three modalities (calcium, exercise, and estrogen) have received the greatest attention in the prevention of menopause- and age-related bone loss. Calcitonin, sodium fluoride, and other treatment strategies are usually reserved for therapy of established disease.

Calcium

The utility of dietary calcium in preventing bone loss is controversial. A Yugoslavian study[27] demonstrated higher bone mass and a lower hip fracture rate in women from a region of high dietary calcium intake as compared with women from a region of low dietary calcium intake. The effect of calcium was postulated to be on maximizing peak bone mass, as no differences in bone loss rates were observed between the two groups. Therapeutic intervention studies have revealed reductions in cortical but not in trabecular bone loss in postmenopausal women given calcium supplements. No studies of calcium supplementation have demonstrated a reduction in fracture incidence. These conflicts in the data may be related to skeletal compartment-specific effects of calcium, differing measurement techniques, failure to account for lifelong differences in calcium intake, age and menopause status differences in the populations studied, and insufficient length of follow-up.[28] All studies comparing calcium supplementation with estrogen replacement therapy have demonstrated the superior efficacy of estrogen in preventing bone loss. One Danish study found no change or continued loss of bone mineral in 70-year-old women randomized to calcium supplementation alone.[29]

It is, however, clear from animal models that calcium deficiency can lead to osteoporosis and it is well known that North American women have an average daily dietary calcium intake well below the recommended daily allowance of 800 mg. To whatever extent a component of calcium deficiency is contributing to increased bone loss, it is reasonable and safe to supplement in order to prevent this added risk. A National Institutes of Health Consensus Development Conference (April 1984) on osteoporosis recommended (based on data of Heaney et al[30]) a daily intake of 1 g of elemental calcium in premenopausal women and 1.5 g in postmenopausal women, from nutritional and/or supplemental sources. Patients must be informed that calcium supplementation alone is not sufficient to prevent either menopausal or age-related bone loss. Risks of calcium supplementation are minimal, but persons with a personal or family history of kidney stones must be screened with 24-hour urinary calcium measurement, and many older patients suffer from constipation and/or rebound gastric hyperacidity when taking calcium carbonate supplements (40% elemental calcium). Calcium citrate (21% elemental calcium) is not associated with these gastrointestinal side effects and may be better tolerated in elderly patients, particularly those with evidence of achlorhydria.

Exercise

It is evident from multiple studies that immobility and disuse (bed rest, weightlessness, casted limbs, paralysis) may lead to accelerated bone loss and osteoporosis. Similarly, in vitro and in vivo evidence is accumulating to suggest that increased demands on the muscles of the skeleton lead to bone remodeling and positive increments in new bone formation. Correlations have been shown between muscle mass and bone density, athletes have higher bone mass in skeletal regions of greatest exertion, and several prospective controlled studies in menopausal women have demonstrated increases in bone mass, total body calcium, and improved calcium balance in the exercising group.[31]

However, it is also clear that exercise is less critical than gonadal hormone sufficiency in the prevention of bone loss, as excess weight loss in premenopausal female marathoners leads to amenorrhea, bone loss, and fractures.[32] In addition, compliance with exercise recommendations (usually at least 45 minutes three times per week) is difficult to achieve in clinical practice, and there is some evidence that exercise-induced gains in bone mass are lost within months after the regimen is discontinued.[31] Clear age-appropriate guidelines for exercise prescription are needed; in their absence, reasonable recommendations include walking, jogging, aerobic exercise, or racquet sports on a regular basis with gradual increases in exertion until a schedule of 45 minutes of exercise three times a week can be maintained. Elderly patients may require stress testing before initiation of a new exercise program.

Estrogen

The critical role of estrogen status on the development of postmenopausal osteoporosis has been demonstrated by numerous studies documenting (1) accelerated bone loss as ovarian function ceases,[33] (2) inhibition of bone loss with initiation of estrogen replacement therapy,[18,34] and (3) resumption of bone loss when estrogen replacement is terminated.[35] The mechanism of estrogen's effect in preventing bone loss probably lies in the recent identification of estrogen receptors in bone osteoblasts.[10,11] Other theories advanced to account for the effect of estrogen deficiency on bone include increased sensitivity to the resorptive effects of parathyroid hormone, decreased renal synthesis of 1,25-dihydroxyvitamin D, subsequent decreases in gastrointestinal calcium absorption, increased urinary calcium losses, and inhibition of (or decreased sensitivity to) calcitonin secretion. Clinical studies have documented rapid bone loss and fractures in young amenorrheic women with anorexia nervosa or excess weight loss due to physical activity.[32,36] Both prospective trials and case control studies have shown prevention of bone loss and reduction in fracture risk with estrogen replacement therapy. When treatment is begun early in menopause (in the first 5 years) and continued for at least 5 years, the incidence of hip fracture is reduced by 50%,[37-40] and significant reductions in distal radial and vertebral fracture have also been observed.

Several studies have concluded that the minimum effective daily dose of oral conjugated estrogens is 0.625 mg or its equivalent. The recent availability of transdermal estrogen formulations (which avoid the first-pass effect of oral estrogens on hepatic protein synthesis) may prove useful in patients with hepatic disease, coagulopathies, renin-dependent hypertension, or congestive heart failure. It is not clear that the transdermal formulation reduces the bile lithogenicity observed with oral estrogens. The minimum transdermal estrogen dose necessary to inhibit bone loss has not yet been determined.

Other benefits of estrogen replacement therapy besides inhibition of bone loss and reduction in fracture risk include prevention of vasomotor flushes and night sweats and relief of symptoms of vaginal atrophy, including dysuria, dyspareunia, bladder infections, and incontinence. Estrogen replacement therapy has been associated in several prospective and case-control studies with a reduction in cardiovascular morbidity and mortality and overall mortality, and with an increase in the high-density lipoprotein cholesterol fraction.[41,42] A notable exception to these investigations, the Framingham study, revealed no morbidity or mortality benefit from estrogen replacement and instead found a higher risk of stroke and heart disease in estrogen-treated cigarette smokers.[43] Until further-longitudinal studies resolve these conflicts in the data, estrogens should not be prescribed for the purpose of reducing cardiovascular disease, and caution should be exercised when considering estrogen replacement in smokers. The long-term effects of estrogen and progestin use on lipid status are unknown, prohibiting definite treatment recommendations and mandating prospective randomized studies to clarify the ultimate effect of menopausal hormone replacement on overall morbidity and mortality (see Chapter 22).

Side effects of estrogen replacement include an increased risk of endometrial hyperplasia and carcinoma in patients treated with unopposed postmenopausal estrogen,[44] although some authors believe that the studies that found such effects suffered from methodologic problems of ascertainment bias,[45] leading to a false inflation of risk. Other studies have shown no increase in mortality in women with estrogen-related endometrial cancer.[46] The 5-year survival rate for patients with endometrial cancer is 70%, with a low annual incidence in the general population of 0.1%, and the annual risk of estrogen-associated endometrial hyperplasia is 0.5%. Cycling with oral medroxyprogesterone (a commonly recommended cycling regimen includes 0.625 mg/d of oral conjugated estrogen on days 1 to 25, 10 mg/d of medroxyprogesterone acetate on days 12 to 25, and nothing on days 26 to 31) leads to monthly shedding of the endometrium and appears to reduce the risk of endometrial cancer to, or below, baseline levels.[47] Of some concern is the adverse effect of progestational agents on high-density lipoprotein cholesterol concentrations, but until the long-term effects of sex hormones on blood lipids is better understood, routine cycling is recommended. More than 90% of women under age 60 years and 60% of women over 65 years will have monthly withdrawal bleeding when cycled with estrogen and progesterone, a side effect of considerable concern, particularly among elderly women.[48] If midcycle bleeding occurs in an estrogen-treated patient, an endometrial biopsy to rule out carcinoma must be undertaken. The utility of routine pretreatment endometrial biopsy and regular biopsies during cycled treatment with estrogen and progesterone is unknown, but such biopsies may be a reasonable precaution, particularly in women at high risk of endometrial carcinoma (history of infertility or obesity). Patients within 10 years of menopause who do not undergo monthly withdrawal bleeding during estrogen cycling should be considered for biopsy, as a higher dose of the progestational agent may be required to prevent endometrial hyperplasia.

Widespread concern regarding the risk of breast cancer from menopausal estrogen replacement is not corroborated by available evidence. Several prospective and case-control studies have shown no increased risk,[49,50] while subgroup analysis in a few studies have shown a small increment in relative risk in women with benign breast disease or with very long durations of therapy.[51,52] Methodologic problems of research design compromise the validity of many of these studies,[50] but the preponderance of the evidence is against any significant increased risk of breast cancer in estrogen-treated patients. Nonetheless, a previous history of breast cancer is an absolute contraindication, and a positive family history in a first degree relative is a relative contraindication, to the use of estrogen replacement therapy.

Other side-effects of estrogen replacement therapy include breast tenderness, increased risk of cholelithiasis, and (uncommonly) worsening of hypertension or congestive heart failure. Contraindications to the use of menopausal hormone replacement are listed in Table 15.4. Patients requiring close monitoring during estrogen replacement include those with seizure disorders, congestive heart failure, high blood pressure, uterine fibroids, migraine headache, endometriosis, and cholelithiasis.

Optimally, hormone therapy for purposes of preventing bone loss should be begun soon after menopause as possible in order to inhibit the accelerated loss

Table 15.4. Contraindications to postmenopausal estrogen replacement therapy

Absolute contraindications:
  History of breast cancer
  Recurrent or recent vascular
    thrombosis or embolism
  Unexplained vaginal bleeding
  Acute liver disease
Relative contraindications:
  Positive family history of breast
    cancer (in patient's mother,
    sister, maternal aunt, or
    daughter)
  Poorly controlled hypertension
  Congestive heart failure
  History of coagulopathy, venous
    thrombosis, or pulmonary
    embolism
  Chronic liver disease

occurring in the first 4 to 6 years after cessation of ovarian function. When estrogens are given during this phase of rapid bone resorption and remodeling, some patients may actually gain new bone mass, as bone formation can transiently exceed bone resorption.[18] Thereafter, bone mass is stabilized or the rate of loss is slowed until treatment is discontinued, whereupon rapid demineralization once again begins. Thus, while estrogens theoretically should be given indefinitely, every year of use delays the onset of clinically important osteopenia, as demonstrated by the reduced hip fracture incidence seen in elderly women treated in the distant past with several years of hormone replacement.[18,39,40,53] A single study randomizing elderly, previously untreated women to treatment with estrogen versus calcium and/or vitamin D showed highly significant increases in bone mass after 1 year of therapy with estrogen and progestin, suggesting that benefit may be conferred from hormone replacement well beyond the immediate postmenopausal period.[29] While estrogen replacement will prevent further age-related bone loss, there are no prospective studies documenting the efficacy of estrogen replacement in preventing fractures in elderly women, and treatment risks and benefits must be carefully individualized in this age group.

Calcitonin

Calcitonin is a peptide hormone synthesized and secreted from the C cells of the thyroid. Specific calcitonin receptors have been identified in bone osteoclasts and kidney. Calcitonin is a potent inhibitor of osteoclastic bone resorption and leads to decreased tubular reabsorption of calcium and phosphate, increased 1,25-dihydroxyvitamin D synthesis, and augmented intestinal calcium absorption. Calcitonin deficiency has been implicated in the pathogenesis of osteoporosis because of variable reports of lower calcitonin levels (1) with increasing age, (2) in women as compared with men, and (3) in osteoporotic patients as compared with controls. Technical problems of study design and the poor sensitivity and specificity of calcitonin bioassays have compromised these studies, and recent data suggests no significant etiologic role of calcitonin in the development of osteoporosis.[54]

The utility of calcitonin as a therapeutic agent in disease states of accelerated bone resorption has been clearly demonstrated in Paget's disease and hypercalcemia of malignancy. Several prospective controlled trials have documented stabilization of bone mass—with modest short-term increases in some cases—in osteoporotic patients treated for 2 years or less.[55,56] Some investigators have observed an escape phenomenon whereby bone loss resumes after 1 to 2 years of treatment; thus, long-term follow-up is required to clarify the ultimate effect of calcitonin therapy on the magnitude and rate of bone loss as well as on the fracture rate. Analgesic effects of calcitonin (presumably via inhibition of osteoclastic bone resorption and reduction in microfractures) have been documented in multiple studies of patients with vertebral fracture, but these studies failed to use appropriate control groups. The utility of calcitonin as a preventive therapy for osteoporosis is poorly understood, but several preliminary studies have reported stabilization of bone mass in calcitonin-treated subjects as compared with controls.[54]

The major drawbacks to calcitonin therapy include its high cost and the need for parenteral administration; alternate routes of administration (nasal spray and rectal suppositories) are under investigation. Its major side effect is transient mild nausea and vomiting, which may be effectively reduced by bedtime administration of the daily calcitonin injection and/or treatment with low-dose metoclopramide. Other side effects include flushing and local irritation of the injection site. These symptoms usually subside with continued therapy.

In view of the limited duration of follow-up in studies of calcitonin therapy for established osteoporosis, the lack of studies establishing a diminished fracture risk after calcitonin therapy, and inadequate data supporting calcitonin's preventive efficacy, its use probably should be reserved for patients with contraindications or nonresponsiveness to established gonadal hormone regimens.

Sodium Fluoride

Fluoride is the only currently available agent capable of specifically stimulating new bone formation via increased osteoblastic activity. Biopsy specimens of fluoride-treated bone demonstrate increased trabecular volume and thickness and increased osteoid surfaces without significant increases in resorption surfaces. Initially the new bone formed may be poorly mineralized, woven bone which is eventually replaced by a lamellar bone structure.

Epidemiologic studies have shown lower rates of hip fracture and higher bone mass in areas of fluoridated water supply. Prospective and retrospective clinical trials have demonstrated both decreased and unchanged vertebral fracture risk in fluoride-treated osteoporotic patients.[57,58] Similarly, bone mass measurements have shown both increased axial (largely trabecular) bone mineral content and decreased or unchanged appendicular (largely cortical) bone mineral content and total body calcium. This suggests that fluoride therapy may result in preferential axial new

bone formation with associated appendicular mineral loss and a theoretical increased risk of appendicular fracture at sites high in cortical bone, such as the hip.

An increased risk of microfracture, presumably due to intense regional bone remodeling has been observed by several investigators, and may explain the variable observation of increased hip fracture rates in some fluoride-treated patients. It has been proposed that fluoride may either cause microfractures due to intense new bone formation or impair healing of stress microfractures that normally occur in osteoporosis, either of which could increase the risk of major appendicular fractures.[59,60] Consistent with this observation, a common side effect of fluoride therapy is lower-extremity (ankle, knee, and plantar fascial) pain[57,61] probably due to a high rate of bone remodeling and local stress fractures, which may be documented by increased uptake on bone scan. Other side effects of fluoride include a probable increase in fracture rate during the 1st year of therapy and gastrointestinal symptoms such as nausea, vomiting, peptic ulcer, and gastrointestinal bleeding in 20% to 60% of treated patients.[57,62] Both lower-extremity pain and gastrointestinal side effects may reverse spontaneously with dose reduction or discontinuation of treatment.[62] Some investigators have reported worsening of osteoarthritis from fluoride therapy. Osteomalacia may occur with fluoride treatment, resulting in a need for concomitant calcium supplementation with 1,500 mg/d of elemental calcium and adequate vitamin D. Many investigators have observed a substantial subgroup of patients who are unresponsive to fluoride, but factors determining responsiveness have not been clarified and at least 1 year of treatment is required to assess responsiveness.

Fluoride remains an experimental drug and has not yet been approved by the Food and Drug Administration for the treatment of osteoporosis. In view of its substantial side effects, the possible increased risk of appendicular (hip) fracture, and the high proportion of nonresponders, fluoride use should be reserved for severe cases of vertebral fracture syndrome unresponsive to other forms of therapy. It may also have some application in the treatment of corticosteroid-induced osteopenia, but control data in support of this indication are not available. Two randomized double-blind controlled studies of fluoride therapy are nearing completion and should indicate the long-term benefits and risks of this approach to treatment.

Other Treatment Strategies

Thiazides have a known positive effect on calcium balance through the inhibition of urinary calcium excretion. Uncontrolled clinical trials have demonstrated increased bone mass and improved calcium balance in patients treated with thiazides.[63,64] Prospective randomized control studies are necessary to confirm these observations. In view of the possible risks of thiazide therapy (glucose intolerance, adverse effect on lipid status and electrocardiographic findings, hypercalcemia, hypokalemia, hyperuricemia, possible risk of orthostasis and falls, central nervous system side effects),[65,66] routine use of thiazides to prevent or treat osteoporosis cannot currently be recommended.

Diphosphonates have proved antiresorptive efficacy in the treatment of Paget's disease, and preliminary data from uncontrolled studies also suggest utility in the treatment of osteoporosis.[18] Anabolic steroids are also potent antiresorptive agents[67] but androgenic side effects, adverse lipid changes, and hepatotoxicity limit their use to the treatment of severe osteoporosis in men, or severe corticosteroid-induced osteoporosis.

Low doses of the 1-34 amino terminal peptide of human parathyroid hormone have been shown in preliminary uncontrolled studies to increase trabecular bone volume and spinal bone mass by stimulating bone turnover and formation. In combination with the active metabolite of vitamin D (calcitriol,) substantial increases in spinal bone mass have been demonstrated.[68] Calcitriol promotes intestinal calcium absorption and improves calcium balance. While decreased gastrointestinal absorption of calcium and diminished synthesis of 1,25-dihydroxyvitamin D_3 have been observed in elderly persons,[69] no clear evidence of the therapeutic efficacy of calcitriol when used alone in osteoporosis has emerged from multiple clinical trials.[70] The risks (hypercalcemia, hypercalciuria, decreased glomerular filtration rate) and cost of calcitriol therapy, combined with the lack of evidence as to its efficacy, suggest that it should not currently be used in the prevention or treatment of osteoporosis.

Pulse or ADFR therapy (*activate, depress, free, repeat*) is a sequential regimen using simultaneous stimulation of bone remodeling units (with parathyroid hormone, calcitriol, or phosphate) followed by depression of bone resorption (with calcitonin or diphosphonate) to permit a net increment in new bone formation.[71] To date, clinical trials have been limited by a failure to use appropriate control groups, and some investigators believe that more basic science and animal research is needed before additional human studies of the ADFR regimen are attempted.

Phosphates can decrease bone resorption, increase mineralization rate, stimulate osteoblast function, and increase matrix synthesis. With continuous or high dosages phosphates can lead to nephrocalcinosis, hypocalcemia, secondary hyperparathyroidism, and increased bone resorption. The use of phosphate in the treatment of osteoporosis remains experimental.

Treatment of Secondary Osteoporosis

Few studies of therapeutic measures for primary osteoporosis have assessed their utility in treating secondary osteoporosis. Wherever possible, the underlying primary disease process leading to osteopenia should be treated. When this is not possible, routine calcium and low-dose vitamin D supplementation, and in women, estrogen therapy, may be of benefit, though no definitive data support this recommendation. In the commonly encountered corticosteroid-induced osteopenia, reasonable, but unproved preventive measures include minimization of corticosteroid dose, topical instead of oral administration, calcium supplementation, and 25-hydroxyvitamin D (calcifediol) supplements (to maintain serum vitamin D concentrations at the upper limit of normal) to counter the corticosteroid-induced inhibition of calcium absorption.[72,73] If hypercalciuria (due to corticosteroids and/or vitamin D supplements) occurs, hypocalciuric diuretics such as hydrochlorothiazide and/or amiloride may be added (with careful monitoring for hypercalcemia). Treatment of patients with established corticosteroid-induced fractures may require the above measures, or in men, treatment with anabolic steroids. Limited studies with fluoride, calcitonin, and diphosphonates suggest benefit, but control data are lacking and treatment must be carefully individualized.

Osteoporosis in Men

The prevalence of osteoporosis in men is increasing as the population ages. Recent studies suggest a higher prevalence of secondary osteoporosis in men than in women. Specifically, over one third of men presenting with osteoporotic vertebral fractures have a secondary cause (such as exogenous hypercortisolism, hypogonadism, gastrectomy, and hypercalciuria with nephrolithiasis) and a high incidence of cigarette smoking, alcoholism, and low body weight.[74] Clearly, careful evaluation for secondary and potentially remediable causes of osteoporosis is mandatory in male patients.

Treatment of osteoporosis in men has been poorly studied, and control trials are lacking. Replacement of testosterone in hypogonadal patients has lead to increased bone mass, but there is no experimental basis for such therapy in eugonadal osteoporotic men. Routine supplementation with calcium and low-dose vitamin D and weight-bearing exercise are reasonable and safe measures, but their efficacy is not yet supported by controlled studies. Similarly, calcitonin, sodium fluoride, and anabolic steroids may be of use in selected osteoporotic men with fracture who have no treatable secondary cause and have failed to respond to more conservative measures. Prospective control trials are required to establish the efficacy of these therapeutic options.

Osteomalacia

Osteomalacia is a metabolic bone disease characterized by a mineralization defect leading to bone deformity, fracture, and bone pain. Because of routine vitamin D supplementation of dairy and other products in the United States, frank osteomalacia is a relatively rare cause of clinical fracture syndromes (< 5% overall). In view of its amenability to appropriate treatment, however, it is critical that osteomalacia be carefully considered in the differential diagnosis. The most common cause of osteomalacia in the older adult is vitamin D deficiency of various etiologies. Prevalent causes of vitamin D deficiency include nutritional or sunlight deficiencies, hepatic disease with secondary failure of 25-hydroxyvitamin D synthesis, and chronic renal disease with secondary failure of 1,25-dihydroxyvitamin D synthesis. Phosphate-deficient osteomalacia may be caused by excess ingestion of aluminum-containing (phosphate-binding) antacids. Table 15.5 lists causes of osteomalacia to be considered in any evaluation of metabolic bone disease in elderly patients.[75]

Bone histomorphometry in osteomalacia reveals increased osteoid surfaces and width. While vitamin D deficiency is clearly associated with osteomalacia, it appears to be the presence of hypocalcemia or hypophosphatemia per se that leads to abnormal osteoblas-

Table 15.5. Causes of osteomalacia

   I. Vitamin D deficiency
      A. Insufficient intake
         1. Inadequate exposure to sunlight
         2. Decreased gastrointestinal absorption
            a) Nutritional deficit
            b) Malabsorption
            c) Gastrectomy, small intestine resection
            d) Pancreatic insufficiency
         3. Increased skin pigment (?)
      B. Decreased metabolic conversion
         1. Chronic renal disease
         2. Hepatic disease
  II. Phosphate deficiency
      A. Phosphate binders (aluminum-containing antacids)
      B. Hyperphosphaturia
 III. Drugs
      A. Diphosphonates
      B. Sodium fluoride
      C. Cholestyramine
      D. Phenytoin, barbiturates

tic regulation of osteoid maturation. Vitamin D deficiency also may lead to secondary hyperparathyroidism and osteoporosis. Elderly persons are at particular risk of vitamin D deficiency because of diminished exposure to sunlight, diminished dermal conversion of 7-dihydrocholesterol plus ultraviolet light to vitamin D_3, diminished dietary intake of foods containing vitamin D_2, and diminished gastrointestinal absorption of dietary vitamin D_2.[76]

Clinical and Laboratory Presentation

The clinical presentation of advanced osteomalacia typically includes diffuse bone tenderness, weakness, fatigue, and depression.[75] Skeletal pain is largely due to microfractures that may not be visible on plain radiographs and are evident as areas of increased uptake on bone scan. Vertebral compression and long-bone fractures also may occur. Laboratory abnormalities include hypocalcemia, hypophosphatemia, increased alkaline phosphatase levels, secondary increases in parathyroid hormone levels, and hypocalciuria. In vitamin D–deficient states, serum concentrations of vitamin D metabolites are usually diminished. In later stages, bone densitometry may reveal low bone mineral content, but this is of no use in distinguishing osteomalacia from other causes of osteopenia, and in mild osteomalacia, bone density may remain normal owing to the relative preservation of cortical bone. In more advanced cases of osteomalacia, bone scans reveal generalized increased skeletal uptake due to microfractures and increased osteoblastic osteoid formation. In osteoporosis, in the absence of recent fracture, bone scans are normal. Late radiographic changes include pseudofractures (lucent areas surrounded by callus) and bone deformities. Double tetracycline–labeled bone histomorphometry reveals a decreased uptake of the label in the mineralization front, prolonged mineralization lag time, and increased osteoid width and surface. In the absence of the typical clinical and laboratory characteristics of osteomalacia described above, bone biopsy may be necessary to distinguish more clearly between osteoporosis and mild or moderate osteomalacia when osteomalacia is strongly suspected clinically.

Treatment

Vitamin D replacment is the mainstay of treatment in vitamin D–deficient osteomalacia, with a goal of normalized serum and urine calcium concentrations and bone healing.[77] Appropriate vitamin D formulation and doses are listed in Table 15.6. Supplemental calcium (1,000 to 2,000 mg/d of elemental calcium) should also be given. End points to note in follow-up

Table 15.6. Treatment of vitamin D–deficient osteomalacia*

	Elemental calcium (1,000–2,000 mg/d)
Nutritional and sunlight deficiency	PLUS vitamin D (1,000 IU/d)
Hepatic disease	Calcifediol (25-hydroxyvitamin D$_3$) (25–50 μg/d) or vitamin D (5,000 IU/d)
Renal disease	Calcitriol (1,25-dihydroxyvitamin D$_3$) (0.1–0.5 μg/d)

*Frequent monitoring of serum and 24-hour urinary calcium concentrations, creatinine clearance, and serum vitamin D (25-hydroxy- and/or 1,25-dihydroxy-metabolite) concentrations is mandatory during pharmacologic vitamin D replacement.

include clinical resolution of symptoms and normalization of biochemical indexes and radiographic findings. Close monitoring of 24-hour urinary calcium excretion (not to exceed 250 mg/d) and serum calcium levels must be maintained to prevent hypercalcemia, nephrocalcinosis, and nephrolithiasis. Renal function and serum vitamin D concentrations should also be monitored. Evidence of hypercalciuria or hypercalcemia mandates reduction or discontinuation of vitamin D supplements. Because of the risks of toxicity from vitamin D, which is stored in adipose tissue and has a half-life of months, consideration should be given to use of shorter-half-life (and more expensive) forms of vitamin D in deficiencies caused by hepatic or renal disease. Calcifediol (25-hydroxyvitamin D) has a 10-day half life and calcitriol (1,25-dihydroxyvitamin D) has a 1-day half-life, permitting a relatively rapid return of normocalcemia once supplements are discontinued.

Hypophosphatemic osteomalacia requires oral neutral phosphate salt replacement, with monitoring of dosages to avoid diarrhea. In some patients, vitamin D replacement will also be necessary to prevent hypocalcemia as a complication of phosphate replacement.

Primary Hyperparathyroidism

Primary hyperparathyroidism is a metabolic bone disorder secondary to excess secretion of parathyroid hormone from hyperplastic or adenomatous parathyroid glands, and it is manifested early by hypercalcemia. Increased used of multichannel autoanalyzers has lead to greater and earlier detection of asymptomatic hypercalcemia due to hyperparathyroidism. Twenty-five percent to 50% of cases occur between the ages of 60 and 90 years, and the distinction between the myriad manifestations of the disease and other common ailments of old age presents a major clinical challenge.[78]

Skeletal manifestations of primary hyperparathyroidism include osteoporotic fracture, dental problems, arthralgias, and bone pain. Gastrointestinal and renal signs and symptoms include peptic ulcer, pancreatitis, constipation, nausea and vomiting (with severe hypercalcemia), hypercalciuria, nephrolithiasis, and diminished glomerular filtration rate.[79] Hypertension is more prevalent among patients with hyperparathyroidism. Neuromuscular manifestations include muscle weakness, paresthesia, and fatigue. Finally, and of great importance in elderly persons, primary hyperparathyroidism may be manifested by memory loss, delirium, personality changes, or depression.[80] Thus, while as many as 50% of hyperparathyroid patients are reported to be asymptomatic, many manifestations of the disease may have been wrongly attributed to the aging process alone.

Diagnosis

The diagnosis requires the presence of hypercalcemia (which may be intermittent), in association with a confirmatory elevation of parathyroid hormone concentration. Other laboratory findings may include hypophosphatemia, hyperchloremia, hypercalciuria, elevated urinary excretion of cyclic adenosine monophosphate, and elevated serum levels of alkaline phosphatase.[79]

The differential diagnosis of hypercalcemia includes various neoplasms (especially lung, breast, gastrointestinal tract, and kidney neoplasms and multiple myeloma), vitamin D intoxication, hyperthyroidism, sarcoidosis, tuberculosis, and immobilization (especially in active Paget's disease). Thiazide diuretics may cause small elevations in serum calcium levels, which should resolve on discontinuation of the drug. Severely elevated serum calcium concentrations and/or suppressed or normal parathyroid hormone concentrations suggest a diagnosis of neoplasm as opposed to primary hyperparathyroidism, although these diagnoses may coexist. Thorough evaluation to rule out these causes of hypercalcemia must precede a diagnosis of primary hyperparathyroidism.

Treatment

The treatment of hyperparathyroidism remains controversial. For patients whose disease is manifested by substantial hypercalcemia (with serum calcium levels >1 mg/dL over the upper limit of normal values) or who have clear signs and symptoms of disease, appropriate management requires surgical exploration of the neck and removal of the adenomatous or hyperplastic tissue. In asymptomatic patients with milder hypercalcemia, general recommendations include appropriate hydration, exercise, and avoidance of diuretics. Restriction of dietary calcium has not been shown to be of clear benefit and should not be employed unless this measure results in reduced serum and urine calcium levels without concomitant rise in parathyroid hormone concentration. Studies attempting to inhibit parathyroid hormone secretion with β-adrenergic blockers or histamine$_2$ receptor antagonists have yielded inconclusive results.[81]

Patients who refuse or are poor candidates for surgery should be considered for efforts to inhibit the effect of parathyroid hormone on bone. Possible agents for this purpose include oral phosphate (which requires careful monitoring because of risk of ectopic calcification), calcitonin, and diphosphonates. Several recent studies of estrogens in the treatment of postmenopausal women with primary hyperparathyroidism have observed biochemical evidence of diminished bone turnover and decreased serum and urinary calcium without change in parathyroid hormone concentration.[82,83] Estrogen's effects on bone mass, fracture risk, and other manifestations of hyperparathyroidism require long-term controlled studies.

In one 10-year study, 23% of untreated asymptomatic patients required surgery because clinical manifestations of disease developed.[84] Indications for considering surgery in these patients include declining renal function, hypercalciuria, nephrolithiasis, poorly controlled hypertension, a rise in serum calcium levels (> 1 mg/dL above the upper limit of normal values), a rapid decline in bone density, and the appearance of osteoporotic fractures, peptic ulcer disease, or altered mental status. In the absence of these manifestations, continued conservative management and careful observation is a reasonable alternative. A long-term controlled study of surgery versus medical management in asymptomatic patients is necessary to identify definitively the optimal management strategy in this group of patients.

The risk of neck exploration is greatly reduced by the presence of a highly experienced surgeon and pathologist. Postoperative hypocalcemia and tetany occur rarely, primarily in patients with severe bone disease or hyperplastic glands, mandating frequent monitoring and replacement of calcium, magnesium, and vitamin D as needed to restore normocalcemia. Marked improvement in subtle symptoms of fatigue or memory loss may follow surgery.

Paget's Disease of Bone

Paget's disease of bone is a chronic focal disorder of the skeleton that is asymptomatic in the vast majority of affected individuals. It is characterized by an early period of sharply defined areas of bone resorption, followed by rapid formation of disorganized new bone, resulting in histologically abnormal bone, skeletal deformity, and an increased risk of fracture.

Epidemiology

Paget's disease of bone affects 1% to 4% of persons over age 40 years and more than 10% of those over age 80 years. It is common in Northern European (except Scandinavia) and North American temperate regions and rare in tropical and Asian nations. A slight male predominance has been observed, and some familial clusters have been reported, suggesting a genetic (autosomal dominant) susceptibility to the disease.[85]

Pathophysiology

The early pagetic lesion is characterized by a well-defined area of osteolytic bone resorption, resulting from the proliferation of large multinucleated osteoclasts. These abnormal osteoclasts contain typical nuclear and cytoplasmic inclusions in a random or paracrystalline microfilament array, resembling the nucleocapsids of the paramyxovirdae virus and suggestive of a slow viral etiology of the disease. This pathologically increased osteoclastic activity is associated with greatly increased physiologic osteoblast activity, with enlarged osteoblasts lining lacunae within the bone, which result from the osteoclastic resorptive phase. Pagetic bone has a mosaic pattern resulting from simultaneous appearance of disordered and accelerated bone resorption and formation, and replacement of displaced hematopoietic marrow with fibrovascular connective tissue and ''burned out'' lesions (areas in which accelerated osteoclastic and osteoblastic activity have ceased). The etiology of the disease is unknown.[85]

Clinical Characteristics

Paget's disease of bone is typically asymptomatic, requiring treatment in less than 1% of affected patients. It is usually detected because of an incidental elevation of serum alkaline phosphatase levels or an abnormal radiograph of the axial or weight-bearing skeleton. The disease may be mild or severe, localized or in multiple skeletal locations, resulting in a variety of possible clinical presentations. Deformity of skull and clavicle, bowing and fracture of weight-bearing bones, and associated mild to moderate bone pain, are typical signs and symptoms. Severe bone pain in a patient with Paget's disease should suggest coexisting arthritis, acute fracture, neurologic impairment, or sarcomatous degeneration of a bone lesion. Enlargement of skull structures may lead to headache, cranial nerve deficits (vertigo, tinnitus), and hearing loss, and pressure on the base of skull may result in diplopia, incontinence, abnormal gait, slurring of speech, and abnormal swallowing. Involvement of spinal vertebrae with subsequent nerve root entrapment may also be observed.

Neoplastic transformation occurs in less than 1% of patients, is characterized by a rapid increase in alkaline phosphatase levels, severe bone pain, or accelerated deformity, and requires bone biopsy for diagnosis. Other complications include ectopic calcification (of vessels, heart valves, joints, and Bruch's membrane with angioid streaks), high-output congestive heart failure caused by increased blood flow to bone, and hyperuricemia and gout caused by increased cell turnover. Hypercalcemia and hypercalciuria with nephrolithiasis secondary to immobilization after a pathologic fracture or neurologic complication also occur. These symptoms and complications are indications for aggressive therapy.

Diagnosis

Elevation in serum osteoblastic alkaline phosphatase levels is an early herald of the disease, correlates well with the extent of bone involvement, and is a reliable indicator of disease activity and response to therapy. Elevation of urinary hydroxyproline levels is a measure of increased osteoclastic activity and is also a useful indicator of response to therapy. Serum and urinary calcium and phosphorus levels are normal unless immobilization of a patient with active disease occurs, or unless neoplasm supervenes.[85-87]

Radiographs characteristically reveal early well-defined lucent areas (osteoporosis circumscripta) that may be adjacent to areas of dense or mottled sclerosis in later stages of disease. Bowed and thickened irregular long bones with an advancing V-shaped osteolytic front, thickened ileopectineal line, sclerotic vertebral margins, and honeycomb-or cotton wool–like mottling of the skull may also occur. Scintigraphic findings are highly sensitive, but not specific, for Paget's disease and are useful in defining the activity and skeletal distribution of disease.[87]

Differential diagnosis requires consideration of diseases resulting in substantial elevations of serum alkaline phosphatase levels, including metastatic prostate carcinoma, osteogenic sarcoma, and Paget's disease of bone. Osteoporotic fractures and accompanying pain may present some difficulties in the differential diagnosis. However, the postfracture elevation in alkaline phosphatase levels is usually mild and transient and the radiographic characteristics of simple osteopenia are not typical of Paget's disease. The two diseases may occur simultaneously in the elderly persons. Distinguishing osteoarthritis from Paget's disease is also difficult because of the frequent coexistence of these conditions. Appropriate radiographic and laboratory studies will usually clarify the etiology of the pain. Treatment may require both anti-inflammatory agents for the arthritis and specific therapy of Paget's disease.

Treatment

Indications for active treatment of Paget's disease include skeletal pain, bone deformity, neurologic complications (including hearing loss), medical complications (such as high-output congestive heart failure, hypercalcemia, and hypercalciuria), and preparation for orthopedic surgery. Preventive intervention in asymptomatic patients with active disease is of uncertain utility. The efficacy of therapy depends on reducing osteoclast and osteoblast activity, and response is indicated by reduction in pain and other symptoms, reduced alkaline phosphatase and urinary hydroxyproline levels, and improved radiographic findings. Surgical intervention may be required in patients with symptoms of bone pressure on brain or spinal cord, severe hip dysfunction, and long-bone bowing sufficient to precipitate fracture.[87]

Calcitonin

Treatment with calcitonin is followed by a rapid decrease in urinary hydroxyproline and a slower decline in serum alkaline phosphatase levels, healing of bone lesions, and a reduction in symptoms and complications of the disease. Calcitonin is the preferred drug in patients with active osteolytic lesions and in those undergoing preparation for orthopedic surgery. Treatment may be discontinued after 1 year of therapy, and symptoms may not recur for months to years thereafter. Response to calcitonin appears to plateau after roughly a 50% reduction in disease activity, for reasons which are not well understood. More than half of treated patients develop antibodies to salmon calcitonin, which may result in resistance to therapy. Human calcitonin does not appear to cause antibody formation and may be used if responsiveness to salmon calcitonin is lost; however, a similar plateau effect of uncertain cause has also been observed with human calcitonin treatment.[88]

Calcitonin must be administered by subcutaneous or intramuscular injection (a nasal spray form is in investigational use) and is extremely costly. Side effects occur in 10% to 20% of patients and include nausea and vomiting, flushing, polyuria, hypercalciuria, paresthesias, and local irritation of the injection site. Hypersensitivity reactions are rare, but a dilute initial test dose is recommended by the manufacturer. Continuation of a reduced dose usually resolves these problems. Administration of calcitonin at bedtime, in combination with a low dose of metoclopramide if necessary, has been reported to reduce gastrointestinal intolerance in most patients. For dosage and method of administration, see Table 15.7.

Diphosphonates

Diphosphonates are analogues of pyrophosphate, a constituent of bone important to mineralization. They inhibit bone resorption and formation by uncertain mechanisms. Etidronate disodium is the diphosphonate in widest current usage. Clinical effects of etidronate are dose related and include relief of bone pain and complications of disease, as well as reduced levels of urinary hydroxyproline and serum alkaline phosphatase. Unlike calcitonin, etidronate does not heal osteolytic lesions and thus is not a preferred therapy in patients with extensive pagetic osteolysis. Treatment for 6 months is usually sufficient to achieve remission or a biochemical plateau, and symptoms may not recur for variable periods thereafter. A drug-free interval of 6 months is recommended. Recurrent signs and symptoms of disease are indications for another course of therapy. Side effects are seen less often with etidronate than with calcitonin, and include (uncommonly) diarrhea, nausea, and, with high doses, hyperphosphatemia and mineralization defects. High-dose etidronate is more effective in reducing disease activity but may be associated with mineralization defects,

worsening of osteolysis, and pathologic fracture. Thus, high-dose etidronate should be used only if the response to lower doses is poor and should be given for shorter intervals (1 to 3 months). Combination therapy with etidronate and calcitonin has been reported to prevent progression and permit healing of osteolytic areas.[89] Dosages and methods of administration are listed in Table 15.7.

Mithramycin

Mithramycin is a cytotoxic antibiotic that effectively inhibits osteoclast activity and results in suppression of disease activity and relief of pain. Its use is limited by toxicity affecting bone marrow, kidney, and liver. Thus, it is usually avoided unless other regimens have failed.

Other Therapies

Bone pain may be relieved by aspirin and other nonsteroidal anti-inflammatory agents. Surgical intervention for decompression of neurologic deficits, total hip replacement, tibial and fibular osteotomy, or fracture fixation may be complicated by hemorrhage. Presurgical treatment with calcitonin for 3 months to achieve a 50% reduction in biochemical indexes of disease usually is sufficient to prevent major bleeding. Fracture and postoperative healing in Paget's disease generally is excellent.[87]

Table 15.7. Treatment regimens for Paget's disease of bone

Drug	Dosage*
Salmon calcitonin	0.25–0.50 μg (50–100 MRC units) IM or SC at bedtime every other or every day†
Human calcitonin	0.5–1 mg IM or SC at bedtime every other or every day†
Etidronate disodium	5–20 mg/kg body weight, taken orally every day‡
Mithramycin§	10–50 μg/kg body weight/wk IV

*IM indicates intramuscularly; SC, subcutaneously; IV, intravenously.
†Higher daily doses may be required in patients with active or extensive disease. With stabilization, a lower dose administered three times a week is usually sufficient.
‡Higher doses may lead to defective mineralization, osteomalacia, and fracture.
§Use is limited by severe nausea and marrow, renal, and hepatic toxicity.

References

1. Riggs BL, Melton LJ III. Involutional osteoporosis. *N Engl J Med* 1986;314:1676–86.
2. Gallagher JC, Riggs BL, Eisman J, et al. Intestinal calcium absorption and serum vitamin D metabolites in normal subjects and osteoporotic patients: effect of age and dietary calcium. *J Clin Invest* 1979;64:729–734.
3. Cummings SR, Kelsey JL, Nevitt MC, O'Dowd KJ. Epidemiology of osteoporosis and osteoporotic fractures. *Epidemiol Rev* 1985;7:178–208.
4. Jensen GF, Christiansen C, Boesen J, et al. Epidemiology of postmenopausal spinal and long bone fractures: a unifying approach to postmenopausal osteoporosis. *Clin Orthop* 1966;45:31–36.
5. Owen RA, Melton LJ, Johnson KA, et al. Incidence of Colle's fracture in a North American community. *Am J Public Health* 1982;72:604–607.
6. Gallagher JC, Melton LJ, Riggs BL. Epidemiology of fractures of the proximal femur in Rochester, Minnesota. *Clin Orthop* 1980;150:163–171.
7. Melton LJ, Ilstrup M, Riggs B, et al. Fifty year trend in hip fracture incidence. *Clin Orthop* 1982;62:144–149.
8. Wallace W. The increasing incidence of fractures of the proximal femur: an orthopedic epidemic. *Lancet* 1983;2:1413–14.
9. Riggs BL, Melton LJ. Evidence for two distinct syn-

dromes of involutional osteoporosis. *Am J Med* 1983; 75:899–901.

10. Eriksen EF, Colvard DS, Berg NJ, et al. Evidence of estrogen receptors in normal human osteoblast-like cells. *Science* 1988;241:84–86.

11. Komm BS, Terpening CM, Benz DJ, et al. Estrogen binding, receptor mRNA, and biologic response in osteoblast-like osteocarcoma cells. *Science* 1988; 241:81–84.

12. Cummings SR. Epidemiology of osteoporotic fractures: selected topics. In Roche AF, ed. *Osteoporosis: Current Concepts—Report of the 7th Ross Conference on Medical Research.* Columbus, Ohio: Ross Laboratories; 1987:3–8.

13. Williams AR, Weiss NS, Ure Cl, et al. Effect of weight, smoking, and estrogen use on the risk of hip and forearm fractures in post-menopausal women. *Obstet Gynecol* 1982;60:695–699.

14. Heaney RP, Gallagher JC, Johnston CC, et al. Calcium nutrition and bone health in the elderly. *Am J Clin Nutr* 1982;36:986–1013.

15. Hull RD, Raskob GE, Hirsh J. Prophylaxis of venous thrombembolism: an overview. *Chest* 1986(suppl);89: 374S–383S.

16. Riggs BL, Wahner HW. Bone densitometry and clinical decision-making in osteoporosis. *Ann Intern Med* 1988;108:293–295.

17. Cummings SR, Black D. Should perimenopausal women be screened for osteoporosis? *Ann Intern Med* 1986; 104:817–823.

18. Lindsay R. Osteoporosis. *Clin Geriatr Med* 1988;4:411–430.

19. Bohr H, Schaadt O. Bone mineral content of the femoral bone and the lumbar spine measured in women with fracture of the femoral neck by dual photon absorptiometry. *Clin Orthop* 1983;1979:240–245.

20. Pacifici R, Susman N, Carr PL, et al. Single and dual energy tomographic analysis of spinal trabecular bone: a comparative study in normal and osteoporotic women. *J Clin Endocrinol Metab* 1987;64:209–214.

21. Cummings SR. Bone mineral densitometry (position paper, Health and Public Policy Committee, American College of Physicians.) *Ann Intern Med* 1987;107:932–936.

22. Cameron JR, Mazess RB, Sorenson JA. Precision and accuracy of bone mineral determination by direct photon absorptiometry. *Invest Radiol* 1968;3:141–150.

23. Silverberg S, Shane E, delaCruz L, et al. Skeletal disease in primary hyperparathyroidism. *J Bone Miner Res* 1988;3(suppl 1):89. Abstract.

24. Riggs BL, Wahner HW, Dunn WL, et al. Differential changes in bone mineral density of the appendicular and axial skeleton with aging. *J Clin Invest* 1981;67:328–335.

25. Wahner WH, Riggs BL. Methods and application of bone densitometry in clinical diagnosis. *CRC Crit Rev Clin Lab Sci* 1986;24:217–233.

26. Cann CE. Quantitative computed tomography for bone mineral analysis: technical considerations. In: Genant HK, ed. *Osteoporosis Update.* San Francisco, California: Radiology Research and Educational Foundation; 1987:131–144.

27. Matkovic V, Kostial K, Simonovic I, et al. Bone status and fracture rates in two regions of Yugoslavia. *Am J Clin Nutr* 1979;32:540–548.

28. Heaney RP. Calcium, bone health and osteoporosis. *Bone Miner Res* 1986;4:255–301.

29. Finn Jensen G, Christiansen C, Transbol I. Treatment of postmenopausal osteoporosis: a controlled therapeutic trial comparing o estrogen/gestagen, 1,25 dihydroxy vitamin D$_3$ and calcium. *Clin Endocrinol* 1982;16:515–524.

30. Heaney RP, Recker RR, Saville PD. Calcium balance and calcium requirements in middle-aged women. *Am J Cin Nutr* 1977;30:1603–1611.

31. Dalsky GP, Stocke KS, Ehsani AA, et al. Weight bearing exercise training and lumbar bone mineral content in post menopausal women. *Ann Intern Med 1988;108:824–828.*

32. Drinkwater BD, Nilson KC, Chestnut CH. Bone mineral content of amenorrheic and eumenorrheic athletes. *N Engl J Med* 1984;311:277–281.

33. Heaney RP, Recker RR, Saville PD. Menopausal changes in bone remodeling. *J Lab Clin Med* 1978; 92:964–970.

34. Nachtigall LE, Nachtigall RH, Nachtigall RD. Estrogen replacement therapy, I: a 10 year prospective study in the relationship of osteoporosis. *Obstet Gynecol* 1979;53: 277–284.

35. Lindsay R, Hart DM, MacLean A, et al. Bone response to termination of oestrogen treatment. *Lancet* 1978;1: 1325–1327.

36. Marcus R, Cann C, Madvig P, et al. Menstrual function and bone mass in elite women distance runners. *Ann Intern Med* 1985;102:158–163.

37. Ettinger B, Genant HK, Cann CE. Long term estrogen therapy prevents bone loss and fracture. *Ann Intern Med* 1985;102:319–324.

38. Hutchinson TA, Polansky JM, Feinstein AR. Postmenopausal oestrogens protect against fracture of the hip and distal radius. *Lancet* 1979;2:705–709.

39. Kreiger N, Kelsey JL, Holford TR. An epidemiological study of hip fracture in postmenopausal women. *Am J Epidemiol* 1982;116:141–148.

40. Smith DM, Khairi MRA, Johnston CC. The loss of bone mineral with aging and its relationship to risk of fracture. *J Clin Invest* 1975;56:311–318.

41. Bush TL, Barrett-Connor E. Noncontraceptive estrogen use and cardiovascular disease. *Epidemiol Rev* 1985; 7:80–104.

42. Stampfer MJ, Willett WC, Colditz GA. A prospective study of postmenopausal estrogen therapy and coronary heart disease. *N Engl J Med* 1985;313:1044–1049.

43. Wilson PWF, Garrison RJ, Castelli WP. Postmenopausal estrogen use, cigarette smoking, and cardiovascular morbidity in women over 50: the Framingham study. *N Engl J Med* 1985;313:1038–1043.

44. Shapiro S, Kelley JP, Rosenberg L. Risk of localized and widespread endometrial cancer in relation to recent and discontinued use of conjugated estrogens. *N Engl J Med* 1985;313:969–972.

45. Horowitz RI, Feinstein AR. Alternative analytic methods for case control studies of estrogens and endometrial cancer. *N Engl J Med* 1978;299:1088–1094.

46. Chu J, Schweed AI, Weiss NS. Survival among women with endometrial cancer: a comparison of estrogen users and non users. *Am J Obstet Gynecol* 1982;143:569–573.

47. Gambrell RD, Massey FM, Castaneda TA, et al. Reduced incidence of endometrial cancer among postmenopausal women treated with progestogens. *J Am Geriatr Soc* 1979;27:389–394.

48. Gambrell RD. The menopause: benefits and risks of estrogen-progestogen replacement therapy. *Fertil Steril* 1982;37:457–477.

49. Wingo PA, Layde PM, Lee NC, et al. The risk of breast cancer in postmenopausal women who have used estrogen replacement therapy. *JAMA* 1987;257:209–215.

50. Horowitz RI, Feinstein AR. Effect of clinical features on the association of estrogens and breast cancer. *Am J Med* 1984;76:192–198.

51. Hoover R, Glass A, Finkle WG, et al. Conjugated estrogens and breast cancer risk in women. *JNCI* 1981; 67:815–820.

52. Kelsey JL, Fischer DB, Holford TR, et al. Exogenous estrogens and other factors in the epidemiology of breast cancer. *JNCI* 1981;67:327–333.

53. Ettinger B, Genant HK, Cann CE. Long term estrogen therapy prevents bone loss and fracture. *Ann Intern Med* 1985;102:319–324.

54. McDermott MT, Kidd GS. The role of calcitonin in the development and treatment of osteoporosis. *Endocr Rev* 1987;8:377–390.

55. Gruber HE, Ivey JL, Baylink DL, et al. Long term calcitonin therapy in postmenopausal osteoporosis. *Metabolism* 1984;33:295–303.

56. Mazzuoli GF, Passeri M, Gennari C, et al. Effects of salmon calcitonin in postmenopausal osteoporosis: a controlled double-blind clinical study. *Calcif Tissue Int* 1986;38:3–8.

57. Riggs BL, Seeman E, Hodgson SF, et al. Effect of the fluoride/calcium regimen on vertebral fracture occurence in postmenopausal osteoporosis. *N Engl J Med* 1982; 306:446–450.

58. Inkovaana J, Heikinheimo R, Jarvinen K, et al. Prophylactic fluoride treatment and aged bones. *Br Med J* 1975;3:73–74.

59. Einhorn TA, Vigorita VJ. Unique histology of the fracture callus in a sodium fluoride-treated osteoporotic patient with hip fracture. In: Christiansen C, ed. *Osteoporosis 1987*. Copenhagen, Denmark: Osteopress ApS; 1987: 262–265.

60. Gutteridge DH, Price RJ, Nicholson GC, et al. Fluoride in osteoporotic fractures-trabecular increase, vertebral protection, femoral fractures. In: Christiansen C, et al, eds. *Osteoporosis 2*. Copenhagen International Symposium Osteo, June 1984.

61. O'Duffy JD, Wahner HW, O'Fallon WM, et al. Mechanism of acute lower extremity pain syndrome in fluoride-treated osteoporotic patients. *Am J Med* 1986;80:561–566.

62. Baylink DJ, Ivey JL. Sodium fluoride for osteoporosis: some unanswered questions. *JAMA* 1980;245:463–464.

63. Wasnich RD, Benfante RJ, Yano K, et al. Thiazide effect on the mineral content of bone. *N Engl J Med* 1983;309:344–347.

64. Transbol I, Christensen GF, Jensen GF, et al. Thiazide for the postponement of postmenopausal bone loss. *Metabolism* 1982;31:383–386.

65. Christiansen C, Christensen MS, Hagen C, et al. Effects of natural estrogen-gestagen and thiazide on coronary risk factors in normal postmenopausal women. *Acta Obstet Gynecol Scand* 1981;60:407–412.

66. Multiple Risk Factor Intervention Trial Research Group. Multiple risk factor intervention trial: risk factor changes and mortality results. *JAMA* 1982;248:1465–1477.

67. Chestnut CH, Ivey JL, Gruber HE, et al. Stanozolol in postmenopausal osteoporosis: therapeutic efficacy and possible mechanisms of action. *Metabolism* 1983;32:571–580.

68. Slovik DM, Rosenthal D, Doppelt SH, et al. Restoration of spinal bone in osteoporotic men by treatment with human parathyroid hormone (1–34) and 1,25 dihydroxyvitamin D. *Bone Miner Res* 1986;1:377–381.

69. Slovik DM, Adams JS, Neer RM, et al. Deficient production of 1,25 dihydroxyvitamin D in elderly osteoporotic patients. *N Engl J Med* 1981;305:372–374.

70. Jensen GF, Meinecke B, Boesen J, et al. Does $1,25(OH)_2D_3$ accelerate spinal bone loss? *Clin Orthop* 1985;192:215–221.

71. Frost HM. 'Coherence' treatment of osteoporosis by ADFR scheme. In: DeLuca HF, Frost HM, Lee WS, et al, eds. *Osteoporosis: Recent Advances in Pathogenesis and Treatment*. Baltimore, Md, University Park Press; 1981:393–396.

72. Hahn TJ, Halstead LR, Teitelbaum SL, et al. Altered mineral metabolism in glucocorticoid-induced osteopenia: effect of 25-hydroxyvitamin D. *J Clin Invest* 1979; 64:655–665.

73. Reid IR, Ibbertson HK. Calcium supplements in the prevention of steroid-induced osteoporosis. *Am J Clin Nutr* 1986;44:287–290.

74. Seeman E, Melton LJ, O'Fallon WM, et al. Risk factors for spinal osteoporosis in men. *Am J Med* 1983;75:977–983.

75. Frame B, Parfitt AM. Osteomalacia: current concepts *Ann Intern Med* 1978;89:996–982.

76. Holick MF. Vitamin D requirements for the elderly. *Clin Nutr* 1986;5:121–129.

77. Parfitt AM, Frame B. Treatment of rickets and osteomalacia. *Semin Drug Treat* 1972;2:83–115.

78. Heath H, Hodgson SF, Kennedy MA. Primary hyperparathyroidism: incidence, morbidity and potential economic impact in a community. *N Engl J Med* 1980; 302:189–193.

79. Mallette LE. Primary hyperparathyroidism: clinical and biochemical features. *Medicine* 1974;53:127–146.

80. Karpati G, Frame B. Neuropsychiatric disorders in primary hyperparathyroidism. *Arch Neurol* 1964;10:387–397.

81. Bilezikian JP. The medical management of primary hyperparathyroidism. *Ann Intern Med* 1982;96:198–202.

82. Marcus R, Madvig P, Crim M, et al. Conjugated estrogens in the treatment of postmenopausal women with hyperparathyroidism. *Ann Intern Med* 1984;100:633–640.

83. Selby PL, Peacock M. Ethinyl estradiol and norethin-

drone in the treatment of primary hyperparathyroidism in postmenopausal women. *N Engl J Med* 1986;314:1481–1485.

84. Scholz DA, Purnell DC. Asymptomatic primary hyperparathyroidism: 10 year prospective study. *Mayo Clin Proc* 1981;56:473–478.

85. Singer FR. *Paget's Disease of Bone*. New York, NY: Plenum Medical Book Co; 1977.

86. Frame B. Paget disease: a review of current knowledge. *Radiology* 1981;141:21–24.

87. Singer FR. Paget's disease of bone. In: Martin TJ, Raisz LG, eds. *Clinical Endocrinology of Calcium Metabolism*. New York, NY: Marcel Dekker Inc; 1987:369–402.

88. Singer FR, Fredericks RS, Minkin C. Salmon calcitonin therapy for Paget's disease of bone: the problem of acquired clinical resistance. *Arthritis Rheum* 1980;23:1148–1154.

89. Fleisch H. Biphosphonates: mechanisms of action and clinical applications. In: Peck WA, ed. *Bone and Mineral Research Annual 1*. Amsterdam, the Netherlands: Excerpta Medica; 1983:319–357.

16

Rheumatology

Leif B. Sorensen

By all demographic projections, the population 65 years of age and older will increase rapidly in absolute and relative numbers through the year 2020 and beyond. Although in the future the majority of older individuals will be healthy and able to function independently, a significant fraction will develop chronic health problems varying in degree from relatively minor difficulties to severe disabilities. Chronic diseases, and among those arthritis, will contribute prominently to disability. In a survey conducted in 1984 by the National Center for Health Statistics, arthritis ranked first among the 10 most prevalent chronic health problems, with a prevalence of 473 per 1,000 individuals 65 years and older and 495 per 1,000 individuals age 75 and above.

The prevalence of the common types of arthritis increases with age. This is especially true for osteoarthritis. Numerous epidemiological studies have shown an exponential increase in osteoarthritis with advancing years. The strong association between aging and osteoarthritis has raised questions on the relationship of osteoarthritis to aging. Age-related changes do occur in articular cartilage and bone, but the changes are not those of osteoarthritis. The hypothesis that osteoarthritis is a result of aging of joint tissues largely has been abandoned. However, biochemical changes in senescent cartilage or changes in joint biomechanics may facilitate the development of the osteoarthritic process.

Age-Related Changes in the Joint

Normal adult hyaline cartilage is avascular, alymphatic, and aneural. Chondrocytes make up only 5% of its volume, while water constitutes 70 to 80% of the cartilage by weight. The extracellular matrix is principally a mixture of proteoglycans and type II collagen. The chondrocyte is extremely active metabolically. Not only is it responsible for the synthesis of proteoglycans, collagen, link protein, and hyaluronic acid, but it also releases a variety of degradative enzymes. While collagen is metabolically inert in normal cartilage, proteoglycan turnover is a normal remodelling process.

Aging of cartilage is associated with specific biochemical changes. The content of water decreases—a finding that is in contrast to the increased water content of osteoarthritic cartilage. Total proteoglycan content remains unchanged, but both composition and structure of the proteoglycan molecule undergo alterations. Chondroitin sulfate content decreases, whereas keratan sulfate content increases. The cell density is lower in adult than in young cartilage, but the cell count alters little in aging articular cartilage once adulthood is reached.

With age, joints become increasingly congruent in shape. The basis for this increase in congruity is unknown, but it may be due to a progressive diminution in blood flow at the osteochondral junction, with a consequent decrease in the rate of remodelling at this site.

Osteoarthritis

Osteoarthritis is by far the most common form of arthritis in the elderly. In the US, more than 50 million people suffer from pain and limitation of motion, and an estimated 180,000 people are bed or wheel chair bound from osteoarthritis. Also known as osteoarthrosis and degenerative joint disease, osteoarthritis is characterized by a slowly progressive deterioration of a joint in which localized loss of cartilage occurs in association with subchondral sclerosis, cyst formation, osteophytosis, and capsular and synovial thickening. Traditionally, osteoarthritis has been divided into two main types: a primary or idiopathic form and secondary osteoarthritis in which some underlying condition is present. This classification may at times be somewhat artificial. For example, many cases of osteoarthritis of the hip, thought to be primary, may in fact be secondary to childhood anatomic abnormalities such as congenital hip dysplasia, Legg–Calve–Perthes disease, or slipped femoral epiphysis.

All epidemiological studies have shown that the prevalence of osteoarthritis increases progressively with age. Autopsy surveys have shown that by age 40, 90% of all persons have histologic evidence of osteoarthritis, while in the tenth decade, the process has become universal, but such investigations define earlier disease than do clinical studies based on symptoms and signs. In a survey of roentgenograms of hands and feet, 37% of all adults in the U.S. had some evidence of osteoarthritis. The prevalence rose from 4 per 100 among persons 18 to 24 years of age to 85 per 100 at 75 to 79 years. In the Framingham study[1] radiographic evidence of osteoarthritis increased with age, from 27% in subjects younger than age 70 years to 44% in subjects aged 80 years and older. Our own study[2] of a representative sample of 79-year-olds in Gothenburg, Sweden, demonstrated radiographic evidence of osteoarthritis of the hands in 65% of 81 individuals, whereas 14% had osteoarthritis of the knees, defined radiographically as both joint space narrowing and sclerosis of adjacent bone.

Biochemical and Structural Changes in the Osteoarthritic Joint

The prevailing view is that the earliest events in osteoarthritis occur in the cartilage.[3] Multiple etiologic factors are thought to result in biochemical and metabolic changes in cartilage: decreased total proteoglycan content, shortening of the glycosaminoglycan branches, and a decrease in the length of the subunit coreprotein. As the disease advances, the hyaluronate binding region becomes defective, resulting in lack of aggregation.

The total content of collagen in cartilage does not change in osteoarthritis. However, the collagen fibers are less uniform in size and the weave is looser. Eventually the supporting collagen network is disrupted, allowing the proteoglycan molecules to expand and imbibe water. This exposure of water-binding proteoglycans explains the increased water content in osteoarthritic cartilage and its swelling when immersed in water.

Chondrocytes do not normally divide, but in osteoarthritis—once the continuity of the surface of cartilage is disrupted—the cells can divide, forming clusters of chondrocytes, so-called "brood capsules." These are readily seen under the microscope along the clefts of fibrillated cartilage. The changes in anabolic and catabolic activities of chondrocytes in osteoarthritis have been extensively studied. Most investigators have noted substantially increased synthesis and release of degradative enzymes, including acid cathepsins, neutral proteases, sugar-splitting enzymes, and sulfatases. Collagenase enzyme activity, which is difficult to demonstrate in normal cartilage, was positively correlated with the severity of human osteoarthritic lesions based on histologic criteria. Concurrently with this accelerated breakdown of cartilage matrix, the chondrocyte increases its synthesis of proteoglycan, type II collagen, and hyaluronic acid, in an attempt to reverse the depletion of matrix constituents. The products of regenerating cartilage appear to differ slightly in structure and function from their normal counterparts. Nevertheless, at least for a time, the chondrocyte is successful in its attempt to repair the breakdown caused by the degradative processes. Eventually, the disease progresses to a stage where tissue changes are so severe that the chondrocyte "fails" and synthesis of matrix constituents diminishes.

Fibrillation is the earliest gross change of cartilage in osteoarthritis. As fibrillated cartilage is abraded, focal erosions are formed. These erosions coalesce with progressive denudation of underlying sclerotic bone. Proliferation of bone occurs at the joint margins to form osteophytes and in subchondral bone, especially in areas denuded of cartilage. The term eburnation applies to the glistening appearance of the polished sclerotic bone surface.

Whereas most authorities believe that the earliest events in osteoarthritis occur in cartilage, a divergent view suggests that changes in subchondral bone precede measurable changes in the cartilage. It is postulated that the earliest lesions are trabecular fractures in cancellous bone. The healing of these fatigue fractures results in thickening of the trabeculae, leading to an increase in the density of bone with a consequent reduction in its ability to absorb energy. With loss of this functional role of bone, energy absorption is shifted toward the overlying cartilage whose collagen fibers sustain fatigue fractures, eventually leading to deterioration of cartilage. Cyst formation is commonly seen in the juxtaarticular bone, probably a result of tissue breakdown related to focal areas of microfracture in the ischemic subchondral bone.

Focal, chronic, synovitis, characterized by lymphocyte and mononuclear cell infiltration, is frequently seen in osteoarthritis. This probably is due to release of hydroxyapatite or calcium pyrophosphate crystals, inflammatory mediators initiated by cartilage breakdown components, and/or the presence of immune complexes in the surface of the cartilage.

Etiologic Factors

The nature of the events that initiate osteoarthritis is poorly understood. Aging alone does not cause osteoarthritis, but matrix alterations that occur with aging may facilitate the process. Trauma, especially in the form of excessive repetitive impulse loading over many years, is likely to be an important contributory factor. Certain occupations are associated with a high incidence of osteoarthritis in specific joints which are otherwise rarely involved in osteoarthritis. Chronic malalignment and laxness of ligamentous structures predispose to osteoarthritis. Genetic factors play a role in the development of Heberden's nodes. The genetic mechanism appears to involve a simple autosomal gene, sex influenced, dominant in women and recessive in men. Certain metabolic diseases, eg, alkaptonuria, hemochromatosis, and crystal deposition diseases, cause alterations in matrix structure that predispose to osteoarthritis. In certain patients with calcium pyrophosphate deposition disease, crystal deposition clearly antedates osteoarthritis, whereas in other patients, osteoarthritis is present for a long period and crystal deposition disease occurs later in the disorder. Thus changes in osteoarthritic cartilage seem to facilitate precipitation and deposition of crystals. There is considerable evidence that endocrine factors may initiate and accelerate the process. The arthropathy complicating acromegaly is an example of damage to articular cartilage by somatotropin, through somatomedin-induced stimulation. Insulin stimulates chondrocyte synthesis of proteoglycans. Diabetic patients have a higher incidence of osteoarthritis than nondiabetics. The association between obesity and osteoarthritis is unclear. Obesity is not a contributing factor to osteoarthritis of the hip. Previous cross-sectional studies that found an association of obesity with knee osteoarthritis failed to clarify whether obesity follows osteoarthritis because a person with disease is less active and consequently more likely to become obese, or whether osteoarthritis follows obesity because of the extra stress on the joints imposed by the excessive weight. However, a recent survey[4] of a subset of the Framingham Heart Study cohort demonstrated a strong association between obesity and the later development of knee osteoarthritis. Finally, there is evidence of immunological mechanisms being operative in osteoarthritis—if not as a primary event, then certainly later in the destructive stage of the disease. Because cartilage is isolated from the rest of the body under normal conditions, the immune system may not recognize antigenic determinants of cartilage itself. A number of cartilage components are known to have immunogenic properties.

Clinical Features

The joints commonly affected in osteoarthritis are the distal and proximal interphalangeal joints of the hands, the first carpometacarpal joint, the first metatarsophalangeal joint, the hip, the knee, and the spine. For reasons that are unclear, the wrist, elbow, shoulder, and ankle are spared except with previous trauma or congenital anomaly.

Symptoms and signs that are common to osteoarthritis in general are morning stiffness that lasts less than 30 minutes; stiffness after periods of inactivity during the day, so-called gelling; pain on motion and later also at rest; limitation of motion due to incongruity of joint surfaces, muscle, or capsular contracture, or mechanical block from osteophytes or loose bodies; and acute flares of crystal-induced synovitis in response to calcium phyrophosphate or hydroxyapatite crystals. Objectively, local tenderness may be elicited, especially if synovitis is present. Pain on passive motion, and crepitus, a crackling sound or sensation as the joint is moved, are common findings. Joint enlargement may result from proliferative synovitis, an increase in synovial fluid, or osteophyte formation. Osteophytes can often be palpated along the margins of affected joints. In the late stages, gross deformities and subluxation ensue. In addition to these general symptoms, the clinical picture depends on the particular joint involvement.

Heberden's nodes are characterized by bony enlargement of the dorsolateral and dorsomedial aspects of the distal interphalangeal joints of the fingers. Flexor and lateral deviation of the distal phalanx is common. Similar nodes at the proximal interphalangeal joints are known as *Bouchard's nodes*.

As discussed previously, Heberden's nodes are prevalent in the elderly. They may be single, but they usually are multiple. In most patients they develop slowly over months or years, giving rise to little or no pain. In a few patients, they evolve rapidly with redness and tenderness. Small gelatinous cysts sometimes appear over the dorsal aspects of the joint. These cysts, which morphologically resemble ganglia, may disappear spontaneously or persist indefinitely. In some cases they communicate with the joint itself.

Involvement of the *first carpometacarpal joint* is common and is frequently symptomatic. Marked osteophytosis at this site leads to a characteristic squaring appearance of the hands.

Erosive inflammatory osteoarthritis is a variant of osteoarthritis of the hands. This entity, which most often affects postmenopausal women, involves the distal and proximal interphalangeal joints and less often the metacarpophalangeal joints. Painful inflammatory episodes eventually lead to joint deformities and sometimes to ankylosis. After years of intermittent acute flares, the joints become quiescent. The clinical picture may be confused with rheumatoid arthritis. Radiographic findings include loss of joint cartilage, spur formation, subchondral sclerosis, and bony erosions, usually in the central portion of the joints. Rheumatoid factor tests are negative, and the sedimentation rate is normal or only slightly elevated. The presence of immune complexes in the synovium and a frequent association with the sicca syndrome suggest that immune mechanisms may be at work in this subset of osteoarthritis.

Osteoarthritis of the *acromioclavicular joint* is frequently overlooked. Motion of the shoulder, albeit frequently of normal range, elicits shoulder pain.

Osteoarthritis of the *knee* may be localized to one or more of its three anatomic compartments, the patellofemoral, and the medial and lateral femerotibial compartments. In primary osteoarthritis, there is usually disproportionate degenerative change in the medial and lateral compartments. Most often, the medial compartment is most involved, giving rise to a genu varus deformity. When the changes predominate in the lateral compartment, genu valgus is likely to be present. The knee should be examined for ligamentous laxity. The physical examination should include observation of the gait, checking for an antalgic limp, in which the patient spends less time on the involved leg.

Spontaneous osteonecrosis of the knee must be considered in the differential diagnosis of an acutely painful knee in the elderly. This condition is characterized clinically by acute onset of pain, usually in the medial compartment, aggravated by weight bearing. Usually the patient requires a cane and moderate doses of analgesics. A knee effusion and localized tenderness of the involved femoral condyle or tibial plateau are found on examination. Radiographic changes do not develop until several months after onset of symptoms. The bone scan is positive early on. The most common site of involvement is the medial femoral condyle, less frequently the medial tibial plateau, and rarely the lateral

femoral condyle. Superficially, the radiograph may resemble osteochondritis dissecans of the young, and, in the earlier literature, the conditon was reported as osteochondritis dissecans of the elderly (see Figure 16.1). In a study[5] of 66 patients with spontaneous osteonecrosis of the knee, the mean age of onset was 68 years and the majority were female. The structural changes alter biomechanics of the joint and may lead to development of severe osteoarthritis in less than a year. Clinical and radiologic healing occurs in some patients.

Osteoarthritis of the *hip* is primarily confined to older individuals. It may be unilateral or bilateral. True hip pain is usually located in the groin, lateral thigh area, or along the inner aspect of the thigh. It may be referred to the buttock or along the obturator nerve to the knee. At times, the pain in the knee so dominates the picture that the diagnosis may be missed. Conversely, in the evaluation of pain in the hip area, other causes must be considered. Disorders of the lumbar spine at the L2–L3 level may refer pain into the groin, and at the L5–S1 level into the buttock. Trochanteric bursitis also may be confused with intraarticular hip disease. Physical examination shows loss of internal rotation and abduction early in the disease process. Flexion contrac-

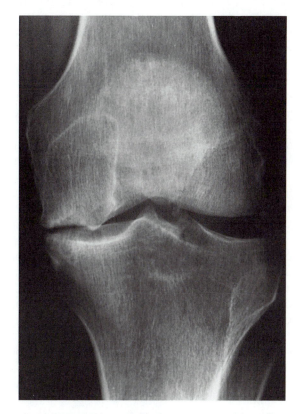

Fig. 16.1. Spontaneous osteonecrosis of outer portion of the medial femoral condyle. The radiograph shows a well demarcated subchondral radiolucent lesion with a sclerotic border.

ture may be determined by using the Thomas test, in which the knee of the uninvolved leg is drawn to the chest to flatten the lumbar lordosis. If a flexion contracture exists, the involved leg will flex off the examining table. On gait examination, the patient may demonstrate an antalgic gait limp or a gluteus medius lurch in which the torso leans over the involved weight-bearing hip. This move reflects an unconscious attempt to place the center of gravity over the painful hip, thereby decreasing the forces across that joint. In advanced disease, the leg is often held in external rotation with the hip flexed and adducted. Functional shortening of the leg may result in a short-limb limp.

Degenerative joint disease of the spine results from involvement of the intervertebral discs, vertebral bodies, or the posterior apophyseal articulations. Narrowing of the discs may cause subluxation of the posterior apophyseal joints. The term *spinal osteoarthritis* describes the changes in the apophyseal joints, whereas *degenerative disc disease* applies to the changes in the intervertebral synchondrosis.

Impingement on the nerve roots by spurs that comprise the intervertebral foramina is particularly common in the neck because of the small size of foraminal spaces in this location. In patients with involvement of the lower cervical spine, pain in the neck radiates to the shoulder, and sometimes to the arm and hand. Paresthesias and reflex changes are common in the distribution of the involved nerve root.

Osteophytes in the uncovertebral (Luschka) joints may compress the neighboring vertebral arteries as they traverse the transverse processes of the cervical spine, leading to signs and symptoms of basilar artery insufficiency. Narrowing of the vascular lumen is most marked during rotation of the head. Symptoms that frequently present in an intermittent pattern include vertigo, headache, blurring of vision, diplopia, and defects in visual field. Sudden loss of strength in an extremity has been reported. Nystagmus and ataxia may be demonstrated on examination. Angiographic studies serve to confirm the diagnosis.

Large spurs arising anteriorly from the vertebral bodies are prevalent. They rarely give rise to symptoms, but dysphagia due to external compression of the esophagus and respiratory symptoms in the form of coughing and hoarseness have been reported.

Large posterior spurs protruding into the spinal canal may compress the spinal cord leading to upper-motor-neuron and other long-tract signs. Compression of the anterior spinal artery may produce a central cord syndrome.

Nerve root compression in the dorsal spine causing radicular pain around the chest wall is less common. Involvement of the nerve roots in the lumbosacral area is associated with low back pain and neurologic signs and symptoms in the distribution of the involved roots. Since all the nerve roots have different dermatomes, determining the location of pain by careful history taking and demonstration of sensory or reflex changes in the limbs will indicate the nerve root involved and will locate the level of the disc lesion.

The lumbar and sacral roots, collectively called the cauda equina, have a long course in the spinal canal, since the end of the spinal cord, the conus medullaris, lies at the level of the first lumbar vertebra. *Lumbar spinal stenosis* is characterized by narrowing of the spinal canal, nerve root canals, and/or intervertebral foramina. A combination of degenerative changes such as disc protrusion, osteophyte formation, spondylolisthesis, ligamentous hypertrophy, and thickening of the nerve roots reduces the space needed for the spinal cord and the lumbar and sacral roots. All diameters of the canal may be reduced, and the cross-sectional configuration assumes a triangular shape. Lumbar stenosis is being recognized with increasing frequency in the elderly population. The acquired form of spinal stenosis affects primarily men and has a peak incidence in the 7th decade. Pseudoclaudication is the most frequent symptom, defined as discomfort in the buttock, thigh, or leg on standing or walking that is relieved by rest. Because of the relationship of pain, numbness, or weakness to walking and evidence of comprised vascular supply to the cauda equina, the condition has been called "claudication of the cauda equina." Bodily positions that flex the lumbar spine tend to relieve the pain, whereas positions that extend the spine make the pain worse. The patient may stand with knees, hips, and lumbar spine flexed (simian stance). Most patients have concomitant back pain, and sphincter dysfunction may be present. Unlike the situation in isolated disc protrusion, straight leg raising is usually not painful. Routine roentgenograms are usually inadequate for diagnostic purposes. Computerized axial tomography or magnetic resonance imaging, as well as electromyography, yield important diagnostic information. Extensive decompressive surgery yields good to excellent results in two-thirds of patients with lumbar stenosis.[6]

A variant form of spinal osteophytosis seen in the elderly is the *ankylosing hyperostosis of Forestier*. This condition is characterized by large spurs or marginal proliferations that fuse to form flowing ossifications along the anterolateral aspects of vertebral bodies. The process extends to the connective tissue surrounding the spine, including the anterior longitudinal ligament. The distal thoracic spine is the site of predilection, but other levels of the spine may be affected.

Radiographic criteria include the presence of flowing calcifications and ossifications along the antero-lateral aspects of at least four contiguous vertebral bodies, relative preservation of the intervertebral disc height, and absence of ankylosis of the sacroiliac and apophyseal joints (see Fig. 16.2). It is estimated that 5 to 10% of persons over 65 years meet the radiologic criteria for establishing a diagnosis of Forestier's disease. Despite extensive anatomic abnormalities, the patients are either free of symptoms or they complain of modest pain and stiffness and mild restriction of motion. The term *diffuse idiopathic skeletal hyperostosis* is applied when the vertebral condition is accompanied by extraspinal manifestations. Those changes include irregular new bone formation or "whiskering" commonly seen in the paraacetabular, tarsal and metatarsal areas, large bone spurs on the olecranon process, calcaneus and patella, and ligament calcification and ossification, in particular of the sacrotuberous and ileolumbar ligaments. Heel pain may be a prominent symptom. Dysphagia related to cervical osteophytosis has been reported.

Generalized osteoarthritis is seen predominantly in middle-aged to elderly women. Presenting complaints may be limited to one joint only and then spread to other sites. An acute inflammatory phase may precede chronic articular symptoms. The typical distribution of generalized osteoarthritis involves the distal and proximal interphalangeal joints, the first carpometacarpal joints, the base of the large toes, knees, hips, and the cervical and lumbar spine. The concept of primary generalized osteoarthritis as a distinct subset has been questioned by some. It may be that these cases represent a more severe form of ordinary osteoarthritis, differing only in the number and severity of joints involved.

The natural history of osteoarthritis is not one of inevitable progression of pain and disability. Involvement of weight-bearing joints or the spine is more likely to lead to symptoms. Severe involvement of critical joints such as knees or hips can lead to significant disability.

Laboratory and Radiographic Findings

There are no diagnostic laboratory abnormalities in primary osteoarthritis. The erythrocyte sedimentation rate is usually normal; slight elevation may be seen in generalized osteoarthritis and in erosive osteoarthritis. Rheumatoid factor tests are negative. Laboratory studies become more important in excluding other rheumatic diseases. Synovial fluid analysis typically reveals a noninflammatory, translucent fluid. Viscosity is good, the mucin clot is firm, and the cell count is slightly increased. Calcium pyrophosphate and/or hydroxyapatite crystals may be present.

X-ray findings reflect the anatomic changes. Joint space narrowing is a result of cartilage degeneration. Subchondral bone sclerosis correlates with proliferation of bone in the subchondral tissue; marginal osteophytes occur as a result of proliferation of cartilage and bone at the periphery of the joint. Cysts, varying in size from a few millimeters to several centimeters, are seen

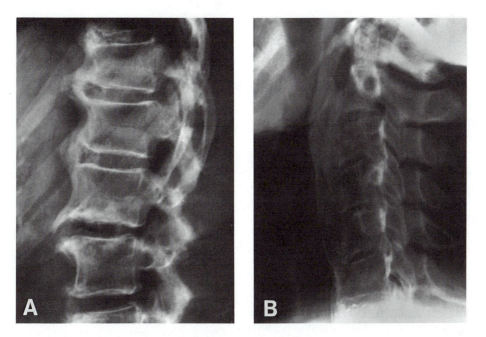

Fig. 16.2. Forestier's disease. *A.* Dorsal spine, lateral projection. Note flowing calcifications anteriorly, and preservation of the intervertebral disc spaces. *B.* Cervical spine of an elderly man with restricted neck motion. There is massive ossification of the anterior ligament bridging the bodies of the cervical vertebrae.

as translucent areas in juxtaarticular bone. In advanced cases, there is gross deformity and subluxation. Osteoporosis is not a feature of osteoarthritis. Both diseases are common in the older age group, but no association exists between these senescent processes. Some authors claim that osteophytes correlate with aging, and that they are not by themselves a sign of osteoarthritis. According to this view, joint space narrowing or changes in subchondral bone are required to make a diagnosis of osteoarthritis radiologically. Ankylosis is not a feature of osteoarthritis except in erosive osteoarthritis and ankylosing hyperostosis.

There are large discrepancies between radiologic incidence of osteoarthritis and clinical complaints. In the Framingham Study[1] of elderly subjects referred to earlier, the prevalence of radiographic changes of osteoarthritis in the knee was 34% in women and 31% in men. Yet, only 11% of all women and 7% of all men had symptomatic disease. The discordance between symptoms and radiographic findings of osteoarthritis in the lumbar spine is striking. At age 50, 87% of adults have radiographic evidence of lumbar spondylosis, and almost 70% of asymptomatic persons have degenerative disc disease on spine films.[7] Because of the frequency of osteoarthritic changes on radiologic examination of the lower spine, it must never be assumed that they are the cause of back pain until proven.

Differential Diagnosis

In most patients, the diagnosis of osteoarthritis is not difficult. Erosive osteoarthritis may resemble rheumatoid arthritis, but osteophytosis is rarely seen in seropositive rheumatoid arthritis. Calcium pyrophosphate deposition disease may simulate osteoarthritis when crystal shedding occurs at a low rate on a continuing basis. Neurologic symptoms that are secondary to spinal osteoarthritis must be differentiated from those that result from primary neurologic disorders. Neurologic complications of osteoarthritis of the cervical spine may be confused with amyotrophic lateral sclerosis, spinal cord tumors, and basilar artery disease. The differential diagnosis is also complicated by the high prevalence of x-ray evidence of osteoarthritis in the elderly. Various pain symptoms may be misdiagnosed as osteoarthritis with resulting delays of the diagnosis and treatment of the actual underlying problem.

Treatment

The specific treatment regimen to be selected for the patient with osteoarthritis must be individualized. Many patients who present with mild disease need only reassurance that the disease process is not likely to become generalized or crippling.

Physical Measures

Of special benefit to patients with mild to moderate disease are physical measures that decrease the patient's pain, improve the range of motion, and increase the individual's ability to live independently and carry out activities of daily living. Measures to decrease joint loading should be recommended. Strenuous exercises and stair climbing should be avoided whenever possible. A body-toning exercise program such as regular swimming is an excellent alternative. If the patient is obese, weight reduction should be prescribed. Activities that require loading of the involved joint should be fractionated. For example, several short periods of walking are preferable to sustained walking for the patient with osteoarthritis of the hip or knee. Rest periods in the morning and afternoon are to be encouraged. A cane, held in the opposite hand, is helpful if hip or knee involvement is unilateral. If bilateral, crutches or a walker are more desirable. Knee cages or elastic supports may provide some stability when ligamentous laxity is present. Pillows should never be placed under the knees at night, because of the risk of developing flexion contracture. Flexion contracture of the hip may be prevented, and mild ones may be corrected by having the patient lie prone for 30 minutes twice daily. Patients with involvement of the cervical spine and evidence of nerve root compression or muscle spasm will benefit from a cervical collar or traction. A lumbosacral corset and a firm mattress or a board placed under the mattress are helpful measures in treating osteoarthritis of the lumbar spine.

Physical therapy, an important component of the treatment program, relieves pain and associated muscle spasm and maintains and regains joint range of motion. It involves, principally, the use of heat or cold and an exercise program tailored to the individual. The simpler, less expensive forms of heat therapy, such as plain hot water soaks or a warm tub bath, are more likely to be utilized and are as effective as more complex measures. Caution must be exercised when prescribing heat treatment to a patient who also has peripheral vascular disease. The exercise program is designed to preserve or to improve the range of motion and to strengthen periarticular muscles. Isometric exercises, in which the muscles are strengthened against weight resistance while the joint is kept in a normal anatomic position, maintain muscle function and strength. Isotonic exercises, in which joints are put through a range of motion while being exercised should in general be used without resistance.

Drug Therapy

Analgesic or antiinflammatory agents are added when the basic program fails to provide the desired relief. In patients with mild or moderate pain without clinical evidence of inflammation, analgesic agents such as acetaminophen, diflunisal, or aspirin, 650 mg, taken with food every 8 hours may be used on a continuous or as needed basis. At the indicated dose, aspirin has analgesic properties, but little antiinflammatory effect. Codeine may be required for acute radicular pain of spinal osteoarthritis, but it should not be prescribed for a prolonged period in the elderly with chronic disease.

When synovitis is present, judicious use of higher doses of aspirin or one of the newer nonsteroidal antiinflammatory drugs (NSAIDs) may be extremely helpful. In addition to possessing analgesic and antipyretic properties, these drugs reduce symptoms and signs of inflammation. The beneficial effects—and for that matter many of the adverse effects—of NSAIDs are related to their inhibition of the membrane-bound cyclooxygenase, which leads to a reduction in the synthesis of prostaglandins.

In prescribing NSAIDs to older patients, it is important to keep in mind the physiological changes that occur with aging and which may profoundly alter patient response to therapy (see Chapter 7). Drug interactions are more likely in the elderly who frequently take multiple medications. Thus potential drug interactions of NSAIDs with some of the most commonly used drugs in the elderly (anticoagulants, hypoglycemic drugs, digoxin, antihypertensives, and diuretics) should be kept in mind when prescribing these drugs.

In order to obtain the antiinflammatory effect of aspirin, it is necessary to prescribe a dose of 975 mg three or four times daily. The aim is to obtain a salicylate concentration in the vicinity of 20 mg/100 ml. The development of tinnitus is a less reliable clue to mild salicylate toxicity than it is in the younger age group; measurement of plasma salicylate level is more reliable. In general, aspirin is less well tolerated in the elderly than it is in young adults. The incidence of gastrointestinal and central nervous system symptoms increases with age. Enteric-coated aspirin and the nonacetylated salicylate compounds, such as Disalcid, cause less gastric distress than unbuffered aspirin.

The newer NSAIDs have efficacy similar to aspirin, but are generally better tolerated and have less tendency to cause side effects, especially from the gastrointestinal tract. The choice between the various NSAIDs is largely empirical. Compounds with a short biological half-life, such as ibuprofen and ketoprofen, are preferable to those with prolonged half-lives. NSAIDs that are principally excreted in the urine, eg, azapropazone, should be given in a lower dose to patients with age-related reduction in renal function. There is no rationale for combining NSAIDs. On the contrary, the antiinflammatory effect may be reduced, and the risk for development of adverse reactions increased. Individual variability in patient response to different NSAIDs is a well recognized clinical experience.

The salient points to remember when prescribing NSAIDs in the elderly are: it is not possible to predict which NSAID will be most effective for a particular patient; the starting dose should be lower than that recommended for younger adults; stepwise adjustments should be made until optimal therapeutic response is obtained; and maximum tolerated dose may well be lower than that for younger individuals. Most NSAIDs are bound to plasma proteins. In elderly patients with low serum albumin concentration and in patients who are treated with other drugs that bind to plasma protein, concomitant treatment with an NSAID will require a reduction in dose.

Because of the high prevalence of rheumatic diseases in older persons, it is not surprising that this age group consumes a proportionately higher share of these drugs than the population at large. The widespread use and greater susceptibility of the elderly to toxic effects of drugs place them at significant risk of adverse effects from NSAIDs. The major toxicities occur in the gastrointestinal tract, central nervous system, kidney, liver, skin, and hematopoietic system.

Aspirin and all the newer NSAIDs have been shown to cause gastrointestinal lesions varying from diffuse gastritis to superficial erosions to large ulcer craters. Slow occult blood loss or massive gastrointestinal bleeding with severe symptoms of acute hemorrhagic anemia may occur. NSAID-gastropathy is frequently a silent disease until the sudden onset of acute bleeding or perforation. There is a mounting evidence that older persons taking NSAIDs are more prone to develop serious complications of ulcer disease than younger populations. A recent study[8] demonstrated that elderly patients who were taking prescription NSAIDs were over four times more likely to die from upper gastrointestinal hemorrhage or perforation than were nonusers. The use of gastroprotective agents, such as H-2 blockers, sucralfate, or antacids should be considered in patients most at risk who do require an NSAID.

Reversible depression of renal function may occur in situations when renal blood flow is dependent on local prostaglandin synthesis. Renal production of vasodilatory prostaglandins is stimulated by vasoconstrictor substances, such as angiotensin II and catecholamines, and is markedly inhibited by NSAIDs. The effects of loss of prostaglandins on the function of normal kidneys appear to be small, but when intrinsic renal disease is present or when hyperreninemic conditions associated with a contracted or functionally ineffective plasma volume exist, prostaglandins become essential to the maintenance of adequate renal blood flow and glomerular filtration rate. Under these circumstances, treatment with NSAIDs may precipitate acute renal failure. Patients at risk for NSAID-induced renal insufficiency include those with reduced cardiac output associated with congestive failure, liver disease with cirrhosis and ascites, renal ischemia due to low perfusion pressure as in hemorrhagic hypotension and septic shock, diuretic-induced volume depletion, salt depletion, and chronic parenchymal disease. Patients of advanced age alone, presumably because of subclinical renal disease, have also been reported to be at greater risk of renal failure secondary to NSAIDs. The elderly also are more susceptible to the development of other renal complications induced by NSAIDs, such as acute interstitial nephritis presenting as nephrotic syndrome, papillary necrosis, hyperkalemia, and sodium retention with edema.

Aspirin and other NSAIDs have been reported to be hepatotoxic. Approximately 4% of patients on NSAIDs have abnormalities of one or more liver function tests. Advanced age, decreased renal function, and multiple drug use are risk factors for the development of hepatotoxicity. In view of possible hepatotoxicity, it has been recommended that transaminases be monitored at regular intervals during the first year of treatment with an NSAID.

Central nervous system adverse effects associated with NSAIDs are not uncommon. Reversible hearing loss and tinnitus occur in patients who are placed on high doses of aspirin. As mentioned above, tinnitus may be absent in the elderly, especially those with presbycusis, in the presence of a high salicylate level. Confusion, hyperactivity, slurred speech, hallucinations, generalized seizures, and coma may dominate the clinical picture. In an elderly patient who is taking aspirin, it is important to recognize that these symptoms may signal salicylate intoxication.

Skin reactions, blood dyscrasias, and hypersensitivity reactions are similar in young and old, and do not appear to occur more frequently in the older age group.

Aspirin and most other NSAIDs bind firmly to plasma proteins. In so doing, they may displace other drugs from their binding sites, or may themselves be displaced by other drugs. As a result of such displacement, the fraction of free drug in the plasma increases with consequent enhancement of the activity and/or toxicity of drugs that bind strongly to plasma proteins, eg, coumarin derivatives, phenytoin, sulfonylurea hypoglycemic agents, and sulfonamides.

Systemic adrenal corticosteroid analogues are not recommended in the management of osteoarthritis. Clinical results with these drugs are equivocal and are outweighed by their potential side effects. On the other hand, the occasional selective intraarticular administration of adrenal corticosteroid may be beneficial. The over-use of joints following pain relief and a direct deleterious effect upon cartilage metabolism may aggravate joint deterioration. In general, intraarticular injections of corticosteroid into a weight-bearing joint should be given no more than once or twice a year. The patient should be cautioned to avoid joint loading for 7 to 10 days following the intraarticular injection. Pericapsular and ligamentous injections into areas of tenderness around involved joints may produce excellent relief of symptoms while avoiding the potential hazards of the intraarticular route.

Our current knowledge of the pathogenesis of osteoarthritis has directed attention toward the development of new drugs that stimulate chondrocyte matrix formation or inhibit degradative enzyme release. None of these investigational agents have been shown to alter the natural history of osteoarthritis in a controlled study. Nevertheless, vigorous efforts in this exciting area may well result in a significant breakthrough in the medical treatment of this disease.

For patients with advanced disease who have intractable pain and severe disability, *surgical treatment* may be the answer. For further discussion of the variety of surgical procedures available to the patient with arthritis, the reader is referred to Chapter 17.

Sexuality

Sexual function is often impaired in patients with arthritis. It is important for the physician to evaluate a dysfunction in this area and to advise the patient of measures aimed at overcoming handicaps. Many elderly continue to be sexually active into advanced age, and their sexual needs are not diminished with disability or disease. Patients with osteoarthritis of the hips, knees, or spine frequently have problems with sexual intercourse due to pain or mechanical problems. Despite these limitations, sexual activity can be undertaken with the use of analgesics beforehand. Patients should be encouraged to try a variety of experimental procedures and positions that allow the successful performance of intercourse. The Arthritis Foundation's pamphlet "Living and Loving with Arthritis" describes a variety of sexual problems and suggested solutions.

Crystal Deposition Disease

The main types of salts implicated in crystal deposition, in addition to urate, are calcium pyrophosphate dihydrate, hydroxyapatite, and other basic calcium phosphates. The prevalence of crystal deposition diseases increases with age. Deposits of calcium pyrophosphate and hydroxyapatite are often seen in association with osteoarthritis. Although most often asymptomatic, articular manifestations of this group of diseases are extremely common in the geriatric population.

Deposition of Crystals—the Relationship to Aging and Osteoarthritis

The precise mechanisms by which crystals are deposited are imperfectly understood, but increased concentrations of metastable calcium salts and sodium urate, the unmasking of activators of crystal nucleation and crystal growth, or a decrease in concentration of inhibitors of crystal nucleation may act singly or together to promote crystal formation. In idiopathic or sporadic calcium pyrophosphate dihydrate (CPPD) deposition disease seen in the elderly, isolated elevation of pyrophosphate in synovial fluid is due to local abnormalities. Increased pyrophosphate production has been demonstrated in osteoarthritic cartilage and is probably due to enhanced breakdown of nucleotides mediated by the chondrocytic ectoenzymes, 5'-nucleotidase and nucleoside triphosphate pyrophosphohydrolase. The increased activity of these metabolic processes is an attempt by chrondrocytes to repair damaged cartilage. Ultrastructural studies have demonstrated deposits of CPPD in chondrocyte lacunae in areas of damaged matrix and activated chondrocytes. Aggregated proteoglycans are potent inhibitors of crystal formation. Deaggregation of proteoglycans in aged and osteochondritic cartilage would lead to a loss of natural calcium crystal inhibitor. Fibrils of senile amyloid have been shown to have a special affinity for calcium and inorganic pyrophosphate.

It would appear that deposits of CPPD and monosodium urate can form in the absence of osteoarthritis. The familial cases of chondrocalcinosis and gout in younger persons are examples of deposition of crystals in seemingly normal cartilage. On the other hand, biochemical changes in osteoarthritic cartilage may predispose to crystal deposition, which in turn may contribute to further joint deterioration. In this latter setting, crystal deposition is a secondary, opportunistic process in damaged cartilage. Aging alone appears to be the major factor leading to formation of CPPD in fibrocartilaginous structures.

The simultaneous finding of mixtures of crystal deposits in the same joints of elderly patients is further evidence of their susceptibility to intraarticular and periarticular crystal deposition. A variety of species of crystals or mixtures thereof have the propensity to accumulate in osteoarthritic cartilage that has reduced concentrations of inhibitors of crystallization. A positive association exists between gout and CPPD deposition disease, and between CPPD and hydroxyapatite formation. Mixtures of different basic calcium phosphates have also been reported.

Crystal-Induced Synovitis

It is generally believed that preformed microcrystals are shed from cartilage or synovium. Crystals that are associated with arthritis possess a negative surface charge and avidly bind proteins, including immunoglobulins, albumin, lysosomal enzymes, complement, and lipoproteins. Urate crystals have a strong affinity for IgG. The molecular orientation of IgG on the crystal surface leaves the Fc portion exposed and free to interact with the Fc cell membrane receptors on leukocytes, monocytes, synovicytes, and platelets. The interaction between cells and crystals causes the cells to become activated, with release of a host of inflammatory mediators. Coating of the crystal surface with IgG greatly enhances phagocytosis and complement activation. Monocytes and polymorphonuclear leukocytes release a potent chemotactic factor that causes rapid accumulation of polymorphonuclear leukocytes. Phagocytosis induces release of oxygen radicals and lysosomal enzymes. Monosodium urate crystals induce release of interleukin-1 from monocytes, an observation that may explain the fever of acute gouty arthritis.

Some crystals, e.g., monosodium urate, are membranolytic. After digestion of their protein coating in the phagolysosome, the uncoated crystal causes rupture of the phagolysosome with release of its enzymes into the cytoplasm, resulting in cellular autolysis, increased permeability of the cell wall, and release of intracellular enzymes into the surrounding medium. Coating of the crystals with hyaluronic acid and certain proteins, viz. albumin or lipoprotein, may inhibit or prevent crystal-induced inflammation. Crystals are often found in the joint fluid after the inflammatory reaction has subsided or even in the absence of any detectable inflammation. A plausible explanation for this finding is that products in the synovial fluid provide a coating of the surfaces of the crystals that protects them from being phagocytized.

Study of synovial fluid by polarized light microscopy provides clinicians with a precise method of identifying monosodium urate and CPPD when the crystals are more than 1 μm in size. The findings by plane polarized light are augmented by using a first-order red plate compensator which allows one to determine the sign of birefringence.

Non-birefringent apatite and other basic calcium phosphate crystals are so minute that they cannot be identified by ordinary light microscopy. They tend to aggregate into non-birefringent microspherules that are difficult to differentiate from cell detritus and fat droplets. Alizarin red S stain of fresh synovial fluid has been used as a simple screening test to detect calcium-containing particles such as bone fragments and crystals of calcium salts. Definitive identification of apatite and other basic calcium phosphates requires sophisticated techniques.

Plain radiographs identify macroscopic deposits of radioopaque calcium containing salts. Hydroxyapatite deposits are frequently seen in periarticular and capsular distribution, while CPPD deposition disease is associated with characteristic punctate and linear calcifications in fibrocartilagenous and hyaline cartilage.

Gout

New onset of gouty arthritis is common among the elderly. Most of these patients have hyperuricemia on the basis of decreased urinary excretion of uric acid, related to the effects of diuretic therapy, mild renal failure, hypertension, or hypertriglyceridemia. It has been estimated that about half of all patients presenting with their initial attack of acute gouty arthritis are taking a diuretic. With the widespread use of these drugs in the elderly population it is hardly a surprise that diuretic use is a major cause of gout in this age group. Less commonly, gout is secondary to overproduction of uric acid due to increased turnover of cells, as in myeloproliferative disorders.

The presentation of gout in the elderly differs from the more classic picture in younger men. The pattern is frequently polyarticular, subacute, or chronic, and men and women appear to be affected with the same frequency. In women the first manifestations of gout may be acute arthritis in finger joints, sometimes presenting as inflamed Heberden's or Bouchard's nodes. Elderly women are particularly prone to develop diuretic-induced polyarticular gout. Many have underlying osteoarthritis; concomitant tophi and osteoarthritic changes in the same joint have been described. The appearance of asymptomatic tophi in Heberden's and Bouchard's nodes in elderly women in the absence of synovitis has been highlighted in several recent reports.[9,10]

Chronic polyarticular gout with tophi can be misdiagnosed as rheumatoid arthritis with rheumatoid nodules, resulting in improper treatment and otherwise preventable disability. To add to the confusion, rheumatoid factor tests are positive in about 30% of patients with tophaceous gout, a finding that relates to the coating of urate crystals by IgG.

The diagnosis of gout can be readily established by the study of synovial fluid or tophaceous material by polarized light microscopy. Needle-shaped negatively birefringent crystals of monosodium urate are seen in 95% of patients with acute gouty arthritis and are a sine qua non for establishing a definitive diagnosis. Hyperuricemia, common in the elderly, is less reliable as a diagnostic test. Furthermore, serum urate level is within normal limits at the time of the acute attack in

7% of the cases. Calcium pyrophosphate dihydrate crystals can coexist with urate crystals, and isolated cases of bacterial arthritis superimposed on gouty arthritis have been reported. If the clinical picture is suspicious of a septic joint, synovial fluid must be cultured.

The management of gout in the elderly is guided by the same principles that apply to a younger age group. The acute attack is treated with colchicine or one of the nonsteroidal antiinflammatory drugs (NSAIDs). The cautious use of NSAIDs has been discussed under osteoarthritis. A patient with decreased renal function whose gout is precipitated by administration of a diuretic is at risk of developing renal insufficiency if a NSAID is used to treat acute gouty arthritis. Colchicine has a low therapeutic margin and should be administered with caution. It is given in hourly doses of 0.6 mg, for a total of four to eight doses dependent on the patient's physical constitution. The drug must be stopped promptly at the first sign of loose stools to avoid the consequences of dehydration and potassium loss. Renal, hepatic, and myocardial impairment and the presence of cardiac arrhythmias enhance the risk for colchicine toxicity. Colchicine may be administered slowly into a large vein in a dose of 2 mg. Great caution must be exercised to avoid extravasation, which may result in tissue necrosis and sloughing of the skin. Intraarticular injection of corticosteroid is helpful when gout involves an accessible joint. Oral administration of corticosteroids or injection of ACTH is also effective, but because of a tendency of gouty arthritis to rebound, concomitant administration of a maintenance dose of colchicine or a NSAID is necessary.

Drugs to lower serum urate should be initiated once the acute attack has subsided. Since acute gouty arthritis may occur during the initial treatment with a hypouricemic drug, it is advisable to use colchicine prophylactically in a dose of 0.6 mg twice daily for several weeks. Uricosuric drugs are effective as long as the creatinine clearance exceeds 50 ml per minute. Probenecid and sulfinpyrazone are the principal uricosuric drugs. Diflunisal in a dose of 500 mg two times daily is weakly uricosuric and may be worthwhile trying in a patient who also requires an analgesic drug for symptomatic osteoarthritis. Aspirin abolishes the effect of uricosuric drugs and should not be given concomitantly. Allopurinol is the drug of choice in patients with overproduction of uric acid or with significant reduction in renal function, or in those who require continuous treatment with aspirin, diuretics, or other drugs that interfere with the tubular secretion of urate. The dose of allopurinol in elderly patients with diminished uric acid excretion is smaller than in overproducers of uric acid. The goal is to prescribe the lowest dose of allopurinol that will maintain serum urate between 5 and 6 mg/dl. Frequently 100 or 200 mg allopurinol given in a single morning dose will suffice. Serious toxicity includes agranulocytosis, granulomatous hepatitis and exfoliative dermatitis. Many cases of prolonged hypersensitivity reactions characterized by an erythematous maculopapular rash, eosinophilia, fever, liver function abnormalities, and progressive renal failure have been recorded. Another concern in using allopurinol is the observation of an increased incidence of severe hypersensitivity reactions from coadministered drugs, eg, penicillin and ampicillin.

Calcium Pyrophosphate Dihydrate Deposition Disease

Calcium pyrophosphate dihydrate (CPPD) causes the most common crystal-associated arthritis in the elderly. In 1962, McCarty reported an acute arthritis mimicking gout, and therefore termed pseudogout, in elderly patients with chondrocalcinosis. He further identified the crystals in synovial fluid and cartilage as calcium pyrophosphate dihydrate ($Ca_2P_2O_7,2H_2O$). Metabolic conditions that predispose to calcium pyrophosphate crystal deposition include hyperparathyroidism, hypothyroidism, hypophosphatasia, hypomagnesemia, hemochromatosis, ochronosis, gout, Wilson's disease, and senile amyloidosis. The idiopathic or sporadic form is by far the most common type of CPPD deposition disease. The prevalence increases in stepwise fashion with age. It is rare before age 50, but increases from 10 to 15% in those aged 65 to 75 to 30 to 60% in those over 85 years. Ellman[11] studied the prevalence of knee chondrocalcinosis in hospital and clinic patients older than 50 years and found an overall prevalence of 9.6%. In a representative sample of 79-year-olds in Gothenburg, radiographic evidence of chondrocalcinosis in knees and/or hands was present in 16%.[2]

The majority of patients with chondrocalcinosis are free of symptoms. Radioopaque densities are noted in fibrocartilage (especially menisci, radiocarpal joint, symphysis pubis, shoulders, and hips and in the midzonal layer of hyaline cartilage, giving rise to punctate or linear calcifications (see Figure 16.3).

Acute synovitis, or pseudogout, is the most dramatic clinical manifestation. It presents as an acute monoarthritis, most often located at the knee, but also commonly seen in the wrist, shoulder, or ankle. As in gout, surgery, trauma, or serious medical illness may trigger an acute attack. About 10% of patients have oligoarticular involvement or a migratory pattern involving several joints successively, sometimes over a course of many weeks or months. About half of the symptomatic patients present with clinical and radiographic features that are reminiscent of low-grade osteoarthritis, except

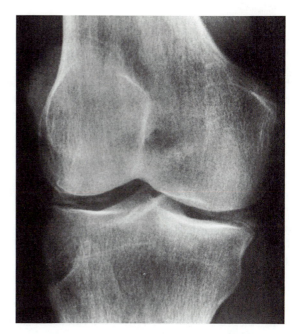

Fig. 16.3. Chondrocalcinosis. Punctate calcifications in menisci and midzonal layer of hyaline cartilage.

that joint involvement is that of pseudogout rather than generalized osteoarthritis. The patients complain of chronic pain and stiffness and restricted movement of the knees, wrists, shoulders, elbows, metacarpophalangeal joints, hips, and ankles. Minor acute attacks may be superimposed on chronic symptoms. Acute and chronic tenosynovitis may be present. Wrist involvement may produce a carpal tunnel syndrome. The chronic polyarticular arthropathy may be confused with rheumatoid arthritis. A number of reports[12] have described a severe destructive arthropathy similar to a Charcot joint and affecting almost exclusively elderly women in association with calcium pyrophosphate deposition, involving the shoulder, elbow, or wrist, in addition to knees or hips. In addition to the typical x-ray findings of calcifications in articular cartilage described above, calcifications may be seen in the joint capsule, synovium, bursae, and in tendons, especially the Achilles, triceps, quadriceps, and supraspinatus tendons.

The diagnosis is confirmed by presence of weakly positively birefringent calcium pyrophosphate crystals in synovial fluid and characteristic radiologic findings. In acute arthritis, polymorphonuclear leukocytes predominate. Total synovial fluid WBC counts range from 4,000 to 50,000 per mm^3. Triclinic, rhomboid crystals are found within leukocytes and extracellularly. In chronic arthritis the leukocyte count is lower and mononuclear cells more numerous. CPPD synovitis is a prevalent disease, and one should always keep in mind the possible coexistence of another joint disease.

Treatment of acute synovitis is with nonsteroidal antiinflammatory drugs, aspiration of joint fluid, and intraarticular injection of corticosteroid. The effect of colchicine is less reliable than in acute gouty arthritis. Chronic CPPD arthritis is managed in much the same way as osteoarthritis. The principles and potential hazards of using NSAIDs have been discussed in the section on osteoarthritis.

Apatite Deposition Disease

Apatite and other basic calcium phosphates, which comprise the mineral phase of bone and teeth, make up the majority of ectopic or extraskeletal calcifications. Ectopic calcifications can be divided into dystrophic types, which occur in tissue that has been injured, and metastatic calcifications, which are related to increased calcium and phosphate concentration. Examples of dystrophic lesions are the calcifications that may occur in scleroderma, dermatomyositis, ochronosis, tophi, and following local injections of corticosteroids. Metastatic calcifications may be seen in hyperparathyroidism, sarcoidosis, and end-stage renal disease managed with chronic hemodialysis.

Idiopathic periarticular apatite deposition occurs commonly in bursae and tendons. More recently, apatite crystals have been found in synovial fluid in a high percentage of patients with osteoarthritis and less often in patients with other types of arthritis. Because of their minute size (75–250 Å in diameter), individual apatite crystals cannot be identified by ordinary or polarized light microscopy. Their precise identification requires electron microscopic techniques, microprobe, or x-ray diffraction analysis.

Apatite crystals can cause acute inflammation of tendons and bursae. The common rotator tendon is one typical site. The etiology of calcific tendinitis is unknown; presumably trauma leads to tissue damage with calcium deposition in the form of hydroxyapatite occurring at the site of tissue injury. In calcific periarthritis the skin is often warm and red over the affected joints; the tissues are boggy and tender, but effusion is absent. Periarthritic calcification is visible on radiographs.

Apatite-containing particles can be found in approximately 30 to 50% of knee effusions from patients with osteoarthritis.[13] Apatite crystals have been shown to have phlogistic properties and have been implicated as a cause of the flares of synovitis seen in osteoarthritis, in which cases there is a tendency to higher synovial fluid cell count and a more severe course.

Apatite-associated destructive arthritis is an unusual form of rapidly progressive destructive osteoarthritis of large joints of elderly patients that is associated with apatite crystals in the synovial fluid. Although the shoulder is a typical site (so-called "Milwaukee shoulder")[14] it is well recognized today that similar destructive changes can occur in other large joints such as the knee, hip, and ankle, and even in small joints. Almost all of the patients with apatite-associated destructive arthritis have been elderly women. Rapid joint destruction leading to instability and large, noninflammatory, often hemorrhagic effusions, containing large amounts of apatite particles and joint detritus, are cardinal clinical features. Radiographs show characteristic changes. Marked attrition of bone and cartilage on both sides of the joint; little or no osteophytosis, subchondral sclerosis, or cyst formation; scalloping pressure defects; and periarticular calcifications are typical findings (see Figure 16-4). The pathogenesis of this destructive arthropathy has not been fully delineated, but activated collagenase and neutral protease play a major role in accelerating chondrolysis and joint destruction.

Other Crystals and Particles

A variety of other birefringent materials may occasionally cause synovitis. Calcium oxalate crystal deposition can be seen in elderly patients with end-stage

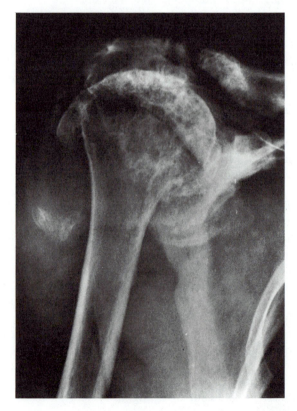

Fig. 16.4. Apatite-associated destructive arthropathy. Radiograph of right shoulder showing upward subluxation of the humeral head, attrition of bone on both sides of the acromioclavicular joint, and soft tissue calcifications.

renal disease who are maintained on chronic hemodialysis. Positively birefringent, bipyramidal, and polymorphic calcium oxalate crystals have been demonstrated in cartilage, synovium, and synovial fluid. Radiographically, deposits in cartilage cannot be distinguished from calcium pyrophosphate deposition. Involvement of metacarpophalangeal and proximal interphalangeal joints are common. Joint disease in chronic renal failure may be associated with either apatite or calcium oxalate deposition.

Cryoglobulins found in essential cryoglobulinemia and multiple myeloma can precipitate in crystalline form in a variety of tissues, including the synovium. Rare cases of cryoglobulin crystal-associated arthritis have been reported. Cholesterol crystals are mainly seen in chronic inflammatory effusions. Crystalline depot corticosteroid preparations may occasionally induce a transient inflammation hours after intraarticular injection (post-injection flare). Corticosteroid crystals can appear as positively or negatively birefringent rods, similar in size to urate or CPPD, as granules, or as irregular debris. Finally, particles of wearing surgical articular implants can be associated with a chronic detritic synovitis in elderly patients who have undergone partial or total joint replacement.

Polymyalgia Rheumatica and Giant Cell Arteritis

Temporal arteritis and polymyalgia rheumatica are closely related diseases in that they affect only the elderly, frequently occur in the same individual, and may produce constitutional symptoms in the form of malaise, fatigue, weight loss, anemia, and elevated levels of acute-phase reactants. Furthermore, in both syndromes, a rapid response to glucocorticoids is seen regularly.

Temporal arteritis and polymyalgia rheumatica are nosological terms used to define typical clinical syndromes, whereas giant cell arteritis denotes a specific pathologic process. The question of the relationship between temporal arteritis and polymyalgia rheumatica is still a valid one. Some consider the two to be syndromes at either end of the spectrum of one disease, with temporal arteritis the more severe and polymyalgia rheumatica the less severe expression of an underlying giant cell arteritis. Others believe that a common etiologic agent produces either a proximal synovitis leading to symptoms of polymyalgia rheumatica, or a giant cell arteritis leading to symptoms of temporal arteritis.

The association of polymyalgia rheumatica with giant cell arteritis is striking. Most series have shown that 40 to 60% of patients with giant cell arteritis have symptoms of polymyalgia rheumatica, which may be the initial presentation in one-third of the patients. Conversely, biopsy of the temporal artery has demonstrated giant cell arteritis in 15 to 30% of patients with polymyalgia rheumatica who had no symptoms or signs of arteritis.

The term polymyalgia rheumatica was coined by Barber in 1957 to describe a syndrome characterized by myalgias and stiffness of the shoulder and pelvic girdles, neck, or torso for a duration of one month or more, accompanied by constitutional symptoms and an elevated erythrocyte sedimentation rate in patients who have no underlying disease to explain the symptoms. The syndrome is extremely rare in patients under the age of 50 years. Despite widespread awareness of the condition in the US, the first report in the American literature did not appear until 1963.

Giant cell arteritis, clinically also known as temporal arteritis or cranial arteritis, is a form of granulomatous vasculitis, typically with presence of giant cells, that most often causes occlusion of the branches of the external and internal carotids, but may involve many medium- and large-sized arteries throughout the body, including the aorta.

Epidemiology

Polymyalgia rheumatica and giant cell arteritis are relatively common diseases in the elderly. Hunder et al.[15,16,17] have conducted epidemiological studies of these entities in Olmstead County, Minnesota, which comprises an urban population in Rochester and a surrounding rural population. The mean annual incidence of polymyalgia rheumatica over a 10-year span (1970–1979) was 53.7 per 100,000 population 50 years of age and older. This may be compared to an incidence of rheumatoid arthritis of 77 per 100,000 in the same age group. The prevalence of polymyalgia rheumatica on January 1, 1980 was estimated at 550 per 100,000 aged 50 and older. The average annual incidence of giant cell arteritis in the period between 1950 and 1983 was 16 per 100,000 population 50 years and over, with a slightly higher figure at 21.7 for the most recent period between 1975 and 1983. The age-specific incidence rate rose from 1.4 per 100,0000 population aged 50 to 59 years, to a maximum of 44.7 per 100,000 population older than 80 years. On January 1, 1984, the prevalence of persons with a history of temporal arteritis was 234 per 100,000 population aged 50 and older. This compares with a prevalence of 135/100,000 population for ankylosing spondylitis in the same community. The incidence rates of polymyalgia rheumatica and giant cell arteritis for women were significantly higher than for men. A prospective epidemiological study[18] conducted recently in Ribe County, Denmark, comprising a population of 200,000, identified 46 new cases of temporal arteritis and polymyalgia rheumatica within one year. The corresponding incidence rate was 76.6 per 100,000 population 50 years and older. Autopsy studies suggest that giant cell arteritis is even more prevalent. In a prospective study,[19] Östberg found giant cell arteritis in 1.6% of 889 postmortem cases in which sections of the temporal arteries and two transverse sections of the aorta were made.

Etiology and Pathogenesis

The cause of polymyalgia rheumatica and giant cell arteritis is not known, nor has its striking prevalence in older people been elucidated. No association with class I HLA antigens has been detected. More recent studies have focused on the role of class II antigens in polymyalgia rheumatica and giant cell arteritis because class II-restricted T helper cells have been found in the wall of affected vessels. In one study,[20] using pooled analysis, HLA-DR4 was significantly increased in patients with giant cell arteritis and polymyalgia rheumatica, but not in patients with giant cell arteritis alone. The association of polymyalgia rheumatica with HLA-DR4 may explain the lower incidence of giant cell arteritis and polymyalgia rheumatica in blacks. This antigen is found in only one-fourth as many blacks as whites. Until recently, temporal arteritis was considered rare in blacks. Our own experience in a hospital that provides medical care for a population about equally divided between blacks and whites conforms to the more recent impression that polymyalgia rheumatica and giant cell arteritis are more common in blacks than had been appreciated previously.

Pathology

The pathologic diagnosis of giant cell arteritis is based on the presence of typical histologic changes in each arterial layer. The changes tend to affect the arteries in a patchy fashion with abnormal segments of the artery interspersed between normal segments. A distinctive fibromyxoid intimal proliferation causing variable degree of luminal compromise with or without thrombus formation is seen in almost all patients. Giant cells are often intimately associated with elastic lamina fragmentation. The media shows patchy degeneration, dropout of smooth muscle cells, and granulomas containing lymphocytes, histiocytes, epithelioid cells, and multinucleated giant cells. Giant cells are not seen in all sections, and their presence is not required to make the diagnosis if the remainder of the histologic findings are characteristic.

Giant cell arteritis has a predilection for the vessels that originate from the arch of the aorta, but involve-

ment of almost every medium and large-sized artery has been reported. The intracranial arteries are involved less often.

In polymyalgia rheumatica, muscle biopsies have been normal or at most have shown nonspecific type II muscle atrophy, but a number of ultrastructural abnormalities have been observed. Arthroscopy and biopsy of shoulder and knee joints have demonstrated synovitis, which, histologically, is characterized by mild inflammation with lymphocytes and a few polymorphonuclear leukocytes, but without evidence of vasculitis. Granulomatous myocarditis and hepatitis have also been reported.

Clinical Picture

The mean age at onset of both giant cell arteritis and polymyalgia rheumatica is about 70 years. Both diseases occur twice as often in women as they do in men. In terms of diagnosis and treatment, it is useful to recognize four patient groups: (1) patients with polymyalgia rheumatica; (2) patients with temporal arteritis; (3) patients with symptoms of both polymyalgia rheumatica and temporal arteritis; and (4) patients without local symptoms of arteritis or muscular symptoms, but with systemic symptoms such as fever, malaise, and weight loss.

The onset of polymyalgia rheumatica usually is insidious, but can be abrupt. The most common symptoms are aches and stiffness involving the proximal muscle girdles and the neck. The discomfort usually extends to the proximal portion of the arms and thighs, and to the axial musculature. The stiffness is prominent in the morning and after prolonged inactivity. Pain is accentuated by movements of the joints. Pain and stiffness may be so incapacitating that the patient cannot get out of bed in the morning without the assistance of another person. Generalized systemic complaints may include low grade fever, night sweats, anorexia, weight loss, and depression.

Physical signs are conspicuously few. Muscular strength is not impaired. Tenderness, when present, is felt mostly around the shoulders. Active range of motion may be limited due to elicitation of pain, but passive motion is normal. Concurrent synovitis is present in 15% of the patients and is most often detectable in the sternoclavicular joint, the acromioclavicular joint, the wrist, and the knee.

Giant cell arteritis is also often insidious in onset and is associated with symptoms and signs that are dictated by the anatomic involvement. Most of the clinical features can be related to vasculitis and occlusion of the cranial branches of arteries originating from the aortic arch. The most common symptom is headache that is usually boring or lancinating in nature. Scalp tenderness along the course of the superficial temporal, posterior auricular, or occipital arteries is a prominent finding. The temporal artery may be swollen and pulseless. Tender nodules are sometimes felt. Rarely, occlusion leads to areas of gangrene of the scalp. Jaw claudication is often considered pathognomonic, but occurs in less than half of the patients. Temporal arteritis may present with unusual manifestations, and the diagnosis should be considered in elderly patients who complain of pain with deglutition, throat or tongue pain, hoarseness, cough, ear pain, or sudden loss of hearing when no obvious cause for these symptoms can be found.

A well recognized and serious complication of giant cell arteritis is ocular involvement, leading to partial or complete visual loss in 15 to 20% of the patients. This is a lower incidence than found in older studies and may reflect earlier recognition and treatment of the disease. Even though the dramatic manifestations of ocular involvement may appear suddenly, most patients have various complaints relating to the eyes for some time before loss of vision occurs, ie, transient blurring and diplopia, ptosis, or other manifestations of ophthalmoplegia. Impaired visual acuity is due to ischemic optic neuritis that is secondary to involvement of the ophthalmic or the posterior ciliary arteries that supply the nerve. Occlusion of the central retinal artery is rarely a cause of blindness in temporal arteritis.

Clinical evidence of involvement of large arteries occurs in 15% of cases. Arteritic lesions of the aorta may lead to aortic valve incompetence or a dissecting aneurysm and rupture of the aorta. Involvement of the large arteries to upper extremities is considerably more common than disease of the legs. Upper extremity claudication, Raynaud's phenomenon, paresthesias, bruits over the large proximal arteries, and decreased or absent pulses and blood pressure are common manifestations. Lower extremity involvement, when it occurs, presents as leg claudication. Visceral manifestations include myocardial infarction, abdominal angina, and neurological symptoms due to vertebral arteritis. Fever and high erythrocyte sedimentation rate in patients with myocardial infarction, cerebrovascular accident, or aortic aneurysm may signal giant cell arteritis.

Instead of the classic symptoms of arteritis, patients may present with prominent constitutional symptoms, such as fever, weight loss, malaise, and depression. In a retrospective study[21] of 100 patients with biopsy-proven temporal arteritis, 15 fulfilled the criteria for fever of unknown origin. In eleven of the fifteen patients, manifestations suggesting giant cell arteritis were eventually recognized, but in four patients the giant cell arteritis was discovered only after a random temporal artery biopsy. Therefore, temporal artery bi-

opsy must be considered strongly in an elderly patient who presents with fever or unexplained anemia. The survival rate for patients with giant cell arteritis is not altered compared with the general population of the same age. However, large artery involvement resulting in a fatal outcome does occur.[22] All patients with giant cell arteritis should be examined carefully for large artery lesions, since early recognition and treatment may prevent arterial occlusion, rupture, and death.

Diagnostic Studies

Polymyalgia rheumatica and giant cell arteritis characteristically are associated with a very high erythrocyte sedimentation rate and elevation of other acute-phase reactants, such as CRP, fibrinogen, platelet count, and complement level. Westergren's sedimentation rate in giant cell arteritis is frequently more than 100 mm in 1 hour. Rare cases of normal sedimentation rate in untreated patients have been reported. A moderate normochromic anemia is a characteristic finding. The leukocyte count is generally normal. Abnormal liver function tests, especially elevation of alkaline phosphatase, are present in one-third of the cases. Various alterations in immunoglobulin profile may be present. Rates of positive rheumatoid factor and antinuclear antibody tests do not differ from those in control populations of elderly patients. The synovial fluid is mildly inflammatory with a cell count between 1,000 and 8,000 per cubic millimeter, of which 40 to 50% are polymorphonuclear leukocytes. Synovial fluid complement level is normal. Technicium 99^m diphosphonate scintigrams show increased uptake in central joints, such as shoulders and hips, in patients with polymyalgia rheumatica.

The diagnosis of giant cell arteritis may be confirmed by superficial temporal artery biopsy, but since this condition is segmental and often has skip areas, it is necessary to remove a 2 to 3 cm segment of the artery and perform serial sections. If the first biopsy is normal, and suspicion of giant cell arteritis remains strong, a contralateral biopsy should be considered. The posterior auricular or the occipital arteries may be chosen for biopsy when tenderness is marked along their distribution. Miniarteriography has been used to locate a suitable area of the temporal artery for biopsy, but the method is nonspecific and inconsistent, and is not advocated for routine use. In patients with aortic arch syndrome, angiographic studies should be performed, especially because temporal artery biopsy is not always diagnostic of giant cell arteritis.

The need for temporal artery biopsy in all cases of polymyalgia is debatable. An acceptable course of action would be to follow carefully without biopsy those patients who show a rapid response to corticosteroid treatment in terms of symptomatic relief and normalization of the sedimentation rate. On the other hand, biopsy should be performed in cases where clinical evidence for giant cell arteritis is present. It is well recognized that symptoms of giant cell arteritis may occur suddenly in a patient who was originally thought to have pure polymyalgia and who is being treated with small doses of prednisone sufficient to control all symptoms of polymyalgia and to normalize the sedimentation rate.

Differential Diagnosis

The differential diagnosis of polymyalgia rheumatica includes other inflammatory and noninflammatory rheumatic diseases, malignant neoplasms, and occult infections. About a quarter of patients with elderly-onset rheumatoid arthritis present with synovitis involving shoulder and hip, absence of rheumatoid nodules, an erythrocyte sedimentation rate greater than 50 mm per hour, and a negative test for rheumatoid factor. This presentation resembles that of polymyalgia rheumatica, and it may not be until later in the course that a clear differentiation between the two can be made. Polymyositis can be distinguished from polymyalgia rheumatica by its characteristic muscular weakness, elevated muscle enzymes, and abnormal electromyogram. An occasional prolonged viremia or chronic bacterial infection, such as subacute bacterial endocarditis, may present with polymyalgia-type symptoms. The elevated sedimentation rate in polymyalgia rheumatica is helpful in differentiating noninflammatory rheumatic diseases, such as fibromyositis, tendinitis, and capsulitis.

The diagnosis of giant cell arteritis is not difficult in the presence of classic symptoms. It is important to keep this diagnosis in mind when an elderly patient presents with fever and marked constitutional symptoms.

Treatment

Pure polymyalgia rheumatica is best treated with 10 to 15 mg prednisone given in the morning. Usually, the patient obtains dramatic, symptomatic relief within a few days. A prompt response to corticosteroids can be regarded as additional confirmation of the diagnosis. In contrast, polymyalgia-like symptoms of a paraneoplastic syndrome respond poorly to corticosteroid treatment. Prednisone dosage should be slowly tapered in relation to symptomatic relief and the decrease in the erythrocyte sedimentation rate. When the 10 mg daily dose level is reached, further reduction should be done in 1-mg decrements. Polymyalgia rheumatica shows considerable variability in its course. There may be two populations of patients, one with a self-limited illness requiring prednisone for 1 to 2 years, and another with a more persistent process requiring long-term therapy. In one study,[23] 40 percent of the patients required treatment for more than 4 years. Relapses accompanied by new elevation of the sedimentation rate are usually caused by too rapid reduction of corticosteroid dosage. In such a situation, prednisone dosage will have to be increased temporarily, and subsequent reductions may have to be made in smaller decrements at longer intervals. Milder cases of polymyalgia rheumatica have been treated with aspirin or nonsteroidal antiinflammatory drugs, but the response has been less dramatic, and many patients initially treated in this way have had to be eventually switched to prednisone.

The manifestations of giant cell arteritis respond favorably to high dose corticosteroid. Treatment should begin with 60 to 80 mg of prednisone in divided daily doses. Constitutional symptoms resolve within 24 to 48 hours after initiation of treatment. Localized symptoms of arteritis usually improve after 2 to 4 weeks. However, visual loss, once it occurs, is rarely reversible. In patients with threatening vascular complications, corticosteroid therapy should be initiated while awaiting arterial biopsy. Changes of inflammation of the arterial wall can be recognized for at least a week after corticosteroid treatment has been started. Once reversible symptoms have subsided and laboratory tests have reverted to normal, the dose of prednisone may be tapered slowly to a maintenance dose of 7.5 to 10 mg daily with careful attention to readjustment of dosage if symptoms recur. Stepwise reduction of the corticosteroid dose should be done in decrements of 10%. Treatment should be continued for at least 2 years. In general, the prognosis is quite good with optimal corticosteroid treatment. Most patients will achieve complete remission that is often maintained after withdrawal of treatment.

Adverse side effects of corticosteroid treatment occur in one third of the patients, including cushingoid appearance, symptomatic vertebral compression fractures, proximal muscle weakness, subcapsular cataracts, and, in patients with diabetes mellitus, increased insulin resistance.

Rheumatoid Arthritis

Rheumatoid arthritis (RA) is the most common type of chronic inflammatory arthritis, estimated to affect more than 6 million Americans or about 3% of the adult population. The etiology of RA is still unknown. A genetic predisposition is strongly suggested because the frequency of HLA-DR4 among seropositive RA patients is about twice that of the general population. The prevailing hypothesis is that an unknown initiating agent causes immunologic reactions and inflammation in the presence of a certain genetic makeup. The peak incidence of rheumatoid arthritis is between the 35th and 45th year, but onset of disease in higher age groups is not infrequent. Several surveys have shown that the incidence of rheumatoid arthritis in the 60 or older age group is 10–20% of the total rheumatoid population. As a result of new cases being added to those carrying residua from prior onset, the prevalence of rheumatoid arthritis rises with age. The prevalence among 537 79-year-olds in Gothenburg, Sweden was 10%. [2] Other surveys have found the prevalence to be even higher.

Clinical Features

The clinical course and prognosis of RA in adults vary widely, ranging from a mild pauciarticular disease to a progressive destructive polyarthritis associated with systemic vasculitis. The pattern is influenced by sex, rapidity of onset, presence of rheumatoid factor, and genetic and endocrine factors. In general, patients whose sera contain high titers of rheumatoid factor fare less well. Abrupt onset portends a more favorable prognosis. Age also is of significance, and when onset occurs before the age of 16 years, the difference in clinical presentation is recognized by its separate classification as juvenile rheumatoid arthritis. Changes in the pattern of disease in old age are less well recognized. Nevertheless, the few studies that have addressed the onset of RA after age 60 have noted a greater frequency of acute onset, systemic symptoms, and large joint involvement, as well as less rheumatoid factor seropositivity, than in younger patients and a better prognosis for seronegative elderly onset rheumatoid arthritis.

Most elderly patients with RA have lived with their disease since youth or middle years. In many cases, the disease is no longer active, and the patient presents with functional deficits from deformities or with symptoms and signs of superimposed osteoarthritis. However, some patients continue to show evidence of active synovitis or they develop serious extraarticular and systemic complications.

When rheumatoid arthritis has its onset after the age of 60, the clinical picture conforms more often than not to the pattern seen in younger patients. Constitutional symptoms such as fatigue, weight loss, and generalized stiffness may precede or accompany the insidious onset of arthritis in the small joints of hands and feet, wrists, and knees. Symmetrical swelling of the 2nd and 3rd metacarpophalangeal joints (MCPs), fusiform swelling of the fingers, and prolonged morning stiffness of the inflamed joints are characteristic. Later, arthritis may spread to involve more central joints. As the disease progresses, erosions of bone of the MCP and PIP joints of the hands, the wrists, and the MTP joints of the feet are visible on radiographic examination (see Figure 16.5). Progressive joint damage leads to the development of characteristic deformities. This presentation is usually associated with rheumatoid factor positivity, and rheumatoid nodules are seen in approximately 25% of the patients. Unlike early onset RA, extraarticular manifestations, particularly vasculitis, are uncommon in RA that has its onset in later years.

At least a quarter of patients with elderly onset RA (EORA) exhibit a clinical picture that is less often seen in younger age groups. This subgroup is characterized by acute and florid onset, early and more severe involvement of large joints, especially the shoulder joint, prominent constitutional symptoms, very high sedimentation rate, and a near equal sex distribution in contrast to the usual 3:1 female preponderance.

The clinical course of EORA has been the subject of three recent studies[24,25,26] that have included a younger onset rheumatoid arthritis (YORA) group for direct comparison. These studies have confirmed earlier observations. When comparing groups with similar disease duration,[26] abrupt onset occurred nearly twice as often in the EORA group. Younger patients were twice as likely to have small joint disease, while elderly patients tended to have more arthritis in hips and shoulders. Patients with EORA had higher initial sedimentation rate and were more likely to be negative for rheumatoid factor. A polymyalgia rheumatica-like presentation was observed in 23% of the EORA group compared with only 5% of the YORA group. Both groups received nearly identical treatment. Patients with EORA had significantly better outcome than younger patients after a disease duration of 2.5 years and at the end of the study some 5 years after the disease onset. These outcome differences persisted when patients with polymyalgia-like presentations were excluded from the analysis.

A syndrome of remitting seronegative symmetrical synovitis with pitting edema, believed to represent a distinct subset of seronegative RA, was reported recently by McCarty et al.[27] This syndrome, which has a predilection for elderly persons, is characterized by sudden onset of symmetrical synovitis of peripheral joints and flexor tendons associated with pitting edema of the dorsum of hands and feet. Rheumatoid factors were consistently absent and radiologically evident erosions did not develop. Leukocyte counts of joint fluid were low relative to those found in seropositive RA. A benign course with complete remission from 3 to 36 months after onset was observed in all cases.

A case[28] of adult onset juvenile RA in a 70-year-old women who presented with a 2-year history of quo-

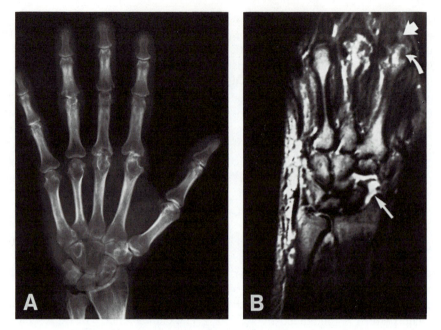

Fig. 16.5. Rheumatoid arthritis. *A.* Fine-detail radiograph showing marginal erosions of the ulnar styloid, the second and third metacarpal heads, and distal aspect of the second, third, and fourth interphalangeal joints. *B.* Magnetic resonance imaging of the same hand showing erosion (curved arrow), proliferating synovium (thick arrow), and synovial fluid accumulation (thin arrow).

tidian fever, rash, pleuritis, and mild joint manifestations suggests that this entity is not limited to young adults, but occasionally may have its debut at an advanced age.

Laboratory Diagnosis

A normocytic, normo- or hypochromic anemia, elevated erythrocyte sedimentation rate, and increases in alpha$_2$ and gamma globulin represent nonspecific features associated with inflammation.

Approximately 75% of adult patients with RA have circulating rheumatoid factors in their sera. In the clinical laboratory, rheumatoid factors are detected by agglutination procedures that use sheep red blood cells sensitized with rabbit anti-sheep cell antibodies or latex particles coated with human IgG on their surface. The sensitized sheep cell test is more specific for RA. A positive test does not necessarily imply that the patient has RA, since rheumatoid factors may also be found in other diseases that have chronic antigenic stimulation as a common denominator. Depending on the sensitivity of the test procedure used, rheumatoid factors are found in 1 to 5% of normal subjects, the incidence increasing with advanced age. The latex fixation test especially may be positive in a low titer in a high proportion of elderly individuals without rheumatoid disease, and there is general agreement that this test is less useful as a diagnostic indicator in elderly patients. As mentioned earlier, EORA has a higher frequency of rheumatoid factor negativity than RA in earlier life.

HLA-DR4, a B lymphocyte-related antigen, has been shown to be associated with seropositive rheumatoid arthritis. In contradistinction, no association has been found between this genetic marker and seronegative rheumatoid arthritis.

Differential Diagnosis

RA, when it occurs in its typical form, rarely presents a problem in diagnosis. The difficulties lie in distinguishing seronegative RA from other seronegative arthritides that meet the American Rheumatism Association's 1958 criteria for a diagnosis of definite rheumatoid arthritis. This set of criteria has formed the basis for classification of RA in clinical studies during the past 30 years. Quite recently, the ARA has proposed revised criteria (ARA 1987)[29] which differ from the old ones by eliminating pain and tenderness and by stressing swelling of three or more joint regions, with special emphasis on wrists, MCP, and PIP joints. The classification of RA into classical, definite, and probable categories has been abolished. A consequence of the revised criteria is that some patients who meet the 1958 criteria do not satisfy the 1987 criteria and vice versa.

When a patient presents with constitutional symptoms, marked shoulder synovitis and a high ESR, it is often difficult to differentiate polymyalgia rheumatica (PMR) from EORA. The two diseases have many manifestations in common. PMR is actually an axial synovitis, primarily of hips and shoulders, but peripheral synovitis is seen in a third of the patients, most frequently involving knees, wrists, carpal tunnels, and metacarpophalangeal joints. It is not surprising, therefore, that the literature contains many reports of patients who after an initial diagnosis of PMR, months or years later develop small joint involvement typical of rheumatoid arthritis.

Amyloid arthropathy may be mistaken for RA. Amyloid of the primary variety and that which occurs in association with multiple myeloma may infiltrate the synovium of joints and periarticular structures, causing joint swelling and sometimes a carpal tunnel syndrome. Prolonged stiffness is not a feature of amyloid arthritis. Other conditions that need to be excluded include erosive osteoarthritis of the hands, polyarticular gout and other crystal diseases, and cancer-related syndromes, including pulmonary osteoarthropathy.

The discussion of EORA would not be complete without making reference to an ongoing debate over the validity of seronegative RA as a clinical diagnosis. The lack of an increase in frequency of HLA-DR4 in seronegative RA raises the question whether seronegative RA represents an immunologic subset in the broader spectrum of clinical RA, which includes the seropositive form, or whether it represents a separate immunogenetic disease. The issue is further complicated because special methods of detecting rheumatoid factors have uncovered hidden* rheumatoid factors in a high proportion of seronegative juvenile R.A. and in a few adult patients who test negative by agglutination assays. It has been further argued that seronegative RA represents a group of syndromes. This notion grew out of the experience with HLA-B27 testing, which led to reclassification of several syndromes previously believed to be ''rheumatoid arthritis variants'' as genetically distinct seronegative types of arthritis that are closely associated with HLA-B27. Remitting seronegative symmetric synovitis with pitting edema, which is strongly associated with HLA-B7, may represent a separate entity. Similarly, at least a portion of the subgroup of EORA presenting with prominent constitutional symptoms, shoulder arthritis, and high ESR may in fact be the synovitis of polymyalgia rheumatica or a related inflammatory syndrome. With increasing knowledge of the correlation of genetic markers with various arthritis syndromes one may expect that subsets of patients with conditions currently diagnosed as seronegative RA will become better defined and differentiated from seropositive disease. On the basis of our present knowledge, the clinical concept of seronegative RA is justified when the clinical findings are

otherwise typical of rheumatoid arthritis. The existence of true seronegative RA will not be definitively understood until the causes of RA and similar syndromes are identified.

Treatment

The treatment of RA arising de novo in the elderly follows the same guidelines as in younger patients. The main objectives are to reduce or suppress inflammation, relieve pain, and preserve muscle and joint function. Appropriate drug treatment in concert with systemic and local rest, good nutrition, physical and occupational therapy, use of appropriate appliances and special equipment, and orthopedic evaluation and corrective surgery are the mainstays of the management program. Every patient with RA should have a physical exercise program tailored for optimum activity and rest. Patients must learn that both excessive rest and excessive exercise can lead to increased joint stress. Prescribed individual exercises alternating with specific rest periods are required to maintain good muscle tone and avoid fatigue.

Drug Treatment

A patient with new onset rheumatoid arthritis should be started on aspirin or one of the newer nonsteroidal antiinflammatory drugs. The cautious use of these drugs has been discussed under osteoarthritis. Many elderly do not tolerate aspirin in the doses required for its anti-inflammatory effect as well as do younger patients. Patients with presbycusis may experience a further reduction in hearing ability without developing tinnitus. Gastrointestinal bleeding from erosive gastritis or a frank ulcer may have serious pathophysiological consequences in the elderly, who tolerate blood loss poorly.

Patients who develop erosive disease are candidates for more aggressive therapy. Most patients who develop erosions do so within 2 years of onset of joint symptoms. It is important to identify these patients in a very early stage so that proper therapy can be initiated. The indications for commencing disease modifying antirheumatic drugs (DMARDs) are not different in elderly patients. Experience to date suggests that DMARDs are as effective in the older age groups as in younger patients, but that elderly are at increased risk of developing adverse effects—in part as a consequence of altered pharmacokinetics and reduced functional reserve of organ systems. The most commonly used DMARDs are hydroxychloroquine, gold salts, D-penicillamine, azathioprine, and sulfasalazine.

Sulfasalazine, a drug commonly used to treat inflammatory bowel disease, has been recently approved by the FDA for use in rheumatoid arthritis. Because of

---

*Rheumatoid factor activity is hidden in routine assays due to avid binding of autologous IgG to IgM-rheumatoid facor, but becomes detectable upon complex dissociation under mildly acidic conditions.

its convenience, relative safety, and fairly rapid onset of action, sulfasalazine is an appropriate choice for early and mild cases of RA before use of other DMARDs. The starting dose is one or two 500 mg-tablets daily for the first month. The dose is raised by 500 mg each month, administered twice daily, up to a maintenance dose of 3 g. Within a few weeks, there is generally some indication of tolerance and efficacy. Most studies have shown that sulfasalazine suppresses rheumatoid inflammation to a degree comparable with standard DMARDs. Adverse reactions are frequent, but rarely serious or life-threatening. Gastrointestinal side effects, skin rash, fever, cytopenias, and hemolytic anemia or methemoglobinemia are the most common drug complications and result in discontinuation of treatment in about one quarter of the patients. Blood counts should be done biweekly for the first 3 months and monthly thereafter.

There is no contraindication to the use of hydroxychloroquine in the elderly. A careful eye examination, including visual field testing, must be performed prior to initiating treatment to exclude macular degeneration. The retinopathy of antimalarials is similar in appearance to macular degeneration, both causing loss of central acuity. The recommended dose of hydroxychloroquine is 200 mg daily. Follow-up examination of visual fields should be performed every 4 to 6 months.

Gold salts—the standard-bearer among DMARDs—have been used parenterally since 1929, and more recently auranofin, an oral gold preparation, has become available. Gold therapy suppresses inflammation and slows progression of the disease, as measured radiologically. The principles of intramuscular administration of gold salts are the same as those that apply to younger patients. It is now standard to continue treatment beyond a total dose of 1 g given over a course of some 20 weeks. The frequency of gold injections is gradually tapered to every 4th week. There is no specific time limit to gold therapy and many patients have been on continuous gold therapy for many years. Some studies have suggested that bone-marrow toxicity occurs more often with advancing age, but this has not been substantiated in others. Side effects are quite common, necessitating discontinuation of treatment in one third of the patients. Blood counts and urinalysis should be performed prior to each injection. The usual dose of auranofin is 6 mg daily. Adverse drug reactions of oral gold therapy are similar to those observed with parenteral preparations. In addition, gastrointestinal complaints, especially diarrhea, are quite common.

Penicillamine has efficacy and toxicity similar to injectable gold compounds. Kean et al.[30] found that elderly patients responded to the drug as well as younger patients with RA, with an overall response rate of 75% in both groups. For the elderly rheumatoid patient,

they recommend that D-penicillamine dosage be started at 250 mg/day and increased to 500 mg/day after 2 months. If favorable response is observed at this dosage, no further increase is recommended. The most common adverse drug reactions are rash, taste abnormalities, proteinuria, thrombocytopenia, gastrointestinal intolerance, mouth ulcers, and leukopenia. Rare side effects include myasthenia gravis, drug-induced SLE, and pemphigus. In the study by Kean, skin involvement, in the form of rash or pemphigoid-like reactions and abnormal taste sensation was significantly more common in the elderly compared with the younger group, but the incidence of other side effects was not markedly different.

Azathioprine should be restricted to patients with severe, active, and erosive disease that has not responded to other DMARDs. The initial dose should be approximately 1.0 mg/kg. Therapeutic response usually occurs after 6 to 8 weeks of treatment. The dose may be increased after several weeks, if there are no toxicities and the initial response is suboptimal. Dose increments should be 0.5 mg/kg daily up to a maximum dose of 2.5 mg/kg/day. Patients not improved after 12 weeks can be considered refractory. The drug may be continued long-term in patients with clinical response, but patients should be monitored carefully, and gradual dosage reduction should be attempted to reduce risk of toxicities. The principal and potentially serious side effects of azathioprine are hematologic and gastrointestinal.

Methotrexate is gaining widespread use as an immunosuppressive drug in various rheumatic diseases, particularly psoriatic arthritis, dermatomyositis, and more recently rheumatoid arthritis. Spectacular remission of active erosive disease has been obtained with a dose of 7.5 to 10 mg per week. Methotrexate has recently been approved by the FDA for use in rheumatoid arthritis.

The use of high dose corticosteroids administered orally or parenterally in RA can be life-saving in elderly patients with serious systemic complications such as vasculitis. In smaller doses, corticosteroids are helpful in maintaining mobility and reducing long-term disability. This beneficial effect of corticosteroids is particularly useful in the elderly who may have other conditions affecting ambulation and for whom superimposed RA might become the final event leading to a sedentary existence. The ability to remain ambulatory and active will more than offset the risk of osteoporosis and compression fracture due to steroid therapy. From a purely practical standpoint, the ease of administration, low cost, and relative safety of low doses make corticosteroids a reasonable alternative for the elderly with persistent disabling systemic manifestations refractory to other therapeutic modalities. The recommended dose is 5 to 10 mg of prednisone given once daily in the morning. Alternate-day regimens are not effective in RA because symptoms often are too pronounced on the "off" days. Prednisone also is useful as a therapeutic bridge between the first-line drugs, such as aspirin and other nonsteroidal antiinflammatory drugs, and the second-line DMARDs, which may not become effective for several months. Finally, it is reasonable to treat the subgroup of elderly onset RA with constitutional symptoms and proximal joint involvement in the same way as one would polymyalgia rheumatica, ie, an initial dose of prednisone of 10 to 15 mg/day. As constitutional symptoms subside and the ESR falls, prednisone is tapered slowly to the lowest dose that will control symptoms. Although not proven to be of benefit, many recommend supplemental vitamin D (50,000 units once weekly) and supplemental calcium (1 g/day of elemental calcium). The side effects of corticosteroids are legion. Adverse reactions that pertain particularly to the elderly include compression fractures, osteonecrosis, skin changes of steroid atrophy and purpura, electrolyte disturbances and fluid retention, glaucoma, and increased risk of sepsis.

Intraarticular injection of "depot" corticosteroids is a useful adjunct for synovitis limited to a few joints. Repeat injections into the same joint can be associated with necrosis and collapse of bone. For this reason, injections into a single joint should be spaced not less than 6 months apart, and no joint should be injected more than five times.

Prognosis

Rheumatoid arthritis is not thought of as a fatal disease. Nonetheless, rheumatoid patients have a reduced life expectancy. The shortened survival is restricted to patients with more severe disease. Most patients die from the same causes as the general population, though at an earlier age. Rheumatoid patients have an increased susceptibility to bacterial infections. The mortality from malignancy and cardiovascular disease is the same as in the general population. In a carefully conducted study of more than 1,000 patients with rheumatoid arthritis in the Canadian province of Saskatchewan, Mitchell et al[31] identified 233 deaths over a mean period of 12 years, 79 more than expected in a matched control population. Survival in rheumatoid arthritis was diminished by 4 years in men and 10 years in women. Of the 79 excess deaths, 18 were caused by infection, particularly pneumonia and sepsis. Twenty were directly related to rheumatoid arthritis, including vasculitis, rheumatoid lung disease, and cervical subluxation, while eight could be attributed to complications of drug therapy, mainly gastrointestinal bleeding and perforation. Only one

death was due to drug-induced blood dyscrasia. Amyloidosis and renal failure appear to cause death in rheumatoid arthritis patients four to five times more frequently in Finland than in North America.[32]

Systemic Lupus Erythematosus

Systemic lupus erythematosus (SLE) is a chronic inflammatory disease of unknown etiology with a wide spectrum of both clinical and serologic manifestations. A greater clinical awareness combined with wider use of laboratory techniques to identify characteristic autoantibodies have enlarged the diagnostic spectrum of SLE. In unselected series, elderly onset SLE comprises from 6 to 18% of the SLE populations; yet, SLE is often not considered in the differential diagnosis of a debilitating illness in elderly patients.

Several studies[33-37] dealing with "late-onset" SLE" have addressed age-related differences in the clinical picture at onset, course, survival, and serological characteristics. In these studies, the division between "old" and "young" was set at either 50 or 55 years, defined either as onset of symptoms or time of clinical diagnosis. Difficulties in comparing these series arise from differences in geographic region, racial distribution, age-related entry, and case selection of a relatively small number of patients in each study. Despite these variances, on examining the data collectively there is convincing evidence that age modifies the clinical expression of SLE.

Most studies indicate that female predominance is less marked in elderly patients. One study[38] found that the sex ratio between women and men was 2:1 in the older age-group compared to 7:1 in younger patients. The mean age at diagnosis was almost 10 years higher for white men than for white women, and almost one-half of white men were diagnosed at age 55 and later. This difference in age of onset is felt to be related to hormonal factors. The clinical onset is usually more insidious than in younger patients. In one series,[35] the interval from onset of symptoms to time of diagnosis was 4 years when SLE developed after age 55 compared to 2 years in the younger age group.

Age also influences the pattern of organ involvement. Severe renal disease; neurological complications; mesenteric vasculitis; cutaneous vasculitis; Raynaud's phenomenon; and alopecia are far less common in the older group, while polyserositis, especially as a presenting syndrome; interstitial lung disease; and peripheral neuropathy occur more commonly. Some authors have likened the expression of SLE in the elderly to the clinical picture of drug-induced lupus. Two studies[35,36] have identified increased frequency of secondary Sjögren's syndrome and of antibodies to Ro(SS-A) and La(SS-B) in white patients with late-onset SLE. These antibodies are found in approximately one-third of patients with SLE and in a much higher percentage of patients with primary Sjögren's syndrome. Cattogio et al[35] found that 38% of the patients who developed SLE after age 55 developed keratoconjunctivitis sicca; 88% had anti-Ro antibodies and 62% had anti-La antibodies compared to only 36% in younger patients.

Several reports have emphasized that late onset SLE represents an overall milder disease than that seen in patients with early onset disease. This impression is partly based on the reduced steroid requirement in patients with older-onset SLE and the longer time lag between onset of symptoms and diagnosis. The perception of SLE being a benign disease in older individuals may have to be revised in view of recent data on the survival in SLE. Thus, Studenski et al[38] could not show evidence of improved outcome with age. These authors examined the effects of age, race, sex, and socioeconomic status on clinical outcome and survival in 411 patients with SLE, almost equally divided between whites and blacks, utilizing multivariate analytic techniques. Black race and low economic status had independent negative effects on survival. The authors suggest that previously reported findings of improved survival rate with age may have been confounded by racial differences in age and mortality; viz., if younger groups were heavily weighted with blacks, and older age groups were weighted with whites, age would appear, incorrectly, to be related to improved survival in pooled groups.

Laboratory Diagnosis

Antinuclear antibodies (ANA) are present in almost all patients with SLE. Antibodies to nuclear material may react with nucleoprotein, denatured and native DNA, Smith antigen, nuclear RNP, Ro and La antigens, and histones and other basic proteins. Antibodies to nucleoproteins react with the entire nuclear substance, and when fluorescent methods are used to demonstrate these antibodies, nuclei stain in a homogenous pattern. This pattern is the most common one, but it is also the least specific. It can be demonstrated in 70% of patients with connective tissue diseases, in an assortment of other clinical entities, and in a low titer in about one-third of all "normal" elderly persons. Antibodies to double stranded DNA and the Smith antigen are of great importance in the diagnosis of SLE. Since antibodies to Ro and La are found with high frequency in elderly onset SLE they become useful in the diagnosis as well, although they cannot serologically distinguish SLE from primary Sjögren's syndrome. Antibodies to

double-stranded DNA and to Ro and La are not a feature of antibodies that occur with increased frequency in the normal elderly population. Some studies have reported a lower frequency of antibodies to dsDNA in elderly patients with SLE, but this has not been substantiated in other studies. Hypocomplementemia is more common in younger patients with SLE.

HLA-DR2 and DR3 are weakly associated with SLE, HLA-DR2 occurring more frequently in young onset SLE than in older-age onset, and DR3 showing the reverse relationship. Further analysis has shown that the association between HLA phenotypes and antibodies to Ro and La are stronger than HLA correlations with SLE itself.[36] In fact, when Ro and La antibody populations were removed from a group of 113 white SLE patients, the frequency of HLA-DR2 and DR3 were similar to that in normal Caucasians.

Drug-Induced Lupus

In contrast to idiopathic SLE, the incidence of drug-induced lupus (DIL) increases with age, in part reflecting the increased usage in the elderly of drugs that can produce a lupus-like syndrome. It is estimated that about 50,000 cases, or 10% of all patients with SLE, are drug-related. In the United States symptomatic DIL is rare among blacks. At this writing, some 50 drugs have been reported to be associated with drug-induced autoimmunity or symptomatic lupus. Drug-induced autoimmunity refers to induction of ANA which is much more common than symptomatic DIL. Two categories of drugs can be recognized: an unambiguous group that includes procainamide, hydralazine, phenytoin, quinidine, isoniazid, methyldopa and chlorpromazine; and an ambiguous group of drugs for which anecdotal reporting has suggested a possible association. Procainamide and hydralazine pose the greatest risk of inducing both ANA and DIL. Use of procainamide will cause positive ANA in 80 percent of the patients. About a quarter of this group will manifest clinical symptoms. Women are at greater risk of developing procainamide and hydralazine-induced lupus. The male-to-female ratio of 2:1 in symptomatic procainamide-treated patients is accounted for by the disproportionate use of procainamide in men. Approximately one-fifth of patients treated with isoniazid, methyldopa, or chloropromazine develop positive ANA during treatment, but the incidence of a lupus-like syndrome induced by these drugs is less than 1%.

In order to make a diagnosis of DIL, it is necessary to exclude preexisting SLE. Symptoms typically occur after several months or years of drug therapy. ANA are invariably present. Following withdrawal of the offending drug, there should be rapid improvement in the clinical symptoms and a gradual fall in the antinuclear antibodies. The most common features of DIL include fever, myalgias, arthralgias, and polyserositis. CNS and renal involvement is highly unusual. Severe cytopenias, butterfly rash, discoid lesions, and mucosal ulcerations are observed less often than in idiopathic SLE. A strong association between acetylator phenotype and the incidence of autoantibodies and DIL has been noted for procainamide and hydralazine. ANA appear more quickly in slow acetylators, and clinical symptoms occur earlier and predominantly in patients with this phenotype. However, slow acetylator phenotype is not a general predisposing factor underlying autoimmunity as indicated by a lack of association between acetylator phenotype and induction of ANA by isoniazid or by captopril as well as in idiopathic SLE.

The major laboratory abnormalities in DIL are ANA, which are antihistone antibodies and are responsible for the positive LE cell phenomenon, and deoxyribonucleoprotein binding. Different drugs are associated with different antihistone profiles. Antibodies to denatured DNA are seen less often. Antibodies to native, double stranded DNA are not seen in procainamide or hydralazine-induced lupus, but they may occasionally be present in DIL induced by quinidine, penicillamine, and captopril. Hypocomplementemia is rare in DIL, but in vivo complement activation can often be detected by measuring the cleavage products of C4.

Other Connective Tissue Diseases

Dermatomyositis/polymyositis, progressive systemic sclerosis, and polyarteritis nodosa have their peak onset earlier in life, but may occur in the older age group. There are no data in the literature to support age-related modulation of the clinical expression of these diseases.

Dermatomyositis and *polymyositis* have long been considered to be accompanied by a higher incidence of malignancy than in the general population. The association is stronger with dermatomyositis than polymyositis, and it increases with age. In the Veterans Administration Hospital system's survey, based on discharges during 1963–1968, there were 141 definite or probable cases of dermatomyositis/polymyositis. Dividing the cases into 21 to 40, 41 to 60, and 61 to 80 age groups, cancers were present, respectively, in 5.4, 15.1, and 41.9% of the cases. The highest association was between dermatomyositis and cancer in the 51 to 70 age group: 16 of 32 cases, ie 50%.[39] No unusual concentration of one type of cancer has been observed. The most common tumor types associated with dermatomyositis are breast, lung, ovary, colon, stomach, and uterus in that order. The temporal relationship of ma-

lignancy and myositis is such that in about one-third of the cases myositis precedes the tumor by several years, in one-third they occur concomitantly, and in one-third myositis follows tumor by many years. Concurrent beginning, improvement of dermatomyositis with tumor therapy, and relapse with recurrence of the tumor suggest a causal relationship. Since the association of dermatomyositis and cancer is high in the elderly, a search for cancer is justified in this age group. The most common malignancies occur in areas that can be evaluated by physical examination or fairly simple radiologic procedures such as chest x-ray and mammography. Finally, a lack of response of myositis to treatment with prednisone or other modalities should result in a more extensive search for malignancy.

Sjögren's syndrome has been estimated to be the second commonest autoimmune rheumatic disease, affecting about 2% of the adult population. This disorder may occur alone (primary Sjögren's syndrome) or in association with other autoimmune diseases, primarily rheumatoid arthritis and systemic lupus erythematosus. Secondary Sjögren's syndrome parallels the age distribution of the associated diseases, while primary Sjögren's syndrome predominates in the older age group. More than 90% of the patients are women. Age does not modify the clinical picture.

The clinical hallmark is the sicca syndrome (keratoconjunctivitis and xerostomia). The underlying process is a lymphocyte-mediated destruction of exocrine glands that leads to diminished or absent glandular secretions and mucosal dryness. In addition to lacrimal and salivary glands, other exocrine glands may be affected. Involvement of the upper and lower respiratory tract leads to dry nose, throat, and trachea, clinically presenting as chronic nonproductive cough and hoarseness. Upper gastrointestinal involvement may cause dysphagia, and atrophic gastritis with achlorhydria. Vaginal involvement causes dyspareunia and pruritus. Dry skin due to immunologic injury of the exocrine glands of the skin is a common complaint.

In about a quarter of the patients, there is evidence of extension of lymphoproliferation to extraglandular sites, such as lymph nodes, lung, kidney, the central nervous system, and bone marrow. The lymphoid infiltrates may be benign or malignant. The term pseudolymphoma describes tumor-like clusters of lymphoid cells that do not meet the histologic criteria for malignancy. In the kidney, the histopathologic lesion is interstitial lymphocytic infiltration with tubular atrophy and fibrosis, which clinically presents as hyposthenuria and renal tubular acidosis. Involvement of the lungs leads to diffuse interstitial pneumonitis or fibrosis. In patients with primary Sjögren's syndrome a nondeforming or nonerosive polyarthritis and Raynaud's phenomenon are the most common extraglandular manifestations. Within the last few years, it has been pointed out that many patients with primary Sjögren's syndrome frequently have involvement of the central nervous system.[40,41] The neuropsychiatric manifestations are protean. Sensory changes are the most common, followed by spasticity, optic neuritis, cerebellar ataxia, hemiplegia, and cranial neuropathy. Spinal cord involvement can result in neurogenic bladder and paraparesis secondary to transverse myelitis or chronic progressive myelopathy. Psychiatric disturbances, such as depression, hysterical symptoms, and cognitive dysfunction, are frequently associated with neurologic abnormalities, suggesting an organic basis for psychiatric dysfunction. Neurologic events may be transient and self-limited initially, but later on, they tend to become fixed. The neurologic findings may closely resemble those of multiple sclerosis. The cerebrospinal fluid findings include a mild mononuclear cell pleocytosis, elevated total protein and IgG, and oligoclonal bands on agarose gel electrophoresis. In contrast to multiple sclerosis, which usually has between two and ten bands, patients with Sjögrens syndrome generally have only one or two bands. Peripheral nerve involvement in the form of motor and sensory polyneuropathy or entrapment neuropathy occurs in 40% of patients with CNS disease.

About 20% of patients with primary Sjögren's syndrome develop vasculitis, which presents with purpura and other cutaneous manifestations, myositis, or mononeuritis multiplex. Histopathologic studies have shown this to be a mononuclear cell or less often a neutrophilic vasculitis. A strong association exists between vasculitis and active CNS disease. An immune complex glomerulonephritis has also been reported.

The risk of lymphoma in the Sjögren syndrome population is 6.4 cases per 100 cases per year, or 44 times greater than the expected incidence in the general population.

Common laboratory findings include polyclonal hypergammaglobulinemia, positive rheumatoid factor, and antinuclear antibodies that on fluorescent staining yield a homogenous or speckled pattern. The incidence of anti-Ro(SS-A) and anti-La(SS-B) antibodies is very high and serves as a reliable diagnostic marker for Sjögren's syndrome in its primary form or when it occurs in association with systemic lupus erythematosus. Less often seen are circulating immune complexes, cryoglobulins, cold agglutinins, antisalivary duct antibodies and hypocomplementemia. A Coomb's positive autoimmune hemolytic anemia has been reported. Mild anemia and leukopenia are common findings, but thrombocytopenia is unusual. Patients with primary Sjögren's syndrome do not have antibodies directed against Sm antigen, nuclear ribonucleoprotein, or native DNA.

Xerostomia is a fairly common symptom in otherwise healthy elderly women. Definite sicca syndrome occurs in 3.5% of women and 2.8% of men over the age of 80 years. The absence of autoantibodies suggests that senile atrophy of exocrine glands rather than immunological injury is the etiologic basis for sicca complaints.

Extraglandular manifestations may dominate the clinical picture although subclinical inflammation of the salivary glands always can be documented. The Schirmer test, rose bengal or fluorescein staining to document filamentary keratitis, measurements of salivary flow rates, and lower lip biopsy are important diagnostic aids in the sicca syndrome. The characteristic serologic profile assists in confirming the diagnosis.

Sjögren's syndrome occurs more commonly than estimated previously. This diagnosis should be considered in elderly patients with unexplained neuropsychiatric dysfunction, interstitial lung disease, and polyarthritis. Patients with Sjögren's syndrome can fall anywhere along a spectrum ranging from benign sicca syndrome with local disease of exocrine glands to extracellular spread of benign lymphoproliferation and symptoms secondary to various organ involvement to frank lymphoreticular malignancy.

Local measures for relief of sicca symptoms include artificial tears for keratoconjunctivitis, oral lubricants containing a carboxymethyl cellulose base (Xerolube, Saliva Substitute), and K-Y jelly for sicca vaginitis. Early recognition of extraglandular involvement is important, since prompt institution of treatment with prednisone frequently leads to symptomatic improvement or stabilization.

Amyloidosis

Amyloidosis is a syndrome characterized by extracellular deposits of insoluble proteinaceous amyloid fibrils in tissues that result in pressure atrophy with dysfunction of the affected organs. Despite their very different protein components, all amyloid deposits have the following in common: fibrillar structure when examined by electron microscopy; a green birefringence when observed with Congo red stain under polarization microscopy; and an unusual beta pleated structure when examined by x-ray diffraction. The modern classification of amyloidosis is based on the biochemical composition of the amyloid fibrils. The fibrils of primary amyloidosis and of amyloidosis associated with multiple myeloma consist of portions of immunoglobulin light chains and are called AL. Amyloid deposits of secondary amyloidosis associated with chronic inflammatory and infectious diseases show immunochemical homology with portions of the acute-phase reactant serum amyloid A and are called AA. In some of the familial forms of amyloidosis, AF, the fibrils are immunologically identical to prealbumin. Several different types of senile amyloid found in the heart and brains of elderly patients are designated AS. Amyloid deposits of endocrine origin, AEO, occurring in or adjacent to endocrine glands, are closely related to polypeptide hormones, their precursors or breakdown products.

Amyloidosis is relevant to rheumatic disease because it occurs as a potentially fatal complication of longstanding chronic inflammatory disease, such as rheumatoid arthritis; or amyloid may be deposited in periarticular and synovial tissues causing joint pain and restricted motion.

In secondary amyloidosis, deposits of amyloid AA accumulate predominantly in kidneys, spleen, adrenal gland, and liver, resulting in dysfunction of the organs. Death as a consequence of amyloidosis complicating rheumatoid arthritis is not uncommon in Europe. Although this type of amyloidosis is found at postmortem examination in 10% of RA cases in the United States, it is rarely of clinical significance.

Amyloid arthropathy is caused by deposition of amyloid AL, and occurs, therefore, in multiple myeloma and in a disorder of immunoglobulin, previously known as primary amyloidosis. Amyloid arthropathy can affect any joint. Small and large joints are involved with equal frequency. When the small joints are involved, amyloidosis can be easily mistaken for rheumatoid arthritis, but joint inflammation is less conspicuous and the swelling distinctly firmer on palpation. Flexion contractures of the hand joints may appear early in the illness. Subcutaneous amyloid deposits may be mistaken for rheumatoid nodules. Amyloid arthropathy may present as massive deposition at an isolated site; an example is the so-called Hercules look in which amyloid deposition in or around the shoulder joint produces the characteristic "shoulder pad sign." Occasionally, amyloidosis results in punched-out lytic lesions in bone; large tumefactions in bone may be complicated by pathological fractures.

Synovial fluid analysis reveals a non-inflammatory fluid with mononuclear cells predominating. Examination of centrifuged Congo red-stained sediment from synovial fluid under polarization microscopy may reveal the typical apple green birefringence of amyloid fibrils.

Carpal tunnel syndrome occurs in approximately 25% of the cases. When elderly men present with idiopathic carpal tunnel syndrome, the possibility of amyloidosis should be entertained. The diagnostic yield from biopsy of the carpal ligament approaches 100%.

Paraneoplastic Syndromes

Certain musculoskeletal syndromes have a close temporal relationship to the onset of a malignancy. Hypertrophic pulmonary osteoarthropathy is perhaps the best known entity. This condition is most often associated with pleuropulmonary disease, in particular lung cancer and mesothelioma. The term "pulmonary" is somewhat misleading, because certain extrathoracic diseases such as nonneoplastic liver diseases and inflammatory bowel disease may be associated with hypertrophic osteoarthropathy.

The age distribution of hypertrophic pulmonary osteoarthropathy coincides with that of lung cancer, about one half of which occurs above the age of 60 years. Approximately 10% of patients with lung cancer develop symptoms and signs of hypertrophic osteoarthropathy. Patients complain of pain in the ankles, knees and wrists. On examination the most conspicuous, but also the least specific sign is clubbing of the fingers and toes. Diffuse periarticular tenderness is present on palpation, and knee effusion is not unusual. The skeletal symptoms may precede clinical manifestations of lung cancer by many months. When this occurs, hypertrophic osteoarthropathy may be mistaken for rheumatoid arthritis. The diagnosis is confirmed by bone scan or x-ray examination which demonstrate periostitis with subperiosteal new bone formation along the distal and/or proximal ends of long bones.

Carcinomatous polyarthritis is characterized by a close temporal relationship between onset of seronegative arthritis and the discovery of malignancy. Most cases occur in the elderly age group. Clinically, it has certain similarities with rheumatoid arthritis, but is less likely to be symmetric. The onset may be explosive or insidious. Characteristically, the arthropathy remits when the tumor has been resected, and reappears with recurrence of the neoplasm. In contrast to hypertrophic pulmonary osteoarthropathy, the association with carcinomatous arthritis is not limited to intrathoracic solid tumors. Women with this syndrome have a high incidence of breast cancer. The association of palmar fasciitis and polyarthritis with ovarian carcinoma in postmenopausal women has been reported recently.[42] Because of the prominent shoulder and hand involvement, this syndrome has a certain similarity to reflex sympathetic dystrophy; however, arthritis may involve elbows, wrists, knees, and ankles, joints which are not affected in reflex sympathetic dystrophy. Palmar fasciitis and tendon sheath thickening leading to flexion contractures of the fingers are prominent features.

A variety of miscellaneous musculoskeletal syndromes have been described as a manifestation of underlying malignancy. The Eaton-Lambert syndrome that commonly presents with weakness of the pelvic girdle musculature has a strong association with small cell carcinoma of the lung. Carcinomatous neuromyopathy is characterized by symmetrical proximal muscular weakness out of proportion to the loss of muscle mass. Involvement of pelvic girdle muscles cause gait disturbances and difficulty in climbing stairs. These syndromes must be distinguished from polymyositis and polymyalgia rheumatica. The diagnosis is best established by electromyography.

Dermatomyositis/polymyositis that has a close temporal relationship in onset and a parallel course with a malignancy can be considered a paraneoplastic syndrome. Rarely, malignancy may present as a lupus-like syndrome. In at least some of these cases, autoantibodies are directed against nuclear antigens that are distinct from those recognized in patients with idiopathic SLE.[43]

References

1. Felson DT, Naimark A, Anderson J, et al. The prevalence of knee osteoarthritis in the elderly: The Framingham Osteoarthritis Study. *Arthritis Rheum* 1987; 30:914–918.
2. Bergström G, Bjelle A, Sorensen LB, et al. Prevalence of rheumatoid arthritis, osteoarthritis, chondrocalcinosis and gouty arthritis at age 79. *J Rheum* 1986;13:527–534.
3. Brandt KD. Osteoarthritis. *Clin Geriatr Med* 1988; 4:279–293.
4. Felson DT, Anderson JJ, Naimark A. Obesity and knee osteoarthritis. Ann Intern Med 1988;109:18–24.
5. Houpt JB, Pritzker KPH, Alpert B, et al. Natural history of spontaneous osteonecrosis of the knee (SONK): A review. *Semin Arthritis Rheum* 1983;13:212–227.
6. Hall S, Bartleson JD, Onofrio BM, et al. Lumbar spinal stenosis: Clinical features, diagnostic procedures, and results of surgical treatment in 68 patients. Ann Intern Med 1985;103:271–275.
7. Hult L. Cervical, dorsal and lumbar spinal syndromes. A field investigation of a non-selected material of 1200 workers in different occupations with special reference to disc degeneration and so-called muscular rheumatism. *Acta Orthop Scand* 1954;*Suppl* 17:1–102.
8. Griffin MR, Ray WA, Schaffner W. Nonsteroidal anti-inflammatory drug use and death from peptic ulcer in elderly persons. *Ann Intern Med* 1988;109:359–363.
9. Hollingworth P, Scott JT, Burry HC. Nonarticular gout: Hyperuricemia and tophus formation without gouty arthritis. *Arthritis Rheum* 1983;26:98–101.
10. Shmerling RH, Stern SH, Gravallese EM, et al. Tophaceous deposition in the finger pads without gouty arthritis. *Arch Intern Med* 1988;148:1830–1832.
11. Ellman MH, Brown ML, Levin B: Prevalence of knee chondrocalcinosis in hospital and clinic patients aged 50 or older. *J Am Geriatr Soc* 1981;29:189–192.

12. Menkes CJ, Simon F, Delrieu F, et al. Destructive arthropathy in chondrocalcinosis. *Arthritis Rheum* 1976;19(Suppl):329–348.
13. Reginato AJ, Schumacher HR: Crystal-associated arthropathies. *Clin Geriatr Med* 1988;4:295–322.
14. McCarty DJ, Halverson PB, Carrera GF, et al. Milwaukee shoulder association of microspheroids containing hydroxyapatite crystals, active collagenase and neutral protease with rotator cuff defects. I. Clinical aspects. *Arthritis Rheum* 1981;24:464–473.
15. Hunder GG, Hazleman BL. Giant cell arteritis and polymyalgia rheumatica. In: Kelley WN, Harrris ED, Ruddy S, Sledge CB, edts. *Textbook of Rheumatology.* Philadelphia: W.B. Saunders. 1985, pp 1166–1173.
16. Chuang T-Y, Hunder GG, Ilstrup DM, et al. Polymyalgia rheumatica: A 10-year epidemiologic and clinical study. *Ann Intern Med* 1982;97:672–680.
17. Machado EB, Michet CJ, Ballard DJ, et al. Temporal arteritis: An epidemiologic and clinical study. *Arthritis Rheum* 1987;30:No.4(Suppl) S50.
18. Boesen P, Sørensen SF. Giant cell arteritis, temporal arteritis, and polymyalgia rheumatica in a Danish county: A prospective investigation, 1982–1985. *Arthritis Rheum* 1987;30:294–299.
19. Östberg G: On arteritis with special reference to polymyalgia arteritica. *Acta Pathol Microbiol Scand* 1973;237(Suppl A):1–59.
20. Richardson JE, Gladman DD, Fam A, et al. HLA-DR4 in giant cell arteritis: Association with polymyalgia rheumatica syndrome. *Arthritis Rheum* 1987;30:1293–1297.
21. Calamia KT, Hunder GG. Giant cell arteritis (temporal arteritis) presenting as fever of undetermined origin. *Arthritis Rheum* 1981;24:1414–1418.
22. Säve-Söderbergh J, Malmvall B-E, Andersson R, et al. Giant cell arteritis as a cause of death: Report of nine cases. *JAMA* 1986;255:493–496.
23. Ayoub WT, Franklin CM, Torretti T. Polymyalgia rheumatica: Duration of therapy and long-term outcome. *Am J Med* 1985;79:309–315.
24. Schmidt KL, Frencl V. Die rheumatoide Arthritis mit Beginn im höheren Lebensalter. *Dtsch Med Wochenschr* 1982;107:1506–1510.
25. Terkeltaub R, Esdaile J, Décary F, et al. A clinical study of older age rheumatoid arthritis with comparison to a younger onset group. *J Rheum* 1983;10:418–424.
26. Deal CL, Meenan RF, Goldenberg DL, et al. The clinical features of elderly-onset rheumatoid arthritis. *Arthritis Rheum* 1985;28:987–994.
27. McCarty DJ, O'Duffy JD, Pearson L, et al. Remitting seronegative symmetrical synovitis with pitting edema. *JAMA* 1985;254:2763–2767.
28. Steffe LA, Cooke CL. Still's disease in a 70-year-old woman. *JAMA* 1983;249:2062–2063.
29. Arnett FC, Edworthy SM, Bloch DA et al. The American Rheumatism Association 1987 revised criteria for classification of rheumatoid arthritis. *Arthritis Rheum* 1988;31:315–324.
30. Kean WF, Anastassiades TP, Dwash IL, et al. Efficacy and toxicity of D-penicillamine for rheumatoid disease in the elderly. *J. Am Geriatr Soc* 1982;30:94–100.

31. Mitchell DM, Spitz PW, Young DY, et al. Survival, prognosis, and causes of death in rheumatoid arthritis. *Arthritis Rheum* 1986;29:706–714.

32. Laakso M, Mitru O, Isomäki H, et al. Mortality from amyloidosis and renal disease in patients with rheumatoid arthritis. *Ann Rheum Dis* 1986;45:663–667.

33. Dimant J, Ginzler EM, Schlesinger M, et al. Systemic lupus erythematosus in the older age group: Computer analysis. *J Am Geriatr Soc* 1979;27:58–61.

34. Ballou SP, Khan MA, Kushner I. Clinical features of systemic lupus erythematosus. Differences related to race and age of onset. *Arthritis Rheum* 1982;25:55–60.

35. Catoggio LJ, Skinner RP, Smith G, et al. Systemic lupus erythematosus in the elderly: Clinical and serological characteristics. *J Rheum* 1984;11:175–181.

36. Hochberg MC, Boyd RE, Ahearn JM, et al. Systemic lupus erythematosus: A review of clinico-laboratory features and immunogenetic markers in 150 patients with emphasis on demographic subsets. *Medicine* 1985;64:285–295.

37. Baer AN, Pincus T. Occult systemic lupus erythematosus in elderly men. *JAMA* 1983;249:3350–3352.

38. Studenski S, Allen NB, Caldwell DS, et al. Survival in systemic lupus erythematosus. A multivariate analysis of demographic factors. *Arthritis Rheum* 1987;30:1326–1331.

39. Medsger TA, Personal communication. Benedek TG. Neoplastic associations of rheumatic diseases and rheumatic manifestations of cancer. *Clin Geriatr Med* 1988;4:333–355.

40. Malinow KL, Molina R, Gordon B, et al. Neuropsychiatric dysfunction in primary Sjögren's syndrome. *Ann Intern Med* 1985;103:344–349.

41. Alexander EL, Malinow K, Lejewski JE. Primary Sjögren's syndrome with central nervous system disease mimicking multiple sclerosis. *Ann Intern Med* 1986; 104:323–330.

42. Medsger TA, Dixon JA, Garwood VF. Palmar fasciitis and polyarthritis associated with ovarian carcinoma. *Ann Intern Med* 1982;96:424–431.

43. Freundlich B, Makover D, Maul GG. A novel antinuclear antibody associated with a lupus-like paraneoplastic syndrome. *Ann Intern Med* 1988;109:295–297.

17

Orthopedic Problems

Lawrence A. Pottenger

Musculoskeletal problems are frequently perceived by people as the first concrete signs of aging. The problems tend to be chronic in nature with little or no hope of complete return to the premorbid condition. While the pains are usually not severe, they make people feel tired, which is interpreted as feeling "old." Increased pain with activity accentuates the feeling of aging by forcing people to accept more sedentary life-styles. A patient typically complains that she feels like a "45 year-old woman in an 80-year-old body." Depression, which is associated with all forms of chronic pain, can be particularly severe if the patient relates it to fundamental changes such as decreased mobility and growing old.

Osteoarthritis[1]

Age-related changes in joints are different from those in other musculoskeletal tissues. The strength of cartilage does not appear to decrease with age, but cartilage has very little ability to heal at any age. Injuries to cartilage therefore tend to accumulate with age. Since the function of cartilage is to provide a smooth surface for weight bearing, disruptions of the surface produce friction, which leads to further disruption. Eventually, changes typical of osteoarthritis appear. In a random population of people over age 45 years, 4.1% had osteoarthritis in at least one hip joint.[2] While any one particular joint may have escaped injury throughout life, it is virtually impossible to find someone over

60 years of age who does not have osteoarthritis somewhere in his or her body. Indeed, anthropologists use evidence of degenerative joint changes in human skeletons to determine the age at time of death.

Any irreversible damage to the cartilaginous surface of a joint will proceed to osteoarthritis if the joint continues to function. This includes damage from trauma, infections, and inflammatory arthritis. The rate of progression of osteoarthritis cannot be estimated from a single roentgenogram, because it depends on how much the patient continues to use the joint. If the joint is no longer used, the disease will progress very little, if at all.

Roentgenograms of joints in the early stages of osteoarthritis may show only joint space narrowing where some cartilage has been lost. It is therefore very important to obtain roentgenograms of knees and ankles while the patient is bearing weight on the affected extremity, in order to detect the narrowing. These joints have a tendency to open when not bearing weight. As osteoarthritis progresses, the subchondral bone in areas of stress becomes sclerotic, with cystlike areas filled with fibrofatty tissue. The edges of the joint develop osteophytes, which are areas of new bone formation with new cartilage on the surface that faces the joint.

Osteophytes are thought, by some investigators, to make the joints more stable by broadening the surface of weight bearing.[3] They may also stabilize joints by applying lateral pressure on ligaments that have become slack because of loss of cartilage and bone within the joint. Large osteophytes can limit normal motion and cause fixed angular deformities of the joint.

It is generally agreed that the first lesion seen in osteoarthritis is disruption of the articular cartilage in the area of the joint that sustains the greatest loads. Early cartilage lesions are frequently asymptomatic, because cartilage contains no nerves. It is not surprising to see a patient with only a 2-week history of knee pain who has roentgenographic evidence of advanced osteoarthritis. Pain inevitably arrives when cartilage has disappeared from both sides of the joint in a weight-bearing area, because bone contains nerves.

Early cartilage lesions can become painful for several reasons. Large amounts of cartilage debris within the joint cause inflammation of the synovial lining of the joint, with swelling and generalized aching in the anterior part of the joint. Flaps of undermined cartilage can become painfully caught in the joint and can break off, creating loose bodies that might later become caught in the joint. Osteophytes can also break off the bone to become loose bodies. Pieces of fibrillated cartilage, which are often very long, can also become caught in the joint, even though they are still attached to the bone.

Broken osteophytes that do not separate from the bone can cause pain by rubbing at the point of the fracture. Osteophytes can also cause chronic inflammation if they protrude against tendons, ligaments, or joint capsules that move across the joint during motion. This is frequently seen in the knee joint. The quadriceps expansion on both sides of the patella rubs against osteophytes on the anterior part of the femoral condyles as the joint flexes. The synovium under the expansion becomes inflamed because of the increased pressure. The inflamed area becomes fibrotic. The fibrous tissue causes focal elevations of the synovium, which leads to even greater focal pressures and more inflammation. As the process becomes self-perpetuating, fibrous nodules a centimeter or more in diameter can develop, and the pain can become disabling. This condition can easily be diagnosed by placing a hand on the affected knee as it flexes. One feels crepitus on both sides of the patella. Patients often get dramatic relief from intraarticular corticosteroid injections, which reduce the inflammation and tend to make the nodules melt away. Large nodules occasionally require excision through an arthroscope.

Chronic entrapment of material within the joint causes a "locked joint." This is most often recognized in the knee, although it probably happens in many joints throughout the body. The patient is unable to extend the knee fully and walks with a painful bent knee. Attempts to extend it forcibly cause severe pain

in the anterior part of the knee on the side where the material is caught. Some knees unlock spontaneously as trapped material escapes from the joint. Others require removal with an arthroscope.

A locked knee should be treated with some urgency. Material trapped in the knee can cause further cartilage damage during weight bearing. In addition, patients with osteoarthritis who do not fully extend their knees can develop osteophytes on the anterior part of their femoral condyles, which permanently prevent the knees from extending. The time required for development of anterior osteophytes varies, but it is probably unwise to leave a knee locked for more than a month.

A torn meniscus is a frequent cause of locked knee that may not be associated with osteoarthritis. A tear of the meniscus tends to get caught in the part of the joint where the femoral condyle has direct contact with the tibial plateau. In young patients, the tears are well defined and easily visualized with knee arthrography. Older patients have "degenerative tears" where the end of the tear is frayed like unwound yarn and frequently cannot be seen with arthrography. Tears in the front and midportion of the meniscus lead to locking of the knee. Posterior tears cause pain with knee flexion and can actually prevent full flexion.

There is still much controversy concerning the extent to which tears in the meniscus might initiate cartilage damage leading to osteoarthritis. Although meniscal degeneration and even total loss of the menisci are frequently seen in osteoarthritis, there are also many cases where the femoral and tibial cartilage is severely eroded and the menisci are relatively intact. At arthroscopy, however, focal areas of degeneration of femoral cartilage often are seen directly over a torn meniscus, which appears to indicate that the loss of cartilage was due to abrasion from the piece of torn meniscus trapped in the joint. It is not known if these small areas of cartilage disruption will progress to generalized knee osteoarthritis.

Nonsurgical Treatment

In the early stages of osteoarthritis, one can often mitigate the effects of the disease without medications or surgery. The most important way is to reduce the forces transmitted across the affected joints. In the upper extremity, patients find ways to avoid using painful joints by substituting other motions. In the lower extremities, where all of the joints are used during most activities, the emphasis must be placed on decreasing the forces across the joint by decreasing body weight. For instance it has been estimated that during stair climbing, forces of four to six times body weight are placed across the knee joint. Although it is very difficult to change the eating habits of elderly people, obese patients should at least be told that weight loss could have a very beneficial effect on both the symptoms and the progression of the disease.

A cane to help relieve some of the weight bearing on the affected side can also be very beneficial and is particularly important when medications do not relieve the symptoms. Many patients under 75 years of age refuse to use a cane because they see it as a sign of old age. Some of these patients can be persuaded to use one crutch, as they believe the crutch indicates the presence of a disease rather than an infirmity.

Exercise can also be very beneficial for arthritic patients. Increased activity has both positive and negative influences on the course of arthritic diseases. It causes cartilage wear, but it also keeps muscles and bones strong. With respect to the lower extremities, the best exercises are those that minimize the effects of weight bearing on the joints while promoting muscle strengthening. Swimming, riding a stationary bicycle, and doing low-impact exercises are generally beneficial in moderation and they give the patient a feeling of well-being that counteracts some of the chronic pain. Walking, if it is not painful, is also very beneficial. It is a well-known phenomenon that patients with complete loss of cartilage from their joints have less pain if the bone in their joints is very hard, eburnated bone with few cysts. Such bone is generally found in very active people who appear to be able to tolerate their disease much longer before requiring surgery.

Any exercise that causes joint pain, either at the time of the activity or later, is probably not beneficial. Range-of-motion exercises in moderation are generally good, but it should be kept in mind that joint contractures in osteoarthritis frequently develop because the muscles have restricted movements that would otherwise be painful. Overcoming that restriction can cause the joint to become more painful.

Braces are generally of little help in lower-extremity osteoarthritis. A plastic ankle-foot orthosis that limits ankle motion is sometimes helpful in severe ankle osteoarthritis. Osteoarthritic knee joints tend to collapse toward the most involved side so that eventually all of the weight is carried by that side. The opposite side of the knee often remains relatively free of arthritis. For a brace to be effective, it would have to apply a great deal of pressure in order to transfer the weight to the unaffected side. It would be uncomfortable and would rapidly cause skin problems. Small braces around the knee sometimes can be helpful if there is gross instability, but they cannot take the weight off the diseased side of the joint. Braces are of no value in hip arthritis and are generally not useful for upper-extremity arthritis.

Nonsteroidal anti-inflammatory drugs (NSAIDs) can cause dramatic relief of the symptoms of osteoarthritis, but there is little evidence that they slow the progression of the disease, and they may hasten it by allowing the patients to increase their activity levels to the point of causing increased cartilage degeneration (see Chapter 16). Patients frequently show dramatic relief from a corticosteroid injection. Cortisone effectively treats inflammation, but it also inhibits cartilage repair by slowing the metabolism of chondrocytes. Multiple injections can cause rapid loss of cartilage. The number of injections into any one joint should be very limited unless the joint has degenerated to the point that the only alternative is total joint arthroplasty.

Surgical Treatment

Current surgical methods cannot restore damaged cartilage or recreate the original anatomy of the joint. Surgery is performed for four reasons: to débride areas of symptomatic cartilage, to redirect the load bearing to a relatively unaffected part of the joint, to fuse the joint, and to "replace the joint" by attaching artificial surfaces to the ends of the involved bones.

Arthroscopic Joint Débridement

Flaps of undermined cartilage and frayed cartilage can cause pain and muscle spasm if they become caught in the joint (see above).[4] This is particularly evident in knee arthritis but can also occur in the ankle, hip, and shoulder. Meniscal tears with entrapment are also seen in the older population.[5] Material caught within a joint can cause rapid destruction of the cartilage on both sides of the joint by a process called "three-body wear," which is similar to that seen when a piece of sand is caught in a metal bearing. The treatment for this condition is to remove the symptomatic cartilage arthroscopically.

Arthroscopic débridement is most effective in early osteoarthritis when the symptoms appear to be much greater than would be indicated by the roentgenograms, including chronic effusions in spite of NSAIDs and a sudden decrease in the joint's range of motion (with pain on attempts to increase the range manually). Arthroscopic débridement usually is of little benefit in severe osteoarthritis.

Knee and ankle arthroscopy usually can be performed as an outpatient procedure using only local anesthetic.[6] The risks of a complication are small. The possibility of infection is so small that many orthopedists do not use prophylactic antibiotics. The relatively benign effects of arthroscopy make it tempting to expand the indications for its use. This temptation should be resisted because "exploratory arthroscopies" often are not beneficial to the patient. Arthroscopy should not be performed for osteoarthritis unless the physical examination and roentgenograms indicate a specific condition that is known to benefit from arthroscopic surgery, such as physical entrapment of cartilage. If there is a question concerning the cause of the arthritis, arthroscopy is safe way to obtain synovial biopsy specimens.

Realignment Osteotomies[7]

In the early stages of osteoarthritis of the hip and knee, the weight-bearing areas of the joint are primarily affected. Osteotomies have been used to redirect the weight to areas of cartilage that have remained relatively intact. Hip osteotomies are rarely performed in the United States, because their results are unpredictable, but they continue to be popular in Europe. Knee osteotomies continue to be universally popular, but the effective use of NSAIDs often reduces joint symptoms so that surgery is not considered until the joint has degenerated beyond the point where osteotomy would be beneficial. Knee osteotomy entails removing a wedge of bone from above or below the knee so that the direction of weight bearing is oriented to the unaffected side of the joint.

The advantage of osteotomy over total joint replacement is that it does not involve placement within the joint of artificial material that might wear out or become loose.[8] However, patients with knee osteotomies frequently experience recurrence of their symptoms in 5 to 10 years, and some never experience significant relief of pain.[9] In addition, the recovery time for an osteotomy is much longer than for a routine total joint replacement, because bone healing is required.

Joint Fusion

Joint fusion means to remove the joint and approximate the bones on either side of the joint. Joint fusion has always been the most effective way to eliminate permanently the pain of osteoarthritis. In addition, it is often preferred for manual laborers, because it maintains the strength of the extremity better than arthroplasty and it is not as likely to require future surgery. Fusion is the only surgical treatment possible for many of the small joints of the body that become arthritic.

Patients are frequently unhappy with fusions. Prolonged postoperative periods of immobilization in a cast often are necessary to obtain a solid fusion, and reoperation may be necessary if the fusion is not successful. In addition, fusion of a large joint such as the hip or knee changes the walking pattern, making it difficult to sit in a chair and putting additional stress on other joints. Fusions of the hip and knee are generally reserved for young patients with monoarticular disease. They are contraindicated in the lower extremity if a second joint is arthritic, even mildly so, because the additional stress can cause rapid degeneration of the second joint.

Total Joint Arthroplasty

Total joint arthroplasties are procedures that replace the articular surfaces of joints with one or more artificial substances, including metal, high-density polyethylene, ceramic, and silastic. In most cases, only a small amount of bone is removed in order to install the joint. The ligaments, joint capsule, and muscles continue to hold the two sides of the joint together. Patients frequently think that a joint arthroplasty involves replacement of a large segment of the extremity and are relieved to find how little bone is actually replaced. Hips and knees are the most frequently replaced joints. Less frequently replaced joints include finger and toe joints, shoulders, wrists, and elbows.

Arthroplasties of the hip and knee should not be considered unless the joint is irreversibly damaged, with areas of full-thickness loss of cartilage, and the patient's walking capacity is limited to only a few blocks in spite of intensive medical treatment. Roentgenographic indications of the severity of the disease are not important in the decision to perform an arthroplasty, except to indicate that the arthritic condition is irreversible because areas of the joint have completely lost their cartilage. Many patients have severe roentgenographic changes with only mild symptoms. Delaying surgery until symptoms become worse rarely makes the surgery more complicated. The best indications for surgery are the amount of suffering and the degree to which the patients have had to change their life-styles.

As with all elective surgeries, the final decision as to whether to have an arthroplasty must be made by an informed patient. The potential benefits of arthroplasty have to be weighed against the risks of surgery. Current hip and knee arthroplasties can be expected to last an average of 10 to 15 years. If the patient is young, alternatives such as fusion or osteotomy must be considered. Arthroplasties do not enable people to return to active sports, and rarely do they make the joint feel completely normal. Patients who can barely function prior to surgery are usually extremely pleased with their arthroplasty, but those who have an arthroplasty because of mild pain often are unhappy.

Before considering hip or knee arthroplasty, it is necessary to assess all the joints of both lower extremities. Osteoarthritis that is well controlled with antiinflammatory drugs usually hurts only with activity. Pain in a particular joint is often directly related to the amount of activity. An arthritic right knee may not hurt until a patient has walked more than a block. If the left hip hurts after half a block of walking, the patient may not realize that his right knee is severely arthritic until after the left hip has been replaced. Patients become angry and depressed when they realize that they have undergone a major operation for only a slight improvement in their ambulatory capacity. This situation is particularly true for patients with rheumatoid arthritis because of the frequent occurrence of arthritis in the joints of the foot and ankle. When a person has extensive arthritic damage in many joints, several arthroplasties as well as other procedures may be necessary to improve function significantly. Careful preoperative planning and absolute candidness with the patient are very important for a successful outcome.

Operations for hip and knee replacement usually take from 2 to 4 hours. The patients are usually out of bed the next day and ambulating in physical therapy on the second postoperative day. The length of stay in the hospital averages 7 to 10 days. Patients are discharged when their wounds are healing well and they can walk independently with crutches or a walker. At home, they do muscle strengthening exercises and range-of-motion exercises daily. They continue with protective weight bearing for 1 to 2 months. If a patient has two severely arthritic joints, often it is beneficial to replace both joints during the same hospitalization in order to reduce to total length of disability and maximize the benefits of postoperative physical therapy.

In most cases, four units of blood are required for hip replacement and two for knee replacement. Much of the blood loss is due to the fact that patients must receive prophylaxis for deep vein thrombosis prior to surgery to prevent pulmonary embolism.[10] When medically possible, the patient should be asked to donate blood for autologous transfusion during the operation.

Prophylactic antibiotics are used to reduce the possibility of infection.[11] The antibiotic coverage should include *Staphylococcus aureus* and *Staphylococcus epidermidis*. In uncomplicated cases, the infection rate is less than 2%. Deep wound infections may require removal of the prosthesis. Reimplantation is often possible after the infection is under control.

Most of the newer designs of hip and knee arthroplasties have a coating of porous metal on the side of the prosthesis that faces the bone. The coating is designed to take advantage of the fact that healing bone will grow into porous materials. Loosening of cemented prostheses often occurs at the cement-bone interface with fracture of the cement. A direct bond between the bone and prosthesis eliminates the need for bone cement (methyl methacrylate). Presently, most of the advantages of using cementless prostheses remain theoretical. They have not been implanted long enough to determine if they will last longer than cemented prostheses. Some of the prostheses have fibrous ingrowth into the porous coating rather than bony ingrowth. Others have such good ingrowth that bone in some areas atrophies because it is totally relieved of weight bearing.

Degenerative Arthritis of the Spine

Degenerative arthritis of the spine is a common problem in older people. Both the intervertebral disks and the posterior facet joints are generally involved. There may be a history of trauma, sports injuries, or occupations that have stressed the neck and back, but many cases have no known cause. Intervertebral disk material tends to desiccate and fragment with age. The annulus fibrosus may weaken, allowing disk material to protrude into the spinal canal or laterally into the neural foramina. The posterior facet joints, can develop osteophytes so large that they significantly narrow the foramina.

Pain may be caused by the arthritic joints or by neural impingement. In addition, pain within the spine usually causes reflex spasm of paravertebral muscles, which can also become painful from overwork. Patients with vertebral osteoarthritis tend to restrict their motion in order to relieve the pain. At first the loss of disk material may cause painful joint instability. Later, the ligaments tighten with relief of pain, and the joints become nearly fused. Patients with generalized ligament laxity tend to have much more pain because they cannot tighten their ligaments to prevent pain.

Nearly everyone over the age of 60 years has roentgenographic evidence of osteoarthritis in the spine. Because of the tendency for ligament tightening to reduce the symptoms of arthritis, there is no correlation between the degree of symptoms and the severity of the arthritis as indicated on roentgenograms.[12] Indeed, the worst-appearing spines frequently are asymptomatic. Since there are many different causes of back pain, arthritis should be considered only after other common causes have been ruled out.

Pain from arthritis alone, without nerve compression, can radiate into the shoulder and arm from the neck and into the buttock and thigh from the lumbar spine. The presence or absence of numbness, paresthesias, and specific muscle weakness is very important in differentiating nerve impingement from arthritic pain. Any of these symptoms would suggest nerve root compression. Further workup for nerve root compression can include electromyographic studies to determine which nerve roots are involved and myelographic studies and magnetic resonance imaging to determine the site of compression.

In the neck, the initial treatment of an acute episode of either nerve root compression or arthritis is immobilization with a soft collar. Analgesics, muscle relaxants, and NSAIDs are also helpful. Intermittent cervical traction, which can be used in the home, often can provide dramatic relief of symptoms. Patients with nerve root compression who have persistent symptoms in spite of conservative treatment may require excision of the disk and fusion of the involved vertebrae. Arthritic pain without nerve root involvement usually responds to conservative treatment. Severe, unremitting pain can be treated by diskectomy and fusion if it is localized to one level. Fusion of multiple levels usually is unwise because it increases the demand for motion at the remaining levels.

In the lumbar spine, analgesics, muscle relaxants, and NSAIDs all have been used effectively for acute episodes of both arthritis and radiculopathy secondary to a herniated disk. Muscle strengthening can also relieve symptoms of degenerative spine disease by reducing the amount of weight which is transmitted down the spine. The lumbar spine is arched forward (lordotic) to allow upright ambulation. Weight that has been borne primarily through the vertebral bodies in the cervical and thoracic spine is transferred to the facet joints in the lower lumbar spine because of the arch. With good abdominal muscle tone, approximately half the weight of the upper torso is transmitted through the abdomen to the pelvis by hydrolic pressure; with poor muscle tone, all the weight is transmitted through the spine. Abdominal muscles relax during sitting. Pressures on the spine are therefore greater while sitting than while lying, standing, or walking.

All obese patients with chronic low back pain would benefit from losing weight in order to relieve the pressure on the disks and facet joints. Bed rest is frequently advised for patients with disk disease. It has no proven value in treating lumbar arthritis. Bed rest makes all the muscles of the body weak, including the back muscles, which are then less able to stabilize a painful arthritic spine. If patients have lumbar arthritis primarily in the area of the vertebrae and disks, a combination of bed rest with frequent walking and little or no sitting is probably best. Patients with lumbar arthritis primarily in the area of the posterior facet joints have greater pain standing than sitting because greater weight is transmitted across the facet joints when the spine is lordotic. They should be allowed to sit. After the arthritic pain has abated, it is important to start an exercise program that strengthens both back and abdominal muscles.

Lumbosacral braces function by increasing intra-abdominal pressure, which takes the weight off the spine. If the brace is tight there is some effect even during sitting. The braces also reduce the lumbar lordosis during standing and immobilize the spine to the extent that muscles in spasm may be able to relax. They should not be worn constantly, because they cause rapid atrophy of back and abdominal muscles. In general, older people do not tolerate lumbosacral braces unless they are accustomed to wearing girdles, in which case they may find a brace beneficial during episodes of arthritic pain.

Patients with herniated disks who have not responded to conservative therapy may require surgical diskectomy. Chymopapain injection into the disk has been used as a method to avoid surgery with good results in some patients, but the long-term results are still unknown.[13] In cases where nerve roots are compressed by osteophytes of facet joints, resection of the osteophytes with decompression of the nerve roots may be necessary. There is no effective surgery for painful osteoarthritis of the lumbar spine not associated with nerve compression. Lumbar fusions, which have been performed in the past for osteoarthritis, are now indicated only in situations where pain is caused by instability of the joints.

Cervical Spondylotic Myelopathy[14]

In both the cervical and lumbar regions, degenerative disease of the spine can cause narrowing of the spinal canal. Cervical myelopathy is the result of bone or soft-tissue compression of the spinal cord in the neck. Frequently, it appears in the 5th or 6th decade. Although the signs and symptoms may vary greatly, the most common sign is spasticity of the extremities followed by weakness. Pain is present in less than half of the patients. Numbness, painful paresthesias, fasciculations, and sphincter disturbances also can be present. The patients' symptoms can be so vague that their cause is easily missed if the possibility of myelopathy is not constantly kept in mind. Electromyographic studies are helpful to document the degree of nerve involvement. Magnetic resonance imaging usually can demonstrate the site of compression.

Lumbar Spinal Stenosis[15]

In the lumbar region, bone hypertrophy from osteoarthritis may narrow both the spinal canal and neural foramina. This condition is called spinal stenosis. Although arthritis of the lumbar spine is frequently seen in the 5th and 6th decades, symptoms of spinal stenosis usually appear in the 7th decade. The first symptoms are vague leg pains, paresthesias, and dysesthesias brought on by walking or standing.[16] Patients experience symptoms similar to vascular claudication.

After walking a certain distance, they find that they have to stop because of increasing leg pain that abates rapidly if they sit or stand leaning forward. In severe cases, patients walk bent forward at the waist. By bending forward, they are straightening the lordosis in their lumbar spine so that their spinal canal has a maximal diameter. Neurologic deficits are present at rest only in severely affected patients.

The diagnosis of spinal stenosis is made by means of computed tomography or magnetic resonance imaging.[18] Most patients with intermittent symptoms respond to rest, anti-inflammatory medications, and back and abdominal strengthening exercises. Severely affected patients may require laminectomy and decompression of neural foramina with approximately an 85% chance of a good result.[19]

Pyogenic Osteomyelitis[20]

Bacterial infections in bone can be extremely difficult to eradicate if the circulation to the bone is impaired. Circulation may be disrupted by arterial insufficiency (as in arterial occlusive disease), by fracture of the bone, or by abscesses caused by the infection itself. Without adequate circulation, antibiotics cannot reach the bacteria. The infection cannot be eliminated unless either the circulation is reestablished or the infected bone is removed. Bacteria reach bone by one of three pathways: hematogenous seeding, direct inoculation, or contiguous spread from a nearby soft-tissue infection.

Hematogenous Infection

Hematogenous seeding of the bone by a transient bacteremia frequently is due to an infection elsewhere in the body, such as pneumonia, cutaneous infection, or urinary tract infection. Bacteremias also can occur during dental and urologic procedures.

Vertebral osteomyelitis[21] is the most common type of hematogenous osteomyelitis in adults. Vertebral bodies may be predisposed to hematogenous seeding of bacteria because their marrow is actively producing blood components. The sinusoidal system of the marrow reduces the blood flow greatly and may allow bacteria to move into the tissue. In addition, urologic infections and other pelvic infections can easily spread through Batson's plexus, which is a system of communicating veins that connect the pelvic venous plexus with that of the spine.

Hematogenous seeding of vertebrae is also seen with pneumonia, skin infections, dental infections, and abdominal infections. For many patients, the source of the organism cannot be found. A large majority of patients have *Staphylococcus aureus* infections. Any vertebra can be involved, but the lower thoracic and lumbar vertebrae have the greatest incidence.

All patients have symptoms of back pain, which may have been present for as long as several years. A small percentage have symptoms of septicemia, such as fevers, night sweats, elevated leukocyte counts, and positive blood cultures. Paraparesis due to neural compression may be present. Surgery is indicated for vertebral osteomyelitis if the spine is unstable, if there is a large soft-tissue abscess present, or if the infection has not responded to antibiotic therapy.

Direct Inoculation

Infection from direct inoculation of bacteria commonly results from bites and puncture wounds in hands and feet. In older patients, surgery involving bones also is a common cause. The presence of metallic implants or dead bone can make eradication difficult. Prevention definitely is the best way to treat orthopedic infections. The surgery should be performed with scrupulous aseptic technique, minimal dissection should be performed, prophylactic antibiotics should be used for all major operations involving implantation of foreign materials, and closed drainage systems should be used to prevent hematomas.

Contiguous Spread of Soft-Tissue Infection

Such spread of infection occurs most frequently in areas of poor blood supply, such as decubitus ulcers and ischemia of the lower extremities. Treatment must first be directed toward increasing blood flow to the involved area. This may require arterial bypass procedures or the use of vascularized muscular flaps. Necrotic bone must be completely removed, and intensive soft-tissue wound care must be instituted. If amputation is required, it should be performed at a level that is known to have sufficient blood flow to allow healing.

Fractures

Hip Fractures

Fracture of the hip is a frequent occurrence in elderly people and is one the few orthopedic conditions in this population that is associated with significant mortality. In a recent study, 22% of patients died within 1 year of sustaining a fractured hip.[22] Patients seldom die as a direct result of hip fractures, but hip fractures generally occur in debilitated people. Elderly people tend to think of hip fractures as occurring very close to the end of life, because they remember friends and relatives who died shortly after fracturing their hips. If the prognosis for recovery is good, this should be discussed with the patient, because he or she may hold dark thoughts about the future that would delay recovery and rehabilitation.

The possibility of a fractured hip is one of the greatest fears of elderly people who live alone. Establishing a system in which they are contacted every day can be very reassuring.

Hip fractures are considered pathologic fractures because generally they are the result of trivial trauma. Patients often feel their hips break before they fall. Bedridden patients frequently sustain hip fractures falling out of bed. Inactive elderly patients develop disuse osteoporosis, which, superimposed on senile osteoporosis, can cause extreme softening of the bone. In addition, poor diet or malabsorption can cause osteomalacia with further softening (see Chapter 15).

Immediate medical evaluation of a patient with a fractured hip is very important. Hip fractures can cause rapid loss of several units of blood into the thigh, which can lead to hypotension and possible cardiac ischemia. In addition, the patient may have fallen as the result of a hypotensive event caused by a cardiac arrythmia. By the time the patient arrives at the hospital, he or she may no longer be hypotensive but should still be examined for the possibility of myocardial damage immediately after the fracture.

People who sustain hip fractures usually require surgery to stabilize the fracture and allow early ambulation. Some types of hip fractures have almost no chance of healing without surgery, while other types would heal only after weeks or months of bed rest. The potential morbidity and mortality of bed rest in elderly, debilitated patients usually is greater than the risks of surgery, but bed rest may be the only option for severely ill patients. Each patient must be evaluated with both possibilities in mind.

Hip fractures occur primarily in two areas of the proximal femur: the intertrochanteric region and the femoral neck. Fractures in the intertrochanteric area have a high chance of healing because this is a broad cross-sectional area with good blood supply from both sides. However, if surgery is not performed, several weeks of bed rest are required, and the fractures tend to heal in shortened, externally rotated positions.

Femoral neck fractures occur between the trochanters and the femoral head. The blood supply to the femoral head comes from the trochanteric region through the femoral neck and vessels surrounding the femoral neck. Displaced femoral neck fractures often totally disrupt the blood supply to the femoral head. If the blood supply is disrupted, the femoral head will become necrotic even if the fracture is surgically

stabilized. For these fractures, the femoral head usually is replaced by a prosthesis called a hemiarthroplasty, although in younger patients a trial of internal fixation may be indicated if there is a chance that the blood supply is still intact. If the ends of the fracture have not displaced, the blood supply is usually intact and the fracture can be successfully treated with screws to hold the ends of the bones together.

Occasionally, patients have impacted femoral neck fractures in which one side of the fracture becomes stably impacted into the bone of the other side. Patients with these fractures frequently can walk with minimal pain. Sometimes the fractures will come apart later, necessitating surgery. If the fracture has impacted in a good position and is relatively painless, it can be treated with protected weight bearing with crutches or a walker.

The goal of surgery for fractured hips is stabilization of the bones of the fracture so that the patient can be rapidly mobilized after surgery. Patients are usually allowed to sit up the day after surgery. Physical therapy for ambulation with protected weight bearing is started as soon as medically possible, which is usually the 2nd day after surgery.

Vertebral Compression Fractures

Vertebral compression fractures are a major cause of back pain in osteoporotic patients. They are frequently undiagnosed or misdiagnosed as arthritic pain. However, the pain tends to be much more acute and usually is in the middle and upper regions of the back. Some patients give a history of apparently trivial trauma, while others merely note gradually increasing back pain. The pain can be severe and often radiates in the direction of the dermatome at that level. It is exacerbated by sitting, standing, and mild percussion of the spine at the level of the fracture.

The diagnosis is made with lateral roentgenography of the thoracolumbar spine. The silhouettes of the vertebral bodies normally are rectangular. Compression fractures cause wedging of the vertebra with loss of anterior height as compared with posterior height. In mild cases, where the loss of height is minimal, one may see only an increased density of the bone where the collapse has occurred below the end plate of the vertebra. Sometimes, instead of wedging, disk material protrudes through a fracture in the end plate of the vertebra, creating a cystic area within the vertebra, called a Schmorl's node.

It is difficult to determine the age of a compression fracture roentgenographically. Previous roentgenograms, if they exist, are often the only way to determine if a fracture is new, since previous compression fractures may have gone undiagnosed and bone scans

220 Lawrence A. Pottenger

often show increased activity in the area of a fracture for many years. Mild compression fractures and Schmorl's nodes are frequently missed on the original roentgenograms. Patients with clinical indications of a compression fracture should be treated according to the presumptive diagnosis if other causes of the pain have been ruled out.

If there is a history of severe trauma or clinical evidence of a neurologic deficit, computed tomography or magnetic resonance imaging of the spine should be performed to determine whether loss of integrity of the posterior elements of the spine has placed pressure on neural structures. Similar procedures should be performed if there is a significant possibility that the collapse may be due to the presence of tumor.

Osteoporotic compression fractures almost invariably heal, because the collapse increases the amount of bone in the area of the fracture. Treatment is directed toward providing symptomatic relief and preventing possible complications. Initially, the pain may be severe. Patients should be treated with rest in a firm bed until the initial severe pain has abated, which usually takes 3 to 5 days. Strong analgesics may be necessary at first. Patients may have a transient ileus secondary to pain and retroperitoneal hemorrhage. They should not eat if there is abdominal distention or if they are not hungry. Food should be reintroduced with a liquid diet. Routine precautions for bedridden patients to prevent thromboembolic disease should be taken. When the patients can sit comfortably, physical therapy for progressive ambulation should be started, with a walker or crutches used to reduce the weight transmitted through the spine.

Soft-Tissue Injuries

Chronic soft-tissue injuries, also called tendinitis or soft-tissue rheumatism, are a common cause of chronic pain in elderly people. There is a tendency for all musculoskeletal tissues to atrophy with age. This is most apparent with the skin, which slowly becomes thinner and more transparent, and the bones, which show thinning and osteopenia on roentgenograms, but similar phenomena occur with muscles, tendons, ligaments, and other soft tissues that cannot be as readily assessed. The tendency for people to gain weight as they grow older puts increased demands on weakened tissues. Minor injuries in elderly people heal slowly, or sometimes not at all if there is continued stress.

Tendons, ligaments, and other tissues that provide tensile strength have very well-organized collagen bundles for maximum strength. Chronic stresses on these structures cause fatigue disruption of the collagen, which is replaced by relatively weak, poorly

organized scar tissue. With rest, the patient's symptoms often abate completely but later return after episodes of activity that would not have injured to the original tissue, but are sufficient to injure the scarred tissue. The result is permanent tissue weakness frequently accompanied by chronic pain, perhaps intermittent, in a specific soft-tissue structure. Patients know what makes it worse and what makes it better, and they are not surprised to hear that the pain may never completely disappear.

Commonly affected areas in the upper extremity include the biceps tendon and rotator cuff of the shoulder, the origin of the finger and wrist extensors (tennis elbow), and the extensor policis longus and abductor policis brevis tendons (de Quervain's). In the back, the fascial attachment of the erector spinae muscles and the interspinous ligaments are common sites of soft-tissue injuries. In the lower extremity, the most commonly affected areas in older people are the tendons of the gluteus medius at the greater trochanter, the pes anserinus (conjoint tendons of the sartorius, gracilis, and semitendinosus muscles) on the medial side of the knee, and the insertion of the plantar fascia of the foot onto the calcaneus (heel spur). In each case there is an element of overuse. Tendinitis around the hip and knee is frequently associated with intraarticular pathology. Presumably, the tendon damage is due to increased use of the muscles that protect the joints (Fig 17.1).

The subjective nature of the symptoms of chronic soft-tissue injuries creates multiple problems for physicians trying to treat the diseases. Roentgenograms and laboratory studies usually are not helpful except to rule out other conditions. The patient is often unable to locate the pain,[23] which tends to radiate distally away from its source. The tenderness associated with soft-tissue injuries, however, can be well localized to the injured tissue. The diagnosis is made by means of a physical examination, which requires the patient to describe the area of tenderness and the physician to identify the area with regard to underlying anatomic structures.

In athletes, diagnosing soft-tissue injuries such as tendinitis is relatively simple. The patients are otherwise healthy and the tenderness is localized in one anatomic structure that can easily be palpated. Making the diagnosis in elderly patients is much more difficult. They frequently have multiple problems, including arthritis in the same extremity, and their tendons and bursae are often separated from the skin by a thick layer of adipose tissue that makes the tendons difficult to palpate. For example, 24% of Anderson's 45 patients with trochanteric bursitis had been referred to him with different diagnoses.[24] Patients with roentgenographic signs of arthritis risk having their soft-tissue

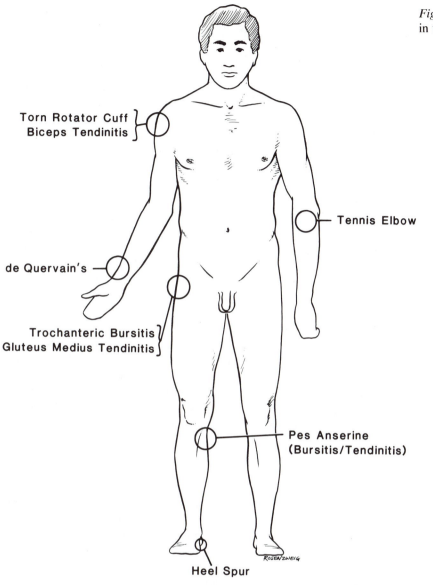

Torn Rotator Cuff
Biceps Tendinitis

Tennis Elbow

de Quervain's

Trochanteric Bursitis
Gluteus Medius Tendinitis

Pes Anserine
(Bursitis/Tendinitis)

Heel Spur

pain diagnosed as "arthritic pain".[25,26] The most frequent reason for misdiagnosis is failure to examine the affected limb. Difficulty in localizing tenderness to specific anatomic structures has led some authors to use the terms tendinitis and bursitis interchangeably,[27,28] while others do not distinguish between tender bursae and nearby tender tendons.[29,30] True bursitis, which is inflammation of a bursa, is much rarer than tendinitis and can usually be cured with a cortisone injection, whereas tendinitis often is a chronic condition.

In the rheumatology literature, the same syndromes have also been called "local fibromyalgia."[31] All forms of tendinitis and bursitis and other localized soft-tissue chronic injuries must be differentiated from generalized fibrositis (also called generalized fibromyaligia), a disease involving multiple tender areas throughout the body and generally seen in younger patients.

When symptoms are severe, patients have a chronic dull pain that becomes sharp to the point of being unbearable when pressure is applied to the affected area. When the disease is relatively quiet, patients may experience pain only when initiating movement of the affected tissues. For example, patients with mild, chronic gluteus medius tendinitis experience pain when getting up from a chair. The pain disappears after a few steps. However, they usually have moderate to severe tenderness in the area of the greater trochanter to the extent that they cannot sleep on the affected side. Patients who appear to be in complete remission continue to have mild to moderate tenderness with deep palpation. Since tendons frequently are tender to deep palpation, it is difficult to diagnose tendinitis unless there is an obvious difference in tenderness between the same tendons on different sides of the body.

Treatment of Tendinitis/Bursitis Syndromes

These syndromes are primarily caused by overuse of specific muscle groups. The history will help to determine if specific activities might have led to excessive stress of the injured tissues. Obesity is a common contributing cause of lower-extremity tendinitis. It may be difficult or impossible to obtain symptomatic relief without weight loss.

Exercise

Frequently, patients want to know what exercises might help their tendinitis. Since tendinitis can appear after excessive exercise, it is important to limit exercises that focus on painful muscle groups. Rest, on the other hand, gives rapid relief of symptoms but also leads to tissue atrophy that renders the tendons more susceptible to future injury when activity is resumed. Gentle muscle strengthening exercises probably are beneficial. Mild stretching exercises are also important to prevent stiffness and contractures that might render the muscles more susceptible to future injuries. In general, any exercise that does not cause increased pain in the affected tendons is probably beneficial.

NSAIDs

A short trial of oral NSAIDs may be of benefit. In view of the potential complications, prolonged use of these drugs is probably not warranted, except in cases of severe, chronic tendinitis, which respond well to NSAIDs.

Corticosteroid Injection

There is an acute form of the disease, which may actually be a different disease, in which the patient experiences sharp, incapacitating pain and tenderness without a prior history of pain in the area. Injection of corticosteroids into the affected area frequently causes permanent relief. This acute form probably is an inflammatory condition with little or no damage to the collagen fibers of the tissue. Patients tend to think that all forms of soft-tissue pain syndromes can be cured with corticosteroid injections, because they know people who have had a good response to the acute form of the disease. However, cortisone injections inhibit tissue repair. Repeated injections into chronically weakened tissues is detrimental. A host of treatments relieve the symptoms of soft-tissue injuries, at least temporarily. These include heating pads, liniments, transcutaneous electrical nerve stimulation (TENS), and ultrasound therapy.

Shoulder Pain

Shoulder pain often is very difficult to diagnose because it can have many different causes, including (1) cervical osteoarthritis or a degenerative disk pain radiating to the shoulder, (2) osteoarthritis of the shoulder or acromioclavicular joint, (3) tendinitis of the long head of the biceps tendon, (4) tears in the rotator cuff, and (5) impingement of soft tissue on the coracoclavicular ligament and anterior border of the acromion (Fig 17.2). Even carpal tunnel syndrome, which is due to compression of the median nerve in the carpal canal, can cause pain radiating to the shoulder. In addition, pain from the diaphragm and heart is often felt in the shoulder and arm, and tumors of the periphery of the lung can present as shoulder and arm pain (Pancoast's syndrome).

Pain from the shoulder joint and surrounding soft tissues tends to be poorly localized. It is frequently most severe along the lateral part of the arm just distal to the insertion of the deltoid muscle. Except in cases of severe inflammation, the pain tends to be dull. It is often exacerbated by specific shoulder movements.

Primary shoulder pain rarely, if ever, radiates to the neck. If there is a history of neck pain, numbness, paresthesias, or muscle atrophy in the arm, the neck should be considered as a source of the pain. Pain from the neck usually is increased with movement of the neck, and there may be tenderness of the paravertebral muscles and trapezius. Significant limitation of neck motion also may be present. Roentgenographic evidence of cervical arthritis, alone, is insufficient to conclude that the shoulder pain is coming from the neck, because even severe cervical arthritis often is asymptomatic.

Osteoarthritis of the shoulder and acromioclavicular joint is seen easily on roentgenograms. Superior displacement of the head of the humerus with respect to the glenoid indicates that the rotator cuff has a significant tear. The area of the lung near the shoulder always should be inspected to rule out Pancoast's syndrome.

Rotator Cuff and Bicepital Tendinitis

Tears of the rotator cuff are frequently seen in the older age groups.[32,33] Patients complain of pain in the shoulder radiating down the lateral part of the arm, pain that is accentuated by abduction or flexion of the shoulder. Combing the hair or putting on a hat can be very painful and sometimes impossible. When there is much inflammation present, the pain, which is nor-

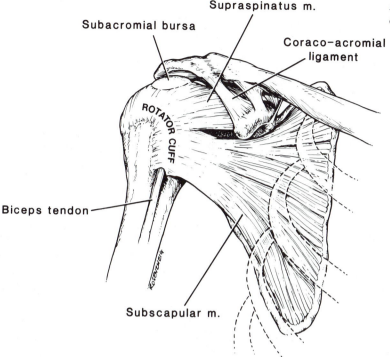

Supraspinatus m.

Subacromial bursa

Coraco-acromial
ligament

ROTATOR CUFF

Biceps tendon

Subscapular m.

Fig. 17.2. Rotator cuff and associated structures commonly involved in pain syndromes.

mally present only with movement, becomes constant. Normal movements of the shoulder during sleep can wake the patient and cause insomnia.

The rotator cuff is formed from the combined tendons of teres minor (from the lateral border of the scapula), infraspinatus (from the dorsal scapular surface below the spine), supraspinatus (from the dorsal scapular surface above the spine), and subscapularus (from the ventral scapular surface). The tendons converge to form the rotator cuff, which covers the top and sides of the humeral head superficial to the joint capsule. Laterally, the rotator cuff inserts into the greater tuberosity. The tendon of the long head of the biceps courses in the bicipital grove of the humerus anteriorly and then into the shoulder joint under the rotator cuff, where it inserts onto the scapula, just above the glenoid rim.

Many factors appear to contribute to degeneration of the rotator cuff. The area of the cuff near its insertion on the greater tuberosity has a very limited blood supply, which may at times be insufficient to sustain the cuff.[34] In addition, with flexion of the shoulder the rotator cuff tends to impinge upon the acromion and coracoacromial ligament, causing local abrasion and thinning. Actual tearing of the cuff may be the result of many years of the trauma of repetitive impingement. The biceps tendon can be similarly damaged. Tenderness of the tendon often is the first sign of impingement. Crepitus is frequently felt over the anterior part of the shoulder when it is put through

a full range of motion, and impingement can be demonstrated by forcibly flexing the shoulder when the arm is in neutral rotation.[35]

The muscles of the rotator cuff function to maintain the head of the humerus in the glenoid during arm motion. Tears of the rotator cuff allow the head of the humerus to sublux superiorly during contraction of the deltoid, which would normally cause abduction of the arm. If the tear is large, the superior subluxation of the humeral head can be noted on a roentgenogram of the shoulder. The space between the bottom of the acromion and the top of the head of the humerus is occupied by the joint capsule and rotator cuff. If the space is greatly diminished, the cuff must be torn. Small tears of the rotator cuff can be demonstrated by leakage of dye out of the shoulder joint during arthrography.

The treatment of shoulder impingement and rotator cuff tears must be closely tailored to the individual. Patients presenting with shoulder pain who have no loss of motion should be treated with rest, oral anti-inflammatory medications, and gentle range of motion and muscle strengthening exercises. Corticosteroid injections into the space between the rotator cuff and the acromion can be tried if oral anti-inflammatory medications are ineffective. Surgical resection of the anterior acromion and coracoacromial ligament should be considered for those patients with prolonged pain that is unresponsive to conservative treatment.

If the patient has recently developed limitation of

motion, arthrography should be performed to determine if the rotator cuff is torn. Large tears should be repaired if the patient's condition permits. Patients with small tears often improve with conservative therapy. Chronic, asymptomatic rotator cuff tears in people over 70 years of age frequently are seen on chest roentgenograms as superior subluxation of the humeral head. Although these people usually have limited shoulder abduction and flexion, the remnants of their rotator cuffs are so atrophic that surgical reconstruction would be of little benefit.

Frozen Shoulder[36]

The first symptom of frozen shoulder is insidious onset of dull shoulder pain, usually with no prior history of trauma. The pain is worse at night and with activity. Patients often have trouble sleeping and tend to hold the arm tightly against the side. At first, with some encouragement, the shoulder can be put through a full range of motion. Later, all directions of motion become restricted and the pain subsides as long as the shoulder is not moved.

Frozen shoulder is a diffuse inflammation of the rotator cuff. Frequently, there is degeneration of the intraarticular portion of the biceps tendon.[37] Contracture of the subscapularis tendon limits abduction and external rotation of the shoulder. Eventually, the shoulder capsule itself becomes contracted. Arthrography shows decreased volume of the joint and obliteration of the normal synovial folds and recesses that allow motion.

Frozen shoulder tends to be a self-limiting disease, with spontaneous recovery for most patients within 2 years. Early physical therapy probably reduces the length of disability. Patients often are very reluctant to move the joints. The patient should use a sling to rest the shoulder. Gentle range-of-motion exercises should be performed in the sling to maintain motion. Pendulum exercises, in which the patient bends forward and lets the arm sway in a circular motion like a pendulum, are particularly good because they do not require shoulder muscle activity, and the natural feeling of the sway tends to relieve apprehension about moving the arm.

Oral NSAIDs may help to reduce the pain and stiffness. Occasionally injections of corticosteroid into the subacromial bursa are helpful. Gentle manipulation of the shoulder under anesthesia may be necessary in patients who are not responding to physical therapy.

Carpal Tunnel Syndrome[38]

Compression of the median nerve at the wrist causes a constellation of signs and symptoms known as carpal tunnel syndrome. The median nerve transverses the carpal canal in conjunction with the long flexor tendons of the fingers. The volume of the carpal canal is limited by the carpal bones dorsally, medially, and laterally and by the flexor retinaculum ventrally. Swelling of the synovium of the tendons increases the pressure within the canal, which causes nerve compression.

Patients most often complain of painful burning and paresthesias of the first four fingers, which is usually most severe at night and often causes insomnia. They report that they have to shake their heads to relieve the tingling. They may say that all of their fingers feel numb, but examination demonstrates that numbness, if present, is confined to the first three fingers and the radial side of the fourth. The thenar muscles can be atrophic as a result of compression of the motor branch of the median nerve. Pain will occasionally radiate up the arm to the shoulder.

The most sensitive provocative test for carpal tunnel syndrome is the Phalen test.[39] The patient is asked to completely flex his or her wrist. Within 1 minute, numbness and tingling will be produced, or exaggerated if already present. This test is positive in only 75% of patients. When Tinel's sign (shocklike sensations on percussion of the median nerve at the wrist) is present, the likelihood of carpal tunnel syndrome is great, but absence of Tinel's sign does not preclude the possibility of carpal tunnel syndrome. Electromyography should be performed if the Phalen test is negative in the presence of a high clinical suspicion of carpal tunnel syndrome or if surgery is being contemplated. Slowing of the nerve conduction velocities is seen when compression of the median nerve is present.[40]

Many diseases are known to cause carpal tunnel syndrome, including all of the common chronic inflammatory arthritides, amyloidosis, hypothyroidism, diabetes, and acromegaly. The syndrome is also frequently seen during pregnancy. An acute form of carpal tunnel syndrome is seen in people who abruptly increase their wrist usage, such as when using crutches. In a large percentage of patients, no cause can be found. If the cause is apparent, therapy should be focused on correcting the problem, if possible.

Cock-up splints prevent wrist flexion, which causes further compression of the carpal canal. They can be worn at night and also during the day in severe cases. Injection of the carpal canal with corticosteroids often will dramatically relieve the symptoms. If the symptoms are not relieved by injection or if they continue to return after multiple injections, surgical release of the flexor retinaculum should be considered. Atrophy of the thenar muscles is an indication for early surgical intervention, because patients often have poor return of muscle strength even after surgery.

Foot Problems

Foot problems often are a major source of concern for elderly people. Diseases of aging that affect the musculoskeletal system frequently are first seen in the foot. Osteoarthritis may be first manifested as a bunion of the first metatarsal phalangeal joint. Muscle weakness appears as loss of strength of the interosseous muscles of the foot leading to claw toes. Arterial insufficiency often appears first as pain in the feet and dry gangrene of toes. Diabetic vasculopathy and neuropathy often become clinically significant first in the feet.

Shoe wear

Many chronic foot problems are due to inappropriate footwear. Bunions are not seen in populations who do not wear shoes. High heels can cause contractures of the Achilles tendon and claw toes. Shoes with narrow toes can cause corns and bunions. Shoes with hard soles cause calluses on the bottom of the feet.

The time to start wearing appropriate shoes is before the foot deformities appear. After a deformity is present, shoes may reduce its effect but cannot correct it. Fortunately, shoe companies are beginning to make shoes that are both comfortable and acceptable in most social settings.

Shoe soles of soft material, such as polyurethane, have several beneficial effects. They prevent calluses on the bottom of the foot where the soft-tissue padding under bony prominences has been lost. They also reduce the amplitude of the forces transmitted from the ground through the foot during walking (ground reactive forces). Reduction of these forces has a mitigating effect on hip and knee osteoarthritis and all types of musculoskeletal low back pain. It also may prevent primary foot osteoarthritis.

Tarsal Tunnel Syndrome[41]

Compression of the posterior nerve at the ankle causes burning pain on the plantar aspect of the foot, known as tarsal tunnel syndrome. The burning is often accompanied by tingling and numbness that is poorly localized. In most patients it is aggravated by activity, but it also may be severe at night. It appears to be analogous to carpal tunnel syndrome in the hand.

Usually patients have Tinel's sign, which is a feeling of electrical shocks when the injured part of the nerve is percussed. The tarsal canal extends around the medial malleolus into the plantar aspect of the foot.

Tinel's sign may be present anywhere within the tunnel and is sometimes present along the distal calf, proximal to the medial malleolus. The diagnosis is established by demonstrating decreased nerve conduction velocities of the posterior tibial nerve or one of its branches.

Tarsal tunnel syndrome can often be treated by local injection or oral NSAIDs. Casting for short periods is occasionally beneficial. If conservative methods fail, the tarsal tunnel can be surgically released, but patients should be warned that symptoms may persist after the release.

Hallux Valgus (Bunion)[42]

Bunions are medial protuberances of the first metatarsal phalangeal joints that appear if the first toes deviate laterally. Frequently, the joints have roentgenographic signs of osteoarthritis. Pressure from shoe wear causes the medial capsule of the joint to become thickened and inflamed and an exostosis develops on the head of the metatarsal. Superficial nerves that course over the top of bunions often become inflamed, causing feelings of numbness along the medial side of the great toe. In older people, the great toe may cross above or below the second toe. This can lead to painful sores or areas of maceration. Interposition of a pad between the two toes is helpful.

Although proper footwear helps prevent the appearance of bunions,[43] it cannot correct bunions after they have formed. Abnormal pull of the tendons around the deformed joint with contracture of the joint capsule prevent return of the toe to its correct position. If a bunion is painful and disabling, surgical reconstruction may be necessary. Bunionectomies usually can be performed under local anesthesia, often without hospitalization of the patient. If the bone deformities are mild, removal of the exostosis and soft-tissue realignment may be sufficient. More complicated bunions require osteotomy of the metatarsal or first phalanx as well.

A "bunionette" or "tailor's bunion" is a prominence along the lateral side of the forefoot due to lateral protrusion of the head of the fifth metatarsal bone. At least some prominence of the fifth metatarsal head is a normal finding in most people. The prominence is accentuated by wearing shoes with narrow toes. The fifth toe is pushed medially, and the prominence becomes irritated by direct pressure from the shoe. A callus forms on the skin over the prominence, and a bursa often forms between the skin and fifth metatarsal phalangeal joint. In general, bunionectomies can be successfully treated by wearing shoes with wide toes and by placing padding over the painful prominence.

Claw Toes

Claw toes is a common foot deformity that appears to be due to ineffective action of the intrinsic muscles of the foot. Although the leg muscles provide most of the strength of the toes, the lumbricals and interosseous muscles of the foot help to keep the toes elongated during flexion by flexing the metatarsal phalangeal joints and extending the interphalangeal joints. Without the intrinsic muscles, flexion of the toes by the leg muscles alone causes hyperextension of the metatarsophalangeal joints and flexion of the interphalangeal joints, which is claw toes. Painful corns develop over the hyperflexed proximal interphalangeal joints, and calluses develop on the tips of the toes, which are pushed into the sole of the shoe while walking. Claw toe deformities usually involve all the toes of the foot, including the great toe. The deformity of claw toes may be accentuated by wearing high-heeled shoes or shoes that are too tight at the toe. Conservative treatment for claw toes includes shoes with broad toes and soft soles to distribute the pressure. Metatarsal bars may be necessary to lessen the pressure of weight bearing on the toes. In severe cases, surgery to straighten the toes may be necessary.

Heel Spur

Pain in the heel during weight bearing often is due to inflammation where the plantar aponeurosis attaches to the tuberosity of the calcaneus. As with other forms of tendinitis, the point of attachment to bone appears to be the weakest area and the one most likely to be chronically inflamed, presumably due to microscopic tears. Prolonged inflammation leads to accretion of new bone, called a spur. Tenderness is usually found at the point where the plantar aponeurosis attaches to the calcaneus, in the middle of the bottom of the heel.

The distal part of the plantar aponeurosis attaches to the base of the proximal phalanges. Dorsiflexion of the phalanges during normal gait accentuates the arch and therefore shortens the foot. If the heel is everted and the arch is relatively flat, large stresses are put upon the aponeurosis with toe dorsiflexion. The stresses can be relieved by wearing soft-soled shoes with good arch supports. If pain persists, many conservative approaches are possible, including foot orthotics to keep the heel inverted, oral NSAIDs, and local injection of corticosteroid. When pain is unremitting despite conservative measures, surgical excision of the spur often is beneficial.

Foot Problems in Diabetics[44]

Foot infection is the most common infection in diabetics that requires hospitalization.[45] Almost all patients with long-standing diabetes have peripheral neuropathies that lead to severe arthropathies (Charcot's joints), because the patients are unable to perceive when their joints are being damaged.[46] As the joints are destroyed, the bones around the joints become deformed and often form protuberances below the skin. The foot ulcers appearing over the protuberances inevitably become colonized with bacteria, which penetrate the foot because the vascular status of the foot is so poor that it is unable to form a protective barrier against bacterial invasion. Ischemia of the foot appears to be due to both atherosclerotic narrowing of large arteries[47] and diabetic microangiopathy.[48] Leukocytes from diabetic patients do not appear to function normally,[49] and increased concentrations of glucose in foot tissues may promote bacterial growth.

Treatment of diabetic patients with serious foot conditions is very complicated, requiring the expertise of many different medical and surgical specialists including diabetologists, orthopedists, vascular surgeons, general surgeons, and infectious disease specialists.[50] The major determinant in the healing of a diabetic foot ulcer appears to be blood supply. If the arterial blood pressure at the ankle is greater than half the brachial artery pressure, the lesions have an excellent chance of healing. Treatment consists of excision of infected bone, joints, and soft tissue. Intensive wound treatment and intravenous antibiotics often require prolonged hospitalization for the best results. Skin grafting may be required for lesions larger than 2 cm in diameter. Future lesions often can be prevented by padding bony prominences[51] and wearing soft shoes with a wide forefoot area.[52]

References

1. Pottenger LA. Pathobiology of osteoarthritis. In: Dante G. Scarpelli DG, Migaki G, eds. *Comparative Pathobiology of Major Age-Related Diseases*. New Yor, NY: Alan R Liss Inc; 1983:159–174.
2. Pogrund H, Rutenberg M, Mankin M, et a. Osteoarthritis of the hip joint and osteoporosis. *Clin Orthop* 1982;164:130–135.
3. Marshall JL, Olsson S-E. Instability of the knee: a long-term experimental study in dogs. *J Bone Joint Surg Am* 1971;53:1561–1570.
4. Hubbard MJS. Arthroscopic surgery for chondral flaps in the knee. *J Bone Joint Surg Br* 1987;69:794–796.
5. Svend B, Hansen H. Arthroscopic partial meniscectomy in patients aged over 50. *J Bone Joint Surg Br* 1986;68:707.
6. McDiarmid AA. Outpatient arthroscopy under local anaesthesia. *J Bone Joint Surg Br* 1986;68:678.
7. Poss R. The role of osteotomy in the treatment of osteoarthritis of the hip. *J Bone Joint Surg Am* 1984;66:144–151.

8. Insall JN, Joseph DM, Msika C. High tibial osteotomy for varus gonarthrosis. *J Bone Joint Surg Am* 1984;66:1040–1048.

9. Vainionpaa S, Laike E, Kirves P, et al. Tibial osteotomy for osteoarthritis of the knee: a five to ten-year follow-up study. *J Bone Joint Surg Am* 1981;63:938–946.

10. Collins R, Scrimgeour A, Yusuf S, et al. Reduction in fatal pulmonary embolism and venous thrombosis by preoperative administration of subcutaneous heparin. *N Engl J Med* 1988;318:1162–1173.

11. Scheller AD, Turner RH, Lowell JD. Complications of arthroplasty and total joint replacement in the hip. In: Epps CH Jr, ed. *Complications in Orthopaedic Surgery.* 2nd ed. Philadelphia, Pa: JB Lippincott; 1986;2:1059–1108.

12. Lawrence JS, Bremner JM, Bier F. Osteoarthritis: prevalence in the population and relationship between symptoms and X-ray changes. *Ann Rheum Dis* 1966;25:1–24.

13. Norby EJ. Chymopapain in intradiscal therapy. *J Bone Joint Surg Am* 1983;65:1350–1353.

14. Crandall PH, Batzdorf U. Cervical spondylotic myelopathy. *J Neurosurg* 1966;25:57–66.

15. Spengler DM. Degenerative stenosis of the lumbar spine. *J Bone Joint Surg Am* 1987;69:305–308.

16. Verbiest H. Pathomorphologic aspects of developmental lumbar stenosis. *Orthop Clin North Am* 1975;6:177–196.

17. Herkowitz HN, Garfin SR, Bell GR, et al. The use of computerized tomography in evaluating non-visualized vertebral levels caudad to a complete block on a lumbar myelogram. *J Bone Joint Surg Am* 1987;69:218–224.

18. Crawshaw C, Kean DM, Mulholland RC, et al. The use of nuclear magnetic resonance in the diagnosis of lateral canal entrapment. *J Bone Joint Surg Br* 1984;66:711–715.

19. Hall S, Bartleson JD, Onofrio BM, et al. Lumbar spinal stenosis: clinical features, diagnostic procedures, and results of surgical treatment in 68 patients. *Ann Intern Med* 1985;103:271–275.

20. Wald ER. Risk factors for osteomyelitis. *Am J Med* 1985;78(suppl 6B):206–212.

21. Sliverthorn KG, Gillespie WJ. Pyogenic spinal osteomyelitis: a review of 61 cases. *NZ Med J* 1986;99:62–65.

22. White BL, Fisher WD, Laurin CA. Rate or mortality for elderly patients after fracture of the hip in the 1980's. *J Bone Joint Surg Am* 1987;69:1335–1340.

23. Swezey RL. Pseudo-radiculopathy in subacute trochanteric burisits of the subgluteus maximus bursa. *Arch Phys Med Rehab* 1976;57:387–390.

24. Anderson TP. Trochanteric bursitis: diagnostic criteria and clinical significance. *Arch Phys Med Rehab* 1958;39:617–622.

25. Brookler MI, Mongan ES. Anserina bursitis: a treatable cause of knee pain in patients with degenerative arthritis. *California Med* 1973;119:8–10.

26. Moschowitz E. Bursitis of sartorius bursa: an undescribed malady simulating chronic arthritis. *JAMA* 1937;109:1362.

27. Gordon EJ. Trochanteris bursitis and tendinitis. *Clin Orthop* 1961;20:193–202.

28. Schein AJ, Lehmann O. Acute trochanteric bursitis with calcification. *Surgery* 1941;9:771–779.

29. Krout RM, Anderson TP. Trochanteric bursitis: management. *Arch Phys Med Rehabil* 1959;40:8–14.

30. Spear IM, Lipscomb PR. Noninfectious trochanteric bursitis and peritendinitis. *Surg Clin North Am* 1952;32:1217–1224.

31. Ynus MB. Fibromyaligia syndrome: need for a uniform classification. *J Rheumat* 1983;10:841–844.

32. Grant JCB, Smith CG. Age incidence of rupture of the supraspinatus tendon. *Anat Rec* 1948;100:666.

33. Nixon JE, DiStefano V. Ruptures of the rotator cuff. *Orthop Clin North Am* 1975;6:423–447.

34. Rathbun JB, Macnab I. Vascular anatomy of the rotator cuff of the shoulder. *J Bone Joint Surg Br* 1970; 52:540–553.

35. Neer CS, Welsh RP. The shoulder in sports. *Orthop Clin North Am* 1977;8:583–591.

36. Macnab I. Rotator cuff tendinitis. *Ann R Coll Surg Engl* 1973;53:271–287.

37. Lippman RK. Frozen shoulder periarthritis, biciptal tenosynovitis. *Arch Surg* 1943;47:283–296.

38. Dorwart BB. Carpal tunnel syndrome: a review. *Semin Arthritis Rheum* 1984;14:134–140.

39. Gellman H, Gelberman RH, Tan AM, et al. Carpal tunnel syndrome. *J Bone Joint Surg Am* 1986;68:735–737.

40. Szabo RM, Gelberman RH, Dimick MP. Sensibility testing in patients with carpal tunnel syndrome. *J Bone Joint Surg Am* 1984;66:60–64.

41. Wilemon WK. Tarsal tunnel syndrome: a 50-year survey of the world literature and a report of 2 cases. *Orthop Rev* 1979;8(11):111.

42. Scranton PE. Principles in bunion surgery. *J Bone Joint Surg Am* 1983;65:1026–1028.

43. Scheck M. Etiology of acquired hammertoe deformity. *Clin Orthop* 1977;123:63–69.

44. Bessman AN. Foot problems in the diabetic. *Compr Ther* 1982;8:32–37.

45. Pratt TC. Gangrene and infection in the diabetic. *Med Clin North Am* 1975;49:987–1004.

46. Lamontagne A, Buchtal F. Electrophysiological studies in diabetic neuropthy. *J Neurol Neurosurg Psychiatry* 1970;33:442–452.

47. Kramer DW, Perilstein, PK. Peripheral vascular complications in diabetes melitus: a survey of 3,600 cases. *Diabetes* 1958;7:384–387.

48. Banson BB, Lacy PE. Diabetic microangiopathy in human toes. *Am J Pathol* 1964;45:41–58.

49. Martin SP, McKinney GR, Green R, et al. The influence of glucose, fructose, and insulin on the metabolism of leukocytes of healthy and diabetic subjects. *J Clin Invest* 1953;32:1171–1174.

50. Jacobs RL, Karmondy AM, Wirth C, et al. The team approach in the salvage of the diabetic foot. *Surg Ann* 1977;9:231–264.

51. Duckworth T, Boulton AJM, Betts RP, et al. Plantar pressure measurements and the prevention of ulceration in the diabetic foot. *J Bone Joint Surg Br* 1985;67:79–85.

52. Mooney V, Wagner FW Jr. Neurocirculatory disorders of the foot. *Clin Orthop* 1977;122:53–61.

18

Diabetes Mellitus

Don Riesenberg

The care of elderly patients with diabetes mellitus requires as much art as science. Today, our understanding of this heterogeneous disease is increasing rapidly. Yet, in the elderly population, the boundary between normal and abnormal glucose tolerance remains unclear, and there exists no perfect therapeutic substitute for glucose homeostasis—the complex interaction between pancreas, liver, and skeletal muscle.[1]

But the treatment of elderly diabetics proves both clinically satisfying and intellectually stimulating for physicians who are familiar with the metabolic hallmarks of, and therapeutic options for, this very common disease. In fact, diabetes mellitus encompasses much of geriatric medicine's knowledge base. The pathologic changes are an accelerated version of what we call biologic aging.

Diagnosis and Etiology

Table 18.1 compares the diagnostic criteria of the National Diabetes Data Group with those of the World Health Organization.[2] For clinical purposes, a person is said to have normal carbohydrate tolerance if the plasma glucose level is less than 140 mg/dL (7.8 mmol/L) both during fasting and 2 hours after oral administration of glucose. Diabetes mellitus is present when the fasting plasma glucose level is over 140 mg/dl (7.8 mmol/L) on *two* occasions or over 200 mg/dL (11.2 mmol/L) 2 hours after oral administration of 75 g of glucose. Impaired glucose toler-

ance is the term applied to persons having intermediate test results: fasting plasma glucose levels less than 140 mg/dL (7.8 mmol/L) but 2-hour levels between 140 mg/dL (7.8 mmol/L) and 200 mg/dL (11.2 mmol/L). Reliance on these criteria obviates the need for formal glucose-tolerance testing in most circumstances.

The utility of the glycosylated hemoglobin level as a diagnostic tool has not been evaluated fully (but see "Assessment of Control," below). Its sensitivity and specificity were 85% and 91%, respectively, in one study of a high-prevalence population.[3] The claim that aging, per se, increases glycosylated hemoglobin levels[4] has been disputed.[5]

Extrapolation from the National Health and Nutrition Examination Survey suggests that, when undiagnosed cases are included, 15% to 20% of Americans between the ages of 65 and 74 years are diabetic (Fig. 18.1).[6] An aberration in the way insulin acts at the level of target issues, also observed in nondiabetic elderly persons, plays a major role in this high prevalence of carbohydrate intolerance. Mean fasting plasma glucose levels rise only 1 mg/dL per decade in adults; however, 2-hour postprandial levels increase by as much as 5 to 10 mg/dL per decade. This suggests that older individuals are less efficient at glucose disposal, which involves (1) secretion of insulin in response to glucose ingestion, (2) insulin-induced suppression of hepatic glucose output, and (3) glucose uptake by skeletal muscle and other target tissues.

The immediate, so-called phase I, insulin response to oral glucose is decreaseed even in nondiabetic

Table 18.1. NDDG and WHO diagnostic criteria.*

	Plasma glucose mg/dL (mmol/L)				
			Oral glucose tolerance test		
Class	Fasting		Midtest		2-hour
NDDG					
Normal	<115 (<6.4)	and	<200 (<11.1)	and	<140 (<7.8)
IGT	<140 (<7.8)	and	≥200 (≥11.1)	and	140–199 (7.8–11.1)
Diabetes†	≥140 (≥7.8)	or	≥200 (≥11.1)	and	≥200 (≥11.1)
WHO					
Normal‡	<140 (<7.8)		. . .	and	<140 (<7.8)
IGT	<140 (<7.8)		. . .	and	140–199(7.8–11.1).
Diabetes†	≥140 (≥7.8)		. . .	or	≥200 (≥11.1)

*From Harris et al.[2] Reproduced with permission from the American Diabetes Association, Inc. NDDG indicates National Diabetes Data Group; WHO, World Health Organization; IGT, impaired glucose tolerance. For the NDDG criteria, all combinations of values other than those listed are considered nondiagnostic. The mmol/L values were determined by dividing the mg/dL values by 18.016 and rounding to the nearest 0.1 mmol/L (NDDG) or by dividing the mg/dL values by 18 and rounding to the nearest 1 mmol/L (WHO).
†The NDDG and the WHO require both the fasting and the 2-hour glucose values to classify a subject, except when the fasting level is ≥140 mg/dL (7.8 mmol/L), which by itself is diagnostic of diabetes.
‡Although the WHO does not define a "normal" result, the term is used here to include subjects who do not meet criteria for diabetes or impaired glucose tolerance.

elderly persons, but by 30 to 60 minutes, insulin secretion catches up with, then exceeds, that of younger subjects (Fig. 18.2). This tardy insulin response in elderly persons results in delayed suppres-

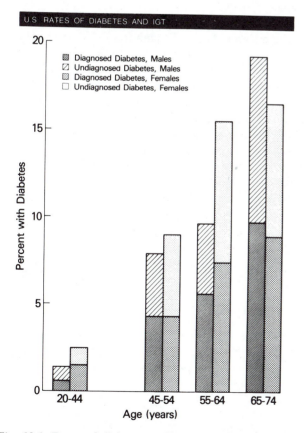

U.S. RATES OF DIABETES AND IGT

▨ Diagnosed Diabetes, Males
▨ Undiagnosed Diabetes, Males
▨ Diagnosed Diabetes, Females
□ Undiagnosed Diabetes, Females

Fig. 18.1. Rates of diabetes mellitus and impaired glucose tolerance in the United States. Reproduced from reference 6 with permission from the American Diabetes Association, Inc.

sion of hepatic glucose output following glucose ingestion.

Of greater etiologic significance is the insulin resistance observed in older individuals. In order for peripheral tissues (most importantly skeletal muscle) to take up glucose, insulin must attach to a specific membrane receptor. The insulin receptor complex initiates a cascade of intracellular actions leading to glucose uptake and metabolism.[7] Careful study has shown that monocytes and adipocytes from elderly subjects have normal numbers of insulin receptors.[8] That observation would seem to localize the abnormality of glucose disposal to one or more rate-limiting postreceptor events.

Finally, there is the adverse effect of hyperglycemia itself on insulin secretion. Chronic elevation of plasma glucose concentration desensitizes the beta cell to an acute glycemic stimulus, so-called glucose poisoning.[1] Figure 18.3 summarizes this complex sequence of events, culminating in the onset of non–insulin-dependent diabetes mellitus (NIDDM), which accounts for at least 90% of diabetes in the elderly population.

Despite understanding of the pathophysiology, finding impaired glucose tolerance in an older individual leaves unanswered important prognostic questions. This is because "hyperglycemia of the elderly" encompasses three very different groups: (1) those in the upper extreme of the normal distribution for glucose tolerance, (2) false-negative diabetics, for whom the diagnostic criteria are not sensitive enough, and (3) individuals in transition from normal to diabetic.[9] Fortunately, the clinical approach is the same for all older persons with impaired glucose tolerance: calorie restriction and increased physical activity, where appropriate, accompanied by periodic re-evaluation.

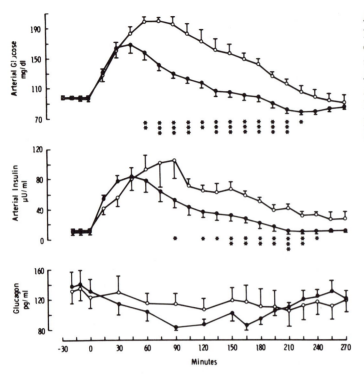

Fig. 18.2. Metabolic response to oral glucose loading in young (closed circles) and elderly (open circles) non-diabetic men. Note delayed, but higher, insulin response in elderly. *P < .05 **P < .01 ***P < .001. Jackson, Rahawani, Roshaniard et. al. Influence of Aging on Hepatic and Peripheral Glucose Metabolism in Humans. Diabetes 1988; 37:119–129. Reproduced with permission from the American Diabetes Association Inc.

For many such patients, further deterioration in glucose tolerance will ensue and will result in the onset of NIDDM, as depicted in Figure 18.3. Presenting symptoms in elderly persons range from none to life threatening. Many patients have long-standing hyperglycemia when they come to the physician's attention. Among the entities encountered at diagnosis are atherosclerosis, visual abnormalities, and neuropathic complaints.

Treatment

Diet

Most physicians agree that dietary manipulation is the cornerstone of therapy for NIDDM in patients of all ages. Recent nutritional guidelines from the American Diabetes Association[10] (Table 18.2) propose a liberalization of carbohydrate content in the diabetic diet (55% to 60% of total calories) with a concomitant reduction in atherogenic fat intake.

The value of the glycemic index has been questioned.[11] Glucose excursions after ingestion of carbohydrate vary not only among individuals but with the content of the rest of the meal. Therefore, predictions about postprandial glycemia based on a meal's carbohydrate content alone are likely to be inaccurate. Study of a small number of type I and type II diabetics has suggested that diets containing fructose, compared with isocaloric diets containing sucrose or starch (between which no differences were demonstrated),

reduce postprandial plasma glucose levels and 24-hour urinary glucose excretion.[12]

Weight reduction is effective in ameliorating insulin resistance but often is difficult to achieve in the elderly diabetic. Contemporaneous administration of insulin or sulfonylurea promotes weight gain through inhibition of lipolysis. Furthermore, many elderly persons have psychological, social, and physical impediments to obtaining and preparing proper meals[13] (Table 18.3). Nevertheless, in view of the evidence that even modest weight reduction (without necessarily achieving ideal body weight) improves control in patients with NIDDM,[14] the patient and family should be taught simple dietary principles, as outlined in Table 18.2.

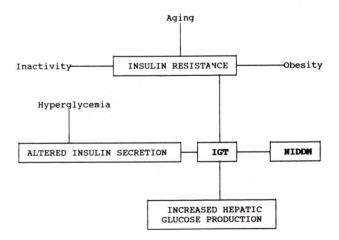

Fig. 18.3. Pathogenesis of non-insulin dependent diabetes mellitus (NIDDM) in elderly persons. Note the common pathway through impaired glucose tolerance (IGT).

Table 18.2. Recommended daily intake.*

Component of diet	Recommended amount
Carbohydrate	≤ 60%
Protein	0.8 g/kg+
Fat	
Polyunsaturated	6%–8%
Saturated	< 10%
Monosaturated	30% − (PUS + S)‡
Cholesterol	<300 mg
Fiber	40 g§

*From American Diabetes Assoc.[10] Reproduced with permission from the American Diabetes Association, Inc. These guidelines are intended to be tailored to individual needs.
+Patients with incipient renal failure may require lower protein intake.
‡PUS indicates the percentage of polyunsaturated fat; S, the percentage of saturated fat. If total fat is reduced, all components should be reduced proportionally.
§Fiber intake should be reduced to 25 g/1,000 kcal for persons on low-calorie diets.

Often, the assistance of a nutritionist, including periodic follow-up, results in greater dietary compliance.

Soluble fibers, such as guar and pectin, have been shown to reduce the glycemic response to carbohydrate-rich meals and improve the lipid profile, but the incremental improvement after achieving optimal diabetic control by other means may be insignificant.[15] Excessive fiber intake in older persons causes gastrointestinal distress (bloating, nausea, possibly bezoar formation), especially in the presence of autonomic neuropathy with gastrointestinal tract involvement. Additionally, dietary fiber may interfere with the absorption of medications (eg, digoxin) and minerals (eg, calcium).

Exercise

Exercise favorably affects the aging cardiovascular and skeletal systems and promotes a sense of well-

Table 18.3. Conditions affecting treatment of diabetes mellitus in elderly persons.*

			Medication	
	Diet	Exercise	Oral	Insulin
Dementia	+	+	+	+
Depression	+	+	+	+
Osteoporosis	−	+	−	−
Arthritis	+	+	−	+
Tremor	+	+	−	+
Visual decline	+	+	+	+
Altered Taste or smell	+	−	−	−
Poverty	+	+	+	+

*A plus sign indicates that treatment is affected by the condition.

being. There is evidence that high-intensity exercise increases insulin sensitivity and decreases lipid levels in older nondiabetics, but even healthy elderly persons (about half the subjects in one investigation[16]) will be unable to sustain the necessary level of exercise. Even if we could extrapolate such data to diabetics and to lower-intensity exercise, Table 18.3 reminds us that comorbidity often interferes. On the other hand, it is possible that greater attention to salutary nutrition and fitness habits in middle age would decrease the alarming prevalence of diabetes in later years.[17]

In diabetics who take insulin, exercise lowers the plasma glucose concentration. The magnitude of this decrease depends on ambient insulin levels, but supplemental calories must be taken in an amount determined by individual response. Additionally, exercise affects the kinetics of insulin absorption. At rest, insulin is absorbed more rapidly from the abdomen than from the arm, and more rapidly from the arm than the leg.[18] However, during activities such as walking or jogging, insulin absorption from the leg may be greatly enhanced, while not affected at other sites.

If dietary manipulation and exercise fail, the physician is faced with a decision regarding treatment with a sulfonylurea or insulin. This, of course, depends on how one defines failure. Some patients, despite reasonable efforts at diet and exercise, will maintain plasma glucose levels above 250 mg/dL (14 mmol/L), which is the average renal threshold for glucose in older persons. This causes symptoms such as polyuria and almost certainly contributes to the development of complications (see below). It has not been demonstrated conclusively that strict control of plasma glucose decreases the risk of diabetic complications; the current Diabetes Control and Complications Trial[19] may suggest an answer, but that study excludes elderly subjects.

Reasons often cited for conservative—if not downright unenthusiastic—treatment of diabetes in elderly patients include decreased life expectancy, poor compliance, increased risk of drug interactions, and the danger of hypoglycemia. These are arguments for the careful approach to treatment that characterizes geriatric medicine. They are not justifications for denying the older diabetic patient relief of symptoms, protection against metabolic derangements during times of physiologic stress, or the possibility of preventing complications.

Sulfonylureas

The sulfonylureas are a group of drugs with multiple pharmacologic actions.[20] They stimulate insulin secretion, except in patients lacking an adequate beta-cell mass (those with type I diabetes or advanced NIDDM with so-called "beta-cell exhaustion"). The sulfonylureas also increase insulin sensitivity in peripheral tissues, through an as yet uncharacterized modification of postreceptor events. Some studies have shown an increase in the density of insulin receptors after sulfonylurea administration. It is not known whether this is a primary drug action or correction of the receptor downregulation seen in untreated NIDDM.

Table 18.4 lists the sulfonylureas commonly used in elderly patients. Chloropropamide is not included, because the risks of prolonged, severe hypoglycemia and hyponatremia (hypersensitization of the nephron to vasopressin) make this drug a poor choice in elderly persons. The second-generation sulfonylureas possess theoretical advantages over their first-generation counterparts, including (1) less dependence on renal excretion; (2) mild diuretic action, as opposed to water retention; (3) once-a-day administration; and (4) decreased interaction with albumin-bound drugs, eg, oral anticoagulants.

The remainder of this section deals with second-generation sulfonylureas, but there is no compelling reason for switching to one of these if an elderly patient's diabetes is well controlled by a first-generation agent.

Both glyburide (known as glibenclamide in Europe) and glipizide may be given once daily; glipizide has a shorter half-life, but appears to undergo enterohepatic recirculation.[21] The usual starting dose of either drug in elderly patients is 2.5 mg/d, but 1.25 mg/d of glyburide is effective in occasional cases. Dosage increases should not be undertaken more often than every 2 weeks—more slowly in the patient with severe hepatic disease—until the fasting plasma glucose is less than 160 mg/dL (9 mmol/L) or the postprandial level is less than 200 mg/dL (11.2 mmol/L). Of course, these targets will vary for the individual patient depending on function, compliance, and comorbidity.

The patient and family should be informed about signs and symptoms of hypoglycemia, including fluctuations in cognition and neurologic function,[22] which replace the more classic adrenergic manifestations in some elderly people. Sustained hypoglycemia can occur with first- and second-generation sulfonylureas;

often this requires hospitalization with bolus and infusion glucose therapy. Plasma glucose levels may fluctuate between normal and low for several days in such instances. The case fatality rate for sulfonylurea-induced hypoglycemia requiring hospitalization is about 5%. In Europe, glibenclamide is a more common cause of severe hypoglycemia than glipizide.[23]

As with the first-generation agents, some patients (perhaps as many as 25%) will not respond initially to glipizide or glyburide, and the secondary failure rate is about 5% per year. Glyburide and glipizide often are ineffective in patients who are no longer controlled on first-generation drugs.[24]

Insulin

As mentioned earlier, hyperglycemia itself may promote further hyperglycemia in some patients with NIDDM. Initiation of insulin therapy can be beneficial in this setting, by reversing insulin resistance.[25] Twice-daily injections of combined regular and intermediate insulins has been instituted rapidly in a group of such patients (mean age, 60 years) during a short hospitalization.[26] However, a randomized, double-blind study has shown no difference in control in NIDDM between glyburide and once-daily intermediate insulin except for higher levels of high-density lipoprotein cholesterol in the insulin group.[27] Insulin therapy in the elderly patient with NIDDM often is begun as a single daily injection of 10 to 20 U of intermediate insulin (eg, NPH). The dose is increased by 5 U every 1 to 2 weeks, based on plasma glucose levels. The "dawn phenomenon" may necessitate a second injection in the evening. This refers to the early morning increase in plasma glucose and insulin requirement, without antecedent hypoglycemia, that occurs in many patients with NIDDM.[28] The mechanism of the dawn phenomenon is poorly understood but probably relates to increased nocturnal hepatic glucose output.

Purified pork and human insulins are of equal efficacy and antigenecity, so cost should be the deciding factor between these two preparations. Both also are useful (injected into the atrophic site) in the treatment of lipoatrophy caused by less highly purified insulin preparations.

Some elderly diabetics have defective counterregulation, the neurohormonal response to hypoglycemia. The decreasing plasma glucose concentration that characterizes an insulin reaction triggers secretion of glucagon, epinephrine, growth hormone, and cortisol. Experimentally, inadequate glucagon production combined with adrenergic blockade or adrenalectomy causes a severe decrement in counterregulatory response.[29] Circumstances propitious to this event ob-

Table 18.4. Sulfonylureas in the United States.

Drug	Dose/d	Duration of action, h
First generation		
Tolbutamide	0.5–3.0 g	6–12
Acetohexamide	0.25–1.5 g	12–24
Tolazamide	0.1–1.0 g	12–24
Second generation		
Glipizide	2.5–40 mg	16–24
Glyburide	1.25–20 mg	12–24

tain in some elderly patients: glucagon secretion is impaired (in the absence of changes in islet-cell morphology), the use of adrenergic-blocking drugs is common, and hypoadrenalism may occur.

Combination therapy with insulin and a sulfonylurea has been tried under strictly controlled conditions, the idea being to provide exogenous insulin and treat insulin resistance simultaneously. The only study of this combination in elderly persons, involving nine subjects, demonstrated lower fasting plasma glucose levels, urinary glucose excretion, and glycosylated hemoglobin levels during the 2-month addition of glyburide to the patients' usual insulin regimens.[30] The investigators did not comment on hypoglycemia, which is a major concern when combining two such powerful hypoglycemic agents.

A number of conditions common in old age can interfere with the self-administration of insulin (Table 18.3). In a study from which persons with neurologic or visual impairment were excluded, the accuracy of self-injected doses by elderly patients varied by ±12%.[31] Premixed insulins, pen-style syringes, jet injectors, and biosynthetic proinsulin ultimately may provide easier access with less risk of hypoglycemia for frail patients, but these modalities have not been studied in elderly diabetics. Patients often choose to use disposable syringes several times before discarding them; this is unlikely to result in skin infection and may yield significant cost savings.[32]

Assessment of Control

The laboratory determination of glycosylated hemoglobin level has enhanced our ability to judge long-term control and should be used to assess control in the diabetic. Normalization of the glycosylated hemoglobin level is the ideal for diabetic management; nonenzymatic glycosylation of other proteins figures in the development of complications (see below). Whether such strict control is attainable in the clinical setting depends on, among other things, the patient's functional status and the frequency of hypoglycemia. Home monitoring of blood glucose levels should be considered for NIDDM patients adhering to agressive insulin regimens. Self-monitoring may help with compliance in selected other patients.

Acute Metabolic Derangements

Hyperosmolar Coma (HC)

HC occurs almost exclusively in the elderly patient with NIDDM. It is a life-threatening state of hyperosmolality caused by marked hyperglycemia. Plasma

glucose levels usually exceed 600 mg/dL (34 mmol/L) and may be as high as 4,000 mg/dL (224 mmol/L). Mild ketosis is often present, but is not a major feature of HC. Lactic acidosis may coexist.

Glycosuria is the diabetic's mechanism for removal of unmetabolized glucose. When an elderly patient becomes dehydrated, especially if the kidneys are already impaired, delivery of glucose to the kidney is decreased and marked hyperglycemia ensues. Limited access to water and decreased thirst conspire in some ill elderly persons to exacerbate the dehydration and hyperglycemia. Intracellular dehydration results, because the underlying insulin resistance and/or deficiency prevents glucose from moving into the intracellular space. Conversely, insulin-independent tissues, such as brain, are subject to intracellular edema during therapy (see below).

Infection, stroke, and other physiologic stresses increase the risk of HC, as they are accompanied by excess cortisol and glucagon secretion. Exactly why elderly patients with NIDDM are more likely to develop HC than ketoacidosis is a matter of conjecture. Contributory factors probably include inhibition of lipolysis (from which is derived free fatty acids) by the hyperosmolality itself, relative glucagon resistance by the aging liver, and the presence of sufficient insulin to inhibit production of ketoacids.

The typical patient presents with an alteration in mental status. In fact only roughly 20% are comatose, but most of the remainder are obtunded to some degree. Many of these patients have had an acute stroke when they are first seen, although HC itself can cause reversible, focal neurologic signs. In some cases the precipitating illness (eg, myocardial infarction) overshadows the hyperosmolar picture. In at least half of all patients with HC, diabetes has not been diagnosed previously.[33] Reported mortality rates vary from 15% to 40%; death is not correlated with the initial plasma glucose level but is correlated with increasing age and osmolality.[34] The latter can be estimated reliably from the following formula:

$$\text{Plasma Osmolality (mOsm)} =$$
$$2(\text{Na}^+ + \text{K}^+) + \text{Glucose (mg/dL)}/18 + \text{BUN (mg/dL)}/2.8,$$

where BUN indicates blood urea nitgrogen.

The average water deficit in HC is 9 L, somewhat greater than in diabetic ketoacidosis (DKA). Deficits of sodium and potassium are sizable but less than in DKA; therefore, replacement of fluid deficit assumes priority in management. Normal saline is well suited for this and may be less likely than hypotonic solutions to precipitate cerebral edema, which can occur during fluid repletion as the excess intracellular glucose in insulin-independent brain tissue draws replaced water intracellularly. In actual practice, cerebral edema in HC is rare, and some experts prefer to use 0.5N saline, believing that correction of the hyperosmolar state is facilitated by giving hypotonic fluids from the outset.

The first 2 to 3 L of fluid should be given in 1 hour, even in elderly patients. Monitoring of the central venous or pulmonary artery wedge pressure is advisable for patients with overt heart disease. When urine flow is established, potassium replacement may commence. Insulin therapy is given intravenously at a rate of 0.1 U/kg/h, after 100 mL is flushed through the infusion set to prevent further insulin absorption by the plastic tubing. Hypotension and erratic absorption prevent reliable use of the intramuscular route in elderly patients with HC. As with DKA, glucose also should be infused once the plasma concentration decreases to approximately 250 mg/dL (14 mmol/L). Bicarbonate supplementation usually is not required unless lactic acidosis coexists. A diligent search for stroke, myocardial infarction, infection, and other precipitating conditions must be undertaken as soon as treatment of HC is underway.

Diabetic Ketoacidosis

Severely uncontrolled DKA occurs in the elderly, but much less frequently than HC. The mortality rate is greater than that of DKA in younger patients but less than the mortality rate of HC.[33] Fluid deficits tend to be somewhat smaller than in HC and sodium and potassium deficits somewhat greater. Nevertheless, fluid, insulin, and potassium therapy are essentially the same as for HC.

Phosphate depletion occurs during DKA and HC, but replacement is controversial. Despite theoretical advantages with regard to red-cell oxygen delivery, cardiac function, and respiratory mechanics, controlled trials have shown no effect on mortality, recovery from hyperglycemia, correction of acidosis, or mental status.[35,36]

Surgery and Diabetic Patients

The physiologic response to surgical stress includes increased secretion of cortisol, catecholamines, growth hormone, and glucagon. Thus, meticulous attention to diabetic control is essential during the perioperative period. For minor surgery, most patients treated with diet or a sulfonylurea will not require insulin. However, if the preoperative plasma glucose level is over 300 mg/dL (17 mmol/L), 15 to 20 U of intermediate-acting insulin before surgery, intraoperative infusion of 5% glucose, and bedside monitoring of blood glucose levels postoperatively should be con-

sidered. A patient with NIDDM who is receiving insulin and undergoes minor surgery may receive half the usual dose of intermediate-acting insulin preoperatively, with intraoperative glucose infusion and postoperative bedside monitoring of blood glucose levels. Alternatively, insulin may be witheld until after surgery, at which time two thirds the usual dose is given.

More aggressive management will be required when major surgery is undertaken, whether or not the patient has been receiving insulin. Subcutaneous administration of short-acting insulin every 4 hours or a constant intravenous infusion should be considered. This requires intraoperative blood glucose monitoring and attention to the potassium level.[37] (See also Chapter 11 for other aspects of perioperative care). Purified pork or human insulin is preferred in cases of temporary administration, to avoid the development of antibodies to insulin.

Complications

Etiology

Data from animal and human investigations suggest a key role for hyperglycemia in the development of diabetic complications. As a consequence of persistently elevated plasma glucose levels, advanced glycosylation products form in vascular basement membrane and sorbitol accumulates in nerve cells and elsewhere.

Excess nonenzymatic glycosylation of proteins, secondary to long-standing hyperglycemia, produces structural abnormalities in the collagen of vascular basement membranes.[38] Matrix protein undergoes irreversible crosslinkage and traps soluble complexes, most importantly low-density lipoprotein cholesterol. Similarly, glycosylation of the low-density lipoprotein itself impairs recognition by its receptors, facilitating accumulation in macrophages, the foam cells of atheromatous lesions.[39]

In tissues where glucose entry is not insulin dependent, hyperglycemia causes elevated levels of intracellular glucose, which is converted to sorbitol by the enzyme aldose reductase. In the lens, high levels of sorbitol result in osmotic damage and contribute to cataract formation. Peripheral nerve function is adversely affected by these events too. Here, sorbitol accumulation may be accompanied by depletion of *myo*-inosotol, a substance essential to neural membrane function. Aldose reductase inhibitors, which improve nerve conduction in diabetic animals, may exert their effect by preventing *myo*-inosotol depletion,[40] although this point remains controversial.[41] Furthermore, the recent attention focused on these interesting phenomena does not negate the importance of other well-known contributors to diabetic complications, such as platelet dysfunction and hyperlipidemia.

Macrovascular Disease

Delineating the influence of diabetes on cardiovascular disease in elderly persons is made more difficult by the prevalence of comorbidity, notably hypertension, cigarette smoking, and hypercholesterolemia. Figure 18.4 calls attention to the interaction of these risk factors in a middle-aged diabetic man, and the relationship holds for elderly persons as well.

In a cross-sectional study, 250 elderly patients with NIDDM (divided more or less equally among those treated with diet only, insulin, and sulfonylureas) were compared with a group of nondiabetic outpatients, who were similar in rates of hypertension, smoking, and hypercholesterolemia. The diabetics had an increased prevalence of coronary artery disease, and diabetes eliminated the usual protective effect of being female.[42] Also, increased prevalences were found for neuropathy, retinopathy, and cataracts, which are discussed below, and impotence (see Chapter 20).

Eye Disease

Diabetic retinopathy is divided into "background" and "proliferative" types, but the two differ only in the latter's being accompanied by new vessel formation. Microangiopathic changes are accompanied by retinal thickening caused by macular edema (see also Chapter 30). Studies of elderly subjects in the United States[43] and Israel[44] link the development of retinopa-

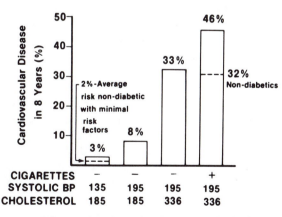

Fig. 18.4. Effects of various risk factors on the incidence of cardiovascular disease in diabetic men 40 years of age. Reproduced with permission from Feingold KR, Siperstein MD: Diabetic vascular disease. *Adv Intern Med* 1986; 31:309–340, Copyright © 1986, by Yearbook Medical Publishers.

thy to both severity of hyperglycemia and duration of disease. Older diabetics are more likely to have central angiopathy and macular edema. Therefore, ophthalmologic consultation is required for every diabetic patient. Early photocoagulation alleviates clinically significant macular edema, even when the retinopathy is mild and not accompanied by proliferative changes.[45]

Diabetes mellitus is thought to accelerate the formation of senile cataracts and to cause osmotic damage to the lens secondary to sorbitol accumulation. A patient offered cataract surgery should be informed that retinopathy may be present behind the cataract and may frustrate the hope of improving vision. Oculomotor nerve palsy occurs with some frequency in the elderly population. Because it is a vascular event, the central portion of the nerve, and with it pupillary function, often is spared.

Nephropathy and Hypertension

Although diabetic nephropathy probably is the most common cause of renal failure among adults in the United States, end-stage disease is not seen frequently in elderly persons, possibly owing to the presence of serious comorbidity and earlier death in these patients. The glomerular dysfunction of diabetic nephropathy is related to basement membrane thickening and increased permeability, a consequence of glomerular hyperfiltration and basement membrane glycosylation.

Older age at onset of NIDDM correlates with the development of persistent proteinuria.[46] Microalbuminuria, defined as the excretion of 30 to 140 $\mu g/mL$ of albumin (detectable by means of radioimmunoassay, not by dipstick), predicts both the subsequent development of proteinuria and increased mortality in older persons with type II diabetes.[47] Microalbuminuria can be eliminated in many patients with NIDDM by strict glycemic control,[48] but whether control influences the progression of renal disease in such patients is unknown.

Often hypertension coexists with NIDDM. Recent findings suggest that this association may be more than coincidental. Using the euglycemic insulin clamp technique, investigators have demonstrated peripheral insulin resistance in young, nonobese, untreated hypertensives.[49] A cause-effect relationship remains to be demonstrated and this will be difficult in older hypertensives, who can be insulin resistant as a consequence of aging.

Hypertension in the presence of diabetic nephropathy requires careful, but assertive management. Here the case for diet is doubly strong. Weight reduction and sodium restriction clearly are beneficial, but often antihypertensive medication also is required. The special pharmacologic considerations in these patients have been summarized recently.[50] Reduction of glomerular hypertension by captopril, an inhibitor of angiotensin-converting enzyme, has been demonstrated conclusively only in type I diabetics. Caution must be exercised when choosing such agents for elderly hypertensive diabetics, because hyporeninemic hypoaldosteronism often is present and, with it, a tendency toward hyperkalemia. The potential of thiazides for decreasing glucose tolerance is well known. Intravenous contrast material should be used in these patients only after careful consideration of potential benefits, as there is a high risk of adversely affecting renal function.

Neuropathy

Diabetic peripheral neuropathy can be disabling. The lower extremities most often are involved, and sensory function is more commonly affected than motor. Symptoms range from mild tingling to excrutiating lancinating pain. An extreme example is diabetic amyotrophy: pain and muscle atrophy in the hip girdle and lower extremities in elderly men, which resolve spontaneously within 1 to 2 years.

There is little doubt that amitriptyline can ameliorate the pain of diabetic peripheral neuropathy. Some have questioned whether this effect is due to the relief of concomitant depression, but a recent, double-blind crossover study suggests that the drug's action is independent of mood improvement.[51] Aldose reductase inhibitors are most likely to find clinical application in the treatment of diabetic neuropathy. These drugs improve nerve conduction velocity,[52] but symptomatic relief has been unpredictable, and few elderly subjects have been tested.

Diabetic autonomic neuropathy affects numerous systems, none more seriously than the cardiovascular. Loss of cardiovascular reflexes is quite serious in older patients, who are prone to dysrythmias and postural hypotension. Evaluation of the degree of involvement can be accomplished in the office with nothing more than an electrocardiogram and a blood pressure cuff.[53] Management varies from such simple measures as slow arising (especially from bed) and use of elastic stockings to administration of fludrocortisone acetate (0.1 mg twice daily, in the absence of conditions predisposing to congestive heart failure).

Gastrointestinal manifestations of autonomic neuropathy include gastroparesis (with a tendency to bezoar formation), constipation, and diarrhea. The first two regularly respond to metoclopramide hydrochloride, but the dosage must be reduced in elderly patients (eg, 2.5 mg of the syrup two or three times daily), because of central nervous system side effects ranging from irritability to extrapyramidal reactions.

Diarrhea also can be a troublesome symptom in the diabetic. Treatment depends on the etiology (see Chapter 27).

Foot Ulcers

Diabetic ulcers on the foot are usually neuropathic in origin. Certainly, peripheral vascular disease coexists in many affected patients, but even the failure to marshal surrounding inflammatory erythema can be secondary to disease of the nociceptive nerve fibers.[54] Patients should check their feet daily, avoid going barefoot, use a bland lubricating lotion when required, and cut the toenails horizontally. Physicians ought to examine the feet at *every* office visit.

An early foot ulcer may respond to avoidance of weight bearing and wet to dry saline dressings. Soaks are inadvisable, because they macerate the skin and can spread infectious agents. Deep or infected foot ulcers require hospital admission. Osteomyelitis may be present in the absence of radiographic changes. Cultures should be obtained from soft tissue and/or bone specimens, not from a swab of the ulcer crater; false-positive and false-negative results are common with the latter. Infections are often mixed, with *Staphylococcus, Enterococcus,* and *Bacteroides* the most frequent pathogens. Appropriate cultures, intravenous antibiotic therapy, and absolute avoidance of weight bearing may prevent or limit amputation.[55]

Cognition

A study of patients with type II diabetes between the ages of 55 and 74 years has shown impairment of memory retrieval compared with age-matched, nondiabetic controls[56] Cognitive impairment was correlated with duration of hyperglycemia and the glycosylated hemoglobin level. However, many study patients were taking insulin or sulfonylureas, introducing hypoglycemia as a possible confounder. Trials of cognitive function in untreated type II diabetics would be informative.

Although hypoglycemia should be avoided assiduously, its contribution to cognitive deterioration in the individual patient is difficult to gauge, because we lack a reliable measure of frequency and severity. Hypoglycemia is not a common cause of dementia among outpatients presenting for evaluation of cognitive decline.[57]

Summary

Diabetes mellitus in elderly persons usually is of the non–insulin-dependent variety. Physicians must keep in mind certain vagaries of diagnosis and treatment of this disease when confronted with the hyperglycemic, aged patient. However, there is no reason to believe that the same benefits will not accrue to the older diabetic receiving careful, persistent management as to a younger counterpart. Patient (in both its meanings) education is one of the most effective interventions in this disease. Diabetes mellitus provides those who care for older persons an opportunity to focus on quality of life by combining expertise with sensitivity. From head (ophthalmology consultation) to toe (examination of the feet at each office encounter), management of diabetes in elderly persons is the essence of geriatric medicine.

References

1. DeFronzo RA. The triumvirate: beta-cell, muscle, liver: a collusion responsible for NIDDM. *Diabetes* 1988; 37:667–687.
2. Harris MI, Hadden WC, Knowler WC, et al: International Criteria for the diagnosis of diabetes and impaired glucose tolerance. *Diabetes Care* 1985;8:562–567.
3. Little RR, England JD, Wiedmeyer HM, et al: Relationship of glycosylated hemoglobin to oral glucose tolerance. *Diabetes* 1988;37:60–64.
4. Arnetz BB, Kallner A, Theorell T. The influence of aging on hemoglobin A¹c (HbA¹c). *J Gerontol* 1982;37:648–650.
5. Kabadi UM. Glycosylation of proteins: lack of influence of aging. *Diabetes Care* 1988;11:429–432.
6. Harris MI, Hadden WC, Knowler WC, et al: Prevalence of diabetes and impaired glucose tolerance and plasma glucose levels in U.S. population aged 20–74 yr. *Diabetes* 1987;36:523–534.
7. Rosen OM. After insulin binds. *Science* 1987;237:1452–1458.
8. Fink RI, Kolterman OG, Griffin J, et al. Mechanisms of insulin resistance in aging. *J Clin Invest* 1983;71:1523–1535.
9. Stern MP. Type II diabetes mellitus: interface between clinical and epidemiological investigation. *Diabetes Care* 1988;11:119–126.
10. American Diabetes Association. Nutritional Recommendations and principles for individuals with diabetes mellitus: 1986 *Diabetes Care* 1987;10:126–132.
11. Hollenbeck CB, Coulston AM, Reaven GM. Comparison of plasma glucose and insulin responses to mixed meals of high-, intermediate-, and low-glycemic potential. *Diabetes Care* 1988;11:323–329.
12. Bantle JP, Laine DC, Thomas WJ. Metabolic effects of dietary fructose and sucrose in types I and II diabetic subjects. *JAMA* 1986;256:3241–3246.
13. Lipson LG. Diabetes in the elderly: diagnosis, pathogenesis, and therapy. *Am J Med* 1986;80(suppl 5A): 10–21.
14. Wing RR, Koeske R, Epstein LH, et al. Long-term effects of modest weight loss in type II diabetic patients. *Arch Intern Med* 1987;147:1749–1753.
15. Holman RR, Steemson J, Darling P, et al. No glycemic benefit from guar adminstration in NIDDM. *Diabetes Care* 1987;10:68–71.
16. Seals DR, Hagberg JM, Hurley BF, et al. Effects of endurance training on glucose tolerance and plasma lipid levels in older men and women. *JAMA* 1984;252:645–649.
17. Reaven GM, Reaven EP. Age, glucose intolerance, and non-insulin-dependent diabetes mellitus. *J Am Geriatr Soc* 1985;33:286–290.
18. Kovisto VA, Felig P. Alterations in insulin absorption and in blood glucose control associated with varying insulin injection sites in diabetic patients. *Ann Intern Med* 1980;92:59–61.
19. The DCCT Research Group. The diabetes control and complications trial (DCCT): design and methodologic considerations for the feasibility phase. *Diabetes* 1986;35:530–545.
20. Melander A. Clinical pharmacology of sulfonylureas. *Metabolism* 1987;36(suppl 1):12–16.
21. Groop L, Groop PH, Stenman S, et al. Comparison of pharmacokinetics, metabolic effects and mechanisms of action of glyburide and glipizide during long-term treatment. *Diabetes Care* 1987;10:671–678.
22. Yoo J, Peter S, Kleinfeld M. Transient hypoglycemic hemiparesis in an elderly patient. *J Am Geriatr Soc* 1986;34:479–481.
23. Ferner RE, Neil HAW. Sulphonylureas and hypoglycaemia. *Br J Med* 1988;296:949–950.
24. Lev JD, Zeidler A, Kumar D. Glyburide and glipizide in treatment of diabetic patients with secondary failures to tolazamide or chlorpropamide. *Diabetes Care* 1987; 10:679–682.
25. Scarlett JA, Gray RS, Griffin J, et al. Insulin treatment reverses the insulin resistance of type II diabetes mellitus. *Diabets Care* 1982;5:353–363.
26. Clements RS, Bell DSH, Benbarka A, et al. Rapid insulin initiation in non-insulin-dependent diabetes mellitus. *Am J Med* 1987;82:415–419.
27. Nathan DM, Roussell A, Godine JE. Glyburide or insulin for metabolic control in non-insulin-dependent diabetes mellitus. *Ann Intern Med* 1988;108:334–340.
28. Bolli GB, Gerich JE. The "dawn phenomenon": a common occurrence in both non-insulin-dependent and insulin-dependent diabetes mellitus. *N Engl J Med* 1984;310:746–750.
29. Cryer PE. Glucose counterregulation in man. *Diabetes* 1981;30:261–264.
30. Kyllastinen M, Groop L. Combination of insulin and glibenclamide in the treatment of elderly non-insulin dependent (type 2) diabetic patients. *Ann Clin Res* 1985;17:100–104.
31. Puxty JAH, Hunter DH, Burr WA. accuracy of insulin injection in elderly patients. *Br Med J* 1983;287:1762.
32. Alexander WD, Tattersall R. Plastic insulin syringes: reuse or waste L8m a year. *Br Med J* 1988;296:877–878.
33. Gale EAM, Dornan TL, Tattersall RB. Severely uncontrolled diabetes in the over-fifties. *Diabetologia* 1981;21:25–28.
34. Wachtel TJ, Silliman RA, Lamberton P. Prognostic factors in the diabetic hyperosmolar state. *J Am Geriatr Soc* 1987;35:737–741.

35. Fisher JN, Kitabchi AE. A randomized study of phosphate therapy in the treatment of diabetic ketoacidosis. *J Clin Endocrinol Metab* 1983;57:177–180.

36. Wilson HK, Keuer SP, Lea AS, et al. Phosphate therapy in diabetic ketoacidosis. *Arch Intern Med* 1982;142:517–520.

37. Pezzarossa A, Taddei F, Cimicchi MC, et al. Perioperative management of diabetic subjects: subcutaneous versus intravenous insulin administration during glucose-potassium infusion. *Diabetes Care* 1988;11:52–58.

38. Brownlee M, Cerami A, Vlassara H. Advanced glycosylation end products in tissue and the biochemical basis of diabetic complications. *N Engl J Med* 1988;318:1315–1321.

39. Lopes-Virella MF, Klein RL, Lyons TJ, et al. Glycosylation of low-density lipoprotein enhances cholesteryl ester synthesis in human monocyte-derived macrophages. *Diabetes* 1988;37:550–557.

40. Greene DA, Lattimer SA, Sima AAF. Sorbitol, phosphoinositides, and sodium-potassium-ATPase in the pathogenesis of diabetic complications. *N Engl J Med* 1987;316:599–606.

41. Dyck PJ, Zimmerman BR, Vilen TH, et al. Nerve glucose, fructose, sorbitol, *myo*-inositol, and fiber degeneration and regeneration in diabetic neuropathy. *N Engl J Med* 1988;319:542–548.

42. Nathan DM, Singer DE, Godine JE, et al. Non-insulin-dependent diabetes in older patients: complications and risk factors. *Am J Med* 1986;81:837–842.

43. Nathan DM, Singer DE, Godine JE, et al. Retinopathy in older type II diabetics: association with glucose control. *Diabetes* 1986;35:797–801.

44. Yanko L, Goldbourt U, Michaelson IC, et al. Prevalence and 15-year incidence of retinopathy and associated characteristics in middle-aged and elderly diabetic men. *Br J Ophthalmol* 1983;67:759–765.

45. Early Treatment Diabetic Retinopathy Study Research Group: photocoagulation for diabetic macular edema: Early Treatment Diabetic Retinopathy Study report number 1. *Arch Ophthalmol* 1985;103:1796–1805.

46. Ballard DJ, Humphrey LL, Melton JL III, et al. Epidemiology of persistent proteinuria in type II diabetes mellitus. *Diabetes* 1988;37:405–412.

47. Mogensen CE. Microalbuminuria predicts clinical proteinuria and early mortality in maturity-onset diabetes. *N Engl J Med* 1984;310:356–360.

48. Luetscher JA, Kraemer FB. Microalbuminuria and increased plasma prorenin: prevalence in diabetics followed up for four years. *Arch Intern Med* 1988;148:937–941.

49. Ferrannini E, Buzzigoli G, Bonadonna R, et al. Insulin resistance in essential hypertension. *N Engl J Med* 1987;317:350–357.

50. Working Group on Hypertension in Diabetes. Statement on hypertension in diabetes. *Diabetes Care* 1987;10:764–776.

51. Max MB, Culnane M, Schafer SC, et al. Amitriptyline relieves diabetic neuropathy pain in patients with normal or depressed mood. *Neurology* 1987;37:589–596.

52. Judzewitsch RG, Jaspan JB, Polonsky KS, et al. Aldose reductase inhibition improves nerve conduction velocity in diabetic patients. *N Engl J Med* 1983;308:119–125.

53. Ewing DJ, Clarke BF. Diagnosis and management of diabetic autonomic neuropathy. *Br Med J* 1982;285:916–918.

54. Parkhouse N, Le Quesne PM. Impaired neurogenic vascular response in patients with diabetes and neuropathic foot lesions. *N Engl J Med* 1988;318:1306–1309.

55. Bamberger DM, Daus GP, Gerding DN. Osteomyelitis in the feet of diabetic patients: long-term results, prognostic factors, and the role of antimicrobial and surgical therapy. *Am J Med* 1987;83:653–660.

56. Perlmuter LC, Hakami MK, Hodgson-Harrington C, et al. Decreased cognitive function in aging non-insulin-dependent diabetic patients. *Am J Med* 1984;77:1043–1048.

57. Larson EB, Reifler BV, Sumi SM, et al. Diagnostic tests in the evaluation of dementia: a prospective study of 200 elderly outpatients. *Ann Intern Med* 1986;146:1917–1922.

19

Thyroid Disorders

David S. Cooper

Thyroid problems in the elderly are commonly encountered and challenging to diagnose and treat. In the geriatric population, the prevalence of certain thyroid diseases (eg, nodules, goiter, hypothyroidism) is high, and some thyroid disorders (eg, hyperthyroidism), may have subtle or atypical presentations. In older patients with common associated nonthyroidal illnesses, thyroid function tests may be altered, making their interpretation all the more difficult. Finally, therapy may be more complex than in younger patients, due to the presence of underlying chronic illness, especially cardiac disease, and because of altered thyroid hormone metabolism.

Regardless of age, thyroid disorders can be conveniently categorized as functional (hyperthyroidism and hypothyroidism), inflammatory (thyroiditis), or neoplastic (nodules, carcinoma). For unknown reasons, virtually all thyroid problems occur more commonly in women. Before discussing thyroid diseases in depth, however, it is necessary to review normal thyroid function and to emphasize the alterations in thyroid structure and function that occur in the elderly. Fundamental but unanswered questions are whether such changes are part of normal senescence and whether they contribute materially to the aging process itself.

Aging and Thyroid Anatomy and Physiology

Thyroid Anatomy

During normal aging, atrophy and fibrosis of the thyroid occur.[1] There is a corresponding reduction in thyroid weight, making palpation of the normal thyroid more difficult. To an unknown extent, these anatomic and histological changes reflect autoimmune phenomena, since the prevalence of antibodies to thyroglobulin and microsomal antigens approaches 20% in women over age 60 years.[2] In addition, the prevalence of microscopic and macroscopic thyroid nodules rises with age, with a marked increase in clinically palpable disease. However, there does not appear to be a correlation of thyroid weight or histology with thyroid function,[3] at least as assessed by circulating thyroxine concentrations.

Thyroid Physiology

Control of Thyroid Function

The hypothalamic-pituitary-thyroid axis functions as a classic negative feedback system (Figure 19.1). Thyrotropin-releasing hormone (TRH), a hypothalamic tripeptide, stimulates the thyrotropes in the pituitary to synthesize and release thyroid-stimulating hormone (TSH, thyrotropin). In turn, TSH binds to specific receptors on thyroid follicular cells, to stimulate virtually all aspects of thyroid growth and function, from the trapping of iodide from the blood to the synthesis and secretion of the thyroid hormones thyroxine (T_4) and triiodothyronine (T_3).

Circulating thyroid hormone exerts negative feedback at the pituitary level, and, as has been recently elucidated, at the hypothalamic level as well. Thus, a rise in thyroid hormone concentrations suppresses TSH and, quite likely, TRH biosynthesis and secretion. On the other hand, a fall in serum thyroid hormone levels stimulates pituitary TSH (and presumably hypothalamic TRH) biosynthesis and secretion.

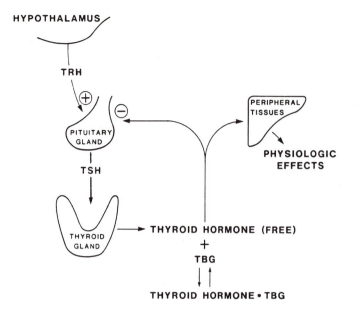

Fig. 19.1. Regulation of TSH and thyroid hormone secretion. The relationship between bound and free thyroid hormones in the serum is depicted, emphasizing the importance of the free thyroid hormone concentration in the feedback control of TSH release and in peripheral tissues.

The hypothalamus and pituitary both respond to changes in thyroid hormone concentrations with exquisite sensitivity. Thus, serum TSH levels can fall or rise in response to seemingly minor reciprocal changes in thyroid hormone concentrations, often still within the normal range and not drastic enough to cause clinical evidence of altered thyroid function. For this reason, serum TSH levels are extremely valuable in diagnosing subtle disturbances in thyroid function, which are particularly common in the elderly.

While the hypothalamic-pituitary unit is of primary importance in the overall control of thyroid function, there is solid evidence that iodide also serves as a regulator of thyroid hormone biosynthesis and secretion. In pharmacologic doses (>30 mg), iodide inhibits thyroid hormone release and blocks thyroidal iodide uptake. Iodide also causes a transient decrease in thyroid hormone biosynthesis, the so-called Wolff-Chaikoff effect. These actions of iodide are probably important in protecting the organism against hyperthyroidism in the event of large iodide loads. Because of its inhibitory effects on thyroid function, iodide occasionally is used to treat hyperthyroidism, but, as will be discussed, it also can cause either hyperthyroidism (the Jod-Basedow phenomenon) or hypothyroidism, given the appropriate clinical substrate.

Thyroid Hormone Synthesis and Transport

Thyroid hormone synthesis is a multistep process that begins with the trapping of iodide by the thyroid follicular cell. Iodide is an essential nutrient and is abundant in the diet of most Western countries. In the United States, the average daily iodine intake is 500 to 1,000 μg/d, and iodine deficiency does not exist, even in elderly individuals who may be poorly nourished. Trapped iodide is oxidized and bound to tyrosine residues in the large protein thyroglobulin, via a process known as "organification." The next step is the "coupling" of two iodinated tyrosines to form the *iodothyronines*, T_4 and T_3. Following synthesis, T_4 and T_3 are stored as colloid in the follicular lumen. With TSH stimulation, the colloid (ie, thyroglobulin) is hydrolyzed inside vacuoles and the free thyroid hormones are released into the bloodstream. The daily T_4 secretion is 10 to 20-fold greater than T_3 secretion (75 to 100 vs 5 to 10 μg/d). Once secreted, they are bound (>99.9%) to transport proteins, principally thyroid-binding globulin (TBG), thyroid-binding prealbumin, and albumin. It is believed that only the unbound, or free, hormone is available to enter cells and exert its metabolic effects. Because of the tight binding of thyroid hormones to serum proteins, their clearance is prolonged significantly: the half-life of T_4 is approximately 7 days; because it is less firmly bound, T_3 has a shorter half-life, approximately 1 day.

It is important to emphasize that quantitative and qualitative changes in the binding proteins alter the serum *total* T_4 and T_3 concentrations but do not affect free thyroid hormone levels. Thus, situations in which thyroid-binding proteins are altered may be confused with true thyroid dysfunction if only total thyroid hormone concentrations are considered.

Thyroid Hormone Metabolism

Although thyroid hormones are metabolized in a variety of ways, the deiodination pathway is the most

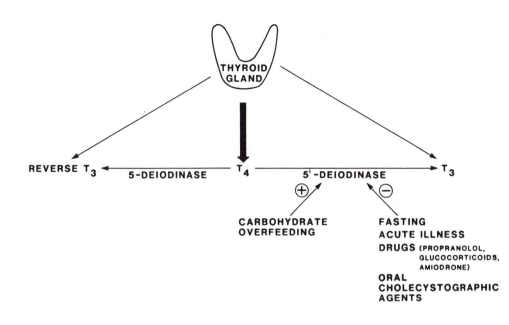

Fig. 19.2. Peripheral metabolism of T_4 and factors that influence the tissue conversion of T_4 to T_3.

relevant clinically (Figure 19.2). Via this route, approximately 50% of the daily T_4 production is converted to T_3 by removal of a single iodine atom from the outer ring of the T_4 molecule. This reaction is catalyzed by a ubiquitous enzyme, 5′ or outer-ring deiodinase, which also degrades the nonbiologically active compound, reverse T_3 (rT_3) to another inert product, T_2. About 80% of the daily T_3 production derives from T_4 deiodination in the peripheral tissues. Since T_3 is the more metabolically active hormone, it has been hypothesized that T_4 is merely a "prohormone" for T_3, but the question has not been resolved. It is clear, however, that most of the biologic effects of thyroid hormone can be accounted for by the actions of T_3 alone.

A variety of clinical states can decrease the conversion of T_4 to T_3 via inhibitory effects on outer-ring deiodinase activity. Starvation, systemic illness, and certain drugs (propranolol, amiodarone, iodinated contrast agents) all cause a fall in serum T_3 concentrations and a reciprocal rise in serum rT_3, due to a fall in T_4 to T_3 conversion and in catabolism of rT_3. The fall in T_3 concentration reduces protein catabolism and tissue oxygen consumption, which may be beneficial to the organism during periods of illness or decreased caloric intake.

Age-Related Changes in Thyroid Function and Metabolism[4]

A number of studies suggest that thyroid function declines with advancing age. In the elderly, plasma iodide levels increase, but thyroidal iodide accumulation actually decreases. The fall in thyroidal iodine uptake is accompanied by a decrease in iodine release, and by inference, in T_4 secretion. However, decreased T_4 secretion in the elderly is not necessarily indicative of thyroid failure, since it is not accompanied by elevations in serum TSH. Furthermore, most studies show little, if any, change in circulating T_4 or free T_4 levels in the blood. Accordingly, studies of elderly men [4,5] have revealed reductions in the T_4 metabolic clearance rate.

Possible alterations in serum T_3 concentrations are more controversial. While several studies have shown age-related reductions in serum T_3 levels, particularly after age 60 years, others have found no significant decline over the 5th through the 9th decade.[6] One explanation for the discrepancies among the various reports is the inclusion of individuals with subclinical illness in the study populations. Thus, the reported decline in serum T_3 noted by some investigators may be secondary to the presence of subtle infirmities associated with aging, rather than the aging process itself.

Despite the tentative conclusion drawn by many investigators that serum T_3 levels do not fall with age, it is clear that T_3 levels often are low in randomly selected elderly individuals without obvious illness. Since the major source of daily T_3 production derives from outer-ring deiodination of T_4, one possible explanation for the low T_3 levels is a decrease in the T_4 deiodination rate, which is the hallmark of systemic illness or decreased caloric intake. However, if a fall in deiodination were the explanation, a reciprocal rise in rT_3 would be expected, and this has not been observed in elderly persons. Thus, the fall in serum T_3 may be due to the decrease in T_4 production by the thyroid gland, discussed above.

As noted earlier, the decline in thyroidal T_4 secretion is not accompanied by an elevated serum TSH level, which is the most sensitive indicator of thyroid hypofunction. However, numerous studies of TSH levels in elderly persons do suggest that mean TSH levels are higher than values observed in younger individuals. Because most studies have shown that elderly women more often have high-normal or frankly elevated TSH levels and that antithyroid antibodies are often (although not always) present in such patients, it is reasonable to conclude that the slight elevation in mean TSH noted in most reports results from the inclusion in the study population of patients with subclinical autoimmune thyroiditis.

Thyroid Hormone Action

Thyroid hormones enter the cell by diffusion and bind to specific receptors located in the nucleus. One of the exciting recent developments in thyroidology is the discovery that the thyroid hormone receptor is the protein product or products of a family of oncogenes (erb-A).[7] The thyroid hormone receptor protein acts to modify DNA transcription and the synthesis of new proteins by the cell (eg, angiotensin-converting enzyme, sex hormone–binding globulin, the β-adrengeric receptor, factor VIII), while it inhibits the synthesis of TSH and TRH.

Virtually all tissues contain thyroid hormone receptors in varying amounts; the degree to which a tissue responds to thyroid hormone is proportional to the thyroid hormone receptor density within that tissue. Clinical observations suggest that elderly persons have decreased responsiveness to thyroid hormones. This is particularly striking in the older patient with thyrotoxicosis, as discussed in the next section. One recent study suggested that the thyroid hormone response of erythrocyte Ca^{++}/adenosine triphosphatase (a non–receptor-mediated activity) falls with age,[8] and another found a decrease in lymphocyte nuclear thyroid hormone receptors with age.[9]

Thyroid Function Testing

The many recent advances in the laboratory measurement of thyroid function have greatly simplified the evaluation of thyroid dysfunction. Even subtle forms of hypo- and hyperthyroidism can be diagnosed easily, and thyroid hormone therapy can be adjusted with great precision.

Table 19.1. Clinical situations associated with abnormal TBG concentrations.

TBG excess	TBG deficiency
Estrogen therapy	Androgen therapy
Acute hepatocellular disease	Chronic liver disease
	Severe catabolic illness
	Congenital X-linked deficiency

Measurement of Thyroid Hormone Concentrations

Radioimmunoassays for T_4 and T_3 are routinely available, with rapid turnaround times. It must be recalled that alterations in TBG affect the total T_4 and T_3 concentrations but not the circulating *free* thyroid hormone concentrations. Thus, patients with TBG excess or deficiency have high or low T_4 and T_3 concentrations, respectively, but are clinically and biochemically euthyroid (Table 19.1). It behooves the clinician to determine the true thyroid status of the patient in order to avoid erroneous diagnoses and inappropriate therapy. Although direct measurement of TBG and or free T_4 is possible, the traditional method for determining the thyroid status is the free T_4 index, which is the product of total T_4 and the T_3 resin uptake (T_3RU). The T_3RU is an indirect approximation of TBG binding capacity, and, when used in concert with the total T_4 concentration, it permits one to distinguish true thyroid disease from perturbations in TBG concentration. It is important not to confuse the T_3RU, which uses radioactive T_3 in vitro, with the direct assay of serum T_3 (the T_3 radioimmunoassay).

Low Serum Total T_4 Levels

Hypothyroxinemia is characteristic of hypothyroidism, but other conditions also must be considered (Table 19.2). A decrease in serum total T_4 often is due to TBG deficiency or to inhibition of T_4 binding to TBG by drugs (high-dose salicylates, anticonvulsants) or endogenous factors. A circulating inhibitor of T_4 binding to TBG has been described in nonthyroidal

Table 19.2. Major causes of abnormal serum T_4 concentrations in elderly patients.

Increased T_4	Decreased T_4
Hyperthyroidism	Hypothyroidism
Increased protein binding	TBG deficiency
TBG excess	Serious illness
Anti-T_4 antibodies	
Abnormal binding proteins	
Acute illness (transient)	

illness, and probably accounts for the often extraordinarily low serum T_4 values (<3 $\mu g/dL$) observed in critically ill patients. As would be expected, free T_4 levels are normal or even slightly elevated in such circumstances, and patients are considered to be euthyroid because of their normal serum TSH levels. This severe hypothyroxinemia has been termed the "euthyroid sick syndrome" and is invariably accompanied by extremely low serum T_3 levels.

High Serum Total T_4 Levels

Hyperthyroxinemia is seen in most patients with hyperthyroidism. Approximately 10% of such patients, however, have T_3 toxicosis, with normal serum T_4 but elevated serum T_3 levels. This circumstance is particularly common in patients with toxic nodules and toxic multinodular goiter. Interestingly, elderly thyrotoxic patients often also develop "T_4 toxicosis," with normal serum T_3 levels, a finding that is rare in younger hyperthyroid patients. This is discussed in more detail in the section on hyperthyroidism.

Euthyroid hyperthyroxinemia (Table 19.2), ie, a high total T_4 level due to elevations in TBG or other binding proteins, is commonly confused with biochemical hyperthyroidism. However, estimation of the TBG level with the T_3RU generally permits the correct interpretation of an elevated serum T_4 level. In rare patients, such elevation will be due to elevations or abnormalities of the other T_4-binding proteins (thyroid-binding prealbumin and albumin). These disorders can be extremely difficult to diagnose, because the T_3RU is normal. They should be suspected if the serum T_3 and TSH levels are normal.

Measurement of Free T_4 Concentrations

The direct measurement of free T_4 occasionally is necessary when the total T_4 level, the T_3RU, and other data yield conflicting or uncertain results. Equilibrium dialysis is the "gold standard" for measuring free T_4, but a variety of more direct, but somewhat less reliable, methods have been devised. The best test for assessing thyroid function in critically ill patients is the serum TSH level, although the free T_4 level, measured by equilibrium dialysis in a reliable laboratory, is also valid. The serum rT_3 level, which rises in illness, has been proposed as an additional way of distinguishing patients with nonthyroidal illness from those with hypothyroidism. However, the assay is not routinely available.

Measurement of TSH

The pituitary gland is exquisitely sensitive to changes in circulating thyroid hormone concentrations. Serum TSH levels will therefore be elevated even in mild primary hypothyroidism and, theoretically, TSH levels should be low in virtually all forms of hyperthyroidism. Of course, the serum TSH level will be inappropriately low in hypothyroid patients with pituitary or hypothalamic failure, and in the rare patient with a TSH-secreting pituitary adenoma causing hyperthyroidism, the TSH level will be inappropriately elevated or normal.

In recent years, TSH assays have been refined, with improvements in their level of sensitivity. Modern techniques, sometimes called "high-sensitivity" or "ultrasensitive" TSH assays, can distinguish the low TSH levels in hyperthyroidism from normal TSH levels, which is not possible with conventional TSH assays. This important modification permits the clinician to diagnose hyperthyroidism (which should yield low or undetectable TSH levels) with greater ease. Previously, patients with borderline or equivocal T_4 and T_3 results required TRH testing for the diagnosis of hyperthyroidism to be established. In this test, TRH is administered intravenously and TSH release by the pituitary is measured. In normal individuals, TRH stimulates pituitary TSH release, whereas the pituitary response in hyperthyroidism is flat or markedly attenuated due to negative feedback by T_4 at the pituitary level. With the availability of the new, more sensitive TSH assays, TRH testing is no longer necessary in most situations. This is particularly important in older patients, since the TSH response to TRH is blunted in some healthy elderly patients, especially men.

Radionuclide Evaluation of Thyroid Structure and Function

The thyroid gland traps iodide and other ions, permitting glandular morphology and function to be assessed with isotopes of iodine (^{123}I and ^{131}I) and technetium ($^{99m}TcO_4$). Technetium is used frequently to image the thyroid, because it is inexpensive and convenient (imaging after 20 minutes). But since it is trapped but not organified (unlike iodide), it cannot provide as much useful information about overall thyroid function as does iodide, with imaging after 6 to 24 hours.

Unfortunately, the radioiodine uptake (RAIU) is only occasionally helpful in diagnosing hypo- or hyperthyroidism. Since the normal 24-hour RAIU is lower than in previous decades (normal, 5% to 25%), there is a great deal of overlap between normal and hypothyroid values. Furthermore, many elderly hyperthyroid patients, especially those with toxic nodular goiter, have 24-hour RAIU values in the normal range. Additionally, some hypothyroid patients with Hashimoto's thyroiditis can actually have elevated RAIU, while patients with hyperthyroidism due to thyroiditis have low RAIU. Thus, the test is very nonspecific. Stable iodide blocks the uptake of radioactive iodide by the thyroid; therefore, isotopic studies should not be performed within several weeks of receiving iodinated contrast dyes.

Although the 24-hour RAIU is of limited usefulness, thyroid scanning is helpful in determining the size and location of thyroid tissue and the functional nature of thyroid nodules. Thyroid scanning is also invaluable in the diagnosis of functioning metastases from well-differentiated thyroid cancer.

Other Thyroid-Related Tests

Antithyroid antibodies are important in establishing the diagnosis of autoimmune thyroid disease. Thyroglobulin is released from the thyroid in a host of thyroid disorders, and its measurement is most useful in the follow-up of patients with well-differentiated thyroid cancer. Thyroid needle biopsy, thyroid ultrasonography, and neck computed tomography will be discussed in the section on thyroid neoplasia and goiter.

Disturbances of Thyroid Function

Thyrotoxicosis

Thyrotoxicosis is being recognized with increasing frequency in the elderly. While most reports indicate that the peak incidence is in the 2nd and 3rd decades of life, one recent prospective study found that, of 49 cases of thyrotoxicosis diagnosed over a 3-year period, 28 (57%) were in individuals over the age of 60 years.[10] Graves' disease is the most common cause of thyrotoxicosis in all age groups, but the proportion of patients with toxic multinodular goiter (Plummer's disease) increases with age. Since the prevalence of thyroid nodularity in general is higher in the elderly, some older patients with preexisting nontoxic nodules undoubtedly develop thyrotoxicosis due to Graves' disease, accounting for diagnostic difficulty. On the other hand, 20% to 30% of elderly thyrotoxic patients have nonpalpable thyroid glands, also making the diagnosis more obscure. In a recent study of hyperthyroidism in 21 individuals over age 75 years, only three had a palpable gland.[11]

Clinical Features

In contrast to the classic symptoms and signs of hyperthyroidism in younger individuals, elderly patients typically display few of the sympathomimetic features that are characteristic of the thyrotoxic state. Thus, the apt term "masked" or "apathetic" thyrotoxicosis has been applied to the elderly thyrotoxic patient who presents with depression, lethargy, weakness, and cachexia. However, most older patients *do* have symptoms that should bring the diagnosis to mind. Agitation and confusion ("thyrotoxic encephalopathy") can mimic cerebrovascular disease. Unexplained weight loss, nervousness, palpitations, and tremulousness are present in well over half the patients, with weight loss occurring in up to 80%.[12] In contrast to younger thyrotoxic patients however, elderly patients frequently (but not invariably) have a poor appetite, and constipation is present in one third of them. The combination of weight loss and diminished appetite often triggers a fruitless evaluation for occult malignancy.

It is well known that the cardiovascular system retains its sensitivity to thyroid hormone action in the elderly. This, coupled with a high prevalence of atherosclerotic coronary disease, probably is the explanation for palpitations, worsening angina, and, more rarely, symptoms of congestive heart failure. Atrial fibrillation, often with a relatively slow ventricular response, is the presenting feature in up to 20% of patients, and the development of atrial fibrillation should always prompt a thorough screen for thyrotoxicosis. A recent study of nursing home residents over age 65 years found that 11% of men and 31% of women with atrial fibrillation were thyrotoxic.[13]

Despite the fact that Graves' disease is the most common form of thyrotoxicosis in the elderly, infiltrative ophthalmopathy is present in less than 10% of patients. The reasons for this are unknown. However, lid lag and lid retraction, reflecting the hyperadrenergic state, are seen in approximately one third of affected individuals.

Laboratory Testing

In contrast to the ease with which the laboratory diagnosis of thyrotoxicosis is made in younger patients, thyroid function test interpretation in the elderly can be a vexing problem. As in younger patients, the serum T_4 level, the free T_4 index or free T_4 level, and the T_3 level all are elevated in the average patient. However, "T_3 toxicosis" is common in patients with solitary toxic nodules and toxic multinodular goiter. Since these diagnoses occur more frequently in the elderly, the possibility of thyrotoxicosis with normal serum T_4 and free T_4 levels, but an elevated T_3 level, must be kept in mind. Even more problematic is "T_4 toxicosis," which typically occurs in elderly hyperthyroid patients who have concurrent nonthyroidal illness. The decrease in T_4 to T_3 conversion, brought about by the illness, produces normal or even low serum T_3 values. While the serum T_3 level is virtually always elevated in younger thyrotoxic patients, it is normal in one third of elderly thyrotoxic patients. However, it is of great importance to distinguish "T_4 toxicosis" from "euthyroid hyperthyroxinemia."[14] It should also be recognized that the serum T_4 and T_3 levels may actually be normal in debilitated elderly thyrotoxic patients, due to a decrease in serum TBG and a decrease in T_4 to T_3 conversion, respectively. Although the free T_4 index should correct for changes in TBG, it is frequently unreliable, and direct measurement of free T_4 may be necessary.

The measurement of TSH and the TSH response to TRH are of great value in distinguishing true thyrotoxicosis from euthyroid hyperthyroxinemia. In the former situation, TSH levels will be low, and the TSH response to TRH will be absent or severely blunted, while in the latter circumstance, TSH levels should be normal, with a normal TSH response to TRH. As noted above, new, highly sensitive TSH assays have been developed that can clearly distinguish the low TSH levels of thyrotoxicosis from the normal values seen in euthyroidism, making TRH testing unnecessary in diagnosing hyperthyroidism. Unfortunately, a low serum TSH or a blunted TSH response to TRH are not always unequivocal; some "euthyroid" individuals with nontoxic multinodular goiter may have "subclinical hyperthyroidism" with normal T_4, free T_4, and T_3 levels, but suppression of the hypothalamic-pituitary axis. Whether such individuals require therapy is controversial. The TSH levels also may be low in critically ill patients, but such patients usually have low rather than high serum T_4 levels, and hypothyroidism is the diagnostic problem, rather than hyperthyroidism.[15]

The 24-hour RAIU is normal in up to 30% of elderly patients with Graves' disease and in over two thirds of elderly individuals with Plummer's disease.[16] Repeated thyroid function testing (to rule out transient euthyroid hyperthyroxinemia), the measurement of serum T_3 in patients with normal serum T_4 levels, and the use of high-sensitivity TSH assays all should facilitate the laboratory evaluation and maximize diagnostic accuracy.

Differential Diagnosis

Before initiating a therapy for the thyrotoxic patient, the etiology of hyperthyroidism must be known (Table 19.3). As stated earlier Graves' disease is the most frequent cause (in 50% to 70% of cases), followed by toxic multinodular goiter. Together, these two account for well over 95% of cases. Two uncommon forms of thyroiditis are transient and self-limited. Subacute thyroiditis (De Quervain's) typically presents with severe anterior neck pain, fever, and general malaise

Table 19.3. Causes of thyrotoxicosis in elderly patients.

Thyroid hormone hypersecretion
  Graves' disease
  Toxic adenoma and toxic nodular goiter
  Iodine-induced hyperthyroidism (rare)
  Metastatic follicular carcinoma (rare)
  Pituitary TSH-secreting tumor (rare)
Follicular disruption
  Subacute thyroiditis
  Painless thyroiditis (rare)
  Radiation thyroiditis, especially after ^{131}I therapy
Exogenous thyroid hormone
  Iatrogenic hyperthyroidism
  Factitious hyperthyroidism

and is thought to be viral in origin. Thyroid function test results are elevated due to release of stored hormone into the blood, but the 24-hour RAIU is *low,* because of damage to the thyroid gland as well as suppression of endogenous TSH by the high thyroid hormone levels. Treatment consists of antiinflammatory agents (salicylates and other nonsteroidal antiinflammatory agents, glucocorticoids in severe cases) and β-adrenergic blocking drugs for symptomatic relief. Painless ("silent") or lymphocytic thyroiditis, rare in the elderly, presents with thyrotoxicosis and small painless goiter.[17] It can be extremely difficult to distinguish from Graves' disease by laboratory testing, except that, as in subacute thyroiditis, the 24-hour RAIU is very low. Therapy is limited to the use of β-adrenergic blockers until the thyrotoxicosis has resolved.

Another diagnosis that should be considered in the elderly patient with thyrotoxicosis is the possibility of a TSH-secreting pituitary tumor. The hallmark is the presence of serum TSH levels that are inappropriate given the elevations in serum T_4 and T_3 levels (ie, instead of being suppressed, TSH levels are normal or high). A full discussion of inappropriate TSH syndromes is beyond the scope of this chapter, but is the subject of a recent review.[18]

Finally, iodine-induced thyrotoxicosis (Jod-Basedow phenomenon) occurs in individuals exposed to iodide or iodide-containing compounds who have an underlying multinodular goiter. The problem is becoming more common with the recent introduction of amiodarone, an iodinated antiarrhythmic agent. Although iodine-induced thyrotoxicosis is self-limited, it can be very severe, requiring large doses of antithyroid drugs.

Treatment

The three treatments for hyperthyroidism are antithyroid drugs, radioactive iodine, and surgery. In elderly patients, surgery is rarely employed because of its attendant morbidity, unless a large toxic multinodular goiter is present and causing local symptoms (dysphagia and/or dyspnea). Antithyroid drugs (propylthiouracil and methimazole) often are used as primary therapy for Graves' disease in younger patients, for a variety of reasons, including the possibility of spontaneous remission and theoretical but unproved concerns about long-term consequences of radioiodine. In elderly patients, late complications of radioiodine are less relevant and the major goal is definitive therapy with permanent cure. Thus, radioiodine ablation is the treatment of choice for virtually all older thyrotoxic patients.

It must be emphasized, however, that radioiodine therapy cannot be given with impunity to elderly patients. A major concern is possible exacerbation of thyrotoxicosis after radioiodine treatment, due to the release of preformed thyroid hormone into the circulation from radiation-induced thyroiditis. This problem can be life-threatening in the elderly thyrotoxic patient, particularly in the presence of underlying cardiac disease. Therefore, many thyroidologists render such patients biochemically euthyroid with antithyroid drugs prior to the administration of radioiodine. These drugs impair the biosynthesis of thyroid hormone, but not its release. Thus, within 4 to 8 weeks, the thyroid is depleted of hormonal stores, and radioiodine can be given safely. Traditionally, antithyroid drugs are discontinued for 3 to 5 days prior to radioiodine administration and are not resumed for 3 to 5 days afterward, so as not to interfere with the intrathyroidal accumulation of radioiodine. The dosage of the antithyroid drug is tapered over the ensuing months, as the effects of radioiodine are becoming manifest.

Antithyroid drugs cause fever, rash, and arthralgias in 1% to 5% of individuals. Agranulocytosis occurs in approximately one in 300 to 500 patients (usually in the first 2 months of treatment) and may be more common in elderly patients.[19] Methimazole in low doses (<30 mg/d) may pose less of a risk of agranulocytosis than propylthiouracil and has the added advantage of being a once-a-day agent, which improves compliance. Patients beginning antithyroid drug therapy should be warned that if fever or oropharyngitis develops, the medication should be stopped immediately and the physician contacted.

The β-adrenergic blocking agents are an important adjunct in the management of thyrotoxicosis. Rapid and almost complete resolution of cardiac and neuromuscular symptoms can be accomplished with agents in this class. They do not normalize oxygen consumption or reverse the negative nitrogen balance that typifies the thyrotoxic state, and they should therefore not be used as sole therapy except in those rare patients with self-limited disease due to thyroiditis. These agents are extremely useful before and after antithyroid drug and radioiodine therapy, because euthyroidism generally is not attained for 1 to 2 months after antithyroid drugs are started or for up to 12 months after radioiodine. Propranolol, with its short serum half-life, is not as useful as nadolol. Atenolol and metoprolol, two long-acting cardioselective agents, also are used frequently. The β-blockers are contraindicated in patients with asthma and congestive heart failure (unless rate related) and should be used cautiously in patients with diabetes treated with oral hypoglycemic agents or insulin.

Following radioiodine therapy, patients must be followed up expectantly for the development of iatrogenic hypothyroidism. This complication occurs almost inevitably in patients with Graves' disease but is quite rare in toxic nodular goiter, presumably due to the failure of radioiodine to be concentrated in suppressed regions of the gland. Posttherapy hypothyroidism develops within 12 months in 40% to 50% of patients with Graves' disease and then occurs at a rate of 2% to 3% per year thereafter.

Atrial fibrillation, especially when present for a relatively short time (less than 6 months), frequently spontaneously converts to normal sinus rhythm with control of thyrotoxicosis. In one study,[20] 62% of patients converted, with 75% converting within 3 weeks of becoming euthyroid; no patient converted after euthyroidism had been established for 4 months. Although age was not predictive of spontaneous conversion in this study, other reports suggest that spontaneous conversion occurs less frequently in elderly patients. Embolic stroke is a recognized complication of atrial fibrillation in thyrotoxicosis, although a recent report, using age-matched controls, did not find that atrial fibrillation was a risk factor for stroke in elderly persons.[21] Routine anticoagulation has been recommended for patients with atrial fibrillation due to thyrotoxicosis, but therapy must be individualized, and no firm recommendations can be made. If anticoagulation is undertaken, it should be recognized that thyrotoxic patients are *more* sensitive to the effects of coumarin derivatives than are euthyroid patients.

Severe Hyperthyroidism and Thyroid Storm

For those patients who are so severely ill with thyrotoxicosis that hospitalization is required, more rapid control of the disease is desirable. Large doses of antithyroid drugs are typically employed (eg, 200 mg/6h of propylthiouracil or 40 to 80 mg/d of methimazole as a single dose), which theoretically blocks thyroid hormone production completely. However, since thyroid hormone release is unaffected by antithyroid drugs, other agents must be employed to achieve an expeditious resolution of the thyrotoxic state. Traditionally, potassium iodide (as SSKI, containing 35 mg of iodide per drop or Lugol's solution, containing 8 mg of iodide per drop) has been used for this purpose, because iodine is a potent inhibitor of thyroid hormone release. Doses range form 100 to 500 mg/d in divided doses; iodide should be given only after the patient has been started on antithyroid drugs.

More recently, the iodinated contrast agents sodium ipodate and sodium iopanoate have been used in dosages of 1 to 2 g daily in divided doses. These compounds have two beneficial effects. First, they release free iodide into the circulation which, in turn, inhibits thyroid hormone secretion. Second these compounds are potent inhibitors of T_4 to T_3 conversion, and they rapidly lower serum T_3 levels toward normal. Thyroxine has a half-life in serum of about 7 days; blocking both synthesis and release does not improve symptoms and signs due to hormone already present in the circulation. By lowering the serum T_3 levels, the iodinated contrast agents are very useful in this regard. The β-adrenergic blockers also are efficacious in reversing sympathomimetic symptoms and signs due to circulating thyroid hormone. For life-threatening tachyarrhythmias, 1 mg of propranolol hydrochloride can be given slowly intravenously, with the dose repeated every 5 minutes. For those patients in atrial fibrillation in whom β-blockers are contraindicated, verapamil can be used.

Thyroid storm is a state of decompensated thyrotoxicosis, defined by severe hypermetabolism, fever, neuropsychiatric changes, and, often, congestive heart failure. Thyroid function test results are no different in patients with thyroid storm than in those with less severe clinical disease. Rather, the ability to deal with the hypermetabolic state is compromised, often by the superimposed stress of acute illness (eg, infection) or trauma (eg, surgery). Therapy consists of fluid and electrolyte support, active cooling, and large doses of antithyroid drugs, iodide or iodinated contrast agents, and β-blockers. Additionally, stress doses of glucocorticoids are usually employed. Due to the relatively more apathetic presentation of hyperthyroidism in elderly patients, they tend to have a better prognosis than younger patients in thyroid storm.[22]

Hypothyroidism

Approximately 70% of hypothyroid patients are over age 50 years at the time of diagnosis.[23] The prevalence of hypothyroidism in the population depends on how the condition is defined: if a low serum T_4 or free T_4 level is the criterion, approximately 0.5% of individuals (largely women) over age 65 years will be found to be overtly hypothyroid.[2] If the more liberal definition of an elevated serum TSH level with or without a low T_4 level is employed, up to 17.5% of individuals over age 75 years will have mild hypothyroidism.[2,24] This latter situation may be more appropriately termed "subclinical hypothyroidism," since serum T_4 and free T_4 levels are still within the broad range of normal.

Etiology

The most common cause of hypothyroidism in the elderly is autoimmune thyroid failure (Hashimoto's thyroiditis, chronic lymphocytic thyroiditis, Table 19.4). Over two thirds of patients with thyroid failure have antithyroid antibodies.[25] Two types of antithyroid antibodies have been described in Hashimoto's thyroiditis: antimicrosomal and antithyroglobulin. Antimicrosomal antibodies are highly specific for autoimmune thyroiditis. Antithyroglobulin antibodies, on the other hand, are not specific for autoimmune thyroid disease, and their presence in the absence of antimicrosomal antibody is not sufficient to establish the diagnosis.

Iatrogenic hypothyroidism is an additional important, though less frequent, cause of thyroid failure. Radioiodine and surgical therapy for Graves' disease can lead to permanent hypothyroidism. Additionally, several studies suggest that permanent hypothyroidism is a late phase in the evolution of drug-treated Graves' disease. Not surprisingly, external beam radiotherapy to the head and neck region also can cause late thyroid hypofunction. Iodine-containing medications can provoke hypothyroidism; this has become an increasing problem with the recent introduction of amiodarone, an antiarrhythmic used widely in older patients.[26] Finally, many patients with subacute or painless thyroiditis have mild transient hypothyroidism following hyperthyroidism, but this rarely requires therapy.

Diagnosis

The diagnosis of hypothyroidism is not difficult in a young patient with typical symptoms of fatigue, weight gain, dry skin, cold intolerance, and constipation. In

Table 19.4. Causes of hypothyroidism in elderly patients.

Primary hypothyroidism
   Chronic lymphocytic (Hashimoto's) thyroiditis
   Iatrogenic hypothyroidism
      Radioiodine or surgery for hyperthyroidism
      External radiation
      Drugs (antithyroid drugs, iodine, lithium)
Secondary hypothyroidism
   Pituitary disease
   Hypothalamic disease

elderly patients, however, these same complaints are attributed all too often to the aging process itself. The problem is further complicated by the insidious development of symptoms, often over a period of years, and by patients who present in an atypical manner. Thus, it behooves the physician to be creative and vigilant and to resist the stereotypical image of the "normal aging process."

Certain findings on physical examination should alert the clinician to the possibility of hypothyroidism. Hypertension, for example, can be a presenting sign, as can bradycardia and, surprisingly, various tachyarrhythmias. Hypothermic patients always should be evaluated for hypothyroidism, hypoglycemia, and sepsis. Although nonpitting edema of the face and limbs is a hallmark of hypothyroidism, pitting edema also is frequently found, possibly due to a lowered glomerular filtration rate and decreased cardiac output. Frank congestive heart failure is unusual in hypothyroidism, and cardiomegaly more often is due to the presence of pericardial effusion; while the pericardial effusions in hypothyroidism are usually not hemodynamically significant, tamponade has been described. Pleural effusions and ascites also can be seen.

In contrast to younger hypothyroid patients, older individuals rarely have a goiter. Whether this represents the natural history of goitrous autoimmune thyroiditis or a separate, atrophic variant of autoimmune thyroiditis is unclear. Ophthalmopathy also may be present, even in the absence of a history of Graves' disease. Neuropsychiatric signs, including depression, lassitude, and poor memory, are common; muscle cramps, peripheral neuropathy (carpal tunnel syndrome), and cerebellar ataxia are additional features of hypothyroidism, along with ileus, urinary retention, and sleep apnea.

Sometimes hypothyroidism is found serendipitously because of abnormal laboratory data. Elevations in serum cholesterol levels (when previously normal) and high creatine kinase levels are hallmarks of hypothyroidism and are due to decreased clearance. Hyponatremia commonly is seen in elderly patients and should always prompt an evaluation of thyroid status. Its origin is controversial but probably relates to both decreased glomerular filtration and the inappropriate secretion of vasopressin. A normochromic normocytic anemia, possibly due to decreased erythropoetin secretion, commonly is seen in hypothyroidism, and pernicious anemia occurs frequently in association with autoimmune thyroid disease.

Laboratory Diagnosis

Hypothyroidism is perhaps the simplest thyroid functional abnormality to diagnose. The hallmark of primary hypothyroidism is a low serum T_4 and free Thyroxine Index or free T_4, with concomitant elevation of the serum TSH. As previously noted, "subclinical" hypothyroidism is characterized by normal serum T_4 levels with only minimal to modest increases in TSH levels (eg, 5 to 20 U/L, with normal values <5 U/L). Measurement of T_3 is of little use in the diagnosis of hypothyroidism, because normal serum levels are often maintained until severe hypothyroidism supervenes. This may be related to a shift from T_4 and T_3 secretion by the thyroid gland, under intense stimulation by high levels of TSH.

Several pitfalls in the laboratory diagnosis of hypothyroidism deserve mention. First, patients with *secondary* hypothyroidism (ie, due to hypothalamic or pituitary disease with TSH *deficiency*) will have low T_4 values with inappropriately low or normal serum TSH levels. Recent studies suggest that in hypothalamic-pituitary disease, the pituitary secretes TSH that is immunologically active in the radioimmunoassay but has lower than normal bioactivity.[27] Thus, if hypothyroidism is suspected clinically and serum T_4 values are low, evaluation of hypothalamic and pituitary anatomy and function is indicated, even if the serum TSH level is "normal." Generally, other hormonal deficits will be present in this clinical circumstance (eg, adrenal insufficiency, hypogonadism).

A second problem that confounds the diagnosis of hypothyroidism is severe illness.[28] Thus, it may be extremely difficult to distinguish a critically ill patient with low T_4 and normal TSH levels from one with secondary hypothyroidism (see above). To further complicate matters, serum TSH levels occasionally *rise* during the recovery phase of illness, often to levels consistent with primary hypothyroidism. In this circumstance, repeating the TSH measurement after recovery is complete is the appropriate strategy.

Treatment

Once the diagnosis of primary hypothyroidism is made, therapy with thyroxine should be initiated; patients with chronic fatigue or obesity who are not hypothyroid should never be treated with this drug. Thyroxine is well absorbed from the gastrointestinal tract and has a long serum half-life, thus producing nonfluctuating serum levels. Cholestyramine interferes with its absorption and should not be taken concurrently. As in healthy untreated individuals, much of the orally administered thyroxine is deiodinated to T_3, at a rate determined by the patient's clinical status (ie, decreased in illness or starvation). Thyroxine is available in proprietary forms (Synthroid and Levothroid) and in generic form. While most generic brands probably are equivalent to the proprietary preparations, some clearly are inferior with respect to hormonal content and/or bioavailability. Unfortunately, it is often quite difficult to determine the ultimate manufacturer of a generic product. Therefore, most endocrinologists prefer the proprietary forms of thyroxine for their proved reliability.

The dictum "start low, go slow" should be followed in elderly patients when initiating thyroxine therapy, since rapid increases in myocardial oxygen consumption theoretically could trigger or worsen angina. Therefore, it is best to be prudent and initiate treatment with doses of 25 to 50 μg/d, with monthly monitoring of thyroid function. The biochemical goal of therapy is the normalization of serum TSH levels; in a high-sensitivity TSH assay, the TSH level should not be below the normal range, which would suggest overreplacement. As discussed above, the daily T_4 production rate declines with age, and consequently, as has been noted by most investigators, the daily thyroxine replacement dose is approximately 10% lower in elderly patients than in young or middle-aged adults.[29] In general, doses of 0.8 to 1.2 μg/kg of lean body mass are sufficient to normalize serum TSH levels in patients over age 70 years. The thyroxine replacement dose for elderly patients can be predicted by the following formula[30]:

$$T_4 (\mu/d) = 3.6 \times LBM - 30,$$

where LBM (males) = $(79.5 - 0.24M - 0.15 \times A)$ M/73.2, LBM (females) = $(69.8 - 0.26M - 0.12 \times A)$ M/73.2, M indicates body weight in kilograms, and A indicates age in years. Overreplacement is to be avoided, not only because of untoward cardiac effects, but also because of recent data showing that even mild asymptomatic iatrogenic hyperthyroidism can be associated with accelerated bone loss.[31] The dose requirement may be higher in patients with malabsorption or in those taking anticonvulsants.

A large and potentially bewildering number of thyroid hormone preparations are available (Table 19.5). They are traditionally classified as "synthetic" or "biologic." As described above, synthetic thyroxine is the therapy of choice. Another synthetic preparation, liotrix, is a combination of T_4 and T_3 (Euthroid,

Table 19.5. Thyroid hormone preparations.

Preparation	Available forms
Synthetic	
Thyroxine (T_4)*	Synthroid, Levothroid, generics
Triiodothyronine (T_3)	Cytomel
Liotrix (T_4 plus T_3)	Euthroid, Thyrolar
Biologic	
USP thyroid	Generic, Armour
Thyroglobulin	Proloid

* Drug of choice.

Thyrolar). This product was developed decades ago, before it was known that T_3 arose from peripheral conversion of T_4, rather than from direct thyroidal secretion. It is now clear that providing T_3 to the patient is unnecessary and theoretically could raise serum T_3 levels to above normal, causing palpitations, anxiety, and other bothersome symptoms. Furthermore, liotrix is more expensive, and its use makes monitoring of therapy more difficult and expensive, because of the necessity of measuring serum T_3 levels as well as T_4 levels. An additional synthetic thyroid hormone, pure L-triiodothyronine (Cytomel), should never be used for long-term replacement therapy. It is often used for short periods in patients with thyroid cancer preparing for radioiodine scanning.

The "biologic" thyroid hormone preparations include desiccated thyroid (generic and Armour) and thyroglobulin (Proloid), a more highly purified version of desiccated thyroid. These drugs are derived from the thyroid glands of slaughterhouse animals. The generic biologic preparations are notorious for their lack of standardization. The proprietary preparations have better quality control but suffer from the same problem as liotrix and T_3, ie, they contain T_3, which is an undesirable drug for chronic replacement therapy. Most endocrinologists agree that the biologic preparations are of historical interest only; patients who are taking them should be switched to synthetic thyroxine at doses of 0.05 to 0.1 mg/d.

Special Therapeutic Considerations

Hypothyroid Patients with Severe Coronary Artery Disease

Elderly hypothyroid patients not infrequently have concomitant coronary artery disease. Indeed, long-standing hypothyroidism, with its attendant hypercholesterolemia, may be an important contributing factor in the development of atherosclerosis. In this setting, it may be difficult to replace thyroxine fully without provoking or exacerbating angina. Every effort should be made to maximize the antianginal regimen medically. If that fails, and if the patient remains clinically hypothyroid because of the inability to prescribe an adequate dosage of thyroxine, coronary artery bypass surgery should be considered.[32] Open heart surgery, and, indeed, any surgery, can be performed safely in patients with severe hypothyroidism,[33] so long as scrupulous attention is paid to patients' pulmonary status and fluid balance in the perioperative period. In the untreated hypothyroid patient with unstable angina, it is probably best to send the patient to surgery rather than risk myocardial infarction by treating the hypothyroidism and delaying surgery.[32]

Subclinical Hypothyroidism

Subclinical hypothyroidism is defined biochemically as normal serum T_4 and free T_4 levels with an elevated serum TSH level. As noted earlier, it is one of the most common thyroid disorders among elderly persons, being present in up to 14% of women over age 60 years.[24] Most patients have circulating antithyroid antibodies, suggesting that the condition is autoimmune in nature. Some patients have a history of Graves' disease, while others are taking drugs (lithium or iodide-containing compounds) that are known to inhibit thyroid function, especially in the presence of underlying autoimmune thyroid disease.

A central question is whether patients with subclinical hypothyroidism, who are seemingly asymptomatic and appear to be suffering solely from a biochemical abnormality, should be treated. Although no definite answer can be provided at this time, one study indicated that patients with subclinical hypothyroidism do have subtle symptoms consistent with mild thyroid failure.[34] Furthermore, treatment with small doses of thyroxine (50 to 100 μg/d) resulted in a statistically significant symptomatic improvement compared with placebo treatment. On the basis of these data, therapy can be justified, if there are no contraindications (eg, severe angina).

Replacement therapy also can be used as prophylaxis against overt hypothyroidism. Several studies have shown that those patients with subclinical hypothyroidism who also have circulating antithyroid antibodies are likely to develop overt hypothyroidism; in the elderly, the rate may be as high as 20% per year.[35]

If it is elected not to treat a patient with subclinical hypothyroidism, it would be reasonable to test for antithyroid antibodies, since careful monitoring for thyroid failure is necessary if they are present. It should be pointed out, however, that hypothyroidism can develop even in the absence of antithyroid antibodies,[25] so that continuous monitoring of thyroid function is necessary in all untreated patients with subclinical hypothyroidism.

Myxedema Coma

Myxedema coma, like its hyperthyroid counterpart thyroid storm, results from the physiologic decompensation of a hypothyroid individual. Generally, there is a precipitating factor, most often an undiagnosed infection. Patients with myxedema "coma" are not necessarily comatose and can present with stupor, seizures, or psychotic manifestations. Myxedema coma is most often a disease of elderly hypothyroid individuals and generally occurs in the winter months.

Hypothermia is a frequent, but not invariable, manifestation; its absence should suggest an occult infection.

The diagnosis of myxedema coma usually is difficult, although it is made easier if there is a history of thyroid disorder or a neck scar or proptosis on physical examination. If the diagnosis is considered, therapy should be initiated, since the mortality approaches 50%, even with treatment. Optimal management consists of scrupulous attention to the patient's pulmonary, cardiovascular, gastrointestinal, and renal status. Often intubation and ventilatory assistance are necessary because of carbon dioxide retention. Active warming is contraindicated, because severe hypotension may supervene. A search for infection and prompt treatment is mandatory. Hyponatremia is common, and free water must be administered judiciously. Sedatives and narcotics should be avoided because of the risk of further respiratory depression.

Thyroxine should be administered intravenously, since gastrointestinal absorption may be altered because of hypomotility. Initial doses of 0.3 to 0.5 mg is recommended to replace the total body thyroid hormone pool, with daily doses of 0.1 mg thereafter. It has been suggested that T_3 therapy might be preferred, because T_3 is the active thyroid hormone; in the presence of severe illness, insufficient quantities of T_4 might be converted peripherally to T_3. However, it can also be argued that the body's controlled formation of T_3 and T_4 is more desirable than a sudden and dramatic increase in serum T_3. Indeed, a number of deaths have been attributed to T_3-induced cardiac arrhythmias. Current guidelines, therefore, recommend thyroxine rather than T_3 for myxedema coma.[22]

Thyroid Neoplasia and Goiter

Thyroid nodularity increases in frequency with age. Autopsy data suggest that 90% of women over age 70 years and 60% of men over age 80 years have one or more thyroid nodules.[3] Clinically significant nodules, ie, those that come to medical attention because they are palpable, are also more prevalent in the elderly, with approximately 5% of adults having a palpable nodule in the Framingham study population.[36] As would be expected, palpable nodules are also much more common in women than in men (6% vs 2%).

It is clear from surgical or thyroid scanning data that at least one quarter of nodules that are thought to be solitary on palpation are, in reality, part of a multinodular gland. Nevertheless, it is useful to distinguish clinically solitary nodules and so-called dominant nodules (nodules that are larger than the others that may be palpably present within the gland), since these have a greater likelihood of being malignant. Fortunately, malignancy is present in only about 10% of nodules, a frequency that is no higher and is perhaps lower than in younger patients with thyroid nodules. Given the low likelihood of malignancy, it is a challenge to diagnose and treat those nodules that are cancerous while at the same time avoiding unnecessary surgery in the 90% of patients who have benign disease.

Thyroid Nodules

Clinical Assessment

Although excision of all nodules would be simultaneously diagnostic and curative, surgery, particularly in the elderly, is associated with excess morbidity as well as great potential expense. Although a number of historical features (male sex, rapid growth, compressive symptoms) and physical findings (firm or rock-hard consistency, fixation to underlying neck structures, and cervical adenopathy) are important clues that suggest malignancy, there is considerable overlap in findings with benign nodules. Indeed, only a distinct minority of malignant nodules have a "classic" clinical presentation.

A history of head, neck, or upper thoracic radiation in childhood or adolescence is important to elicit. From the 1920s through the early 1960s, several million people received radiation for thymic enlargement, tonsillitis, mastoiditis, acne, and a host of other benign conditions. Many thousands of irradiated patients who are now in the geriatric population are at excess (three- to 10-fold) risk for the development of thyroid cancer, as well as benign nodular disease. In addition, it is becoming clear that radiation for malignancies that included the thyroid gland in the radiation port, eg, the mantle area for Hodgkin's disease, can also be associated with thyroid carcinoma. Thus, a history of radiation exposure warrants a prompt and definitive evaluation.

Differential Diagnosis

While most thyroid nodules are, in fact, benign tumors, any generalized thyroid disease can present as a thyroid nodule. Thus, the various forms of thyroiditis (subacute, Hashimoto's) are not infrequently asymmetric in their involvement and can mimic a solitary nodule. Other rare causes of an apparent thyroid nodule include hemiagenesis of the opposite lobe of the thyroid, cystic hygromas, and teratomas. Thyroid cysts and neoplasms (benign follicular adenomas, colloid nodules, nodular adenomatous hyperplasia, and carcinomas) comprise the majority of all nodules, however. Although most forms of thyroid cancer (papillary, medullary, anaplastic) are easily diagnosed by means of biopsy, follicular lesions are notoriously difficult to evaluate cytopathologically. While the majority of follicular neoplasms are benign, it can be extremely difficult to distinguish a more atypical benign tumor from a minimally invasive follicular carcinoma. Hürthle cell tumors, a variety of follicular adenoma once thought to always be malignant, are usually benign. Rarely, thyroid nodules are due to metastatic spread of cancer to the thyroid gland.

Laboratory Evaluation

Although a large number of blood tests and radiologic procedures are available to aid in the evaluation of thyroid nodules, most are, unfortunately, of little practical use. Results of routine thyroid function tests are almost always normal but are worth obtaining to find the rare patient with hyperthyroidism due to an autonomously functioning nodule, and to enable the diagnosis of hypothyroidism, which would suggest Hashimoto's thyroiditis as the underlying disease process.

Other blood tests should be used more selectively. A serum calcitonin determination should be obtained only if there is a family history of medullary thyroid carcinoma or other condition suggestive of multiple endocrine neoplasia syndrome, type 2. Antithyroid antibody assays might be performed if the serum TSH level is elevated, suggesting Hashimoto's thyroiditis. Serum thyroglobulin levels are nonspecifically elevated in a host of thyroid diseases, and this determination is used mainly in the follow-up of patients with thyroid cancer.

Traditionally, after routine blood tests, thyroid scanning with radioiodine or technetium has been the next step in the workup of a thyroid nodule. Nodules that concentrate the radionuclide ("hot" nodules) are, for practical purposes, never malignant, and require no further evaluation other than to be sure that hyperthyroidism is not present. On the other hand, hypofunctioning nodules ("cold" nodules) require further evaluation with needle biopsy.

Although categorizing nodules as "hot" or "cold" is intellectually satisfying, it is not cost-effective, since at least 90% of all nodules are hypofunctioning. An approach that is gaining wider acceptance is the performance of needle biopsy as the initial diagnostic step.[37] The advantage of this scheme is that patients do not have to wait for a scan, and, perhaps more importantly, that a scan becomes unnecessary for 90% of patients. The disadvantage is that the 10% of patients with "hot" nodules undergo biopsy needlessly. On the other hand, the fine-needle aspiration biopsy is a relatively painless procedure with virtually no morbidity (see below).

Thyroid ultrasonography, once considered a valuable tool in the evaluation of thyroid nodules, is being used with less frequency nowadays. Although purely cystic lesions are not malignant, pure cysts of the thyroid are rare. In fact, over 95% of nodules are either solid or complex (having solid and cystic components), the latter having the same clinical implications as a solid lesion. Thus, routine ultrasonography is not a cost-effective initial diagnostic test. It can be a useful technique for monitoring the size of nodules, particularly those that are difficult to palpate.

Needle Biopsy of Thyroid Nodules

Thyroid needle biopsy, and more specifically, fine-needle aspiration biopsy, has revolutionized the care of patients with thyroid disease.[38] Its diagnostic accuracy depends on the skill of the person performing the procedure, and, even more importantly, on the expertise of the cytopathologist who is interpreting the aspirate. For malignancy, the false-negative rate is low (<10%), although the specificity is only about 70% (if suspicious nodules are included). Most series report that 60% to 70% of lesions are benign and 5% are malignant.[37] About 25% are "indeterminate" or "suspicious," and these include less well-differentiated benign follicular adenomas, Hürthle cell neoplasms, and follicular carcinoma. Only 15% of suspicious lesions prove to be malignant at the time of surgery.[39]

Management of Thyroid Nodules

If the nodule is *benign,* then no further diagnostic evaluation is necessary, although continued follow-up is important and suppression therapy with thyroxine is reasonable. Malignant nodules, or course, require surgery. If a nodule is suspicious cytologically, the next step would be a thyroid scan, if it had not been performed prior to the biopsy, since suspicious lesions can be functioning ("hot") follicular adenomas. If the nodule is "hot," then additional laboratory studies should be performed to rule out hyperthyroidism. If the suspicious nodule is "cold," then excision is generally recommended. An alternate approach would be a 3- to 6-month trial of suppression therapy with thyroxine. If the nodule fails to decrease in size, then surgery is indicated. If the nodule shrinks, then close follow-up with continued thyroxine therapy is reasonable.

The rationale for suppression therapy with thyroxine is the belief that thyroid growth is dependent upon continued stimulation by TSH. Theoretically, when pituitary TSH secretion is suppressed with exogenous thyroid hormone, both the thyroid and benign nodules should decrease in size. Unfortunately, many benign nodules do not shrink with thyroxine therapy and there have been rare but well-documented instances of

cancers responding to TSH suppression with a decrease in size. Despite these drawbacks, suppression therapy for benign and suspicious thyroid nodules is an attractive approach in elderly patients, in whom coexisting disease makes surgery less appealing.

It should be recognized, however, that suppression therapy is effective in only 30% to 50% of patients, at most. Thus, the failure of a nodule to decrease in size with a suppressive dose of thyroxine (1 to 2 μg/kg of body weight) is not necessarily an indication of malignancy and, in the presence of a benign biopsy, should not be an indication for surgery. If the biopsy is suspicious, however, surgery should be more strongly considered. Continued enlargement despite adequate suppression, even with a benign biopsy specimen, should prompt reevaluation, including repeated biopsy or surgical excision. It should also be noted that suppression therapy can be hazardous in elderly patients, because of the intentional production of mild iatrogenic hyperthyroidism. This problem can be compounded if the nodule is part of a multinodular goiter, in which areas of autonomous (ie, nonsuppressible) function are present. Recent data on bone loss in patients undergoing thyroid hormone suppression[31] may prompt a reevaluation of this form of therapy for benign disease in elderly patients.

Goiter (Diffuse or Nodular)

Goiter, or a generalized enlargement of the thyroid, is a common problem in the elderly. Indeed, large, nodular, compressive goiters are seen almost exclusively in this age group. Goiters are termed "diffuse" or "nodular," depending on their surface characteristics on physical examination. A significant minority of goiters are caused by Hashimoto's thyroiditis, but most are idiopathic. Pathologically, most idiopathic multinodular goiters consist of areas of nodular adenomatous hyperplasia, interspersed with hemorrhagic cysts, fibrosis, and calcification.

Goiters usually are discovered at physical examination or visualized on routine chest radiographs as a mass in the anterior superior mediastinum. Mild tracheal deviation is frequent and does not necessarily indicate respiratory compromise. Goiter uncommonly causes symptoms by compressing adjacent neck structures (eg, dysphagia, respiratory difficulty, superior vena cava syndrome). It should be emphasized, however, that such symptoms are most often due to benign disease and not thyroid cancer. A history of rapid growth is worrisome, although benign hemorrhagic cysts frequently present in this manner, often with concomitant pain radiating to the ear. Even recurrent laryngeal nerve paralysis can be caused by benign thyroid enlargement, rather than malignancy.

Aside from the history and physical examination, routine thyroid function tests, including a serum T_3 and/or a high-sensitivity serum TSH determination, should be performed in all patients with goiter, because of the possibility of subtle thyrotoxicosis. Antithyroid antibodies are also valuable in this situation, especially in patients whose goiter is diffuse and firm on palpation. Computed tomography of the neck and chest can be helpful in delineating the extent of the goiter in the thorax, but generally it is unnecessary.

Aside from the question of thyroid function, the central issues in the patient with a large goiter are (1) whether malignancy is present and (2) whether there is clinically significant compression of adjacent neck structures. Regarding malignancy, if there is any suggestion of a recently enlarging goiter or if there is a dominant nodule within a multinodular goiter, a biopsy should be performed. With respect to esophageal or tracheal compression, a history of dysphagia or dyspnea is usually obtained. It should be emphasized, however, that upper-airway compromise may be subtle or asymptomatic, or may present as "asthma" or wheezing. Pulmonary function testing, with evaluation of upper-airway function by means of flow-volume loops, should be performed in all patients with large goiters who have suggestive respiratory symptoms or evidence of tracheal compression, even in the absence of symptoms.

The indications for surgery in elderly patients with large goiters are more stringent than in younger individuals. Obviously, malignancy or significant esophageal, tracheal, or venacaval compression mandate surgery. Certainly, there is no reason to remove a large asymptomatic goiter simply because "it is there" and may cause trouble "in the future," especially if it is cytologically benign. Suppressive therapy with thyroxine usually is of no benefit in long-standing large goiter and may be potentially hazardous in elderly patients. One recent report suggested that compressive symptoms can be improved with radioiodine ablation, even in patients who are euthyroid,[40] but this has not been the experience of most thyroidologists.

As indicated earlier, patients with nontoxic multinodular goiter are susceptible to iodine-induced thyrotoxicosis. Iodine-containing compounds, including iodinated contrast media, should be avoided, if possible, in such patients.

Thyroid Cancer

Thyroid cancer in elderly patients shares many features with that seen in younger patients, but there are dramatic differences as well. The histologic types (papillary, follicular, medullary, anaplastic, lymphoma) all occur, but with a shift in histologic type from the more indolent (papillary) to the more aggressive (medullary, anaplastic, Fig. 19.3). Even within a histologic category, advanced age portends a far worse prognosis.[41]

Papillary Carcinoma

Papillary carcinoma and mixed papillary-follicular carcinoma are the most common kinds of thyroid malignancy in the elderly. The tumor often involves ipsilateral cervical lymph nodes, without affecting the prognosis. Although the outlook is generally good, this form of cancer can be aggressive in elderly patients, with local invasion into the trachea or lung metastases. Primary therapy consists of near-total thyroidectomy, whereas in younger patients less extensive surgery is acceptable. Postoperatively, whole-body radioiodine scanning establishes whether residual thyroid tissue or local or distant metastases are present. Radioiodine is administered if the scan is positive. Patients usually succumb from recurrent local disease, rather than from distant metastases. All patients require life-long suppressive doses of thyroxine, with doses sufficient to suppress serum TSH to undetectable levels in a high-sensitivity TSH assay. Theoretically, patients who have undergone total thyroidectomy and who do not have distant metastases should have undetectable thyroglobulin levels (<5 μg/L). Thyroglobulin levels above 50 μg/L suggest recurrent or metastatic disease. Details regarding the specifics of management of papillary carcinoma are discussed elsewhere.[42]

Follicular Carcinoma

Follicular carcinoma comprises about 20% of thyroid cancer in the elderly. Tumors tend to spread hematogenously to bone, lungs, and liver. Approximately one third of patients present with metastases (usually to the bone) as the initial manifestation of disease. The prognosis of follicular cancer is worse in elderly patients, especially in those with metastatic disease. The management is similar to that outlined for papillary cancer.

Medullary Cancer of the Thyroid

Medullary cancer of the thyroid arises from the calcitonin-producing "C" cells in the thyroid, rather than the follicular cells. This tumor is sporadic in approximately 75% of older patients, with only a minority of tumors being associated with multiple endocrine neoplasia syndrome, type 2 (medullary cancer of the thyroid, pheochromocytoma, hyperparathyroidism).[43] Medullary cancer of the thyroid is almost always metastatic to regional cervical nodes at the time of diagnosis, and it frequently metastasizes to

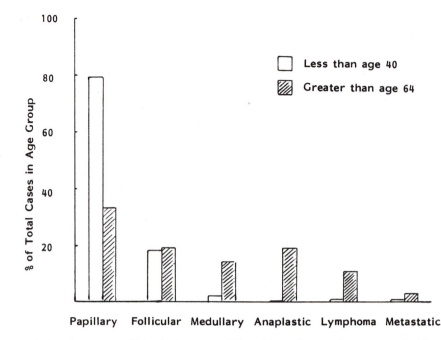

Fig. 19.3. Relative frequency of histologic types of thyroid carcinomas in young and older populations.

the liver and bone. The diagnosis is usually made by means of needle biopsy or after surgical removal of a suspicious nodule. The tumor is frequently bilateral, and a total thyroidectomy is mandatory. Since it is a neoplasm of calcitonin-producing cells, serum calcitonin can be used as a tumor marker to detect recurrence and to monitor therapy. Carcinoembryonic antigen is also frequently secreted by medullary cancer of the thyroid and is another useful tumor marker. Since the tumor does not arise from the follicular cells of the thyroid, it does not concentrate radioiodine. Furthermore, suppressive doses of thyroxine are not indicated, since the tumor is not dependent upon TSH for growth. Screening of family members for this tumor is indicated, since the patient could be the index case of a kindred with multiple endocrine neoplasia syndrome, type 2. Family screening generally involves measuring serum calcitonin basally and after stimulation with pentagastrin or calcium.

Lymphoma of the Thyroid

Thyroid lymphoma was once thought to represent a distinct form of "small cell" cancer. It is now known that lymphoma may arise primarily within the thyroid and that it is often, but not always, associated with disseminated extrathyroidal lymphoma.[44] Typically, thyroid lymphoma presents as a rapidly enlarging neck mass in an elderly woman with a history of Hashimoto's thyroiditis; however, there may be no previous thyroid disease, and antithyroid antibodies are often negative. The diagnosis of thyroid lymphoma is difficult to make with needle biopsy, since the cytologic appearance is similar to that of lymphocytic thyroiditis; open biopsy with special immunohistochemical stains often is necessary to establish the diagnosis. Staging for disseminated disease is indicated for all patients. Treatment consists of local radiotherapy and combination chemotherapy.

Anaplastic Thyroid Cancer

Anaplastic thyroid cancer is one of the most aggressive malignancies of man.[45] It occurs almost exclusively in elderly persons, often arising in preexisting goiters or in patients who previously have been treated for well-differentiated cancer. Anaplastic cancer presents as a rapidly enlarging mass that quickly produces compressive symptoms. There is no effective treatment.

References

1. Irvine RE. Thyroid disease in old age. In: Brocklehurst JC, ed. *Textbook of Geriatric Medicine and Geronotology.* New York, NY: Churchill Livingstone Inc; 1973:435–458.
2. Tunbridge WMG, Evered DC, Hall R, et al. The spectrum of thyroid disease in a community: the Wickham survey. *Clin Endocrinol* 1977;7:481–493.
3. Denham MJ, Wills EJ. A clinico-pathological survey of thyroid glands in old age. *Gerontology* 1980;26:160–166.
4. Gregerman RI. Intrinsic physiologic variables. In: Ingbar SH, Braverman LE, eds. *Werner's The Thyroid. 5th ed.* Hagerstown, Md: Harper & Row; 1986:361–381.
5. Gregerman RI, Gaffney GW, Shock NW, et al. Thyroxine turnover in euthyroid man with special reference to changes with age. *J Clin Invest* 1962;41:2565–2574.

6. Kabadi UM, Rosman PM. Thyroid hormone indices in adult healthy subjects: no influence of aging. *J Am Geriatr Soc* 1988;36:312–316.

7. Weinberger C, Thompson CC, Ong ES, et al. The c-erb-A gene encodes a thyroid hormone receptor. *Nature* 1986;324:641–646.

8. Davis PJ, Davis FB, Blas SD, et al. Donor age-dependent decline in response of human RBC Ca^{++}/ATPase activity to thyroid hormone in vitro. *J Clin Endocrinol Metabol* 1987;64:921–925.

9. Kvetny J. Nuclear T4 and T3 binding in mononuclear cells in dependence of age. *Horm Metab Res* 1985;17:35–38.

10. Ronnov-Jessen V, Kirkegaard C. Hyperthyroidism: a disease of old age? *Br Med J* 1973;1:41–43.

11. Tibaldi JM, Barzel US, Albin J, et al. Thyrotoxicosis in the very old. *Am J Med* 1986;81:619–622.

12. Nordyke RA, Gilbert FI, Harada ASM. Graves' disease. Influence of age on clinical findings. *Arch Intern Med* 1988;184:626–631.

13. Cobler JL, Williams ME, Greenland P. Thyrotoxicosis in institutionalized elderly patients with atrial fibrillation. *Arch Intern Med* 1984;144:1758–1760.

14. Borst GC, Eil C, Burman KD. Euthyroid hyperthyroxinemia. *Ann Intern Med* 1983;98:366–378.

15. Wehmann RE, Gregerman RI, Burns WH, et al. Suppression of thyrotropin in the low-thyroxine state of severe nonthyroidal illness. *N Engl J Med* 1985;312:546–552.

16. Caplan RH, Glasser JE, Davis K, et al. Thyroid function tests in elderly hyperthyroid patients. *J Am Geriatr Soc* 1978;26:116–120.

17. Gordon M, Gryfe CI. Hyperthyroidism with painless subacute thyroiditis in the elderly. *JAMA* 1981;246:2354–2355.

18. Weintraub BD, Gershengorn MC, Kourides IA, et al. Inappropriate secretion of thyroid-stimulating hormone. *Ann Intern Med* 1981;95:339–351.

19. Cooper DS, Goldminz D, Levin AA, et al. Agranulocytosis associated with antithyroid drugs: effects of patient age and drug dose. *Ann Intern Med* 1983;98:26–29.

20. Nakazawa HK, Sakurai K, Hamada N, et al. Management of atrial fibrillation in the post-thyrotoxic state. *Am J Med* 1982;72:903–906.

21. Petersen P, Hansen JM. Stroke in thyrotoxicosis with atrial fibrillation. *Stroke* 1988;19:15–18.

22. Nicoloff JT. Thyroid storm and myxedema coma. *Med Clin North Am* 1985;69:1005–1117.

23. Davis PJ, Davis FM. Hypothyroidism in the elderly. *Compr Ther* 1984;10:17–23.

24. Sawin CT, Chopra D, Azizi F, et al. The aging thyroid: increased prevalence of elevated serum thyrotropin levels in the elderly. *JAMA* 1979;242:247–250.

25. Sawin CT, Bigos ST, Land S, et al. The aging thyroid: relationship between elevated serum thyrotropin level and thyroid antibodies in elderly patients. *Am J Med* 1985;79:591–595.

26. Martino E, Safran M, Aghini-Lombardi F, et al. Environmental iodine intake and thyroid dysfunction during chronic amiodarone therapy. *Ann Intern Med* 1984;101:28–34.

27. Beck-Peccoz P, Amr S, Menezes-Ferreira MM, et al. Decreased receptor binding of biologically inactive thyrotropin in central hypothyroidism: effect of treatment with thyrotropin-releasing hormone. *N Engl J Med* 1985;312:1085–1090.

28. Tibaldi JM, Surks MJ. Effects of nonthyroidal illness on thyroid function. *Med Clin North Am* 1985;69:899–911.

29. Sawin CT, Herman T, Molitch ME, et al. Aging and the thyroid. Decreased requirement for thyroid hormone in older hypothyroid patients. *Am J Med* 1983;75:206–209.

30. Cunningham JJ, Barzel US. Lean body mass as a predictor of the daily requirement for thyroid hormone in older men and women. *J Am Geriatr Soc* 1984;32:204–207.

31. Cooper DS. Thyroid hormone and the skeleton: a bone of contention. *JAMA* 1988;259:3175.

32. Hay ID, Duick DS, Vlietstra RE, et al. Thyroxine therapy in hypothyroid patients undergoing coronary revascularization: a retrospective analysis. *Ann Intern Med* 1981;95:456–457.

33. Ladenson PW, Levin AA, Ridgway EC, et al., Complications of surgery in hypothyroid patients. *Am J Med* 1984;77:261–266.

34. Cooper DS, Halpern R, Wood LC, et al. L-thyroxine therapy in subclinical hypothyroidism. A double-blind, placebo-controlled trial. *Ann Intern Med* 1984;101:18–24.

35. Rosenthal MJ, Hunt WC, Garry PJ, et al. Thyroid failure in the elderly: microsomal antibodies as discriminant for therapy. *JAMA* 1987;258:209–213.

36. Vander JB, Gaston EA, Dawber TR. The significance of nontoxic thyroid nodules. *Ann Intern Med* 1968;69:537–540.

37. Rojeski MT, Gharib H. Nodular thyroid disease: evaluation and management. *N Engl J Med* 1985;313:428–436.

38. Miller JM. Evaluation of thyroid nodules: accent on needle biopsy. *Med Clin North Am* 1985;69:1063–1077.

39. Gharib H, Goellner JR, Zinsmeister AR. Fine-needle apsiration biopsy of the thyroid: the problem of suspicious cytologic findings. *Ann Intern Med* 1984;101:25–28.

40. Kay TWH, d'Emden MC, Andrews JT, et al. Treatment of nontoxic multinodular goiter with radioactive iodine. *Am J Med* 1988;84:19–22.

41. Hamburger JI. The presentation of thyroid malignancy in the geriatric patient. *Henry Ford Hosp Med J* 1980;28:158–160.

42. Leeper RD. Thyroid cancer. *Med Clin North Am* 1985;69:1079–1096.

43. Saad MF, Ordonez NG, Rashid RK, et al. Medullary carcinoma of the thyroid: a study of the clinical features and prognostic factors in 161 patients. *Medicine* 1984;63:319–342.

44. Hamburger JI, Miller JM, Kini SR. Lymphoma of the thyroid. *Ann Intern Med* 1983;99:685–693.

45. Nel CJC, van Heerden JA, Goellner JR, et al. Anaplastic carcinoma of the thyroid: a clinicopathologic study of 82 cases. *Mayo Clin Proc* 1986;60:51–58.

20

Male Sexual Function

John E. Morley, Fran E. Kaiser, and L.E. Johnson

Sexual function decreases markedly with advancing age. In a survey of an outpatient clinic population, Slag et al[1] found that one in three patients over 40 years of age had erectile dysfunction. Half of these patients wanted treatment for their impotence. Kinsey et al[2] found that the frequency of intercourse decreased from an average of once per week at 65 years of age to once every 10 weeks by the age of 80 years. The reasons for the decline in sexual function with advancing age are multifactorial and include psychological, physiologic, and pathologic processes. The exact role played by each of these processes varies from individual to individual. In addition, a number of changes occur in male hormonal function with advancing age. The effects of these changes on male sexuality are ill defined, and they may also play a role in a number of changes commonly associated with aging, such as decreased muscle strength and osteopenia.

Physiologic Changes in Sexual Function

Our knowledge of the physiologic changes that occur in sexual function with advancing age is based on studies by Masters and Johnson[3] of a relatively small number of men over the age of 50 years. Masters and Johnson have described four stages of sexual response: excitement, plateau, orgasm, and resolution. All four phases are altered during aging.

During the excitement phase, there is a significant delay in erectile attainment with aging. The erection is also often less full (though this could be related to concomitant vascular disease, as discussed below). It is important to realize that the older man who loses his erection without ejaculation may not be able to regain it. This secondary refractory period is rare in men younger than 50 years of age. Vasocongestion of the scrotal sac is less obvious, and normal "tensing" of the scrotal sac does not occur. There may be little, if any, testicular elevation. Cremasteric vascular tone decreases with age. The normal vasocongestive increase in testicular size is rarely present.

The plateau phase tends to last longer in older men than in younger ones. In general, control of ejaculation demand is much better in 50- to 70-year-olds than in 20- to 40-year-olds. There is either an absence or marked reduction of preejaculatory fluid emission (Cowper's gland secretion) with advancing age.

In contrast to the plateau phase, the orgasmic phase is much shorter. Usually, the older man does not experience a recognizable first phase (ie, ejaculatory inevitability), during which the ejaculation is felt coming but can no longer be controlled. In those who do have a recognizable first phase, only one or two prostatic contractions will be recognized and the phase will last only 1 or 2 seconds, compared with 2 to 4 seconds in younger men. Some older men will experience a prolonged first phase, in which the prostate, instead of contracting cyclically at 0.8-second intervals, contracts spastically for several seconds before returning to the rhythmically expulsive contractions. It has been suggested that the lack of a recognizable first stage in orgasmic experience may be related to low testosterone levels.[4]

In the second phase of orgasm, there are only one or two expulsive contractions of the penile urethra. Ejaculatory force is decreased, so that seminal fluid travels only 3 to 12 in from the urethral meatus, rather than the 12 to 14 in seen in younger men. In a young man who abstains from ejaculation for 24 to 36 hours, the seminal fluid volume is 3 to 5 mL, compared with 2 to 3 mL in men over 50 years of age. Despite these physiologic changes, most older men do not differ in their subjective interpretation of the level of sensate pleasure during orgasm.

The refractory period following ejaculation lasts for a number of hours before a full erection can again be obtained. Following ejaculation, the older man's erection may be lost within a few seconds, compared with minutes or hours for a younger man. Similarly, testicular descent is very rapid although involution of the smaller amount of vasocongestion is slowed.

These changes in sexual response in older men are summarized in Figure 20.1. It is important that older men and their partners be aware of these age-related changes in order to decrease performance anxiety problems that may occur with aging.

Nocturnal penile tumescence (NPT) has been used as the "gold standard" to measure penile erectile function. With aging, there is increasing evidence that NPT is diminished. Kahn and Fisher[5] reported full or moderate nocturnal erections in 45% of healthy elderly male volunteers, compared with 82% of younger men. Karacan et al[6] reported that older men had reduced frequency and duration of maximal tumescent episodes. Schiavi and Schreiner-Engel[7] found that the frequency and duration of NPT, but not penile circumference during tumescent episodes, decreased with age independently of age-related sleep variations (Fig 20.2). In men over the age of 60 years, the penis was less rigid during tumescent episodes, despite adequate increases in circumference. These findings suggest that NPT cannot be used in diagnosing impotence in older men and fit with our clinical experience suggesting that normal NPT (as defined in young control subjects) is rarely seen in older patients.

Sexuality and Aging

The frequency of intercourse decreases markedly with advancing age. In a study of 70-year-old Swedish men, Persson[8] reported that 46% of men were still having intercourse. Reasons for decreasing sexual activity included bereavement, mental health problems, and low sex drive. Pfeiffer et al[9] reported that 95% of men

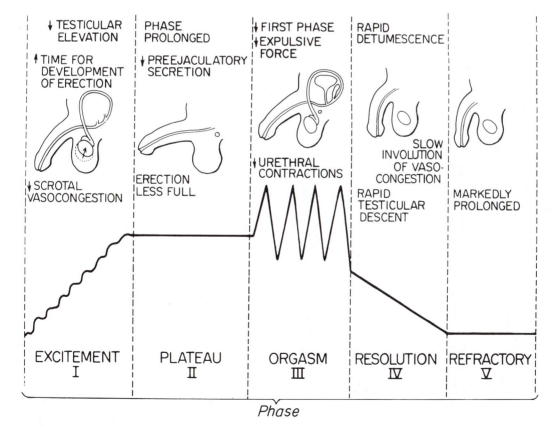

Fig. 20.1. Changes in sexual response with age in men.

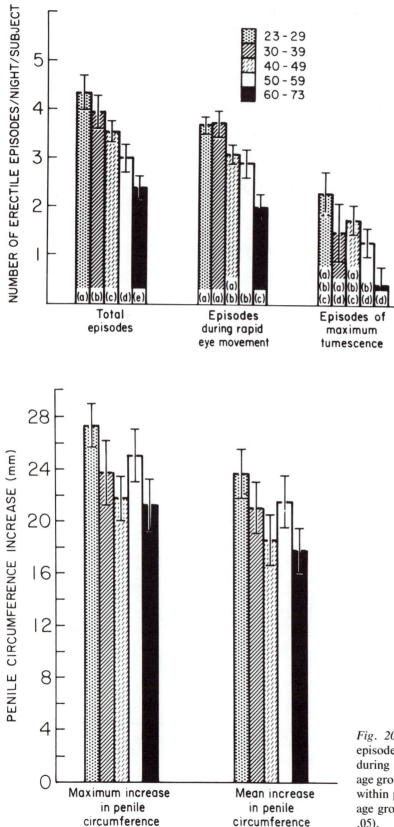

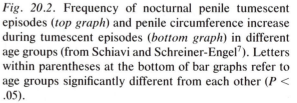

Fig. 20.2. Frequency of nocturnal penile tumescent episodes (*top graph*) and penile circumference increase during tumescent episodes (*bottom graph*) in different age groups (from Schiavi and Schreiner-Engel[7]). Letters within parentheses at the bottom of bar graphs refer to age groups significantly different from each other (*P <* .05).

aged 46 to 50 years had intercourse once a week, while in the 66- to 71-year-old group, only 28% were having intercourse once a week and 24% had no intercourse at all. In a follow-up study by the same group, only 20% of subjects remained sexually active by the age of 78 years.[10] In a community study in Michigan of persons 60 years old or older, 63.5% of married and 38.8% of unmarried males were sexually active.[11] Lack of sexual activity was correlated with reduced physical activity, sedative use, and respiratory and bowel problems. Less strong correlations included history of heart attack, diabetes mellitus, paraplegia, genital and rectal surgery, and urinary catheter use.

The Starr-Weiner report[12] on subjects over 60 years of age attending senior citizen centers found that only 7% of these men were not sexually active and 90% had sex more than once a month. Approximately 55% had sex at least once a week. Of these men, 50% considered orgasm the most important experience, 23% cited foreplay, 11% love, 10% intercourse, and 6% satisfying their partner. The majority (76.3%) believed that masturbation was an acceptable way to relieve sexual tensions, but only 43.6% masturbated themselves. Of those who masturbated, 28.6% did it at least once a week. Only 26% disapproved of older men and women without partners going to prostitutes to satisfy sexual needs. The ideal lover was characterized as being over 60 years of age by 19% of those surveyed, 45 to 59 years by 12%, and under 44 years by 21% of men over 60 years of age. Reasons for not having sexual relations included lack of an available partner (21%), poor health (26%), impotence (8%), and lack of desire (15.6%). Sex was considered an inappropriate activity for older people by 23.4% of the respondents. Only 54% of men had an orgasm every time they had intercourse, and 60% reported difficulty in obtaining an erection. Fifty-one percent of older men thought that they would like to try new sexual experiences that they had heard or read about. Overall, this comprehensive study of sexual attitudes in older men clearly established that sexuality remains an important part of life for many of them. Many older persons have "liberal" attitudes toward sex outside marriage, alternative sexual practices, and masturbation within their own age group.

Bretschneider and McCoy[13] studied a group of healthy men over 80 years of age. Twenty-nine percent of men were having intercourse at least weekly; 38% were not having intercourse at all. Enjoyment of sexual intercourse was characterized as moderate or great by 63%. Forty-one percent reported masturbating at least once a week. The main sex problems reported were fear of poor performance (37%), inability to achieve or maintain an erection (28% to 33%), inability to reach orgasm (28%), insufficient opportuni-

ties for sexual encounters (23%), and partner's vaginal pain or lack of lubrication (23%). Overall, this group of senior citizens appeared to have a highly satisfactory sexual life compared with other reported groups.

Sexuality and Long-Term Care

Admission to a hospital and/or nursing home is often associated with little attention to the sexual needs of the resident. In many cases, the male residents are expected to make their bodies available to the probing hands and eyes of caregivers of the opposite sex. In these instances, development of an erection can be embarrassing for the patient and caregiver and, on occasion, may be misunderstood by the caregiver. When the caregiver is particularly attentive to a resident, this may be misunderstood by the resident, leading to sexual approaches. A few demented patients develop hypersexuality, and in such cases other residents must be protected and the staff must be trained to handle this behavioral problem without open expressions of disgust. Masturbation may be carried out in open view of staff and other residents.

In a study of attitudes of staff and residents toward sexuality in a nursing home,[14] residents were more likely than staff to disapprove of sex. Many residents felt that masturbation was unhealthy. Lack of privacy was seen as a major reason for limitation of sexual activity. Over 60% of the residents did not feel sexually attractive. Another study in a nursing home found that 39% of men and 53% of women did not consider sex appropriate for someone of their age.[15] Of the men, 42% believed that masturbation was harmful or immoral. Major reasons for no longer being sexually active included lack of a partner (27%), poor health (19%), inability to perform (15%), and loss of interest (8%). Male residents tended to have a better factual sexual knowledge than did female residents.

Elderly persons in a long-term care setting often are sexually oppressed. The expression of sexuality in the nursing home often is poorly accepted by the staff. It is essential to provide staff education on sexuality to prevent this "emotional malnutrition" from occurring in the nursing home. All nursing homes should provide a "quiet room" or some other form of privacy where sexually active, consenting adults can spend time together. If sexual visitation rights are given to prisoners, surely the same consideration should be available when only one partner is institutionalized. Hugging and lying next to one another may be all the sexual expression desired, but for many elderly persons these behaviors require privacy. Masturbation also requires privacy. Some residents may wish to view pornographic or "sexy" movies in private. Complex ethical issues arise when older, cognitively impaired residents become romantically involved. Nursing homes need to develop an open attitude toward sexuality. Education of staff and patients should be aimed at developing a healthy environment where the many different sexual viewpoints expressed by older individuals can be accepted.

Regulation of Male Hormones

The testes have two anatomic components: (1) the interstitial or Leydig cells, which are involved in steroid hormone synthesis and secretion and (2) the seminiferous tubule component which consists of developing sperm in the germinal epithelium and Sertoli cells. The hypothalamic-pituitary-testicular axis is predominantly under the regulation of the pulsatile release of gonadotropin-releasing hormone (GnRH). This decapeptide then stimulates the synthesis and release of luteinizing hormone (LH) and follicle-stimulating hormone (FSH) from the pituitary. This leads to LH being released into the circulation in a pulsatile manner every 30 to 90 minutes. Both the number and amplitude of the pulses determine the effectiveness of LH in stimulating the synthesis and secretion of testosterone from the Leydig cells. The activated LH receptor promotes the formation of cyclic adenosine monophosphate as a second messenger to stimulate testosterone secretion. Testosterone then feeds back at both the pituitary and the hypothalamic levels (where it is aromatized to estradiol) to inhibit the release of LH and GnRH[16] (Fig 20.3).

The secreted testosterone shows a marked circadian variation in younger men, with values rising between 8 and 10 AM and falling dramatically in the afternoon. Approximately 5 mg of testosterone is secreted daily. Of this, 0.3% is aromatized to estradiol and 6% to 8% is converted to plasma dihydrotestosterone (DHT) by 5α-reductase. These steroid hormones bind to receptors in the cytoplasm of androgen-responsive tissues and are then translocated to the nucleus where they initiate the transcription of selected messenger RNA molecules.

Actions attributed to testosterone can be due to testosterone itself or to estradiol or DHT. The remaining testosterone is acted on by 17β-OH-steroid dehydrogenase to form 17-ketosteroids, by hydroxylases (forming diol or triol metabolites), or by conjugating enzymes. These compounds represent the excretory metabolites of testosterone.

Gonadotropin-releasing hormone also stimulates the release of FSH, but the pulsatile nature of its secretion is less obvious because of its longer circulating half-

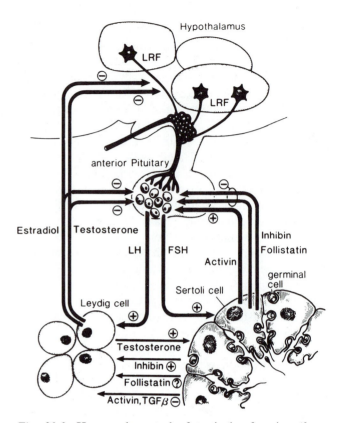

Fig. 20.3. Hormonal control of testicular function (from Ying[16]). LRF indicates gonadotropin-releasing factor, TGF β, transforming growth factor β.

life. Luteinizing hormone and FSH do not respond identically in all situations, a fact that could be explained by differential feedback effects or by the existence of a separate FSH-releasing factor. Follicle-stimulating hormone binds to cell membranes of Sertoli cells and activates adenylate cyclase and protein kinase activity. This leads to the stimulation of the synthesis of a number of proteins, including androgen-binding protein. This protein concentrates testosterone in the lumen of the seminiferous tubules and increases the available androgen to act on the developing spermatozoa. Follicle-stimulating hormone can also up-regulate the number of LH receptors. Sertoli cells also produce inhibin, a peptide hormone that feeds back to inhibit FSH release from the pituitary. Two inhibins, A and B forms, have been isolated. Inhibin also acts directly on the testes to modulate the proliferation of testicular cells. Activins are peptide hormones that are produced by the testes and closely related to inhibin but that stimulate rather than inhibit FSH secretion from the pituitary. Activins also inhibit Leydig cell androgen biosynthesis.

Gonadotropin-releasing hormone is under the control of the limbic system. Norepinephrine stimulates the secretion of GnRH, which is also under the tonic inhibition of β-endorphin. Blockade of endogenous opiates with the opiate antagonist, naloxone, leads to an increase in LH secretion. Animal studies have shown that stressors lead to a decrease in LH and testosterone. This decrease appears to be due to release of corticotropin-releasing factor (CRF), which inhibits LH release. The low values of testosterone seen in depressed and/or stressed patients may be secondary to CRF release.

Aging and the Hypothalamic-Pituitary-Testicular Axis

Steroid Hormones

Aging has marked effects on the hypothalamic-pituitary-testicular axis (Table 20.1). Advancing age is associated with a decreased testosterone level in the majority of cases[17,18] (Fig 20.4). This fall is most marked in the morning, as older subjects have attenuation of the morning testosterone peak.[19] Most circu-

Table 20.1. Age-related changes in the hypothalamic-pituitary-testicular axis.

Steroid levels
   Decrease in testosterone
   Decrease in BT
   Decrease in dihydrotestosterone
   Increase or no change in estradiol
   Increase or no change in SHBG
Gonadotropin levels
   Failure of LH to elevate in response to low BT
   Increase in LH (late)
   Increase in FSH
   Decrease in LH response to GnRH
   Increased ability of testosterone to lower LH
Sertoli cells
   Fewer Sertoli cells
   Decrease in inhibin

lating testosterone is bound to sex hormone–binding globulin (SHBG). There is a tendency for the level of SHBG to increase slightly in older individuals,[18] which would lead to a spurious increase in total testosterone. The testosterone available to tissues is determined by

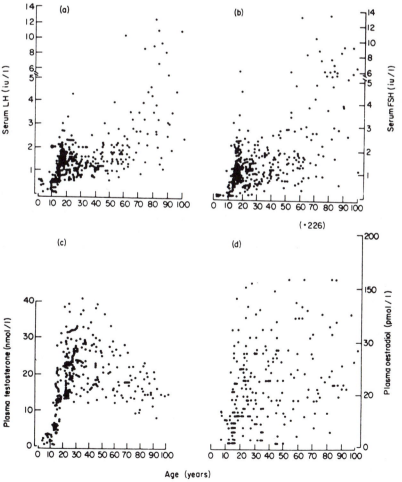

Fig. 20.4. Serum LH **(a)**, serum FSH **(b)**, plasma testosterone **(c)**, and plasma estradiol **(d)** levels as a function of age in healthy men (from Baker et al[17]).

measuring bioavailable testosterone (BT), which is testosterone that is free or weakly bound to albumin. Both free testosterone and BT levels are reduced in older subjects.[20,21] In many cases, this reduction is clearly established by 50 years of age.[22] The BT levels of 60-year-old men are about half of those seen in men under 40 years of age.[22] As is the case with testosterone, older men do not show the circadian variation in BT levels that is seen in young men. The DHT levels also are reduced with advancing age.[18] In contrast, estradiol levels do not fall or increase slightly with advancing age.[18] Peripheral conversion of androstenedione to estrone increases with age.[18]

The fall in circulating BT is compatible with the decrease in total number of Leydig cells seen with advancing age.[23] Testosterone production rate is decreased in subjects over 70 years of age (mean, 4 mg/24 h) compared with subjects under 50 years of age (6.6 mg/24 h).[24] In addition, there is impaired Leydig cell responsiveness to human chorionic gonadotropin (HCG) stimulation,[18] suggesting a decrease in testicular reserve.

Gonadotropins

Numerous studies have found that certain individuals have markedly increased gonadotropin levels with advancing age and that mean levels of gonadotropins also are increased.[18] These elevations have been reported to occur as early as 40 years of age,[25] although in very healthy monks, elevations were not seen until the 60s.[26] The increments in FSH usually precede those in LH. These findings are in keeping with the concept that the primary defect in aging is testicular failure, with a secondary rise in gonadotropin levels.

We have recently examined the relationship of BT and LH levels in a group of healthy men between 51 and 91 years of age (unpublished observations). In this group, only one subject had primary hypogonadism, and none had compensated hypogonadism. Low BT levels were present in over half of these patients, low LH levels in 70%. These data show that LH levels are not appropriately elevated in response to the fall in BT that occurs with advancing age. Thus, in addition to a testicular defect, aging is also associated with abnormal responsiveness of the hypothalamic-pituitary axis. The reason for the failure of the hypothalamic-pituitary axis to respond adequately to the fall in BT levels with advancing age is unclear. However, older men have been shown to have an enhanced suppression of LH in response to exogenous testosterone administration.[27]

The effects of aging on LH pulse characteristics are summarized in Table 20.2.[20,28–30] In vitro studies have shown that hypothalami from old rats show reduced basal and norepinephrine- and naloxone-stimulated

Table 20.2. LH pulse characteristics in young and elderly men.

Source, y	Age of subjects, y	N	Frequency/h	Amplitude, (mIU/mL)
Winters and Troen,[28] 1984	18–32	14	0.48*	8.6
	65–80	14	0.59*	5.6
Deslypere et al,[29] 1987	27–55	27	0.25*	3.15
	65–87	21	0.39*	3.15
Tenover et al,[20] 1987	22–35	14	0.60	16 ng/mL†
	65–84	14	0.58	15 ng/mL†
Kaiser et al,[30] 1987	22–32	7	0.95	2.8*
	65–84	6	0.73	4.4*

* Significant difference between elderly and young subjects.
† Using LER 907 standard.

GnRH release. Older human subjects have a blunted LH response to GnRH[18] and a mild age-related decline in the ratio of LH bioactivity to immunoreactivity.[31] In one study of older men, the antiestrogen tamoxifen failed to increase the 12-hour mean bioactive LH concentrations and bioactive LH peak amplitudes to the same degree as in younger men.[32] These studies support the concept of hypothalamic or pituitary exhaustion with old age.

Spermatogenesis

Testicular size decreases with age. Histologic changes include thickening of the basement membrane, peritubular fibrosis, and impaired spermatogenic maturation. Testicular degeneration occurs in a patchy distribution, allowing normal spermatogenesis to be present in over half of men at age 70 years.[33] Sperm output is either slightly decreased or normal with advancing age,[18] but sperm motility is decreased and morphology is altered with aging.[34] In an in vitro study, sperm production was greater than 200 million sperm per day in men under age 40 years and lower than this in most older men.[23] The highest FSH levels were seen in men with the lowest sperm production.

The number of sertoli cells decreases in older men.[35] Those aged 65 to 85 years have lower levels of inhibin than do younger men[36] (Fig 20.5). Clomiphene citrate administered for 1 week increased inhibin levels by 71% in young men but by only 24% in elderly men. Thus, normal aging results in a decreased ability of Sertoli cells to secrete inhibin.

Testosterone and Aging

There is little information available on the effects of the decreased BT that occurs with aging. Table 20.3 lists the effects common to both testosterone lack (hypogo-

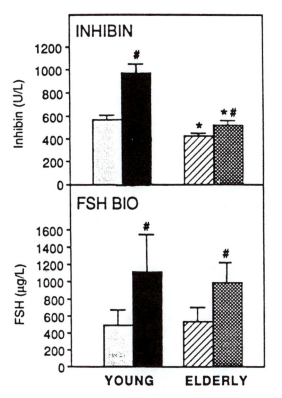

Fig. 20.5. Mean (± SEM) serum inhibin and bioactive FSH levels in 11 young and 13 elderly men before (▭ and ■) and after (▨ and ▧) 1 week of clomiphene citrate administration. (from Tenover et al[36]). Asterisk indicates $P < .01$ compared with young men; number sign, $P < .01$ compared with baseline.

nadism) and normal aging. However, to our knowledge, no controlled intervention trials have examined the effects of testosterone replacement on the organ changes associated with aging. When patients with clear-cut hypogonadism are excluded, there is limited evidence that testosterone affects libido or sexual function in older men. There is a major need for double-blind controlled studies on the role of testosterone in the changes seen with normal aging. The availability of transscrotal testosterone patches should allow these studies to be undertaken with physiologic, rather than pharmacologic, doses of testosterone.

Table 20.3. Effects common to both testosterone lack (hypogonadism) and normal aging in men.

Decrease in muscle mass
Decrease in growth hormone secretion
Mild decrease in red blood cell mass
Osteopenia
Decrease in food intake
Decrease in facial hair growth
Increase in adipose tissue

Gonadal Dysfunction and Systemic Disease

Aging is often associated with the development of a variety of disease processes.[37] Many of these diseases have a direct effect on gonadal function. Table 20.4 lists some of the diseases that commonly alter the activity of the hypothalamic-pituitary-testicular axis.

Systemic disease can alter hormonal release and metabolism at multiple levels. The effects of systemic disease include direct toxic effects on the testes, pituitary damage, hypothalamic disease, and altered hormonal metabolism. Renal failure is an example of a disease that has multiple effects on gonadal function, including hypothalamic dysfunction (increased prolactin level), pituitary dysfunction (occasional flat response to GnRH), and testicular dysfunction (elevated LH level and decreased testosterone level with decreased responsiveness to HCG). Chronic obstructive pulmonary disease is associated with low testosterone levels.[38] This decrease appears to be related to hypoxia, with serum testosterone levels falling below normal when the PaO_2 drops below 55 mm Hg.

Endocrine disorders often affect gonadal function. Hyperthyroidism leads to an increase in SHBG, LH, and total testosterone levels but to a decrease in BT levels. Microadenomas producing prolactin are associated with decreased testosterone levels and impotence. However, testosterone therapy alone does not restore potency until prolactin levels have been lowered by a dopamine agonist, eg, bromocriptine. Prolactin appears to interfere with the action of the tissues involved in the erectile process as well as decrease the testicular production of testosterone.

Protein energy metabolism decreases testosterone by effects both at the gonadal and the pituitary level. Obesity is associated with decreased SHBG and testosterone and increased estradiol levels. Zinc deficiency leads to decreased testosterone levels and impotence and may particularly be seen in patients taking diuretics or with diabetes mellitus.

Table 20.4. Systemic diseases associated with disruption of the hypothalamic-pituitary-testicular axis

Renal failure
Chronic obstructive pulmonary disease
Cirrhosis
Hemochromatosis
Myotonia dystrophica
Hyperthyroidism
Hypothyroidism
Prolactinoma
Sarcoidosis
Temporal lobe epilepsy
Depression

Gynecomastia and Aging

The incidence of gynecomastia (palpable breast tissue) increases with advancing age.[39] Gynecomastia is associated with an increase in the estrogen-to-androgen ratio. Most of the diseases that alter hypothalamic-pituitary-gonadal function also produce gynecomastia. In addition, numerous drugs, such as the androgen-receptor antagonist spironolactone, cytotoxic agents that directly damage the testes, and digoxin, can be associated with breast enlargement.

From the practical perspective, unilateral gynecomastia has the same significance as bilateral gynecomastia. Painful gynecomastia usually represents new-onset, rapidly expanding breast growth causing stretching of the surrounding tissues. In male patients, any question that breast enlargement may be due to carcinoma is best settled by removal of the unwanted tissue. It should be remembered that ectopic HCG production by oat cell carcinomas of the lung can lead to gynecomastia in men.

Impotence

Impotence is defined as the inability to obtain or maintain an erection adequate for sexual intercourse. Multiple studies have demonstrated a marked increase in the prevalence of impotence with increasing age. While psychogenic causes of impotence are more common in younger men, an organic cause is frequently found when impotence occurs in older men. It should be remembered, however, that any patient who fails at sexual intercourse may experience secondary psychological problems associated with his failure. These problems may play a major role in the continued failure to obtain an adequate erection ("performance anxiety"), or the patient's anxiety over his sexual failure may prevent the physician from identifying treatable organic disease.

Physiology of Normal Erections

An erection is the product of the complex interaction of the central and peripheral nervous system, the vascular supply, and the hormonal milieu. Two separate parts of the spinal cord are involved in normal erectile function. Sympathetic impulses from T-12 to L-1, via hypogastric nerves, are responsible for constriction of cavernosal arteries and sinusoidal spaces, and parasympathetic impulses from S-2 to S-4, via pelvic nerves, influence arterial dilatation. Erections due to psychogenic stimuli are mediated through the thoracolumbar spinal center, while erections due to direct penile stimulation are mediated through the sacral nerve center via the pudendal nerve. Decreased penile sensitivity to vibration and light touch occurs with aging, which may explain why elderly men require more direct penile stimulation to achieve an erection. The relaxed introitus and vagina in postmenopausal women may no longer provide adequate stimulation to sustain an erection in such men.

Penile blood supply arises from the paired internal iliac arteries through the internal pudendal arteries[40] (Fig 20.6). The deep cavernosal arteries are responsible for tumescence. The dorsal arteries supply the glans and penile skin; the urethral arteries supply the glans, corpus spongiosum, and urethra; and the bulbar arteries supply the proximal urethral bulb and Cowper's glands. In addition to obstruction of the arterial supply, a failure to obtain full erections or sustain an erection may be related to venous insufficiency.

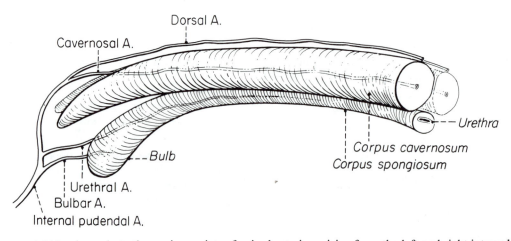

Fig. 20.6. The arterial blood supply to the penis consists of paired arteries arising from the left and right internal iliac arteries (from Johnson and Morley[40]; reprinted from the November 1988 issue of *American Family Physician*, published by the American Academy of Family Physicians).

Etiology and Diagnosis of Impotence

The causes of impotence are illustrated in Figure 20.7.[40-42] Vascular disease is the most common cause of impotence in older men, being implicated in up to 50% of cases in men over 50 years. The gold standard for diagnosing an arterial disorder is penile arteriography. However, in most cases the diagnosis of arterial disease can be made by comparing cavernosal arterial blood pressures, the so-called penile-brachial index (PBI). A value below 0.75 is highly suggestive of vasculogenic impotence, while a PBI between 0.75 and 0.9 represents an uncertain gray area. Accuracy improves if the PBI is obtained following exercise of the lower extremities, as patients with a "steal syndrome" will then show a drop in penile systolic pressure. A similar "steal syndrome" may also occur during the exercise associated with sexual intercourse, causing detumescence. Intracavernosal injection of papaverine may be more sensitive than PBI alone in differen-tiating vasculogenic from psychogenic and neurologic impotence. More accurate assessment of penile blood flow may be made by penile pneumoplethysmography, ultrasonic Doppler pulse wave analysis, or duplex sonography.

Recently, we have reported that impotence due to vascular disease is highly predictive of later myocardial infarction or cerebrovascular accident (CVA).[43] In impotent men with a PBI of less than 0.65 followed for up to 3 years, 12% had a myocardial infarction, 16% had a CVA, and 10% died. In comparison, among men with a PBI greater than 0.66, only 1.5% had a myocardial infarction, 3% had a CVA, and 1.5% died. In a follow-up study, preliminary data show that a low PBI is highly predictive of an abnormal electrocardiographic response to exercise stress testing. Those findings have led us to manage cardiovascular risk factors aggressively in patients with vasculogenic impotence.

Venous leakage may be associated with a less rigid erection or an inability to sustain the erection. Venous leakage is diagnosed by infusing saline into the corpora cavernosa and measuring the pressure necessary to maintain a full erection. Instillation of a radiopaque dye permits demonstration of the leak, which may then be repaired by a urologist.

Medications are implicated in producing impotence in approximately one quarter of all patients (Table 20.5). Sixteen of the top 200 prescription drugs in the

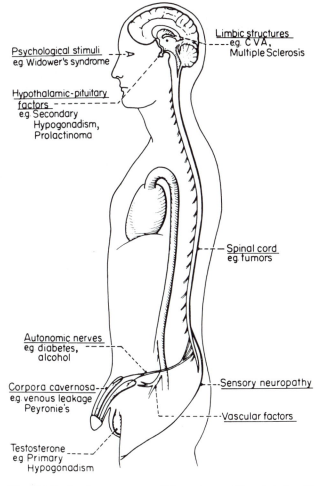

Fig. 20.7. Various causes of impotence (Reprinted with permission from the American Geriatrics Society, Sexual Dysfunction in the elderly male, by Morley et al.[42] Journal of the American Geriatrics Society, 1987;35:1014–1022).

Table 20.5. Drugs commonly associated with impotence.

Antihypertensive agents
  Diuretics
  Methyldopa
  β-blockers
  Reserpine
Centrally active agents
  Heterocyclic antidepressants
  Monoamine oxidase inhibitors
  Phenothiazines
  Butyrophenones
  Barbiturates
  Phenytoin
  Carbamazepine
Cancer chemotherapeutic agents
Testosterone receptor antagonists
  Spironolactone
  Cimetidine
Estrogenlike drugs
  Diethylstilbesterol
  Digoxin (?)
Drugs of abuse
  Tobacco
  Heroin
  Cocaine
  Alcohol

United States have been shown to cause impotence. Thiazide diuretics and antihypertensive drugs are the most common pharmacologic causes of impotence. Up to 43% of patients treated for hypertension will have erectile difficulties. Among the antihypertensive agents, angiotensin-converting enzyme inhibitors, vasodilators, calcium channel antagonists, and the more selective β-adrenergic antagonists are less likely to produce impotence; if impotence occurs during treatment with other agents, substitution may be tried. When impotence develops, it can be a major cause of noncompliance with medication.

Nonprescription drug use and abuse (eg, alcohol, heroin, cocaine) can lead to sexual dysfunction. Smoking is related to impotence both chronically by accelerating atherosclerosis and acutely by directly inhibiting the erection process.

A number of central nervous system disorders can result in impotence. These include CVAs and temporal lobe epilepsy. Up to 50% of men with multiple sclerosis develop impotence, which may be intermittent.

Depression causes a decrease in erectile capability. The "widower's syndrome" is an occasional cause of impotence. In this syndrome, the man experiences impotence during the bereavement phase following his wife's death, after suddenly being pressured to engage in intercourse with another woman.

Hypogonadism in elderly men has been discussed in detail above. The exact role in the pathogenesis of

impotence is uncertain. Diabetes mellitus tends to produce impotence at a younger age. The causes of impotence in patients with diabetes mellitus are the same as those in the general population: vascular, neurologic, hormonal, and pharmacologic. Rarely, zinc deficiency may be the cause of impotence.

Treatment of Impotence

An approach to the treatment of impotence is given in the flow diagram in Figure 20.8.[40] Treatment in older men has been improved by the introduction of vacuum tumescence devices. These devices consist of a hollow cylinder, one end of which is placed over the penis. The opposite end is connected to a vacuum pump (Fig 20.9). Negative pressure is produced around the penis, leading to blood flow into the penis and subsequent erection. A constricting band is placed around the base of the penis to prevent venous outflow and to maintain the erection following removal of the cylinder. The constricting band is kept in place during intercourse but should be removed within 30 minutes. Patient satisfaction is high in selected individuals with cooperative partners. Mild bruising is an occasional complication. The system requires manual dexterity, often necessitating help of the partner. We have had success with these systems in patients with poor blood flow and even in patients who have had penile prostheses removed.

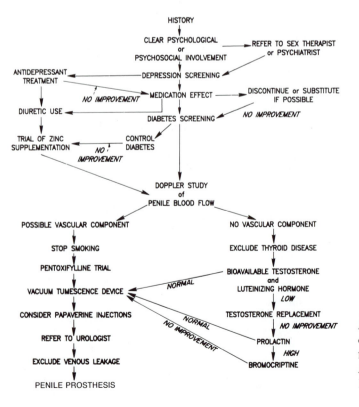

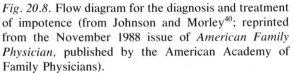

Fig. 20.8. Flow diagram for the diagnosis and treatment of impotence (from Johnson and Morley[40]; reprinted from the November 1988 issue of *American Family Physician,* published by the American Academy of Family Physicians).

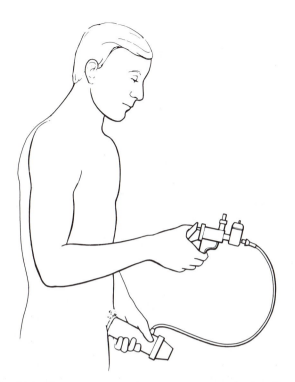

Fig. 20.9. The vacuum erection or tumescence device shown in place with the hand-held vacuum pump.

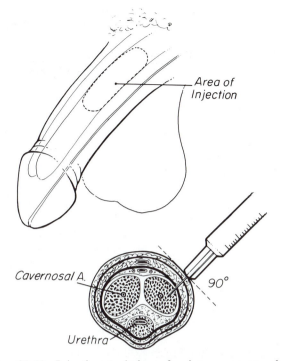

Fig. 20.10. Injection technique for intracavernous drug administration (from Johnson and Morley[40]; detailed instructions can be found in that reference. Reprinted from the November 1988 issue of *American Family Physician*, published by the American Academy of Family Physicians).

Intracavernous injections of many drugs can produce erections (Fig 20.10). The most common drug combination used is papaverine and phentolamine. Patients have been taught to inject themselves at home prior to intercourse. Complications include severe bruising, urethral bleeding, priapism, fibrosis, and systemic hypotension. Alprostadil (prostaglandin E_1) may produce fewer side effects after intracorporal injection. The development of external pastes that can be absorbed through the penile skin and produce an erection is an option for the future. Nitroglycerine paste will produce erections in some individuals but is often associated with severe headaches. Some patients with a vascular cause of impotence will respond to a 3-month trial of pentoxifylline.

Testosterone therapy should be reserved for those patients with clear hypogonadism. Oral testosterone preparations are absorbed erratically and have a propensity to cause hepatotoxicity; they are therefore not recommended. Testosterone enanthate or cypionate (150 to 300 mg every 2 to 3 weeks) given intramuscularly is the treatment of choice. Testosterone patches, placed on the scrotum, may produce physiologic levels of the hormone, but at a substantially higher price than injections. The initial response to testosterone often is reasonable but usually declines over time, probably due to the presence of coexisting causes of impotence, such as vascular disease.

Testosterone therapy can lead to prostate growth (necessitating rectal examinations every 6 months and instructions to discontinue therapy and consult the physician if difficulty in urination occurs), gynecomastia, increased hematocrits (all patients should have hematocrits checked every 6 months), water retention leading to worsening hypertension or heart failure, and an increase in low-density-lipoprotein cholesterol levels. Testosterone is contraindicated in patients with prostatic carcinoma.

The surgical placement of a penile prosthesis remains a permanent cure for impotence. Age is no barrier to the insertion of a prosthesis. Approximately 80% of patients who have a prosthesis inserted are satisfied with the operation. Overall, we prefer the use of malleable rods or hinged prostheses in older patients, as they are the simplest devices, the least likely to develop complications, and the least expensive (Fig 20.11). A number of inflatable hydraulic prostheses are now available. These are of two types: those having reservoirs implanted in the pelvis and scrotum and the more modern ones, that are self-contained within the penis (Figs 20.12, 20.13). Inflatable prostheses may be preferred if future transurethral instrumentation is anticipated or when decreased penile sensation occurs. They are particularly difficult for arthritic patients to use.

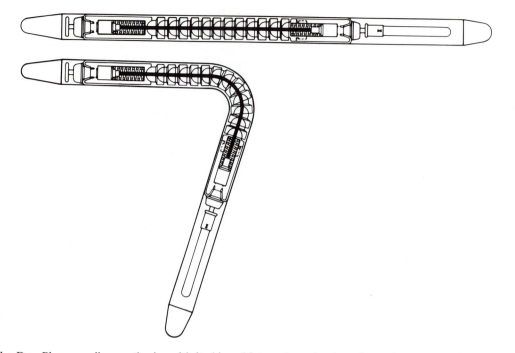

Fig. 20.11. The DuraPhase penile prosthesis, with its hinged internal mechanism shown in cross section. This prosthesis is rigid when straight but is bent downward when the patient is not having sexual intercourse (by permission from Dacomed Corp, Minneapolis, Minn).

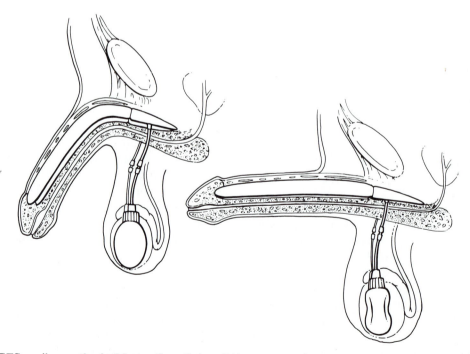

Fig. 20.12. The GFS penile prosthesis (Mentor Corp Goleta CA) represents the new generation of penile inflatable implants, in which the pelvic reservoir is eliminated. The penile rods, placed in the corpora cavernosa, are inflated by squeezing the bulb located beside one testicle. Compressing the release ring above the scrotal bulb causes deflation (from: Johnson and Morley[40]; reprinted from the November 1988 issue of *American Family Physician,* published by the American Academy of Family Physicians).

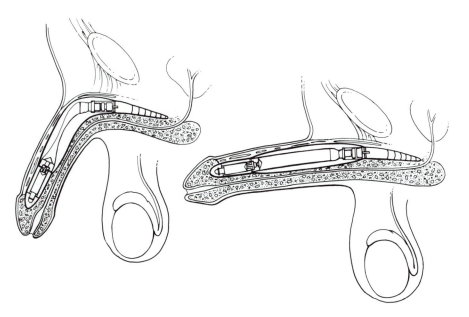

Fig. 20.13. The Surgitek Flexi-Flate II (Medical Engineering Corp) is a completely self-contained inflatable penile implant. The prostheses, inserted into the corpora cavernosa, are activated by several firm compressions of the distal tips, located behind the glans. The erection is deflated by bending the erect penis in half (from: Johnson and Morley[40]; reprinted from the November 1988 issue of *American Family Physician,* published by the American Academy of Family Physicians).

In conclusion, the issue of sexual dysfunction should be raised in all elderly male patients, since there are now treatment modalities to enhance function in nearly all cases.

References

1. Slag MF, Morley JE, Elson MK, et al. Impotence in medical clinic outpatients. *JAMA* 1983;249:1736–1740.
2. Kinsey A, Pomeroy W, Martin C. *Sexual Behavior in the Human Male.* Philadelphia, Pa: WB Saunders Co; 1948.
3. Masters W, Johnson V. *Human Sexual Response.* Boston, Mass: Little Brown & Co Inc; 1966.
4. LoPiccolo J, Stock WE. Treatment of sexual dysfunction. *J Consult Clin Psychol* 1986;54:158–167.
5. Kahn E, Fisher C. REM sleep and sexuality in the aged. *J Geriatr Psychiatry* 1969;2:181–199.
6. Karacan I, Williams RL, Thornby JI, Salis PJ. Sleep-related tumescence as a function of age. *Am J Psychiatry* 1975;132:932–937.
7. Schiavi RC, Schreiner-Engel P. Nocturnal penile tumescence in healthy aging men. *J Gerontol Med Sci* 1988;43:M146–M150.
8. Persson G. Sexuality in a 70-year-old urban population. *J Psychosom Res* 1980;24:335–342.
9. Pfeiffer E, Verwoerdt A, Wang HS. Sexual behavior in aged men and women. *Arch Gen Psychiatry* 1968;19:735–758.
10. Pfeiffer E, Verwoerdt A, Davis GC. Sexual behavior in middle life. *Am J Psychiatry* 1972;128:1262–1267.
11. Diokno AC, Bromberg J, Herzog R, et al. Correlates of sexual dysfunction in the elderly. *J Urol* 1988;139:496A.
12. Starr B, Weiner M. *The Starr-Weiner Report on Sex and Sexuality in the Mature Years.* New York, NY: Stein & Day Publishers, 1981.
13. Bretschneider JG, McCoy NL. Sexual interest and behavior in healthy 80- to 102-year-olds. *Arch Sex Behav* 1988;17:109–129.
14. Kass MJ. Sexual expression of the elderly in nursing homes. *Gerontologist* 1978;18:372–378.
15. Wasow M, Loeb MB. Sexuality in nursing homes. *J Am Geriatr Soc* 1979;27:73–79.
16. Ying SY. Inhibins, activins and follistatins: Gonadal proteins modulating the secretion of follicle-stimulating hormone *Endocr Rev* 1988;9:267–293.
17. Baker HWG, Burger HY, de Kretser DM, et al. Changes in the pituitary testicular system with age. *Clin Endocrinol* 1976;5:349–372.
18. Morley JE, Kaiser FE. Testicular function in the aging male. In: Armbrecht HJ, ed. *Endocrine Function and Aging.* New York, NY: Springer-Verlag NY Inc. In press.
19. Zumoff B, Strain GW, Kream J, et al. Age variation of the 24-hour mean plasma concentrations of androgens, estrogens and gonadotropins in normal adult men. *J Clin Endocrinol Metab* 1982;54:534–538.
20. Tenover JS, Matsumoto AM, Plymate SR, et al. The effects of aging in normal men in bioavailable testosterone and luteinizing hormone secretion: response to clomiphene citrate. *J Clin Endocrinol Metab* 1987;65:1118–1125.
21. Nankin HR, Calkins JH. Decreased bioavailable testosterone in aging normal and impotent men. *J Clin Endocrinol Metab* 1986;63:1418–1420.
22. Kaiser FE, Viosca SP, Morley JE et al. Impotence and

aging: clinical and hormonal factors. *J Am Geriatr Soc* 1988;36:511–519.

23. Tillenger KG. Testicular morphology. *Acta Endocrinol Suppl (Copenh)* 1957;24:1–192.

24. Vermeulen A, Reubens R, Verdonck L. Testosterone secretion and metabolism in male senescence. *J Clin Endocrinol Metab* 1972;34:730–735.

25. Stearns EL, MacDonnell JA, Kaufman BJ, et al. Declining testicular function with age. *Am J Med* 1974;57:761–766.

26. Deslypere JP, Vermuelen A. Leydig cell function in normal men: effect of age, lifestyle, residence, diet and activity. *J Clin Endocrinol Metab* 1984;59:955–962.

27. Winters SJ, Sheins RJ, Troen P. The gonadotropin-suppressive activity of androgen is increased in elderly men. *Metabolism* 1984;1052–1059.

28. Winters SJ, Troen P. Evidence for the role of endogenous estrogen in the hypothalamic control of gonadotropin secretion in men. *J Clin Endocrinol Metab* 1985;61:842–845.

29. Deslypere JP, Kaufman JM, Vermeulen T, et al. Influence of age on pulsatile luteinizing hormone release and responsiveness of the gonadotropins to sex hormone feedback in men. *J Clin Endocrinol Metab* 1987;64:68–73.

30. Kaiser FE, Viosca SP, Mooradian AD, et al. Impotence and aging: alterations in hormonal secretory patterns with age. *Clin Res* 1988;36:96A. Abstract.

31. Blackman MR, Tsitouras PD, Harman SM. Reproductive hormones in aging men, III: basal and LH-RH-stimulated serum concentrations of the common alpha-subunit of the glycoprotein hormones. *J Gerontol* 1987;42:476–481.

32. Urban RJ, Veldhuis JD, Blizzard RM, et al. Attenuated release of biologically active luteinizing hormone in healthy aging men. *J Clin Invest* 1988;81:1020–1029.

33. Engle ET. The male reproductive system. In: Lansing AI, ed. *Cowdry's Problems of Aging*. 3rd ed. Baltimore, Md: Williams & Wilkins; 1952:708–729.

34. Natoli A, Riondino G, Brancati A. Studio delta funizone gonadale ormonia e spermatogenetica nel corso della senescenza muschille. *G Gerontol* 1972;20:1103–1119.

35. Johnson L, Zune RS, Petty CS, et al. Quantification of the human Sertoli cell population: its distribution, relation to germ cell numbers, and age related decline. *Biol Reprod* 1984;31:785–789.

36. Tenover JS, McLachlan RI, Dahl KD, et al. Decreased serum inhibin levels in normal elderly men: evidence for a decline in Sertoli cell function with aging. *J Clin Endocrinol Metab* 1988;67:455–459.

37. Morley JE, Melmed S. Gonadal dysfunction in systemic disorders. *Metabolism* 1979;28:1051–1073.

38. Semple PD'A, Beastall GM, Brown TM, et al. Sex hormone suppression and sexual impotence in hypoxic pulmonary fibrosis. *Thorax* 1984;39:46–51.

39. Niewoehner CB, Nuttal FQ. Gynecomastia in a hospitalized male population. *Am J Med* 1984;77:633–638.

40. Johnson LE, Morley JE. Impotence in the elderly. *Am Fam Physician* 1988;38:225–240.

41. Morley JE. Impotence. *Am J Med* 1986;80:897–905.

42. Morley JE, Korenman SG, Mooradean AD, Kaiser FE. Sexual dysfunction on the elderly male. *J Am Geriatr Soc* 1987;35:1014–1022.

43. Morley JE, Korenman SG, Kaiser FE, et al. Relationship of penile brachial pressure index to myocardial infarction and cerebrovascular accidents in older males. *Am J Med* 1988;84:445–448.

21

Diseases of the Prostate

Gerald W. Chodak

Benign Prostatic Hypertrophy

Benign prostatic hypertrophy (BPH) is a common enlargement of the prostate gland that affects a high percentage of aging men. Its cause is not known, although there may be some association with high-fat diets. As a result of this enlargement patients frequently develop obstructive voiding symptoms, termed prostatism, which include decreased urinary flow rate, hesitancy, nocturia, and dribbling. Long-standing BPH may lead to acute or chronic urinary retention, bladder stone formation, hydroureteronephrosis, urinary tract infections, or renal failure. Urinary frequency or incontinence also may be associated with BPH; this often occurs when patients have chronic urinary retention.

Clinical Diagnosis

The most common method for detecting BPH is the digital rectal examination. However, it is important to realize that the findings on digital rectal examination may not correlate with the presence or absence of prostatism. Some patients with a small gland may develop obstructive voiding symptoms, and many with a large gland may have no urinary complaints. In the absence of voiding symptoms, patients with an enlarged prostate usually do not require any therapy. Furthermore, diagnostic tests are rarely indicated in the absence of symptomatic complaints unless objective findings are present. These objective findings include urinary retention, hematuria, urinary tract infections, and renal insufficiency.

If patients present with obstructive voiding symptoms, the clinician is faced with deciding which patients require therapy and which patients can simply be observed. Until recently, the primary therapy for prostatism was a simple prostatectomy, performed either transurethrally or by an open procedure. In the past several years, however, nonoperative treatments have been used or are under investigation and offer the patient alternatives to surgery.

The initial evaluation of a patient with voiding symptoms includes a physical examination, a urinalysis, and a urinary flow rate determination. The physical examination should be performed after the patient urinates in order to determine if a large residual urine is present. If urinary retention is suspected, abdominal ultrasound may be performed or the patient may be catheterized. Ultrasound may be the safer procedure because it is noninvasive and has no complications, whereas the patient may develop a urinary infection or urinary retention following catheterization. The prostate is examined for size, shape, and consistency. Normally, the prostate gland is smooth and symmetric, measuring approximately 2 cm in thickness, 3 cm in width, and 4 cm in length. If induration, asymmetry, or a palpable nodule is detected, then a prostate biopsy should be performed before any treatment is undertaken for the prostatic enlargement.

The urinalysis may show white and/or red blood cells. If white cells are present, a urine culture and an intravenous pyelogram should be performed. If red cells are found, intravenous pyelography and cystourethroscopy should be performed to determine if a tumor is present.

The easiest method for detecting outlet obstruction is to measure the urinary flow rate. This noninvasive test is performed by having a patient void into a urine container that records the volume as a function of time. Nomograms for the mean and peak flow rate have been established for each voided urine volume.[1] Outlet obstruction is diagnosed when the peak and mean flow rates are significantly below normal. Because an abnormal flow rate could be caused by either an enlarged prostate or a urethral stricture, either cystourethroscopy or retrograde urethrography should be performed to determine the cause of the problem. In the absence of a history of gonorrhea or urethral trauma, an abnormal flow rate in a man aged 50 years or older is most likely due to an enlarged prostate.

In the past few years, there has been considerable debate over the role of radiologic testing in patients with BPH.[2,3] The most common method for evaluating the kidneys is intravenous pyelography, which yields information about upper tract functioning as well as residual urine, bladder enlargement, and diverticuli formation. The incidence of adverse effects from the iodine dye is low, but severe reactions still occur. Newer contrast media are associated with fewer allergic reactions.

An alternative study is abdominal ultrasonography, which can also provide information about upper urinary tract abnormalities and bladder distention. Its primary advantage is that it has no known side-effects. Therefore, if a radiologic study is indicated, then ultrasound should be selected initially unless hematuria is present. A controversy currently exists, however, over the need for any radiologic studies in patients with symptoms of prostatism.[2] Renal function may be adequately assessed by measuring the serum creatinine level. One of the arguments used to support radiologic testing in these patients is the fear of missing a kidney, renal pelvic, or ureteral tumor. Several studies have shown that this argument is invalid because the incidence of these tumors in patients with BPH is identical to the incidence in the general population.[2,4] Routine screening of these patients is not justified. This applies, however, only to patients who have normal renal function and no pyuria or hematuria. Another reason to limit the use of radiologic tests is that the ultimate decision to offer therapy for BPH rarely is based on the results of the these studies.

Indications for Surgery

The most important reason to perform surgery in a patient with BPH is that the patient is unhappy with his symptoms.[5] Many men do not like losing sleep as a result of nocturia and find it unpleasant that urination

is difficult or time consuming. This is purely a subjective evaluation. Whereas some patients cannot cope with urinating twice during the night, others do not mind getting up three or four times. Careful questioning may identify patients whose nocturia is due in part to a large fluid intake just prior to going to bed, and simply decreasing the volume and time of drinking may markedly reduce their symptoms. There is no good evidence to show that patients with nocturia are at risk for developing acute urinary retention or renal insufficiency in the near future. Patients should be counseled about potential changes in symptoms so that they do not wait too long to seek help.

In the absence of significant voiding complaints, therapeutic intervention is still warranted in several circumstances: acute urinary retention, chronic urinary tract infections, hydroureteronephrosis, diverticuli formation, or the presence of bladder calculi. A less well-defined indication is moderate residual urine in the range of 100 to 150 mL. If surgery is not performed in patients with this indication, careful follow-up is necessary because a decompensated bladder may gradually develop.

Chronic Urinary Retention

Some patients with a long-standing history of prostatism may present with a large amount of residual urine (>500 mL). Immediate surgery may not be appropriate in these patients because they are unlikely to be able to empty their bladders immediately after surgery. The chronic distention results in an atonic bladder, which can be documented with cystometrography. The initial treatment is placement of an indwelling urethral catheter for several days to allow the bladder to regain its tone. Some patients may develop postobstructive diuresis, because the concentrating mechanism of the kidney may be impaired. Usually, these patients can be managed by allowing oral fluid intake ad libitum; in some cases, however, intravenous fluid replacement may be necessary. This is a marked change from the previous approach to managing this problem, in which set percentages of hourly urine output were replaced by intravenous fluids. That practice is no longer necessary. Patients with chronic urinary retention often have an elevated serum creatinine level, which usually decreases rapidly after a catheter has been placed. After several days, another cystometrogram can be obtained to determine if bladder function has returned. At that time, a prostatectomy may be performed, provided that patients have normal sensation and can generate bladder contractions. In many cases, however, bladder function does not improve. Under those circumstances the patient must be taught to perform intermittent catheterization at approximately 4-hour intervals. Avoiding overdistention is most important for eventual improvement. Surgery generally is not performed unless the patient has difficulty performing the catheterization or unless significant bleeding occurs due to the prostatic enlargement.

Simple Prostatectomy

A transurethral prostatectomy, the most common approach used for this operation, has a high success rate and a low complication rate. Generally, patients are hospitalized for 2 to 4 days. An open prostatectomy usually is reserved for very large glands (>80 g). Following an open prostatectomy, patients are usually hospitalized for 5 to 7 days.

Patients who are considering surgery should be counseled that the operation will often cause retrograde ejaculation. In addition, approximately 7% of patients report decreased erections following surgery, an effect which is not easily explained. These results are not well documented, however, because potency is rarely tested objectively prior to surgery. Nevertheless, patients should be informed of this possibility. Another potential long-term complication is the development of a urethral stricture or bladder neck contracture. This occurs within several weeks or months of the operation and can usually be treated by means of urethral dilation. patients also should be told that symptomatic prostatic enlargement may occur again, with approximately 10% of patients requiring a second operation.[5] All patients should be aware that a simple prostatectomy does not prevent prostate cancer. Thus, annual digital examinations should be performed following surgery.

Alternatives to Surgery

The prostate gland is innervated by the sympathetic nervous system, with α-adrenergic receptors found in the prostate, prostatic capsule, and bladder neck. Several controlled studies have shown that α-adrenergic blockers can improve the obstructive complaints associated with BPH.[6,7] Phenoxybenzamine was the first drug used for this purpose, although postural hypotension or dizziness may develop in 20% of patients.[6] More recently, prazosin, which produces fewer side effects, has been used.[7] Appropriate candidates for this therapy include patients who are poor surgical risks or who refuse to undergo surgery.

A less desirable alternative is medical or surgical castration, which causes a reduction in prostatic size because prostate size is influenced by testosterone. Symptomatic improvement may not occur until several weeks after therapy is initiated. Therefore, this treatment probably is not appropriate for patients with acute urinary retention. A side effect of this therapy is loss of libido, which is unacceptable in most sexually active men. Medical castration can be achieved by administering the same luteinizing hormone releasing hormone (LH-RH) agonists that are used to treat prostate cancer.[8] This may be a reasonable second-line choice in patients who are not sexually active and do not tolerate one of the α-blockers. The advantages of the LH-RH agonists is that surgery is avoided and libido can be restored by discontinuing the medication.

The most recent alternative to prostatectomy is balloon dilation of the prostatic urethral and bladder neck. Preliminary data suggest that this method provides short-term relief of symptoms in some cases.[9] Further investigation is underway to identify the ideal candidates and determine the long-term success rate for this procedure.

Carcinoma of the Prostate

Prostate cancer is now the third most common cancer in men in the United States. The number of deaths from prostate cancer and the number of new cases diagnosed each year has gradually increased. In 1988, approximately 96,000 new cases were diagnosed, and 28,000 men died of the disease.[10]

The causes of prostate cancer are unknown, although diet may play a role. This is partly demonstrated by a 10-fold higher incidence among Japanese men living in the United States compared with Japanese men living in Japan.

Over the past few years, there have been significant changes in the diagnosis, treatment, and management of this disease. Prostate cancer, like most malignancies, causes few symptoms during its early stages. As the tumors become more advanced, patients may develop obstructive urinary symptoms that include slowing of the stream, hesitancy, and nocturia. Although these symptoms are the same for BPH, patients with prostate cancer tend to have a more rapid change in their voiding pattern. Other symptoms associated with prostate cancer include bone pain caused by metastases.

Diagnosis

Presently, the best method for detecting prostate cancer is the digital rectal examination. Over the past few years, there has been an increased awareness of the abnormalities associated with less advanced tumors. The classic findings of prostate cancer are a stony, hard prostate, asymmetry, induration, and discrete nodules. A biopsy is indicated in patients with any of these findings. Induration, which is defined as a loss of tissue resiliency, may be very slight. Nevertheless, further evaluation is warranted regardless of how slight the abnormality. Following prostate surgery, the prostate is more difficult to evaluate because it may lose its normal consistency and symmetry. Consequently, detecting prostate cancer becomes more difficult in postsurgical patients. Unfortunately, the digital examination cannot be standardized and is not easily taught. It is likely that many small tumors are not detected because of the variable expertise of the physicians performing the examinations. The best advice is to approach the examination with a heightened awareness of the physical signs of prostate cancer, even if it results in an increased number of patients who are referred for biopsy. Induration may be the most subtle finding, and this is best detected by comparing similar areas in the right and left lobe to assess whether focal differences are present. other physical findings associated with prostate cancer include raised or flat nodules. Prostate cancer can be confirmed only by biopsy. Therefore, a prostate biopsy should be recommended for every patient who has the slightest abnormality on digital examination.

During the past few years, substantial discussion has occurred about the use of transrectal ultrasonography in diagnosing prostate cancer. This test is performed by passing an ultrasound probe into the rectum (Fig. 21.1). It yields better results that transabdominal ultrasound. The sensitivity of ultrasound in detecting prostate cancer is approximately 85% to 90%.[11,12] Most important, ultrasound may enable the diagnosis of nonpalpable tumors.[13,14] As a result, many centers around the country are encouraging the use of routine ultrasound in all men above a certain age in order to detect more tumors while they are potentially curable. The argument in favor of screening with ultrasound is that it appears to be better than screening with the digital examination. Unfortunately, there is still no proof that routine screening will decrease the mortality rate from prostate cancer. Until such a benefit is demonstrated, annual sonography should not be routinely performed.

Biopsy Methods

The most common methods of detecting prostate cancer are transurethral, transperineal, and transrectal biopsy. Transurethral biopsy probably is least effective, because 80% of the tumors develop in the peripheral portion of the prostate and transurethral biopsies do not adequately sample that area of the gland. The transrectal core biopsy offers the most direct access to a palpable lesion; however, fever and sepsis may occur even when antibiotics and enemas are used.[15-17] Traditionally, a 16-gauge needle has been used for the core biopsy. This needle also may be used to perform a transperineal biopsy, in which case the infection rate is lower compared than for transcrectal biopsy, but a local or regional anesthetic is necessary. A fundamental problem with the core biopsy is the high false-negative rate, which ranges between 10% and 20%.[18,19] Therefore, biopsy should be repeated if the results are initially negative, to avoid missing a tumor.

Transrectal fine-needle aspiration biopsy (FNAB) is another biopsy method becoming more popular in the United States. Recent data have shown that the results of FNAB are comparable with or better than those

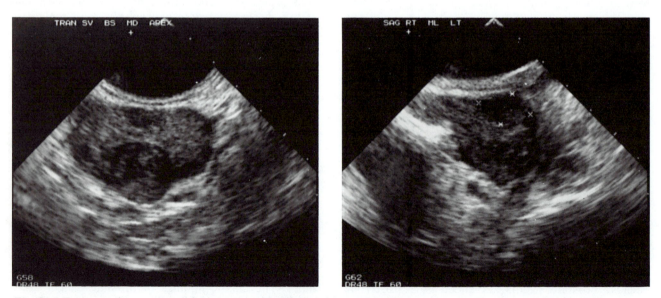

Fig. 21.1 Transrectal sonograms of the prostate in patients with nonpalpable prostate cancers. Hypoechoic lesion is seen on transverse (**left photo**) and longitudinal (**right photo**) scans.

obtained with other biopsy methods.[20] The major advantage is that no anesthesia, enemas, or antibiotics are necessary. Thus, the procedure can be performed in the office, which makes it convenient and inexpensive for the patient. The procedure has an infection rate of less than 0.01%, which avoids the need for antibiotics or enemas.[21] The major disadvantages are that both the urologist and cytopathologist must gain experience with this method in order to use the results as a basis for initiating treatment.

All of the above biopsy methods are essentially "blind," in that the needle is directed digitally into an area of suspected abnormality. Directed biopsies can now be guided by means of transrectal ultrasonography.[22] The advantage of this approach is that an abnormal area visualized on the sonogram can be accurately sampled.

Serum Tumor Markers

Two excellent markers are available for prostate cancer. These are serum acid phosphatase and serum prostate-specific antigen (PSA).[23] Both measurements have been suggested as possible screening tests, but neither is justified for this purpose. Although some unsuspected tumors may be detected in asymptomatic men by these means, their sensitivity and specificity are too low to justify their routine use. Thus, neither test should be performed routinely as part of an annual checkup, nor should they be ordered when a patient has a palpable lesion. Rather these tests should be performed only after a diagnosis of prostate cancer has been proved by biopsy. Both markers may be elevated by a digital examination, a transurethral prostatectomy, a prostatic massage, or an acute prostatic infection.[23] The appropriate use for both tests is in the staging and monitoring of known cases of prostatic carcinoma. Of the two markers, PSA is becoming more widely used because it has a better correlation with the course of the disease. The major role for acid phosphatase is in determining the likelihood of extracapsular tumor in untreated patients. If the acid phosphatase level is elevated, the carcinoma probably is not curable by radical surgery. The predictive value of PSA for extracapsular disease is too low to be reliable, but this may change with additional investigation. Although very high PSA levels usually indicate advanced disease, therapy should not be based solely on the PSA value. The PSA level is most useful for assessing the response to radical surgery, and it should drop to undetectable levels within 3 weeks after operation.[23] If the PSA level remains measurable or rises soon after surgery, the patient has residual disease. Progressive disease may also be better assessed with PSA levels than with acid

phosphatase levels. A rise in PSA indicates that the patient's disease is progressing. The optimum interval between PSA measurements in patients with localized prostate cancer has not yet been defined, but it may be reasonable to repeat the test 3 to 6 months after initial treatment. No PSA levels should be obtained within several days after a digital examination.

Staging

The traditional staging system in the United States is the Whitmore-Jewett system, whereas in Europe the TNM system is preferred (Table 21.1). In the former system, stage A cancer refers to nonpalpable tumors that are detected at the time of a simple prostatectomy. Stage A tumors are divided into A1 and A2. Although the definition of these categories is not uniform, stage A1 is defined as well-differentiated tumor that is found in three prostate chips or 5% of the tissue obtained during a transurethral prostatectomy. In contrast, stage A2 tumors are not well differentiated and they occupy a greater volume. The distinction is important because it is believed that patients who have stage A1 tumors do not require treatment.

If a tumor is palpable, it is further classified into stage B, C, or D. Stage B1 tumors occupy only one lobe or are less than 1.5 cm in diameter. Stage B2 tumors are greater than 1.5 cm in diameter or occupy both lobes. Stage C tumors are either extracapsular

Table 21.1. Staging method for prostrate cancer.

Description of tumor	Stage	
	TNM system	Whitmore-Jewitt system
Nonpalpable, ≤3 foci of well-differentiated cancer	T0a	A1
Nonpalpable, moderately or ≤3 foci of poorly differentiated cancer	T0b	A2
Palpable, involving one lobe ≤1.5 cm in diameter	T1a or T1b	B1
Palpable, involving both lobes or >1.5 cm diameter but confined within gland	T1c or T2	B2
Involving prostatic capsule	T3	C1
Involving seminal vesicles	T3	C2
Invading adjacent organs or prostate fixed to periprostatic tissues	T4	
Invades pelvic lymph nodes	TX, N+	D1
Distant metastases into bones or other organs	TX, NX, M+	D2

(C1) or extend into the seminal vesicles (C2). If the patient has no evidence of metastatic disease, but the acid phosphatase level is elevated, the stage is D0. Micrometastases likely are present in these patients. Stage D1 is defined as metastatic tumor into the lymph nodes, and stage D2 is defined as other sites of metastases, including bones, lung, liver and brain.

Before treatment is initiated, patients undergo staging chest radiography, bone scanning, and measurements of serum acid and alkaline phosphatase and PSA. Other tests performed may include computed tomography, transrectal ultra-sonography, a cystoscopy and an intravenous pyelogram, although compelling arguments can be made to omit these latter studies. Even when all of these are performed, a high percentage of cases are not staged accurately, because pelvic lymph node metastases and extracapsular or seminal vesicle invasion are difficult to assess preoperatively. Approximately 50% of the patients who undergo surgery are found to have either lymph node metastases or extracapsular tumors.[24,25] Initial studies suggest that the staging accuracy may be improved with the use of transrectal ultrasonography.[26,27] Nevertheless, all patients should be counseled that if they select surgery there is a possibility that the tumor will not be completely removed.

Treatment

Presently, there is no consensus on the optimum therapy for patients with prostate cancer.[28] This may be explained by a paucity of randomized prospective studies and the inability to stage the disease accurately with clinical tests alone. The various options for treatment are presented below (Table 21.2).

Stage A1

In most cases, no additional treatment is necessary for patients with Stage a1 disease. Presently, transrectal ultrasonography is being studied to determine if some patients with stage A1 disease have more extensive

Table 21.2. Treatment options for carcinoma of the prostate.

Stage	Treatment options
A1	Observation or radical prostatectomy
A2, B, B2	Radical prostatectomy or external beam-radiation
C	Radiation therapy with or without radical prostatectomy
D1	Hormone therapy, alone or with radiation therapy or radical prostatectomy
D2	Hormone therapy, observation, or focal radiation therapy

tumors. Younger patients may warrant more careful re-evaluation to ensure that more extensive disease has not been overlooked.

Stage A2

Aggressive therapy is needed for patients with stage A2 prostate cancer. Unfortunately, approximately 30% of these patients have metastases to the pelvic lymph nodes at the time of diagnosis.[25] The optimum therapy for patients with this stage of disease is either radical prostatectomy or external-beam radiation therapy. These treatments appear to yield comparable 10-year results; however, no long-term randomized clinical trials have been performed to compare the two treatments. An alternative therapy that was popular until recently is interstitial implantation of radioactive iodine seeds (^{125}I) directly into the prostate at the time of a lymph node dissection. This method appears to be less effective than either radical surgery or external-beam therapy.[28]

Stage B

Similar to stage A2 disease, stage B disease may be treated with either radical surgery or external beam radiationtherapy. One of the problems with selecting the optimum therapy is the inability to stage disease accurately. The optimum candidate for radical surgery is a patient whose tumor is confined entirely within the gland. Despite the available staging methods, approximately 20% to 50% of patients with stage B disease are found to have extracapsular tumor following surgery.[25] Recent data show that a high percentage of patients with tumors larger than 4 cm^3 have extracapsular disease.[29] Therefore, as newer methods, such as transrectal ultra-sonography, are developed for assessing tumor volume, only the most appropriate patients will be selected for radical surgery.

If extracapsular disease is discovered following radical prostatectomy, adjunctive radiation therapy may be indicated.[30] Residual disease may be indicated by the serum PSA level. Approximately 3 weeks following surgery, the PSA level should be undetectable. If not, additional therapy may be appropriate.

Stage C

The optimum treatment for stage C disease is not known. Therapeutic options include radical surgery, radiation therapy, and hormone therapy. Early hormone therapy may delay progression to stage D disease.[31] However, there is insufficient evidence to show that survival is prolonged by this approach. Further investigation is needed.

Stage D

In 1964 a Nobel prize was awarded to Dr Charles Huggins for showing that patients with metastatic prostatic cancer derived both subjective and objective improvements from the lowering of serum testosterone levels.[32] Circulating testosterone enters the prostatic cells, where it is converted to dihydrotestosterone. It is then transported into the nucleus, where it binds to a receptor and then acts on DNA to stimulate cell division. Lowering the testosterone level interferes with the process and produces a reduction in tumor size, as well as bone pain. It has never been conclusively determined, however, whether hormone treatment improves survival. Consequently, there is a continuing debate over the optimum timing for hormone therapy in asymptomatic patients who have metastatic disease. Some clinicians argue that hormone therapy should be withheld until symptoms develop, whereas others believe that more cells may be responsive if treatment is initiated early. The problem with hormone therapy is that many tumor cells are hormone independent, which means that they continue to grow in the absence of testosterone. As tumors grow larger, they become more poorly differentiated and less dependent on hormones.[33] Therefore, more cells will be responsive to this therapy early. The only disadvantage to early therapy is the potential side effects of the treatment.

Until recently, the most common approach to hormonal manipulation was a bilateral orchiectomy. This operation causes little morbidity and does not require hospitalization. The primary disadvantages are a reduction in libido and the possible development of hot flashes and decreased potency.[34] There is no conclusive evidence that a bilateral orchiectomy renders men impotent. Hot flashes may be quite bothersome to some patients and, unfortunately, no treatment for this problem has been approved in the United States. The other disadvantage to bilateral orchiectomy is psychological.

For those men who do not want their testicles removed there are now two alternatives. Diethylstilbestrol has been shown to produce results equivalent to those of surgery.[31] The usual dosage has been 1 mg three times daily, which produces maximal suppression of testosterone. Unfortunately, this dosage results in a cardiovascular complication rate of approximately 7%.[35] Other side effects include myocardial infarction, pulmonary embolism, congestive heart failure, breast enlargement, breast tenderness, and edema. Usually, breast tenderness and enlargement may be suppressed by two or three radiation treatments to the breast. Although more complete hormone suppression is obtained with a dosage of 1 mg three times daily, there is no evidence that it will provide better results than a dosage of 1 mg/d.[36] The lower dosage appears to have fewer cardiovascular side effects. Before a patient is given this drug, he should be warned of the potential adverse effects.

Recently, another method for suppressing testosterone has been developed. Testosterone production is regulated by luteinizing hormone releasing hormone (LH-RH), a decapeptide produced in the hypothalamus that causes the pituitary to stimulate the release of luteinizing hormone. This in turn causes the testes to produce testosterone. The LH-RH agonists are as effective as diethylbestrol.[35] Importantly, no cardiovascular side effects are caused by LH-RH agents.

Several LH-RH agonists are currently available which are administered by the patient as a daily subcutaneous injection. During the first 2 weeks following injection of an LH-RH agonist, the serum testosterone level increases, which can produce a flare of symptoms.[37] Therefore, before this treatment is administered, patients who have significant spinal metastases with a potential for spinal cord compression should receive focal radiation to the involved areas of the spine. Alternatively, 1 mg/d of diethylstilbestrol can be administered during the first 3 weeks in order to prevent the flare. The LH-RH agonists are generally well tolerated by patients, regardless of their age. The most common side effects are hot flashes and decreased libido. Several long-acting LH-RH agonists currently being tested will only require one injection per month.

Once patients are administered hormone therapy, they should be seen approximately every 3 to 4 months. The latest approach to monitoring patients is to obtain a serum PSA level, performing a bone scan only if bone pain or the PSA level increases. Approximately 7% of patients will develop progressive disease in the face of a stable PSA level.

When progressive disease develops, the choice for second-line therapy is not clear. Chemotherapy may be less well tolerated in elderly patients and not very effective, with objective response rates of only 10% to 20%.[38] If patients suffer from severe bone pain, focal radiation to the involved bones may reduce the symptoms. Unfortunately, many such patients experience a slow deterioration in their condition. Adequate pain control is essential for these individuals. Further studies are needed to assess the optimum approach to treatment of hormone-refractory prostate cancer.

References

1. Siroky MB, Olsson CA, Krane RJ. The flow rate nomogram, II: clinical correlation. *J Urol* 1980;123:208–210.
2. Bauer DL, Garrison R, McRoberts W. The health and

cost implications of routine excretory urography before transurethral prostatectomy. *J Urol* 1980;123:386–389.

3. Pollack HM, Banner MP: Current status of excretory urography. *Urol Clin North Am* 1985;12:585–601.

4. Christoffersen I, Moller I. *Eur Urol* 1980;7:65–67.

5. Barry MJ, Mulley AG, Fowler FJ, et al. Watchful waiting vs. immediate transurethral resection for symptomatic prostatism. *JAMA* 1988;259:3010–3017.

6. Caine M, Perlberg S, Meretyk S. A placebo-controlled double-blind study of the effect of phenoxybenzamine in benign prprostatic obstruction. *Br J. Urol* 1978;50:551–554.

7. Hedlund H, Andersson KE, Ek A. Effects of prazosin in patients with benign prostatic obstruction. *J Urol* 1983;130:275–278.

8. Peters C, Walsh P. The effect of nafareline acetate: a luteinizing hormone releasing hormone agonist on benign prostatic hyperplasia. *N Engl J Med* 1987;317:559–604.

9. Klein LA, Leeming BL: Balloon dilatation for prostatic obstruction; long term follow-up. *J Urol* 1988;139:273A.

10. American Cancer Society. *Cancer Facts and Figures, 1988.* New York, NY American Cancer Society; 1988.

11. Brooman PJC, Griffiths, GJ, Roberts E, et al. Perirectal ultrasound in the investigation of prostatic disease. *Clin Radiol* 1981;32:669–676.

12. Chodak GW, Wald V, Parmer E, et al. Comparison of digital examination and transrectal ultrasonography for the diagnosis of prostatic cancer. *J Urol* 1986;135:951–954.

13. Cooner WH, Eggers GW, Lichtenstein P. New hope for early diagnosis. *Ala Med* 187;56:13–16.

14. Lee F, Littrup PJ, Torp-Pedersen ST, et al. Prostate cancer: comparison of transrectal US and digital rectal examination for screening. *Radiology* 1988;168:389–394.

15. Davidson P, Malament M: Urinary contamination as a result of transrectal biopsy of the prostate. *J Urol* 1971;105:545–546.

16. Fawcett DP, Eykyn S, Bultitude MI. Urinary tract infection following trans-rectal biopsy of the prostate. *Br J Urol* 1975;47:679–681.

17. Wendel RG, Evans AT. Complications of punch biopsy of the prostate gland. *J Urol* 1967;97:122–126.

18. Kline TS, Kelsey DM, Kohler FP. Prostatic carcinoma and needle aspiration biopsy. *Am J Pasthol* 1977;67:131–133.

19. Zincke H, Campbell JT, Utz DC, et al. Confidence in the negative transrectal needle biopsy. *Surg Gynecol Obstet* 1973;136:78–80.

20. Chodak GW, Steinberg GD, Bibbo M, et al. The role of transrectal aspiration biopsy in the diagnosis of prostatic cancer. *J Urol* 1986;135:299–302.

21. Esposi PL, Elman A, Norlen H. Complications of trans-rectal aspiration biopsy of the prostate. *Scand J Urol Nephrol* 1975;9:208–213.

22. Rifkin MD, Kurtz AB, Goldberg BG. Sonographically guided transperineal prostatic biopsy: preliminary experience with a longitudinal linear-array transducer. *Am J Radiol* 1983;140:745–747.

23. Stamey T, Yang N, Hay AR, et al. Prostate specific antigen as a serum marker for adenocarcinoma of the prostate. *N Engl J Med* 1987;317;909–916.

24. Catalona WJ, Stein AJ. Staging errors in clinically localized prostate cancer. *J Urol* 1982;127:452–456.

25. Stamey TA. Cancer of the prostate. *Monogr Urol* 1983;4:68–92.

26. Pontes JE, Eisenkraft S, Watanabe H, et al. Preoperative evaluation of localized prostatic carcinoma by transrectal ultrasonography. *J Urol* 1985;134:289–291.

27. Salo JO, Kivisaari L, Rannikko S, et al. Computerized tomography and transrectal ultrasound in the assessment of local extension of prostatic cancer before radical retropubic prostatectomy. *J Urol* 1987;137:435–438.

28. Consensus Conference. The management of clinically localized prostate cancer. *JAMA* 1987;258:2727–2730.

29. McNeal JE, Kindrachuk RA, Freiha FS, et al. Patterns of progression in prostate cancer. *Lancet* 1986;1:60–62.

30. Lange PH, Reddy PK, Medini E, et al. Radiation therapy as adjunctive treatment after radical prostatectomy. *NCI Monogr* 1988;7:141–150.

31. Veterans Administration Cooperative Urological Research Group. Estrogen treatment for cancer of the prostate: early results with three doses of diethylstilbestrol and placebo. *Cancer* 1970;26:257–261.

32. Huggins, C, Hodges CV: Studies on prostatic cancer, I: the effect of castration, estrogen and androgen injections on serum phosphatases in metastatic carcinoma of the prostate. *Cancer Res* 1941;1:293–297.

33. Benson MC, Coffey DS. Prostate cancer research: current concepts and controversies. *Semin Urol* 1983;1:323–330.

34. Resnick MI. Hormonal therapy in prostatic carcinoma. *Urology* 1984;24:18–23.

35. Leuprolide Study Group. Leuprolide versus diethylstilbestrol for metastatic prostatic cancer. *N Engl J Med* 1984;311:1281–1286.

36. Byar DP. The Veterans Administration Cooperative Urological Research Group's studies of cancer of the prostrate. *Cancer* 1972;32:1126–1130.

37. Schally AV, Kastin AJ, Coy DH. LH-releasing hormone and its analogues: recent basic and clinical investigations. *Int J Fertil* 1976;21:1–30.

38. Eisenberg MA. Chemotherapy for prostate cancer. *NCI Monogr* 1988;7:151–163.

The Menopause and Beyond

Fran E. Kaiser and John E. Morley

Menopause is the permanent cessation of menses. In the United States, the mean age at menopause is approximately 51 years, with the majority of women experiencing menopause at 45 to 55 years of age. The age at which menopause occurs has not altered substantially since the first available records, which placed it at 50 years in medieval Europe. The major change has been that, with increasing longevity, women now live approximately a third of their total life span after menopause. Menstruation beyond age 55 years increases the possibility of endometrial hyperplasia and/or malignancy and requires that an endometrial biopsy be performed. The age at menopause is not altered by use of oral contraceptives, age at or number of pregnancies, age at menarche, race, body habitus, or socioeconomic conditions. The major environmental factor altering the age at onset of menopause is cigarette smoking, which causes, menopause to occur 1 to 2 years earlier than might be predicted. The hormonal basis of menopause is decreased ovarian steroidogenesis, which occurs in the face of adequate gonadotropin stimulation.

The physiologic period during which ovarian function declines is referred to as the climacteric. Although the climacteric and menopause are normal physiologic states, they are often associated with a cluster of symptoms and consequences that can clearly be considered pathologic. This was pointed out in 1877 by Borner; who said that "ill-defined are the boundaries between the physiological and pathological in this field of study."[1] It is important that physicians focus on discrete physiologic symptoms, rather than on some general "menopausal syndrome," thus avoiding negative connotations of the menopause as "a disease" while recognizing the veracity of menopause-associated complaints. When dealing with climacteric symptoms, physicians should include the patient as part of the health care team making decisions regarding pharmacologic interventions. Decisions should be made only when a woman is fully aware of the relative risks and benefits of any intervention. To carry on a meaningful dialogue with patients experiencing the climacteric, physicians should be aware of the content of popular books on the menopause, such as Budoff's *No More Hot Flashes and Other Good News*[2] and *Menopause: A Guide for Women and the Men Who Love Them* by Cutler et al.[3]

Endocrinology of the Menopause

Gamete Physiology

At 20 weeks of gestational age, the number of ooctyes available to any female is fixed at a range of 5 to 7 million.[4] Oocyte number then delines to 1 to 2 million at birth, and by puberty only 300,000 to 400,000 primordial follicles are present. The decrease in primordial follicles then continues more slowly until the age of 45 years, when there are less than 10,000 remaining. Only 300 to 400 follicles are lost through ovulation, the majority being lost without significant follicular maturation. This explains why gonadotropin suppression with oral contraceptives fails to prolong the reproductive life span. Similarly, unilateral oopho-rectomy does not alter the age at which menopause occurs. At least 80% of ovarian tissue must be removed to alter the reproductive life span significantly.

Histologically, the menopausal ovary shows a disappearance of primordial ova and follicles, with loss of granulosa and thecal cells, blood vessel wall thickening, and generalized fibrosis. Stromal cells may be unchanged or may occasionally become hyperplastic.

Premature ovarian failure may occur due to autoimmune oophoritis, viral oophoritis, lack of gonadotropin secretion or action, 17α-hydroxylase deficiency, or galactosemia. The major environmental gametotoxic agent is cigarette smoking. Both polycyclic aromatic hydrocarbons and carbon monoxide have been incriminated as gametic toxins.[5]

Menstrual Changes

With aging, there is a shortening of the follicular phase of the menstrual cycle. As menopause approaches, cycles become irregular, with both long and short intervals between menstruation. Short cycles have a normal luteal phase, with a shortened follicular phase and decreased estrogen secretion. Long cycles are anovulatory, with low or absent progesterone secretion. These changes in menstrual regularity are often associated with the onset of climacteric symptomatology. After approximately 5 years of irregular cycles, menopause occurs.

Ovarian Hormones

The ovarian stroma produces predominantly ovarian androgens (viz., androstenedione and testosterone) but has the biosynthetic enzymes necessary to produce estrogens and progesterones as well.[4] Overall, the stromal production of hormones is considerably less than the production by the theca and granulosa cells. The theca produces primarily androgens and a small amount of estrogen under the control of luteinizing hormone (LH). The granulosa cells lack 17,20 desmolase and therefore cannot convert C-21 progestogens to C-19 androgens. Estrogens, in turn, are synthesized by aromatization from androgenic precursors. Thecal androgens are provided to the granulosa cells, where they undergo aromatization to estrogens by a follicle-stimulating hormone (FSH)–inducible aromatase. This process leads to a high estrogen concentration, which that allows normal granulosa cell mitosis and oocyte maturation. Androstenedione is converted to estrone, and testosterone is converted to estradiol. In premenopausal women, about one third of the estrone is produced by periph-eral aromatization of adrenal and ovarian androstenedione, while almost all of the estradiol is produced by the ovary. Progesterone is produced after ovulation by luteinized granulosa and thecal cells.

With the onset of the perimenopausal years and domination of anovulatory cycles, estrone replaces estradiol as the major circulating estrogen. There is a marked decrease in estradiol with the menopause, but the ovary continues to secrete some estradiol into the circulation for up to 4 years thereafter (Table 22.1). The ovarian stroma continues to be major source of testosterone production throughout the menopausal years, resulting in an increased androgen-estrogen ratio in the postmenopausal years. Adipose tissue plays a significant role in the peripheral aromatization of estrogens from androgens in postmenopausal women[6] (Fig. 22.1). This fact explains the increased prevalence of endometrial hyperplasia in obese postmenopausal women. Postmenopausal women with cirrhosis of the liver also have increased estrogen levels as well as an increased prevalence of endometrial hyperplasia and cancer.

Hypothalamic-Pituitary Axis

With the degeneration of granulosa and thecal cells in the perimenopausal years, there is a decreased production of inhibin, which leads to an increase in FSH. At this time, there is also a mild decrease in circulating estradiol levels, but there is no change in LH or progesterone levels.[7] With a further decline in estradiol levels, there is eventually an increase in LH levels[7] (Fig. 22.2). In the postmenopausal years, FSH concentrations are always increased to a greater extent than LH levels. These increments represent augmented pituitary production of gonadotropins, as the clearance rates of LH and FSH are not significantly altered postmenopausally.[8] However, the relative increase in FSH compared with LH could be due, in

Table 22.1. Hormonal alterations that occur with the menopause.

Hormone	Direction of change	Degree of change
Ovarian		
Estradiol	Decrease	4- to 40-fold
Estrone	Decrease	1 1/2- to 70-fold
Testosterone	Mild decrease	1 1/2-fold
Androstenedione	Mild decrease	1 1/2-fold
Progesterone	No change	. . .
Pituitary		
LH	Increase	7-fold
FSH	Increase	8-fold
Prolactin	Decrease	1–2 ng/mL

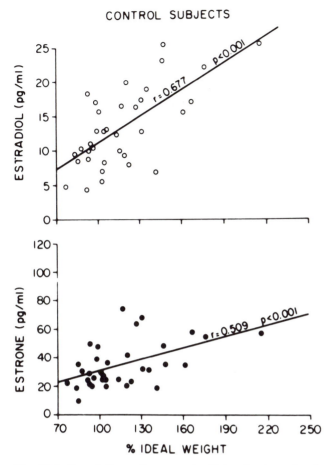

Fig. 22.1. Correlations of serum estradiol and estrone levels with percentage of ideal weight in 35 healthy postmenopausal women (from ref. 6. Reprinted with permission of C.V. Mosby Company).

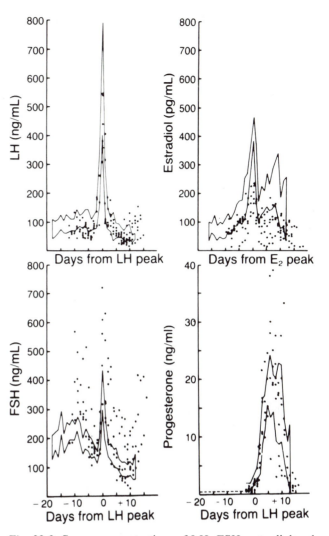

Fig. 22.2. Serum concentrations of LH, FSH, estradiol and progesterone in eight cycles from perimenopausal women (from Sherman et al[7]). Enclosed area represents mean ± 2 SEs in 10 normal ovulatory cycles from women under age 30 years.

part, to its longer clearance time. In postmenopausal women, LH and FSH secretion occurs in pulses every 60 to 90 minutes, and these pulses appear to reflect the pulsatile release of gonadotropin-releasing hormone (GnRH) from the arcuate nucleus of hypothalamus.[9] Postmenopausal women demonstrate an exaggerated response to exogenously administered GnRH.[9] Scaglia et al[9] studied four age groups of postmenopausal women, by decades from 60 to 100 years. No differences in LH or FSH concentrations could be discerned (Fig. 22.3). These findings suggest that the site of the "menopausal clock" in humans is the ovary rather than the hypothalamus.

The postmenopausal increase in LH levels appears to be partly due to the lack of estrogen, which in turn, leads to a decrease in opioid inhibitory tone of GnRH secretion.[10] The estrogen effect on endogenous opioids (which normally inhibit GnRH) appears to be mediated through a decrease in central nervous system dopaminergic activity.[11] The hormonal changes that occur with menopause are summarized in Figure 22.4.

Vasomotor Symptoms

Vasomotor symptoms, ie, hot flushes or flashes and night sweats, are the pathognomonic symptoms of the menopause. They occur in 65% to 76% of women undergoing spontaneous menopause and continue for more than a year in 80% of women who experience them.[12] Rarely do hot flashes last for more than 5 years. Obesity is somewhat protective against the development of hot flashes. Postmenopausal women with hot flashes have lower estrone and estradiol levels and lower concentrations of non–sex hormone–binding globulin-bound estradiol.[13] However, flashes are related more to estrogen withdrawal (relative rate of change) than to absolute estrogen levels.

The hot flash often starts as a sensation of pressure

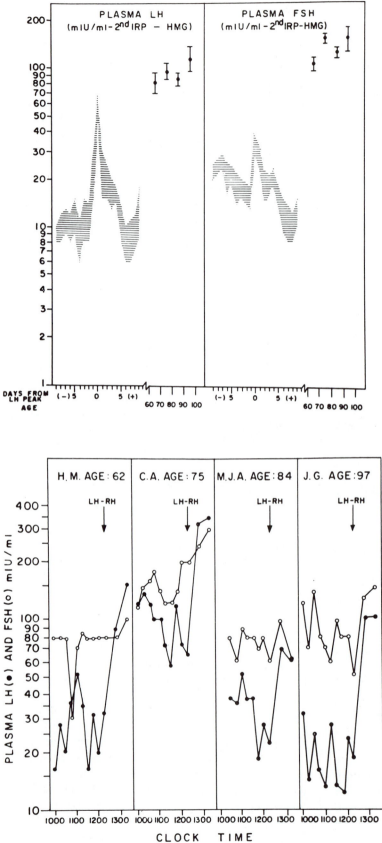

Fig. 22.3. (*top chart*) Plasma levels of immunoreactive LH and FSH (± SEM) in four groups of postmenopausal women, compared to levels observed throughout the normal menstrual cycle (results expressed in milli-international units per milliliter). (*bottom chart*) Episodic fluctuations in plasma gonadotropins and pituitary responsiveness to exogenous GnRH in postmenopausal women of advanced age (from ref. 9 with permission).

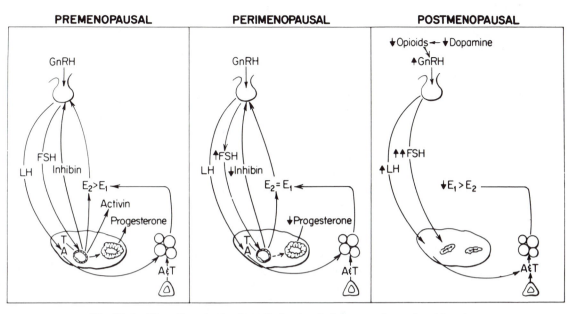

Fig. 22.4. Alterations in the hypothalamic-pituitary-ovarian axis with aging.

in the head. This is followed by the flash, which usually begins in the head and neck and passes in waves over the body. This is followed by diaphoresis, predominantly over the upper torso. The flashes are often accompanied by a transient tachycardia that can be experienced as palpitation. The duration of most flashes is about 30 minutes. Approximately 20% of women have more than one flash per day. Flashes often occur at night and are sufficiently severe to produce sleep disturbances.

Physiologically, the hot flash is characterized by a prodromal period during which there is a subjective feeling of "flushing," which can last for up to four minutes. An alteration in skin conductance represents the first measurable sign of the flash. This is followed by an increase in digital perfusion and skin temperature, is accompanied by tachycardia and an increase in LH, growth hormone, epinephrine, dehydroepiandrosterone, corticotropin (ACTH), and cortisol levels. Levels of neurotensin, a vasodilatory peptide, are also increased during the hot flash.[14] Heat loss by radiation and sweating causes the core temperature to decline by about 0.2°C and return to normal after about 30 minutes. These physiologic changes can continue for some minutes after subjective symptoms have abated.[15,16] There are no changes in the levels of FSH, estrogens, or norepinephrine during the flash. Flashes can occur in women who have undergone pituitary ablation, suggesting that the changes in LH and other pituitary hormones that occur with the hot flash are not involved in the pathogenesis of the flush.

The pathogenesis of the hot flash is poorly understood. The major factors involved appear to originate in the central nervous system. Alterations in the activity of the noradrenergic neurons in the locus ceruleus have been suggested to play a central role in the pathogenesis of the flash.[17] The α_2-adrenergic agonist clonidine attenuates the development of the flash, but not to the same extent as estrogens.[18]

The temperature regulation center is in the preoptic area of the hypothalamus. Cox and Lee[19] have shown that ovariectomy in rodents disrupts intrahypothalamic dopaminergic neuronal activity. Recently, veralipride, an antidopaminergic agent, has been shown to alleviate of vasomotor symptoms significantly.[20] This would suggest that surges of excess dopaminergic activity play a role in the pathogenesis of the hot flash. Other neurotransmitters, that may play a role in the pathogenesis of the hot flash are endogenous opioids and prostaglandins.

The most effective treatment for vasomotor symptoms is estrogen replacement. Progestogens represent a viable alternative to estrogens in treating the menopausal syndrome.[21] However, the contraindications for estrogens and progestogens are almost identical (see below). Other agents that can be used in subjects who have contraindications to estrogens and progestogens include clonidine hydrochloride (0.1 mg three times a day),[22] veralipride,[20] and Bellergal (a mixture of phenobarbital, ergotamine, and belladonna alkaloids). The opioid antagonist naloxone has also been reported to decrease the severity of hot flashes, but these results are controversial.[23]

In advising women how to deal with hot flashes, physicians should ask them to look carefully for factors that trigger the flash, such as caffeine-containing drinks, alcohol, spicy or hot foods, and very large meals. Stress may trigger hot flashes, and stress alleviation techniques may be helpful. If hot flashes interrupt sleep, naps should be taken to reduce fatigue. Dressing in layers and removing some clothes at the start of the flash may be helpful, as is the use of a hand-held fan. Moving to a cool spot, drinking something cool, or placing something cool on the wrists, temples, or forehead may help at the start of the flash. Informing those who are around that a hot flash is occurring and breaking the taboos against menopause by talking about it has been found helpful by some women.

A number of herbs have been used by women from many cultures for menopausal symptoms. These include ginseng, black cohosh, damicera, dong quai, licorice root, sarsaparilla and yerba buena (spearmint). The scientific efficacy of these "home" remedies is, for the most part, neither proved nor disproved. Physicians need to know whether their patients are using any of these herbs. Ginseng can produce hypertension, and it and black cohosh both contain estrogens. The physiologic and hormonal changes that occur during hot flashes are summarized in Figure 22.5.

Other Menopausal Symptoms

Besides hot flashes, a cluster of other symptoms occurs during menopause. It is uncertain whether these symptoms are primary—that is, related to estrogen deficiency per se—or secondary to the hot flashes and sleep disturbances. Estrogen therapy has improved hot flashes, insomnia, irritability, headaches, urinary frequency, anxiety, cognitive disturbances, and vaginal dryness.[24] Estrogen had no effect on arthralgias, backache, vaginal discomfort, or skin condition.

Urogenital Atrophy

Following menopause, the myometrium shrinks, with uterine weight falling from 120 g to between 25 and 30 g. Postmenopausally, the endometrium can be atrophic or weakly proliferative, hyperplastic (cystic or adenomatous) or neoplastic. Endometrial estrogen receptors lose their ability to translocate to the nucleus.[25]

There is shortening and thinning of the vagina, with loss of rugal folds. The vulvar epithelium also becomes thin and may be irritated and subject to infection. Continued intercourse is said to be somewhat protective against these changes. The integrity of the lower urinary tract mucosa and the trigone of the bladder is

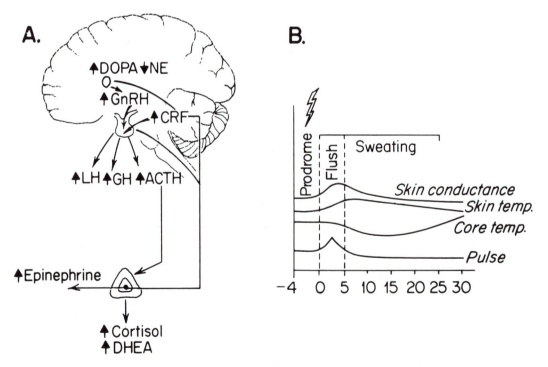

Fig. 22.5. The hormonal and physiologic changes involved in a hot flash. Horizontal axis in (B) is minutes.

dependent on estrogens, and postmenopausal urethral atrophy can occur. The symptoms associated with urogenital atrophy are outlined in Table 22.2.

Hysterectomy and Ovarian Removal

By the age of 60 years approximately one third of women in the United States have undergone a hysterectomy.[26] The major reasons for hysterectomy are fibromyomas (27%), prolapse (21%), endometriosis (15%), and cancer (10%). In 1984, bilateral oophorectomy was concurrently performed in 41% of hysterectomies. The justification for the increase in bilateral oophorectomy has been that ovarian cancer occurs in 1% of women, is difficult to detect at an early stage by means of routine pelvic examination, and is associated with a poor survival rate. The prevalence of hysterectomy in the United States by age 60 years is much higher than in the United Kingdom (13%) and France (9%). At present, there are insufficient grounds for either accepting or rejecting the somewhat cavalier attitude to hysterectomy and bilateral oophorectomy in the United States. The major quality-of-life issue appears to be the potential effects on sexuality. This has led to the development in Europe of supracervical hysterectomies, which are claimed to better preserve sexual function but involve the continued risk of carcinoma of the cervix.[27] Women need to understand the alternatives to hysterectomy, such as myomectomy, endometrial resection for submucous fibroids, and conservative treatments for endometriosis. The cardiovascular, oncologic, and sexual implications of hysterectomy and prophylactic ovarian removal need to be discussed, and decisions on treatment should be made in a true collaboration between a women and her gynecologist.

Sexuality

"Fun and enjoyment are not luxuries; they are necessities of mental health. Depending on his or her value system, a person's fun may or may not include sex. There are ample forms of fun without sex, but sex is a natural body function and our society has grossly distorted it, especially with the older generation."

—Shearer and Shearer, 1977[28]

The classic study of the effects of aging on orgasm was by Masters and Johnson.[29] The excitement phase is decreased with aging. Breast vasocongestion and vaginal lubrication are reduced, the vaginal orifice expands to a lesser degree, and the labia majora fail to flatten and separate. In the plateau phase, areolar engorgement is less intense, as is vasocongestion of the vaginal orgasmic platform. Tenting of the transcervical vagina and uterine elevation are less marked. Clitoral size decreases in the 6th decade, and there is less fullness of the clitoral hood and the fat pad over the mons. During orgasm, there is reduced frequency of uterine contractions; in some women, spastic, painful orgasmic contractions may occur. During resolution, clitoral tumescence is rapidly lost and retraction occurs more quickly than in younger women. Despite these changes, many women report continued enjoyment of sexual intercourse in older age.

During midlife, approximately one third of women complain of sexual difficulties.[30,31] The most common complaints are decreased libido, infrequent orgasm, vaginal dryness, and dyspareunia. Stress incontinence is strongly associated with sexual problems, but neither gynecological surgery nor menopausal symptoms have been correlated with sexual dysfunction. McCoy and Davidson[32] studied the frequency of intercourse longitudinally in a group of women around the time of menopause. Coital frequency and sexual thoughts declined significantly in the postmenopausal compared with the premenopausal period (Fig. 22.6). Testosterone levels correlated more closely with coital frequency than did estrogen levels.

A number of studies have examined sexual activity in older women. All studies have shown a decrease in sexual function with advancing age. Starr and Weiner[33] reported that the frequency of sexual intercourse was 1.39 times per week for women aged 60 to 91 years, which was the same frequency that Kinsey et al[34] had reported for 46- to 50-year-olds 28 years previously. Three recent studies have shown that a substantial percentage (26% to 43%) of women

Table 22.2. Symptoms associated with urogenital atrophy.

Genital atrophy, age-related vaginitis
   Burning
   Pruritus
   Dryness
   Dyspareunia
   Vaginal bleeding
   Leukorrhea
   Vaginismus
   Decreased libido
   Infection
Urethral syndrome
   Dysuria
   Frequency of urination
   Urgency of urination
   Nocturia
   Dribbling after urination
   Urethral caruncles

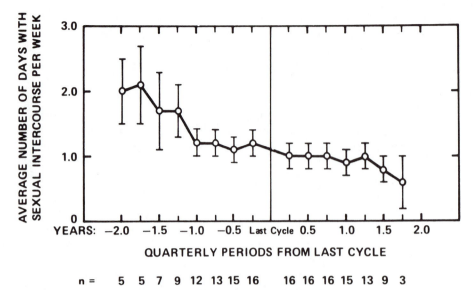

Fig. 22.6. Average number of days with sexual intercourse per week (± SE), by 13-week periods before and following the last menstrual cycle (Reproduced with permission from McCoy and Davidson[32]). Maturitas 1985;7:203–210.

over 75 years old are anorgasmic.[33,35,36] In a Swedish study, the major factors that correlated with reduced sexual activity included an older spouse, poor mental or physical health, marital difficulties, previous negative sexual experiences, and negative attitudes toward sexuality in older people.[37] Masturbation is practiced by 40% to 50% of females over 60 years, with about 8% masturbating at least once a week.[33,36] A diminished need to fantasize may occur with the use of vibrators. Both paraclitoral stimulation and vaginal insertion can produce sexual arousal in older women. The repeated mechanical stimulation of masturbation can lead to cystitis.

In women over 80 years of age, the following sexual problems were reported: anorgasmy (30%), decreased libido (23%), partner's impotence (30%), poor vaginal lubrication (30%), and insufficient opportunities for sexual encounters (25%).[36] In the Starr-Weiner[33] report on women over 60 years of age anorgasmy occurred in 23% and dyspareunia in 17.6%. Up to one third of women expressed dissatisfaction with their sexual experiences.

Therapeutic approaches to sexual dysfunction in older women include giving "permission," providing information, and making specific suggestions. Permission from the physician (as "authority" figure) to indulge in sexual fantasies or to assume a different sexual position may be sufficient to solve the problem. In some cases, the provision of graded erotic exercises may be helpful. It is vital, however, to be sensitive to the older patient's cultural background and beliefs. In addition, in patients complaining of sexual dysfunction, it is important to screen fro depression, which can interfere with sexual functioning at multiple levels.

As early as 1943, testosterone was reported to improve libido in females.[38] Subsequent studies have

been controversial, with androgens found to have some added effect over estrogens or to be ineffective.[39] While androgens may improve libido in some postmenopausal women, the lack of long-term studies makes it impossible to recommend this therapy as a treatment for the common problem of lack of sexual desire.

There is almost no scientific literature on the problems, or lack of them, experienced by older lesbians. In *Long Time Passing: Lives of Older Lesbians,* Mary Adelman has provided a sometimes moving set of anecodotal stories of the problems that beset older lesbians.[40] The Gay and Lesbian Outreach to Elders in San Francisco is an example of a social service organization developed to provide advice to older lesbians.

Sexuality is an important issue for many postmenopausal women. The physician needs to be sensitive to the needs of postmenopausal women and to provide them with opportunities to discuss sexual issues. It is also important, however, that the physician be aware of the patient's cultural background and beliefs and not to impose his or her viewpoint of sexual normality on the patient.

Sexual Assault and the Elderly Women

Sexual assault is not limited to younger women. In a study of 78 women over 50 years of age who were raped, physical force was used in 97%; actual beating occurred in half the cases.[41] In most cases, rape was associated with robbery. The elderly victim of sexual assault is humiliated, frightened, and often severely injured. The entire vagina should be examined with a narrow-blade speculum to exclude vault tears. Prophylaxis against veneral disease should be provided routinely. Counseling and support are essential for the rape victim.

Menopause and Heart Disease

The exact role of the menopause and estrogens in the development of atherosclerosis and myocardial infarction is uncertain. There is a marked increase in the incidence of myocardial infarction following menopause. Overall, it appears that unopposed estrogen therapy decreases the rate of mortality from cardiovascular disease[42,43] although not all studies have reached this conclusion.[44] It should be remembered that Japanese, Bantu, and black American females have relatively little increase in atherosclerosis related to the menopause.

The cardioprotective effect of estrogens has been related to the decreasing levels of low-density lipoproteins (LDLs) and increasing levels of high-density lipoproteins (HDLs). Estrogens produce particularly marked increases in HDL_2 and in apoprotein AI and AII levels.[45] The addition of a progestogen to estrogen, while still allowing LDL levels to fall, negates the positive effects of estrogens on HDL and HDL_2.[46] The studies showing beneficial effects of estrogens on heart disease have all used unopposed estrogens, so it would seem prudent to administer the lowest dose of progestin that inhibits the hyperplastic activity of estrogen on the endometrium.

Osteoporosis

It is clear that there is a rapid loss in bone mass following the menopause and that this rate of loss is markedly attenuated by estrogen replacement. Bone loss is greater in white and oriental women than in black women. (The role of estrogens in the treatment of osteoporosis is discussed in detail in Chapter 15.)

Cancer and Estrogens

Epidemiologic studies have suggested that there is a three-to sevenfold risk of endometrial cancer in postmenopausal women taking estrogen.[12] These original studies probably overestimated the risk of endometrial cancer, as most of patients with endometrial cancer were taking high doses of estrogens (1.25 mg of conjugated estrogen daily). The risk of developing endometrial cancer while taking estrogen was one in 500 in these epidemiologic studies, but autopsy studies have suggested that, of women dying of other causes, one in 300 have undiagnosed endometrial cancer.

Collins et al[47] found that the 10-year survival for women with endometrial cancer who were not receiving estrogen approached 50%, compared with 90% for those who were taking estrogens and then developed endometrial cancer. The latter rate was actually better than the 80% survival in women without endometrial cancer who were not taking estrogens. Overall, it appears that endometrial cancer that occurs in women taking estrogen is well differentiated and can be treated effectively by means of hysterectomy. It is also possible that women taking estrogens receive better surveillance than those not taking estrogens.

Progesterone and synthetic progestins decrease the synthesis of estrogen receptors and thus suppress the proliferative effect of estrogens on the endometrium. A number of studies have suggested that a progestin given for at least 9 days will decrease the occurrence of endometrial cancer in women receiving estrogens.[48]

As some breast cancers are estrogen sensitive, it was hypothesized that estrogen replacement therapy would increase the incidence of breast cancer. However, the available studies appear to indicate that this is not the case in postmenopausal women.[49] Women receiving estrogen replacement should have yearly mammograms. Women who have already had breast cancer should not receive menopausal estrogen replacement.

Hypertension, Glucose Tolerance, and Gallbladder Disease

Synthetic estrogens may induce hypertension in a small subset of susceptible individuals. This form of hypertension is associated with an increase in plasma renin activity, renin substrate, and aldosterone secretion. Overall, postmenopausal estrogen replacement is rarely associated with hypertension, but occasional idiosyncratic hypertension due to replacement estrogen warrants routine blood pressure measurements.

Estrogens may produce mild abnormalities in glucose tolerance. However, they do not appear to induce frank diabetes mellitus.

There is a 2.5-fold risk of gallbladder disease in women aged 45 to 49 years who are receiving replacement estrogen.[50] All women taking estrogens should be informed of the symptoms of gallbladder disease and warned of this risk.

Hormonal Replacement

Current prescribing practices suggest that three quarters of postmenopausal women receive estrogens for at least 10 years.[51] Many women also take a progestin.

In view of this, it should be remembered that there have been no long-term studies on combination therapy in the postmenopausal years. The major reasons for estrogen replacement are the treatment of hot flashes and other perimenopausal symptoms and the prevention of osteoporosis and, possibly, cardiovascular disease.

The contraindications to estrogen therapy are listed in Table 22.3. While estrogens increase fibrinogen and decrease antithrombin III levels, evidence that they increase thromboembolic disease during the postmenopausal years is lacking. there appears to be a slight decrease in cerebrovascular accidents and thromboembolic disease.[52,53] The contraindications for progestogens are similar to those for estrogen.

The side effects of estrogens include breast tenderness, edema or bloating, premenstrual syndrome–like symptoms, nausea, and headaches. Progesterone side effects include breast tenderness, premenstrual syndrome–like symptoms, depression, irritability, mood swings, lethargy, and abdominal bloating. Symptoms of water retention often respond to a diuretic given for 7 to 10 days before the menses. Resumption of menses occurs in 97% of women until age 60 years and about 60% of women after age 65 years when combination estrogen-progesterone therapy is used. The periods are frequently shorter (3 to 4 days), lighter, and less painful. Abnormal bleeding requiring curettage occurs in 23% of women not taking hormones in 14% of those taking only estrogen, and in 4% of those receiving estrogen-progestogen combinations.[54]

Examples of the available oral estrogens are listed in Table 22.4. Most women require 0.625 mg/d of conjugated estrogens or an equivalent dosage of other oral estrogen preparations. Occasionally, higher dosages may be necessary to inhibit hot flashes, especially in women undergoing surgically induced menopause. Conjugated estrogens consist of a mixture of sodium estrone sulfate, sodium equilin sulfate, sodium equilenin sulfate, and sodium estradiol sulfate.

A variety of vaginal creams are available and provide the quickest relief for symptoms of atrophic

Table 22.3. Contraindications to estrogen replacement in postmenopausal women.

| 1. Known or suspected breast cancer |
| 2. Vaginal bleeding of unknown origin |
| 3. Known or suspected estrogen-dependent neoplasia (eg, uterus, kidney, melanoma) |
| 4. Active or previous thromboembolic disorder (particularly if associated with estrogen use) |
| 5. Porphyria |
| 6. Liver disease |

Table 22.4. Examples of available oral estrogens and equivalent dosages.

Type	Example	Equivalent dosages mg/d
Conjugated	Premarin	0.625
Natural	Micronized estradiol	1
Synthetic	Ethinyl estradiol	0.02
	Quinestrol	0.1

vaginitis. Oral estrogens are usually started simultaneously with 1 g/d of Premarin cream (0.625 mg of conjugated estrogens per gram); in many cases, the vaginal estrogen creams can be reduced to three times per week or discontinued after 2 to 4 weeks. Some women, however, do not respond to oral estrogens alone and require continuous vaginal cream applications. Vaginal estrogens are absorbed into the systemic circulation. After vaginal administration, estradiol is poorly converted to estrone, in contrast to the rapid conversion that occurs after oral administration.

Transdermal estrogen replacement therapy is now available. These systems also increase estradiol more than they increase estrone and have less effect on hepatic protein synthesis (ie, on renin substrate, sex hormone–binding globulin, ferroxidase (ceruloplasmin), cortisol-binding globulin, and antithrombin III) than do oral preparations. However, these preparations also fail to have beneficial effects on HDL cholesterol levels. It should be remembered that progesterone must still be administered along with transdermal estrogen.

Cyclic administration of a progestogen for 10 to 15 days each month is commonly used to prevent the development of endometrial cancer. C-21 progestogens (eg, medroxyprogesterone acetate, 5 to 10 mg/d) are best used in women with a history of breast disease, but 19-norprogestogens (eg, norethindrone acetate, 1mg/d) may be more effective in women with a history of heavy menstrual periods. There is not firm evidence that progesterone therapy is beneficial in women who have had a hysterectomy.

Besides receiving hormonal therapy, all postmenopausal women should be advised to abstain from smoking, which decreases circulating estrogen levels even in women receiving replacement estrogen. Smoking also accelerates osteoporosis and atherosclerosis and increases the risk of cancer. It seems prudent to have all postmenopausal white and oriental women take between 1 and 1.5 g/d of calcium. The recent studies suggesting no effect of calcium supplementation (elemental calcium) on bone mass in the perimenopausal years should be viewed cautiously, as they have all been short term and have ignored the potential long-term benefits of calcium supplementation on age-related osteopenia. Regular physical exercise should be recommended to all postmenopausal women. Postmenopausal women with a contraindication to estrogens may consider taking injectable or intranasal calcitonin for its protective effects on bone.

To summarize, there is mounting evidence that oral estrogen replacement therapy, most probably in combination with progesterone, is beneficial and cost-effective for most postmenopausal women. However, the final choice of whether or not to take hormonal therapy rests with the woman herself, who should make her own decision after being fully informed of the facts concerning replacement therapy. All women should be informed that there have been no long-term studies of combination therapy with progestogens and, therefore, that while such therapy theoretically appears reasonable, women who choose this option are, in fact, entering themselves into an uncontrolled clinical trial. Similarly, the only-recent availability of transdermal estrogen patches makes their long-term use experimental. Whether groups at low risk for osteoporosis and atherosclerosis benefit from postmenopausal estrogen replacement is unknown.

References

1. Borner E. The menopause. In: *Cyclopaedia of Obstetrics and Gynecology*. New York, NY: William Wood; 1887.
2. Budoff PW. *No More Hot Flashes and Other Good News*. New York; NY: GP Putnam's Sons; 1983.
3. Cutler WB, Garcia CR, Edwards DA. *Menopause: A guide for Women and the Men Who Love Them*. New York; NY: Norton; 1983.
4. Haney AF. The 'physiology' of the climacterium. *Clin Obstet Gynecol* 1986;29:397–405.
5. Jick H, Porter J, Morrison AS. Relation between smoking and age of natural menopause: report from Boston Collaborative Drug Surveillance Program, Boston University Medical Center. *Lancet* 1977;1:1354–1356.
6. Judd HL, Davidson BJ, Frumar AM, et al. Serum androgens and estrogens in postmenopausal women with and without endometrial cancer. *Am J Obstet* 1980;136:859–871.
7. Sherman BM, West JH, Korenman SG. The menopausal transition: analysis of LH, FSH, estradiol and progesterone concentrations during menstrual cycles of older women. *J Clin Endocrinol Metab* 1976;42:629–636.
8. Kohler PO, Ross GT, Odell WD. Metabolic clearance and production rates of human luteinizing hormone in pre- and post-menopausal women. *J Clin Invest* 1968;43:381–388.
9. Scaglia H, Medina M, Pinto-Ferreira Al, et al. Pituitary LH and FSH section and responsiveness in women of old age. *Acta Endocrinol* 1976;81:673–679.
10. Petraglia A, Porro C, Facchinetti F, et al. Opioid control of LH secretion in humans: menstrual cycle, menopause and aging reduce effect of naloxone but not of morphine. *Life Sci* 1986;38:2103–2110.
11. Melis GB, Cagnacci A, Gambacciani M, et al. Chronic bromocriptine administration restores luteinizing hormone response to naloxone in post-menopausal women. *Neuroendocrinology* 1988; 47:159–163.
12. Mishell DR, Jr, Brenner PF. Menopause. In: Mishell DR, Jr, Davajan V, eds. *Infertility, Contraception, and Reproductive Endocrinology*. 2nd ed. Oradell, NJ: Medical Economics Books; 1986:179–202.
13. Erik Y, Meldrum DR, Judd HL. Estrogen levels in post-menopausal women with hot flashes. *Obstet Gynecol* 1982;59:403–411.
14. Kronenberg M, Carraway RE. Changes in neurotensin-like immunoreactivity during menopausal hot flashes. *J Clin Endocrinol Metab* 1985;60:1081–1086.
15. Jaffe RB. The menopausal and perimenopausal period. In: Yen SSC, Jaffe RB, eds. *Reproductive Endocrinology*. Philadelphia, Pa: WB Saunders Co; 1986.
16. Tataryn IV, Meldrum DR, Lu LH, et al. LH, FSH, and skin temperature during the menopausal hot flash. *J Clin Endocrinol Metab* 1979;49:152–158.
17. Svenson TH. Clonidine treatment in vegetative dysfunction: experimental reationales. *Acta Obstet Gynecol Scand Suppl* 1985;132:23–28.
18. Hammar M, Berg G. Clonidine in the treatment of menopausal flushing. *Acta Obstet Gynecol Scand Suppl* 1985;132:29–31.
19. Cox B, Lee TF. Further evidence for a physiological role for hypothalamic dopamine in thermoregulation in the rat. *J Physiol* 1980;300:7–12.
20. David A, Don R, Tajchner G, et al. Veralipride: alternative antidopaminergic treatmtne for menopausal symptoms. *Am J Obstet Gynecol* 1988;158:1107–1115.
21. Paterson MEL. Randomized double-blind crossover trial into the effect of norethisterone on climateric symptoms and biochemical profile. *Br J Obstet Gynecol* 1982; 89:464–472.
22. Laufer LR, Erlik Y, Meldrum DR, et al. Effect of chlonidine on hot flashes in postmenopausal women. *Obstet Gynecol* 1982;60:583–586.
23. Lightman SL, Jacobs HS. Naloxone suppresses menopausal hot flushes. *Lancet* 1979;2:1071–1074.
24. Campbell S. Double-blind psychometric studies on the effects of natural estrogens on post-menopausal women. In: Campbell S, ed. *Management of the Menopause and Post-Menopausal Years*. Lancaster, England: MTP Press Ltd; 1976:152–163.
25. Strathy JH, Coulam CB, Spelsburg TC. Comparison of estrogen receptors in human premenopausal and postmenopausal uteri: indication of biologically inactive receptor in postmenopausal uteri. *Am J Obstet Gynecol* 1982;142:372–376.
26. Greenwood S. Hysterectomy and ovarian removal: a major health issue in the perimenopausal years. *West J Med* 1988;149:771–772.
27. Kikku P, Gronroos M, Hirvonen T, et al. Supravaginal uterine amputation vs. hysterectomy: effects on libido

and orgasm. *Acta Obstet Gynecol Scand* 1983;62:147–152.

28. Shearer MR, Shearer ML. Sexuality and sexual counseling in the elderly. *Clin Obstet Gynecol* 1977;20:197–208.

29. Masters W, Johnson V. Human sexual response. Boston; Mass: Little Brown & Co Inc, 1970.

30. Garde K, Lunde I. Female sexual behavior in a random sample of 40-year-old women. *Maturitas* 1980;2:225–240.

31. Osborn M, Hawton K, Gath D. Sexual dysfunction among middle-aged women in the communuity. *Bri Med J* 1988;296:959–962.

32. McCoy NL, Davidson JM. A longitudinal study of the effects of menopause on sexuality. *Maturitas* 1985;7:203–210.

33. Starr BD, Weiner MB. *On Sex and Sexuality in the Mature Years*. New York; NY: Stein & Day Publishers, 1981.

34. Kinsey AC, Pomeroy WB, Martin CE. *Sexual Behavior in the Human Female*. Philadelphia, Pa: WB Saunders; 1953.

35. Newman G, Nichols CR. Sexual activities and attitudes in older persons. *JAMA* 1960;173:33–35.

36. Bretschneider JG, McCoy NL. Sexual interest and behavior in healthy 80- to 102-year-olds. *Arch Sex Behav* 1988;17:109–129.

37. Persson G. Sexuality in a 70-year-old urban population. *J Psychosom Res* 1980;24:137–154.

38. Salmon TJ, Geist SH. Effect of androgens on libido in women. *J Clin Endocrinol Metab* 1943;3:235–238.

39. Studd JWW, Collins WP, Charkrvati S. Oestradiol and testosterone implants in the treatment of psychosexual problems in the postmenopausal women. *Br J Obstet Gynaecol* 1977;84:314–316.

40. Adelman M. *Long Time Passing: Lives of Older Lesbians*. Boston; Mass: Alyson Publications Inc; 1986.

41. Davis LJ. Rape and older women. In: Warner CG, ed. *Rape and Sexual Assault Management and Intervention*. Rockville, Md: Aspen Publishers; 1980:94–118.

42. Ross RK, Paganini-Hill A, Mack TM. Menopausal oestrogen therapy and protection from death from ischemic disease. *Lancet* 1981;1:858–862.

43. Bush TL, Barrett-Connor E, Cowan LD, et al. Cardiovascular mortality and non-contraceptive use of estrogen in women: results from the Lipid Research Clinics Program Follow-up Study. *Circulation* 1987;75:1102–1109.

44. Colditz GA, Willett WC, Stampfer MJ, et al. Menopause and the risk of coronary heart disease in women. *N Engl J Med* 1987;316:1105-1110.

45. Ottosson UB, Carlstrom K, Johansson BG, et al. Estrogen induction of liver proteins and high-density liporpotein cholesterol: comparison between estradiol valenate and ethinyl estradiol. *Gynecol Obstet Invest* 1986;22:198–205.

46. Farish E, Fletcher CD, Hart DM et al. The effects of conjugated equine oestrogens with and without a cyclical progestogen on lipoproteins and HDL subfractions in postmenopausal women. *Acta Endocrinol* 1986;113:123–127.

47. Collins J, Donner A, Allen LH, et al. Oestrogen use and survival in endometrial cancer. *Lancet* 1980;2:961–963.

48. Varma TR. Effect of long-term therapy with estrogen and progesterone on endometrium of postmenopausal women. *Acta Obstet Gynecol Scand* 1985;64:41–46.

49. Wingo PA, Layde PM, Lee NC, et al. The risk of breast cancer in postmenopausal women who have used estrogen replacement therapy. *JAMA* 1987;257:209–215.

50. Boston Collaborative Drug Project: Surgically confirmed gallbladder disease, venous thromboembolism, and breast tumors in relation to postmenopausal estrogen therapy. *N Engl J Med* 1974;290:15–19.

51. Barrett-Connor E. Postmenopausal estrogens: current prescribing patterns of San Diego gynecologists. *West J Med* 1986;144:620–621.

52. Hammond CB, Jelovsek FR, Lee KL, et al. Effects of long-term estrogen replacement therapy, I: metabolic. *Am J Obstet Gynecol* 1979;133:525–536.

53. Nachtigall L, Nachtigall RH, Nachtigall RD, et al. Estrogen replacement, II: a prospective study in the relationship t carcinoma and cardiovascular and metabolic problems. *Obstet Gynecol* 1979;54:74–79.

54. Gambrell RD Jr, Castaneda TA, Ricci CA. Management of postmenopausal bleeding to prevent endometrial cancer. *Maturitas* 1978;1:99–106.

23

Gynecology

Lane J. Mercer

The average age of surgical menopause in the United States is 45.5 years, and that of natural menopause is 51.4 years. Therefore, for many women the postmenopausal period is now longer than time of reproductive function. During the postmenopausal years, many problems of the female reproductive tract can affect a woman's daily functioning, influence her longevity, and alter her feelings of self-esteem. In recent years, awareness of the postmenopausal woman's needs has increased, and the scope of gynecologic health care has expanded to meet her expectations.

History

Care must be taken in eliciting the gynecologic history from an older woman, as important symptoms may range from the subtle to the obvious. Many symptoms and complaints may be mild and long-standing yet reflect a real threat to the patient's well-being. A history must begin with questions regarding menarche, reproduction function, and regularity of menses, even though these events may seem distant to an elderly woman. Irregularities of menses or reproductive dysfunction earlier in life may place the patient at a higher risk for endometrial disease in later years. A careful review of gynecologic or breast surgery may reveal a potential for a disease process that places the patient at higher risk for a subsequent lesion or recurrence in later years. Seemingly minor details of a patient's history, such as loss of height or change in posture, which many patients may consider normal processes of aging,

can indicate signficant osteoporosis. The patient should be asked specifically about vulvar burning, dryness, and itching, which may be symptoms of estrogen deficiency but may also indicate the presence of a carcinoma of the vulva or vulvar dystrophy. Vaginal discharges must be inquired about, not only because of the discomfort they cause but because they may indicate the presence of underlying pathology. Vaginal bleeding of any nature or of any amount is an important historical point in this age group. As the volume of bleeding does not reflect the severity of an underlying lesion, all vaginal bleeding or bloody discharges need to be completely evaluated. Although often overlooked and rarely brought up voluntarily by the patient, symptoms of urinary dysfunction, should be inquired about, including incontinence, dysuria, hematuria, and urgency. By taking a careful history, one may be able to attribute urinary incontinence to medication, functional disabilities, or primary bladder dysfunction. Questions regarding prolapse of the pelvic organs, including the presence of pelvic pressure, the timing of the occurrence of this pressure, or the feeling of a protruding mass from the vagina, may suggest a diagnosis that would be missed when examining a patient in the lithotomy position.

Last, a sensitive but thorough sexual history must be taken to ascertain the extent of sexual activity, whether pain or discomfort is experienced with sexual intercourse, whether this pain is limiting or preventing sexual intercourse, and the patient's wishes regarding treatment of these problems. The embarrassment over such questions will often lead to denial. However, with sensitive questioning and reassurance, an accurate sexual history can be obtained.

Examination

Breasts

Examination of the breasts must be included in all complete gynecologic examinations. Although all patients should be encouraged to do breast self-examinations, these must not take the place of a thorough examination by a physician. This examination should be performed with the patient in both the supine and upright positions and should include palpation of the entire breast, including the tail of the breast and the axilla. The breast should be squeezed gently but firmly, in an attempt to express fluid from the nipples. A small amount (one drop) of serous fluid may be considered normal, but cytologic examination of the fluid is warranted if there is any suspicion of abnormality. This can be performed simply by placing a glass slide against the nipple, streaking the discharge onto the slide, and treating it with fixative as for cervical cytology. Bloody discharge from the nipple is particularly worrisome, as it may represent intraductal carcinoma. Other abnormal discharges should be further evaluated with cytology and mammography.

Any palpable mass warrants further investigation; so-called "benign masses," such as changes attributed to fibrocystic breast condition in the premenopausal woman, are rare in the postmenopausal age group. If a mass is palpated during examination, special attention should be paid to the contralateral breast in the "mirror image" position, as the rate of bilaterality of carcinoma is highest in this area. Mammographic evaluation will also allow characterization of the mass as to relative risk of malignancy and the presence of other foci. Should mammography reveal an area of possible malignancy that is not palpable during physical examination, needle localization can be performed with a local anesthetic. A radiologist, using stereotaxic views to localize the mass, can direct a thin guide wire into the breast toward the vicinity of the lesion. The surgeon can then use this wire to locate the lesion, resecting the tissue surrounding the needle tip. This specimen biopsy then undergoes mammographic comparison with the original lesion to ensure that the abnormal area has indeed been removed. This technique allows for accurate localization of the lesion, reduces the incidence of hemimastectomy for evaluation of nonpalpable lesions, and allows the procedure to be performed with local anesthesia. As mammography has a false-negative rate of approximately 10% to 15% in the detection of a malignancy, the liberal use of biopsy, particularly with local anesthetic, is justified in patients with new breast masses or masses suspected of malignancy.

Vulva

Normal changes of the vulva in the estrogen-deficient postmenopausal woman include thinning of the tissue to a pale appearance, petechiae, and the loss of normal vulvar architecture whereby the labia minora may appear to be diminished or absent. While petechiae may be a normal finding, particularly in a sexually active older woman, ulcerations or nonhealing fissures sugest early invasive carcinoma of the vulva and should be liberally sampled for biopsy. Likewise, hypertrophic or thickened, gray-appearing lesions of the vulva may represent carcinoma in situ and should undergo biopsy. Papillary lesions of the vulva include simple achrochordon as found in any other areas of the skin. However, verrucous-appearing lesions are uncommon in this age group and unlikely to represent condylomata acuminata as they do in premenopausal women. These may represent a a locally invasive squamous cell carcinoma variant, verrucous carcinoma. Therefore, biopsy with wide incision of any new-appearing verrucous lesion should be undertaken. As with other skin surfaces of the body, common lesions can be seen on the vulva. Seborrheic keratoses, nevi, and psoriasis are not unusual on the vulva and should be treated as they would be at other sites.

Biopsy of the vulva can be performed easily in an office setting with minimal discomfort to the patient. After preparing the biopsy site with local antiseptic, 1% lidocaine is infiltrated with a 26-gauge needle. A biopsy specimen is then taken by means of a Keyes punch biopsy, an elliptical excision with a scalpel blade, or a cervical biopsy forceps, such as the Tischler forceps. Rarely are sutures necessary for hemostasis. Topical hemostatics, such as silver nitrate or ferric subsulfate (Monsel's solution), may be applied to stop bleeding. If suturing is necessary, this can be accomplished with a small, absorbable suture, negating the need for removal at a later date.

The most common vulvar symptoms are pruritis, burning, and discharge. Pruritis usually reflects the atrophic changes associated with estrogen deficiency. The classic findings of small petechial hemorrhages, thin-appearing mucosa, and loss of local architecture support this diagnosis. The application of topical estrogens can relieve many of these symptoms and should do so relatively soon (1 to 2 weeks) after the initiation of therapy. The patient should be told that topical estrogens are also absorbed systemically, leading to many of the symptoms seen with estrogen replacement therapy, such as breast tenderness. A patient with an intact uterus may need progestrone therapy to counteract the potential carcinogenic effects of the estrogen on the endometrium (see Chapter 22). Vulvar pruritis may also reflect an infectious process, most commonly that due to *Candida albicans,* characterized by a thin white coating on the vulva. It is unusual, however, for a patient with estrogen deficiency to develop vulvar candidiasis without underlying glucose intolerance, or prednisone or recent antibiotic therapy. Patients with recurrent candidal infections should undergo evaluation of their glucose tolerance.

The diagnosis is based both on the clinical symptoms and the microscopic presence of hyphae in scrapings of the vulva mounted in potassium hydroxide. Lichen sclerosis can also lead to severe itching of the vulva. Although frequently mistaken for estrogen deficiency, it is a distinct entity that must be treated very differently. Lichen sclerosis is characterized by a loss of local architecture of the vulva, which tends to be more severe than that seen with estrogen deficiency. The labia majora and minora in the most severe cases may appear to be totally absent. A wrinkled ''cigarette paper'' quality to the vulvar skin is classically described though infrequently found. Most commonly, the diagnosis is made by means of a biopsy after failure of topical estrogen therapy. Lichen sclerosis is treated with topical testoserone. A combination of 2% testosterone proprionate in a petrolatum base is applied sparingly to the affected area every day for 2 weeks and then intermittently as needed for maintenance. Care should be taken to avoid application to the clitoris, as hypertrophy may rarely occur. When this mixture is used sparingly, side effects are few. However, the prescribing physician must be aware that increased libido is occasionaly reported with the use of this mixture, and the patient should be reassured that this is a temporary situation. In some cases, underlying chronic inflammation from previous treatment and local excoriation may make topical steroids necessary for immediate symptomatic relief. A 1% hydrocortisone cream can be applied to the vulva, alternating with the testosterone mixture. However, under no circumstances should a corticosteroid ointment be used by itself, as this tends to thin the skin and worsen symptoms.

Burning, particularly on contact with urine, is a symptom commonly attributed to estrogen deficiency. However, if the vulvar skin appears thickened with areas of hyperkeratosis, biopsy must be performed. The thickening may represent a hyertrophic dystrophy of the vulva. These lesions may be seen contemporaneously with a carcinoma in situ of the vulva and may themselves display cytologic atypia, which many believe to have a malignant potential. Biopsies are performed on the thickest-appearing areas. A solution of 1% toluidine blue can be painted on the vulva, allowed to dry for 1 to 2 minutes, and then washed with a 1%

acetic acid solution. The remaining stained areas represent concentrations of nucleic acids, indicating cellular atypia and directing biopsy to that site. Treatment is dependent on the biopsy results. If severe intraepithelial neoplasia or carcinoma in situ is identified, either local excision or ablation with a laser is indicated. However, if hypertrophic dystrophy alone is diagnosed, then treatment with a mild topical fluorinated corticosteroid twice a day will relieve symptoms within 1 to 2 weeks. Maintainance therapy calls for a milder steroid, such as 1% hydrocortisone, to prevent further stricture of the vulva.[1]

Paget's disease of the vulva is also characterized by burning. Although it is a relatively rare lesion, the physician must be aware of its occurrence in this age group. It is characterized by a beefy red appearance of the vulva. Frequently the patient will have been treated for yeast infections without success. Biopsy must be performed to diagnose this cancer of the apocrine sweat glands. Treatment for Paget's disease is wide excision. However, recurrences appear in as many as 20% of the patients. Invasive squamous cell carcinoma of the vulva occurs synchronously with Paget's disease in a significant number of patients,[2] and careful evaluation must be undertaken in order to determine the proper therapy.

Vulvar discharge usually reflects a vaginal condition. However, fistulas from the lower gastrointestinal tract may appear on the vulva or perineal body and should be sought in patients with this complaint. Previous history of radiation therapy, Crohn's disease, or cancer of the colon should further alert the physician to this problem.

The urethra, like the vulva, is an estrogen-dependent organ and is markedly affected by estrogen deficiency. Total circumferential prolapse of the urethra can occur, appearing as a reddened meatus. This urethral mucosa is extremely friable and may be a source of postmenopausal bleeding. Congested mucosa may become strangulated, causing severe pain and dysuria. This is a simple diagnosis to make, as the urethral meatus apears dusky blue in early stages and necrotic in later stages. Simple palpation with a cotton swab is very painful. A urethral caruncle or polyp is a small extrusion of urethral tissue, usually at the 6 o'clock position. Both of these lesions respond to estrogen replacement therapy. Lack of resolution with topical estrogen warrants further investigation and biopsy to rule out urethral carcinoma.

Bartholin's glands, located at the posterior vulva at approximately the 5 and 7 o'clock positions, are unusual sources of vulvar inflammation in elderly women. However, this area should be palpated during routine examinations to identify any enlargement or thickening of the glands. Adenocarcinoma of Bartholin's gland, although rare, frequently is fatal because of the aggressive nature of the lesion and the failure to make a timely diagnosis. Any newly palpable mass in this area should be investigated with a biopsy or excision.

Vagina

Examination of the vagina in the elderly woman must be performed with care, because many of the changes associated with estrogen deficiency and aging make such an examination uncomfortable and difficult. Initially, a finger should be placed on the perineal body and, with gentle downward pressure, the vagina should be examined for evidence of prolapse. The patient is asked to bear down, at which time either a rectocele or a cystocele may be noted. This pressure also may cause some leakage of urine in patients suffering from genuine stress incontinence. A speculum examination is then performed. As many patients have a foreshortened vagina because of surgery or aging, care must be taken not to inflict pain by inserting the speculum too far or too vigorously into the vagina. A smaller Pederson speculum has advantages over the standard Graves speculum in older patients, in that the blades are narrower and vary in length. As the epithelium of the atrophic vagina is very thin, special attention must be paid to the opening of the speculum, so as not to cause bleeding or excessive irritation.

The most common cause of vaginal discharge in the postmenopausal woman is atrophic vaginitis. The creamy white discharge, often mistaken for recurrent monilial or "yeast" vulvovaginitis, does not have a foul odor and is microscopically characterized by a paucity of microorganisms and a large number of basal cells (small round cells with large nuclei). A thicker white discharge with severe itching is more characteristic of "yeast" vaginitis. Characteristically, this causes a thick, curd-like discharge noted during speculum examination; hyphae are noted on microscopic examination of the discharge suspended in 10% potassium hydroxide. A bloody discharge may result from trauma to the atrophic vagina. However, it must be ascertained with certainty that this bleeding is not of uterine origin. Other infectious organisms, such as *Trichomonas vaginalis* and *Gardnerella vaginalis,* can be seen in sexually active postmenopausal women and should be sought when evaluating vaginal discharge.

Atrophic vaginitis is treated with estrogen. Although oral estrogen is an effective long-term treatment, the acute application of topical conjugated estrogen will provide both adequate levels of estrogen and soothing relief to the affected area. Many preparations currently are available, and there is no advantage to a particular formulation. A dosage of conjugated estrogen equivalent to 0.625 mg/ml is standard. It must be remembered that in the vagina estrogen is rapidly absorbed, with the patient exhibiting all the symptoms and sequelae of systemic estrogen replacement therapy.[3]

The treatment of candidal or yeast vaginitis requires evaluation for underlying pathology, including glucose intolerance. Many preparations are currently available. Because of some increased resistance by candidal strains to older antifungal preparations (clotrimazole), newer and more effective regimens (miconazole, terconazole, butoconazole) are available. A patient with recurrent yeast infections is problematic. If systemic causes of recurrence are ruled out or treated, an oral preparation of ketaconazole (200 mg for 7 days) often is effective. However, one must monitor hepatic function at the start and at completion of therapy.

Cervix

The cervix often is difficult to visualize in a postmenopausal patient. Atrophy of the vagina may limit visual access, the cervix may be flush with the upper vagina, and the cervical os may be stenotic, making it difficult to distinguish from the vaginal apex. Care must be taken to locate the cervix for adequate gross and cytologic evaluation. Although cervical carcinoma occurs in greatest frequency in a younger age group, it can occur in the postmenopausal years. Any questionable lesions should undergo biopsy. Cytologic examination or Pap smears of the cervix have been shown to be cost-effective in the geriatric population.[4] Care must be taken to ensure an adequate endocervical sampling. As the endocervical os is often tight and the squamocolumnar junction has receded well within the endocervical canal, one must attempt to sample the endocervical canal thoroughly. In the estrogen-deficient patient, it is often difficult to obtain enough cells to interpret the Pap smear accurately. The interpretation of a Pap smear in this age group is far from routine. With a predominance of basal cells from the vagina, as well as inflammatory changes associated with the postmenopausal years, the cytologic findings may be overinterpreted as atypia or early dysplasia. A patient with a Pap smear of class III or greater, clearly showing dysplasia, should undergo colposcopic evaluation for localization and histopathologic analysis of the lesion. However class IIA smears, as well as those showing mild dysplastic changes or those with atypia, may reflect the above-mentioned changes. Therefore, a short course (4 weeks) of topical estrogen therapy is used before another smear is obtained. If the second smear shows these abnormalities, then further evaluation with colposcopy is warranted.

Uterus

A bimanual examination should be performed to evaluate the uterus and adnexae. However, this may be difficult due to the atrophic vagina, obesity, or previous surgery foreshortening the vagina. A single-digit examination may suffice in a cooperative, thin patient. However, a rectal examination to palpate the pelvic organs may be necessary in some patients when adequate vaginal examination is prohibited. The uterus after menopause is usually small, so retrodisplacement of this organ presents no clinical problems. Enlargement of the uterus has many different causes, and it must be ascertained whether it predates the menopause. Leiomyomata uteri or fibroid tumors that are present before menopause will persist after it. Although some may decrease in size, total shrinkage to a normal-sized uterus is uncommon. Enlargement of a fibroid tumor in an estrogen-deficient woman must make one suspicious of leiomyosarcoma, leading to further investigation and exploratory laparotomy. Other causes of increased fibroid tumors include exogenous estrogen therapy and an endogenous estrogen-secreting tumor of the ovary. Blood levels of estradiol should be measured and ultrasonography of the ovaries should be performed in patients with increasing fibroid tumors who are not receiving estrogen replacement therapy, in order to exclude ovarian neoplasm. Even in patients receiving hormone supplementation, all other causes of an enlarging uterine mass must be excluded before attributing these changes to exogenous estrogen.

As the amount of bleeding does not necessarily reflect the severity of the lesion, gynecologic bleeding of any amount should alert the health care provider to the possibility of a malignancy. Evaluation of gynecologic bleeding should include careful inspection of the vagina for atrophic vaginitis, trauma to the vagina from sexual activity, and cervical lesions. Evaluation of the uterus must include endometrial sampling. Although transvaginal ultrasonography can be useful in diagnosing endometrial polyps or evaluating endometrial thickening, it is only with tissue diagnosis that one can totally exclude malignancy. Various office endometrial sampling techniques have been developed, and their results correlate highly with those of traditional dilation and curettage.[5] The use of a Novack curette for single-pass sampling may be inadequate in postmenopausal women, in whom focal disease may occur. Other aspiration techniques are more successful and can be performed with minimal discomfort in the office. While some patients can tolerate the procedure without anesthesia, a paracervical block is particularly useful in the patient with a stenotic cervical os. Often, it is diffi-cult to do outpatient sampling in postmenopausal women, because visualization is difficult and the cervical os is tightly closed. A short course of oral conjugated estrogen (0.625 mg orally for 7 days) may allow softening of the cervical os and entry of a probe into the uterus. However, some physicians are reticent to use estrogens even briefly in a patient with possible malignancy.

An inadequate endometrial sampling, due to inability to perform the technique or insufficient tissue for interpretation, necessitates the use of fractional dilation and curettage. With today's techniques, general anesthesia is rarely necessary for this procedure. Paracervical anesthesia and intravenous sedation permit this procedure to be performed safely and cost-effectively on an outpatient basis. Samplings from the endometrium should be fractionated, separated into an endocervical and an endometrial portion to help stage carcinoma should it be found.

Endometrial carcinoma is the most common malignancy of the lower female reproductive tract in the United States today. Peaking in incidence between the ages of 50 and 65 years, this lesion is believed in most cases to be the result of unopposed estrogen. Other risk factors include menopause after the age of 52 years, obesity, nulliparity, estrogen-producing ovarian tumors, and a history of polycystic ovarian disease. Unopposed estrogen can also result in other hyperplastic lesions of the endometrium, not all of which have premalignant potential. Cystic hyperplasia or marked dilatation of the endometrial glands is not considered to be a premalignant lesion. Dilation and curettage of a patient with this lesion will produce extremely large amounts of endometrium, which can lead the unsuspecting physician to diagnose cancer without pathologic confirmation. Adenomatous hyperplasia is described as an alteration in appearance of the glands of the endometrium. Without cytologic or architectural atypia, this is not considered to be a premalignant lesion and can be treated medically. Atypical adenomatous hyperplasia is characterized by marked cellular and architectural atypia, making it difficult to distinguish it from a well-differentiated endometrial carcinoma. This lesion may have premalignant potential, and therapy is necessary. The end stage of atypical adenomatous hyperplasia may be termed carcinoma in situ of the endometium and is characterized by severe cytologic atypia. Therapy for mild to moderate atypical adenomatous hyperplasia includes dilation and curettage, followed by prolonged progestational therapy. Such therapy can include medroxyprogesterone (10 mg for 10 days every month) or a combination of estrogen and progesterone therapy with monthly withdrawal bleeding. Abnormal bleeding of any nature during such therapy should warrant repeated biopsy to exclude occult malignancy. After 1 year of successful therapy, repeated endometrial sampling is necessary to rule out a recurrence once again.

Patients whose endometrium shows hyperplasia with severe cytologic atypia or carcinoma in situ generally require hysterectomy. If surgery is medically contraindicated, alternative therapy with long-term, high-dose progestational therapy, such as megestrol acetate to a total dose of 320 mg/d, has been shown to be effective.[6] Endometrial sampling every 6 months is advised to evaluate the efficacy of this therapy.

The prognosis of endometrial cancer is predicated on the stage, grade of differentiation, and depth of myometrial invasion. With the proper use of radiation therapy and surgery, treatment of endometrial carcinoma is very successful. Indeed, although the most common of all gynecologic malignancies, it results in the lowest percentage of deaths of all neoplasms of the female reproductive tract. During the 1960s and 1970s, a sudden increase in the incidence of adenocarcinoma of the endometrium was noted following the use of unopposed exogenous estrogens as hormone replacement therapy. In spite of the great increase in frequency of this disease, no significantly increased mortality was noted.[7] This has been attributed to the well-differentiated nature of the lesion as well as to rapid and successful management.

Ovaries

Ovarian cancer continues to cause more deaths than any other gynecologic neoplasm. The death rate rises with age and continues to increase until early in the 8th decade of life. As no adequate biochemical screening method is available, the health care provider must rely on physical examination for the early diagnosis of this cancer. The postmenopausal ovary usually is not palpable bimanually. Any enlargement of the ovary, even to the normal premenopausal size must be interpreted as potentially malignant. This "postmenopausal palpable ovary syndrome" has been shown to be an effective means of diagnosing early cancer of the ovary.[8] The likelihood of malignancy increases with the age of the patient and the size of the mass. Sonography may be useful in following a 1- to 2-cm cyst in a geriatric patient, with repeated examination in 6 weeks. Any mass 3 cm or larger should be acted on without hesitation. Diagnosis may be aided with computed tomography or magnetic resonance imaging, but neither modality has proved uniformly successful, and the ultimate value of these tests is uncertain. A true diagnosis can be made only by means of histopathology. Although laparos-

copy and ultrasonography may confirm the presence of a frankly malignant lesion, they cannot enable the diagnosis of a benign lesion. Exploratory laparotomy with excision of the ovary is necessary. Indeed, the risk of a malignancy in a primary ovarian tumor rises to approximately 33% in women over 45 years of age.

Though there are five types of ovarian tumors, epithelial tumors are the most common in the geriatric age group. Mucinous cystadenoma is the most common benign tumor, serous cystadenocarcinoma the most common malignant tumor. Bilaterality occurs in one third to two thirds of all identified cases. Primary therapy consists of surgical debulking followed by radiation therapy or, more commonly, chemotherapy. Surgical therapy consists of total abdominal hysterecomy with bilateral salpingo-oopherectomy, omentectomy, and sampling of the diaphragms and peritoneal fluid for evidence of metastatic disease. Survival rates remain poor, particularly when the tumors are diagnosed at later stages, with a 5-year survival of approximately 10% for stage III epithelial malignancies and approximately 5% for stage IV. Therefore, it is imperative that the physician maintain a high level of suspicion and monitor any adnexal mass to rule out malignancy as early and as efficiently as possible.

Additional causes of adnexal masses are related to the proximity of other organs within the pelvis. Unilateral left-sided masses must always bring to mind diverticulitis with scarring or abscess formation. Colonic cancer may be first detected either as a primary adnexal mass or as metastatic disease to the ovary. In an elderly patient, the atypical presentation of an appendiceal abscess may lead to the discovery of a right-sided adnexal mass. A rare finding in the postmenopausal patient is tubo-ovarian abscess. The cause of such abscesses in this age group is unknown, but they may result from the rupture of a diverticulum with infection of the adjacent fallopian tube or ovary. Rarely are these abscesses considered to be sexually transmitted, as the microorganisms recovered usually resemble those of the bowel more closely than those found in sexually transmitted diseases.

Fallopian tube carcinoma is the rarest of all gynecologic malignancies, occurring most commonly in the 5th decade of life; however, cases are reported well beyond that age. Although usually diagnosed as an incidental finding during pelvic surgery, fallopian tube carcinoma can cause a profuse watery discharge, hydrops tubae profluens. Although cytologic findings are positive in only approximately 10% of cases, the presence on a Pap smear of adenocarcinoma cells, without any other explainable cause, requires further investigation to rule out this diagnosis.

Pelvic Prolapse

Although pelvic prolapse is often thought of as a single entity, it is actually a number of different processes leading to similar symptoms. The uterus is held in position by the cardinal and uterosacral ligaments. The vagina maintains its position with the apex attached to the lower supporting ligaments of the uterus, the middle third supported by the levator ani muscles, and the lower third in proximity to the urogenital pelvic diaphragms. Detachment or injury to these ligaments or supporting attachments can lead to descent of the uterus or vagina and to the commonly associated symptoms. The etiology of pelvic prolapse is not well delineated. Various hypotheses have been provided, but few have been substantiated. Loss of striated muscle associated with aging, loss of tissue turgor with estrogen deficiency, damage during birthing processes, and destruction of the neuromuscular junction with aging or trauma all have been put forth as the cause of pelvic prolapse.

The most common symptoms of pelvic prolapse are a protruding mass from the vagina, pelvic pressure exacerbated in the upright position and alleviated in the supine, and dysfunction of defecation or micturition. Prolapse is graded by degrees. In first-degree prolapse, the organ has descended from its normal position; in second-degree prolapse, the organ is approaching the introitus; and in third-degree prolapse, the organ is either at or protruding from the introitus. With a simple examination, it often is difficult to ascertain exactly what is prolapsing. Using a normal bivalve speculum, false support can be added to the tissues, thereby obscuring the true nature of the descensus. It is best either to use a small Sims speculum or to separate the standard bivalve speculum into two parts and use the blades independently, retracting anteriorly and posteriorly.

Prolapse of the anterior wall of the vagina forms a cystocele, prolapse of the posterior vagina with accompanying rectum is a rectocele, and an internal herniation of the small bowel into the septum between the rectum and the vagina is referred to as an enterocele. Uterine prolapse is easily identified by downward displacement of the cervix, often with protrusion through the vaginal introitus. In patients who have undergone hysterectomy, prolapse of the vaginal apex may occur independently. It is necessary to differentiate this condition from a rectocele or cystocele, as the corrective measures differ. Uterine prolapse often is accompanied by marked cystocele and rectocele and almost always by enterocele, because the descent of the uterus widens the rectovaginal septum, promoting internal herniation.

Frequently, the examiner discovers asymptomatic pelvic relaxation. The finding of a large cystocele-rectocele does not necessarily indicate that surgery is warranted. However, careful history and examination must be performed before these findings are deemed nonsignificant. The presence of a cystocele may result in a large postvoiding residual urine volume, leading to chronic bacteriuria and recurrent urinary tract infections. Therefore, the postvoiding residual urine volume should be measured in patients with signficant anterior vaginal wall relaxation. As the cystocele will often prolapse below the urethra, the operator must be careful to insert his or her fingers into the vagina during catheterization to elevate the bladder base above the neck of the urethra, thus ensuring an accurate assessment of urine volume. Many patients with large cystoceles have no complaints of urinary incontinence. This is because the large cystocele protrudes toward the introitus resulting in a "kinking" of the urethra (see Chapter 38). During sudden increases in intra-abdominal pressure, such as occur with coughing or sneezing, the cystocele effectively blocks urine leakage. But this can lead to incomplete emptying of the bladder, a large residual urine volume, and urinary frequency.

Patients with a rectocele may have difficulty defecating and may have to exert pressure on the perineal body or place a digit into the posterior vagina to aid evacuation. An undiagnosed enterocele can present as intermittent lower abdominal pain and pressure worsened with standing or walking and relieved with lying down. Because most patients are more mobile as the day progresses, the pain progressively worsens until bedtime. As patients often sit in a physician's office prior to examination, the entrocele can be reduced and not diagnosed during examination in the supine position. Patients with symptoms suggestive of an enterocele should be examined while standing with one leg elevated on a small stool. The physician should examine the pelvis with one finger in the rectum and one finger in the vagina, having the patient bear down so that a sliding loop of the small bowel can be palpated between the rectum and vagina.

The approach to total pelvic prolapse is either supportive or surgical. Supportive therapy consists of the use of pessaries, vaginal appliances designed to reduce prolapse and restore normal anatomy. Many types of pessaries exist, and each one is designed for specific types of prolapse. The choice of type or size is best left to a practitioner experienced in fitting pessaries. An overly large pessary can cause urethral constriction and prevent complete emptying of the bladder. Similarly, rectal pressure can cause dificulty in voiding or displacement of the pessary with bowel movement. Pessaries that require support from the pelvic diaphragm or the bony structure of the pelvis to remain in the proper position may not fit correctly in women with marked prolapse or atrophy of the vagina. Care of the pessary is important; proper hygiene will allow continued usage and patient acceptance. The pessary should be removed and cleansed weekly to prevent pressure ulcers and foul discharge. At the time of removal, the vagina should be carefully inspected for evidence of irritation or pressure necrosis. If a patient is capable of inserting and cleansing the pessary herself, this is of course preferable. As pessaries have been associated with primary vaginal cancer, routine gynecologic care must include cytologic examination of the vagina and treatment of underlying discharge. Often it is necessary to give the patient supplemental estrogen to thicken the vaginal mucosa enough for the patient to tolerate repeated removal and cleansing of the pessary. Any ulcerations or lesions appearing during the use of the pessary should be evaluated fully and not just assumed to be the result of the pessary. These ulcerations should be allowed to heal completely before the pessary is replaced.

The surgical approach to pelvic prolapse is dependent on the extent of prolapse and the patient's sexual functioning. Complete uterovaginal prolapse can be treated with vaginal hysterectomy and suspension of the vagina. Vaginal suspension can be carried out either through the vagina, with a sacrospinous suspension, or through the abdomen, with various techniques. There appear to be benefits and risks to both procedures, with no critical advantage of one technique over the other. Sacrospinous suspension is more often associated with urinary dysfunction following the procedure, and follow-up of this technique has not been extensive enough to ascertain the long-term results. Abdominal suspensions require opening of the peritoneal cavity, with the subsequent morbidity and mortality associated with this major surgery. In the patient who is not sexually activity or who is unable to undergo an operative procedure involving opening of the peritoneal cavity, colpocleisis is an alternative. In the patient with uterine prolapse, a LeFort colpocleisis with inversion of the uterus and closure of the vagina often is successful, can be carried out with local anesthetic, and is usually completed in under 40 minutes. It is necessary to ensure that no uterine disease is present, because this procedure prevents further access to the uterus for sampling or cytology. Colpocleisis in a patient without a uterus is the closure of the vagina, leaving the patient with a small nonfunctional "perineal dimple." Both of these colpocleisis techniques are successful and useful alternatives to vaginal hysterectomy and suspension, and recovery is rapid since the peritoneal cavity need not be opened. The risk of hemorrhage in these cases is minimal, because no major blood vessels need be ligated. Anterior and posterior colporrhaphy is the most common approach to vaginal prolapse without uterine prolapse or in the absence of the uterus. Although only a cystocele or rectocele may be present, it is usual to repair the anterior and posterior vagina simultanously, to prevent subsequent prolapse and further surgery. At the time of colporrhaphy, it is important for the operator to search for and identify the enterocele sac in order to prevent herniation and further discomfort from the pelvic prolapse.

Estrogen Replacement Therapy (see also Chapter 22)

Many women suffer from symptoms related to estrogen deficiency following the menopause. While some of these symptoms, such as vasomotor instability and mood alterations, occur only shortly after the onset of menopause, others are long-term sequelae, such as urinary incontinence, pelvic prolapse, and osteoporosis. In order to prevent many of these symptoms and to improve the general well-being of the older woman, hormonal replacement therapy has been advocated. This replacement takes the form of estrogen alone, estrogen in combination with an androgen or progesterone, or a progestational agent alone. In the United States today, estrogen with or without a progestational agent is the most commonly prescribed replacement therapy. Prior to the initiation of such therapy, a careful history must be taken for contraindications to estrogen therapy, which include breast or endometrial carcinoma, chronic or acute liver disease, a history of acute vascular thrombosis, neuroophthalmologic vascular disease, estrogen-related hypertension, undiagnosed vaginal bleeding, and estrogen-related cholestasis. Other conditions that may be adversely affected by estrogen replacement therapy include cholelithiasis, leiomyomata uteri, fibrocystic breast condition, endometriosis, and familial hyperlipidemia. While caution should be used in prescribing hormones for such patients, successful replacement therapy can be achieved with proper counseling and close monitoring.

Controversy exists as to the need for endometrial biopsy prior to the onset of estrogen replacement therapy. The low incidence of endometrial hyperplasia or cancer in an asymptomatic woman,[9] the difficulty in performing such a biopsy in a woman with urogenital atrophy, and the lack of patient acceptance of this procedure prevent the biopsy from being used as a standard of practice. An alterntive technique is the use of progestational withdrawal to induce uterine bleeding prior to initiation of hormone replacement therapy. A patient with an unstimulated endometrium will not have withdrawal bleeding in response to withdrawal of progestational therapy, while patients with an estrogen-stimulated endometrium will have vaginal bleeding. Therefore, only a select population of patients with proved estrogen stimulation of the endometrium will undergo biopsy. The efficacy of this technique is still unproved.

The most common forms of estrogen given today are conjugated estrogens and their equivalents. These are preferred because of their beneficial effects on blood lipids, their relatively minimal effect on coagulation parameters, and their inexpensiveness. It is imperative in older women to avoid nonsteroidal estrogens and synthetic estrogens, such as those found in oral contraceptives, because of their adverse effect on blood lipid levels and their association with an increased incidence of thrombosis. Newer forms of estrogen delivery systems, such as transdermal patches or gels, show initial beneficial effects with minimal adverse effects. The use of a delivery system that bypasses the "first pass" effect on the liver ameliorates the elevated coagulation factors associated with oral therapy, but the effects on serum lipids remain uncertain. Transvaginal estrogen application also is an acceptable route of estrogen replacement therapy. Its benefits include high dose and rapid relief of vaginal symptoms. It must be remembered that vaginally applied estrogen is absorbed systemically and exerts its primary effect through delivery to target cells by the circulation.[3]

The use of unopposed estrogen replacement therapy in a woman with an intact uterus has been shown to be associated with a two- to eightfold increase in the relative risk of endometrial carcinoma.[10] Although a minimum of 2 to 4 years' use of the estrogen is necessary to achieve this risk, it is currently recommended that a progestational agent be added in such patients in order to prevent endometrial hyperplasia or cancer. Interestingly, these lesions associated with estrogen replacement therapy tend to be early and well differentiated and do not adversely affect the mortality rates of the women receiving these hormones. It is not advocated that one use estrogen without progestational therapy, but a history of such usage should not exclude continued therapy with a combination estrogen-progestational regimen after adequate endometrial sampling.

A progestational compound added to estrogen replacement therapy has been clearly shown to be advantageous in preventing endometrial hyperplasia in women with intact uteri. However, side effects are encountered and may be dose related.[11] Adverse effects upon blood lipids, with a lowering of high-density lipoprotein levels and a raising of low-density lipo-protein levels, are noted in patients receiving medroxyprogesterone acetate. This appears to be more significant effect at 10 mg/d than at lower dosages. Water retention, acne, and depression all have been related to the intake of progestational agents. While the symptoms are rare and usually mild, in rare instances they can be debilitating and alter patient compliance. The use of a progestin in a woman after hysterectomy remains controversial. A recent review shows no clear-cut benefit of the use of progesteronelike compounds to prevent breast cancer. Early data show an additive effect of progesterone to the prevention of osteoporosis by estrogen alone. Therefore, the risks and benefits of the addition of progesterone in the postmenopausal patient must be weighed, particularly in patients with hypercholesterolemia or a history of heart disease.

Androgens also have been used as hormonal replacement therapy. Theoretically, they provide relief of vasomotor symptoms and prevention of osteoporosis, without the side effect of migraine headaches and other estrogen-related problems. Another benefit attributed to androgens is an increase in sexual responsiveness and arousability, though this has not been well studied. The disadvantages of androgenic therapy include adverse effect on serum lipids, increased hirsutism, and depression. While androgens may serve as an alternative therapy for patients intolerant of estrogen or progesterone, they are not considered a primary choice for hormonal replacement.

Oral estrogens are the most commonly prescribed replacement therapy. A starting dosage equivalent to 0.625 mg/d of conjugated estrogen is usual. The exact type of oral estrogen (estrone, estradiol) probably makes little physiologic difference. Symptoms following initiation of therapy include breast tenderness and fullness, which usually resolve spontaneously in 2 to 4 weeks, mild weight gain, and an exacerbation of migraine headaches in susceptible patients. The addition of progesterone therapy in the patient with an intact uterus is fairly standard today. The two most commonly used preparations are medroxyprogesterone acetate and norethindrone acetate. A minimum of 10 to 14 days per month administered in a cyclic manner, is recommended. Care must be taken to assure that adequate absorption of oral progesterone is achieved, as many preparations may have as much as a 50% variance in serum levels between patients receiving similar dosages. While it is important to minimize the dosage of progestin, adequate levels must be achieved to prevent endometrial pathology. A typical starting regimine consists of 0.625 mg/d of conjugated estrogen for the first 25 days of the month, with 5 mg/d of medroxyprogesterone acetate or norethindrone acetate during days 16 through 25. With this regimen, a small but important number of patients can be expected to have withdrawal bleeding. Should the patient be long past menopause and have bleeding in response to the combination therapy, edometrial sampling is warranted following the first such incident. Any bleeding other than that following subsequent progestin withdrawal and any excessive or prolonged bleeding is considered abnormal, warranting endometrial sampling. Some patients cannot tolerate the drug-free interval at end of each month becoming markedly symptomatic during that time. Continuous therapy with 0.625 mg/d of conjugated estrogen and a progestin for the first 14 days of the month is recommended in such patients. Recent reports have indicated that the incidence of vaginal bleeding can be reduced by giving continuous estrogen and progesterone, such as conjugated estrogen at a dosage of 0.625 mg/d and medroxyprogesterone at a dosage of 2.5 mg/d.[12] It has recently been noted by physcians that patients receiving successful hormone replacement therapy with conjugated estrogen may suddenly become symptomatic once again. In many cases, this effect has been linked to generic substitutions or a change in formulation of the estrogen. Although physiologically equivalent in animal models, absorption rates in actual patients may vary between preparations and lead to new onset of symptoms of estrogen deficiency. Therefore, a patient who was doing well on therapy but then develops estrogen-deficiency symptoms again should return to the original formulation before an increase in the amount of estrogen is considered.

Newer preparations of transdermal estrogen are being used in Europe and are under investigation in the United States. A transdermal patch system for delivery of estrogen has been shown to be effective in relieving menopausal symptoms. It offers the advantage of decreasing the massive "first pass" effect of estrogen on the liver that is experienced with oral preparations. Theoretically, this will decrease the incidence of thrombosis and cholestasis. However, it also negates some of the beneficial effects of oral estrogen on serum lipids, and the long-term efficacy of this preparation in preventing osteoporosis is not well established.

Patients with absolute contraindications to estrogen replacement may benefit from progestational supplementation alone. The use of progestin has been shown to relieve vasomotor symptoms and possibly prevent osteoporosis. However, the physician must monitor the side effects commonly associated with the intake of progestational agents (see above).

References

1. Droegemueller MD, Herbst AL, Mishell DR, et al. Premalignant and malignant diseases of the vulva. In: *Comprehensive Gynecology*. St Louis, Mo: CV Mosby Co; 1987:876–900.
2. Lee SC, Roth LM, Ehrlich C, et al. Extramammary Paget's disease of the vulva: a clinicopathologic study of 13 cases. *Cancer* 1977;39:2540–2549.
3. Rigg LA, Hermann IT, Yen SSC. Absorption of estrogens from vaginal creams. *N Engl J Med* 1978;298:195.
4. Mandelblatt JS, Fahs MC. The cost-effectiveness of cervical cancer screening for low-income elderly women. *JAMA* 1988;259:1409.
5. Bibbo M, Kluskens L, Aziz F, et al. Accuracy of three sampling techniques for the diagnosis of endometrial cancer and hyperplasias. *J Reprod Med* 1982;27:622.
6. Gal D, Edman CD, Vellios F, et al. Long-term effect of megestrol acetate in the treatment of endometrial hyperplasia. *Am J Obstet Gynecol* 1983;146:316.
7. Collins J, Donner A, Allen LH, et al. Oestrogen use and survival in endometril cancer. *Lancet* 1980;2:961.
8. Barber HRK, Graber EA. The PMPO syndrome (postmenopausal palpable ovary syndrome). *Obstet Gynecol* 1971;38:921.
9. Koss LG, Schreiber K, Oberlander SG, et al: Detection of endometrial carcinoma and hyperplasia in asymptomatic women. *Obstet Gyecol* 1984;64:1.
10. Smith DC, Prentice R, Thompson DJ, et al. Association of exogenous estrogen and endometrial carcinoma. *N Engl J Med* 1975;293:1167.
11. Ottosson VE, Johansson BG, VonSchultz B. Subfractions of high-density lipoprotein cholesterol during estrogen replacement therapy: a comparison between progestogens and natural progesterone. *Am J Obstet Gynecol* 1985;151:746.
12. Luciano AA, Turksoy RN, Carleo J, et al. Clinical and metabolic responses of menopausal women to sequential versus continuous estrogen and progestin replacement therapy. *Obstet Gynecol* 1988;71:39.

Nephrology/Fluid and Electrolyte Disorders

Sharon Anderson

The biologic price of aging includes progressive deterioration of the anatomic structure and filtration function of the kidney, and the changes in renal function during normal aging are among the most dramatic of any organ system. This chapter considers the functional and structural changes that occur with normal aging; more detailed reviews may be found in several recent publications.[1–4]

Age-Related Changes in Renal Function and Structure

The glomerular filtration rate (GFR) is low at birth, approaches adult levels by the end of the second year of life, and is maintained at approximately 140 mL/min/1.73 m^2 until the fourth decade. Thereafter, the GFR declines by about 8 mL/min/1.73 m^2 per decade,[5,6] an effect that is accelerated in the presence of systemic hypertension.[7] The age-related reduction in creatinine clearance is accompanied by a reduction in the daily urinary creatinine excretion, due to reduced muscle mass.[6] Accordingly, the relationship between the serum creatinine level (S_{Cr}) and creatinine clearance changes. The net effect is near-constancy of the S_{Cr} level, whereas the true GFR and creatinine clearance decline and, consequently, substantial reductions of the GFR despite a relatively normal S_{Cr} level. The creatinine clearance in mL/min in adult males may be estimated from the S_{Cr} level with the following formula:

$$\text{Creatinine clearance} = (140 - \text{age})(\text{weight in kilograms})/(72 \times S_{Cr})$$

and, in females, by multiplying this value by 0.85.[8]

Parallel changes in renal blood flow (RBF) occur, so that RBF is well maintained at about 600 mL/min until approximately the fourth decade, and then it declines by about 10% per decade.[9,10] The reduction in RBF is not entirely due to a loss of renal mass, as xenon washout studies have demonstrated a progressive reduction in blood flow per unit kidney mass with advancing age.[10] The decrease in RBF is most profound in the renal cortex; redistribution of flow from the cortex to the medulla may explain the slight increase in the filtration fraction seen in elderly persons.[9,10]

Studies in laboratory rats, in which age-related renal changes resemble an accelerated version of those in humans, suggest that another functional abnormality in aging is an increase in the glomerular basement membrane (GBM) permeability, leading to an increase in urinary total protein excretion, accompanied by increasing percentages of albumin and higher molecular weight proteins.[11] Studies in aging humans demonstrate decreased sulfation of the GBM glycosaminoglycans,[12] which would be expected to render the GBM more permeable to macromolecules. Age-related changes in proteinuria in humans have not been extensively studied, but the incidence of proteinuria in elderly persons may be minimally elevated.[13]

The renal mass increases from about 50 g at birth to over 400 g during the fourth decade, after which it declines to under 300 g by the ninth decade. The loss of renal mass primarily is cortical, with relative sparing of the medulla.[14] The glomerular number decreases, while the size of the remaining glomeruli tends to increase.[15,16] The glomerular shape changes as well,[15] with the spherical glomerulus in the fetal kidney developing lobular indentations as it matures. With aging, lobulation tends to diminish, and the length of the glomerular tuft perimeter decreases relative to the total area. The GBM undergoes progressive folding and then thickening.[17,18] This stage is accompanied by glomerular simplification, with the formation of free anastomoses between a reduced number of glomerular capillary loops. Frequently, dilatation of the afferent arteriole near the hilum is seen at this stage. Eventually, the folded and thickened GBM condenses into hyaline material with glomerular tuft collapse. Degeneration of cortical glomeruli results in atrophy of both afferent and efferent arterioles, with global sclerosis. In the juxtamedullary glomeruli, glomerular tuft sclerosis is accompanied by the formation of direct channels between the afferent and efferent arterioles, resulting in aglomerular arterioles.[17,18] These aglomerular arterioles, which presumably contribute to the maintenance of medullary blood flow, are rarely seen in kidneys from healthy young persons; their frequency increases both in aging kidneys and in the presence of intrinsic renal disease.[18]

The incidence of glomerular sclerosis increases with advancing age. Sclerotic glomeruli constitute fewer than 5% of the total under the age of 40 years; thereafter, the incidence increases so that sclerosis involves as much as 30% of the glomerular population by the eighth decade.[19,20] Thus, both diminished glomerular lobulation and sclerosis of glomeruli tend to reduce the surface area available for filtration and, therefore, contribute to the observed age-related decline in the GFR.[15]

Age-Related Alterations in Fluid and Electrolyte Homeostasis

Advancing age is not characterized by any specific changes in serum electrolyte or acid-base parameters in healthy subjects. However, the aging kidney demonstrates an impaired ability to respond to perturbations of fluid and electrolyte balance, and these complications are frequently encountered in the presence of intercurrent illness. In concert with the loss of functioning glomeruli, evidence of tubular dysfunction is found as well, with deterioration of several proximal tubular functions, including maximum excretion of p-aminohippurate[21] and iodopyracet (Diodrast)[5] and maximal absorption of glucose.[22] The most prominent abnormalities are found in renal handling of sodium and water.

Disorders of Sodium Balance

In the absence of acquired renal disease, the aging kidney is able to adjust sodium handling appropriately in the face of extracellular sodium deficiency or excess; however, the response time is impaired, and management of these disorders is accordingly complicated. The renal response to dietary sodium deprivation in elderly persons is blunted. When challenged with an acute reduction in sodium intake (from 100 to 10 mEq/d), elderly subjects are able to conserve sodium and achieve sodium balance, but at a slower rate than in younger subjects. A short-term study of dietary sodium restriction found that the half-time for reduction in urinary sodium after salt restriction was 17.6 hours in young persons, but was prolonged to 30.9 hours in older subjects.[23] In a more chronic state of sodium deprivation, administration of a 50-mEq/d sodium diet led to urinary sodium conservation and achievement of sodium balance after 5 days in younger subjects, whereas elderly patients did not return to sodium balance after 9 days despite a weight loss of 1.4 kg.[24] Studies in the segmental handling of sodium in elderly patients suggest that sodium handling is fairly normal in the proximal tubule, but that the capacity to reabsorb sodium in the ascending limb of the loop of Henle is markedly impaired.[25] The reduced loop capacity to reabsorb sodium has two important consequences: (1) the amount of sodium delivered to the more distal segments increases, and (2) the capacity to concentrate the medullary interstitium is reduced, thereby also contributing to the inability to concentrate the urine.

Age-related abnormalities in the renin-angiotensin-aldosterone axis are likely to play a role in this impaired ability to conserve sodium. Plasma renin levels and blood and urinary aldosterone levels are significantly reduced in the elderly population, and responses to appropriate stimuli, such as sodium restriction, are blunted.[23,26,27] In addition, the tubular response to the administration of aldosterone is reduced.[28] Accordingly, the impaired response to sodium deprivation (or relative "salt wasting") renders the elderly patient more susceptible to developing a cumulative sodium deficit and its attendant systemic complications.

Similarly, the renal response to a sodium load is sluggish in elderly patients. Natriuresis is impaired both by the reduction in the GFR, leading to a reduced delivery of sodium to the nephron, and by abnormalities in tubular handling of sodium as well, leading to difficulties in the management of disorders associated with sodium excess.

Disorders of Water Balance

Renal concentrating and diluting abilities are also impaired in the aging kidney.[29,30] In response to water deprivation, studies in healthy elderly patients indicate that both the maximal decrease in urine volume and the maximal increase in urine osmolality are significantly diminished as compared with responses in younger subjects; the changes are not completely explained by the reduced GFR.[31]

The mechanisms that underlie the impaired concentrating capacity have been extensively explored. The reduced number of functioning nephrons may contribute to an obligatory solute diuresis in the remaining intact nephrons, as occurs with chronic renal failure. In addition, the effect of age on the renal response to exogenous antidiuretic hormone (ADH) has been studied. While age-related differences in response to submaximal ADH infusions were not found, a defect in concentrating response was found when higher doses of ADH were infused.[32] One explanation for these differences may be the relative sparing of medullary blood flow in the aging kidney; this might contribute to a "washout" of the medullary osmotic gradient necessary for urine concentration by the countercurrent multiplier system.

In addition to altered responsiveness to exogenous ADH, the release of endogenous ADH in response to appropriate stimuli is abnormal in elderly subjects. Morphologic studies have indicated no evidence of age-related degenerative changes in the supraoptic and paraventricular nuclei, the sites of ADH production.[33] The increase in plasma ADH levels after infusion of hypertonic saline (an osmolar stimulus) is higher in elderly than in younger subjects, incidating enhanced osmoreceptor sensitivity in elderly subjects.[34] In contrast to the response to an osmolar stimulus, however, the ADH response to volume-pressure stimuli (assumption of an upright posture after overnight dehydration) is markedly impaired in some elderly subjects.[35] A portion of the afferent limb of this reflex arc is the vasomotor center. In elderly subjects, plasma norepinephrine levels were comparable in those who did and who did not respond appropriately to the pressure-volume stimulus, suggesting that the defect in the afferent limb must exist between the vasomotor center and the hypothalamic area that controls ADH release. This reflex arc is inhibitory to ADH secretion, and a defect in this area would result in a lesser dampening of osmotically stimulated ADH release. These studies suggest that baroreflex input at the hypothalamic level during aging modulates osmotically mediated ADH release and, thus, may alter water balance.

Plasma ADH levels under basal conditions do not change with advancing age,[34] and there are no differences in exogenously administered ADH pharmacokinetics after adaptation to high- or low-sodium diets between young and elderly subjects.[36] However, these studies found the secondary increases in ADH that were enhanced in magnitude during low-sodium intake to be absent in elderly subjects. Taken together, these results indicate that ADH is present in elderly subjects, and that provocative stimuli can both accentuate its release and reduce its suppressibility; the mechanisms underlying these observations, as well as the consequences of attenuation of secondary ADH release, remain incompletely defined.

Similarly, the aging kidney demonstrates a modest inability to dilute urine appropriately, as determined by the maximal excretion of free water after water loading.[37] This is most likely due to the reduced GFR and renal perfusion, as well as to functional impairment in the diluting segment of the nephron.[25,37]

Hyponatremia

Serum sodium levels generally are within the normal range in healthy elderly individuals, but the defective sodium and water homeostatic mechanisms render this population markedly susceptible to perturbations. Hyponatremia is the most common electrolyte disorder in elderly patients, occurring in as many as one quarter of all hospitalized or institutionalized elderly patients.[24,38] Numerous mechanisms contribute to the susceptibility to hyponatremia and may be identified after clinical evaluation. The most common underlying mechanisms of geriatric hyponatremia are (1) a decreased ability to excrete water, (2) water intoxication in the setting of diuretic therapy, and (3) oversecretion of ADH.

As in patients of any age, evaluation of the hyponatremic patient begins with confirmation of true hyponatremia, a hypo-osmolar state.[30,39] Pseudohyponatremia may be found in the setting of marked hyperglycemia, hyperlipidemia, and hyperproteinemia. Measurement of plasma osmolality confirms this diagnosis, as plasma osmolality is normal in pseudohyponatremia, but reduced in true hyponatremic states. Further evaluation requires estimation of extracellular fluid volume status by physical examination and measurement of the urinary sodium concentration. Hyponatremia may be associated with extracellular volume depletion (due to renal or extrarenal losses); with extracellular volume excess (due to cardiac failure, nephrotic syndrome, cirrhosis, or renal failure); or with normal to slightly increased extracellular volume in the absence of edema (endocrine disorders, drugs, and excess ADH secretion).

Elderly patients may suffer from any of these disorders and, in fact, carry a disproportionate burden of illness associated with extracellular fluid volume deficit and excess.[39] Extracellular volume depletion is common, particularly after administration of diuretics; in one series of 77 elderly patients, diuretic therapy accounted for two thirds of all cases of hyponatremia.[40] Three age-related abnormalities are likely to contribute to this increased susceptibility: volume depletion, potassium depletion, and inhibition of urinary dilution. Diuretic-induced hyponatremia occurs almost exclusively with thiazide diuretics, which interfere with urinary diluting but not concentrating ability and therefore may engender defects in free-water excretion, particularly in the presence of ADH. Clinically significant hyponatremia may occur as early as the first few days of diuretic administration, and the frequency of life-threatening hyponatremia is increased in the elderly population.[41,42] Therapy consists of discontinuation of the drug and restriction of water intake. In the setting of severe central nervous system symptoms, administration of intravenous hypertonic saline is warranted.

Hypervolemic hyponatremia also is common in elderly persons, with congestive heart failure being the most common cause of this disorder. The reductions in renal perfusion and, thus, the GFR that accompany congestive heart failure at any age may be more dangerous in elderly persons, in whom values for the GFR are only half those of younger persons when cardiac function is optimal. Congestive heart failure may be accompanied by increased plasma ADH levels, particularly in elderly patients.[43] Therapy consists of water restriction and treatment of congestive heart failure with loop diuretics (rather than thiazides) and the other usual modalities.

Relatively isovolemic hyponatremia also is common in elderly persons, who may exhibit elevations in plasma ADH levels in the absence of recognizable stimuli for ADH secretion.[44] Elderly individuals seem to be particularly susceptible to hyponatremia in the setting of the syndrome of inappropriate ADH due to pulmonary disease, central nervous system disorders, paraneoplastic syndromes, pain, narcotics, and drugs that cause the syndrome. For example, elderly patients account for most of the cases of hyponatremia associated with chlorpropamide administration.[45] The presence of excessive levels of ADH, together with the impaired ability to excrete free water, render elderly persons prone to hyponatremia in numerous clinical settings, especially postoperatively and in the presence of narcotic administration or large amounts of intravenous hypotonic fluids. In one large series of elderly patients, excessive administration of hypotonic intravenous fluids was responsible for 14% of the cases of hyponatremia.[40]

Hypernatremia

Hypernatremia also is particularly prominent in advanced age. The major defense against hypernatremia is thirst, and so the populations at highest risk for hypernatremia are those with impaired access to water: the very young, the very old, and the very sick. A group at particularly high risk is that of institutionalized older patients with cognitive impairments, resulting in a failure to recognize thirst and/or an inability to obtain fluids. Additional evidence, while not entirely unequivocal, suggests that hypodipsia, or the failure to recognize thirst despite substantial elevations in serum osmolality, may be more common in elderly patients.[30,46] Cerebrovascular disease also may inhibit thirst, as well as limiting physical access to fluids. These problems, together with the inability of the aging kidney to conserve water maximally, render elderly patients at higher risk for the development of hypernatremia.

Hypernatremia may result from the following factors: the loss of sodium and water with predominant water loss and low total-body sodium levels; water losses with normal total-body sodium levels (from nephrogenic or central diabetes insipidus, or inadequate water intake in the presence of normal water losses); and sodium addition with increased total-body sodium levels (endocrine disorders, intravenous or oral sodium administration). Clinical evaluation and measurement of urinary sodium usually will disclose the cause. Therapy consists of administration of hypotonic saline in the setting of low total-body sodium levels; water in the setting of normal total-body sodium levels; and diuretics and water replacement in the setting of high total-body sodium levels.

Alterations in Potassium Balance

Plasma potassium concentrations in elderly persons remain within the normal range in the absence of certain stresses. However, significant abnormalities in cellular and total-body potassium levels do occur with advancing age. The erythrocyte potassium concentration (a reflection of the general intracellular potassium content) is decreased, and the total exchangeable body potassium concentration is reduced by about 20% as compared with younger subjects.[24,47] Several mechanisms for this reduction in the total-body potassium concentration have been proposed, including decreased muscle mass, alterations of cell membrane characteristics, nutritional deficiencies, and an inability of the kidney to conserve potassium.[24] Renal potassium excretion has been noted to be reduced in elderly subjects, but when corrected for the reduction in the GFR, the fractional excretion of potassium actually may be higher.[24]

Hypokalemia

Hypokalemia is the most common potassium abnormality in the elderly population; in one series, it was found in 11% of elderly patients who visited an emergency room, regardless of the reason for the visit.[48] The most prominent cause of hypokalemia in the elderly population probably is diuretic therapy; aging patients appear to be more susceptible to the hypokalemic effects of these drugs.[40]

Hyperkalemia

Hyperkalemia is relatively uncommon in elderly patients in the absence of renal disease or administration of potassium-sparing diuretics, despite evidence in aging experimental animals of an impaired ability to excrete a potassium load.[49] The reduction in total-body potassium stores may serve to offset the reduced GFR, thus protecting against significant hyperkalemia. However, the reduced activity of the renin-angiotensin-aldosterone system in older persons (see above), and the predisposition to the syndrome of hyporeninemic hypoaldosteronism (type IV renal tubular acidosis) may serve to limit potassium excretion, thus enhancing the risk of hyperkalemia in the presence of excessive potassium loads or drugs that predispose to hyperkalemia.

Disorders of Acid-Base Balance

Abnormalities in both pulmonary and renal acid-base mechanisms may contribute to disorders in elderly patients. Despite evidence for substantial deterioration in lung and kidney function with advancing age, acid-base balance is remarkably well maintained in elderly persons, who generally are able to maintain normal values for serum pH, carbon dioxide pressure, and bicarbonate concentrations.[50–52] Although these systems adequately dispose of the normal daily acid load, studies of ammonium loading in elderly patients indicate a reduced ability to excrete an acute exogenous acid load. However, when corrected for the reduced values for the GFR, the response of the elderly subjects is similar to that in younger subjects, indicating that nephron loss rather than tubular dysfunction probably accounts for this difference.[53,54] More chronic acid loading, however, may be associated with a delayed restoration of normal serum pH and bicarbonate concentrations,[55] and the response to alkali loading also may be delayed in elderly subjects. Although relatively few data are available that address the clinical outcomes of various acid-base disorders in the elderly population, it seems to be possible that the numerous causes of acidosis and alkalosis (particularly those due to drugs) may result in more frequent, profound, and long-lasting acid-base disorders in this population.[50,51]

Renal Disease in Elderly Persons

By itself, an age-related loss of functioning nephrons poses little threat to well-being, since even 50% of the normal GFR is ample for sustaining renal excretory function. However, the gradual loss of renal function that accompanies normal aging may be greatly accelerated when surgical loss of renal mass or acquired intrinsic renal disease is superimposed on this process.

The incidence of primary renal disease in elderly persons is not significantly different from that in young adults,[4,56] although the relative frequency of specific forms of glomerular injury varies in different age groups. Several recent, large series of renal biopsies undertaken in elderly patients have indicated the prevalence of the major forms of glomerular injury[57–61] and are summarized in Table 24.1. For comparison, the prevalence of various glomerular diseases in patients older than and younger than the age of 60 years in one representative study is depicted in Table 24.2.[61]

Although differences in reporting classification make exact comparisons difficult, several general trends are apparent from these studies. In each of these series, approximately two thirds of the patients were found to have primary glomerular disease, with the remainder exhibiting glomerulopathies secondary to systemic or primary tubulointerstitial diseases. Of the primary glomerular diseases, membranous glomerulonephritis was the most frequent, followed in varying rank by proliferative or rapidly progressive glomerulonephritis and focal glomerular sclerosis. Of note, most of these series found a substantial proportion of minimal-change disease; although most frequently considered to be a disease of children, in whom it constitutes the vast majority of glomerular disorders, this condition occurs in every age group, including elderly persons. Other primary glomerular diseases were found to be relatively infrequent. Thus, in the elderly population, membranous glomerulonephritis is the most common cause of nephrotic syndrome, and rapidly progressive glomerulonephritis is the most common cause of an acute nephritic syndrome.

The incidence of renal disease secondary to systemic illness, such as atherosclerosis, hypertension, cardiac failure, diabetes, and malignancy, clearly increases with advancing age.[4] The causes of glomerular diseases secondary to systemic disease are also depicted in Table 24.1. Hypertensive nephrosclerosis, which was not

Table 24.1. Renal biopsy diagnoses in elderly patients.*

	Study prevalence, %			
	Moorthy and Zimmermann[57] (n=115)	Kingswood et al[59] (n=143)	Ramirez and Saba[60] (n=277)	Glickman et al[61] (n=244)
Primary glomerular disease				
Membranous GN	13	17	21	12
Minimal-change disease	8	1	6	4
Focal glomerular sclerosis	13	1	4	8
Idiopathic crescentic GN	17	6	6	11
Focal proliferative GN	6	11	} 7	10
Diffuse proliferative GN	4	16		5
Chronic GN	4	. . .	. . .	5
Membranoproliferative GN	2	3	5	3
Systemic disease				
Vasculitis	10	6	2	3
Amyloidosis	4	13	7	8
Nephrosclerosis	. . .	7	. . .	14
Collagen vascular disease	3	. . .	4	2
Diabetic nephropathy	. . .	. . .	5	8
Other or nonglomerular disease	13	16	32	5

* GN indicates glomerulonephritis.

listed as an independent category in all series, may be the most frequent, followed by vasculitis and amyloidosis, which are relatively infrequent in younger patients. Particularly prominent in elderly persons are deposition diseases, including amyloidosis, light-chain deposition disease, and fibrillary glomerulonephritis.

Table 24.2. Pathologic diagnoses in patients undergoing biopsies.*

	Patient Age, y	
Diagnosis	≥60 (n=244)	≤60 (n=875)
Nephrosclerosis	13.9	10.7
Membranous GN	11.9	7.5
Crescentic GN	11.1	4.1
Focal glomerular sclerosis	7.8	5.6
Amyloidosis	7.8	2.2
Diabetic nephropathy	7.8	8.1
Chronic GN	4.5	6.4
Acute GN	4.5	3.8
Focal GN	4.1	6.7
Minimal-change disease	3.7	8.3
Membranoproliferative GN	2.9	6.3
Vasculitis	2.5	2.1
Systemic lupus erythematosus	2.0	6.6

* GN indicates glomerulonephritis. Prevalence values are given as percentages (adapted from Glickman et al[61] with permission).

End-Stage Renal Disease in Elderly

The number and relative frequency of elderly patients who enter end-stage renal disease programs, and the average age of patients who undergo dialysis, are increasing each year in the United States, reflecting the aging of the population in general. In a detailed analysis of the Medicare End-Stage Renal Disease Program in the United States for the years 1978 to 1980, both the incidence of new patients per million population and the rate of increases in the incidence between the years 1978 and 1980 were higher in patients older than 55 years than in younger patients.[62,63] In a representative series of 2,000 patients older than the age of 65 years treated at the Northwest Kidney Center in Seattle, Wash, the cause of chronic renal failure was nephrosclerosis (presumably secondary to hypertension) in about 25% and chronic glomerulonephritis in 16.8%, followed by other causes. In patients aged 15 to 64 years, the most common causes were diabetic nephropathy (28.9%), chronic glomerulonephritis (23.7%), and nephrosclerosis (10.2%).[64] Similar percentages were found in a study of 87 elderly patients in the Medicare ESRD Program in Virginia, of which 36.8% had underlying hypertensive nephrosclerosis, 25.3% had diabetic nephropathy, and 12.6% had crescentic glomerulonephritis.[61]

Thus, elderly patients constitute an ever-increasing percentage of the patients enrolled in treatment for the Medicare ESRD Program. The incidence of secondary renal disease is higher in this population, which is at higher risk for acquired systemic illness and (because of an underlying age-related loss of renal function) for developing severe renal failure after various renal insults, such as exposure to nephrotoxins.

Acute Renal Failure in Elderly Patients

Elderly patients are likely to suffer all of the causes of acute renal failure seen in the general population, although the evidence for enhanced susceptibility is not entirely clear.[65-67] Presumably, elderly patients may be at higher risk for prerenal causes of acute renal failure because of a tendency toward hypodipsia and reduced sodium intake, diuretic administration, and an inability to conserve sodium, thus predisposing to underlying dehydration and/or sodium depletion. A representative study of the causes of acute renal failure in 67 young and 298 elderly patients is depicted in Table 24.3,[67] in which volume depletion was deemed to be primarily responsible in 23.4% of cases. Obviously, preexisting volume depletion also would enhance the risk of acute renal failure after administration of contrast agents or nephrotoxic drugs as well.

Whether advanced age is an independent risk factor for mortality associated with acute renal failure is not entirely clear.[67] Certain causes of acute renal failure certainly are more frequent in elderly patients; these include multiple myeloma, carcinoma leading to obstruction, humoral abnormalities, nephrotoxicity from chemotherapeutic interventions, polypharmacy with or without inappropriate drug dosing (which fails to take into account the marked reduction in the GFR in elderly patients), obstructive uropathy due to prostatic disease, and atheroembolic renal disease.[67]

Table 24.3. Causes of acute renal failure.*

	%	
Cause	Young patients (n=67)	Elderly patients (n=298)
Nephrotoxic	6.8	10.8
Volume depletion	15.1	23.4
Septic shock	20.5	25.8
After surgery	8.2	5.1
Cardiogenic shock	11.0	5.8
Multifactorial	15.1	11.9
Obstructive	5.5	10.5
Hepatorenal syndrome	4.1	1.0
Glomerular disease	5.5	0.7
Other	8.2	5.8

* Adapted from Macias Nunez and Sanchez Tomero[67] with permission.

Experimental Considerations and Implications for Further Research

The potential mechanisms associated with the normal age-related loss of renal function have been explored in experimental animals, which also exhibit age-related declines in renal blood flow and the GFR in association with progressive glomerular sclerosis. The adaptive response to the loss of functioning nephrons consists of increases in the glomerular capillary pressures and flows in the remaining functional nephrons, a compensation that serves to preserve the total GFR. In the extreme case of extensive surgical removal of renal mass in the rat, the increased filtration in the surviving nephrons is accompanied by systemic hypertension, progressive azotemia, proteinuria, and glomerular sclerosis.[68-70] By using this analogy, the presumed sequential changes in single-nephron function that occur during normal aging are depicted in Fig 24.1.[71] The bottom panel shows the nephron population that is

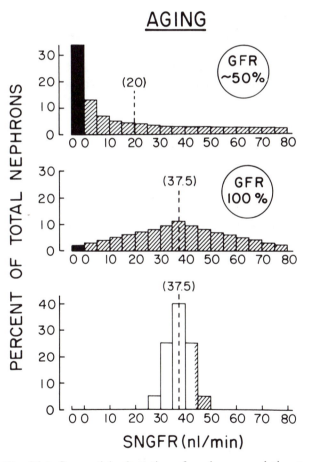

Fig. 24.1. Sequential adaptation of nephron population to normal aging. SN indicates single nephron; GFR, glomerular filtration rate. See text for discussion (from Brenner[71] with permission).

typical of the healthy young rat, and presumably of the healthy young human as well. Single-nephron glomerular filtration rates follow a relatively narrow gaussian distribution, with the mean value depicted by the broken line. With increasing age and the solute load engendered by the western protein-rich diet, a fraction of the glomeruli at the upper end of the function scale (the shaded area in the bottom panel) are burdened by relative hyperfiltration. Over time, these glomeruli develop progressive glomerular sclerosis and eventually fail, giving rise (as shown in the middle panel) to populations of nonfunctioning and poorly functioning nephrons. In consequence, more normal glomeruli hyperfilter to accommodate an unchanged solute load in the face of fewer functioning nephrons. Single-nephron filtration rates therefore widen considerably in distribution and, in doing so, all glomeruli operate at higher levels, as indicated by the marked expansion of the shaded area. Despite the heterogeneity in single-nephron GFR values, the distribution still is largely gaussian, and the average single-nephron GFR is unchanged from that in the bottom panel. Since the total nephron number remains constant, the total GFR remains at 100% of the starting value. Eventually, the stage depicted in the top panel is reached. The previously most burdened glomeruli cease to function, yielding a large population with single-nephron GFR values essentially equal to zero (black bar) and an increasing fraction of the total nephron population with single-nephron GFR rates below normal. The total GFR also must now decline. In this example, the serum creatinine value would still be under 2 mg/dL, but the total GFR would be reduced by 50%.

Observations in aging humans and experimental animals are highly reminiscent of changes observed in the setting of acquired renal disease and lend support to the hypothesis that hemodynamic factors in the aging kidney operate in a similar, albeit slower, fashion to injure and ultimately destroy the glomerular population. As schematized in Fig 24.2,[72] this formulation suggests that an age- or disease-related reduction in functioning renal mass, systemic hypertension, conventionally treated diabetes, and ad libitum protein intake all lead to unrelenting vasodilatation. The resulting long-term elevations in glomerular pressures and flows promote hyperfiltration, impair the permselective properties of the glomerular wall, and injure the component cells of the glomerulus. The resulting glomerular sclerosis exerts a positive feedback stimulus to compensatory hyperfiltration in less affected glomeruli, contributing in turn to their eventual destruction. Numerous dietary, endocrine, and toxic factors that may accelerate nephron loss with normal aging or renal disease have been identified,[71-74] and certain dietary manipulations (particularly dietary protein restriction and total food restriction) have been demonstrated to retard the progression of age-related renal disease in laboratory animals.[75,76] Given the vulnerability of the aging kidney to acceleration of renal insufficiency after acquired injury, it remains imperative to pay attention to those risk factors (volume depletion, nephrotoxic insults, uncontrolled hypertension, and diet) that may contribute to the loss of renal function. Recent clinical studies have provided encouraging preliminary evidence that dietary protein restriction[77] and control of systemic hypertension, particularly with agents that may prevent glomerular capillary hypertension,[78-80] may slow the decline of renal function in patients with chronic renal insufficiency. Although little information is available that specifically addresses these interventions in the elderly population, it seems likely that these hemodynamically protective in-

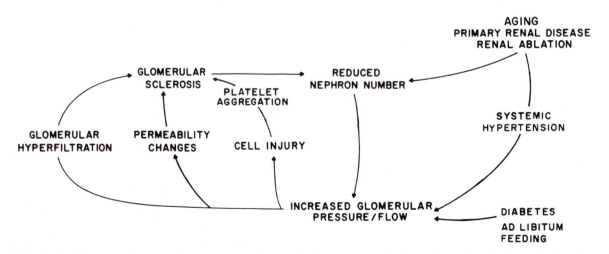

Fig. 24.2. Role of increased glomerular pressures and flows in development of glomerular sclerosis. See text for discussion (from Anderson[72] with permission).

terventions will prove to be efficacious in this population as well. With the ever-increasing number of elderly patients entering Medicare ESRD Programs, clinical studies that evaluate these therapeutic interventions in this population at great risk are certainly warranted.

References

1. Macias Nunez JF, Cameron JS, eds. *Renal Function and Disease in the Elderly*. Stoneham, Mass: Butterworths; 1987.
2. Oreopoulos DG, ed. *Geriatric Nephrology*. Dordrecht, the Netherlands: Martinus Nijhoff Publishers; 1986.
3. Zawada ET Jr, Sica DA, eds. *Geriatric Nephrology and Urology*. Littleton, Mass: PSG Publishing Co Inc; 1985.
4. Samiy A. Renal disease in the elderly. *Med Clin North Am* 1983;67:463–480.
5. Davies DF, Shock NW. Age changes in glomerular filtration rate, effective renal plasma flow, and tubular excretory capacity in adult males. *J Clin Invest* 1950;29:496–507.
6. Rowe JW, Andres R, Tobin JD, et al. The effect of age on creatinine clearance in men: a cross-sectional and longitudinal study. *J Gerontol* 1976;31:155–163.
7. Lindeman RD, Tobin JD, Shock NW. Association between blood pressure and the rate of decline in renal function with age. *Kidney Int* 1984;27:553–557.
8. Cockcroft DW, Gault MH. Prediction of creatinine clearance from serum creatinine. *Nephron* 1976;16:31–41.
9. Wesson LG. Renal hemodynamics in physiological states. In: Wesson LG, ed. *Physiology of the Human Kidney*. New York, NY: Grune & Stratton; 1969:96–108.
10. Hollenberg NK, Adams DF, Solomon HS, et al. Senescence and the renal vasculature in normal man. *Circ Res* 1974;34:309–316.
11. Bolton WK, Benton FR, Maclay JG, et al. Spontaneous glomerular sclerosis in aging Sprague-Dawley rats. *Am J Pathol* 1976;85:227–302.
12. Cohen MP, Ku L. Age-related changes in sulfation of basement membrane glycosaminoglycans. *Exp Gerontol* 1976;18:447–450.
13. Van Zonneveld RJ. Some data on the genito-urinary system as found in old age surveys in the Netherlands. *Gerontol Clin* 1959;1:167–173.
14. Tauchi H, Tsuboi K, Okutomi J. Age changes in the human kidney of the different races. *Gerontologia* 1971;17:87–97.
15. McLachlan MSF. The ageing kidney. *Lancet* 1978;2:143–146.
16. Goyal VK. Changes with age in the human kidney. *Exp Gerontol* 1982;17:321–331.
17. Ljungqvist A, Lagergren C. Normal intrarenal arterial pattern in adult and ageing human kidney: a microangiographical and histological study. *J Anat* 1962;96:285–300.
18. Takazakura E, Sawabu N, Handa A, et al. Intrarenal vascular changes with age and disease. *Kidney Int* 1972;2:224–230.
19. Kaplan C, Pasternack B, Shah H, et al. Age-related incidence of sclerotic glomeruli in human kidneys. *Am J Pathol* 1974;80:227–234.
20. Kappel B, Olsen S. Cortical interstitial tissue and sclerosed glomeruli in the normal human kidney, related to age and sex: a quantitative study. *Virchows Arch A* 1980;387:271–277.
21. Watkin DM, Shock NW. Agewise standard values for C_{In}, C_{PAH} and TmPAH in adult males. *J Clin Invest* 1955;34:969–976.
22. Miller JH, McDonald RK, Shock NW. Age changes in the maximal rate of renal tubular reabsorption of glucose. *J Gerontol* 1952;7:196–200.
23. Epstein M, Hollenberg NK. Renal 'salt wasting' despite apparently normal renal, adrenal and central nervous system function. *Nephron* 1979;24:121–126.
24. Macias Nunez JF, Bondia Roman AB, Rodriguez Commes JL. Physiology and disorders of water balance and electrolytes in the elderly. In: Macias Nunez, JF, Cameron JS, eds. *Renal Function and Disease in the Elderly*. Stoneham, Mass: Butterworths; 1987:67–93.
25. Macias Nunez JF, Garcia-Iglesias C, Tabernero-Romo JM, et al. Renal management of sodium under indomethacin and aldosterone in the elderly. *Age Ageing* 1978;9:165–172.
26. Weidmann P, De Myttanaere-Bursztein S, Maxwell MH, et al. Effect of aging on plasma renin and aldosterone in normal man. *Kidney Int* 1975;8:325–333.
27. Epstein M, Hollenberg NK. Age as a determinant of renal sodium conservation in normal man. *J Lab Clin Med* 1976;87:411–417.
28. Ceruso D, Squadrito G, Quartarone M, Parisi M. Comportamento della funzionalita renale e degli elettroliti ematici ed urinari dopo aldosterone in soggetti anziani. *Giornale Gerontologia* 1970;18:1–6.
29. Shannon RP, Minaker KL, Rowe JW. Aging and water balance in humans. *Semin Nephrol* 1984;4:346–353.
30. Sica DA, Harford A. Sodium and water disorders in the elderly. In: Zawada ET Jr, Sica DA, eds. *Geriatric Nephrology and Urology*. Littleton, Mass: PSG Publishing Co Inc; 1985:127–156.
31. Rowe JW, Shock NW, de Fronzo RA. The influence of age on the renal response to water deprivation in man. *Nephron* 1976;17:270–278.
32. Lindemann RD, Lee TD, Yiengst MJ, et al. Influence of age, renal disease, hypertension, diuretics and calcium on the antidiuretic response to suboptimal infusions of vasopressin. *J Lab Clin Med* 1966;68:206–223.
33. Frolkis VV, Bezinkov W, Duplinko YK, et al. The hypothalamus in aging. *Exp Gerontol* 1972;7:169–184.
34. Helderman JH, Vestal RE, Rowe JW, et al. The response of arginine vasopressin to intravenous ethanol and hypertonic saline in man: the impact of aging. *J Gerontol* 1978;33:39–47.
35. Rowe JW, Minaker KL, Sparrow D, et al. Age-related failure of volume-pressure-mediated vasopressin release. *J Clin Endocrinol Metab* 1982;54:661–664.
36. Engel PA, Rowe JW, Minaker KL, et al. Stimulation of

310   Sharon Anderson

vasopressin release by exogenous vasopressin: effect of sodium intake and age. *Am J Physiol* 1984;246:E202–E207.

37. Dontas AS, Karkeros S, Papanayioutou P. Mechanisms of renal tubular defects in old age. *Postgrad Med J* 1972;48:295–303.

38. Kleinfeld M, Casimir M, Borra A. Hyponatremia as observed in a chronic disease facility. *J Am Geriatr Soc* 1979;27:156–161.

39. Narins RG, Jones ER, Stom MC, et al. Diagnostic strategies in disorders of fluid, electrolyte, and acid-base homeostasis. *Am J Med* 1982;72:496–520.

40. Sunderam SG, Mankikar GD. Hyponatremia in the elderly. *Age Ageing* 1983;12:77–80.

41. Booker JA. Severe symptomatic hyponatremia in elderly outpatients: the role of thiazide therapy and stress. *J Am Geriatr Soc* 1984;32:108–113.

42. Ashraf N, Locksley R, Arieff A. Thiazide-induced hyponatremia associated with death or neurologic damage in out-patients. *Am J Med* 1981;70:1163–1168.

43. Rondeau E, de Lima J, Caillens H, et al. High plasma antidiuretic hormone in patients with cardiac failure: influence of age. *Miner Electrolyte Metab* 1982;8:267–274.

44. Goldstein CS, Braunstein S, Goldfarb S. Idiopathic syndrome of inappropriate antidiuretic hormone secretion possibly due to advanced age. *Ann Intern Med* 1983;99:185–188.

45. Weissman P, Shenkman L, Gregerman R. Chlorpropamide hyponatremia. *N Engl J Med* 1971;284:65–71.

46. Mukherjee AP, Coni NK, Davison W. Osmoreceptor function among the elderly. *Gerontol Clin* 1973;15:227–233.

47. Lye M. Distribution of body potassium in healthy elderly subjects. *Gerontology* 1981;27:286–292.

48. McCarthy ST. Body fluid, electrolytes and diuretics. *Curr Med Res Opin* 1982;7:87–95.

49. Bengele HH, Mathias R, Perkins JH, et al. Impaired renal and extrarenal adaptation in old rats. *Kidney Int* 1983;23:684–690.

50. Goodkin DA, Waldman R, Narins RG. Acid-base disorders in the elderly. In: Zawada ET Jr, Sica DA, eds. *Geriatric Nephrology and Urology*. Littleton, Mass: PSG Publishing Co Inc; 1985:157–174.

51. Taberno Romo JM. Proximal tubular function and renal acidification in the aged. In: Macias Nunez JF, Cameron JS, eds. *Renal Function and Disease in the Elderly*. Stoneham, Mass: Butterworths; 1984:143–161.

52. Shock NW, Yiengst MJ. Age changes in the acid-base equilibrium of the blood of males. *J Gerontol* 1950;5:1–4.

53. Adler S, Lindeman RD, Yiengst MJ, et al. Effect of acute acid loading on urinary acid excretion by the aging human kidney. *J Lab Clin Med* 1968;72:278–289.

54. Agarwal BN, Cabebe RG. Renal acidification in elderly subjects. *Nephron* 1980;26:291–295.

55. Hilton JG, Goodbody MF, Kruesi OR. The effect of prolonged administration of ammonium chloride on the blood acid-base equilibrium of geriatric subjects. *J Am Geriatr Soc* 1955;3:697–703.

56. Murray BM, Raij L. Glomerular disease in the aged. In: Macias Nunez JF, Cameron JS, eds. *Renal Function and Disease in the Elderly*. Stoneham, Mass: Butterworths; 1987:298–320.

57. Moorthy AV, Zimmerman SW. Renal disease in the elderly: clinicopathologic analysis of renal disease in 115 elderly patients. *Clin Nephrol* 1977;14:223–229.

58. Zech P, Colon S, Pointet S, et al. The nephrotic syndrome in adults aged over 60: etiology, evolution and treatment of 76 cases. *Clin Nephrol* 1982;18:232–236.

59. Kingswood JC, Banks RA, Tribe CR, et al. Renal biopsy in the elderly: clinicopathological correlations in 143 patients. *Clin Nephrol* 1984;22:183–187.

60. Ramirez G, Saba SR. Primary glomerulonephritis in the elderly. In: Zawada ET Jr, Sica DA, eds. *Geriatric Nephrology and Urology*. Littleton, Mass: PSG Publishing Co Inc; 1985:49–66.

61. Glickman JL, Kaiser DL, Bolton WK. Aetiology and diagnosis of chronic renal insufficiency in the aged: the role of renal biopsy. In: Zawada ET Jr, Sica DA, eds. *Geriatric Nephrology and Urology*. Littleton, Mass: PSG Publishing Co Inc; 1985:485–508.

62. Eggers PW, Connerton R, McMullan M. The Medicare experience with end-stage renal disease: trends in incidence, prevalence and survival. *Health Care Financing Rev* 1984;5:69–88.

63. Blagg CR, Wahl PW, Lamers JY. Treatment of chronic renal failure at the Northwest Kidney Center, Seattle, from 1962 to 1982. *ASAIO Trans* 1983;6:170–175.

64. Blagg CR. Chronic renal failure in the elderly. In: Oreopoulos DG, ed. *Geriatric Nephrology*. Dordrecht, the Netherlands: Martinus Nijhoff Publishers; 1986:117–126.

65. Oken DE, Wolfert AI, Sica DA. Acute renal failure in the elderly. In: Zawada ET Jr, Sica DA, eds. *Geriatric Nephrology and Urology*. Littleton, Mass: PSG Publishing Inc; 1985:91–116.

66. Lameire N, DeKeyzer K, Pauwels W, et al. Acute renal failure in the elderly. In: Oreopoulos DG, ed. *Geriatric Nephrology*. Dordrecht, the Netherlands: Martinus Nijhoff Publishers; 1986:103–116.

67. Macias Nunez JF, Sanchez Tomero JA. Acute renal failure in old people. In: Macias Nunez JF, Cameron JS, eds. *Renal Function and Disease in the Elderly*. Stoneham, Mass: Butterworths; 1987:461–484.

68. Hostetter TH, Olson JL, Rennke HG, et al. Hyperfiltration in remnant nephrons: a potentially adverse response to renal ablation. *Am J Physiol* 1981;241:F85–F93.

69. Hostetter TH, Meyer TW, Rennke HG, et al. Chronic effects of dietary protein on renal structure and function in the rat with intact and reduced renal mass. *Kidney Int* 1986;30:509–517.

70. Anderson S, Rennke HG, Brenner BM. Therapeutic advantage of converting enzyme inhibitors in arresting progressive renal disease associated with systemic hypertension in the rat. *J Clin Invest* 1986;77:1993–2000.

71. Brenner BM. Nephron adaptation to renal injury or ablation: mechanisms, benefits and risks. *Am J Physiol* 1985;249:F324–F337.

72. Anderson S. Decline of renal function with age: mechanisms, risk factors and therapeutic implications. In: Ore-

opoulos DG, ed. *Geriatric Nephrology*. Dordrecht, the Netherlands: Martinus Nijhoff Publishers: 1986:57–71.

73. Brenner BM, Meyer TW, Hostetter TH. Dietary protein intake and the progressive nature of kidney disease. *N Engl J Med* 1982;307:652–660.

74. Anderson S, Meyer TW, Brenner BM. Mechanisms of age-associated glomerular sclerosis. In: Macias Nunez JF, Cameron JS, eds. *Renal Function and Disease in the Elderly*. Stoneham, Mass: Butterworths; 1987:49–66.

75. Saxton JA Jr, Kimball GC. Relation of nephrosis and other diseases of albino rats to age and to modifications of diet. *Arch Pathol Lab Med* 1941;32:951–965.

76. Gehrig JJ Jr, Ross J, Jamison RL. Effect of long-term, alternate day feeding on renal function in aging conscious rats. *Kidney Int* 1988;34:620–630.

77. Mitch WE. The influence of diet on the progression of renal insufficiency. *Annu Rev Med* 1984;35:249–264.

78. Bauer JH, Reams GP, Lai SM. Renal protective effect of strict blood pressure control with enalapril therapy. *Arch Intern Med* 1987;147:1397–1400.

79. Heeg JE, de Jong PE, van der Hem GK, et al. Reduction of proteinuria by angiotensin converting enzyme inhibition. *Kidney Int* 1987;32:78–83.

80. Mann J, Ritz E. Preservation of kidney function by use of converting enzyme inhibitors for control of hypertension. *Lancet* 1987;2:622.

25

Immunology and Infectious Disease

Edith A. Burns and James S. Goodwin

Immunologic function declines with age. Indeed, most physiologic functions decline with age. Why, then, has so much attention been given to the study of immunologic changes in elderly humans and laboratory animals? Immunologic function probably is the most intensively studied physiologic process in gerontology. Part of the reason has to do with the rapid growth in all aspects of immunologic research in the past 3 decades. In addition, immunocytes (lymphocytes, monocytes, and polymorphonuclear leukocytes) are the most easily obtained tissue specimens in humans. A tube of venous blood provides the immunologist with millions of cells with which to study antibody production, cytotoxicity, proliferation, migration, and other characteristics that are necessary for the continued health and survival of an organism.

There are more fundamental reasons, however, why the study of immunology is particularly relevant to gerontology. Concomitant with the decline in immune function, there is a rise in the incidence of many infections and malignancies with age. There is greater morbidity and mortality associated with common infections in adults over age 65 years. An understanding of immunologic changes might be important not only in understanding the aging process, but also in developing potential strategies to prevent some of the morbidity and other changes that occur with age.[1] In this chapter, the changes seen in the aging immune system will be described along with data supporting various mechanisms to account for these changes. The declines in humoral immune function that are seen result in decreased responses of elderly subjects to immunizations against common infections such as influenza and pneumococcal pneumonia. These infections also will be reviewed, along with others where the presentation, treatment, or outcome is substantially different in adults over the age of 65 years than in younger age groups.

Relevance of the Issues

Evidence that links depressed or disordered immune function in humans to subsequent morbidity and/or mortality is scarce. Most authorities simply have assumed that a decline in immune function is deleterious, or they have used theoretical arguments to support this belief. One example is the idea of "immune surveillance," which was first conceptualized by Erlich,[2] named by Burnet,[3] and popularized by Thomas,[4] and others. It proposes that the cellular immune system is the first defense against cancer. The most enthusiastic proponents of immune surveillance contended that new malignancies were popping up every day, only to be eliminated by the ever-vigilant immune system. A corollary of this theory is that clinical cancer represents a failure of immune surveillance. Thus, elderly persons or other individuals with a depressed immune function should have a higher incidence rate of malignancy. More recently, the lack of a generalized increase in most malignancies among immunosuppressed humans and experimental animals has thrown this theory into relative disrepute.

However, the rejection of the immune surveillance theory does not mean that intact immune function is unimportant for continued health. One lesson of the AIDS epidemic is the disastrous consequences of impaired immunity. The question of whether decreased cellular immune responses contribute to morbidity and mortality in elderly persons has been addressed in several ways. Roberts-Thompson et al[5] placed five delayed-type hypersensitivity skin tests for common antigens on 52 octogenarians and correlated the response with survival after 2 years. Of those subjects who responded to none or only one antigen (the "anergic" group), 80% were dead within 2 years, compared with 35% of those who responded to two or more antigens (Table 25.1). The octogenerian subjects in this series were not well characterized as to the presence of medical illnesses at the time of initial skin testing.

While the investigators used their data to suggest that anergy was a risk factor for subsequent mortality, an equally plausible explanation was that the underlying medical condition ultimately responsible for death also contributed to the depressed cellular immunity in these individuals. Perhaps the least controversial conclusion from this study is that octogenaraians do not live long, regardless of their immune status. Actually, the overall 65% death rate during the 2-year follow-up in this Australian study contrasts sharply with the mean life expectancy of 8 years for all men and women 80 to 85 years of age in the United States.[6] This again suggests that the population studied had serious underlying illnesses.

A more recent study examined the in vitro correlate of delayed hypersensitivity skin testing, lymphocyte proliferation in response to mitogens, in a group of 403 adults over the age of 65 years.[7] In this group of community-living adults seen in an outpatient geriatric clinic, 18% had lymphocytes that did not respond to any of three mitogens. A 3-year follow-up found a significantly greater mortality rate among those with a negative response than among those with a positive response, 26% versus 13%. The increase in overall mortality was not due to an increase in one particular cause of death, such as infection or malignancy, and this increase remained significant after the investigators controlled for medication use, an indirect indicator of health status.

Since 1979, we have been following up a group of healthy elderly individuals in New Mexico. Entry criteria included age greater than 65 years, no medication use, and the absence of medical illness. These 300 individuals underwent a number of immunologic tests, including mitogen responsiveness and delayed hypersensitivity skin testing. Approximately one third were anergic at initial testing.[8] The anergic group had an approximately twofold higher mortality rate and also a twofold higher incidence of pneumonia during 8 years of follow-up.[9] Both these differences were statistically significant.

The other body of evidence that links disordered immune function to disease and death concerns the possible role of autoantibodies and circulating immune complexes in the etiology of atherosclerosis. While it had been recognized for many years that circulating immune complexes produced by repeated injections of a foreign antigen could cause an acute arteritis, only within the last 2 decades has evidence accumulated to suggest that autoimmunity might contribute to atherosclerosis. The combination of injections of foreign proteins and atherogenic diets in rabbits results in more atherosclerosis than an atherogenic diet alone.[10] In addition, the histologic type of atherosclerosis produced in these rabbits closely resembles that found in humans.[10] Similar data were obtained in baboons.[11] Chronic stimuli for circulating immune complex formation will lead to atherosclerosis even in animals on a nonatherogenic diet. The most striking evidence that links autoimmunity to atherosclerosis in experimental animals comes from a study of the long-term effects of vasectomy on rhesus monkeys.[12] Vasectomy can be seen as a mild stimulus for autoantibody and circulating immune complex formation. Antisperm antibodies develop in about 50% of all vasectomized human males and experimental animals.[13] Clarkson and Alexander demonstrated that vasectomies led to accelerated atherosclerosis in monkeys who were fed a high-fat diet.[12] They then showed that monkeys vasectomized and maintained on a very low-fat, no-cholesterol diet (fruit and commercial monkey chow) had an increased incidence of atherosclerosis at autopsy 9 to 14 years later compared with nonvasectomized control monkeys.[12] Thus, a very mild stimulus for autoantibody formation leads to accelerated atherosclerosis even without an atherogenic diet. This evidence provides a strong theoretic basis for proposing that autoantibodies and the resultant circulating immune complexes in humans,

Table 25.1. Response to delayed-type hypersensitivity skin testing and 2-year survival rate in 52 subjects over 80 years of age.*

No. of positive skin tests	No. of subjects	No. dead at 2 y	% Dead at 2 y
0	21	17	80
1	14	11	
2	10	2	35
3	3	2	
4	4	2	

* Adapted from Roberts-Thompson et al.[5]

by causing a low level of chronic irritation in blood vessels, contribute to the development of atherosclerosis.

In addition to the studies in experimental animals, there also are some epidemiologic data in humans that support a link between autoimmunity and atherosclerosis. Mackay and his colleagues measured a variety of autoantibodies in serum samples from most of the adult population of the town of Busselton in western Australia.[14] There was an association between the presence of autoantibodies and the presence of cardiovascular diseases. In addition, the presence of autoantibodies in 1969 (the time of the comprehensive survey) was associated with an increased risk of death due to vascular disease and cancer during the period of 1970 to 1975. As in the study summarized in Table 25.1, the association of disordered immune function (in this case autoantibodies) and subsequent mortality rate may have been due to both phenomena being secondary to a serious medical illness that was present when the subjects were first tested.

Specific Changes in Immune Function with Age

Problems of Methodology

There are two major methodologic questions that plague gerontologists. First, do age-related changes found in short-lived species such as mice or guinea pigs have any relevance to age-related changes in humans? Are the processes responsible for making a mouse old at 3 years of age the same as those that make a human old at age 75 years? Second, is a given physiologic change that is found in a majority of aging organisms secondary to the aging process per se, or is it secondary to one of the many diseases whose prevalence increases with age? Concern about the first question would tend to move investigators away from experimental animals to the study of aging humans, while concern about the second question would tend to push investigators in the opposite direction.

The problems raised by these questions are real; many reported investigations on immunologic changes with age do not deal with these issues rigorosly.[15] It is not at all uncommon to see articles on the differences in some immunologic response in "young" versus "old" mice based on data obtained in 2-month-old versus 1-year-old animals. These would be analogous to 4-year-old and 25-year-old humans. Even when truly aged experimental animals are used, there are few parallels between the physiologic changes, diseases, and causes of death in these animals and humans. Conversely, few studies of immunologic changes in elderly persons rigorously define their subjects in terms of underlying disease, medication status, occupational exposure history, and so on. It is surprising how many widely accepted immunologic changes in aging humans were based on studies of hospitalized, potentially malnourished, and psychologically stressed men and women taking a great variety of prescription medications and suffering from a great variety of acute and chronic diseases. A sentence commonly encountered in the "Methods and Materials" sections is that "the subjects studied had no diseases and were taking no medications known to affect the immune system." This is an empty promise, for most medications have not been studied for their effect on immunologic function. Even experimental animal studies may label as an age-related change something that in reality is secondary to stress, chronic disease, or diet.

Given all the reservations expressed above, it still is possible to reach a consensus on some changes in immune function that would seem to occur as a result of age (Table 25.2). The following sections in this chapter will describe those changes, as well as the mechanisms thought to cause them. When possible, the emphasis will be on data from human rather than experimental animal studies.

Changes in Cellular Immunity

The immune system classically has been divided into the cellular and humoral components, with monocyte and granulocyte function treated separately. The cellular immune response is responsible for rejecting grafts of foreign tissues, for killing virus-infected cells, for protecting against fungi and some intracellular parasites and bacteria, and (possibly) for defense against the growth of tumors. The function of the humoral immune system is the production of antibodies, which are the main defense against bacteria and other infectious agents that gain entry into an organism. Cells of the monocyte-macrophage series, in addition to ingesting and/or killing foreign material that may or may not have been previously opsonized with antibodies, also play an important regulatory role in both humoral and cellular immune responses. Table 25.3 summarizes

Table 25.2. Changes in the immune system associated with aging.

Thymic involution and decline in thymic hormone production

Decreased response to delayed hypersensitivity skin testing

Increase in circulating autoantibodies

Increase in circulating immune complexes

Decreased antibody response to specific antigen challenge

Table 25.3. Changes in cellular immune function
with aging.

I. Increased incidence of anergy
II. Decreased lymphocyte proliferation in response to
mitogen or antigen stimulation
  1. Fewer mitogen-responsive cells
  2. Decreased vigor of the proliferative response
  3. Decreased response to endogenous, cytoplasmic
    signals for proliferation
  4. Decreased production of interleukin-2
  5. Decreased density of interleukin-2 cell surface
    receptors
  6. Decreased expression of messenger RNA for
    interleukin-2

changes in cellular immune function associated with
aging.

A depression of cellular immune responses is the
most universal and easily demonstrated age-related
change in immune function. The incidence of anergy
(lack of a delayed-type hypersensitivity response to
intradermal testing with a battery of common antigens)
increases in adults over 60 years of age.[5,8,14,15] This
increase in anergy with age occurs even in healthy,
well-nourished populations taking no medications.[8]
Analogous findings have been reported in mice, which
manifest a decreased ability to reject foreign skin grafts
with age.[1]

The in vitro correlate of delayed-type hypersensitivity skin testing is the proliferative response of lymphocytes that are cultured with specific antigens or nonspecific mitogens. Lymphocytes are isolated from the
peripheral blood and cultured in media with specific
antigens such as *Candida* or streptokinase, or with
mitogens such as phytohemagglutinin (PHA) or
pokeweed mitogen, which nonspecifically activate
most lymphocytes. The degree of the proliferative response can be quantitated by adding radiolabeled thymidine to the cultures, harvesting the cells, and measuring the amount of radioactivity incorporated into
the lymphocyte DNA. Most investigators have reported that antigen- or mitogen-stimulated cultures of
lymphocytes from persons over 65 years of age incorporate less radiolabeled thymidine,[5,7,16-18] but there
also are conflicting reports.[16,19] Czlonkowska and
Korlak[16] reported a decreased lymphocytic proliferative response to PHA—but not to other mitogens or to
antigens—in 30 subjects over 60 years of age, compared with young subjects. Portaro et al[19] studied 200
healthy, working persons 21 to 70 years of age and
found no age-related decrease in response to several
concentrations of PHA. The authors noted that their
group of subjects was better characterized as to health
status than previously reported subjects in whom a
decline in the PHA response had been found. On the

other hand, the oldest subjects in this study were only
70 years of age, and the number of subjects in the two
oldest categories (61 to 65 years [n = 11] and 66 to 70
years [n = 14]) may have been too small to reflect
substantial differences in PHA responses. The study of
300 healthy elderly people by Goodwin et al showed a
substantial decrease in PHA response with age.[8] The
mean response of the elderly subjects was significantly
less than the mean response of the young control subjects to all mitogen doses ($P \leq .0001$). To pursue the
distinction between age-related changes due to chronic
illnesses or medications that frequently accompany aging, we also measured the PHA responses of 24
chronically ill patients over 65 years of age who had a
variety of life-threatening medical conditions and who
were receiving a number of medications. The PHA
responses of this chronically ill group were not different from those of the healthy group. Thus, age per se,
and not an accompanying illness, was the major determinant of a depressed cellular immunity in this population. Within the healthy elderly group, there was a
significant decrease in PHA response with age ($r =
-.23$, $P \leq .0001$).

Mechanism of Decreased Cellular Immunity

The causes of depressed cellular immune responses
with age are certainly multiple, and they may differ
depending on the aspect of cellular immune function
that is examined. For example, anergy to delayed-type
hypersensitivity skin testing could represent problems
with antigen recognition, T-cell proliferation, lympho-
kine production, lymphocyte or monocyte chemotaxis,
vascular response to inflammatory mediators, or a multitude of other steps that are required to produce induration after an intradermal challenge with antigens (Fig
25.1). Given the complexity of the in vivo system, it is
understandable that immunologists who are searching
for mechanisms have turned to in vitro assays, in which
specific cell functions can be more or less studied in
isolation. Such investigations have, as expected, resulted in the identification of several, specific age-
related lesions in cellular immune functions.

Hyporesponsiveness to PHA of lymphocytes from
aging humans has been demonstrated to be a sum of at
least two deficiencies.[17] First, the number of mitogen-
responsive cells is reduced in lymphocyte preparations
from elderly persons. Second, the mitogen-responsive
cells from elderly persons do not proliferate as vigorously after exposure to PHA as do lymphocytes from
young persons.

Lymphocytes from healthy subjects over 70 years of
age are reported to be significantly more sensitive to
inhibition by prostaglandin E_2 in mitogen-stimulated
cultures.[18,20] Because prostaglandin E_2 acts as a nor-

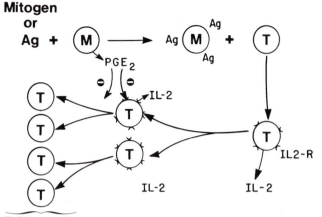

Fig. 25.1. Model of the cellular immune system. Ag indicates antigen; IL-2, interleukin-2; IL2-R, interleukin-2 receptor; M, macrophage/monocyte; PGE$_2$, prostaglandin E$_2$; T, T-cell, −, inhibition.

mal endogenous feedback inhibitor of cellular immune responses in vitro and in vivo,[21] an increased sensitivity to this immunomodulator may partially account for the depressed cellular immune responses seen in this group of subjects. Indeed, the addition of drugs that block the production of prostaglandin E$_2$ in PHA-stimulated cultures partially reverses the depressed response of lymphocytes in subjects over 70 years of age.[18] The increased sensitivity with age to prostaglandin E$_2$ would not appear to be part of a general increase in sensitivity to all immunomodulators; for example, lymphocytes from subjects over 70 years of age actually are less sensitive to inhibition by histamine and hydrocortisone than are lymphocytes from young control subjects.[20]

The proliferative response of T cells to mitogens results from a complex set of interactions involving T cells and macrophages or other accessory cells, as outlined in Figure 25.1. Mitogens such as PHA bind to, cross-link with, and thereby activate the T-cell antigen receptor. This results in activation of phospholipase C, cleavage of membrane phosphatidylinositol phosphates, and liberation of inositol bisphosphate and diacylglycerol. Inositol bisphosphate and its metabolite inositol triphosphate raise intracellular free calcium concentrations by releasing bound calcium from intracellular stores and by opening calcium channels. Diacylglycerol binds to and activates protein kinase C, which is further activated by the increased free calcium concentration. Protein kinase C activation then leads to increased transcription and subsequent translation of the gene coding for interleukin-2 (also known as T-cell growth factor) and also of receptors for interleukin-2. Interleukin-2 is thus an autocrine growth fac-

tor, produced by the same cells that respond to it. Exposure of interleukin-2 receptor–bearing T cells to interleukin-2 results in proliferation, though the intracellular second messengers for interleukin-2 action are presently unknown.

Accessory cells help T cells produce and respond to interleukin-2 by cross-linking T-cell receptors. Macrophages secrete interleukin-1 and probably other monokines that provide additional signals necessary for complete activation of T cells. This recently described system has been used to dissect further the age-related defect in cellular immunity. Several laboratories have demonstrated decreased production of interleukin-2[22] after mitogen stimulation and a decreased density of interleukin-2 receptor expression and decreased proliferation of these cells in response to interleukin-2.[23] Additional experiments in rodents suggest that the picture might be more complex, with specific defects in production of or sensitivity to interleukin-2, depending on the immunologic stimulus.[24] Other investigators have shown that lymphocytes from aged rats are defective in their ability to express messenger RNA for interleukin-2.[25]

Other work in humans suggests that functional defects of the lymphocyte nucleus distal to interleukin 2 production may contribute to the decreased proliferative response in aging. A lymphocyte cytoplasmic factor found only in activated cells, and dubbed the "activator of DNA replication" or (ADR), has been described by Gutowski and Cohen.[26] This factor is capable of inducing DNA synthesis in isolated lymphocyte nuclei but not in intact cells, indicating that it is an intracellular modulator of proliferation. Lymphocytes from adults over age 65 years were found to produce ADR at levels comparable to those found in lymphocytes from young adults.[27] However, lymphocyte nuclei from adults over the age of 65 years that proliferated poorly in response to PHA also proliferated poorly when stimulated by exogenous sources of ADR.[27] The lymphocyte nuclei from these elderly individuals did not respond well to a cytoplasmic stimulatory signal for proliferation.

The most obvious change associated with the decline in cellular immunity with age is involution of the thymus. Thymic lymphatic mass, particularly in the cortical area, decreases with age in humans and experimental animals, starting in adolescence. The thymic mass of aging humans and experimental animals is approximately 10% that of a younger thymus.[28] Associated with a loss of thymic mass is a decreased output of thymic hormones, such as thymosin.[28] Thymectomy leads to the acceleration of normal age-related changes in immune function in mice, which suggests that thymic involution may indeed be a central aspect of age-related immunodeficiencies. Moreover, the treatment of aging mice with thymic hormone preparations causes some reversal of the immunodeficiencies.[29,30]

Changes in Humoral Immunity With Age

The distinction between cellular and humoral immunity is, in some ways, artificial, because both B cells (bone marrow derived) and T cells (thymus derived) can participate in each reaction. For example, B cells can act as antigen-presenting cells in cellular immune responses, while T cells are required for the great majority of humoral (antibody) responses. Thus, changes in humoral immunity frequently are secondary to alterations in T-cell function. There is growing evidence that B-cell function also is altered with increasing age. A model of the humoral immune response is presented in Figure 25.2.

A number of age-related defects in humoral immunity have been described (Table 25.4). The number of B cells circulating in humans and splenic B cells in mice does not change with age.[1] However, the functional ability of B cells to mount appropriate antibody responses does change. For example, there are increases in autoantibodies to a variety of endogenous antigens. Specific antibody responses to antigenic challenges are

Table 25.4. Changes in humoral immunity associated with aging.

I. Increase in circulating autoantibodies
II. Increase in circulating immune complexes
III. Decreased antibody production
    A. Decreased response to immunization
        1. Lower peak serum levels
        2. Failure to maintain specific antibody levels in serum
    B. Increased T helper cell function
    C. Decreased T suppressor cell function
    D. Decreased intrinsic B-cell function

decreased in aging animals and humans.[31] Following in vivo immunization with influenza vaccine, serum antibody levels are significantly lower in older than in younger adults.[32,33] A faster decay in these serum antibody levels over time also has been reported. Following immunization with tetanus toxoid, adults over age 65 years had significantly lower peak serum anti–tetanus toxoid antibody titers than adults under age 34 years.[34] In this study, repeated sampling of serum titers over a 10-week period revealed consistently lower levels in the older adults and a more rapid decay in serum titers than in the young control group.

Defects in specific antibody synthesis also have been reported in older adults in response to antigens such as flagellin.[35] In a study of the antibody response to flagellin immunization in subjects of different ages, mean serum titers of IgG and IgM antibodies were similar among the old and young subjects, but there was a failure in the older subjects to maintain levels of IgG antibody over time.

The distinction between T-dependent and T-independent antigens is more clear in mice than humans and is made on the basis of whether there is an absolute requirement for T-cell help in the antibody response. In experimental animals, the decrease in T-dependent antibody responses is more obvious, with an 80% decrease in antibody-forming cells in older animals.[36]

Mechanism of Depressed Humoral Immunity

As described for cellular immunity, a decrease in humoral immune response could be due to a multiplicity of factors, including defects in B-cell or T-cell function, or both. The past decade has brought an appreciation of the importance of suppressor T cells, which modulate normal immune responses and prevent the development of autoimmunity. For example, healthy persons have circulating B cells that are programmed to differentiate into autoantibody-producing plasma cells (producing antinuclear, antithyroid, antimitochondrial, and other antibodies); however, tonic inhibition of this

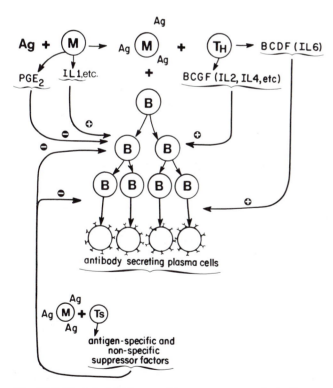

Fig. 25.2. Model of the humoral immune system. Ag indicates antigen; B, B cell; BCDF, B-cell differentiation factor; BCGF, B-cell growth factor; IL, interleukin; M, macrophage/monocyte; TH, T helper cell; TS, T suppressor cell; +, stimulation; −, inhibition.

autoimmune response by suppressor T cells is one mechanism preventing such an immunologic aberration. Several studies employing in vitro cultures of human lymphocytes have addressed the mechanism of age-related decreases in humoral immunity. Lymphocytes from older subjects produce greater amounts of IgG and IgM when cultured with pokeweed mitogen than do lymphocytes from young control subjects.[37] When the lymphocytes are separated into T-cell and B-cell fractions and various combinations of old T cells are cultured with old B cells, old T cells with young B cells, and so on, the old T cells are more capable than the young T cells of supporting immunoglobulin production by either young or old B cells. This increased helper activity of the old T cells could be due to an actual increase in helper activity or a decrease in suppressor activity. The same investigators addressed this question by studying the effects of irradiation of T cells in this system, taking advantage of the fact that suppressor T cells are sensitive to low doses of irradiation while helper T cells are relatively radioresistant. Irradiation of T cells from elderly people resulted in smaller increases in immunoglobulin production in subsequent cultures than did irradiation of T cells from young people.[37] This suggests that the overall increase in T-cell helper function with age actually was due at least in part to a failure of suppressor cell function.

Our laboratory has examined the role of isolated T-cell subsets in the changes in polyclonal immunoglobulin production and the production of IgM rheumatoid factor in elderly humans.[38,39] In isolated T-cell subsets from elderly donors, we found both increased activity of helper cells and decreased activity of suppressor cells. However, the most striking finding was a diminished ability of purified B cells to respond to isolated T helper cells or to T cell–derived helper factors. This finding suggests that the age-related changes in helper and suppressor T-cell function might represent a homeostatic mechanism to maintain immunoglobulin production in the face of a failing B-cell compartment. The concept of a primary failure of B-cell function with age is supported by functional experiments in mice[40] and by studies showing age-related, structural changes in B cells.[41]

Other information on changes in humoral immunity with age come from studies measuring the in vitro antibody response to specific antigens. Kishimoto et al[42] studied specific anti–tetanus toxoid antibody production and also found evidence of declining B-cell function in adults over age 65 years. Purified B cells from elderly or young subjects were cultured with T cells from a young individual who had been immunized with tetanus toxoid a week before. The B cells from the older subjects made significantly less antibody to tetanus toxoid than those from the younger subjects. We

also have examined changes in tetanus toxoid–specific antibody production in elderly humans (unpublished data). Peripheral blood lymphocytes from adults of different ages were stimulated in vitro with tetanus toxoid, and the amount of anti–tetanus toxoid antibody produced was measured. Regardless of the time elapsed since the last booster immunization, the anti–tetanus toxoid serum titers of the older subjects (60 to 88 years of age) were significantly lower than those of the younger subjects (18 to 40 years of age). In addition, the amount of specific anti–tetanus toxoid antibody produced in vitro was significantly less in cultures of lymphocytes of the older subjects. Using limiting dilution assays, we calculated that the number of anti–tetanus toxoid precursor cells in the peripheral blood of the older subjects was more than a log magnitude lower than it was in the younger subjects. Thus, the lack of precursor cells with the ability to respond to a specific antigen was primarily responsible for the decreased specific antibody production against tetanus toxoid.

Arachidonic acid metabolites also have been implicated in age-related changes in humoral immunity. As discussed earlier, prostaglandin E_2 is a feedback inhibitor of T-cell proliferation in humans,[43] and T cells from older adults are much more sensitive to inhibition by prostaglandin E_2.[18] Thus, prostaglandin E_2 may interfere with the expansion of antigen-specific T-cell helper clones. Delfraissey et al have shown that this increased sensitivity to prostaglandin E_2 was responsible for the impaired primary antibody response of lymphocytes from older adults that were cultured with trinitrophenylated polyacrylamide beads (TNP-PA).[44] Lymphocytes from older subjects made substantially less antibody to TNP-PA than lymphocytes from younger subjects. Removing monocytes (the source of prostaglandin E_2 production) or adding indomethacin (a cyclooxygenase inhibitor) restored the antibody response of the older subjects to the level of the younger subjects.

Increase in Autoimmunity with Age

The classic autoimmune diseases generally are associated with young adults. Systemic lupus erythematosus, polymyositis, and rheumatoid arthritis all have a higher incidence in young than in older adults. Nevertheless, the serologic manifestations of autoimmunity (autoantibodies and circulating immune complexes) are much more prevalent in healthy older adults than in young persons. The possible role of the autoantibodies and circulating immune complexes in the pathogenesis of arteriosclerosis was discussed earlier.

Many different investigators have reported an increase in the prevalence of positive tests for various autoantibodies with age (antinuclear antibodies, rheumatoid factors, antithyroid antibodies, anti–smooth muscle antibodies, and antilymphocyte antibodies). The rise in prevalence becomes steep around 70 years of age[8,45] As with the data on age-related decreases in PHA response discussed earlier, some studies did not find an increase in autoantibodies with age, but the great majority of studies did.

The prevalence of antinuclear antibody, lymphocytotoxic antibody, rheumatoid factor, and circulating immune complexes in 278 healthy elderly subjects is given in Table 25.5, along with analogous findings in 100 young control subjects. There is a clear increase in the percentage of serum samples from older subjects that are positive for each test, compared with samples from younger control subjects. The fact that a given serum sample was positive in one of these tests did not increase the chance of its being positive in the remaining tests.[8] Of all the subjects tested, 50% were positive for at least one test, which is exactly the figure predicted if positivity for each test were distributed independently and not clustered in a subgroup of elderly persons. In another study,[45] there was an association between the presence of circulating immune complexes and the presence of one or more autoantibodies in 189 healthy subjects 20 to 70 years of age.

The reason for the increased prevalence of autoantibodies with age is not completely understood. It is important to remember, as stated earlier, that all humans and experimental animals of any age are fully capable of producing autoantibodies (ie, we all have B cells programmed to produce all of the described autoantibodies). Indeed, we all have autoantibodies such as rheumatoid factor, antinuclear antibodies, antithyroid, and so on in our serum, but they are present at low levels that are not detected by means of the standard agglutination or immunofluorescence tests. Therefore, autoimmunity in aging is a matter of degree, and it presumably results from a failure of immunoregulation. The suggestion that the increase in autoantibodies with age is secondary to a loss of the T-cell control of B-cell function was supported by the report of a negative

association between PHA response and the presence of autoantibodies in elderly persons[46] (ie, the higher the proliferation of T cells to mitogens, the lower was the level of autoantibodies).

Stress, Immunity, and Aging

It has long been known that stress affects the occurrence of disease. Investigators in the field of physiologic psychology have described complex and direct links between the perceptual capabilities of the central nervous system and the immune system. For example, it is possible to elicit specific immune responses in animals with sensory cues. Ader and Cohen have performed a series of elegant taste-aversion learning experiments in rats.[47] In one of these studies, a flavored substance, saccharin water, was administered to the animals along with a dose of cyclophosphamide. Several days later, the animals were injected with sheep red blood cells, with or without readministration of the saccharin solution. Animals given the saccharin had profound suppression of hemagglutitin response to the sheep red blood cells.

The neurohumorally mediated effects of stress on the immune system have been well demonstrated in carefully controlled experiments with animals.[48] In primates, levels of cortisol and complement factors are profoundly affected by a single stressful event.[49] Studies in humans have demonstrated similar effects, though it is impossible to achieve the same degree of control as in the animal studies. Correlational studies have found that clusters of illness (from the common cold to cancer) occur around the time of major life changes.[50] More recent studies have found strong correlations between loneliness and decreased proliferative response of lymphocytes to mitogens, decreased natural killer cell activity, and impaired DNA splicing and repair in lymphocytes.[50,51] We found that healthy adults over the age of 60 years with a strong social support system (ie, a close confidant) had significantly lower serum uric acid levels and cholesterol levels,

Table 25.5. Autoantibodies and circulating immune complexes in healthy elderly subjects.*

Assay	Older subject		Young control group	
	Positive/Total tested	(% Positive)	Positive/Total tested	(% Positive)
Antinuclear antibody	50/278	(18)	4/98	(4)
Rheumatoid factor	38/278	(14)	4/98	(4)
Lymphocytotoxic antibody	27/278	(10)	3/93	(3)
Circulating immune complexes	43/197	(22)	5/100	(5)

*Adapted from Goodwin et al.[8] Positive results were defined as follows: for antinuclear antibody, a titer of >1 : 10; for rheumatoid factor, >1 : 20; for lymphocytotoxic antibody, >30% killing in >50% of the samples of peripheral blood lymphocytes from 11 healthy donors; and for circulating immune complexes, >2 SDs above the mean for a panel of normal control sera.

greater total lymphocyte counts, and a stronger immune response (mitogen-induced proliferation of lymphocytes) than those without such a relationship.[52] Being married has been correlated with lower mortality from any cause, in contrast to being single, widowed, or divorced.[53] The beneficial effects of social support appears to act at several different steps. For example, we found that married people with cancer tended to have their disease diagnosed at an earlier stage and were more likely to receive definitive treatment.[53] But even after controlling for stage at diagnosis and type of treatment, married people had a longer survival with cancer than did single, widowed, or divorced individuals.

Quasiexperimental or "natural" experiments also have linked stress to depressed immune function and illness. Several studies found depressed lymphocyte proliferation in response to mitogens after bereavement.[54] The stress of final examinations has been correlated with the recurrence of herpes simplex type I cold sores and rises in serum antibody titers against the virus.[55]

Old age is associated with a greater frequency of major life changes, such as loss of spouse or close friends, and changes in life-style due to retirement. Because of the decreased reserve in immune function with aging, elderly persons may be more sensitive to the effects of these stressful life events.

Infections in Older Adults

Immunizations

After infants and young children, older adults are the group most targeted for preventive immunization. Current recommendations are that adults over the age of 65 years be immunized against influenza, tetanus, and diphtheria on a regular basis and immunized against *Pneumococcus* at least once.[56] However, as noted in the preceding sections, this age group does not respond well to preventive immunizations as compared with adults between the ages of 20 and 40 years. In spite of this, there is evidence to suggest that immunizations can reduce the morbidity and mortality associated with the infections they are meant to prevent.[56] Specific examples will be presented in the following sections.

Influenza

Epidemiology and Clinical Presentation

Influenza is a common and important respiratory illness in elderly patients. The National Center for Health Statistics reported that 80–90% of the excess deaths

from influenza (40,000 per epidemic) from 1957–1986 occurred in adults who were older than 65 years.[57]

Influenza virus infection usually is manifested as a mild upper respiratory illness. In a typical case, the disease begins suddenly with chills, fever, and rhinorrhea. The systemic symptoms usually are more impressive than the respiratory complaints. Gastrointestinal manifestations are uncommon.

Influenza becomes clinically important when it occurs in elderly or debilitated patients and when it is complicated by bacterial pneumonia. Uncommonly, influenza may progress to influenza virus pneumonia. Increasing age and the presence of chronic diseases contribute to the risk of developing pneumonia with an influenza infection.[58] Examples of such chronic conditions are rheumatic or ischemic heart disease, hypertension with cardiac or renal complications, cerebrovascular disease, chronic obstructive pulmonary disease, chronic renal disease, diabetes, cirrhosis, epilepsy, and malignancy. The incidence rate of influenza pneumonia in persons over 45 years of age with no known risk factors is four per 100,000 persons.[59] If one risk factor is present, the incidence rises to 157 per 100,000. With two or more risk factors, the incidence of influenza pneumonia rises to 615 per 100,000. In addition to being a cause of both endemic and epidemic disease in the community, influenza virus infection has also been associated with outbreaks of respiratory illness in long-term care facilities.[59,60] In institutional outbreaks, there is also a correlation between susceptibility to influenza and increasing age.[60]

Prophylaxis and Treatment

The incidence and severity of influenza infections may be reduced by annual immunization or by the use of the antiviral agent amantadine.[57,61-63] The beneficial effects of immunization and amantadine are additive, and the use of both modalities has been suggested in high-risk groups.[61] Immunization is recommended for virtually all patients over 65 years of age and for younger patients with any of the chronic diseases listed above.[57]

Administration of influenza vaccine is clearly efficacious when epidemic and vaccine strains are similar.[57] There is a reduction in the incidence of pneumonia and hospitalization among immunized elderly persons. The mortality from influenza in high-risk, institutionalized elderly persons is reduced by up to 75%.[62] If the antigenic determinants of the wild-type viruses have "drifted" during the span of time it takes to manufacture and administer the vaccine, the incidence of influenza infection is still decreased.[62] Even when the vaccine's efficacy in preventing illness is low, it can still reduce the severity of infection, and reductions in morbidity and mortality remain substantial.[63]

Although approved since 1966 for the prevention of influenza A, amantadine has enjoyed only limited use in the United States. In healthy adults, amantadine is reported to be 70% to 100% effective in preventing clinical influenza. A comparative study of amantadine and rimantadine in a group of 450 volunteers showed that these two agents were similarly efficacious in preventing influenza.[61] Amantadine has also been shown to ameliorate the symptoms of influenza when therapy is started after an infection has occurred.

Unfortunately, side effects from amantadine are commonly seen in elderly persons. The reactions usually consist of mild but often disturbing central nervous system changes, such as dizziness, headache, interference with sleep patterns, and confusion. In a recent trial, 13% of patients stopped taking amantadine because of these adverse reactions. The incidence of side effects with rimantadine appears to be about half that of amantadine.[61]

Either of these drugs can be used in an influenza outbreak, especially in a long-term care institution, to prevent infection in susceptible elderly patients. Although it is reasonable to expect a reduction of both influenza disease and influenza-associated deaths, there are no data that clearly demonstrate the efficacy of these drugs in elderly patients. The recommended adult dosage for both amantadine hydrochloride and rimantadine hydrochloride is 200 mg/d, given in one or two doses. The dosage needs to be reduced in patients with impaired renal function.

Pneumonia

Epidemiology and Pathogenesis

An increased incidence and severity of pneumonia in elderly patients has been recognized for many years. About 50% of all cases of pneumonia that require hospitalization occur in adults over the age of 50.[64] Mortality from pneumonia also is higher in the elderly population. According to the National Center for Health Statistics, of the 65,561 people who died of pneumonia in 1985, 87% were over 65 years of age. An earlier study reported a mortality rate of 8% for patients under age 40 years hospitalized with pneumonia; this increased to 26% for those aged 40 to 69 years and 39% for those aged 70 years or older.[64]

About two thirds of all pneumonias in adults resulting in hospitalization are bacterial.[64] Of these, the overwhelming majority are caused by *Streptococcus pneumoniae*. The remaining third of cases is about equally divided between those in which no cause is identified and those in which nonbacterial (ie, viral, fungal, and protozoal) or mycoplasmal causes are found.

Past studies suggest that the pathogens responsible for pneumonia in elderly persons may be somewhat different than in younger age groups. In one study, 38% of all cases of pneumonia in patients over age 70 years were caused by gram-negative bacilli, compared with 10% in patients under age 40 years.[64] In a retrospective study of community-acquired bacterial pneumonia, the proportion of patients with gram-negative pneumonia was about three times greater in elderly than in younger subjects.[65]

It is thought that most cases of bacterial pneumonia develop after aspiration of minute quantities of saliva from the oropharynx. The aspiration of oral fluids has been shown to occur in healthy individuals during sleep. Other studies have documented the development of a respiratory colonization with gram-negative bacilli during hospitalization. In one study, 45% of 213 patients who were admitted to a medical intensive care unit developed respiratory tract colonization with gram-negative bacilli.[66] In 22% of this group, colonization developed on the first hospital day. A nosocomial respiratory infection occurred in 23% of the colonized patients but in only 3% of the patients not colonized with gram-negative bacilli. Nursing home patients also are at risk for pharangeal colonization with gram-negative organisms, and pneumonias acquired in nursing homes are more likely to be caused by gram-negative organisms.[67]

Clinical Presentation, Treatment, and Prophylaxis

The clinical evaluation of an elderly patient with respiratory illness requires special care, because signs and symptoms may not be as evident as in younger individuals. Tachypnea may be the only clue to lower respiratory infection in elderly patients.[68] Therapy should follow careful clinical evaluation. While most episodes of pneumonia in elderly persons result from infections due to organisms susceptible to commonly used antibiotics, the possibility of gram-negative pneumonia in elderly persons requires broad-spectrum initial therapy, unless there is clear evidence that *S pneumoniae* or *Haemophilus influenzae* is the cause. Therapy can be changed to more specific antibiotics once the results of cultures are available (see also Chapter 28).

Pneumococcal polysaccharide vaccine contains capsular carbohydrates from 23 pneumococcal types that are most often recovered from patients with bacteremic pneumococcal pneumonia. Although pneumococcal vaccine was available in the late 1940s, the introduction of penicillin resulted in an apathetic response to the vaccine by the medical community. A renewed interest in developing a vaccine to prevent pneumococcal diseases followed the observation that early mortality from pneumococcal pneumonia is not greatly affected by administration of antibiotics.[69]

There is general agreement that patients with a variety of chronic illnesses are at an increased risk of mortality from pneumococcal infection. Cardiac disease, chronic pulmonary disease, diabetes, sickle cell anemia, multiple myeloma, chronic renal failure, splenic dysfunction, and cirrhosis usually are cited as conditions that are associated with an increased risk of serious morbidity and mortality from pneumococcal infection. The effectiveness of the vaccine in healthy elderly persons has been a topic of debate for the better part of a decade. Several studies have found little evidence of efficacy.[70,71] However, the incidence of pneumococcal disease in one study was low, resulting in a small sample size.[70] In another, determination of vaccination status was inadequate.[71] Other recent case-control studies have compared elderly adults with culture-proved *S pneumoniae* infection with age- and sex-matched controls and estimated that the vaccine was about 70% effective.[72]

Approximately 50% of all patients immunized with the 23-valent pneumococcal vaccine develop erythema or mild pain at the site of the injection. Other adverse reactions have been uncommon. Unfortunately, significant local reactions following second doses of vaccine have been reported. For these reasons, and because the duration of protection resulting from vaccination is unknown, only a single immunization is recommended for adults at present. Pneumococcal vaccine and influenza vaccine can be given simultaneously without an increased incidence of side effects.

Tuberculosis

Epidemiology

Much of the recent epidemiology of tuberculosis has been described by William Stead of the University of Arkansas. Most of his work has dealt with the population of elderly patients in nursing homes in that state. In the early 1980s, Stead noted that the proportion of cases of active tuberculosis that occurred in adults over age 65 years had been increasing for more than 20 years, while decreasing for younger age groups. In Arkansas from 1981 to 1983, over 50% of all reported cases of tuberculosis occurred in adults over the age of 65 years, making the case rate three times greater than for adults between the ages of 40 and 60 years.[73] From 1977 to 1985, Stead and To[74] noted that the case rate for adults over age 65 years living in nursing homes was nearly five times higher than for adults of the same age living independently. In a survey of nearly all nursing home residents in the state of Arkansas, 12% of newly admitted persons were tuberculin positive.[73] For those

individuals who had been residing in a nursing home for at least 1 month, the percentage of tuberculin-positive responders was just under 21%.[73] For those who initially had a negative skin test, there was a 5% rate of conversion for each year spent living in a nursing home with a known infected case, and a 3.5% conversion rate for each year living in a home without a known infected case. Given these statistics, the recognition and control of the disease in the population of institutionalized adults is of considerable importance to public health workers and clinicians.

Diagnosis and Presentation in Older Adults

The utility of skin testing as a means of identifying tuberculosis infection in elderly persons is not well established. As mentioned previously, patients more than 60 years of age tend to have relative anergy to commonly applied skin test antigens, which implies that the efficacy of skin testing as a technique for detecting cases of tuberculosis in elderly persons may be overestimated.[5,74] A recent study of nearly 50,000 adults[74] supports the use of the two-stage tuberculin skin test. This survey found that 3% of untreated reactors developed clinical disease as opposed to 0.02% of nonreactors, a 150-fold increase. A negative response to high-dose purified protein derivative, (PPD) with positive controls, is good evidence for lack of tuberculosis exposure.

Tuberculosis in elderly persons may present with protean manifestations. Patients may have obscure hematologic findings as the only clue to disseminated disease.[75] Localized pulmonary, renal, gastrointestinal, or bone diseases also may occur.[75] Lymph node tuberculosis, which is particularly common in elderly women, usually presents as an insidious cervical mass that spontaneously begins to drain through the skin. Even uncomplicated pulmonary tuberculosis may present with atypical clinical and radiographic findings in elderly persons.[75] Tuberculosis should always be considered when there is evidence of an obscure infection in elderly patients.

Prophylaxis

In persons less than 35 years of age, preventive therapy for those with positive tuberculin skin tests is widely administered. The administration of isoniazid, at a dosage of 300 mg/d for adults, for a period of 12 months, significantly reduces the likelihood of clinical tuberculosis.[76] In the past, the preventive administration of isoniazid has been limited to younger individuals because of evidence that the risk of hepatitis associated with this drug increases significantly with advancing age.[76] Recently, evidence has been accumulating that preventive therapy with isoniazid is warranted in an older population. In their study of Arkansas nursing homes,[73] Stead et al compared the development of active disease in residents treated with isoniazid and those receiving no therapy. For residents with positive tuberculin skin tests and evidence of old pulmonary disease (ie, apical scarring on chest radiographs) or those receiving systemic corticosteroids, 0.8% treated with isoniazid developed active tuberculosis. For residents with the same characteristics who were not treated with isoniazid, 2.4% developed active disease. For residents who initially had negative tuberculin skin reactions (<10 mm of induration) and converted to positive reactions on retesting (>12 mm of induration), only 0.16% of those treated with isoniazid developed active disease. Of converters who were not treated with isoniazid, 5.9% developed active disease. The incidence of hepatic side effects or other drug intolerance (anorexia, nausea, vomiting, headache, somnolence, fever, rash) interfered with completion of preventive therapy in 10% of cases.[76] There was no evidence that the use of isoniazid contributed to mortality in the 7% of residents who died. The authors noted that the risk of developing clinical tuberculosis can be as high as 12% in elderly men whose tuberculin skin tests convert to positive. Preventive therapy with isoniazid is warranted in this group, or when the size of the tuberculin reaction is greater than 12 mm.[76] If signs of intolerance or hepatic toxicity develop, therapy should be stopped and hepatic function studies checked. If the aspartate aminotransferase level is less than five times the normal level, therapy may be reinstituted once the individual recovers[76] (see also Chapter 8).

Treatment of Active Tuberculosis

For adults with uncomplicated pulmonary tuberculosis, the daily administration of isoniazid and rifampin for a period of 9 months, or daily administration for 1 month followed by twice-weekly administration for another 8 months, is effective in curing the disease.[77] The same regimen appeared to be successful in 95% of patients with extrapulmonary disease.[77]

Screening in Nursing Home Employees and Residents

The recommendations for screening for tuberculosis in employees and residents of nursing homes vary somewhat from state to state. For example, long-term care facilities in Minnesota are required to demonstrate that their employees are free from tuberculosis. An employee must have had a negative Mantoux test within 45 days before employment began. If an individual has a positive tuberculin test or is known to have had a positive reaction to tuberculin skin tests in the past, a chest radiograph is required. The screening of

employees can be done using the two-step tuberculin test with PPD. If the first Mantoux test results in less than 10 mm of induration, a second test is administered 1 week later. The use of two tests is recommended to induce immunologic recall in previously infected persons.[74] The result of the second test is recorded as an employee's baseline. Retesting each year is not required; the interval between tests depends on the likelihood of exposure to tuberculosis within the nursing home.

If the Mantoux reaction is 10 mm or more, a chest radiograph is required. If there is evidence of apical scarring, preventive therapy is appropriate. Employees with positive skin tests and normal chest radiographs who complete either 1 year of preventive therapy or 5 years of annual chest radiographs are considered free of tuberculosis and are exempt from further screening.

For residents of nursing homes and board-and-care facilities, a Mantoux test is also required. As with employees, this enables an identification of current cases of tuberculosis and allows the establishment of a baseline if additional testing is needed. For residents older than 35 years of age, it is currently recommended that both a two-step tuberculin test and a chest radiograph be obtained at the time of admission to a long-term care facility. Repetitive skin testing is not presently recommended, unless patients are exposed to tuberculosis. Patients with positive skin tests or radiographs that are consistent with tuberculosis should be carefully evaluated to rule out active disease.

Septicemia

It has been reported that elderly persons are more vulnerable to sepsis than young persons and are at greater risk of death from such an infection.[78] The incidence rate of bacteremia, mortality from bacteremia, and the predominant organism found varies depending on the population being surveyed. A community-based population study found an increasing incidence of bacteremia with increasing age over 60 years.[79] The mortality rate in this group increased in the presence of serious underlying disease and increasing age over 70 years. The overall mortality rate from bacteremia was 9.1% for adults over the age of 70 years. Gram-negative bacilli acquired from a urinary tract infection accounted for over 50% of bacteremias. Adults over age 70 years are more likely to develop hospital-acquired bacteremias[78] Another study found similar results for adults over 60 years as well as a greater risk of developing a hospital-acquired septicemia during hospital stays longer than 7 days.[80]

Studies of bacteremia in institutionalized adults have found higher incidence rates than in community-dwelling adults and mortality rates of over 15%.[78] Gram-negative bacilli were also the most common organisms found, but polymicrobial infections (associated with a significantly higher mortality rate) were also more common than in community dwelling adults.[78]

Herpes Zoster

A clear age-associated increase in the incidence of infection is present in only two dermatologic infections: postoperative wound infection and herpes zoster. Two studies have demonstrated an increased infection rate in elderly patients with surgical wounds. In 38 hospitals in Great Britain, the incidence rate of surgical wound infections was highest in elderly persons.[81] Similar data also was developed by the National Research Council in this nation more than 20 years ago.

Herpes zoster is the other dermatologic infection that is particularly common in elderly persons. While recognized as a disease of immunocompromised persons, it is especially frequent in elderly individuals. The most extensive data about the epidemiology of herpes zoster were reported in a study conducted in Rochester, Minnesota, over a 15-year period.[82] There was a marked age-associated increase in the incidence of herpes zoster demonstrated in this study (Fig 25.3). The disease clearly is most common in patients over 75 years of age.

Herpes zoster is caused by the varicella-zoster virus that causes varicella, or chickenpox. After recovery from varicella, patients continue to harbor the varicella-zoster virus, probably in the dorsal root ganglia. Clinical evidence of an infection typically is absent for many years after the primary infection. It is likely that the zoster only results from a reactivation of previous varicella-zoster infections. Zoster does not appear to result from exposure to a patient with varicella.

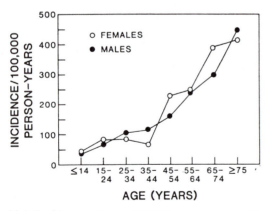

Fig. 25.3. Incidence rate per 100,000 person-years of herpes zoster among residents of Rochester, Minnesota, 1945 to 1959, by age and sex (from Ragozzino et al[86] Population-based study of herpes zoster and its sequelae. Medicine 61:310–316, © by Willams & Wilkins, 1982).

Factors that control the latency of the virus are unknown, but, in both elderly patients and patients with certain malignancies, a reactivation of the virus and development of zoster occurs. Cellular immunity against varicella zoster, as measured by cutaneous delayed-type hypersensitivity, gradually wanes with increasing age, beginning at 40 years.[83] Antibody levels, however, were found to be present in elderly patients. This suggests that the decline in cellular immunity with increasing age might be causally related to the reactivation of a varicella-zoster virus.

The cutaneous eruption in herpes zoster involves the trigeminal nerve, with periocular involvement in approximately 15% to 20% of affected patients. The remaining patients have involvement of the neck, trunk, and abdomen. The rash usually is unilateral and characteristically involves one to three dermatomes. Patients may have a prodrome of radicular pain before the onset of rash. The cutaneous lesion is similar to that of varicella, with a vesicle present on an erythematous base. Although all of the vesicles may appear at once, cutaneous lesions may continue to develop over several days following the initial onset. Particularly in patients with periocular involvement, there is often a confluent erythema with scattered vesicles present on the markedly inflamed skin.

Involvement of the nerves that supply the bladder or the anus may be associated with dysfunction of these organs. Symptoms of bladder involvement (usually those of cystitis or retention) typically occur 1 to 2 weeks after the onset of a rash.[84] Anal involvement may occur in association with bladder disease or as an isolated event. Most patients with involvement of these organs have cutaneous perineal zoster. Complete recovery of function is the rule.[84]

The dissemination of herpes zoster occurs in a minority of both immunocompromised and healthy individuals. Uncommonly, evidence of central nervous system and hepatic involvement may be seen.[85] The occurence of herpes zoster is not evidence of an underlying malignancy. Studies in which patients with zoster have been evaluated for evidence of occult malignancies have not been rewarding.[86]

Zoster is of particular importance in the older patient because of the frequent occurrence and disabling nature of postherpetic neuralgia. This complication is uncommon in patients less than 40 years of age. Over 50% of all persons more than 60 years of age develop postherpetic neuralgia that persists for more than 1 year.[82] A dramatic reduction in postherpetic pain has been reported in patients who were treated with corticosteroids.[87] Prednisolone is recommended at a dosage of 40 mg/d for 10 days, with a stepwise decrease over the next 3 weeks. When treated with prednisolone, 15% of affected patients had pain lasting for more than

2 months. In the control group, 65% of the patients had postherpetic neuralgia.[87] It is appropriate to question the use of corticosteroids in patients with an active viral infection, but the benefits may outweigh the associated risks. In healthy persons more than 50 years of age who develop herpes zoster, the use of glucocorticoids should be considered as a technique for reducing the incidence of postherpetic neuralgia.

Another study evaluated the role of levodopa in 47 patients with herpes zoster.[88] A significant reduction in the occurrence of postherpetic neuralgia was demonstrated 3 weeks after the end of treatment, but not after 60 days.

Tetanus and Diphtheria

Tetanus is a serious and often fatal disease. Of the 70 to 100 cases reported each year in the United States, nearly all occur in unimmunized adults. Elderly persons are at the greatest risk, with over 70% of all cases reported between 1982 and 1986 occurring in adults over the age of 50 years.[57] The overall case-fatality rate was 39%, but this was higher in the older age groups. It is estimated that only 34% to 51% of all adults over the age of 60 years have serum anti–tetanus toxoid antibody levels that are protective against tetanus.[57]

Diphtheria is quite rare, with only one to five cases reported each year in the United States.[57] Again, nearly all of these occur in unimmunized adults. Only 12% to 59% of adults over age 60 years have significant antibody levels against diphtheria toxin. This lack of protective serum antibody levels increases the risk of diphtheria outbreaks.[89]

Vaccination with tetanus toxoid is almost 100% effective in preventing the disease, while vaccination with diphtheria toxoid is at least 95% effective in preventing diphtheria. Physicians providing primary care for elderly individuals should remember that tetanus-diphtheria toxoids need to be administered to elderly patients at the same interval that is recommended for other adults (ie, every 10 years).

Acquired Immunodeficiency Syndrome

The acquired immunodeficiency syndrome, or AIDS, has been in the forefront of the medical news from the early 1980s to the present. The viral pathogen, the human immunodeficiency virus (HIV) attacks the T4 epitope on helper lymphocytes, monocytes, and glial cells.[90] These cells of the immune system provide a reservoir for the virus. Virtually 100% of those shown to be infected with the HIV virus will develop the full-blown syndrome of AIDS, with lag periods of anywhere from several months to 15 years. The clinical syndrome includes infections with organisms that do not normally cause disease in immunocompetent humans, and the occurrence of uncommon malignancies such as Kaposi's sarcoma.

From June 1981 through April of 1988, close to 60,000 cases of full-blown AIDS had been reported, with 51% reported between January 1987 and April 1988.[91] It is estimated that, as of 1988, 1 to 2 million persons in the United States have been infected with the virus. Deaths due to AIDS have led to a 0.7% increase in the overall male mortality rate and a 0.07% increase in the overall female mortality rate. Groups at high risk for infection include homosexual men, hemophiliacs, Haitian immigrants, and intravenous drug abusers, as well as their infants and sexual partners. The rates in blacks and hispanics tend to be three to 12 times greater than for whites with the same risk factors. Estimates of the rate of infection in the general heterosexual population vary widely, from 0% to 2.6%.[91]

While the vast majority of cases occur in individuals under the age of 40 years, a small percentage has occurred in older adults. Table 25.6 gives the percentage of all AIDS cases by deciles in adults over the age of 60 years.

Published reports of AIDS in older adults are sketchy at best.[92–95] Most of these cases are associated with a history of blood transfusion in the period before the national blood supplies were rigorously tested for HIV. In older persons, AIDS can present more subtly, with symptoms that are seen often in this age group. These include rheumatologic complaints, dementia, and wasting syndromes. There is some evidence that the disease progresses more rapidly in elderly persons.[96] AIDS should be added to the differential diagnosis of dementia and delerium in elderly persons and must be considered in the presence of opportunistic infections and evidence of immunocompromise.

Prospects for Therapeutic Intervention in the Age-Related Decline in Immune Function

It is perhaps premature to discuss potential methods of reversing the age-related decline in immune function when it is not clear that depressed immune function is

Table 25.6. Percentage of AIDS cases in adults over age 60 years by deciles.*

Age, y	% of Total AIDS cases
60–70	2.3
70–80	0.6
>80	0.1

*Personal communication from Harold Jaffe, MD, Centers for Disease Control, 1988.

an independent risk factor for anything. The few studies that link a disordered immune function with subsequent morbidity and mortality are suggestive but far from conclusive. One of the major purposes of our longitudinal study of 300 healthy older men and women is to determine if there is a greater risk of death or specific illnesses in persons who are anergic to skin testing or who have high levels of autoantibodies or circulating immune complexes. The above misgivings notwithstanding, we conclude with a brief discussion of the potential ways to stimulate a failing immune system in elderly persons.

Often, the most intriguing scientific discoveries are those that also are without an obvious practical consequence. A prime example was the discovery by McCay and his colleagues in 1935 that caloric restriction of experimental animals markedly prolonged their life span.[97] These investigators reported that restricting the total caloric intake to 50% to 60% of what is required to maintain normal growth in adolescent mice, rats, and guinea pigs resulted in an approximately 50% prolongation of the total life span of animals that survived the 6- to 12-month period of starvation. This interesting medical oddity received little attention over the next 3 decades until other investigators showed that the early starvation of experimental animals resulted in a preservation of normal immune function into old age.[29] The possibility that lesser amounts of caloric restriction, supplemented with essential nutrients, might have a similar beneficial effect in humans is now being seriously discussed,[29] although it has not been formally tested.

Because thymic atrophy seems central to the loss of immunocompetence with aging, an obvious group of strategies to reverse the decline involves injecting extracts of young thymic tissue, administering thymic hormones, or transplanting young thymic tissue into aging animals.[29] A variety of in vivo and in vitro experimental procedures have indicated that, in certain situations, any of the above strategies can lead to a restoration of immunocompetence in some functions of an aging immune system.[98,99] Various preparations of thymic hormones or the active portions of these hormones can be chemically synthesized or produced via recombinant DNA technology, which means that large amounts could be made available if such preparations proved efficacious. It is not yet clear whether thymic hormone administration has any effect on the life span of experimental animals.

Another potential means of preventing age-related declines in immunity is immunopharmacologic—administering drugs that in one way or another stimulate immune function. In this regard, prostaglandin synthetase inhibitors, such as the nonsteroidal anti-inflammatory drugs (NSAID), have received increasing attention. By reducing the production of the feedback inhibitor prostaglandin E_2, NSAIDs stimulate immune responses in vitro and in vivo.[21] For example, two of our patients with an adult-acquired immunodeficiency who were completely anergic became responsive to delayed-type hypersensitivity skin testing when they were treated with the cyclooxygenase inhibitor indomethacin.[100] Such therapeutic strategy might be especially relevant to elderly persons, because their T cells are more sensitive to inhibition by prostaglandin E_2, which partially accounts for the depressed proliferative response to mitogens.[18] Recent evidence suggests that prostaglandin synthetase inhibitors also might reduce the increase in autoantibody production that occurs with age,[101] while stimulating the primary antibody response to new antigens.[45]

The above examples of the potential methods of immunostimulation are representative of the many therapies that have been proposed and/or tested. All these attempts at immunostimulation violate a basic conservative tenet in medicine of leaving well enough alone. It is difficult, if not impossible, to justify intervention in a healthy individual with a disordered laboratory parameter (such as low PHA response or skin test anergy), especially when the intervention is not benign (and no intervention is), unless it has been clearly shown that: (1) the disordered laboratory parameter is associated with an increased risk of morbidity and mortality and (2) this intervention reduces that risk. Neither criterion has been met for the age-related decline in immune function.

References

1. Makinodan T. Biology of aging: Retrospect and prospect. In: Makinodan T, Yunis E, eds. *Immunology and Aging.* New York, NY: Plenum Press, 1977:1–8.
2. Erlich P. Uber den jetzigen stano der karzinomforschung. *Ned Tijdschr Geneeskd* 1909;53:273–290.
3. Burnet FM. The concept of immunological surveillance. *Prog Exp Tumor Res* 1970;13:1–27.
4. Thomas L. Reactions to homologous tissue antigens in relation to hypersensitivity. In: Lawrence HS, ed. *Cellular and Humoral Aspects of the Hypersensitivity States.* New York, NY: Hoeber-Harper; 1959:529–532.
5. Roberts-Thompson IC, Whittingham S, Young-Chaiyud U, et al. Aging, immune response and mortality. *Lancet* 1974;2:368–370.
6. Abridged life tables by color and sex: United States, 1977. *Monthly vital Stat Rep* 1974;4.
7. Murasko DM, Weiner P, Kaye D. Association of lack of mitogen-induced lymphocyte proliferation with increased mortality in the elderly. *Aging: Immunol Infect Disease.* 1988;1:1–6.
8. Goodwin JS, Searles RP, Tung KSK. Immunological responses of a healthy elderly population. *Clin Exp Immunol* 1982;48:403–410.

9. Wayne S, Rhyne R, Garry P, et al. Cell mediated immunity as a predictor of morbidity and mortality in the aged. *J. Gerontol*. In Press.

10. Minick CR, Murphy GE, Campbell WG. Experimental induction of athero-arteriosclerosis by the synergy of allergic injury to arteries and lipid rich diet. *J Exp Med* 1966;124:635–652.

11. Howard AN, Paterski J, Bowyer DE, et al. Atherosclerosis induced in hypercholesterolemic baboons by immunologic injury. *Atherosclerosis* 1971;14:17–29.

12. Clarkson RB, Alexander NJ. Long term vasectomy: effects on the occurrence and extent of atherosclerosis in rhesus monkeys. *J Clin Invest* 1980;65:15–25.

13. Ansbacher R, Keung-Yeung K, Wurster JC. Sperm antibodies in vasectomized men. *Fertil Steril* 1972;23:640–643.

14. Mackay IR, Whittingham SF, Mathews JD. The immunoepidemiology of aging. In: Makinodan T, Yunis E, eds. *Immunology and Aging* New York, NY: Plenum Press; 1977:35–50.

15. Hess EV, Knapp D. The immune system and aging: a case of the cart before the horse. *J Chronic Dis* 1978;31:647–649.

16. Czlonkowska A, Korlak J. The immune response during aging. *J Gerontol* 1979;34:9–14.

17. Inkeles B, Innes JB, Kuntz MM, et al. Immunological studies of aging, III: cytokinetic basis for the impaired response of lymphocytes from aged humans to plant lectins. *J Exp Med* 1977;145:1176–1187.

18. Goodwin JS, Messner RP. Sensitivity of lymphocytes to prostaglandin E2 increases in subjects over age 70. *J Clin Invest* 1979;64:434–439.

19. Portaro JK, Glick GI, Zighelboim J. Population immunity: age and immune cell parameters. *Clin Immunol Immunopathol* 1978;11:339–350.

20. Goodwin JS. Changes in lymphocyte sensitivity to prostaglandin E, histamine, hydrocortisone, and X-irradiation with age: studies in a healthy elderly population. *Clin Immunol Immunopathol* 1982;25:243–251.

21. Goodwin JS, Webb DR. Regulation of the immune response by prostaglandins: a critical review. *Clin Immunol Immunopathol* 1981;15:116–132.

22. Gillis S, Kozak R, Duranke M, et al. Immunological studies of aging: decreased production of and response to T cell growth factor by lymphocytes from aged humans. *J Clin Invest* 1981;67:937–942.

23. Negoro S, Hara H, Miyata S, et al. Mechanisms of age-related decline in antigen-specific T cell proliferative response: IL-2 receptor expression and recombinant IL-2 induced proliferative response of purified Tac-positive T cells. *Mech Ageing Dev* 1986;36:223–241.

24. Gilman SC, Rosenberg JS, Feldman JD. T lymphocytes of young and old rats. *J Immunol* 1982;128:644–650.

25. Wu W, Pahlavani M, Cheung HT, et al. The effect of aging on the expression of interleukin 2 messenger ribonucleic acid. *Cell Immunol* 1986;100:224–231.

26. Gutowski JK, Cohen S. Induction of DNA synthesis in isolated nuclei by cytoplasmic factors from spontaneously proliferating and mitogen-activated lymphoid cells. *Cell Immunol* 1983;75:300–311.

27. Gutowski JK, Innes JB, Weksler ME, et al. Impaired nuclear responsiveness to cytoplasmic signals in lympyhocytes from elderly humans with depressed proliferative responses. *J Clin Invest* 1986;78:40–43.

28. Lewis V, Twomey J, Bealmear P, et al. Age, thymic function and circulating thymic hormone activity. *J Clin Endocrinol Metab* 1978;47:145–152.

29. Walford RL, Meridith PJ, Cheney KE. Immunoengineering: prospects for correction of age-related immunodeficiency states. In: Makinodan T, Yunis E, eds. *Immunology and Aging*. New York, NY: Plenum Press; 1977:183–201.

30. Effros RB, Casillas A, Walford RL. The effect of thymosin-1 on immunity to influenza in aged mice. *Aging: Immunol Infect Dis* 1988;1:31–40.

31. Delafuente JC. Immunosenescence: clinical and pharmacologic considerations. *Med Clin North Am* 1985;69:475–486.

32. Howells CH, Vesselinova-Jenkins CK, Evans AD, et al. Influenza vaccination and mortality from bronchopneumonia in the elderly. *Lancet* 1975;1:381–83.

33. Ershler WB, Moore Al, Socinski MA. Influenza and aging: age-related changes and the effects of thymosin on the antibody response to influenza vaccine. *J Clin Immunol* 1984;4:445–454.

34. Kishimoto S, Tomino S, Mitsuya H, et al. Age-related decline in the in vitro and in vivo synthesis of anti-tetanus toxoid antibody in humans. *J Immunol* 1980;125:2347–2352.

35. Whittingham S, Buckley JD, Mackay IR. Factors influencing the secondary antibody response to flagellin in man. *Clin Exp Immunol* 1978;34:170–178.

36. Gerbase-Delima M, Wilkinson J, Smith G, et al. Age related decline in thymic-independent immune function in a long-lived mouse strain. *J Gerontol* 1974;29:261–268.

37. Kishimoto S, Tomino S, Mitsuya H, et al. Age-related changes in suppressor functions of human T cells. *J Immunol* 1979;123:1586–1592.

38. Cueppens JL, Goodwin JS. Regulation of immunoglobulin production in pokeweed mitogen-stimulated cultures of lymphocytes from young and old adults. *J Immunol* 1982;128:2429–2434.

39. Rodriguez M, Cueppens J, Goodwin JS. Regulation of IgM rheumatoid factor production in lymphocyte cultures from young and old subjects. *J Immunol* 1982;128:2422–2428.

40. Friedman D, Globerson A. Immune reactivity during aging: analysis of the cellular mechanisms involved in the deficient antibody response in old mice. *Mech Ageing Dev*. 1978;7:299–310.

41. Callard R, Basten A, Blanden R. Loss of immune competence with age may be due to a qualitative abnormality in lymphocyte membranes. *Nature* 1979;281:218–221.

42. Kishimoto S, Tomino S, Mitsuya H, et al. Age-related decrease in frequencies of B-cell precursors and specific helper T cells involved in the IgG anti-tetanus toxoid antibody production in humans. *Clin Immunol Immunopathol* 1982;25:1–10.

43. Goodwin JS, Bankhurst AD, Messner RP. Suppression

of human T cell mitogenesis by prostaglandin. *J Exp Med* 1977;146:1719–34.

44. Delfraissey J, Galanaud P, Wallon C, et al. Abolished in vitro antibody response in the elderly: exclusive involvement of prostaglandin-induced T suppressor cells. *Clin Immunol Immunopathol* 1982;24:377–385.

45. Delespesse G, Gausset PH, Sarfati M, et al. Circulating immune complexes in old people and in diabetics: correlation with autoantibodies. *Clin Exp Immunol* 1980; 40:96–102.

46. Hallgren H, Buckley C, Gilbertson V, et al. Lymphocyte phytohemagglutinin responsiveness, immunoglobulins, and autoantibodies in aging humans. *J Immunol* 1973;111:1101–1107.

47. Ader R, Cohen N. Conditioned immunopharmacologic responses. In: Ader R, ed. *Psychoneuroimmunology*. Orlando, Fla: Academic Press Inc; 1981:281–317.

48. Borysenko M, Borysenko J. Stress, behavior and immunity: animal models and mediating mechanisms. *Gen Hosp Psychiatry* 1982;4:59–67.

49. Rosenberg LT, Coe CL, Levine S. Complement levels in the squirrel monkey. *Lab Anim Sci* 1982;32:371–372.

50. Minter RE, Patterson-Kimball C. Life events and illness onset: a review. *Psychosomatics* 1978;19:334–339.

51. Glaser R, Thorn BE, Tarr KL, et al. Effects of stress on methyltransferase synthesis: an important DNA repair enzyme. *Health Psych* 1985;4:403–412.

52. Thomas PD, Goodwin JM, Goodwin JS. Effect of social support on stress-related changes in cholesterol level, uric acid level and immune function in an elderly sample. *Am J Psych* 1985;142:735–737.

53. Goodwin JS, Hunt WC, Kay CR, et al. The effect of marital status on stage, treatment and survival of cancer patients. *JAMA* 1987;255:3125–3130.

54. Schleifer SJ, Keller SE, Camerino M, et al. Suppression of lymphocyte function following bereavement. *JAMA* 1983;250:374–377.

55. Glaser R, Kiecolt-Glaser JK, Speicher CE, et al. The relationship of stress and loneliness and changes in herpes virus latency. *J Behav Med* 1985;8:249–260.

56. Williams WW, Hickson MA, Kane MA, et al. Immunization policies and vaccine coverage among adults. *Ann Intern Med* 1988;108:616–625.

57. ACIP. Prevention & control of Influenza: Part I, Vaccines. *MMWR* 1989;38:297–311.

58. Barker WH, Mullooly JP. Pneumonia and influenza deaths during epidemics: implications and prevention. *Arch Intern Med* 1982;142:85–89.

59. Mathur U, Bentley DW, Hall CB, et al. Influenza A/Brazil/78(H1N1) infection in the elderly. *Am Rev Respir Dis* 1981;123:633–635.

60. Hall WN, Goodman RA, Noble GR, et al. An outbreak of influenza B in an elderly population. *J Infect Dis* 1981;144:297–302.

61. Douglas RG Jr. Amantadine as an antiviral agent in influenza. *N Engl J Med* 1982;307:617–618.

62. Gross PA, Quinnan GV, Rodstein M, et al. Association of influenza immunization with reduction in mortality in an elderly population. *Arch Intern Med* 1988;148:562–565.

63. Arden NH, Patriarca PA, Kendal AP. Experiences in the use and efficacy of inactivated influenza vaccine in nursing homes. In: Kendal AP, Patriarca PA, eds. *Options for the Control of Influenza*. New York, NY: Alan R Liss Inc; 1986:155–168.

64. Sullivan RJ Jr, Dowdle WR, Marine WM, et al. Adult pneumonia in a general hospital. *Arch Intern Med* 1972;129:935–942.

65. Ebright JR, Rytel MW. Bacterial pneumonia in the elderly. *J Am Geriatr Soc* 1980;28:220–223.

66. Johanson WB, Pierce AK, Sanford JP, et al. Nosocomial respiratory infections with gram-negative bacilli: the significance of colonization of the respiratory tract. *Ann Intern Med* 1972;77:701–706.

67. Irwin RS, Whitaker S, Pratter MR, et al. The transiency of oropharyngeal colonization with gram-negative bacilli in residents of a skilled nursing facility. *Chest* 1982;81:31–35.

68. McFadden JP, Price RC, Eastwood HD, et al. Raised respiratory rate in elderly patients: a valuable physical sign. *Br Med J* 1982;284:626–627.

69. Austrian R, Gold J. Pneumococcal bacteremia with especial reference to bacteremic pneumococcal pneumonia. *Ann Intern Med* 1964;60:759–776.

70. Forrester HL, Jahnigen DW, LaForce FM. Inefficacy of pneumococcal vaccine in a high-risk population. *Am J Med* 1987;83:425–430.

71. Simberkoff MS, Cross AP, Al-Ibrahim M, et al. Efficacy of pneumococcal vaccine in high-risk patients: results of a Veterans Administration Cooperative Study. *N Engl J Med* 1986;315:1318–1327.

72. Sims RV, Steinmann WC, McConville JH, et al. The clinical effectiveness of pneumococcal vaccine in the elderly. *Ann Intern Med* 1988;108:653–657.

73. Stead WW, Lofgren JP, Warren E, et al. Tuberculosis as an endemic and nosocomial infection among the elderly in nursing homes. *N Engl J Med* 1985;312:1483–1487.

74. Stead WW, To T. The significance of the tuberculin skin test in elderly persons. *Ann Intern Med* 1987;107:837–42.

75. Slavin RE, Walsh TJ, Pollack AD. Late generalized tuberculosis: clinical pathologic analysis and comparison of 100 cases in the preantibiotic and antibiotic era. *Medicine* 1980;59:352–366.

76. Stead WW, To T, Harrison RW, et al. Benefit-risk considerations in preventive therapy for tuberculosis in elderly persons. *Ann Intern Med* 1987;107:843–845.

77. Dutt AK, Moers D, Stead WW. Short-course chemotherapy for extrapulmonary tuberculosis: nine years' experience. *Ann Intern Med* 1986;104:7–12.

78. Hontanosas A, Cohen Z, Rudman D. Bactermia in a veteran's administration extended care facility. *Prog Clin Biol Res* 1988;264:243–253.

79. McCue JD. Gram-negative bacillary bacteremia in the elderly: incidence, ecology, etiology, and mortality. *J Am Geriatr Soc* 1987;35:213–218.

80. Saviteer SM, Samsa GP, Rutala WA. Nosocomial infections in the elderly: increased risk per hospital day. *Am J Med* 1988;84:661–666.

81. Ayliffe GAJ, Brightwell KM, Collins BJ, et al. Surveys

of hospital infection in the Birmingham region, I: effect of age, sex, length of stay and antibiotic use on nasal carriage of tetracycline-resistant *Staphylococcus aureus* and on postoperative wound infection. *J Hyg (Camb)* 1977;79:299–314.

82. Ragozzino MW, Melton LJ III, Kurland LT, et al. Population-based study of herpes zoster and its sequelae. *Medicine* 1982;61:310–316.

83. Burke BL, Steele RW, Beard OW, et al. Immune responses to varicella-zoster in the aged. *Arch Intern Med* 1982;142:291–293.

84. Jellinek EH, Tulloch WS. Herpes zoster with dysfunction of bladder and anus. *Lancet* 1976;2:1291–1222.

85. Mazur MH, Dolin R. Herpes zoster at the NIH: a 20 year experience. *Am J Med* 1978;65:738–744.

86. Ragozzino MW, Melton LJ III, Kurland LT, et al. Risk of cancer after herpes zoster: a population-based study. *N Engl J Med* 1982;307:393–397.

87. Keczkes K, Basheer AM. Do corticosteroids prevent post-herpetic neuralgia? *Br J Dermatol* 1980;102:551–555.

88. Kernbaum S, Hauchecorne J. Administration of levodopa for relief of herpes zoster pain. *JAMA* 1981;246:132–134.

89. Karzon DT, Edwards KM. Diphtheria outbreaks in immunized populations. *N Engl J Med* 1988;318:41–43.

90. Gallo RC, Wong-Staal F. A human T-lymphotrophic retrovirus (HTLV-III) as the cause of AIDS. *Ann Intern Med* 1985;103:679–689.

91. Curran JW, Jaffe HW, Hardy AM, et al. Epidemiology of HIV and AIDS in the United States. *Science* 1988;293:610–616.

92. Chamberland ME, Castro KG, Haverkos HW, et al. Acquired immunodeficiency syndrome in the United States: an analysis of cases outside high-incidence groups. *Ann Intern Med* 1984;101:617–623.

93. McCormick A, Tillett H, Bannister B, et al. Surveillance of AIDS in the United Kingdom. *Br Med J* 1987;295:1466–1469.

94. Baker L, Kelen GD, Sivertson KT, et al. Unsuspected human immunodeficiency virus in critically ill emergency patients. *JAMA* 1987;257:2609–2611.

95. Lennox, JL, Redfield RJ, Burke DS. HIV Antibody screening in a general hospital population. *JAMA* 1987;257:2914.

96. Steel M. IVth International AIDS Conference. *Lancet* 1988;2:54–55.

97. McCay C, Crowell M, Maynard L. The effects of retarded growth upon the length of life span and upon the ultimate body size. *J Nutr* 1935;10:63–79.

98. Duchateau J, Servais G, Vreyens R, et al. Modulation of immune response in aged humans through different administration modes of thymopentin. *Surv Immunol Res* 1985;4:(suppl 1):94–101.

99. Ershler WB, Moore AL, Hacker MP, et al. Specific antibody synthesis in vitro, II: age-associated thymosin enhancement of antitetanus antibody synthesis. *Immunopharmacology* 1984;8:69–77.

100. Goodwin JS, Bankhurst A, Murphy S, et al. Partial reversal of the cellular immune defect in common variable immunodeficiency with indomethacin. *J Clin Lab Immunol* 1978;1:197–199.

101. Cueppens J Rodriguez M, Goodwin JS. Nonsteroidal anti-inflammatory drugs inhibit the production of IgM rheumatoid factor in vitro. *Lancet* 1982;1:528–531.

26

Hematology

Melinda A. Lee and John R. Walsh

Anemia, monoclonal gammopathies, chronic lymphocytic leukemia (CLL), and myeloproliferative disorders are more common in elderly people. Despite an increasing prevalence, their detection may be delayed because many signs and symptoms may be attributed by both patients and providers to the aging process itself.

Anemia

The prevalence of anemia increases with each decade. Estimates of prevalence range from 12% to 20% in elderly persons,[1,2] compared with 2% for all ages. Studies suggest that the underlying causes of anemia are distributed differently in the elderly than in the young adult population. Symptoms may be more severe in elderly patients or may be expressed in unusual ways. Despite research in the area, many questions about the effects of age on bone marrow function and reserve capacity remain unanswered.

Adult men with a hemoglobin concentration below 14 g/dL or women with a concentration below 12 g/dL are considered at risk for anemia. A decrease of 1 to 2 g/dL below this value is accepted as probably normal in men older than 70 years of age, because of decreased androgen function. With this exception, the normal adult red blood cell (RBC) parameters are considered to apply to elderly individuals, based on studies in healthy, ambulatory elderly persons.[1,3] Earlier studies, showing a decrease in the mean RBC count, hemoglobin concentration, and hematocrit of aging persons,[2,4] may have included patients with chronic disease or nutritional problems. Even in younger persons, there is an overlap at the lower end of the hemoglobin and hematocrit range between values that signify disease and those that do not, because the distribution curves are skewed toward the lower end.

Anemia should be considered a sign of underlying disease in adults of all ages. Iron deficiency and chronic disease have been reported to account for the majority of anemias in elderly persons, followed in prevalence by vitamin B_{12} and folate deficiency anemias. The remaining cases are sideroblastic, myelophthisic, aplastic, and hemolytic anemias, or anemia due to protein-calorie malnutrition. Recent work suggests that, after extensive evaluation, most cases of anemia remain unexplained in this age group.[5,6] Whether age itself, subclinical nutritional deficiency, or undetected chronic disease is responsible for unexplained anemia in elderly persons is not known at this time.

Symptoms characteristic of anemia, such as fatigue, weakness, and dyspnea, may be nonspecific in elderly persons because of the declining functional reserve capacity of other organ systems. Because of this decline in functional reserve, anemia may produce symptoms at higher hemoglobin concentrations in elderly persons than in young persons. For example, a person with underlying cognitive impairment may experience confusion or memory loss with even mild anemia. Coexisting diseases, such as congestive heart failure, coronary artery disease, and postural hypotension, can be aggravated by anemia in older individuals. Moreover, functional disability may be induced or worsened by fatigue and weakness from anemia.

Evaluation of the elderly patient with anemia begins with a complete blood cell count, including RBC indexes, a reticulocyte index, and examination of the peripheral smear. The stool should be examined for occult blood. Based on the RBC indexes and/or appearance of the erythrocytes, the anemia is categorized as microcytic, normocytic, or macrocytic. The finding of a microcytic anemia suggests iron deficiency, chronic disease, or sideroblastic anemia. A normocytic anemia is consistent with chronic disease, protein-calorie malnutrition, and sideroblastic, hemolytic, or hypoproliferative anemia. Macrocytic indexes stimulate a search for folate or vitamin B_{12} deficiency, but may also occur in hypothyroidism, liver disease, or sideroblastic anemia. The appropriate tests of serum iron, total iron-binding capacity (TIBC), ferritin, folate, vitamin B_{12}, or overall nutritional status are obtained, as indicated. A specific diagnosis always should be sought. If iron deficiency is the cause, a source of blood loss should be located and corrected, if possible. If no specific diagnosis is found to explain the anemia, the clinician must continue to follow up the patient at appropriate intervals for evidence of underlying disease. At the present time, there is insufficient evidence to attribute anemia solely to the effects of aging in elderly persons.

Iron Deficiency Anemia

Iron deficiency is characterized by symptoms not only of reduced hemoglobin synthesis, but also of impaired function of iron-dependent tissue enzymes, particularly with exercise. For this reason, minimal decreases in the hemoglobin concentration due to iron deficiency may cause profound functional disabilities in an elderly patient. Several studies suggest that impaired physical performance due to iron deficiency improves with iron replacement even before the hemoglobin concentration increases.[7,8] This improvement is attributed to changes in α-glycerophosphate–mediated phosphorylation, rather than to muscle cytochrome or myoglobin concentrations.

Severe iron deficiency anemia is characterized by hypochromia, a low reticulocyte index, and evidence for depleted bone marrow iron stores. In young adults and in many older patients, this includes a low serum iron level, high transferrin level or TIBC, low transferrin saturation, low serum ferritin level, and absent bone marrow iron stores. These guidelines may be misleading in some elderly persons, however, since the serum iron level has been reported to decrease progressively

with each decade and in the presence of a neoplasm, infection, or inflammation, even when bone marrow iron stores are normal.[9] A recent study of healthy, ambulatory persons older than 65 years of age found no significant decrease in the serum iron level with age, suggesting that undetected chronic disease, rather than age, may account for the findings in previous studies.[10] The serum transferrin level may be decreased in elderly persons,[10] presumably due to coexisting chronic disease or protein-calorie malnutrition. As a consequence of these changes in both the serum iron and transferrin values, the transferrin saturation may be greater than 15%, the value below which iron deficiency is considered to be likely in younger individuals.

The serum ferritin level reflects storage iron and, like bone marrow stores, increases with age.[10,11] The increase in the serum ferritin level is greatest in postmenopausal women. The serum ferritin level is also elevated in inflammatory states, liver disease, iron-overload states, and neoplastic diseases. Although the serum ferritin level occasionally may be normal in the presence of low or absent marrow stores, when it is low, the ferritin level reliably predicts depleted bone marrow stores.[12] A serum ferritin level below 12 μg/L may be the most specific test for iron deficiency in elderly persons, with a cutoff value of 50 μg/L suggestive of iron deficiency anemia in the setting of known inflammatory disease.[13]

Iron deficiency anemia in elderly persons infrequently is due to dietary causes. The iron content of the US diet ranges from 10 to 20 mg/d.[10,14] Several studies have demonstrated that iron intake in most older persons is adequate, although it may be below the recommended dietary allowance (RDA) of 10 mg in certain subgroups, such as institutionalized persons or black women older than 59 years of age.[14] With aging, the dietary sources of iron shift from meat to cereal.[14] When healthy elderly persons without gastrointestinal disease were studied, there was no impairment of iron absorption from the gut with aging, but uptake of iron by RBCs was decreased, suggesting an element of ineffective erythropoiesis in this population.[15] Iron absorption is enhanced by anemia, hypoxia, and chronic liver disease and is also affected by substances in the diet: oxalates in tea and phosphates in antacids complex with iron and inhibit absorption, while ascorbic acid and meat proteins improve absorption.

In both elderly and younger adults, iron deficiency usually is a result of blood loss, and the finding of iron deficiency mandates a search for a bleeding lesion. Chronic gastrointestinal blood loss in older patients commonly is from benign upper tract lesions, gastrointestinal cancer, vascular malformations, diverticular disease, and inflammatory bowel disease. In addition, many drugs frequently consumed by elderly patients, such as aspirin, nonsteroidal anti-inflammatory agents, alcohol, and steroids, may cause gastrointestinal bleeding.

The safest treatment for iron deficiency anemia is oral iron replacement. Ferrous sulfate, 300 mg three times each day, is the least expensive oral preparation and is tolerated well by many older people. At this dose, ferrous sulfate supplies 180 mg of elemental iron. Gastrointestinal upset may be minimized by having the patient take iron supplements with meals and by gradually increasing from one to three doses per day during 3 weeks. If tablets are not tolerated, ferrous sulfate elixir or pediatric solution may be given. The anemia should correct within 6 weeks, although therapy should continue for 6 to 12 months to replenish iron stores. Parenteral therapy with iron dextran (Imferon) is indicated only when patients are noncompliant, intolerant of oral therapy, have continuous bleeding from an uncorrected source, or have gastrointestinal disease that interferes with oral iron absorption. Older patients are more prone to the adverse effects of parenteral iron, such as anaphylactoid reactions, hypotension, urticaria, and the syndrome of delayed lymphadenopathy, myalgia, and headache. Iron dextran (50 mg/mL) is given intramuscularly or, in some instances, intravenously. Patients who have suffered acute blood loss may receive some iron replacement as transfused RBCs. Packed RBCs contain 1 mg of iron per milliliter.

Anemia of Chronic Disease

Anemia may be associated with chronic inflammatory diseases, neoplastic diseases, and chronic infections. The anemia usually is mild to moderate, with hematocrit values ranging from 27% to 35%. Red blood cells are most often normocytic, but, in some instances, are hypochromic. Anemia of chronic disease (ACD) is due to both a shortened RBC life span and a production defect in the marrow. Phagocytes release lactoferrin into plasma during inflammatory states under the influence of interleukin 1. Lactoferrin binds iron, removes it from transferrin, and delivers it to mononuclear phagocytes, thereby interfering with its incorporation into erythrocyte precursors for hemoglobin synthesis. The reticulocyte index is decreased in ACD. Serum iron and TIBC levels are low, and transferrin saturation is usually 15% to 30%. The increased iron stored in reticuloendothelial cells is reflected in an elevated serum ferritin level. Treatment of uncomplicated ACD involves treatment of the underlying disorder. Because these patients have sufficient iron stores, they do not require iron therapy.

Iron deficiency and chronic inflammation may coexist, however, especially in elderly patients. Patients with chronic inflammatory disease, liver disease, or malignant neoplasms have serum ferritin values over 50 μg/L unless iron deficiency is present concomitantly. Most patients with ferritin values above 50 μg/L have stainable bone marrow iron.[16] When the serum ferritin level is less than 25 μg/L in a patient with ACD, associated iron deficiency is highly likely. A 2-month trial of iron replacement may be justified even in a patient with ACD whose serum ferritin level falls below 50 μg/L. A rise in the hemoglobin level would justify a full course of iron replacement therapy.

A diagnosis of ACD may be overused in elderly persons with unexplained anemia who lack an identifiable underlying disorder. Further clarification is needed to explain whether an age-related defect in hematopoiesis exists in some people, or whether the underlying disorders simply remain occult at the time of diagnosis of ACD in some elderly patients.

Hypoproliferative Anemia

Renal failure and hypothyroidism are prominent conditions in elderly patients, producing anemia characterized by normochromic-normocytic RBCs, a low reticulocyte index, and a reduction of erythrocytic precursors in the bone marrow.

The anemia of chronic renal failure may be due not only to decreased RBC production but also to hemolysis and gastrointestinal blood loss. Inadequate erythropoiesis in response to either hemolysis or bleeding is due to insufficient renal production of erythropoietin or to inhibitors of erythropoiesis in uremic serum, or both. The severity of the anemia correlates with the severity of renal function in patients whose creatinine clearance is less than 40 mL/min/1.73 M^2.

Dialysis has been shown to remove an inhibitor of erythropoiesis. In addition, androgens are effective in some patients who are undergoing dialysis. Erythropoietin replacement therapy looks promising, but it has not yet been shown to be effective in the presence of uremic inhibitors of erythropoiesis.

In patients with chronic renal failure, a serum ferritin level below 50 μg/L is highly suggestive of a coexisting iron deficiency.[16] Patients who are undergoing maintenance dialysis with ferritin levels below 100 μg/L should be given 60 to 100 mg of elemental iron daily.[16] Hemosiderosis can be prevented by monitoring bone marrow iron stores via serum ferritin levels.

Anemia commonly is present in patients with hypothyroidism. The mechanism is unclear, although thyroid hormones are known to stimulate erythropoiesis, probably via erythropoietin. This anemia is usually mild and normochromic, but it may be hypochromic or macrocytic. If normocytic, the anemia is due to ineffective erythropoiesis, and the treatment is thyroid hormone replacement. With replacement, the anemia may take months to correct. The serum iron level and TIBC may be low, but iron stores are normal. The iron turnover rate is decreased. If indexes are hypochromic, concurrent bleeding and iron deficiency must be ruled out. Hypothyroidism impairs gastrointestinal iron absorption. If macrocytic, pernicious anemia should be considered, as these autoimmune conditions coexist in 10% of patients with hypothyroidism.

Anemia of Protein-Calorie Malnutrition

Elderly persons are at risk for protein-calorie malnutrition, particularly those who are hospitalized, reside in nursing homes, or are disabled and living alone. Protein-calorie malnutrition decreases hematopoietic stem-cell proliferation, resulting in a normocytic, normochromic anemia, a decreased neutrophil response to infection, and impaired cell-mediated immunity. Shortened RBC survival, decreased erythropoietin secretion by the kidney, and concurrent deficiencies of iron, pyridoxine, and folate contribute to the anemia.[17]

The diagnosis should be suspected in patients with decreased muscle mass and a low serum albumin level. In addition to anemia, patients exhibit low lymphocyte counts and cutaneous anergy. Both the serum iron level and TIBC are reduced, with the latter proportionately lower than the former. All hematologic abnormalities, including the anemia, improve within 6 weeks after the correction of nutritional deficiencies.

Vitamin B_{12} and Folate Deficiency Anemias

Macrocytic anemia in an elderly patient raises the possibility of vitamin B_{12} or folic acid deficiency. The mean corpuscular volume (MCV) rises slightly with age and can be greater than 100 μm^3 in heavy smokers, alcohol users, or persons with chronic liver disease, hypothyroidism, or hemolysis. The findings of an MCV over 100 μm^3, anemia, thrombocytopenia, and leukopenia, with macro-ovalocytes and hypersegmented neutrophils on the peripheral blood smear constitute the classic picture of anemia due to vitamin B_{12} or folate deficiency. Additional laboratory abnormalities may include elevations of the serum lactic acid dehydrogenase and bilirubin levels due to intramedullary hemolysis. In recent years, it has been recognized that folate and vitamin B_{12} deficiency frequently do not present this classic picture. The MCV is normal in some patients with confirmed vitamin B_{12} or folate deficiency, especially when complicated by a coexisting iron deficiency or thalassemia.

Vitamin B_{12}, or cobalamin, is essential for DNA synthesis. The deficiency state, therefore, affects rapidly dividing cells, such as hematopoietic and mucosal

tissues. Cobalamin also has an essential but poorly understood role in the metabolism of the nervous system. Therefore, cobalamin deficiency may be manifested as megaloblastic anemia and glossitis, neurologic disease affecting the brain or spinal cord (combined system disease), or both.

Vitamin B_{12} cannot be synthesized by the human body. It is found only in foods of animal origin. Because of vast body stores of vitamin B_{12}, primarily in the liver, it may take years to develop a deficiency state, even on a strict vegetarian diet. The RDA is 3 μg, and the typical American diet contains 5 to 30 μg of vitamin B_{12}. Intrinsic factor (IF), a glycoprotein secreted by gastric parietal cells, is required for intestinal absorption. There are specific receptors for the IF–vitamin B_{12} complex in the terminal ileum, where cobalamin absorption occurs. After transport across the mucosa, cobalamin is bound primarily to transcobalamin II (TCII), which is the transport protein responsible for delivery of most cobalamin from the gut to tissues.

With the use of the new, sensitive radiodilution assay techniques, prevalence of a vitamin B_{12} level below 200 pg/mL in community-dwelling elderly persons ranges from 3% to 7%.[18–20] Whether the low vitamin B_{12} level in these studies always reflects a true deficiency state is unclear, because many subjects had no hematologic manifestations of vitamin B_{12} deficiency, or had nonspecific neurologic findings. The usual causes of vitamin B_{12} deficiency in elderly patients are pernicious anemia or total gastric resection, which result in the absence of IF. However, other causes of malabsorption, such as pancreatic insufficiency, resection or disease of the terminal ileum, and blind loop syndrome, also result in vitamin B_{12} deficiency. Patients with deficient gastric acid secretion after partial gastrectomy or vagotomy and pyloroplasty or even those patients in the early stages of atrophic gastritis may have sufficient IF to absorb radioactive vitamin B_{12} (Schilling test); yet, these patients have a vitamin B_{12} deficiency because of difficulty with extracting protein-bound cobalamin from food.[21]

The neurologic manifestations of vitamin B_{12} deficiency include peripheral neuropathy and mental changes. The neuropathy is characterized by paresthesias, ataxia, muscle weakness, and impaired vibratory and proprioceptive sensation, indicating posterior column involvement. The mental changes can include fatigue, irritability, depression, personality or mood changes, and impairment of memory or other modalities of cognition consistent with dementia. In a recent study of neuropsychiatric disorders in patients with documented vitamin B_{12} deficiency, nearly 30% had normal blood cell counts at presentation, but most had macro-ovalocytes and hypersegmented neutrophils on examination of the peripheral smear.[22] Two studies have documented low serum vitamin B_{12} levels in up to 30% of patients whose conditions were diagnosed clinically as primary degenerative dementia,[23,24] suggesting that these two processes together account for dementia in some patients, that altered vitamin B_{12} metabolism may play a role in the pathophysiology of Alzheimer's disease, or that cobalamin deficiency is often overlooked as a causal factor in progressive dementia.

The diagnosis of cobalamin deficiency is based on a serum vitamin B_{12} level below 200 pg/mL in the presence of anemia, macrocytosis, and hypersegmented polymorphonuclear leukocytes or typical neurologic findings (Fig. 26.1). An abnormal urinary excretion of radiolabeled vitamin B_{12} (Schilling test) is confirmatory. The Schilling test confirms the diagnosis of pernicious anemia or aids in the identification of cobalamin malabsorption due to bacterial overgrowth of the ileum. However, a normal Schilling test in the setting of a low serum vitamin B_{12} level does not necessarily indicate that the vitamin B_{12} level is artifactually low, but may reflect decreased cobalamin-binding sites on TCII in elderly persons; this is a common finding in this age group that is of no physiologic significance.[20] On the other hand, these findings may reflect true defi-

ciency due to the inability to extract cobalamin from foodstuffs, which is not detected by a standard Schilling test.[21] Other measures of vitamin B_{12} tissue deficiency, such as an elevated serum methylmalonic acid or total homocystine level, increased urinary methylmalonic acid excretion, or an abnormal bone marrow deoxyuridine suppression test, may be more specific for confirming cobalamin deficiency, but are limited to research use at this time.

Vitamin B_{12} deficiency is treated with intramuscular hydroxocobalamin or cyanocobalamin, 100 to 1,000 μg every 2 to 3 days for six injections, then 500 to 1,000 μg/mo for cyanocobalamin or every 3 months for hydroxocobalamin. Cyanocobalamin has a higher urinary excretion rate and requires more frequent doses. After initiating treatment with either agent, neutrophil and platelet counts should increase in 5 to 10 days, and the bone marrow should assume a normoblastic appearance in 48 to 72 hours. Potentially life-threatening hypokalemia is an infrequent complication of parenteral vitamin B_{12} therapy, especially in elderly patients. Careful monitoring of the serum potassium level is warranted.

Folate deficiency may be more prevalent in elderly persons than in young control subjects.[25,26] Green leafy

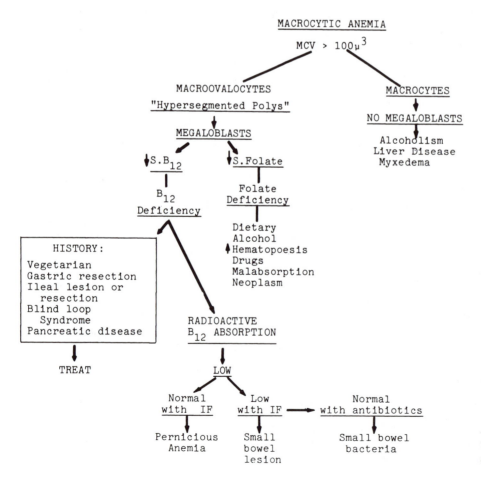

Fig. 26.1. Approach to a differential diagnosis of macrocytic anemia.

vegetables and fruits are the main dietary sources of folic acid. Social isolation, disability, and economic factors may interfere with obtaining and preparing fresh foods. Alcoholism is a major risk factor for folate deficiency. The RDA for folate is 400 μg, easily met by the daily folate content of a normal American diet. Studies suggest that much lower intakes may be adequate to prevent deficiency states.[27] Folates are stored in minimal amounts in the liver. Studies of folate status in elderly patients suggest that although it is not a problem for most elderly persons, some groups are at high risk for folate deficiency, namely, low-income, hospitalized, institutionalized, and alcoholic older persons.[27] In addition, others may be at risk from medications that interfere with folate absorption or utilization, such as phenytoin, sulfasalazine, trimethoprim, antacids, cimetidine, and isoniazid.[27,28]

Reduced serum and RBC folate levels accompany folate deficiency. The RBC level is a better index of tissue folate stores, but most clinicians rely on a low serum folate level and the clinical setting for the diagnosis. Treatment for megaloblastic anemia from folate deficiency is folic acid, 1 mg/d orally for 4 to 6 months, as well as avoidance of alcohol and dietary modification to prevent recurrence. It is important that folate deficiency be carefully distinguished from vitamin B_{12} deficiency, because treatment with folic acid will cause hematologic improvement, but may worsen the neuropathy if the patient is deficient in vitamin B_{12}.

Sideroblastic Anemias

The sideroblastic anemias are a group of disorders characterized by impaired heme synthesis. In sideroblastic anemia, the MCV may be low, normal, or high, but the reticulocyte index is always low. A hypochromic anemia in an elderly person without iron deficiency or chronic disease usually is sideroblastic. Serum iron, transferrin saturation, and ferritin levels all are elevated, reflecting the iron loading that occurs in sideroblastic anemia. On bone marrow examination, erythroid hypoplasia and 15% or more ringed sideroblasts (erythroblasts that contain accumulations of iron) are seen.

Sideroblastic anemia may be primary or secondary to other conditions. The genetic, sex-linked form that frequently responds to pyridoxine usually is diagnosed in younger persons. The acquired form may be a preleukemic condition in elderly persons. Sideroblastic anemia also occurs as a consequence of hematologic malignant neoplasms, rheumatologic disorders, drugs, and toxins, especially lead. Chronic alcoholism is a common cause. Other drugs that may cause sideroblastic anemia include phenytoin, isoniazid, and chloramphenicol.[29]

A patient with sideroblastic anemia should be given a trial of therapy with pharmacologic doses of pyridoxine, 200 mg/d orally for 1 to 2 months. If sideroblastic anemia does not respond to pyridoxine, treatment of the underlying disorder, or removal of the toxic agent, then periodic transfusions may be required.

Evidence for Changes in Bone Marrow Function with Age

Although anemia should always be approached as a sign of disease in elderly individuals, some investigators have questioned whether in some persons anemia may result from an age-related functional decline of the bone marrow. The functional and reserve capacity of other organ systems are known to decline with age. Recent work suggests that many cases of anemia in elderly persons may remain unexplained after standard laboratory evaluation.[5,6] Although it is difficult at this time to separate the confounding effects of inapparent disease, dietary factors, and environmental toxins from the aging process itself, the question of impaired hematopoiesis due to aging is raised when laboratory parameters are consistent with ACD; yet, disorders known to cause anemia are absent.

Various mechanisms could account for a change in bone marrow function with age: a decrease in the number or proliferative capacity of stem cells, a change in the hematopoietic cell response to regulatory factors, altered regulatory function of the hematopoietic microenvironment, or other mechanisms. Bone marrow cellularity is known to diminish with aging in humans[30]; nevertheless, steady-state cell counts remain adequate in most elderly individuals.

In a study of healthy, ambulatory persons older than 65 years of age, both nonanemic elderly subjects and those with unexplained anemia were found to have decreased leukocyte, platelet, and lymphocyte counts compared with young control subjects.[6] In addition, anemic subjects exhibited diminished growth of myeloid and erythroid progenitor cells in culture. Investigations in our laboratory have revealed impaired in vitro production of hematopoietic growth factors by bone marrow stromal cells from healthy elderly donors.[31]

Data from animal studies support the concept of decreased hematopoietic function with aging. Aged mice respond less briskly to hemorrhage with increased RBC production than young mice.[32] The rise in the hematocrit in response to hypoxia is lower and more variable in old vs young mice.[33] In addition, polycythemic aged mice have diminished responsiveness to erythropoietin,[33] which probably represents a diminished erythropoietin response of differentiated erythroid cells in aged mice.[34] In summary, while there is some evidence of decreased bone marrow function, conclusive evidence of diminished hematopoiesis with aging is not presently available in humans or in laboratory animals, but current research promises to delineate further the effect of aging per se on bone marrow function.

Leukemia

Acute Nonlymphocytic Leukemia (ANLL)

Acute nonlymphocytic leukemia accounts for approximately 80% of adult acute leukemias in contrast to acute lymphocytic leukemia, which is predominantly a disease of children. More than 60% of all patients with ANLL are older than 60 years of age. Unlike acute lymphocytic leukemia, ANLL sometimes appears in the wake of another myelodysplastic disorder, such as polycythemia vera (PV), paroxysmal nocturnal hemoglobinuria, agnogenic myeloid metaplasia (AMM), or chronic granulocytic leukemia, and is more likely to follow exposure to radiation therapy, alkylating chemotherapy, or exposure to toxins.[35]

Clinical manifestations often differ in elderly persons. An abrupt onset is characteristic in a young adult, whereas a preleukemic phase introduces the disease in 30% of all elderly patients. Elderly patients have nonspecific complaints of malaise, anorexia, weight loss, and weakness. Fatigue due to anemia, bleeding, and bruising from thrombocytopenia or a disseminated intravascular coagulopathy, fever due to infection, bone and joint pain, lymphadenopathy, and central nervous system symptoms from meningeal infiltration all are part of the clinical inventory of this disorder. Infection is a common serious complication of leukemia and chemotherapy. Neutropenia caused by leukemia or its treatment increases susceptibility to infection. The emergence of unexplained fever (temperature, >38.5°C) in a patient with less than 1,000 neutrophils per cubic millimeter must be managed as life threatening.

Anemia, thrombocytopenia, and granulocytopenia with myeloblasts, monoblasts, or both are typical blood findings. Other prominent features include hypercellular bone marrow composed of myeloblasts, monocytoid granulocytic cells, and occasionally megaloblastic types of erythroid cells and atypical megakaryocytes.

If untreated, the mean duration from the onset of symptoms to death is less than 6 months. The therapeutic goal is establishment of a complete remission, which is defined as the presence of less than 5% blasts in a normocellular bone marrow accompanied by normal peripheral blood cell counts, loss of adenopathy and organomegaly, and return to normal activity. A complete remission in elderly patients occurs less frequently than in younger patients, and there has been no consensus about the treatment of acute leukemia in patients older than 70 years of age.[36,37] Older patients are considered more refractory to therapy and are at greater risk for bleeding and serious infections related to bone marrow aplasia from the chemotherapy. Lower remission rates and a shorter duration of complete remission in older patients have been attributed to many factors, including the inability of aging bone marrow to tolerate aggressive therapy and intrinsic differences in the susceptibility of their neoplasms to cytotoxic therapy, perhaps because acute leukemia in elderly persons often is secondary to other myelodysplastic disorders with lower remission rates. Recent reports of remission induction range from 35% to 76%, and disease-free survival ranging from 1 to 2 years in patients 60 years old and older are encouraging. Age, therefore, is not a contraindication to aggressive therapy for patients with acute leukemia.[36,37]

Judgment about who shall be treated should not be based on age alone. The guiding premise is that acute leukemia without treatment is uniformly fatal; therefore, the patient is entitled to aggressive therapy regardless of age. Yet, a patient with severe physical and mental impairment should not be exposed to the added risks of chemotherapy. With older patients, it is as important to know when not to treat as when to treat. Clear examples prevail at either end of the spectrum, but there continues to be a troubling gray zone where better criteria are needed to aid the clinician in these decisions.

"Smoldering" leukemia in elderly patients is distinguished by mildly elevated white blood cell counts, few myeloblasts, and anemia. There is a risk of infection or hemorrhage in this condition. The progression is slow throughout several years and requires supportive treatment for complications, but no chemotherapy. Eventual progression to an acute stage, however, becomes an indication for antileukemic therapy.

Chronic Lymphocytic Leukemia (CLL)

Chronic lymphocytic leukemia is the most common leukemia found in elderly persons, with 90% of diagnoses occurring in patients older than 50 years of age. It is characterized by proliferation of monoclonal lymphocytes (usually of B-cell origin) in the bone marrow, peripheral blood, lymph nodes, spleen, liver, and sometimes in other organs. The course of this disease is variable, with survival ranging from months to 10 years or longer. Some patients are asymptomatic with mildly or moderately elevated lymphocyte blood counts that persist for many years, while other patients follow an aggressive course with lymphocytic replacement of normal bone marrow cells causing anemia, thrombocytopenia, and neutropenia. Usually, protean symptoms correlate with adenopathy, splenomegaly, and high lymphocyte counts. Therefore, CLL no longer can be viewed as an indolent disease to be ignored by clinicians. A single median survival statistic for a disease with such a varied course is not meaningful.

Classification systems have been designed to aid in the prognosis and to allow a better comparison of therapeutic trials.[40,41] The most widely used is the classification described by Rai et al,[42] which categorizes patients with CLL on the basis of the lymphocyte count, lymphadenopathy, splenomegaly, hepatomegaly, anemia, and thrombocytopenia. Patients with only lymphocytosis (stage 0) and those with associated lymphadenopathy (stage I) have a median survival of greater than 10 years and greater than 8 years, respectively. Patients with hepatomegaly and splenomegaly (stage II), anemia (stage III), or thrombocytopenia (stage IV) have survival times of less than 7 years, 2 to 5 years, and less than 2 years, respectively. A new clinical classification system has been proposed[43] simply to divide patients into low- (stage A), intermediate- (stage B), and high- (stage C) risk groups. Survival of the majority of patients depends on the number of lymph node sites involved. Patients with two or less sites of lymph node enlargement are designated stage A (median survival, >7 years); those with three or more areas of lymphoid enlargement are considered to be stage B (median survival, <5 years); and those with anemia (hemoglobin level, <10 g/dL) or thrombocytopenia (<100,000/μL) are stage C and have the worst prognosis (median survival, ≤2 years).

Clinical and laboratory abnormalities can be attributed to cytopenia and to immunologic deficiencies. Fever, when present, invariably implies infection, and medical attention should be sought immediately. Susceptibility to infection is linked to granulocytopenia, poor cellular immune responses, and hypogammaglobulinemia. Approximately 50% to 75% of patients are hypogammaglobulinemic or agammaglobulinemic,[44] which frequently results in recurrent infections. Intravenous immunoglobulin prevents bacterial infection in selected patients with CLL.[45] Less than 5% of patients with CLL secrete large amounts of IgM, resulting in a paraprotein spike on electrophoresis. Anemia and thrombocytopenia are a consequence of bone marrow replacement with leukemia cells, hypersplenism, autoimmune antibodies, or chemotherapy. Autoimmune hemolytic anemia occurs in about 10% of patients although a positive Coombs' test reveals IgG coating of RBCs in about 20% of patients with CLL.[44] Autoimmune thrombocytopenia occurs in less than 5% of patients with CLL.[44] In those patients who have autoimmune hemolytic anemia and/or thrombocytopenia, corticosteroid therapy achieves good results. The incidence of a second primary neoplasm is high in patients with CLL. These include skin cancers, colorectal cancers, lung cancer, and multiple myelomas.[44] This may be a manifestation of altered immunity in this disorder.

No therapy is indicated for the asymptomatic patient. Those patients with the least clinical involvement (clinical stage A) have survival rates similar to the general population and usually die of other concurrent medical disorders. However, therapy is used during symptomatic or advancing periods of the illness when infections, anemia, lymphadenopathy, and splenomegaly become part of the clinical picture. Symptomatic patients usually are given alkylating agents, such as chlorambucil or cyclophosphamide, which are effective in reducing blood cell counts and shrinking lymphadenopathy, splenomegaly, and hepatomegaly. Prednisone, used with an alkylating agent, is beneficial for cytopenias. A three-drug regimen that consists of cyclophosphamide, vincristine, and prednisone is being evaluated for more aggressive (stage III or IV) or refractory disease. Allopurinol and adequate hydration are essential during chemotherapy or radiotherapy to prevent uric acid stones and nephropathy from excessive uric acid, which is liberated as a result of cell destruction. Radiation therapy is suitable for bulky adenopathy and is indicated for localized lymphocytic infiltration that causes ureteral, bile duct, or bronchial obstruction. Leukapheresis to remove lymphocytes from the circulation is appropriate for management of selected patients with significant anemia and thrombocytopenia from bone marrow failure secondary to previous therapy or for patients who are unable to tolerate chemotherapy.[46] However, responses are brief. None of the present-day treatments cure this disease.

Chronic Myelogenous Leukemia (CML)

Chronic myelogenous leukemia is predominantly a disease of middle age, with the greatest prevalence between the third and sixth decades. However, it has been observed that nearly one third of all patients with CML are older than 60 years of age.[47] The incidence sharply diminishes after 70 years of age. Some patients are asymptomatic and are discovered inadvertently because of changes in the peripheral blood cell counts. Most patients present with a low-grade fever, fatigue, weight loss, and occasional night sweats. Enlargement of the spleen is prominent in most patients. These findings are accompanied by anemia, normal or increased platelets, and a leukocyte count of 20,000 to

50,000/mm³. The peripheral blood smear is characterized by the presence of metamyelocytes, myelocytes, basophilia, and often eosinophilia. A low or absent leukocyte alkaline phosphatase (LAP) is found in the majority of patients, and the Ph¹ chromosome is detectable in 90% of patients.

Chemotherapy produces remissions in nearly all patients with chronic stable CML. The median survival has increased from 19 months for untreated patients to a range of 30 to 45 months for those patients receiving a single agent and 50 to 65 months for those patients treated with intensive chemotherapy.[48] The aim of intensive chemotherapy programs is to reduce or eradicate Ph¹-positive clones to delay the onset of a blast crisis. The combination of chemotherapy with splenectomy has the same goal. However, none of these chemotherapy programs have been curative, and intensive chemotherapy increases toxic side effects and prolongs hospitalization. Radiation therapy to the spleen is no better than chemotherapy alone, and even splenectomy does not alter the incidence of blast transformation.

The transformation from CML to an acute leukemia (blast crisis) occurs in more than 80% of affected patients.[47] It is more common in patients who lack the Ph¹ chromosome.[47] Weakness, fatigue, and increasing splenomegaly accompanied by anemia, thrombocytopenia, myelofibrosis, and an increasing LAP are the most prominent features. The blast transformation is most often myeloblastic, but lymphoblastic transformation has been reported. The blast crisis is extremely resistant to therapy with a complete remission rate of less than 30% and duration of remission short (<3 months).

Monoclonal Gammopathies

The monoclonal gammopathies represent a spectrum of disorders that have in common the clonal proliferation of cells that secrete a homogeneous immunoglobulin or immunoglobulin fragment. The secreted protein has been called an M protein (M for monoclonal), M component, M spike, or paraprotein. The M protein may be an intact immunoglobulin composed of a single class of heavy chain plus a single type of light chain, or it may consist of fragments of either.

The prevalence of monoclonal gammopathies increases with age.[49,50] Recent reports using sensitive techniques estimate the prevalence of monoclonal gammopathies at 7% between the ages of 70 and 79 years, 11% between the ages of 80 and 89 years, and 14% over 90 years of age.[49] The pathophysiology of the age-related increase in clonal proliferation of plasma cells is not known. The proliferation and differentiation of B cells, from which plasma cells originate, is under the influence of T lymphocytes and macrophages. Impairment of several T-lymphocyte functions is known to account for some of the age-related decline in immunocompetence. It is conceivable that the altered control of B-lymphocyte proliferation that results in monoclonal gammopathies may be explained, in part, by these changes in T-cell function (see Chapter 25).[51]

At the time of initial evaluation, approximately one third of patients with monoclonal gammopathy will be found to have multiple myeloma, macroglobulinemia, amyloidosis, or other lymphoproliferative disorders. The remaining two thirds will have benign monoclonal gammopathy, alone or in association with chronic conditions, such as chronic infection, nonhematologic neoplasm, or rheumatologic disorder. This idiopathic, asymptomatic form of the disorder is designated *monoclonal gammopathy of undetermined significance* (MGUS).

MGUS

Monoclonal gammopathy of undetermined significance refers to the presence of a serum M protein in an asymptomatic person who has no evidence of a plasma cell malignant neoplasm. In 10% to 20% of these patients, MGUS will evolve into myeloma, macroglobulinemia, amyloidosis, or CLL during a period of 15 to 20 years.[50] However, at the time of diagnosis of MGUS, there are no features that predict which patients will progress to malignant conditions.

Distinguishing MGUS from multiple myeloma may be difficult, because the boundaries between the two conditions are not clear-cut and some features consistent with a diagnosis of multiple myeloma (anemia, azotemia, and osteoporosis) occur frequently in aged individuals due to disorders that may coexist with MGUS. In current practice, the following features in an asymptomatic individual at the time of initial detection of serum M protein are the best indications that one is dealing with MGUS: (1) levels of monoclonal IgG <3 g/dL or IgM or IgA <1.5 g/dL; (2) normal concentrations of other serum immunoglobulins; (3) bone marrow plasma cells <10%; (4) Bence Jones proteinuria <1 g/d; (5) absence of lytic bone lesions; (6) normal level of serum calcium; (7) hemoglobin level >12 g/dL; and (8) no lymphadenopathy or hepatosplenomegaly.

The distinction between asymptomatic stages of multiple myeloma and MGUS may be particularly difficult. Fortunately, treatment is not indicated for asymptomatic myeloma. If a plasma cell malignant neoplasm has been excluded, or if there is doubt as to the correct diagnosis, careful follow-up with serial quantitation of the M protein is warranted.

Multiple Myeloma

The prevalence of multiple myeloma, like benign monoclonal gammopathy, increases with age. However, multiple myeloma is less common than monoclonal gammopathy. Prevalence rates per 100,000 for multiple myeloma are approximately 11 for the 60-to 69-year-old age group, 27 for those aged 70 to 79 years, and 37 for those older than 80 years of age.[52] Most cases of multiple myeloma are diagnosed after the age of 70 years. The highest rates are found in men older than 80 years of age and women aged older than 70 years. Men outnumber women by a ratio of 3:2. It occurs twice as frequently in blacks as in whites.

The pathogenesis of myeloma is not well understood. There may be familial factors. An association with HLA antigens has been noted.[53] In addition, an increased incidence of myeloma 10 to 30 years after high-dose radiation exposure has been found in atomic bomb survivors.[53] Because B lymphocytes bear surface immunoglobulin of the same idiotype as the M protein in patients with multiple myeloma, neoplastic transformation is thought to occur proximal to the differentiated plasma cell, possibly at a pre–B-cell stage of hematopoiesis.[54]

Multiple myeloma starts in the bone marrow in 93% of cases. Bone marrow involvement may be focal or diffuse, so a single negative bone marrow aspiration does not rule out the diagnosis. In a small minority of cases, multiple myeloma may present as an extramedullary tumor, usually involving the upper airways, but occasionally involving the spleen, lymph nodes, skin, gastrointestinal tract, and, rarely, the breast, vagina, thyroid gland, or testes.[53]

On histologic sections, myeloma cells appear to be relatively uniform, constituting more than 10% of bone marrow cellularity. Cells may appear to be mature, large with increased cytoplasm, or immature with a distinct nucleolus. There may be multinucleate cells. Ninety-eight percent of myelomas secrete an M protein. Fifty percent secrete IgG, 25% produce IgA, 20% produce light chains only, and the remainder secrete IgD, IgE, or IgM. Fully half of all patients with myeloma excrete urinary light chains. In many patients, normal immunoglobulin levels are reduced.

The majority of patients complain of bone pain at presentation. Pain may be located in the back, ribs, or, rarely, the proximal parts of the extremities, and typically is worse during the day, especially with movement. Bone pain characteristically occurs at night only with a change of position. Other presenting symptoms may include pathologic fractures due to lytic lesions or osteoporosis, weight loss, fever, azotemia, anemia, dehydration, or confusion. Abnormal findings due to paraprotein effects may include an elevated erythrocyte sedimentation rate (ESR), rouleaux formation, decreased anion gap, or prolonged bleeding time. In 80% of patients, x-ray films of the skull, spine, and long bones may reveal diffuse osteoporosis, or pathologic fractures due to either of these lesions. Plain x-ray films are the diagnostic procedure of choice for detecting bone lesions, rather than radionuclide bone scans, because of the purely lytic nature of the bone defects. Bone resorption is stimulated by osteoclast activating factor (OAF), which is a secretory product of myeloma cells. Osteoclast activating factor may also produce hypercalcemia, which is a finding in 30% of patients with myeloma.

Azotemia is present in almost 50% of patients, due to a variety of factors, including direct light-chain damage to renal tubules and collecting ducts, obstruction of tubules by protein casts, amyloid or plasma cell infiltration of the kidney, pyelonephritis, and hypercalcemia and dehydration. Hyperuricemia, nephrotoxic antibiotics, and intravenous pyelography may also contribute. Renal involvement by myeloma may present as proximal or distal renal tubular acidosis. Detection of light chains in the urine requires a sulfosalicylic acid precipitation test, because routine urine dipsticks detect only albumin.

Patients with myeloma are at increased risk of infection, the leading cause of death in multiple myeloma. This is due to relative immunosuppression based on several factors, including decreased levels of normal immunoglobulins, a diminished antibody response to some antigens, increased levels of suppressor lymphocytes, chemotherapy-induced neutropenia, and steroid effects. In recent years, gram-negative rods have become the most prevalent organisms that cause pneumonia and urinary tract infection in patients with multiple myeloma, although gram-positive cocci, especially *Staphylococcus aureus* and *Streptococcus pneumoniae* still are commonly involved.[55]

A normochromic, normocytic anemia is found in most patients. Other cytopenias also may occur due to either replacement of normal bone marrow elements by tumor or cytotoxic therapy. Bleeding may result from thrombocytopenia, platelet dysfunction due to M protein coating membranes, or paraprotein interference with clotting factors.

Neurologic complications include radiculopathies from vertebral body collapse, spinal cord compression from extramedullary disease, or sensorimotor peripheral neuropathies from amyloid infiltration. Amyloidosis is present in 30% of cases of multiple myeloma and should be suspected if cardiac enlargement, congestive heart failure, arrhythmias, an enlarged tongue, carpal tunnel syndrome, or peripheral neuropathy is present.

The hyperviscosity syndrome may complicate some

cases of multiple myeloma, particularly those that produce IgM, but also some cases of IgA or IgG myeloma. The signs and symptoms of the hyperviscosity syndrome are listed in Table 26.1. Symptoms are usually associated with a relative serum viscosity above 5. The M components may also aggregate to form cryoglobulins, producing symptoms of pain in the distal parts of extremities on exposure to cold.

Many clinical findings of multiple myeloma are common in elderly patients and may not be recognized as signs of a malignant neoplasm. For instance, osteoporosis, musculoskeletal pain, anemia, an elevated ESR, and a rise in the serum creatinine level all are more prevalent in an aging population. However, complaints of bone pain or several of these features in combination should prompt the clinician to rule out multiple myeloma. Moreover, a change in status, such as confusion, weakness, or drowsiness in an elderly patient with known myeloma should be recognized as a sign of a possible complication, such as hypercalcemia or infection.

The median survival of patients treated for multiple myeloma is approximately 30 months.[53,56] There is typically a chronic phase, during which death may occur due to infection or renal failure, or the disesae may progress to an acute terminal phase, characterized by bone marrow infiltration and failure and, rarely, by plasmacytomas, acute plasma cell leukemia, or ANLL. During the chronic phase, which may last up to 10 years, multiple myeloma usually responds to therapy. However, relapse inevitably occurs, and with each relapse, the regrowth rate is faster.

Clinical staging is based on estimating the tumor cell mass by using the M protein and serum calcium levels and the extent of bony involvement. Renal failure is an independent negative prognostic factor. The widely used staging scheme of Durie and Salmon[57] is shown in

Table 26.2. The tumor cell mass, estimated by this method, correlates well with the prognosis although it does not predict the initial response to chemotherapy. Older patients do not differ significantly from younger patients in response to therapy, remission rates, survival, or toxic side effects from cytotoxic agents.

Asymptomatic myeloma may be classified as "indolent" or "smoldering" if bone marrow plasma cells are less than 30% but greater than 10%, the IgG spike is less than 7 g/dL, the light-chain excretion is less than 1 g/24 h, lytic lesions number less than three, and there is no evidence of infection, anemia, renal failure, or hypercalcemia.[51] The patient with smoldering or indolent multiple myeloma should be followed up closely, but therapy should be reserved until the disease becomes active, because there is no evidence that early therapy for the asymptomatic form delays the onset of disease activity or affects survival.

The initial therapy for multiple myeloma involves alkylating agents, alone or in combination. Most alkylating agents have been proved to be effective

Table 26.1. Hyperviscosity syndrome.

Organ system	Symptoms	Signs
Vision	Blurred vision	Retinal venous engorgement
	Loss of vision	Retinal hemorrhage, papilledema
Neurologic	Lethargy	Somnolence
	Headache	Stupor, coma
	Weakness	Seizures
Hematologic	Epistaxis	Oral, nasal oozing; GI and GU bleeding*; anemia
Cardiac	Dyspnea	Congestive heart failure

*GI indicates gastrointestinal; GU, genitourinary.

Table 26.2. Staging of multiple myeloma.*

Stage	Clinical criteria	Myeloma cell mass
I	All of following: Hemoglobin level, >10 g/dL Serum calcium level, normal Normal bone x-ray films or only a solitary plasmacytoma IgG paraprotein level, <5 g/dL; IgA level, <3 g/dL; and Bence Jones proteinuria, <4 g/24 h	$<0.6 \times 10^{12}$
II	Fitting neither stage I nor stage III	$0.6\text{-}1.2 \times 10^{12}$
III	1 or more of following: Hemoglobin level, <8.5 g/dL Calcium level, >12 mg/dL Advanced lytic bone lesions IgG paraprotein level, >7 g/dL; IgA level, >5 g/dL; Bence Jones proteinuria, >12 g/24 h Subclassification A indicates serum creatinine level less than 2 mg/dL; B, creatinine level greater than or equal to 2 mg/dL.	$>1.2 \times 10^{12}$

*From Durie and Salmon.[57]

against myeloma, including melphalan, cyclophosphamide, and carmustine (BCNU). The most commonly used combination is melphalan and prednisone. This regimen is effective and is well tolerated, even by elderly patients. The long-term risk of ANLL is increased after the use of alkylating agents.

The clinician also must manage the complications of multiple myeloma. Bone pain is treated with analgesic agents to prevent immobility and disability. Localized irradiation may be indicated for intensely painful lytic lesions. Hypercalcemia should be prevented by maintaining adequate hydration. Symptomatic hypercalcemia may be manifested by anorexia, nausea, fatigue, or an altered mental status. If mildly elevated, the serum calcium level may be lowered by normal saline infusion, alone or in combination with furosemide. Prednisone interferes with the action of OAF when given in doses of 60 mg/d, followed by rapidly decreasing doses. If rapid lowering of the serum calcium level is necessary, mithramycin or calcitonin may be used.

Renal failure may be prevented by reducing light-chain excretion with chemotherapy, and by maintaining normal fluid, calcium, and uric acid status. Dialysis occasionally may be necessary as a temporary measure, until disease activity can be brought under control. Infection should be aggressively treated, because of the high associated mortality in this setting. Prevention with pneumococcal and influenza vaccines is appropriate. Spinal cord compression by extramedullary disease should be aggressively investigated, and irradiation should be administered emergently if indicated. Hyperviscosity symptoms may be treated effectively with plasmapheresis.

Other Monoclonal Conditions

Waldenström's macroglobulinemia is a neoplasm of a well-differentiated, lymphoplasmacytic B-cell clone that secretes a monoclonal IgM protein. Waldenström's macroglobulinemia is the diagnosis in half of all cases of IgM monoclonal gammopathy and constitutes 5% of all malignant B-cell disorders accompanied by monoclonal gammopathy. The mean age at presentation is 65 years. Sixty percent of patients are men. The monoclonal protein is responsible for most of the clinical manifestations of Waldenström's macroglobulinemia. The patient most commonly presents with weakness, fatigue, or bleeding from the nasopharynx or gastrointestinal tract. Less commonly, other signs of hyperviscosity, such as neurologic complaints or congestive heart failure, may predominate. On physical examination, hepatosplenomegaly and lymphadenopathy usually are found. Retinal vein engorgement may be seen. A mild-to-moderate normocytic, normochromic anemia is commonly found, due to dilution by an increased plasma volume, bone marrow infiltration, blood loss, or hemolysis by cold agglutinins. Increased serum viscosity in most patients correlates with the IgM level; symptoms are unusual at an IgM level below 3 g/dL or a relative serum viscosity less than 3. Renal abnormalities are less common and less severe than in multiple myeloma. Slight Bence Jones proteinuria, less than 1 g/d, as well as nonspecific proteinuria, may be found. Mixed sensorimotor neuropathy may be due to antimyelin activity of the monoclonal IgM. The differential diagnosis includes IgM myeloma, CLL, lymphocytic lymphoma, mixed cryoglobulinemia, cold agglutinin disease, and MGUS. If the IgM spike is greater than 1.5 g/dL, all of these conditions, except IgM myeloma, are usually ruled out. The IgM myeloma is differentiated from Waldenström's macroglobulinemia primarily by the presence of bony destruction. Treatment of symptomatic macroglobulinemia is aimed at controlling the paraprotein level. An RBC transfusion may be required if anemia is severe due to bone marrow infiltration. Plasmapheresis is indicated for severe dilutional anemia or hyperviscosity symptoms. If plasmapheresis is ineffective, alkylating agents plus prednisone or combination protocols like those used in multiple myeloma may be tried, but, to our knowledge, no systematic studies have been done to compare drugs or schedules in this disease. The mean survival is 50 months from the time of diagnosis.

The heavy-chain diseases are lymphoplasmacytic clonal proliferations marked by secretion of defective heavy chains only. γ–Heavy-chain disease is found mainly in elderly persons, and it is characterized by lymphadenopathy, hepatosplenomegaly, anemia, fever, malaise, and palatal edema and obstruction. A diagnosis is made by the finding of γ heavy chains (>20 g/L), marked hypoglobulinemia on immunoelectrophoresis, and urinary heavy-chain excretion. The course is indolent, ranging from months up to 5 years. Alkylating agents and steroids are not effective.

Myeloproliferative Disorders

Myeloproliferative disorders are characterized by a bone marrow proliferation of pluripotent hematopoietic progenitor cells, including erythrocytes (PV), thrombocytes (essential thrombocythemia), leukocytes (CML), and fibroblasts (myelofibrosis and/or myeloid metaplasia). The myelodysplastic disorder (preleukemia syndrome) and acute myelofibrosis are also included in this category of bone marrow disorders. Many of these chronic disorders undergo a blast crisis, terminating as an acute myeloblastic leukemia.

Myeloid metaplasia is characterized by extramedullary hematopoiesis, splenomegaly, varying degrees of fibrosis of the bone marrow, and a leukoerythroblastic peripheral blood smear. Myeloid metaplasia may be idiopathic (agnogenic myeloid metaplasia), or may evolve from PV into a stage known as postpolycythemic myeloid metaplasia. This latter syndrome occurs in 10% to 12% of patients with PV usually about 10 years after the onset of polycythemia.

Agnogenic Myeloid Metaplasia (AMM)

This disorder, with a peak incidence between 50 and 70 years of age, is due to a proliferation of hematopoietic cells in the spleen, liver, and lymph nodes. A grossly enlarged, firm spleen and abnormal peripheral blood findings are major clues to this diagnosis. The peripheral blood smear shows leukoerythroblastic features, with teardrop-shaped RBCs, nucleated RBCs, immature granulocytes, and large bizarre platelets. The white blood cell count frequently is elevated and may suggest CML, especially if it is greater than $60,000/m^3$. It usually is not as high in AMM. The LAP level is normal or elevated in AMM. Platelet counts may be normal, low, or high. Bone marrow is difficult to obtain and often yields dry taps on aspiration. A bone marrow biopsy specimen shows fibrosis.

Symptoms stem from anemia, thrombocytopenia, an enlarged spleen, or splenic infarcts. Weight loss, sweating, and a low-grade fever are hypermetabolic symptoms of this disorder. Gout occurs from hyperuricemia that is secondary to an increased cell turnover.

The mean life expectancy after diagnosis ranges from 2 to 7 years. Death usually is due to complications, such as infection, hemorrhage, thrombosis, or portal hypertension. Agnogenic myeloid metaplasia may eventuate in a blast crisis that is a transition to acute myeloblastic leukemia. This usually is unresponsive to treatment in elderly persons.

A leukoerythroblastic blood picture also may be found with CML and metastatic carcinoma. The absence of teardrop poikilocytes, increased basophils and eosinophils on the peripheral blood smear, a low leukocyte alkaline phosphatase score, a hypercellular bone marrow, and the presence of the Ph^1 (Philadelphia) chromosome all favor CML. The finding of carcinoma cells on a bone marrow smear or biopsy specimen confirms that diagnosis.

Management of patients with AMM is contingent on symptoms. The asymptomatic patient with splenic enlargement requires no treatment. Anemia associated with AMM may require periodic transfusions. Androgens induce remission of anemia in about a third of patients but do not prolong survival and have side effects, such as cholestatic hepatitis, edema, and virilization in females. Other factors that contribute to anemia, such as deficiencies of iron, folic acid, pyridoxine, and vitamin B_{12}, should be corrected. Prednisone may alleviate hemolytic anemia in some patients.

Patients with thrombocytosis, especially with platelet counts of 1 million per microliter or greater, are at risk for bleeding or thrombosis. Laboratory tests alone are unpredictable in differentiating between these two complications.[58] Aspirin and other antiplatelet agents have been used to treat the hypercoagulable state that is due to thrombocytosis. However, the use of antiplatelet drugs, such as aspirin, is controversial. Aspirin may cause major bleeding complications or unexpected prolongation of the bleeding time. Therefore, a significantly elevated platelet count, by itself, may not be an indication for the use of aspirin since the patient is just as likely to have a complication from bleeding as to have thrombosis.[58]

There are special circumstances in which aspirin and attempts to lower the platelet count with myelosuppressive therapy are indicated. These conditions are microvascular thrombosis causing digital ischemia and transient ischemic attacks of the anterior and posterior cerebral circulation, which are especially prevalent with essential thrombocythemia. In general, a decision to use antiplatelet drugs for patients with thrombocytosis should be made only after carefully weighing the risk of therapy vs the potential value to the patient.

Surgery carries a high risk of serious thrombohemorrhagic complications.[58] Excessive bleeding during surgery and thromboembolic episodes in the postoperative period are potential hazards. Aspirin should be discontinued at least 1 week before surgery. Myelosuppressive therapy to lower the platelet count to less than $500,000/\mu L$ before surgery diminishes the risk of thrombohemorrhagic complications.[59] Splenectomy is reserved for patients with refractory hemolytic anemia and/or thrombocytopenia, splenic infarcts, painful symptoms due to massive splenomegaly, and portal hypertension with bleeding.[60]

Erythrocytosis (Polycythemia)

An elevated hematocrit or blood hemoglobin value, frequently uncovered during an examination performed for other reasons, triggers the diagnostic dilemma of differentiating PV, secondary erythrocytosis, and relative erythrocytosis. The elevated hematocrit is a sign of increased blood viscosity and decreased cerebral blood flow that result in symptoms common to these three groups of disorders.

Initially, the clinician must identify the patient with relative erythrocytosis who has a spurious or falsely elevated hematocrit as a consequence of reduced plasma volume. Hypertension with resultant plasma

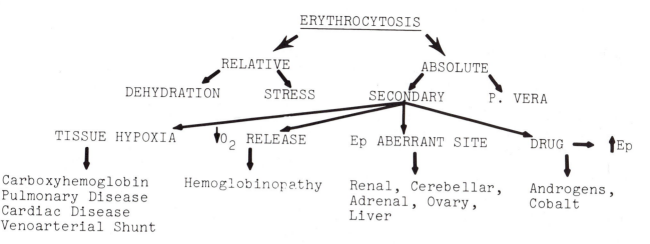

Fig. 26.2. Causes of erythrocytosis. Ep indicates erythropoietin.

volume contraction plays a role. In some patients, chronic alcoholism is involved, and carboxyhemoglobin from cigarette smoking may be implicated. There is an increased prevalence of cardiovascular and cerebrovascular complications,[65] including thromboembolism in 30% of patients with relative erythrocytosis.

The demonstration of an increased RBC volume using RBCs labeled with chromium[51] is essential to confirm absolute erythrocytosis. At sea level, the normal RBC volume for men ranges from 26 to 32 mL/kg and, for women, from 23 to 29 mL/kg of body weight. Polycythemia vera and secondary erythrocytosis are the two major categories of absolute erythrocytosis (Fig. 26.2). Secondary or reactive erythrocytosis is more common than PV. In elderly persons, chronic lung disease, carboxyhemoglobin due to smoking, alveolar hypoventilation due to obesity, and cardiac disease produce tissue hypoxia, resulting in erythrocytosis due to increased circulating erythropoietin.

Before initiating an extensive evaluation to uncover the cause of an increased hematocrit, a history of cigarette smoking should be sought. In cigarette smokers, carbon monoxide attaches to hemoglobin to form carboxyhemoglobin, which cannot bind oxygen. The resultant tissue hypoxia stimulates erythropoietin, which produces an increased hematocrit. Cigarette smoking also reduces the plasma volume, thereby accentuating the increased hematocrit. If cigarette smoking is excluded, an arterial oxygen saturation of less than 92% warrants an investigation of pulmonary and cardiac causes. If the arterial saturation is greater than 92%, a search for other causes of an increased erythropoietin level is indicated. These include renal parenchymal diseases, renal tumors or cysts, hydronephrosis, and

paraneoplastic syndromes related to tumors of the liver, ovaries, adrenal gland, and cerebellum. Rarely, an elderly person may have an abnormal hemoglobin level with an increased affinity for oxygen that leads to tissue hypoxia, increased erythropoietin production, and finally erythrocytosis.

The management of a patient with erythrocytosis is directed at treating the underlying cause. Discontinuation of smoking, oxygen therapy for chronic lung disease, and weight reduction are important considerations to correct erythrocytosis. Therapeutic phlebotomy is considered for all forms of erythrocytosis that have not responded to treatment of the underlying cause, including relative erythrocytosis. There is considerable evidence that the level of the packed cell volume influences blood flow through tissue. Cerebral blood flow diminishes in patients with a hematocrit of 60%, and there is an associated greater risk of thromboembolism.[61-64] High hematocrits that are associated with low cerebral blood flow presumably predispose to transient ischemic attacks and stroke. Phlebotomy produces a significant reduction of whole blood viscosity when the hematocrit is reduced to below 45%, thereby allowing the cerebral blood flow to become normal.[61-64,66] This approach is appropriate even for an elderly patient with modest hematocrit elevation, if the treating clinician is concerned about the risk of cerebrovascular disease.[64] It has been suggested that reduced blood flow from increased blood viscosity associated with a high hematocrit adversely affects collateral blood flow, thereby increasing the size of a cerebral infarct.[67] Interestingly, even patients with relative polycythemia have an increased incidence of vascular disease and, therefore, are good candidates for such therapy.[64] The increase in cerebral blood flow after phlebotomy more than compensates for the calculated decrease in the oxygen-carrying capacity of the blood. This is especially pertinent when considering the effectiveness of this form of therapy in patients with chronic hypoxic lung disease. Until recently, because the elevated RBC volume had been regarded as a compensatory mechanism designed to raise arterial oxygen capacity, therapy to lower it had been considered inappropriate. However, at a hematocrit of approximately 55%, tissue oxygen delivery is compromised more by increased viscosity, so blood flow is improved by lowering the hematocrit. Recent studies of patients with erythrocytosis secondary to chronic obstructive lung disease have shown that using phlebotomy to improve the cerebral blood flow by lowering blood viscosity results in resolution of confusion, headaches, dizziness, lethargy, and drowsiness.[62,63] While a reduction of blood viscosity has resulted in improved cerebral circulation, reduction of hyperviscosity in the peripheral circulation produces uncertain results. Further evidence, therefore, is needed before recommending phlebotomy therapy for treating intermittent claudication.

Polycythemia vera (PV)

Polycythemia vera is a neoplastic clonal proliferation of a pluripotential hematopoietic stem cell that has a peak age at onset of 50 to 60 years. In early stages, there may be no symptoms, and erythrocytosis may be the only clinical finding. When symptoms occur, they are related to hyperviscosity caused by erythrocytosis. As the disease progresses, a leukocytosis (20,000 to 50,000/μL) and/or thrombocytosis with platelet counts sometimes greater than 1 million per microliter may occur. Thrombosis and thromboembolism have been attributed to increased platelet counts; however, these events are more likely related to hyperviscosity caused by erythrocytosis in combination with abnormalities of platelet function. Hemorrhage occurs in about one third of patients but does not correlate with the degree of thrombocytosis.

In addition to an increased RBC mass, criteria for the diagnosis of PV include either splenomegaly (75% of patients with PV) or any two other features, such as thrombocytosis (50% of patients with PV), leukocytosis (60% of patients with PV), increased LAP activity (70% of patients with PV), and increased vitamin B_{12}–binding protein (67% of patients with PV).[68]

Pruritus, often worsened by a warm bath, is attributed to basophil histamine release. Hyperuricemia occurs in about 40% of patients, resulting in gout, renal colic, or hematuria from uric acid stones.[65]

Erythropoietin levels traditionally have been used to distinguish between primary (PV) and secondary polycythemia. In PV, erythropoietin levels are low, while in secondary polycythemias, they are usually elevated due to tissue hypoxia. However, in a recent study,[69] the plasma erythropoietin level was not useful in distinguishing between these two groups. An elevated level may indicate a secondary erythrocytosis, but a normal level has no diagnostic value.

Life expectancy has increased with treatment of PV.[70] The median age at onset is 60 years, with a 10- to 15-year duration of disease associated with prevention of complications. Reduction of the hematocrit to 42% or less by repeated phlebotomy therapy improves cerebral blood flow and relieves the likelihood of a tragic complication.[59] Initially, 500 mL of blood is withdrawn two or three times each week to reach the desired hematocrit, and phlebotomy is then repeated to maintain this hematocrit. Iron depletion eventually results from phlebotomy therapy, reducing the phlebotomy requirement to approximately once every 8 weeks. Older patients tolerate this therapy very well.

Myelosuppressive therapy with phosphorus 32 or chemotherapy is reserved for patients who cannot tolerate phlebotomy because of comorbidity, patients with unbearable pruritus or symptomatic splenic enlargement, and patients for whom the frequency of phlebotomy is unacceptable. A serious disadvantage of myelosuppressive therapy is the increased risk of acute leukemia (ANLL)[70] or a second malignant neoplasm. Phlebotomy, therefore, is the treatment of choice.[71] Nonetheless, the Polycythemia Vera Study Group recommends phosphorus 32 with supplemental phlebotomy for patients older than 70 years of age because of the high incidence of thrombosis in that group.[68]

References

1. Timiras ML, Brownstein H. Prevalence of anemia and correlation of hemoglobin with age in a geriatric screening clinic population. *J Am Geriatr Soc* 1987;35:639–643.
2. Howe RB. Anemia in the elderly. *Postgrad Med* 1983; 73:153–160.
3. Zauber NP, Zauber AG. Hematologic data of healthy very old people. *JAMA* 1987;257:2181–2184.
4. Htoo MSH, Kofkoff RL, Freedman ML. Erythrocyte parameters in the elderly: an argument against new geriatric normal values. *J Am Geriatr Soc* 1979;27:547–551.
5. Lipschitz DA, Mitchell CO, Thompson C. The anemia of senescence. *Am J Hematol* 1981;11:47–54.
6. Lipschitz DA, Udupa KB, Milton KY, et al. Effect of age on hematopoiesis in man. *Blood* 1984;63:502–509.
7. Finch CA, Miller LR, Inamdar AR, et al. Iron deficiency in the rat: physiological and biochemical studies of muscle dysfunction. *J Clin Invest* 1976;58:447–453.
8. Ohira Y, Edgerton VR, Gardiner GW, et al. Work capacity, heart rate and blood lactate responses to iron therapy. *Br J Haematol* 1979;41:365–372.

9. Pirrie R. The influence of age upon serum iron in normal subjects. *J Clin Pathol* 1952;5:10–15.

10. Garry PJ, Goodwin JS, Hunt WC. Iron status and anemia in the elderly: new findings and a review of previous studies. *J Am Geriatr Soc* 1983;31:389–399.

11. Casale G, Bonora C, Migliavacca A, et al. Serum ferritin and ageing. *Age Ageing* 1981;10:119–122.

12. Sharma JC, Roy SN. Value of serum ferritin as an index of iron deficiency in elderly anemic patients. *Age Ageing* 1984;13:248–250.

13. Patterson C, Turpie ID, Benger AM. Assessment of iron stores in anemic geriatric patients. *J Am Geriatr Soc* 1985;33:764–767.

14. Lynch SR, Finch CA, Monsen ER, et al. Iron status of elderly Americans. *Am J Clin Nutr* 1982;36:1032–1045.

15. Marx JJM. Normal iron absorption and decreased red cell iron uptake in the aged. *Blood* 1979;53:204–211.

16. Cook JD. Clinical evaluations of iron deficiency. *Semin Hematol* 1982;19:6–18.

17. Lipschitz DA. Protein calorie malnutrition in the hospitalized elderly. *Prim Care* 1982;9:531–543.

18. Garry PJ, Goodwin JS, Hunt WC. Folate and vitamin B_{12} status in a healthy elderly population. *J Am Geriatr Soc* 1984;32:719–726.

19. Thompson WG, Babitz L, Cassino C, et al. Evaluation of current criteria used to measure vitamin B_{12} levels. *Am J Med* 1987;82:291–294.

20. Grinbrat J, Marcus DL, Hernandez F, et al. Folate and vitamin B_{12} levels in an urban elderly population with chronic diseases. *J Am Geriatr Soc* 1986;34:627–632.

21. Carmel R, Simow R, Siegel ME, et al. Food cobalamin malabsorption occurs frequently in patients with unexplained low serum cobalamin levels. *Arch Intern Med* 1988;148:1715–1719.

22. Lindenbaum J, Healton EB, Savage DG, et al. Neuropsychiatric disorders caused by cobalamin deficiency in the absence of anemia or macrocytosis. *N Engl J Med* 1988;318:1720–1728.

23. Karnaze DS, Carmel R. Low serum cobalamin levels in primary degenerative dementia. *Arch Intern Med* 1987;147:429–431.

24. Cole MG, Prchal JF. Low serum vitamin B_{12} in Alzheimer type dementia. *Age Ageing* 1984;13:101–105.

25. Webster SGP, Leeming JT. Erythrocyte folate levels in young and old. *J Am Geriatr Soc* 1979;27:451–454.

26. Baker H, Frank O, Thind IS, et al. Vitamin profiles in elderly persons living at home or in nursing homes, versus profils in healthy young ones. *J Am Geriatr Soc* 1979;27:444–450.

27. Rosenberg IH, Bowman BB, Cooper BA, et al. Folate nutrition in the elderly. *Am J Clin Nutr* 1982;36;1060–1066.

28. Marcus DL, Freedman ML. Folic acid deficiency in the elderly. *J Am Geriatr Soc* 1985;33:552–558.

29. Gardner FH. Refractory anemia in the elderly. *Adv Intern Med* 1987;32:155–176.

30. Hartsock RJ, Smith EB, Petty CS. Variations with aging of the amount of hematopoietic tissue in bone marrow from the anterior iliac crest. *Am J Clin Pathol* 1965;43:326–331.

31. Lee MA, Segal GM, Bagby GC. The hematopoietic microenvironment in the elderly: defects in IL-1–induced CSF expression in vitro. *Exp Hematol,* 1989;17:952–956.

32. Boggs DR, Patrene KD. Hematopoiesis and aging: anemia and a blunted erythropoietic response to hemorrhage in aged mice. *Am J Hematol* 1985;19:327–338.

33. Upuda KB, Lipschitz DA. Erythropoiesis in the aged mouse: response to stimulation in vivo. *J Lab Clin Med* 1984;103:574–580.

34. Upuda KB, Lipschitz DA. Erythropoiesis in the aged mouse: response to stimulation in vitro. *J Lab Clin Med* 1984;103:581–588.

35. Antin JH, Rosenthal DS. Acute leukemias, myelodysplasia and lymphomas. *Clin Geriatr Med* 1985;1:795–826.

36. Sebban C, Archimband E, Coiffier B, et al. Treatment of acute myeloid leukemia in elderly patients: a retrospective study. *Cancer* 1988;61:227–231.

37. Walters RS, Kantarjian HM, Keating MJ, et al. Intensive treatment of acute leukemia in adults 70 years of age and older. *Cancer* 1987;60:149–155.

38. Reiffers J, Raynal F, Boustet A. Acute myeloblastic leukemia in elderly patients: treatment and prognostic factors. *Cancer* 1980;45:2816–2820.

39. Foon KA, Zighelboim K, Yale C, et al. Intensive chemotherapy is the treatment of choice for elderly patients with acute myelogenous leukemia. *Blood* 1981;58:467–470.

40. Gale RP, Foon KA. Chronic lymphocytic leukemia: recent advances in biology and treatment. *Ann Intern Med* 1985;103:101–120.

41. Foon DA, Gale RP. Staging and therapy of chronic lymphocytic leukemia. *Semin Hematol* 1987;24:264–274.

42. Rai KR, Sarvitsky A, Cronkite EP, et al. Clinical staging of chronic lymphocytic leukemia. *Blood* 1975;46:219–234.

43. Report from the International Workshop on CLL. Chronic lymphocytic leukemia, proposals for a revised prognostic staging system. *Br J Haematol* 1981;48:365–367.

44. Stahl R, Silber R. Chronic lymphocytic leukemia. *Clin Geriatr Med* 1985;1:857–867.

45. Cooperative Group for the Study of Immunoglobulin in Chronic Lymphocytic Leukemia. Intravenous immunoglobulin for the prevention of infection in chronic lymphocytic leukemia: a randomized controlled clinical trial. *N Engl J Med* 1988;319:902–907.

46. Cooper IA, Ding JC, Adams PB, et al. Intensive leukapheresis in the management of cytopenias in patients with chronic lymphocytic leukemia (CLL) and lymphocytic lymphoma. *Am J Hematol* 1979;6:387–398.

47. Maloney WC. Chronic myelogenous leukemia. *Cancer* 1978;41:865–873.

48. Talpaz M, Kantarjian HM, Kurzrock R. Therapy of chronic myelogenous leukemia: chemotherapy and interferons. *Semin Hematol* 1988;25:62–73.

49. Crawford S, Eye MK, Cohen HJ. Evaluation of monoclonal gammopathies in the "well" elderly. *Am J Med* 1987;82:39–45.

50. Kyle RA. Monoclonal gammopathy of undetermined sig-

nificance: natural history in 241 cases. *Am J Med* 1978;64:814–826.

51. Cohen HJ. Monoclonal gammopathies and aging. *Hosp Pract* 1988;30:75–100.

52. Kyle RA, Bayrd ED. *The Monoclonal Gammopathies: Multiple Myeloma and related Plasma-Cell disorders.* Springfield, Ill: Charles C Thomas Publisher; 1976:69.

53. Bergsagel DE, Rider WB. Plasma cell neoplasms. In: DeVita VT, Hellman S, Rosenberg SA, eds. *Cancer: Principles and Practice of Oncology.* Philadelphia, Pa: JB Lippincott; 1985:1753–1795.

54. Cohen HJ. Multiple myeloma in the elderly. *Clin Geriatr Med* 1985;1:827–855.

55. Savage DG, Lindenbaum J, Garrett TJ. Biphasic pattern of bacterial infection in multiple myeloma. *Ann Intern Med* 1982;96:47–50.

56. Cohen HJ. Age and the treatment of multiple myeloma: southeastern cancer study group experience. *Am J Med* 1985;79:316–324.

57. Durie BGM, Salmon SE. A clinical staging system for multiple myeloma. *Cancer* 1975;36:842–854.

58. Schafer AI. Bleeding and thrombosis in the myeloproliferative disorders. *Blood* 1984;64:1–12.

59. Gilbert H. Myeloproliferative disorders. *Clin Geriatr Med* 1985;1:773–793.

60. Silverstein MN, Remine WH. Splenectomy in myeloid metaplasia. *Blood* 1979;53:515–518.

61. Thomas DJ, Marshall J, Ross-Russel RW, et al. Cerebral blood-flow in polycythemia. *Lancet* 1977;2:161–163.

62. Wade JPH, Pearson TC, Ross-Russell RW, et al. Cerebral blood flow and blood viscosity in patients with polycythemia secondary to hypoxic lung disease. *Br Med J Clin Res* 1981;283:689–692.

63. York EL, Jones RL, Menon D, et al. Effects of secondary polycythemia on cerebral blood flow in chronic obstructive pulmonary disease. *Am Rev Respir Dis* 1986; 121:813–818.

64. Humphrey PRD, Marshall J, Ross-Russel RW, et al. Cerebral blood-flow and viscosity in relative polycythemia. *Lancet* 1979;2:873–876.

65. Hocking WG. Primary and secondary erythrocytosis. In: Mazza J, ed. *Manual of Clinical Hematology.* Boston, Mass: Little Brown & Co Inc; 1988:49–64.

66. Pearson TC, Wetherley-Mein G. Vascular occlusive episodes and venous hematocrit in primary proliferative polycythemia. *Lancet* 1978;2:1219–1222.

67. Harrison MJG, Kendall BE, Pollack S, et al. Effect of hematocrit on carotid stenosis and cerebral infarction. *Lancet* 1981;2:114–115.

68. Berk PD, Goldberg JD, Donovan PB, et al. Therapeutic recommendations in polycythemia vera based on polycythemia vera study group protocols. *Semin Hematol* 1986;23:132–143.

69. Cotes PM, Dore CJ, Yin JA, et al. Determination of serum erythropoietin in the investigation of erythrocytosis. *N Engl J Med* 1986;315:283–287.

70. Landaw SA. Acute leukemia in polycythemia vera. *Semin Hematol* 1986;23:156–165.

71. Conley CL. Polycythemia vera diagnosis and treatment. *Hosp Pract* 1987;22:107–136.

Gastroenterology

James B. Nelson and Donald O. Castell

Most disorders of the gastrointestinal (GI) tract found in elderly persons are the same as those seen in the remainder of the adult population. There are, however, distinct differences. One major difference is a dramatic change in the prevalence of certain diseases as the patient's age increases, probably best illustrated by acute GI tract bleeding, which is more likely to be produced by mesenteric ischemia or angiodysplasias in old age. Because of these differences, the differential diagnosis must be altered in the elderly patient. Also, common adult illnesses may present in unusual fashion because of the greater potential for a combination of underlying chronic illnesses. Finally, because of the longer total life span of the elderly patient, there is a greater potential for complications of chronic disorders persisting over longer periods. This seems particularly likely in diseases that have malignant potential, such as ulcerative colitis or atrophic gastritis.

Eating and Swallowing Disorders

Dysphagia, or difficulty in swallowing, can present at any age and may be due to a variety of disorders. In the elderly patient, all of these conditions remain possible, some become more likely, and a few are found exclusively at this stage of life, including age-related alterations in striated muscle fiber size and fiber density.[1]

In addition, eating disorders frequently may result from defects not associated with the GI tract, such as cognitive problems, physical disability of the upper limbs, deterioration of the muscles of mastication, and osteoporosis affecting the mandible.[2,3] Recognizing the etiology of a patient's inability to maintain adequate nutrition is crucial, since it has been shown that eating and swallowing disorders are associated with a particularly bad prognosis in elderly persons.[4] Based on clinical presentation, dysphagia can be divided into two distinct syndromes: that produced by abnormalities of the finely tuned neuromuscular mechanisms controlling movements of the tongue, pharynx, and upper esophageal sphincter (oropharyngeal dysphagia) and that caused by a variety of disorders affecting the esophagus itself (esophageal dysphagia).

Oropharyngeal Dysphagia

Six categories of abnormality are associated with oropharyngeal dysphagia in elderly persons (Table 27.1).

Cerebrovascular Accidents

Patients with major strokes often manifest dysphagia as part of their neurologic deficit, particularly if the lesion involves critical areas in the brain stem affecting the swallowing center. Dysphagia may occur in pseudobulbar palsy or in so-called Wallenberg's syndrome (lesion of the posterior inferior cerebellar artery). In these patients, dysphagia may be the primary symptom, making the specific diagnosis difficult. Patients with poststroke dysphagia occasionally will re-

Table 27.1. Likely causes of oropharyngeal dysphagia in
elderly patients.

Cerebrovascular accidents (particularly with brain-stem
    involvement)
  Major strokes
  Wallenberg's syndrome
  Pseudobulbar palsy
Other neuromuscular disorders
  Parkinson's disease
  Myasthenia gravis
  Hypo- or hyperthyroidism
  Amyotrophic lateral sclerosis
Oropharyngeal tumors
Zenker's diverticulum
Vertebral osteophytes
Cricopharyngeal dysfunction

spond to retraining techniques aimed at rehabilitation
of the physical aspects of swallowing. These approaches are best performed during radiologic assessment of the effects of different foods (liquid, semisolid, solid) on swallowing. More encouraging is the fact that a majority of patients will recover function.[5]

Other Neuromuscular Disorders

A variety of neurologic or muscular disorders that affect movement of the tongue, pharynx, or upper esophageal sphincter may result in oropharyngeal dysphagia. In the elderly patient, likely candidates include Parkinson's disease, myasthenia gravis, hypo- or hyperthyroidism, and amyotrophic lateral sclerosis. These disorders may present as dysphagia without other symptoms. Each must be searched for, particularly hyperthyroidism, which may not have typical manifestations in elderly patients. Other neuromuscular causes of swallowing difficulties include brain-stem tumors, bulbar poliomyelitis, progressive cerebellar degeneration, syringobulbia, tabes dorsalis, myotonic dystrophy oculopharyngeal muscular dystrophy, and mixed connective tissue disease.[6]

Oropharyngeal Tumors

Head and neck tumors are distinct possibilities in the etiology of oropharyngeal dysphagia in elderly patients. Direct laryngoscopy should be performed to search for these lesions.

Zenker's Diverticulum

Transient preesophageal dysphagia may be the earliest symptom of this outpouching of a weak spot (Killian's triangle) in the pharyngeal wall located immediately above the upper esophageal sphincter. When the pha-

ryngeal sac becomes large enough to retain food, patients develop the typical symptoms of coughing, fullness and gurgling in the neck, postprandial regurgitation, and aspiration. Some diverticula become so large that patients must perform various maneuvers to empty them, such as applying pressure on the neck and coughing repeatedly. These sacs can become large enough to produce a visible mass in the neck or to obstruct the esophagus by compression.

The pathogenesis of Zenker's diverticulum is controversial. Both radiographic and manometric studies of patients with these diverticula have shown evidence of premature closure of the cricopharyngeus muscle. A recent manometric study using more refined techniques has failed to show any incoordination between pharyngeal contraction and upper esophageal sphincter relaxation.[7] The preferred therapy is surgical (ie, diverticulectomy). Surgical Myotomy of the cricopharyngeus muscle is controversial.

Cervical Hypertrophic Osteoarthropathy

Dysphagia secondary to compression of the esophagus by hypertrophic spurs of the anterior portion of the cervical vertebrae is unusual, considering the frequency of cervical osteoarthritis. The most common complaint is difficulty in swallowing solid foods, but patients also complain of odynophagia, a foreign-body sensation, coughing, hoarseness, and an urge to clear the throat. Diagnosis can be made by means of barium esophagography (lateral views), although endoscopy should be performed to exclude intraluminal pathology. Other structural lesions interfering with swallowing include inflammatory disorders (pharyngitis), thyromegaly, and tracheoesophageal fistulas.[6]

Cricopharyngeal Dysfunction

The cricopharyngeus muscle, along with adjacent hypopharyngeal musculature, contributes to the high-pressure zone known as the upper esophageal sphincter. Cricopharyngeal dysfunction plays an important role in the development of oropharyngeal dysphagia in a variety of conditions. These abnormalities include hypo- and hypertensive sphincters, incomplete relaxation (cricopharyngeal achalasia), premature closure of the sphincter, and delayed relaxation. In addition, it has been suggested that aging itself decreases the tone of the upper esophageal sphincter.[8]

Diagnostic Approach to Oropharyngeal Dysphagia

Identifying the cause of oropharyngeal dysphagia requires close attention to the history and the findings of physical examination and appropriate diagnostic tests. Barium radiography of the pharynx and upper esophageal sphincter area with videofluoroscopy is the preferred diagnostic approach. Since the sequence of muscular changes occurring in this area requires only about 1 second for the transfer of ingested material from the mouth to the upper esophagus, it is essential that rapid-sequence images be obtained. Manometric studies of the pharynx and upper esophageal sphincter are helpful only occasionally, but improved manometric technics currently are being developed and should provide better diagnostic information.

Treatment

The treatment of patients with oropharyngeal dysphagia obviously depends on the underlying cause. Treatable defects, including Parkinson's disease, myasthenia gravis, and thyroid abnormalities, should receive the appropriate therapy. Tumors should be resected if possible. For the patient with otherwise untreatable neuromuscular disorders, including strokes, rehabilitation procedures are often effective. These include altering the diet and eating with the head held in different positions. These approaches should be determined after consultation with a speech pathologist, including careful radiographic assessment of the patient's ability to swallow various types of food (liquid, semisolid, and solid) while maintaining different head positions.

Esophageal Dysphagia

A variety of neuromuscular (motility) defects or mechanical obstructing lesions can cause esophageal dysphagia by interfering with the transport of ingested material down the esophagus. These two types of disorders usually can be differentiated by means of a detailed history. Motility disorders are more likely to cause dysphagia for both solids and liquids; obstructing lesions usually produce dysphagia for solids only.

Achalasia

Achalasia usually presents between the ages of 20 and 40 years, but a second peak occurs in old age. This disorder is characterized by insidious onset, often with symptoms for months or years prior to diagnosis. The pathophysiologic mechanism of achalasia is neurologic in origin, with defects of the ganglion cells in Auerbach's plexus of the esophageal wall. Clinically, there is slowly progressive dysphagia for solids and liquids and gradual weight loss. Regurgitation of undigested foods and retained secretions can cause nocturnal coughing and aspiration.

Chest radiographs may show a dilated esophagus with an air-fluid level from retained food and saliva, and approximately 50% of cases will not have the normal gastric air bubble. Barium studies reveal a dilated, sometimes tortuous esophagus with a smooth "bird beak" narrowing at the gastroesophageal junction. Esophageal manometry usually provides diagnostic findings of increased lower esophageal sphincter pressure with incomplete sphincteric relaxation during swallowing and an aperistaltic esophagus. These defects result in a major functional obstruction of food passing from the esophagus.

It is particularly important in elderly patients to differentiate between idiopathic achalasia and so-called secondary achalasia, ie, cancer that may rarely produce identical radiographic and manometric findings. Tumors associated with such findings include gastric, pancreatic, and lung cancer, as well as sarcomas. Lymphoma also can present in this manner.[9] Consequently, endoscopy with biopsy of any area suspicious for malignancy is mandatory in all patients with achalasia. Certain radiographic changes also may be helpful in differentiating between primary and secondary achalasia.[10] The clinical triad that may suggest secondary achalasia is age over 50 years, dysphagia for less than 1 year, and weight loss of greater than 15 pounds.[11]

The treatment for achalasia can be medical or surgical. Generally, good results can be obtained with either approach, and the choice should be based on the skills of local physicians, the health of the patient, and the patient's preference after adequate education concerning the techniques, risks, and expected outcomes. Medical management with a pneumatic dilator may be more suitable for older patients in poor health. The dilator is placed in the esophagus, with the center of the bag lying within the lower esophageal sphincter. The bag is then inflated while the dilation is monitored fluoroscopically. Surgical management of achalasia consists of a myotomy of the abnormal sphincter (Heller procedure). When done properly, either procedure is successful in alleviating symptoms in most patients, although surgery is generally associated with a higher incidence of side effects, including gastroesophageal reflux.[12]

Occasionally, sufficient relief of dysphagia can be obtained in the patients with achalasia through regular use of a smooth muscle relaxant given just prior to meals. Either isosorbide or nifedipine is effective when given sublingually just prior to eating. The rapid action of these medications enhances relaxation of the lower esophageal sphincter and may improve dysphagia during the meal. Most patients with achalasia, however, will require the more definitive procedures discussed above to open up the esophagogastric junction. The elderly patient with other serious medical problems may not be a candidate for surgery or pneumatic dilation. In this situation, treatment with smooth muscle relaxants should be considered as possible definitive therapy.

Scleroderma (Progressive Systemic Sclerosis)

Esophageal involvement in scleroderma occurs in over 80% of cases and often is associated with the presence of Raynaud's phenomenon. Scleroderma produces a slowly progressive dysphagia for liquids and solids, as in achalasia; heartburn also is a prominent symptom because of severe gastroesophageal reflux. Up to 40% of these patients develop a peptic esophageal stricture. Manometric findings include decreased peristalsis in the lower esophagus (smooth muscle) in contrast to the upper esophagus (striated muscle), where normal peristalsis continues. In addition, lower esophageal sphincter pressure is very low. Treatment of esophageal involvement in scleroderma should include intensive management of reflux with elevation of the head of the patient's bed and full doses of histamine$_2$ (H$_2$) receptor–blocking agents to suppress acid secretion. Second-line therapy with metoclopramide (Reglan) to enhance gastric emptying needs to be weighed against the potential side effects in elderly patients.[13]

Diffuse Esophageal Spasm and Related Disorders

Diffuse esophageal spasm is an esophageal motility disorder characterized by dysphagia and/or chest pain. Dysphagia usually occurs intermittently for both liquids and solids. Symptoms may be exacerbated by hot or cold foods or drinks and may be induced by stress. The condition may be related to a variety of nonspecific esophageal motility disorders, and it may represent part of a spectrum of disorders that can progress to achalasia. Nutcracker esophagus is another disorder in this spectrum. Patients with nutcracker esophagus have high-amplitude peristaltic contractions (>180 mm Hg) and associated symptoms of dysphagia and/or chest pain.

Treatment of diffuse esophageal spasm and related conditions consists of nitrates, calcium channel blockers (preferably nifedipine or diltiazem), sedatives, muscle relaxants, or anticholinergics. Esophageal dilation also may be helpful, and in severe, refractory cases, esophageal myotomy may be considered. Often, patients benefit from reassurance that their pain is esophageal, not cardiac, in origin and from learning how to cope better with stress. Adjuvant therapy, including the use of anxiolytics and psycho-

tropics, may be needed, with the dose adjusted according to the patient's renal and/or hepatic function.[14]

Esophageal Carcinoma

Patients with this disease generally present with rapidly progressive dysphagia (solids first, then liquids) and weight loss. Typically, they have no history of heartburn, although it may occur. A history of heavy alcohol and tobacco use is common. Barium radiographs often suggest the diagnosis, but endoscopy (with biopsy and cytology) is necessary for a more definitive diagnosis. Treatment depends on the extent of disease, with surgical resection, if possible, the treatment of choice. Computed tomographic (CT) scanning may help determine resectability. Radiation therapy, chemotherapy, or both may be palliative, and laser therapy of obstructing lesions also may be considered. The prognosis, in general, is grim, with 5-year survival rate of less than 5%

Peptic Stricture

This condition is characterized by progressive dysphagia for solids and usually follows a long history of heartburn or other reflux symptoms. The diagnosis is made by means of barium radiography, but endoscopy is mandatory to rule out carcinoma. The strictures are smooth, tapered, and of varying lengths. If they are located above the distal esophagus, Barrett's esophagus (ie, metaplastic columnar epithelium lining the distal esophagus) may be present. Patients with this condition, which is related to chronic gastroesophageal reflux, have an increased risk of cancer. Most peptic strictures can be managed with long-term antireflux therapy, including H$_2$ blockers, head-of-bed elevation, and dietary modifications.[15] Intermittent esophageal dilation is often necessary as well, and occasionally surgery (Nissen fundoplication) is required. While there are some experimental data suggesting disordered peristalsis and abnormal lower esophageal sphincter responses to deglutition in older individuals, there is no increased frequency of spontaneous reflux as measured by ambulatory pH systems.[16,17]

Rings or Webs

These disorders, typically associated with intermittent dysphagia for solids, are best diagnosed by means of barium swallow. Endoscopic evaluation is indicated if there is any question about the diagnosis. Because the first episode frequently occurs while the patient is eating steak and bread, the disorder has been termed the "steakhouse syndrome." The bolus is usually forced down by drinking liquids but occasionally must be regurgitated, after which the meal can be finished without difficulty.

The most common type of structural lesion in this category is Schatzki's ring, composed of invaginated mucosa located at the gastroesophageal mucosal junction. These rings are seen on barium studies about 3 to 4 cm above the diaphragm. They most often produce symptoms when the lumen is narrowed to less than 13 mm. Possible causes include gastroesophageal reflux disease. Treatment consists of one-time dilation of the esophagus with a large-caliber bougie. If the symptoms occur infrequently, more careful eating habits may suffice.

Vascular Causes

Esophageal dysphagia also may be caused by vascular anomalies that produce compression of the esophagus. The most common lesions are congenital aortic arch abnormalities associated with dysphagia presenting early in childhood. Occasionally, symptoms begin in adulthood. Dysphagia aortica is a disorder that occurs in elderly persons and is due to compression of the esophagus by either a large thoracic aortic aneurysm or an atherosclerotic, rigid aorta posteriorly and the heart or esophageal hiatus anteriorly.

Disorders of the Stomach and Duodenum

The most notable change in gastric function in the elderly is decreased acid output with a relative increase in achlorhydria. While gastric acid output decreases, owing to a reduction in parietal cell mass, basal serum gastrin concentrations tend to increase with age.[18,19] Pepsin secretion also appears to decline.[20]

Atrophic Gastritis and Gastric Atrophy

Atrophic gastritis is characterized by increased numbers of inflammatory cells in the stomach wall and variable degrees of atrophy of the mucosa. It is generally believed that this kind of gastritis tends to be progressive and that it may develop into gastric atrophy. It is a diffuse disorder, characterized by a decreased number of secretory cells (both chief and parietal) in the mucosa of the gastric body and fundus, along with an increase in the number of nonparietal cells.[21] Generally, these aging gastric mucosal changes correlate with decreased gastric secretion. Still, some studies have found a lack of correlation between gastric mucosal changes and gastric acid output in up

to a third of achlorhydric patients.[22] Interestingly, recent data suggest an increased frequency of antibodies to *Campylobacter pyloris,* in older individuals a potential cause of gastritis.[23]

Two types of atrophic gastritis have been described. Type A is a more diffuse gastritis with antral sparing, usually associated with circulating parietal cell antibodies, elevated gastrin levels, and other autoimmune disorders. This entity may lead to pernicious anemia. Type B gastritis is a focal (antral) condition associated with less reduction in acid secretion, normal serum gastrin levels, and an absence of parietal cell antibodies.

Patients with these conditions usually are asymptomatic, although benign gastric ulcers may develop. Of major clinical importance is the malignant potential of both atrophic gastritis and gastric atrophy, which share the premalignant feature of pernicious anemia. The management of patients with these conditions, therefore, includes periodic surveillance for carcinoma with endoscopic cytology and/or biopsy. Although the optimal interval for such examinations is not clear, they are generally performed every 1 to 2 years.

Pernicious anemia is the end-stage condition seen in patients with type A chronic gastritis. It presents most often as a hematologic abnormality accompanied by neurologic symptoms; GI symptoms are unusual. The diagnosis, however, is strongly supported by the finding of characteristic achlorhydria, defined as a total absence of gastric acid secretion in response to maximal stimulation. Up to 10% of patients with pernicious anemia will develop carcinoma of the stomach, which is estimated to occur three to five times more often in these patients than in the general population of similar age. A summary of follow-up studies of patients with chronic gastritis indicates an average lifetime incidence of gastric cancer of 5%.[24]

Hypertrophic Gastropathy

The presence of enlarged gastric rugae involving part or all of the stomach has been termed Ménétrier's disease; it is relatively unusual and is not unique to elderly patients. However, a number of conditions that may mimic Ménétrier's disease are more likely to occur in the older population. These include gastric lymphoma, infiltrative carcinoma, granulomatous disorders, such as tuberculosis, and other infiltrative conditions, such as amyloidosis. Clinically, these conditions may be associated with vague epigastric pain and weight loss. Of more importance, however, is edema and hypoalbuminemia secondary to protein loss across the gastric mucosa.

On barium radiographs, all of the conditions described above show large gastric folds, which may appear as polypoid filling defects along the greater curvature of the stomach. Endoscopy with adequate biopsy assists in making the specific diagnosis, upon which treatment depends. Sometimes, anticholinergics decrease the gastric protein loss in Ménétrier's disease. Occasionally, gastrectomy is required.

Peptic Ulcer

Although duodenal ulcer is the predominant form of peptic ulceration in younger individuals, gastric ulcer predominates in the elderly population and is much more likely to result in mortality. The presentation of peptic ulcer occurring later in life may be more acute, including severe hemorrhage, perforation, and obstruction in over half of patients older than 70 years.[25] Aggressive therapy often is necessary in older patients, and surgery should not be delayed or withheld solely because of advanced age. The average mortality for complicated peptic ulcers in elderly persons is 30%, with over three quarters of all ulcer operations in this age group performed on an urgent or emergency basis.[26]

Gastric Ulcer

Ulcers in the stomach of elderly patients often assume unusual characteristics. The "giant gastric ulcer," usually associated with a lesion larger than 3 cm in diameter, is an example. Patients may not have typical ulcer symptoms. Instead they may be pain free or have an unusual pattern of pain, with radiation to the chest, periumbilical region, or lower abdomen. Giant gastric ulcers exhibit high complication and mortality rates, particularly from hemorrhage and perforation, and they have a greater malignant potential: up to five times higher than that of ulcers smaller than 3 cm.[27] Apparently benign ulcers that prove to be malignant occur in 2% to 6% of cases. Concurrence of a duodenal ulcer reduces the malignant potential to 1% to 2%.[27,28] Intense medical therapy should be initiated and the healing process carefully monitored with periodic radiography or endoscopy. An interesting variation of gastric ulcer in elderly persons is the "geriatric ulcer," located high in the gastric fundus, along the lesser curvature. They may present with an unusual form of chest pain, coufounding the diagnosis.

Giant Duodenal Ulcer

Occasionally, elderly men present with upper abdominal pain, often radiating into the back, secondary to large duodenal ulcers. These ulcers, which may exceed 2 cm in diameter, may involve most of the surface of the duodenal bulb. Gastrointestinal tract bleeding occurs frequently, and the lesion can involve contiguous organs, such as the pancreas, gallbladder, or liver. A giant duodenal ulcer is diagnosed with barium radiography. Surgery is often required, as medical healing is difficult and morbidity and mortality rates are high.

Treatment

Therapy for peptic ulcers in elderly patients is similar to that in younger patients. However, certain principles require closer attention when treating older patients.

Antacids. These medications continue to be used frequently for symptoms of peptic ulcer disease. In elderly patients, one must be aware of the sodium content of antacid preparations to avoid sodium overload. Riopan (magaldrate) is the antacid with the lowest sodium content. Other possible side effects in elderly patients are diarrhea and altered absorption of other drugs, including digoxin, quinidine, isoniazid, and broad-spectrum antibiotics.

H₂ Receptor Blockers. The major drugs currently used for the treatment of peptic ulcer disease are the H_2 receptor blockers (cimetidine, ranitidine, famotidine, and nizatidine). All of these may produce mental confusion in the elderly patient, especially when given parenterally. In addition, cimetidine is associated with a number of important drug interactions and may increase blood levels of diazepam, warfarin, theophylline, and phenytoin.

Sucralfate. By enhancing protective mechanisms of the gatric mucosa, sucralfate provides an effective alternative for the treatment of acute peptic ulcer disease. For elderly patients, this drug offers the advantage of being free of the systemic side effects produced by H_2 receptor blockers.

Gastric Irradiation. In the occasional elderly patient with severe peptic ulcer disease who is a poor risk for surgery, acid secretion can be temporarily reduced by gastric irradiation. This treatment decreases or abolishes gastric secretion in up to 90% of patients. However, the secretory capacity usually returns to pretreatment levels within about 1 year.

Zollinger-Ellison Syndrome

This entity comprises the classic triad of (1) recurring peptic ulcer disease, (2) marked gastric hypersecretion of acid, and (3) pancreatic adenoma. The adenoma produces large amounts of gastrin, resulting in continuous stimulation of the parietal cells to produce excessive quantities of acid. Approximately one third of patients with this syndrome are over age 60 years. Therefore, the condition should be considered in any patient with persistent or recurrent peptic ulcer disease and/or diarrhea of unclear etiology. A serum gastrin determination should be obtained and, if the diagnosis of Zollinger-Ellison syndrome remains a possibility, gastric secretory studies should be performed. Patients with Zollinger-Ellison syndrome typically have a basal acid output of more than 15 mEq/h, and maximal stimulation will not double this output. The approach to these patients has changed radically in recent years. Total gastrectomy, once considered *the* essential form of therapy, is no longer performed in most of these patients. With the development of more effective acid suppressing drugs, particularly the H_2 receptor blockers, many patients can be maintained in a pain-free state and recurring ulcers prevented with medical therapy. The dose of H_2 blockers required to suppress hypersecretion in these patients may be as much as ten times the usual daily dose. Newer agents, such as the proton pump blocker omeprazole, also are effacious and now may be the treatment of choice.[29] In addition, vagotomy and antrectomy may be considered to allow effective acid suppression with lower doses of H_2-blocking agents.

Drug-Induced Gastritis

Because of the prevalence of arthritic conditions in the aging population, chronic use of a variety of anti-inflammatory medications is common. These nonsteroidal anti-inflammatory drugs (NSAIDs) share a common potential to produce upper gastrointestinal symptoms and/or lesions of the gastric mucosa. The mechanism by which this injury is produced is believed to be secondary to breakdown of the normal gastric mucosal barrier via inhibition of endogenous prostaglandin. Since all of the available NSAIDs are prostaglandin synthesis inhibitors, they share the potential to produce gastric injury. Endoscopic studies have revealed that aspirin is the worst offender, although the other NSAIDs also can produce varying degrees of gastritis. Enteric-coated agents tend to be the safest. This problem can be managed by switching the patient to the other NSAIDs in an attempt to identify individual tolerance or by adding a mucosal protective agent such as sucralfate. Occasionally, the gastric injury is severe enough to produce frank ulceration and GI bleeding.

Bezoars

Bezoars are seen with increased frequency in elderly patients, especially following vagotomy and/or subtotal gastrectomy, and may be related to reduced gastric motility. They occur frequently in elderly diabetics because of severely abnormal gastric emptying.

In patients without any history of diabetes or underlying GI disease, solid food emptying appears to be unaffected by age, but liquid emptying is impaired.[30] The edentulous patient may be at risk because of the insufficient breaking up of food fibers. Pulpy fruits or vegetables, especially citrus fruits, but also figs, coconuts, apples, green beans, sauerkraut, berries, potato peels, and brussels sprouts, are the more commonly incriminated foods. Barium radiography indicates the presence of a mass lesion in the stomach, which may mimic cancer. Treatment with endoscopy, including attempts to break up the lesion with a biopsy forceps or a jet spray of water, is often successful Chronic use of enzyme preparatious or metoclopramide also may be useful.

Volvulus of the Stomach

This relatively rare condition is seen more often in elderly patients because of relaxation of the ligaments supporting the stomach. A complete twist of the organ can result in strangulation of the blood supply, which can lead to gangrene. Often patients present with an abrupt onset of severe epigastric pain and a history of early vomiting, followed by retching with inability to vomit or belch.

Two types of gastric volvulus are described. The more common organoaxial volvulus involves rotation of the stomach on its longitudinal axis (from cardia to pylorus) and results in the radiographic appearance of an "upside-down stomach" and double air-fluid levels (fundus and antrum). The less common mesenteroaxial volvulus represents rotation around a vertical axis passing through the center of the lesser and greater curvatures. An inability to vomit, upper abdominal pain and distention, and inability to have a nasogastric tube inserted are known as Borchardt's triad. Diagnosis is made by means of abdominal radiography, either plain film or with contrast material enhancement. Acute gastric volvulus requires emergency surgery.

Emphysematous Gastritis

This is also an unusual condition, thought to be due to ischemia with subsequent invasion of the gastric wall by gas-forming organisms. The characteristic appearance on a plain radiograph is mottling of the gastric wall. Once again, emergency surgery is indicated, although mortality rates remain high.

Benign Tumors of the Stomach

A variety of nonmalignant tumors occur in the stomach. Frequently, these are asymptomatic and are found during barium studies or endoscopy for other conditions. If symptomatic, the patient is like to have vague upper GI tract complaints and occasionally will develop upper GI tract bleeding. Larger tumors in the antrum may cause outlet obstruction in rare cases. If a decision for active treatment is made, either endoscopic removal (polypoid lesion) or surgical resection should be considered.

Hyperplastic Polyps

These epithelial polyps comprise up to 90% of polypoid lesions seen in the stomach. They are small (usually <1.5 cm in diameter), uniformly distributed, and not premalignant.[31,32] However, the adjacent epithelium may be susceptible to neoplastic transformation, since independent carcinoma has been reported in the adjacent part of the stomach in many cases.

Adenomatous Polyps

These polyps are true neoplasms that usually occur as isolated lesions in the gastric antrum. They attain a larger size (frequently >4 cm) and often are present in mucosa showing chronic atrophic gastritis with permanent intestinal metaplasia. The incidence of malignancy in adenomatous polyps depends on size; for those with diameters larger than 2 cm, the risk of malignancy is 25% to 50%.[32] The presence of achlorhydria secondary to atrophic gastritis is also associated with an increased risk of malignancy.[33]

Leiomyomas

These tumors of the gastric smooth muscle usually present as solitary lesions, most often in the antrum. In the elderly patient, very large tumors may be leiomyoblastomas, which usually require surgical removal. The outcome is good in localized disease.[34]

Malignant Tumors of the Stomach

Although decreasing in frequency, gastric cancer remains a serious consideration in the elderly patient, especially in Japan. In general, polypoid carcinomas have a more favorable prognosis than ulcerating or infiltrative lesions. Patients with diffusely infiltrating cancers have a particularly poor prognosis because of the condition's poorly differentiated characteristics and tendency to infiltrate extensively through the gastric wall prior to diagnosis (so-called linitis plastica). Superficial spreading carcinoma is rare in the United States (8% to 13% of all gastric cancers); it is seen more commonly in the Orient.[35] If diagnosed early, the disease is potentially curable, although the

5-year survival rate of 40% in patients operated on for cure has not changed over the last several decades.[36] Most gastric carcinomas, however, are incurable by the time symptoms become severe enough to lead to diagnosis. Carcinomas of the signet-ring type occur distally, earlier, and predominantly in women, whereas those of the intestinal type tend to occur proximally and in older men.

Vague epigastric discomfort, anorexia, early satiety, and weight loss are the most frequent symptoms. Other forms of presentation are anemia, the finding of occult blood in the stools, or both. On physical examination, evidence of metastatic spread should be sought in lymph nodes in the left supraclavicular space (Virchow's node) and left axilla. Evidence of hepatomegaly may be present. The diagnosis is usually made by means of barium radiography or gastroscopy, with the latter offering the advantage of diagnostic biopsy. Cytology at endoscopy improves the diagnostic yield, particularly in the patient with an infiltrating tumor. CT can assist in establishing whether the tumor is localized or has spread to adjacent structures and nodes.

Special consideration should be given to patients who have undergone partial gastrectomy or gastroenterostomy for peptic ulcer disease. Such patients have an increased frequency of gastric polyps, epithelial dysplasia, and carcinoma in the remaining gastric pouch, beginning about 10 to 15 years after surgery, with an average risk of 5% for each 5-year period after surgery.[37] The only real potential for cure of gastric cancer is early diagnosis and surgical excision, but surveillance endoscopies in older individuals operated on later in life cannot be advocated, because no studies have clearly identified this group as being at higher risk than a similar group of patients who have not been operated on.[38]

The stomach is a common site of lymphoma of the GI tract.[39] The symptoms are similar to those of gastric carcinoma. The radiographic appearance also may be similar, although the presence of large gastric folds and evidence of infiltration into the duodenum are more typical of lymphoma than of carcinoma. Endoscopy confirms the diagnosis if multiple directed biopsies combined with brush cytology are positive. Because the lesions are submucosal, this technique may be unsuccessful and laparotomy may be required for diagnosis. Therapy consists of wide surgical resection followed by radiation. The prognosis is good with localized disease.

Vascular Lesions of the Stomach

Occult GI bleeding may occur secondary to arteriovenous malformations (*angiodysplasias*) in the mucosa of the stomach or duodenum. These lesions appear more frequently with advancing age. They usually can be identified at endoscopy, but angiographic confirmation may be necessary. Localized lesions may be resected; however, endoscopic therapy with electrocoagulation or laser treatment also may be effective. The use of conjugated estrogens has been advocated in the treatment of angiodysplasias in the stomach and elsewhere in the GI tract.[40]

Disorders of Intestinal Function

The major problems in intestinal function prevalent in aging patients are vascular abnormalities and abnormal motility.

Small-Intestinal Dysfunction and Celiac Disease

Several age-related changes in small-intestinal physiology and anatomy have been shown to occur in both animals and humans. These include shortening and fusion of villi, increased absorption of fat-soluble vitamins, reduced lactase activity, possibly contributing to lactose intolerance, and impairment of vitamin D and calcium absorption.[41] Small-bowel transit appears to be unaffected by aging.

Celiac disease, or gluten-sensitive enteropathy, can occur in elderly patients with up to 25% of cases presenting in patients over the age of 70 years.[42] The classic symptoms of anemia, steatorrhea, and osteomalacia may be absent in elderly patients in whom the disease appears more insidiously, with fatigue, depression, indigestion, or dyspepsia. Low serum folate levels and an increased frequency of small-bowel malignancy, particularly lymphoma, occur in older patients with celiac sprue. Multiple small-intestinal ulcerations also may be present in older patients with celiac sprue.[43] Management is similar to that in younger patients, including maintenance of a gluten-free diet and frequent follow-up visits with a dietician. Calcium, vitamin D, and folate supplementation also may be needed. Failure to respond to gluten withdrawal should alert the clinician to the possibility of collagenous sprue or lymphoma.

Additional age-associated changes in the small intestine include diverticulosis particularly in the duodenum, and often in association with cholelithiasis.[44] Complications of jejunnal diverticula include bacterial overgrowth syndromes manifested by abdominal cramps, distention, diarrhea, steatorrhea, and weight loss.

Also, elderly persons have an increased incidence of small-intestinal ulcerations, which may present as hemorrhage, obstruction, or perforation.[45] Often some form of ischemic insult is the cause, but the use of NSAIDs also may produce the condition.[46]

Intestinal Ischemia

Vascular compromise to either the small or large intestine is usually characterized by abdominal pain with or without the passage of bloody diarrhea. Small-intestinal ischemia is unlikely without significant compromise of two of the three main arterial trunks supplying this organ. The term "abdominal angina" has been used to describe the elderly patient with frequent steady midabdominal pain worsened by eating and progressive weight loss. Although this typical presentation is not common, ischemia must be considered in any elderly patient with abdominal pain, diarrhea, and weight loss. Acute occlusion of the superior mesenteric artery may produce infarction of the small bowel with severe periumbilical pain, often associated with few physical findings until later in the course, when a peritoneal reaction occurs in response to transmural infarction. Diagnostic findings include elevated white blood cell (WBC) counts, fever, and radiographs showing ileus or portal vein air. If this diagnosis is suspected, angiography is indicated to confirm the suspicion and to direct the patient to emergency surgery.

Chronic arterial occlusion, due usually to atherosclerosis in elderly patients, is a rarer form of intestinal ischemia presenting with a longer duration of symptoms. Arteriography followed by revascularization can be done in selected cases.

The potential for episodes of ischemic colitis increases with advancing age. These patients typically have lower abdominal cramping pain and rectal bleeding, often associated with elevated WBC counts and fever. Barium enema studies demonstrate areas of narrowing (frequently showing "thumbprinting") or frank ulcerations. Most cases respond to appropriate therapy, and milder, nongangrenous forms usually resolve spontaneously, with up to one half resulting in asymptomatic strictures. Gangrenous presentations are similar to acute intestinal ischemia and require immediate surgical attention.[47]

Angiodysplasias

An important problem in the elderly patient is recurrent GI bleeding secondary to vascular ectasias, so-called angiodysplasias, in the mucosa of the intestine, predominantly the cecum. These lesions, which increase with increased age, present with a variety of bleeding syndromes, from chronic anemia and the presence of occult blood in stools to frank hematochezia. The patients often are otherwise asymptomatic and show no pertinent physical findings, except for an interesting association with the systolic murmur of aortic stenosis. The etiology is uncertain, although intermittent low-grade obstruction of submucosal veins and antheroembolism are suggested mechanisms.[48] Many of these patients have a history of multiple episodes of GI bleeding, often resolving spontaneously and occasionally requiring transfusions. A specific diagnosis requires colonoscopic evaluation of the large intestine with clear examination of the mucosa of the cecum. Arteriographic findings peculiar to angiodysplasias have been described and may help to localize the lesion prior to surgery.[49] Actively bleeding or suspected lesions often can be treated with electrocoagulation at the time of colonoscopy. Chronic estrogen therapy has been recommended as prophylatic treatment, but this has not been proved effective in a controlled trial.[39] Occasionally, patients will require surgery to remove a recurrently bleeding area.

Diverticular Disease

Diverticula in the colon are estimated to be present in at least one third of all individuals over age 60 years. These are really pseudodiverticula, formed by herniation of mucosa and muscularis through weak areas in the circular muscle layer. They are located primarily in the sigmoid colon and frequently are asymptomatic.[50] Age-associated changes in elastic content of the colon with resultant increased intraluminal pressure may contribute to the development of diverticula, although dietary factors, especially low fiber, are equally important.[50,51] Localized perforation of a diverticulum results in diverticulitis. Patients complain of pain in the left lower quadrant and have tenderness (sometimes accompanied by rebound palpable mass) in this area on physical examination. The diagnosis usually is established by means of abdominal radiography and limited sigmoidoscopic examination to exclude complications or other conditions, such as carcinoma. Most patient will respond to the withholding of food, intravenous fluid replacement, and broad-spectrum antibiotics. One fifth will require surgery, indicated in cases of massive hemorrhage, obstruction, or fistula formation. Bleeding from diverticular disease usually is large in amount.[52] Small rectal bleeds more often are due to hemorrhoids, polyps, or cancer. In the patient with diverticulosis, prevention of complications requires a high-residue diet.

Constipation

A variety of factors may contribute to chronic constipation in the elderly individual, including poor diet, lack of exercise, medications that affect bowel function, intrinsic slowing of large-bowel transit, and decreased fecal water excretion.[53,54] After organic causes have been excluded (usually with barium enema) and medications have been reviewed for anticholinergics, antidepressants, and narcotics, it is important to exclude hypothyroidism. Serious complications of chronic constipation include fecal impaction and intestinal obstruction, megacolon, sigmoid volvulus, and fecal incontinence. Many patients respond to advice regarding adequate fluid intake, the addition of fiber or bulk to the diet, and increased exercise. Artificial bulk-forming agents such as psyllium seed are frequently used, often combined with a stool softener. Intermittent use of gentle laxatives may be necessary, although anthracine purgatives should be discouraged, since their long-term use can lead to degenerative myoneural changes.[55]

Anorectal Incontinence

Several studies have now established that aging is associated with changes in anorectal function, including loss of muscle elasticity, slower stimulated defecation, and, in females, less rectal distention required to produce relaxation of the anal sphincter, along with a reduced obtuse anorectal angle.[56,57] In addition, intrinsic changes in myoneural elements occur with aging, eg, denervation associated with an increase in motor unit fiber density.[58] Thus, older patients, especially women, may be predisposed to develop fecal incontinence. Additional important factors include depressed cerebral function and constipation with resultant "overflow" incontinence. Treatment includes therapy for constipation, pelvic floor exercises, biofeedback, and bowel training with the sequential use of constipating agents and stimulants.[59]

Colorectal Cancer and Polyps

Carcinoma of the colon is the most common malignancy of old age, except for prostatic carcinoma in men. The relationship between carcinoma and polyps is now well-established. Hyperplastic polyps are the most common form of benign tumors of the colorectal region. They are found primarily in the rectum, increase in frequency with age, and generally do not predispose to cancer.[60] The other large group of benign tumors is adenomatous polyps. Many produce signs and symptoms, which include anemia, intermittent bleeding, passage of mucus, and diarrhea. It is these lesions that predispose to cancer, with a frequency of 10% to 40%, the higher frequency occurring with larger polyps.[60] Aside from polyps, other factors also may influence the development of colorectal cancer, including long-standing inflammatory bowel disease (especially ulcerative colitis) and dietary factors (eg, low-fiber diets with reduced dilution of fecal carcinogens such as bile acids). Common clinical presentations of colorectal carcinoma in elderly persons include anorexia, anemia, weight loss, constipation, vomiting, abdominal or rectal mass, change in bowel habits, and abdominal pain. Nonspecific symptoms may predominate; these include a loss of energy and apathy. Diagnostic studies for both polyps and carcinoma should include a barium enema and/or colonoscopy with polypectomy. Surgery remains the only method of curative therapy for carcinoma, with 5-year survival rates dependent on the stage of the lesion. Geriatric patients often present at a later stage and have a higher surgical mortality.[61] Screening for colon cancer is discussed in chapter 8.

Inflammatory Bowel Disease

Crohn's disease has a bimodal presentation, peaking at ages 15 to 35 years and again (a smaller peak) at 60 to 70 years.[62] Older patients more often are female, have less ileal involvement, and are more likely to have disease involving the left colon. Presentation is similar to that of diverticular disease, including abdominal pain, diarrhea, rectal bleeding, abdominal mass, and the development of internal fistulas. Features favoring Crohn's disease include anal lesions, a rectovaginal fistual, or systemic complications such as erythema nodosum, arthritis, uveitis, and pyoderma gangrenosum. Diagnosis is often made by means of a double-contrast barium enema study, which may show characteristic mucosal ulcerations, skip lesions, and terminal ileal involvement. Colonoscopy and biopsy may be necessary and may demonstrate lymphoid aggregates and granulomas. Treatment options include the use of elemental diets, steroids, sulfasalazine, and surgery for complications. Adjuvant treatment includes parenteral nutrition for patients with extensive ileal disease and bile acid–binding agents (cholestyramine) to control the diarrhea. The outlook for elderly patients generally is good.[63]

Chronic ulcerative colitis also has a bimodal presentation and can occur as a new disease late in life, especially in women.[64] The presenting symptom is more likely to be diarrhea in elderly patients and rectal bleeding in young patients. Barium enema and colonoscopy are required to make the diagnosis as well as to exclude other diseases, such as diverticulosis and carcinoma. Conditions that must be differentiated from ulcerative colitis include ischemic colitis and pseudomembranous colitis. Treatment consists of steroids and sulfasalazine. Fewer relapses and a milder course are seen in older patients who survive

the initial stages.[65] Pancolitis with a duration of 10 or more years increases the risk of developing carcinoma, and, therefore, frequent colonoscopic surveillance and/or colectomy is recommended in this group of patients.[66]

Hepatobiliary Disorders

Liver Diseases

Although a decrement in metabolic capacity and regenerative ability occurs in the aging liver, clinical derangements in liver function in elderly persons are minimal. Several changes in liver anatomy and physiology have been identified, including a decrease in size, reduced hepatic blood flow, increased hepatocyte aneuploidy, ductular proliferation, hepatocellular necrosis, reduced protein synthesis, and a reduction in the metabolism of several drugs, especially the benzodiazopines.[67] As a rule, blood chemistry findings remain normal in elderly persons; liver disease must be suspected if they are abnormal. Unlike in younger adults, jaundice in elderly patients is much more likely to represent biliary tract obstruction and to be secondary to malignancy rather than gallstones. Additional causes of cholestatic jaundice are listed in Table 27.2. Hepatitis is less common in elderly patients and is more likely to be drug-induced than secondary to viral infection, although non-A and non-B hepatitis secondary to blood transfusions occurs. Because of these principles, an early approach to the elderly patient with jaundice should include abdominal ultrasound to provide evaluation of the gallbladder, biliary tree, liver, and pancreas. At all ages, elevation primarily in serum aminotransferase levels should favor a diagnosis of hepatocellular disease, with appropriate diagnostic studies including antinuclear antibody titers and hepatitis serology. Liver biopsy may be needed if the

Table 27.2. Causes of cholestatic jaundice.

Medical
    Drug-induced cholestasis
    Congestive heart failure
    Cirrhosis (alcoholic, cryptogenic, primary biliary)
    Cholestatic viral hepatitis
    Primary sclerosing cholangitis
    Miscellaneous (eg, Hodgkin's disease)

Surgical
    Carcinoma of the pancreas
    Metastatic carcinoma of the liver
    Common bile duct stones
    Stricture of the common bile duct
    Common bile duct tumor
    Chronic pancreatitis

diagnosis is unclear or the course is atypical. Since elderly individuals may have many medical diseases and are often taking many medications, drug-induced hepatitis is a frequent consideration. Adverse reactions to medications have been estimated to occur in approximately 25% of patients over age 80 years.[68] Some of the more commonly used drugs having the potential to cause liver toxicity include antihypertensives, antibiotics, anticonvulsants, psychotrophic drugs, hormones, oral hypoglycemics, NSAIDs, antineoplastic drugs, and anesthetics. Usually, drug toxicity stops after withdrawal of the offending agent.

Alcoholic hepatitis is not a common problem in elderly persons but does occasionally occur. In addition, alcoholic cirrhosis peaks in the 7th decade.[69]

It is important to remember that ischemic injury to the liver can occur from any form of circulatory failure, including that occurring after surgery or after an episode of congestive heart failure. Prothrombin times can become prolonged and bilirubin, alkaline phosphatase, and aminotransferase levels can rise. Severe right-sided heart failure, hypotension, or shock can lead to hepatic necrosis, or "shock liver," with serum aminotransferase levels approaching those seen in acute viral hepatitis (over 1,000 IU/mL).[70] Chronic congestive heart failure also may lead to a form of "cardiac cirrhosis" characterized by reverse lobulation.[71]

The complications of cirrhosis of any etiology, including portal hypertension and hepatic encephalopathy, also develop in elderly persons. Vasopressin infusions to control variceal hemorrhage must be used with caution in older patients, as cardiac ischemia and arrythmias can be provoked.

Hereditary (genetic) hemochromatosis, manifested by hepatic iron overload due to enhanced intestinal absorption, is seen in elderly patients, most often presenting as cirrhosis. Phlebotomies help prevent progression of the disease. The importance of making the diagnosis rests in the need for familial screening to identify patients in the precirrhotic stage.

Primary biliary cirrhosis can appear in asymptomatic elderly women as biochemical abnormalities, especially increased alkaline phosphatase levels. Elderly patients with long-standing disease are especially prone to bone abnormalities, including stress fractures and xanthomatous neuropathy. Treatment should include fat-soluble vitamins. Systemic antihistamines may be useful to control symptomatic pruritus.

Pyogenic liver abscess is an important cause of jaundice, fever, and sepsis in elderly persons. The most common causes are septic embolization and biliary tract disease.[72] Delay in making the diagnosis contributes to the high mortality rate.

Finally, the incidence of primary hepatocellular carcinoma peaks at age 50 to 70 years. Most often it is due to underlying cirrhosis, especially with associated hemochromatosis.[73] Treatment is unsatisfactory and the disease usually is fatal. This entity should be suspected in a previously stable cirrhotic patient with suddenly worsening liver function.

Gallbladder and Biliary Tract

Although malignant obstructions of the biliary tract are common, numerous elderly patients have biliary disease secondary to gallstones. These may increase in frequency with age because of an age-associated increase in the lithogenic index of bile.[74,75] As with other diseases, the typical symptoms of biliary colic or acute cholecystitis occur less frequently in elderly patients. More often symptoms are nonspecific (eg, fatigue and anorexia).[76] Other presentations include jaundice or other abnormal liver function test results, septicemia, fever of unknown origin, and pancreatitis. Diagnostic studies should begin with an oral cholecystogram or biliary ultrasound. If the diagnosis remains in doubt, CT, endoscopic retrograde cholangiopancreatography or percutaneous choloangiography may be needed. In the past, surgery has been the mainstay of treatment for symptomatic gallstone disease. There are, however, many new advances and therapeutic approaches to these problems that offer potential for the elderly, high-risk patient. These include the dissolving of gallstones by means of oral bile acid therapy (chenodeoxycholic/ursodeoxycholic acid) or chemicals instilled via a percutaneous catheter placed through the liver (tertbutyl ether), sphincterotomy, endoscopic removal of stones, and shock wave lithotripsy.

Malignant causes are present approximately 50% of jaundiced elderly patients and include pancreatic carcinoma, gallbladder carcinoma, cholangiocarcinoma, and carcinoma of the papilla of Vater.[77] This latter cancer has, in general, the best prognosis, with 5-year survival rates of greater than 20%. The other biliary cancers have a uniformly poor prognosis. Palliation is the goal of therapy, with biliary stents placed either endoscopically or percutaneously to alleviate disabling pruritus.

Pancreatic Disorders

Aging is associated with a definite decline in pancreatic output of bicarbonate and several pancreatic enzymes, including lipase and trypsin.[78] Whether this translates into clinical consequences is doubtful, since over 90% of the pancreas must be destroyed before signs of dysfunction, such as steatorrhea, develop.

There is an increased frequency of pancreatic cancer in elderly persons, presenting as painless jaundice, diarrhea, abdominal pain, or weight loss.

Acute pancreatitis also occurs in elderly persons, especially women. It is often secondary to choledocholithiasis, and its mortality rate is 78% in those over age 60 years versus 9% in younger persons.[79] Two specific age-related causes of acute pancreatitis include embolization of pancreaticoduodenal arteries and complications of translumbar aortography.

Chronic pancreatitis with pain secondary to chronic alcoholism is uncommon in elderly persons. Painless disease, however, occurs not infrequently in older individuals. Presentations include steatorrhea, diabetes, and pancreatic calcifications. Idiopathic forms predominate in elderly persons with painless disease, affect men more often than women, and have a generally good prognosis with enzyme replacement.[80] Chronic primary inflammatory pancreatitis occurs in elderly persons.[81] Developing more often in women, it is characterized by primarily mild abdominal pain and an increased gammaglobulin concentration in over 40% of patients. Weight loss, steatorrhea, and fever may also be noted. Parenchymal atrophy is seen histologically, along with mononuclear infiltration, possibly reflecting an autoimmune etiology. The prognosis is variable; some cases respond favorably to enzyme replacement, whereas others progress rapidly to death.

Summary

Gastrointestinal disorders occur commonly in elderly persons. We have reviewed the etiologies, diagnoses, and treatments of benign and malignant conditions affecting the aging gut. Table 27.3 summarizes differences in the presentation of GI disorders between elderly persons and younger adults.

Table 27.3. Differential clinical aspects of GI tract diseases in elderly vs younger patients.

Clinical condition	Younger adults	Elderly patients
Dysphagia	Esophageal cause	Oropharyngeal cause
Achalasia syndrome	Primary	Secondary
Peptic ulcer	Duodenal	Gastric
Gastric outlet obstruction	Benign	Malignant
Malabsorption	Sprue	Lymphoma or vascular
Colitis	Inflammatory	Ischemic
Jaundice	Hepatocellular	Obstruction
Hepatocellular	Viral hepatitis	Drug induced
Obstructive	Gallstone	Malignant

References

1. Leese G, Hopwood D. Muscle fiber typing in the human pharyngeal constrictors and oesophagus: the effect of aging. *Acta Anat* 1986;127:77–80.
2. Gutmann E. Muscle. In: Finch CE, Hayflick L, eds. *Handbook of the Biology of Aging.* NY: Van Nostrand Reinhold Co; 1977:pp 709–723.
3. Wical KE, Swoope CC. Studies of residual ridge resorption, II: the relationship of dietary calcium and phosphorus to residual ridge resorption. *J Prosthet Dent* 1974;32:13–22.
4. Siebens H, Trupe E, Seibens A, et al. Correlates and consequences of eating dependency in institutionalized elderly. *J Am Geriatr Soc* 1988;34:192–198.
5. Gordon C, Hewer RL, Wade DT. Dysphagia in acute stroke. *Br Med J* 1987;295:411–414.
6. Pelemans W, Vantrappen G. Oesophageal disease in the elderly. *Clin Gastroenterol* 1985;14:635–656.
7. Knuff TE, Benjamin SB, Castell DO. Pharyngoesophageal (Zenker's) diverticulum: a reappraisal. *Gastroenterology* 1982;82:734–736.
8. Pelemans W. *Functie van Defaryngo-Esofagale Overgangszone en Dysfunctie bij Bejaarden.* Thesis, Leuveu, Acco 1983; 128 pp.
9. Kahrilas PJ, Kisak SM, Helm JF. Comparison of pseudoachalasia and achalasia. *Am J Med* 1987;82:439–446.
10. Ott DJ, Gelfand DW, Wu WC, et al. Secondary achalasia in esophagogastric carcinoma: re-emphasis of a difficult differential problem. *Rev Interam Radiol* 1979;4:135–138.
11. Tucker JH, Snape WJ, Cohen S. Achalasia seconary to carcinoma: manometric and clinical features. *Ann Intern Med* 1978;89:315–318.
12. Csendes A, Velasco N, Braghetto I, et al. A prospective randomized study comparing forceful dilatation and esophagomyotomy in patients with achalasia of the esophagus. *Gastroenterology* 1981;80:789–798.
13. Horowitz M, Maddern GJ, Maddox A, et al. Effects of Cisapride on gastric and esophageal emptying in progressive systemic sclerosis. *Gastroenterology* 1987;93:311–315.
14. Nelson JB, Castell DO. Esophageal motility disorders. *DM* 1988;34:297–389.
15. Castell DO, Wu WC, Ott D. *Gastroesophageal Reflux Disease: Pathogenesis Diagnosis, Therapy.* New York, NY: Futura Publishing Co; 1985.
16. Khan TA, Shragge BW, Crispin JS, et al. Esophageal motility in the elderly. *Am J Dig Dis* 1977;22:1049–1054.
17. Spence RAJ, Collins BJ, Parks TG, et al. Does age influence normal gastro-oesophageal reflux? *Gut* 1985;26:799–801.
18. Kekki M, Samloff M, Ihamakci T, et al. Age and sex-related behaviour of gastric acid secretion at the population level. *Scand J Gastroenterol* 1982;17:737–743.
19. McGuigan JE, Trudeau WL. Serum gastrin concentrations in pernicious anemia. *New Engl J Med* 1970;282:358–361.

20. Samloff IM, Liebman WM, Panitch NM. Serum group I pepsinogens by radioimmunoassay in control subjects and patients with peptic ulcer. *Gastroenterology* 1975;69:83–90.

21. Rouoff JH, Leyhe T, Eichhorst UB, et al. Morphologically different biopsy specimens of the human gastric mucosa, I: the use of enzymatic cell isolation for quantitative determination of parietal cells. *Pharmacology* 1986;33:121–130.

22. Bird T, Hall MRP, Schade ROK, et al. Gastric histology and its relation to anemia in the elderly. *Gerontology* 1977;23:309–321.

23. Perez-Perez GI, Dworkin BM, Chodos J, et al. *Campylobacter* antibodies in humans. *Ann Intern Med* 1988;109:11–17.

24. Rosch W. Chronische Gastritis: Mythen and Facten. *Internistische Welt* 1979;10:332–337.

25. Lavrat M, Pasquier J, Lambert R, et al. Peptic ulcer in patients over 60: experience in 287 cases. *J Dig Dis Sci* 1966;11:279.

26. Michel D. Chirurgie des gastroduodenal Ulcus beim alten Menschen. *Chirurg* 1981;52:254–260.

27. Wenger J, Brandborg LL, Spellman FA. The Veterans Administration Cooperative Study on Gastric Ulcer: Cancer, I: clinical aspects. *Gastroenterology* 1971;61:598–621.

28. Ihre BJE, Bar H, Havermark G. Ulcer-cancer of the stomach. *Gastroenterologia* 1964;102:78–91.

29. Olbe L, Berglinoh T, Elander B, et al. Properties of a new class of gastric acid Inhibitors *Scand J Gastroenterol* (Suppl) 1979;14:131–135.

30. Moore JG, Tweedy C, Christian PE, et al. Effect of age on gastric emptying of liquid-solid meals in man. *Dig Dis Sci* 1983;28:340–344.

31. Tomasolo J. Gastric polyps: histologic types and their relationships to gastric carcinoma. *Cancer* 1971; 27:1346–1355.

32. Yamagata S, Hisamichi S. Precancerous lesions of the stomach. *World J Surg* 1979;3:671–673.

33. Laxen F. Gastric carcinoma and pernicious anemia in long-term endoscopic follow-up of subjects with gastric polyps. *Scand J Gastroenterol* 1984;19:535–540.

34. Stout AP. Bizarre smooth muscle tumors of the stomach. *Cancer* 1962;15:400–409.

35. O'Brien M, Burakoff R, Robbins EA, et al. Early gastric cancer. *Am J Med* 1985;78:195–202.

36. Diehl JT, Hermann DE, Cooperman AM, et al. Gastric carcinoma: a ten year review. *Ann Surg* 1983;198:9–12.

37. Offerhaus GJA, Huibregtse K, Deboer J, et al. The operated stomach: a premalignant condition? A prospective endoscopic follow-up study. *Scand J Gastroenterol* 1984;19:521–524.

38. Dougherty SH, Foster CA, Eisenbierg MM. Stomach cancer following gastric surgery for benign disease. *Arch Surg* 1982;117:294–297.

39. Brooks JJ, Enterline HT. Primary gastric lymphoma: a clinicopathologic study of 58 cases with long-term follow-up and literature review. *Cancer* 1983;51:701–711.

40. Brunner MH, Pate MB, Cunningham JT, et al. Estrogen-progesterone therapy for bleeding gastrointestinal telangiectasias in chronic renal failure. *Ann Intern Med* 1986;105:371–374.

41. Holt PR. Gastrointestinal disorders in the elderly: the small intestine. *Clin Gastroenterol* 1985;14:689–723.

42. Swinson CM, Levi AJ. Is coeliac disease underdiagnosed? *Br Med J* 1980;281:1258–1260.

43. Robertson DAF, Dixon MF, Scott BB, et al. Small intestinal ulceration: diagnostic difficulties in relation to coeliac disease. *Gut* 1983;24:565–574.

44. Osnes M, Lotveit T, Larsen S, et al. Duodenal diverticuli and their relationship to age, sex, and biliary calculi. *Scand J Gastroenterol* 1980;16:103–107.

45. Boydstun JS Jr, Gaffey TA, Bartholomew LG. Clinicopathologic study of nonspecific ulcers of the small intestine. *Dig Dis Sci* 1981;26:916–911.

46. Bjarnason I, Price AB, Zanelli G. Clinicopathological features of nonsteroidal anti-inflammatory drug-induced small intestinal strictures. *Gastroenterology* 1988; 94:1070–1074.

47. Marston A. Gastrointestinal disorders in the elderly: Ischemia. *Clin Gastroenterol* 1985;14:847–862.

48. Boley SJ, Sammartano R, Adams A, et al. On the nature and etiology of vascular ectasias of the colon. *Gastroenterology* 1977;72:650–660.

49. Heuverzwyn Van R, Haot J, Dautrebande J. Angiodysplasia and vascular malformations. In: Hellemans J, Vantrappen G, eds. *Gastrointestinal Tract Disorders in the Elderly*. Edinburgh, Scotland: Churchill Livingstone Inc; 1984:125–133.

50. Parks TG. Natural history of diverticular disease of the colon. *Clin Gastroenterol* 1975;4:53–69.

51. Painter N, Burkitt DP. Diverticular disease of the colon: a 20th century problem. *Clin Gastroenterol* 1975;4:3–21.

52. Almy TP, Howell DA. Diverticular disease of the colon. *New Engl J Med* 1980;302:324–331.

53. Brocklehurst JC, Kahn MY. Study of fecal stasis in old age and in the use of "dorbanex" in is prevention. *Gerontol Clin* 1969;11:293–300.

54. Burkitt DP, Walker ARP, Painter NS. Dietary fiber and disease. *JAMA* 1974;229:1068–1074.

55. Smith B. The effect of irritant purgatives on the myenteric plexus in man and mouse. *Gut* 1968;9:139–143.

56. Ihre T. Studies on anal function in continent and incontinent patients. *Scand J Gastroenterol* 1974;9 (suppl 1):1–64.

57. Loening-Baucke V, Anuras S. Effect of age and sex on anorectal manometry. *Am J Gastroenterol* 1985;80:50–53.

58. Percy JP, Neill ME, Kandiah TK, et al. A neurogenic factor in fecal incontinence in the elderly. *Age Ageing* 1982;11:175–179.

59. Jarrat AS, Exton-Smith AN. Treatment of faecal incontinence. *Lancet* 1960;1:925.

60. Brocklehurst JC. Colonic disease in the elderly. *Clin Gastroenterol* 1985;14:725–747.

61. Edwards RTM, Bransom CJ, Crosby DL, et al. Colorectal carcinoma in the elderly: geriatric and surgical practice compared. *Age Ageing* 1983;12:256–262.

62. Kyle J. An epidemiological study of Crohn's disease: in

North East Scotland. *Gastroenterology* 1971;61:826–833.

63. Cooke NT, Mallass E, Prior P, et al. Crohn's disease: course, treatment and long-term prognosis. *Q J Med* 1980;49:363–384.

64. Evans JG, Acheson ED. An epidemiological study of ulcerative colitis and regional enteritis in the Oxford area. *Gut* 1965;6:311–324.

65. Gebbers JO, Otto HF. Ulcerative colitis in the elderly. *Lancet* 1975;2:714–715.

66. Lightdale CJ, Winawer SJ. Polyps and tumors of the large intestine. In: Hellemans J, VanTrappen G, eds. *Gastrointestinal Tract Disorders in the Elderly.* Edinburg, Scotland: Churchill Livingstone Inc, 1984:174–184.

67. Mooney H, Roberts R, Cooksley, et al. Alterations in the liver with aging. *Clin Gastroenterol* 1985;14:757–771.

68. Vestal RE. Drug use in the elderly: a review of problems and special considerations. *Drugs* 1978;16:358–382.

69. James OFW. Gastrointestinal and liver function in old age. *Clin Gastroenterol* 1983;12:671–691.

70. Gibson PR, Dudley FJ. Ischaemic hepatitis: clinical features, diagnosis and prognosis. *Aust N Z J Med* 1984;14:812–815.

71. Dunn GD, Hayes P, Breen KJ, et al. The liver in congestive heart failure: a review. *Am J Med Sci* 1973;265:175–189.

72. Rubin RH, Swartz MN, Malt R. Hepatic abscess: changes in clinical, bacteriologic, and therapeutic aspects. *Am J Med* 1974;57:601–610.

73. Stevens RG, Merkle EJ, Lustbader ED. Age and cohort effects in primary liver cancer. *Intern J Cancer* 1984;33:453–458.

74. Glenn F, McSherry CK. Calculous biliary tract disease. *Curr Probl Surg* 1975;vol. 12. pp. 1–38.

75. Valdivieso V, Palma R, Wunkhaus R, et al. Effect of aging on biliary lipid composition and bile acid metabolism in normal Chilean women. *Gastroenterology* 1978;74:871–874.

76. Cobden I, Lendrum R, Venables CN, et al. Gallstones presenting as mental and physical disability in the elderly. *Lancet* 1984;1:1062–1064.

77. Croker R. Biliary tract disease in the elderly. *Clin Gastroenterol* 1985;14:773–809.

78. Laugier R, Sarles H. Gastrointestinal disorders in the elderly: the pancreas. *Clin Gastroenterol* 1985;14:749–756.

79. Corfield AP, Cooper MJ, Williamson RCH. Acute pancreatitis: a lethal disease of increasing incidence. *Gut* 1985;26:724–729.

80. Amman R, Sulser H. Die 'Senile' chronische Pankreatitis: eine neue nosologische einheit? *Schweiz Med Wochenschr* 1976;106:429–437.

81. Sarles H, Sarles JC, Muratore R, et al. Chronic inflammatory sclerosis of the pancreas: an autonomous pancreatic disease. *Dig Dis Sci* 1961;6:1–7.

28

Pulmonary Diseases

James F. Morris

The bronchopulmonary system is subject to environmental ravages. Every few seconds, the ambient air and all it contains is inhaled and comes in contact with a surface area equivalent in the adult to the size of a tennis court. Perhaps, we are endowed with one extra lung in anticipation of environmental slings and arrows, natural in earlier days and manmade today. With a normal aging process, the bronchopulmonary system should be adequate for about 90 years of continuous functioning. The lungs initially were thought to be designed only for acting as a fluctuating bellows, which results in the transfer of oxygen and carbon dioxide. Additional pulmonary biochemical and immunologic roles have been discovered, revealing a more active metabolic status.

Anatomy

The three main structural elements of the bronchopulmonary system are the airways, the lung parenchyma, and the chest wall. The airways primarily provide a conducting function for the movement of inspired and expired gases. Gas transfer takes place only at or below the level of the respiratory bronchiole. The simultaneous progressive narrowing and branching of the airways produce a marked increase in the total cross-sectional diameter and a resulting decrease in the resistance to airflow. The airways are divided into those with cartilaginous support and those lacking it; the latter are the bronchioles, which are usually 2 mm or less in diameter. The supporting mechanism of the

bronchioles is the tethering effect of the parenchymal elastic tissue. They are, thus, more susceptible to changes in lung inflation and intrathoracic pressure. In addition, airway lumens can be narrowed by a constriction of bronchial muscle, by a loss of supporting epithelium by hypertrophy, edema, or inflammation, and by obstructing bronchopulmonary secretions.

The most easily demonstrable change with aging or environmental damage is the loss of elastic lung parenchyma surrounding small noncartilaginous airways. This causes a premature closure that results in an increase in trapped or residual gas volume and a decrease in forced expired airflows. In the absence of specific lung diseases, aging causes a loss or change in connective tissues, which increases the compliance of the airways, resulting in progressive enlargement of the bronchi, bronchioles, and alveolar ducts. In bronchial walls, aging increases the size of mucous glands and the calcification of cartilage. The enlargement of the airway caliber is negated by the decrease in parenchymal support of the smaller airways, resulting in a net decrease in the diameter of the airways with aging.

Decreased elastic recoil with an increased distensibility causes descent of the diaphragm and expansion of the thorax. A common misconception is that these changes are produced by hyperinflation of the lungs, when, in truth, they are due to the natural tendency of the chest cavity to enlarge unless opposed by the elastic recoil of the lung. The changes in the distribution of parenchymal elastic tissue result in panlobular emphysema, which is characterized by a progressive dilation of alveoli and an eventual disruption of their walls. In contrast to the centrilobular emphysema associated with cigarette smoking, the respiratory bronchioles are minimally involved, there is no inflammatory component, the distribution is predominantly in the lower lobes, the lungs are less compliant, and the changes are not severe. There is a similarity to the panlobular emphysema found in patients with homozygous alpha₁-antitrypsin deficiency, who appear to have accelerated lung senescence. Aging, tobacco smoke and other air pollutants, many pulmonary infections, and deficiency of antiproteases favor the development of various forms of emphysema.

The chest wall has been relatively neglected regarding its contribution to ventilation. Macklem has referred to it as the last unexplored organ in the body.[1] The muscles of respiration consist of the intercostal and accessory muscles, the diaphragm, and the abdominal muscles. During quiet breathing, the diaphragm is responsible for ventilatory work, with the other respiratory muscles helping to stabilize the chest wall and abdomen.[2] During exertion, all the respiratory muscles are needed; the degree of involvement is related to the level of work being done. With aging and a decline in physical activity, muscle atrophy can lead to a diminished exertional capacity. Changes in skeletal portions of the chest wall include calcification of costochondral joints and a decreased chest wall compliance.

Lung Defense Mechanisms

An individual inhales an average tidal volume of 500 mL about 18,000 times daily, or about 9,000 L of ambient air. The lungs have a complex defense system to protect them against inhaled particles, gases, microorganisms, and products of combustion.[3] When these defense mechanisms are overwhelmed or are lacking, respiratory diseases result. In addition to inhaled noxious agents, the lung must defend itself against biochemical substances in the pulmonary capillary blood that can result in damage to the alveolar capillary membrane.

Nonspecific defense mechanisms include the regulation of temperature and humidity, clearance mechanisms, mucus, and cellular defenses. Responses to specific antigens include local antibody production and cell-mediated immunity. Both mechanisms are progressively impaired by the aging process, increasing susceptibility to conditions ranging from viral infections to lung cancer.

Inhaled tobacco smoke blunts the effectiveness of both nonspecific (phagocytic) and specific (immunologic) defense mechanism systems of the lung. This impairment may be responsible for a smoker's increased susceptibility to bronchopulmonary infections; it hampers the handling of other inhaled particulates by the lung. The functions of alveolar macrophages and lymphocytes are adversely affected by cigarette smoke.

Other inhaled particulates and gaseous agents also suppress pulmonary defense mechanisms. Adverse effects of environmental agents include the inhibition of phagocytosis and antibody production, as well as susceptibility to viral and bacterial infections. The effects of cigarette smoke and of environmental pollutants are increased by prolonged exposure and are, thus, worse in older adults.

Chronic diseases of the lungs, heart, kidney, bone marrow, and other organ systems, which are more common in elderly persons, are associated with an increased susceptibility to lower respiratory tract infections. Conditions such as hypoxia, acidosis, malnutrition, uremia, and cold exposure impair alveolar macrophage functions.

Pulmonary Function

A reserve capacity is built into most body organs. Considerable lung disease is required to produce a significant impairment of pulmonary function. As in other organs, diffuse damage results in a greater functional loss than focal damage. The principal symptom of pulmonary function impairment is dyspnea, which represents an awareness of breathing that may or may not mean pulmonary dysfunction.[4] That is, dyspnea may be appropriate for the level of exertion and may result from any deficiency in the entire oxygen transport system.

Ventilation

The principal components of ventilation are lung volumes and airflows. The degrees of inspiratory and expiratory pressures generated by respiratory muscles, as well as age, body position, height, and sex, influence lung volumes. In the upright position, aging decreases the vital capacity and increases the residual volume.[5,6] Only minor changes occur in functional residual capacity and total lung capacity. Increased residual volume represents trapped gas that is probably caused by early airway closure, increased thoracic cage rigidity, and decreased lung elastic recoil.[7]

Expired gas flows are determined by forces that are exerted by respiratory muscular effort and lung elastic recoil and influenced by the airway diameter. As lung volume diminishes, gas flow becomes nearly independent of muscular effort. Conditions that reduce elastic recoil or patency of the airways impair forced expiratory flows. With advancing age, total lung capacity is maintained and contributes to the preservation of large airway diameter,[8] but changes in elastic tissues of the lung result in a decrease in elastic recoil and an increase in compliance or distensibility.

The volume of gas remaining in the lung as airways close is termed the closing volume. As aging results in a reduced elastic recoil, the closing volume increases and, in the supine position, encroaches on the tidal volume.[9] Another force influencing flow is respiratory muscular effort, which decreases with aging. Thus, all flows are reduced, those at high lung volume owing to a diminished elastic recoil and airway diameter.[10]

The five spirometric tests useful in measuring ventilatory function are the FVC, FEV_1, FEF200–1200, FEF25%–75%, and FEF75%–85%[11] (FVC indicates forced vital capacity; FEV_1, forced expiratory volume in 1 second; FEF200–1200, forced expiratory flow rate between 200 and 1200 cm^3; FEF25%–75%, forced expiratory flow rate between 25% and 75% of vital capacity; and FEF75%–85%, forced expiratory flow rate between 75% and 85% of vital capacity.

Figures 28.1 and 28.2 show the age-related decline in four of these measurements based on a cross-sectional study of healthy nonsmoking adults.[12] There are two flaws in such studies; first, a longitudinal study is preferable, but obviously difficult to achieve.[13] Second, normal predicted values are expressed as a linear regression equation, although a curvilinear function is more appropriate. The decrement in flows and vol-

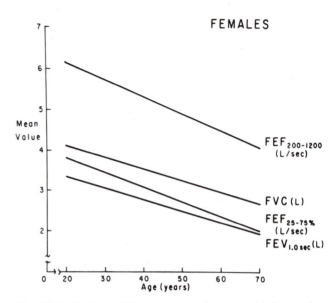

Fig. 28.2. Decline of four spirometric tests with increasing age in women.

umes are not the same for each year of the life span. The difficulty in obtaining an adequate study of representative elderly subjects has yet to be resolved. A normal variation from predicted sample means is substantial despite accounting for sex, height, and respiratory health. Selection of a fixed value such as 1.65 times the mean value may result in negative predicted values for expiratory flows in elderly persons. Serial studies in an individual subject would be preferable for observing the change of pulmonary function, which is influenced not only by age but also by diseases due to smoking, air pollution, and infections.

Table 28.1 lists regression equations that are useful for calculating the equivalent lung age.[14] This represents the age at which the observed test results would be normal for a person of the same age, sex, and height. For example, the FEV_1 of 52-year-old cigarette smoker would be normal for a 75-year-old nonsmoking

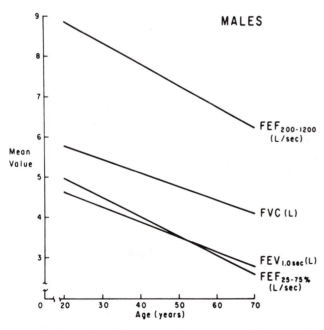

Fig. 28.1. Decline of four spirometric tests with increasing age in men.

Table 28.1. Equivalent lung age.

	Lung age*
Males	
FVC	$5.920H - 40.00(FVC) - 169.640$
FEV_1	$2.870H - 31.250(FEV_1) - 39.375$
$FEV_{200-1200}$	$2.319H - 21.277(FEF_{200-1200}) + 42.766$
$FEF_{25\%-75\%}$	$1.044H - 22.222(FEF_{25\%-75\%}) + 58.444$
Females	
FVC	$4.792H - 41.667(FVC) - 118.833$
FEV_1	$3.560H - 40.000(FEV_1) - 77.280$
$FEF_{200-1200}$	$4.020H - 27.778(FEF_{200-1200}) - 70.333$
$FEF_{25\%-75\%}$	$2.000H - 33.333(FEF_{25\%-75\%}) + 18.367$

*In these equations, FVC, FEV_1 etc, indicate the observed values. H indicates height, in inches.

man of similar height without ventilatory impairment. These calculations may provide a motivation for the cessation of smoking. A variety of spirometers are available, ranging from simple volume displacement devices to computerized electronic systems. The American Thoracic Society has established standards of accuracy to which all devices should conform.[15]

Alveolar Gas Exchange

The essential function of the lungs is to exchange oxygen and carbon dioxide across the alveolar membrane. This process requires not only ventilation and blood perfusion suitable to the metabolic activity of the body but also a matching of ventilation and perfusion that is as perfect as possible.

"Dead space" ventilation represents wasted ventilation. The ratio of dead space to tidal volume increases approximately 0.17% per year in adults from a normal ratio of 25%. In aging lungs, both ventilation and perfusion are distributed unevenly, resulting in a decrease in arterial Po_2 of about 0.42 mm Hg per year in the supine position.[13] Because of earlier airway closure during expiration, arterial Po_2 always is lower in the supine than in the seated position.[16,17] In an upright patient, perfusion of lung bases diminishes with age, which results in an increased ventilation-perfusion (V/Q) ratio. There is no significant change in arterial pH or Pco_2. Other than hypoventilation, elimination of CO_2 is relatively uninfluenced by disease processes that produce a V/Q mismatch, diffusion impairment, or vascular shunting. Aging does not result in CO_2 retention.

Pulmonary Circulation

The pulmonary arteries, containing the venous blood, supply the gas exchange portion of the lung, beginning at the level of the respiratory bronchiole. Pulmonary arteries lack precapillary sphincters common to systemic arterioles. The mean pulmonary arterial pressure at rest is about 19 mm Hg. Because of the ability to recruit collapsed pulmonary capillaries as cardiac output increases, exercise normally produces little rise in mean arterial pressure. Pulmonary capillary blood volume is about 75 mL at rest and 200 mL during exercise, which reflects the cardiac stroke volume. With age, the pulmonary capillary blood volume remains unchanged, as does total lung perfusion. The loss of pulmonary capillaries either from emphysema or from normal aging does not cause pulmonary hypertension. This contrasts with hypoxemia, which induces pulmonary arterial constriction and elevation of pressure.

Perfusion of the lung in the upright position is influenced by gravity, with pressure and perfusion greater in the lower part of the lung (about 70% of the total lung area). Because of this relative increase in pressure, flow in these pulmonary capillaries is independent of alveolar pressure. The decrease in the diffusing capacity for oxygen with advancing age in both men and women presumably is due more to decreasing perfusion at lung bases, with a consequent increase in the V/Q ratio, than to a loss of surface area of the alveolar capillary membrane.

Control of Ventilation

Breathing is regulated by peripheral and central chemoreceptors acting as sensors and central nervous system areas acting as controllers.[18] The primary oxygen sensors are the carotid bodies, which respond to hypoxemia. The control of CO_2 is less clear. Investigators have reported that the peripheral chemoreceptor contribution to regulating the ventilatory response to hypercapnia ranges from 20% to 50%. The central chemoreceptors in the brainstem account for the remainder of the response to abnormal PCO_2. Studies of aging have indicated an overall diminution in response to low oxygen levels, high CO_2 levels, and mechanical loads, which is presumably due to a functional decline of both peripheral and central chemoreceptors.

Sleep Apnea Syndrome

Since 1965, there has been a burgeoning interest in breathing disorders in adults during sleep. As techniques of polysomnography are adapted, the prevalence of sleep apnea syndrome is seen to be wide ranging. Apnea is defined as the cessation of all airflow at the nose and mouth for at least 10 seconds. The syndrome comprises at least 30 such apneic episodes per night, but in elderly subjects, this frequency can be lower. Obstructive apnea results from occlusion of the upper airway in the face of persistent efforts to breathe. Central apnea occurs in the absence of any breathing effort. In mixed apnea, airflow ceases with an early absence of breathing effort, followed by a resumption of unsuccessful ventilatory effort in the latter part of the episode.

Physiologic and clinical consequences may be disastrous and include daytime somnolence, changes in mental status and personality, erythrocytosis, pulmonary hypertension, and cardiac arrhythmias. The incidence is higher in men and postmenopausal women. Risk factors include obesity, older age, and use of central nervous system depressants. Snoring has been identified as a risk factor and an important signal in those with obstructive apnea.[19] Because of the risk of nocturnal mortality and hypoxemia-induced morbidity, symptoms suggesting sleep apnea should be investigated by experts with the experience and facilities to perform polysomnography. (For details of these evaluation methods and therapeutic interventions, see Chapter 43.)

Evaluation of Dyspnea

A common complaint of the aging patient is exertional dyspnea or shortness of breath. This is best defined as an unpleasant sensation of difficulty in breathing. It is truly a sensation and requires peripheral sensors as well as central processing of sensory information and cerebral cortical interpretation.[20] Because the symptom is subjective, it is difficult for both the elderly patient and the physician to measure it, as it is with pain. Another problem is differentiating between deconditioning and the effects of aging, as well as distinguishing between cardiac and pulmonary mechanisms impairing the oxygen transport system. Table 28.2 suggests a general approach to the dyspneic patient. The major diseases causing adult dyspnea include chronic obstructive pulmonary disease (COPD), congestive heart failure, and neurologic disorders. Also, it is important to consider a psychological basis in response to emotional stress or depression.

An exercise test using progressive, incremental mechanical loading is useful for measuring the components of cardiac and pulmonary function. In the presence of clinical obesity or disuse major muscle atrophy, simple measures such as weight reduction and an exercise program may be effective in lessening exertional dyspnea. The two basic approaches to the therapy of dyspnea are to treat the underlying cause (cardiac, pulmonary, anemia, psychogenic) and to provide physical rehabilitation to improve aerobic capacity.[21] In the ambulatory elderly patient, a walking program is the most feasible and safe.

Exercise Training

Exercise capacity usually is measured as the body's maximal oxygen uptake (Vo_2 max). To provide oxygen to the working muscles, the transport system moves oxygen from ambient air to muscle mitochondria. The system includes the interrelationship of the lungs, chest wall, heart, vessels, and hemoglobin.[22] Aging adversely affects all the involved mechanisms to varying degrees, although its effects are difficult to separate from illnesses whose incidence rate increases with

Table 28.2. Evaluation of dyspnea.

1. Medical history
2. Physical examination
3. Chest x-ray films
4. Pulmonary function tests
   (spirometry, hemoglobin, arterial blood gas values, and pH)
5. Cardiac studies (electrocardiography)
6. Exercise testing

age. In younger persons, cardiac output appears to be the limiting factor in endurance performance. The cardiac output decreases by about 8% each decade.

The large reserve in ventilatory capacity has been shown not to be a limitation in exercise performance in young persons. But with age, a stiffening of the chest wall with a loss of compliance combines with decreased muscle strength, vital capacity, and maximum forced expiratory flows to limit exercise capacity.[22] Hemoglobin does not routinely decrease with age sufficiently to impair oxygen transport.

In addition to the effects of aging and disease, the increasingly sedentary life-style common to older people contributes to the loss of aerobic capacity and, thus, endurance function.[23] In a study of healthy older subjects prior to and after endurance conditioning,[24] DeVries showed their trainability in the 7th and 8th decades.[25] Both cardiac and respiratory function improved in terms of improved cardiac output and exercise ventilation. The respiratory pump also can degenerate, a change that can be reversed by training inspiratory muscles.[26]

A study of highly trained, older endurance athletes in comparison with younger athletes revealed a lower maximum heart rate and a Vo_2 max of 15% less in older athletes.[27] The identical oxygen pulse (Vo_2/heart rate) suggested that the reduction in Vo_2 max was due to the lower maximum heart rate than to either the reduced maximum stroke volume or maximum arteriovenous difference. Heath et al estimated that 9% of the Vo_2 max was lost each decade after age 25 years.[27] The average decline in the trained older athletes was 5% per decade; thus, the amount of decline in aerobic capacity and endurance can be reduced by weight control and appropriate exercise (see Chapter 42).

Obstructive Pulmonary Diseases

Chronic obstructive pulmonary disease encompasses a group of diseases having in common an obstruction to expired airflow.[28] Although not a direct major cause of death, COPD does lead to respiratory impairment and cor pulmonale. It results in considerable work disability and hospitalization. As such, it is an important economic burden to individuals and society.

The term COPD generally includes asthma, chronic bronchitis, and emphysema. Other diseases, such as bronchiectasis and cystic fibrosis, are far less common. Asthma, chronic bronchitis, and emphysema may overlap and interact; elements of all three may be present. For clarity, the diseases will be discussed separately.

Asthma

Hyperreactivity of the airways can cause sudden transient attacks of bronchospasm. Other elements of airway obstruction, such as mucus hypersecretion and mucosal edema, may be present. If attacks are neglected, recur frequently, or are complicated by bronchial infections or cigarette smoking, chronic airway obstruction may develop—this end-result may appropriately be termed chronic asthmatic bronchitis. Typical paroxysmal asthma, due to an allergy to specific antigens, occurs at an early age and may wane with maturity. Asthma developing in middle age or later always should be investigated as a possible manifestation of underlying collagen-vascular disease. With advancing age, bronchial hyperreactivity may be provoked by a wider range of stimulants that include cold air, exercise, dust, viral respiratory infections, and others.

Chronic Bronchitis

The essential characteristics are excessive bronchial mucus production and a chronic cough that persists for at least 2 successive years in the absence of any specific disease. This may lead to airflow obstruction via the mechanisms of viscid secretions, mucosal edema, cellular proliferation, smooth muscle spasm, and inflammatory changes in supporting cartilage and connective tissues. Infection and allergy play minor roles, but a major associated factor is inhaled tobacco smoke. The early pathologic changes occur in the small bronchioles and proceed centripetally to the larger bronchi. Thus, bronchiolitis becomes bronchitis. The combination of mucus hypersecretion and inflammation of the bronchial mucosa produces airway obstruction. Because the distribution of bronchial obstruction is nonuniform, V/Q mismatching may occur, which leads first to hypoxemia and later to CO_2 retention. Chronic bronchitis usually precedes parenchymal emphysema, and the diseases coexist. Aging by itself does not cause chronic bronchitis. The greater

the number of smoking "pack-years," the greater the likelihood of having chronic bronchitis.

Emphysema

This process is best defined as enlargement of air spaces that are distal to the terminal nonrespiratory bronchiole, with destruction of alveolar walls. The two principal types are centrilobular and panlobular. As the term suggests, centrilobular emphysema begins as an inflammatory process in the respiratory bronchiole surrounded by alveoli. As the inflammation increases and the bronchiole dilates, the adjacent alveoli also dilate and undergo a disintegration of the walls. A confluence of the destroyed alveoli reduces the elastic forces and the surface area available for gas exchange. Because the bronchioles are held open mechanically by the tethering of the lung parenchyma, the changes of emphysema result in early closure of small peripheral airways during exhalation, especially when forced. Thus, obstruction of airflow can result from an intrinsic blockage due to chronic bronchitis, or a premature airway collapse due to emphysematous destruction.

A second type of emphysema is panlobular. Here, alveolar dilation and destruction occur uniformly throughout the acinus in the presence of normal bronchioles. This form is more prevalent in lower lung areas in contrast to centrilobular emphysema, which favors upper lobes. Panlobular emphysema is associated with aging, but in the absence of specific pulmonary diseases it does not severely impair pulmonary function, due to the reserve capacity of the lungs. Because emphysema does not produce the nonuniform ventilation of chronic bronchitis, it ordinarily does not cause alveolar hypoventilation or V/Q mismatch with abnormalities of the arterial blood gases. As previously mentioned, chronic bronchitis and emphysema, when associated with cigarette smoking, usually coexist; both contribute to abnormalities of gas exchange.

Management

Therapy for elderly patients with COPD is limited and directed toward control of symptoms, an increase in physical activity, independent self-care, and a reduction of hospitalization. These important objectives can benefit greatly the lives of older patients with COPD.

The asthmatic component rarely is atopic or extrinsic, and little effort should be expended in identifying specific allergens and subsequent desensitization. Excellent drugs are available to achieve and maintain satisfactory bronchodilatation (Table 28.3).

Table 28.3. Useful drugs for airway obstruction.

Drug	Route	Dosage
Adrenergic		
Metaproterenol sulfate	Oral	20 mg/8 h
	Inhalation	2 inhalations qid
Albuterol sulfate	Oral	2–4 mg tid or qid
	Inhalation	2 inhalations qid
Terbutaline sulfate	Oral	2.5–5 mg/8 h
	Subcutaneous	0.25 mg/4–8 h
Theophylline (slow release)	Oral	300–600 mg/12 h to maintain plasma level of 10–20 μg/mL
Aminophylline	Intravenous	4–6 mg/kg/d initially
Anticholinergic		
Ipratropium bromide	Inhalation	2 inhalations qid
Glucocorticoids		
Prednisone	Oral	Begin with 60–80 mg/d and reduce to 10–15 mg/d each morning
Methylprednisolone	Intravenous	20–40 mg/8 h
Beclomethasone dipropionate	Inhalation	2 inhalations qid
Triamcinolone acetonide	Inhalation	2 inhalations qid
Flunisolide	Inhalation	2 inhalations bid or qid

Bronchodilators

Theophylline drugs are valuable both for chronic oral dosage and for acute intravenous use. Patient compliance and a consistent control of airway caliber have been achieved by sustained-release preparations. An oral dosage given twice daily has become standard practice. The dosage, however, varies considerably with age, body size, and drug metabolism. Blood levels of 10 to 20 μg/mL are desirable and should be used as guides for therapy. Once an apparently stable dose is achieved, changes in smoking habits and concomitant drugs such as erythromycin and cimetidine may change blood levels of theophylline.

β-Adrenergic Drugs

If maximum ventilatory function is not attained with orally administered theophylline, or if it is poorly tolerated, the use of an inhaled or oral β-adrenergic drug is indicated. Some clinicians prefer to initiate therapy with these drugs. A combination of theophylline and β-adrenergic drugs may produce an optimal ventilation with fewer side effects.

Principal β-adrenergic drugs are metaproterenol, terbutaline, and albuterol. The oral doses may have to be reduced in older patients to minimize side effects, beginning with 2.5 mg of terbutaline sulfate, 2 mg of albuterol, and 20 mg of metaproterenol sulfate, each given three times daily.

The use of a metered-dose inhaler can provide effective bronchodilation with few, if any, side effects. The reason for a lack of maximal effectiveness has been the failure to use such inhalers properly. The two requirements are patient education and proper instructions (Fig. 28.3). The two most important instructions are to inhale the aerosol slowly and to hold the breath at full lung inflation for 10 seconds. Shim and Williams suggest that an inhaled β-adrenergic drug can produce a greater benefit than the same drug taken orally, providing that the inhaled drug is used properly.[29] Spacers may be needed by some patients due to poor coordination or to reduce oropharyngeal drug deposition.

Anticholinergic Drugs

Prior to the release of ipratropium bromide for inhalation therapy of chronic asthmatic bronchitis, atropine sulfate had been nebulized for inhalation. Side effects such as tachycardia and dry mouth were of particular concern in elderly patients. Ipratropium delivered by metered-dose inhaler appears to be more effective than inhaled β-agonist drugs for improving ventilatory function in patients with COPD.[30] The physiologic basis for this superiority could be the predominant mediation of bronchomotor tone by the cholinergic vagus nerve, with only a minor role for the adrenergic system. Side effects from ipratropium have been relatively few due to limited systemic absorption. Most patients with COPD will achieve maximum benefit from ipratropium alone; a small percentage require the addition of an inhaled β-agonist drug.[31] Pulmonary function testing with both types of medications may be informative. Whenever possible, a metered-dose inhaler should be used in preference to the usually less effective nebulizer route of delivery.

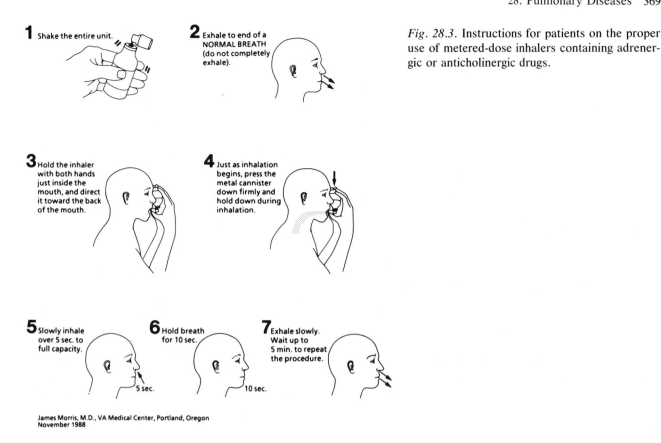

1 Shake the entire unit.

2 Exhale to end of a NORMAL BREATH (do not completely exhale).

3 Hold the inhaler with both hands just inside the mouth, and direct it toward the back of the mouth.

4 Just as inhalation begins, press the metal cannister down firmly and hold down during inhalation.

5 Slowly inhale over 5 sec. to full capacity. 5 sec.

6 Hold breath for 10 sec. 10 sec.

7 Exhale slowly. Wait up to 5 min. to repeat the procedure.

James Morris, M.D., VA Medical Center, Portland, Oregon
November 1988

Fig. 28.3. Instructions for patients on the proper use of metered-dose inhalers containing adrenergic or anticholinergic drugs.

Corticosteroids

Corticosteroids can benefit those persons with reactive airway disease (ie, asthmatic patients) but not those with emphysema. Corticosteroids have not been shown to improve chronic bronchitis, perhaps because of the progression from chronic asthmatic bronchitis to mucous gland hyperplasia and hypersecretion,[32] but may be of value during an acute exacerbation of chronic bronchitis. A major therapeutic advance was the introduction of relatively insoluble, inhaled corticosteroids, chiefly beclomethasone, triamcinolone, and flunisolide. Their effective use helps to reduce or omit systemic corticosteroids as maintenance therapy. They are essentially free from side effects, other than oral candidiasis. Inhaled corticosteroids particularly are beneficial to elderly patients, who are most vulnerable to the side effects of systemic corticosteroids. The use of cromolyn sodium has been of negligible benefit in adult patients.

Nonpharmacologic Therapy

Two therapeutic modalities that have shown demonstrated success have been oxygen therapy and exercise, occasionally used together. Oxygen therapy at home is required by relatively few patients when strict criteria are used (Table 28.4). During sleep, most individuals hypoventilate relative to their waking state. Sleeping patients with COPD commonly develop a serious hypoxia, which may go unrecognized unless monitored with an ear oximeter. Complications, such as sustained pulmonary hypertension with cor pulmonale and congestive heart failure, may develop.[33] The decision to use home oxygen for an elderly patient should be based on firm clinical and laboratory criteria. The major disadvantages are cost, limitation of physical activity, the potential for CO_2 retention, and possible oxygen toxicity. A multicenter study showed an improved survival if oxygen was used continuously rather than for 12 hours daily.[34]

Table 28.4. Indications for outpatient oxygen therapy.

Resting arterial oxygen tension (Pao_2) <56 mm Hg or oxygen saturation (Sao_2) <89%*

Resting Pao_2 > 55 mm Hg with evidence of hypoxic organ dysfunction, including erythrocytosis, cor pulmonale, and sleep or mentation disturbances

Resting Pao_2 > 55 mm Hg or Sao_2 > 88% but Pao_2 < 56 mm Hg during an exercise training program

Hypoxic organ dysfunction or hypoxemia that is benefited by oxygen therapy

*These criteria apply to patients breathing room air at sea level; patients residing at higher altitudes have lower Pao_2 and Sao_2 values.

Less desirable alternatives limit oxygen use to times of sleeping or exercising. Refillable, lightweight, and portable oxygen cylinders are available for increasing the range of activities. Liquid gas containers also provide both home and portable oxygen therapy, but at an increased cost. An alternative to gas cylinder or liquid container oxygen is the oxygen extractor. This device provides a safe, dependable, and relatively economic source of oxygen. Drawbacks include a vulnerability to electrical power failure and the inability to fill portable cylinders.

Various forms of physical therapy are used for patients with COPD, many of which are of dubious value. These include breathing training, postural drainage, and chest percussion or vibration. There is no real controversy regarding the many benefits of exercise training. Because of associated medical problems in elderly persons that may impose limitations, exercise therapy may have to be carefully tailored to the individual patient. Walking, swimming, and bicycling are particularly well suited for an older patient with COPD. The goals are an increased exercise tolerance with less physical dependence and a reduction in exertional dyspnea. For an elderly patient, a return to gainful employment is uncommon. However, reductions in the need for hospitalization and improvement in the quality of life are attainable. An increase in survival and an improvement in pulmonary function are most difficult to prove.

The most important element of patient education is to promote the cessation of smoking; otherwise, the progression of COPD is inevitable. An important component of the smoking cessation program is pulmonary function testing. Confronting older patients with the amount of loss of ventilatory function compared with that in nonsmokers of similar age can motivate them to quit.

As in many chronic illnesses affecting the older patient, realistic goals should be set and directed toward halting further deterioration and promoting a functional performance within limits imposed by structural changes.

Restrictive Pulmonary Diseases

Restricted lung expansion can result from voluntary hypoventilation, such as that due to the pain of breathing, and age-related changes in the muscles or joints of the chest or in the pleura and the lung parenchymal interstitium. Interstitial lung disease causes the greatest physiologic impairment, primarily in gas exchange. Table 28.5 lists the causes of interstitial lung disease, the most common of which is idiopathic pulmonary fibrosis.

Table 28.5. Causes of interstitial lung disease.

Inorganic dusts
Organic dusts
Toxic gases and fumes
Drugs
Poisons
Infections
Chronic heart or kidney failure
Collagen-vascular diseases
Granulomatous diseases
Vasculitides
Idiopathic cases

Idiopathic Pulmonary Fibrosis

This usually is clinically evident in the 6th decade and is manifested by increasing dyspnea on exertion. Dry cough is a common feature. Changes on physical examination and chest x-ray films may be minimal in the early stages. As the disease progresses, inspiratory crackles, increased transmission of breath sounds, prolongation of expiration, and reduced chest expansion develop. The chest x-ray film shows a variety of changes, usually diffuse reticular and reticulonodular patterns. In advanced stages, multiple translucencies may produce a honeycomb appearance.

Measurement of arterial Po_2 and calculation of the alveolar-arterial Po_2 gradient after exercise are the most sensitive measures of intestinal disease impairment.[35] Less consistently, abnormalities are found in lung volumes, expired flows, diffusion capacity, lung compliance, and resting arterial blood gas values.

The assessment for activity of the inflammatory process is critical. The approach to the evaluation and treatment of interstitial lung disease has been systematized.[36] The value of obtaining a lung biopsy specimen depends on obtaining a representative tissue sample of the general pulmonary disease process. Some areas of the lung may show active inflammation, while others are in an advanced fibrotic stage. An initial open-lung biopsy may determine a specific cause of the interstitial lung disease, such as pneumoconiosis or rheumatoid lung disease.

Newer procedures have been advocated to assess inflammatory activity. Gallium-67 scintigraphy is both sensitive and specific for alveolitis. It is valuable in determining the degree of active inflammation, in measuring by serial studies the effectiveness of therapy directed against the alveolitis, and in detecting a relapse. Bronchoalveolar lavage, when properly done, may help determine both the presence and nature of alveolitis. The procedure requires fiberoptic bronchoscopy and is relatively easy and safe to perform. Serial use of both techniques is valuable in monitoring the success of therapy.

Through the methods described above, with special emphasis on postexercise arterial blood gas studies and gallium-67 scintigraphy, an assessment of alveolitis and the degree of physiologic impairment may be made. A major decision is whether there is a specific cause of the interstitial disease or whether it is idiopathic. An inciting exposure to drugs, dusts, or chemicals should be eliminated. In the majority of cases, the cause will be unknown and the choice will be to begin a prolonged aggressive therapy directed toward the prevention of pulmonary fibrosis and loss of functioning acini. In addition to the degree of active inflammation and impairment of pulmonary function, the goals of the patient must be considered. Corticosteroids are the primary drugs currently used to affect the inflammatory and immunologic derangements. Because of the need for high dosages over prolonged periods, the hazards for elderly patients include osteoporosis with vertebral compression fractures, increased susceptibility to infections, and exacerbation of diabetes, hypertension, tuberculosis, peptic ulcer disease, and hypoadrenalism. Therefore, some frail elderly patients with significant disabilities due to other disorders are not treated. There is no accepted regimen for drug therapy, but some clinicians would advocate an aggressive approach.[36]

Alternative drugs, such as cyclophosphamide and azathioprine, have been used in cases of corticosteroid failures. Beside refractoriness to prednisone therapy, relapse is a significant problem and may require repeated courses of antiinflammatory therapy. Progressive worsening of interstitial fibrosis causes increasing hypoxemia that requires inhaled oxygen. Inability to maintain an arterial Po_2 of at least 60 mm Hg may result in the classic sequence of pulmonary hypertension, erythrocytosis, and cor pulmonale.

Bronchopulmonary Infections

Acute Bronchitis

In contrast to chronic bronchitis, acute bronchitis usually is an infectious process, barring acute exposure to irritant chemicals. The cause commonly is nonbacterial. In an older patient, viruses are more common than mycoplasma. Acute bronchitis may be part of a more extensive involvement of respiratory epithelium, such as laryngotracheobronchitis. For patients with a seriously impaired pulmonary function, such as those with COPD, the widespread narrowing of airways due to mucosal inflammation and bronchial secretions may cause severe alveolar hypoventilation

or V/Q mismatch. Therapy is nonspecific in the absence of a bacterial or mycoplasmal cause and includes bronchodilators, systemic hydration, and ventilatory support as needed. The routine use of antimicrobial drugs in acute exacerbations of chronic bronchitis is controversial but appears to offer no convincing benefit.[37]

Bacterial Pneumonia

Bacterial pneumonia has traditionally been more prevalent in elderly persons and is the leading infectious cause of death. In 82% of adult cases of bacterial pneumonia, there are underlying conditions that predispose to bronchopulmonary infection.

In elderly persons, it is assumed that bronchopulmonary clearance mechanisms weaken during the aging process.[38] These include macrophage and mucociliary functions. Decreased production of serum immunoglobulins against certain pathogens, such as pneumococcal serotypes, could partially account for an increased susceptibility to bacterial pneumonias. Most of these pneumonias result from minor aspirations of microorganisms colonizing the nasopharynx. Diminution of the gag reflex with aging could predispose to aspiration. The use of sedative drugs increases this risk.

Diagnosis

The microorganisms to be considered as causes of bacterial pneumonia are listed in Table 28.6. Because an elderly patient may be in a health care facility, hospital, or nursing home, a distinction should be

Table 28.6. Causes of bacterial pneumonia.

Aerobic gram-positive cocci
  Streptococcus pneumoniae
  Staphylococcus aureus
  Streptococcus pyogenes
Aerobic gram-negative bacilli
  Klebsiella enterobacter
  Escherichia coli
  Proteus
  Pseudomonas aeruginosa
  Acinetobacter
  Serratia marcescens
  Legionella pneumophila
  Haemophilus influenzae
  Branhamella catarrhalis
Anaerobic bacteria
  Peptostreptococcus
  Fusobacterium
  Bacteroides

made between community-acquired and nosocomial infection. In the community, infections are most commonly caused by *Streptococcus pneumoniae* throughout the year and influenza A virus during epidemic seasons. In a health care facility, gram-negative bacilli should be suspected as well as pneumococci. *Hemophilus influenzae* commonly colonizes the airway in older patients with chronic bronchitis.[39] These are virtually always nontypable strains that are less likely to cause pneumonia. Because of their presence in bronchopulmonary secretions, they often are mistakenly implicated as causing pneumonia in older patients. Their presence in body fluids (blood, pleural effusion) does establish causation in occasional cases of *H influenzae* pneumonia (see Chapter 25).

The clinical presentation of pneumonia in elderly patients may not be typical. Fever, productive cough, malaise, and physical findings may be muted. Chest x-ray films, however, should reveal airspace consolidation in bacterial pneumonia. Similarly, gram stains of a sputum smear should reveal a predominance of a single aerobic bacterial species. The adequacy of the sputum specimen is verified by finding fewer than 10 epithelial cells and, ideally, more than 25 granulocytes per low-power microscopic field. alternatives to expectorated sputum are invasive. They include nasotracheal suctioning, transtracheal suctioning, fiberoptic bronchoscopic aspiration and brushing, and percutaneous "skinny" needle aspiration. Sputum culture is essential, to enable the definitive identification of microorganisms and the performance of antimicrobial susceptibility tests, especially against *Staphylococcus aureus* and gram-negative bacilli. Blood and pleural fluid cultures are invaluable in indicating the causative bacteria of pneumonia.

Chest x-ray films establish the diagnosis of pneumonia. They also can reveal unusual parenchymal destruction, either necrotizing pneumonia or abscess. Because these are rarely seen in pneumococcal pneumonia, a consideration of infection from staphylococci, gram-negative bacilli, and anaerobic microorganisms is vital. Associated pleural effusion should be aspirated to determine if empyema that requires drainage is present.

Treatment

Because of the potentially high mortality and severe morbidity of bacterial pneumonia in elderly patients, antimicrobial treatment must be prompt and effective, preferably bactericidal. Initial drug therapy should be influenced by the gram-stained sputum smear and modified as cultural and drug susceptibility information becomes available. The large majority of truly community-acquired bacterial pneumonia cases are caused by *S pneumoniae*. Penicillin G given parenterally and penicillin V given orally remain the drugs of first choice. If the patient has a history of penicillin allergy, alternative choices are erythromycin or clindamycin. In patients with bacterial pneumonia acquired in an extended care facility or hospital, treatment is more complex due to greater drug resistance (Table 28.7). The dosage may have to be adjusted in the presence of renal impairment, especially if an aminoglycoside drug is used. Aminoglycosides are potentially more nephrotoxic in the elderly and also have diminished antimicrobial activity in bronchopulmonary infection.

For hospitalized patients, the intravenous route is desirable, at least initially. This is particularly true in older patients who may have inappropriate drug levels when using oral medications because of either un-

Table 28.7. Initial antibiotic regimens for treatment of suspected nosocomial pneumonia in adults.

Pathogen	Antibiotic	Suggested intravenous dosage
Escherichia coli *Klebsiella* species	Second-or-third generation cephalosporin	
Enterobacter/ Serratia species	Aztreonam	2 g/8 h
Pseudomonas aeruginosa	Imipenem	1 g/6–8 h
	Ceftazidime	1 g/8 h
Anaerobic bacteria	Penicillin G	2 million units/4 h
	Clindamycin phosphate	600 mg/8 h
Haemophilus influenzae	Ampicillin	2 g/6 h
	Third- generation cephalosporin	
Branhamella catarrhalis	Erythromycin lactobionate	500 mg/6 h
	Third- generation cephalosporin	
	Trimethoprim- sulfamethoxa- zole	10 mg/kg of TMP
Legionella pneumophila	Erythromycin lactobionate	500 mg/6 h
Staphylococcus aureus	Nafcillin sodium	2 g/4 h
Methicillin sensitive	Cephalothin	2 g/4 h
Methicillin resistant	Vancomycin hydrochloride	500 mg/6 h

dependable absorption from the gastrointestinal tract or erratic ingestion. The duration of antimicrobial therapy varies with the type of infection and the microorganism. For example, most pneumococcal pneumonias require only 5 to 7 days, gram-negative bacilli 2 weeks, staphylococcal infections 4 weeks, and anaerobic lung abscesses 6 weeks. Patients may be switched to intramuscular or oral routes as the infection is controlled.

Prevention

In an older patient, especially one with a chronic impairment, prophylaxis for pneumococcal pneumonia is highly desirable at this time. Two principal measures are immunization with antipneumococcal vaccine (providing 90% protection) and 250 mg of oral penicillin V potassium twice daily (offering 100% protection).[40] For patients at high risk for acute respiratory failure due to pneumococcal pneumonia, both preventive measures should be considered. Recent studies indicate that pneumococcal vaccine provides poorer than expected protection for the chronically ill elderly but good protection against pneumococcal pneumonia in healthy elderly persons.[41]

Despite the availability of effective vaccines, influenza remains a serious cause of morbidity and mortality. Influenza A virus and influenza B virus cause only a fraction of respiratory infections each year but are unique in that they are responsible for periodic widespread outbreaks of febrile respiratory infections in both children and adults. The illness usually produces a fever, chills, headaches, cough, and myalgia. It may last several days or 1 week or longer and usually has a complete recovery. Complications include pneumonia, myocarditis, pericarditis, encephalitis, and aseptic meningitis.

Efforts to prevent or control influenza typically have been directed toward protecting those who are at the greatest risk of death or serious illness. These individuals include those over 65 years of age and chronically ill adults. The mortality rate is one in 100 of those 65 years of age or older in the presence of chronic illness. The chief problem, other than compliance with vaccination, is a variation in the influenza antigens, usually antigen A. This can take the form of antigenic drift, which is a minor change where the vaccine has a real but diminished usefulness. Antigenic shift is seen about every 10 years, when a new vaccine must be prepared. In years without antigenic variation, vaccination can provide up to 85% protection against the viruses contained in the vaccine.[44] Older individuals have a lower antibody response than younger persons. Local reactions, including erythema and induration, are infrequent and mild. Fewer than 1% of persons

vaccinated develop systemic reactions such as fever and myalgia. Considering the hazards of influenza to elderly patients, physicians should encourage annual vaccination.

The use of antiviral agents is limited to influenza A, and both prophylactic and therapeutic effects have been achieved. Amantadine has been available since 1967 and a derivative, rimantadine, is awaiting Food and Drug Administration (FDA) approval. Amantadine has been shown to be 91% effective in preventing influenza A virus infection.[45] It is beneficial for elderly patients or for those with serious chronic illness who are exposed to influenza A virus. It can be used in place of a vaccination or as a supplement. As a therapeutic agent, it has about a 50% ameliorating effect on the course of influenza A virus.[46] There is a 5% rate of central nervous system side effects (usually mild and reversible). With evidence of pneumonia, it is important to distinguish between influenza viral pneumonia and a bacterial suprainfection. Pneumococci and staphylococci account for most of the community-acquired, postinfluenzal bacterial pneumonias (see Chapter 25).

Aspiration Pneumonia

Pulmonary aspiration is a disturbingly common event. In hospitalized patients, it can reproduce different clinical syndromes and frequently is fatal. It occurs commonly in situations accompanied by stupor, coma, alcohol or drug intoxication, nasogastric tube feeding, general anesthesia, seizure disorders, cardiopulmonary resuscitation, and esophageal motility disorders. Frequently, the aspiration is not observed or is overlooked. The damage done by pulmonary aspiration may involve airway obstruction, chemical pneumonitis, or infection. The upper airway is normally protected by gag and cough reflexes. A number of conditions interfere with these defenses, ranging from coma to normal sound sleep. In elderly persons, a diminution in the sensitivity of the cough and gag reflexes weaken these vital defenses, particularly during sleep, and they are further weakened by alcohol, sedatives, and hypnotic drugs.

Clinical Features

Clinical syndromes depend upon the type of material aspirated. They can be separated into nontoxic substances, toxic or acidic substances, and infected oropharyngeal secretions. Nontoxic substances vary in the degree of damage produced. Clear liquids usually produce minimal or transient damage, unless found in large amounts. Large particles (usually poorly chewed food) obviously can obstruct major airways and usually are quickly recognized. Gastric contents are a mixture of partially digested food and gastric secretions and cause chronic injury. The long-term effects of food stuff aspiration seem limited, except for bronchiolitis obliterans.[42] Damage can be done to the lung even when the aspirate is close to neutral in pH. The subsequent administration of corticosteroids can interfere with localization of the lung damage and prolong acute inflammatory changes.

Toxic substances in the lung usually result from aspirating fasting gastric secretions with a pH below 2.5. The normal gastric pH range is 1.5 to 2.4, which can cause severe damage to the alveoli and airways. In an elderly patient, degrees of achlorhydria may result in a gastric secretion with a pH above 2.5, which then falls into the nontoxic substance category. The effects of aspirating toxic substances are similar to a burn injury. Interstitial and alveolar edema result in hypoxemia. Vasodilation and edema of the bronchial epithelium narrows the lumen, causes V/Q mismatch, and contributes to hypoxemia. The end result may be severe fibrosis of the smaller airways and the lung parenchyma.[43] The sequelae of aspirating infected oropharyngeal secretions depend on the predominating bacteria and their numbers. Community-acquired aspiration pneumonia usually is caused by anaerobic bacteria, which are either alone or mixed with aerobes. This particularly is true in patients with gingival infection (periodontitis), which harbors large numbers of anaerobes. Hospital-acquired aspiration pneumonia may be caused by aerobic bacteria (especially gram-negative enteric bacilli) alone or mixed with anaerobes in a dentulous patient.

Chest x-ray films commonly show a nonspecific bronchopneumonia that is segmental rather than lobar, its location corresponding to the dependent area during aspiration. The subsequent course is influenced by the infecting microorganisms; however, in the case of anaerobic bacteria or gram-negative enteric bacilli, necrotizing pneumonia and lung abscesses are common.

Therapy

Some clinicians recommend antimicrobial therapy in all cases of aspiration pneumonia, while others prefer to wait until clear evidence of bacterial infection is obtained. Drugs may be selected according to the following guidelines:

1. Dentulous patients with definite community-acquired pneumonia, especially if necrotizing or with a lung abscess, should be treated for anaerobic infection (4 to 6 weeks of at least 6 million units of penicillin G potassium daily or 600 mg of clindamycin phosphate every 8 hours). If cultures reveal an aerobic bacillary infection, more appropriate antimicrobials are used.
2. Hospital-acquired aspiration pneumonia should be regarded as either an aerobic or mixed aerobic-anaerobic infection. Initially, combination regimens, such as clindamycin phosphate plus a broad-spectrum cephalosporin, are useful until sputum culture findings are definitive.

Tuberculosis

Despite the marked reduction in tuberculosis, it remains the number one fatal communicable disease in the United States. Among all infectious diseases, only pneumonia has a higher annual fatality rate. Modern chemotherapy is extraordinarily effective and should be successful in all cases that are caused by drug-susceptible *Myobacterium tuberculosis*. Why, then, do we continue to see about 22,000 new cases annually resulting in 3,000 deaths? Some of the reasons are noncompliance with therapy regimens, drug-resistant disease, and misdiagnosis.

A unique quality of tuberculosis is that it can remain inactive over decades and then reactivate. The balance between the virulence of the organism and the cell-mediated immunity of the patient determines the course of this lifelong infection. The dimunition of cell-mediated immunity is characteristic of the aging process and may be reflected in a decreased reaction to tuberculin testing. The booster effect of a repeat tuberculin test performed 1 to 4 weeks after a nondiagnostic reaction has been more marked in older populations.[47] Thus, it is not surprising that reactivation tuberculosis increasingly is seen among older individuals.[48] Additional reasons, other than naturally waning immunity, are the development of certain diseases such as diabetes, malignancies, the taking of immunosuppressive drugs such as corticosteroids, malnutrition, and alcoholism.

Diagnosis

As tuberculosis has decreased in prevalence, it has become concentrated in urban areas that are characterized by low social and economic levels. For many physicians, the disease is seen infrequently enough to be easily misdiagnosed. To add to this problem, unusual clinical and x-ray film presentations have become more common. Typically, tuberculosis in adults presents on chest x-ray films as a destructive process located in the upper lobar apical and posterior segments and, less commonly, in the lower lobar superior segments. With progression of the disease, other areas may be affected. With infiltrates elsewhere, a diagnosis may not be made. Finally, the relative infrequency of tuberculosis may result in primary infections in older adults; perhaps this explains the mid and lower lung field involvement and pleural effusion.[49] Miliary disease as a manifestation of reactivation tuberculosis is being observed more frequently in elderly patients.[50]

The definitive diagnosis remains a positive sputum smear for typical acid-fast bacilli, with confirmation by culture. Tuberculin testing via a standard 5-TU Mantoux technique in older persons may result in false-negative reactions, despite positive reactions to control antigens such as mumps, *Candida,* or *Trichophytin.* Two recommended procedures are to repeat the 5-TU test to achieve a booster effect or to repeat it with the second-strength 250 TU test. A negative reaction to a 250-TU test in the presence of a positive control test virtually rules out tuberculous disease.

Therapy

A better understanding of the basic mechanisms of drug action provides a rational basis for currently used therapeutic programs. Principles of therapy include the use of a combination of bactericidal drugs, which affect metabolically different microbial populations by means of specific actions. The current recommendation of the Centers for Disease Control and the American Thoracic Society is 300 mg/d of isoniazid, 600 mg/d of rifampin, and 1500 mg/d of pyrazinamide for 2 months, then isoniazid and rifampin at the same daily doses for an additional 6 months.[51] This is recommended for both pulmonary and extrapulmonary disease (the latter having a surprisingly constant prevalence despite continued decline in pulmonary tuberculosis).

For less compliant patients, a twice-weekly regimen of isoniazid (15 mg/kg) and rifampin (600 mg orally), given for a minimum of 9 months, may be substitute. Because isoniazid, pyrazinamide, and rifampin all are potentially hepatotoxic, patients should be routinely examined for hepatitis or jaundice monthly, with questions regarding hepatitis symptoms and examination for scleral icterus. An aspartate aminotransferase level five times greater than the baseline indicates the need initially to discontinue isoniazide, the toxicity of which increases with the patient's age. The question of when to release a patient from respiratory isolation is unsettled. The most conservative approach is to require three consecutive negative sputum smears for acid-fast bacilli. During therapy, physical activity should be unrestricted. Good nutrition is important, despite the remarkable efficacy of current drug therapy resistance by the *Myobacterium tuberculosis* bacillus continues to remain low in US-born patients of all ages.

Table 28.8. Indications for preventive treatment of tuberculosis.

Household members and other close associates of newly diagnosed patients
Tuberculin skin test converters within the past 2 years
Positive tuberculin skin test reactors with abnormal chest x-ray films consistent with tuberculosis
Positive tuberculin skin test reactors with associated diseases or situations, such as corticosteroid or other immunosuppressive therapy, diabetes, silicosis, and gastric resection with weight loss
Positive tuberculin skin test reactors in patients below age 35 years

Preventive Therapy

The use of isoniazid (300 mg/d for 1 year), recommended for those infected by tubercle bacilli (as shown by a positive tuberculin test without radiologic or microbiologic evidence of disease), is ideally suited to prevent reactivation.[52] Since the recognition that isoniazid can cause serious hepatitis, prophylaxis has become more selective. Toxic hepatitis is distinctly age related. After 35 years of age, the case rate increases until about 64 years of age, where it has a 2.3% rate of occurrence. Therefore, in elderly tuberculin reactors, considering the smaller number of potential years for reactivation and the risk of isoniazid hepatitis, a significant risk factor (Table 28.8) should be required before preventive therapy is given. The otherwise healthy, well-nourished elderly tuberculin reactor faces a greater morbidity and mortality risk with isoniazid than with tuberculosis.

Neoplastic Disease

Bronchogenic Carcinoma

Lung cancer has become infamous as the leading cause of cancer deaths in men and has overtaken breast cancer as the leading cause in women. The annual death rate from lung cancer now exceeds 100,000 in the United States and continues to rise. It also is characterized by a short duration from diagnosis to death. The 5-year survival rate of 5% to 10% has changed little in the past 30 years, despite advances in the diagnosis and treatment. This renders more urgent the necessity of preventing this epidemic disease. Despite minor contributions of occupational and atmospheric exposure, tobacco smoking remains the major cause.

Age is a critical factor in the clinical recognition of lung cancer. Because it probably requires the inhalation of tobacco smoke for at least 20 years, lung cancer rarely occurs in persons younger than 35 years and less than 5% of reported cases are in persons younger than 40 years.[53] The majority of cases manifest in the 6th and 7th decades. Unfortunately, when diagnosed, the tumor has achieved about 80% of its ultimate growth and has a high probability of having produced lymphatic or hematogenous metastases. The major cell types, in order of frequency, are squamous cell carcinoma, adenocarcinoma, small cell carcinoma, and large cell carcinoma. All but adenocarcinoma are closely correlated with cigarette smoking. Adenocarcinoma, including bronchioalveolar carcinoma, has shown the most rapid increase in frequency. The basis for this increase in unknown, but is may be related to environmental pollution such as urban asbestosis.

Diagnosis

A major problem in recognizing lung cancer is that, in the early stages, symptoms may be nonexistent or resemble those of chronic bronchitis. In later stages, symptoms may reflect a distant spread of the tumor. Frequent screening with chest x-ray films has not been shown to improve survival (see Chapter 8). A variety of presentations exist; probably the two most common are the solitary pulmonary nodule and a hilar mass. Body-section x-ray films or laminograms are useful in detecting calcification, localizing the lesion, determining the presence of additional tumor masses, and evaluating the relationship of the tumor to the chest wall. Special views such as 55° hilar laminograms and computerized tomography scans of the mediastinum are useful in the detection of lymph node metastases. Gallium-67 scans have been recommended for the detection of mediastinal metastases, but they have had a limited acceptance because of their lack of specificity.

Sputum cytology is useful for exfoliative endobronchial masses, especially central squamous cell carcinomas, but the false-negative rate is substantial. The fiberoptic bronchoscope, introduced in 1970, has become the most valuable means of obtaining tissue confirmation. Technologic improvements, such as narrower outside diameters, improved optics, and greater tip flexion, have continued to improve its usefulness. Combining endobronchial or transbronchial biopsy and brushing techniques achieves a tissue diagnosis in up to 85% of subsequently proved tumors.[54] In addition, the assessment of the proximity to the main carina, deformity by mediastinal lymph node metastases, and vocal cord paralysis can assist in staging the anatomic extent and determining the potential for surgical resection. Percutaneous needle biopsy procedures have become safer with the development of thin and ultrathin needles.[55] "Liquid biopsy" specimens can be obtained by aspiration, with only a small risk of serious complication. Pneumothorax occurred in 8% of patients undergoing biopsy with ultrathin needles; only two of the four patients required a chest tube.[55] This is an important consideration in a high-risk older patient.

Surgical diagnostic procedures include cervical mediastinoscopy, mediastinotomy, and thoracotomy. The role of mediastinoscopy and, to a lesser extent, mediastinotomy is controversial. A more aggressive removal of hilar and mediastinal nodes in association with a lung resection has brought these two staging procedures into question. They have become less frequently performed as the use of fiberoptic bronchoscopy and percutaneous needle biopsy has increased. If small cell carcinoma is suspected in a centrally located lesion with negative bronchoscopic results, a bone marrow biopsy procedure is indicated before a surgical procedure.[56] If the biopsy specimen is negative, mediastinoscopy or mediastinotomy should precede a thoractomy. The most frequent indication for the two staging procedures is the determination of nonresectability in elderly or impaired patients who are at a high risk for surgical complications. In these patients, the presence of mediastinal metastases provide justification to forego a thoracotomy.

Pulmonary function testing is important before a lung resection in an elderly patient who may have a significant impairment of ventilation or gas exchange. The combination of measuring the FEV_1 and radionuclide perfusion lung scanning has been advocated to help determine operability.[57] Preferably, an FEV_1 of 800 mL should remain after lung resection.

Treatment

Three modalities are available, but with a 5% to 10% 5-year survival rate, success obviously is limited. One study indicates that elderly patients may be more concerned about immediate survival than survival 5 years postoperatively. This contrasts with the attitude of young medical house staff.[58] Failure of the staff to appreciate the values of an elderly patient with lung cancer may seriously impair the quality of his or her remaining life.

Surgery. Particularly in cases of squamous cell carcinoma, pulmonary resection represents the best chance for cure or long term-survival. With adenocarcinoma or large cell carcinoma, surgical cures are fewer because of the greater tendency toward lymphatic and hematogenous spread. This spread is almost uniform with small cell carcinoma, rendering surgery useless except for the possibility of a small peripheral nodule.

The principal limitation of successful surgical resection is unrecognized extrapulmonary spread of the carcinoma. Of additional concern is the operative mortality of patients over 65 years of age, which is reported to be approximately twice that of younger patients undergoing lobectomy or pneumonectomy.[59]

Radiation Therapy. Megavoltage radiation with either cobalt or linear accelerator sources is valuable for palliation of complications. These include pain due to bone metastases, superior vena caval obstruction, central nervous system metastases, and obstructive pneumonia. Postoperative radiation therapy, especially in the presence of hilar or mediastinal nodal metastases, often is done, but without firm evidence of any benefit. Curative irradiation of inoperable tumors also is attempted as a poor alternative to surgery, especially in elderly patients.[60]

Chemotherapy. Single or combination chemotherapy for treatment of non–small-cell carcinoma has been a disappointment in improving the quality and length of survival.[61] It cannot be recommended at this point, except in investigative protocols with new drug regimens. For an elderly patient with a limited life expectancy, a truly informed consent is essential to justify the possible impairment of nutrition and well-being. Small cell carcinoma, however, has emerged as the only cell type with a potential for nonsurgical cure.[62] Aggressive use of combination chemotherapy plus prophylactic brain irradiation is justified for those patients with adequate functional status. Most, if not all chemotherapy can be accomplished on an outpatient basis.

Between 90% and 95% of all patients with lung cancer eventually will die of it. For these approximately 95,000 Americans, the challenge is to provide relief of pain, personal support, encouragement, and realistic discussion of their prospects. For those untold numbers of persons who will develop lung cancer, prevention via cessation of cigarette smoking is a national priority.

Pulmonary Thromboembolism

The prevalence of pulmonary embolism is estimated to be 650,000 cases annually in the United States; 38% of these are fatal.[63] In an autopsy series, only 40% to 60% were recognized antemortem.[64] The source of the emboli is primarily the upper leg, specifically the popliteal, femoral, and iliac veins. Other potential sources are the pelvic veins, calf veins, upper extremity veins, and cardiac chambers. Conditions that predispose to venous thromboembolism are more common in elderly persons. These include immobilization, prolonged bed rest, hip fractures, obesity, congestive heart failure, COPD, and malignancy.

Diagnosis

Clinical manifestations are nonspecific. Some apply to the embolic event, such as dyspnea, tachypnea, and tachycardia. Other manifestations, such as pleuritic chest pain and hemoptysis, pertain to a pulmonary infarction. Electrocardiography may show only a sinus tachycardia. The chest x-ray film usually is normal but less often shows "congestive atelectasis" with elevation of a hemidiaphragm, and pulmonary infarction is seen in only about 10% of the population studied.[63] Hypoxemia may be the only abnormal laboratory value and is present in about 90% of cases. It must be recognized that advancing age reduces arterial Po_2 and increases the alveolar-arterial Po_2 gradient. A perfusion lung scan, if normal, virtually rules out a significant pulmonary embolism. In an older patient, a normal lung scan is much less likely to be obtained because of scarring, panlobular emphysema, or COPD. Classically, a ventilation-perfusion lung scan will show a segmental or greater area of nonperfused lung that is ventilated (Fig. 28.4). This produces the physiologic consequences of wasted ventilation. Unfortunately, even the finding of so-called low-probability scans with less than segmental defects has a frequency of pulmonary embolism between 25% and 40%.[65] Pulmonary angiography is the most reliable diagnostic method but is invasive and carries a small but significant risk. The finding of a filling defect that is larger than a subsegment or the cutoff of a pulmonary arterial branch is characteristic. The confirmation of a pulmonary embolus is essential when anticoagulant therapy will be particularly hazardous, such as in a patient with a potential for bleeding complications.

Because most pulmonary emboli originate in the proximal leg veins, attempts to demonstrate deep venous thrombosis (DVT) are warranted. Effective techniques include (1) contrast venography, (2) radionuclide venography and thromboscintigraphy, and (3) impedance phlebography or plethysmography. The radionuclide venogram can be obtained as part of the perfusion lung scan (Fig. 28.5). It provides good visualization of the deep veins of the lower extremity, without the risk of thrombophlebitis that accompanies contrast venography. A comparison of impedance phlebography with conventional radiographic venography shows excellent agreement.[65] Impedance phlebography has two advantages: it is noninvasive and is a mobile procedure suitable for the bedside, outpatient clinic, or emergency room. It can be used effectively for screening for DVT in the proximal veins of the

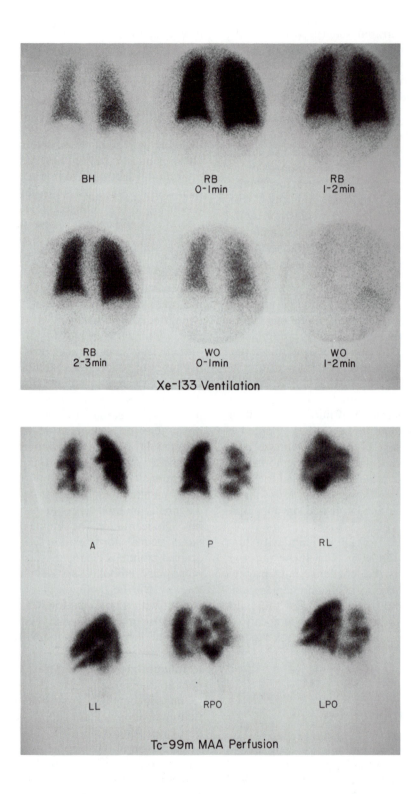

Fig. 28.4. (**top**) Ventilation study with xenon 133 shows normal air entry during breathhold phase (BH), followed by good equilibration (RB) for 3 minutes. There is unifrom clearance of radioactive xenon from both lungs during washout phase (WO). (**bottom**) The perfusion study in the same patient, performed with technetium 99m macroaggregated albumin (MAA), shows multiple bilateral segmental and lobar perfusion defects on the anterior (A) and posterior (P) views, both lateral views (RL, LL), and both posterior oblique (RPO, LPO) views. This is a typical example of multiple pulmonary emboli with V/Q mismatch.

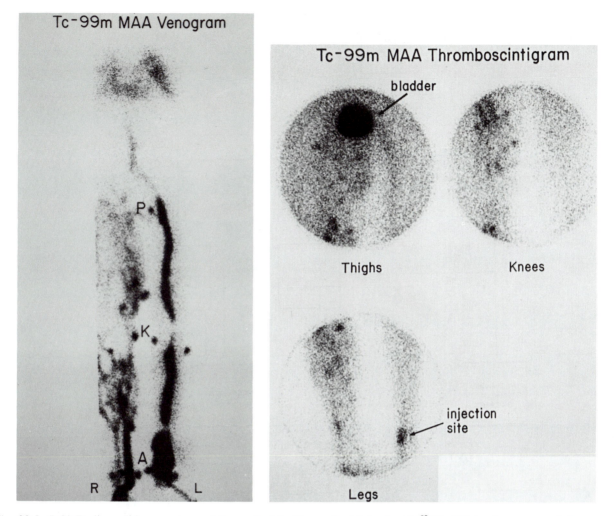

Fig. 28.5. (**left**) Radionuclide venogram of the patient in Figure 4, obtained with ^{99m}Tc MAA, shows normal deep venous system of the left lower extremity (L) as a central single column of radioactivity. The deep venous system of the right lower extremity (R) is replaced by many small collateral veins from the ankle (A) to the pelvis. (K indicates Knees; P, pubis. (**right**) Thromboscintigram obtained with ^{99m}Tc MAA showing clearance of all MAA particles from the normal left lower extremity. Many "hot spots" are seen in the right lower extremity, indicating acute thrombophlebitis.

lower leg (popliteal, femoral, and iliac).[66] Serial testing for 10 to 14 days will demonstrate proximal propogation in 20% of calf vein DVT cases. Figures 28.6 and 28.7 provide diagnostic guidelines for patients with a suspected DVT and/or pulmonary embolism. Individual patients may not be suitable for these algorithms. For example, a critically ill patient at a high risk for bleeding may undergo pulmonary angiography directly. Ultrasonography is a promising new noninvasive approach to detect deep vein thrombosis, either with Doppler or B-mode techniques.[67]

Treatment

The usual treatment of pulmonary embolism is intravenous heparin initially, followed by warfarin. Preventive treatment consists of low-dose subcutaneous hep-

arin sodium at a dose of 5,000 units every 12 hours. This is given to high-risk patients, especially those who remain immobile for at least 48 hours. When a venous thromboembolism is demonstrated, intravenous heparin is given (preferably continuously) in a dosage that maintains a partial thromboplastin time (PTT) of 1.5 to 2.5 times the normal control level. The advantages of continuous over intermittent administration include less bleeding and the ability to monitor PTT without regard to the time of perfusion. Oral warfarin therapy is begun after a few days, but the heparin infusion should be maintained for about 5 days until warfarin is fully effective. The duration of anticoagulant therapy after an initial DVT or pulmonary embolism is controversial. Recommendations range from 10 days to 1 year, but 3 to 6 months is most commonly advised. In a recent study evaluating sub-

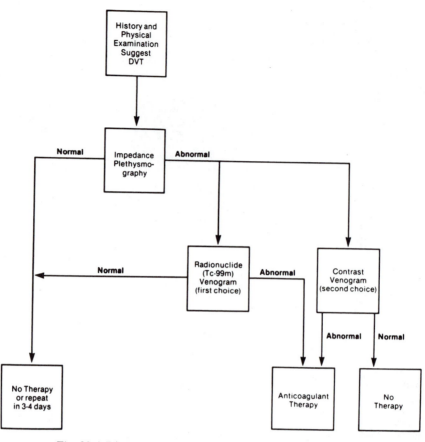

Fig. 28.6. Diagnostic guidelines for patients with a suspected DVT.

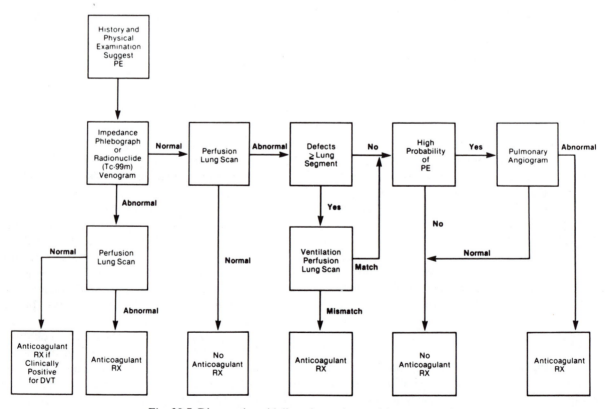

Fig. 28.7. Diagnostic guidelines for patients with a suspected pulmonary embolism.

cutaneous heparin versus oral warfarin in the long-term treatment of DVT, two thirds of the recurrent venous thromboembolism occurred after 3 months of effective anticoagulant therapy.[68] Thrombolytic therapy has not been widely used for pulmonary emboli, perhaps because of its expense and the potential hazards of bleeding. Neither of these problems justify withholding this effective therapy when indications for it exist. The two major indications are an acute, massive pulmonary embolism or serious compromise of circulatory dynamics.[69] Contraindications are conditions predisposing to hemorrhage. All the presently used thrombolytic agents (streptokinase, urokinase, tissue plasminogen activator) activate blood plasminogen. All have advantages, but the ideal agent in terms of efficacy, safety, antigenicity, and cost is yet to come. All three agents, however, do achieve significant clot lysis.

Interruption of the inferior vena cava previously has been technically unsatisfactory. Patients who have recurrent pulmonary emboli despite chronic anticoagulant therapy or in whom such therapy is contraindicated are candidates for an inferior vena cava filter. At present, the Greenfield vena cava filter has proved to be highly efficient, safe (patency of 98%), and effective (4% recurrent pulmonary emboli).[70] Indications include contraindications to anticoagulant therapy and recurrence of pulmonary embolism despite such therapy.

References

1. Macklem PT. Respiratory muscles: the vital pump. *Chest* 1980;78:753–758.
2. Luce JM, Culver BH. Respiratory muscle function in health and disease. *Chest* 1982;81:82–90.
3. Green GM, Jakab GJ, Low RB, et al. Defense mechanisms of the respiratory membrane. *Am Rev Respir Dis* 1977;115:479–514.
4. Pierson DJ, Hudson LD. Evaluation of dyspnea. *Geriatrics* 1981;36:48–62.
5. Kent S. The aging lung, I: loss of elasticity. *Geriatrics* 1978;33:124–130.
6. Manderly JL. Effect of age on pulmonary structure and function of immature and adult animals and man. *Fed Proc* 1979;38:173–177.
7. Jones RL, Overton TR, Hammerlindl DM, et al. Effects of age on regional residual volume. *J Appl Physiol* 1978;44:195–199.
8. Knudson RJ, Clark DF, Dennedy TC, et al. Effect of aging alone on mechanical properties of the normal adult lung. *J Appl Physiol* 1977;43:1054–1062.
9. Dhar S, Shastri SR, Lenoar RA. Aging and the respiratory system. *Med Clin North Am* 1976;60:1121–1139.
10. Kent S. Decline of pulmonary function. *Geriatrics* 1978;33:100–111.
11. Morris JF. Spirometry in the evaluation of pulmonary function. *West J Med* 1976;125:110–118.
12. Morris JF, Koski A, Johnson LC. Spirometric standards for healthy nonsmoking adults. *Am Rev Respir Dis* 1971;103:57–67.
13. Morris J, Koski A, Temple WP, et al. Fifteen-year interval spirmetric evaluation of the Oregon predictive equations. *Chest* 1988;92:123–127.
14. Morris JF, Temple WP. Spirometric "lung age" estimation for motivating smoking cessation. *Prev Med* 1985;14:655–662.
15. Gardner RM, et al. Snowbird workshop on standardization of spirometry: a statement by the American Thoracic Society. *Am Rev Respir Dis* 1979;119:831–838.
16. Sorbini C, Grassi V, Salmas F, et al. Arterial oxygen tension is relation to age in healthy subjects. *Respiration* 1968;25:3–10.
17. Ward RJ, Tolas AG, Benveniste RJ, et al. Effect of posture on normal arterial blood gas tensions in the aged. *Geriatrics* 1966;21:139–143.
18. Berger AJ, Mitchell RA, Severinghaus JW. Regulation of respiration. *N Engl J Med* 1977;297:92–97, 134–143, 194–206.
19. Block AJ. Is snoring a risk factor? *Chest* 1981;80:525.
20. Burki NK. Dyspnea. *Lung* 1987;165:269–277.
21. Mahler DA. Dyspnea: diagnosis and management. *Clin Chest Med* 1987;8:215–230.
22. Wasserman K, Whipp BJ. Exercise physiology in health and disease. *Am Rev Respir Dis* 1975;112:219–249.
23. Astrand PO. Human physical fitness with special reference to sex and age. *Physiol Rev* 1956;36:307–335.
24. deVries HA. Physiological effects of an exercise training regimen upon men aged 52 to 88. *J Gerontol* 1970; 25:325–336.
25. deVries HA. Tips on prescribing exercise regimens for your older patients. *Geriatrics* 1979;34:75–81.
26. Belman MJ, Mittman C. Ventilatory muscle training improves exercise capacity in chronic obstructive pulmonary disease patients. *Am Rev Respir Dis* 1980; 121:273–280.
27. Heath GW, Hagberg JM, Ehsani AA, et al. A physiological comparison of young and older endurance athletes. *J Appl Physiol* 1981;51:634–640.
28. Oregon Thoracic Society. *Chronic Obstructive Pulmonary Disease*. 5th ed. New York: American Lung Association; 1981.
29. Shim C, Williams MH Jr. The adequacy of inhalation from canister nebulizers. *Am J Med* 1980;69:891–894.
30. Tashkin DP, Ashutosh K, Bleeker, ER et al. Comparison of the anticholinergic bronchodilator ipratropium bromide with metaproterenol in chronic obstructive pulmonary disease. *Am J Med* 1986;81(suppl 5A):81–90.
31. Ledoux EJ, Morris JF, Temple WP, et al. Spirometric evaluation of standard and double dose ipratropium bromide and inhaled metaproterenol in patients with chronic obstructive pulmonary disease. *Chest* 1989; 95:1013–1016.
32. Sahn SA. Corticosteroids in chronic bronchitis and pulmonary emphysema. *Chest* 1978;73:389–396.
33. Wynne JW, Block AJ, Hemenway J, et al. Disordered breathing and oxygen desaturation during sleep in patients with chronic obstructive lung disease (COLD). *Am J Med* 1979;66:573–579.

34. Nocturnal Oxygen Therapy Trial Group. Continuous or nocturnal oxygen therapy in hyperemic chronic obstructive lung disease. *Ann Intern Med* 1980;93:391–398.

35. Keogh BA, Crystal RG. Pulmonary function testing in interstitial pulmonary disease. *Chest* 1980;78:856–865.

36. Crystal RG, Gadek JE, Ferrans VJ, et al. Interstitial lung disease: current concepts of pathogenesis, staging and therapy. *Am J Med* 1981;70:542–568.

37. Nicotra MB, Rivera M, Awe R. Antibiotic therapy of acute exacerbations of chronic bronchitis. *Ann Intern Med* 1982;97:18–21.

38. Phair JP, Kauffman CA, Bjornson A, et al. Host defenses in the aged: evaluation of components of the inflammatory and immune responses. *J Infect Dis* 1978;138:67–73.

39. Haas H, Morris JF, Samson S, et al. Bacterial flora of the respiratory tract in chronic bronchitis: comparison of transtracheal, fiberbronchoscopic, and oropharyngeal sampling methods. *Am Rev Respir Dis* 1977;116:41–47.

40. Haas H, Morris J, Samson S. Effect of oral penicillin on pneumococcal carriage in elderly men with chronic bronchitis. *Clin Ther* 1986;8:301–308.

41. Sims RV, Steinmann WC, McConville JH, et al. The clinical effectiveness of pneumococcal vaccine in the elderly. *Ann Intern Med* 1988;108:653–657.

42. Wynne JW, Reynolds JC, Hood IC, et al. Steroid therapy for pneumonitis induced in rabbits by aspiration of foodstuff. *Anesthesiology* 1977;87:466–474.

43. Wynne JW, Modell JH. Respiratory aspiration of stomach contents. *Ann Intern Med* 1977;87:466–474.

44. Williams GO. Vaccines in older patients. combating the risk of mortality. *Geriatrics* 1980;35:55–64.

45. Dolin R, Reichman RC, Madore HP, et al. A controlled trail of amantadine and rimantadine in the prophylaxis of influenza A infection. *N Engl J Med* 1982;307:580–584.

46. VanVoris LP, Betts RF, et al. Successful treatment of naturally occurring influenza A/USSR/77 HlNl. *JAMA* 1981;245:1128–1131.

47. Thompson NJ, Glassroth JL, Snider DE, et al. The booster phenomenon in serial tuberculin testing. *Am Rev Respir Dis* 1979;119:587–597.

48. Stead WW. The pathogenesis of pulmonary tuberculosis among older persons. *Am Rev Respir Dis* 1965;91:811–822.

49. Miller WT, McGregor RR. Tuberculosis: frequency of unusual radiographic findings. *AJR* 1978;130:867–875.

50. Khan MA, Kovnat DM, Bachus F, et al. Clinical and roentgenographic spectrum of pulmonary tuberculosis in the adult. *Am J Med* 1977;62:31–38.

51. American Thoracic Society. Treatment of tuberculosis and tuberculosis infection in adults and children. *Am Rev Respir Dis* 1986;134:355–363.

52. Farer LS. Chemoprophylaxis. *Am Rev Respir Dis* 1982;125(p2):102–07.

53. Matthay RA, Blames JR. Lung Cancer: a persistent challenge. *Geriatrics* 1982;37:109–131.

54. Zavala DC. Diagnostic fiberoptic bronchoscopy: techniques and results of biopsy in 600 patients. *Chest* 1975;68:12–19.

55. Zavala DC, Schoell JE. Ultrathin needle aspiration of the lung in infectious and malignant disease. *Am Rev Respir Dis* 1981;123:125–131.

56. Bruya T, Morris JF, Barker AF. Bronchoscopy and bone marrow examinations: an efficient strategy to establish the diagnosis of small cell carcinoma of the lung. *Chest* 1981;79:423–426.

57. Ali MK, Mountain CF, Ewer MS, et al. Predicting loss of pulmonary function after resection for bronchgenic carcinoma. *Chest* 1980;77:337–342.

58. McNeil BJ, Weichselbaum R, Parker SG. Fallacy of the fiv-year survival in lung cancer. *N Engl J Med* 1978;1397–1401.

59. Peterson BA, Kennedy BJ. Aging and cancer management, I: clinical observations. *CA* 1979;29:322–332.

60. Coy P, Dennelly GM. The role of curative radiotherapy in the treatment of lung cancer. *Cancer* 1980;45:698–702.

61. Spiro SG. The management of lung cancer: *Lung* 1982;160:141–155.

62. Greco FA, Richardson RL, Snell JD, et al. Small cell lung cancer: complete remission and survival. *Am J Med* 1979;66:625–630.

63. Bell WR, Simon TL. Current status of pulmonary thromboembolic disease: pathophysiology, diagnosis, prevention, and treatment. *Am Heart J* 103:239–262.

64. Freiman DG, Suyemoto J, Wessler S. Frequency of pulmonary embolism in man. *N Engl J Med* 1965;272:1278–1280.

65. Hull R, Hirsh J, Sackett DL, et al. Cost effectiveness of clinical diagnosis, venography, and noninvasive testing in patients with symptomatic deep vein thrombosis. *N Engl J Med* 1981;304:1561–1567.

66. Hull RD, Hirsh J, Carter CJ, et al. Diagnostic efficacy of impedance plethysomography for clinically suspected deep vein thrombosis: a randomnized trial. *Ann Intern Med* 1985;102:21–28.

67. Lensing, AWA, Prandoni, P, Brandjes, D, et al: Detection of deep-vein thrombosis by real-time B-mode ultrasonography. *N Engl J Med* 1989;320:342–345.

68. Hull R, Delmore T, Carter C, et al. Adjusted subcutaneous heparin versus warfarin sodium in the long-term treatment of venous thrombosis. *N Engl J Med* 1982;306:189–194.

69. Marder VJ, Sherry S. Thrombolytic therapy: current status. *N Engl J Med* 1988;318:1585–1595.

70. Kanter B, Moser KM. The Greenfield vena cava filter. *Chest* 1988;93:170–175.

29

Dermatology

Michael T. Goldfarb, Charles N. Ellis, and John J. Voorhees

The aging process is most clearly demonstrated in the skin. Since the skin is visible to all, the changes from normal aging and exposure to the physical elements can be disturbing to the elderly, who may seek ways to reverse these cutaneous changes. Also the various dermatologic diseases and growths that may appear with aging are easily noted by both the patient and physician. This chapter will concentrate on the skin changes that occur with aging and the dermatologic diseases that affect primarily the older age groups.

Structure and Physiology of Aging Skin

Epidermis

Even without any damage to the skin by physical elements, it will change and age intrinsically. The epidermal thickness and its rete ridge pattern decreases with aging. The keratinocytes are smaller and have a lower proliferation rate. These changes cause the skin to be sensitive to minor trauma and to heal more slowly. The skin also provides less of a barrier. The number of functioning melanocytes decreases by 10% to 20% each decade, reducing the body's ability to protect itself from ultraviolet light. Langerhans cells, which are epidermal dendritic cells originating from the bone marrow, are responsible for the skin's immune defenses; they are reduced by almost 50% in

the older population, making the skin less sensitive to allergic stimuli and possibly less protected from neoplastic development.[1]

Dermis

Changes in the dermis occur mainly from physical elements, but the dermis also changes intrinsically with aging. The dermis will lose approximately 20% of its thickness, causing the skin to feel thin and become transparent. This thinning is due largely to the loss of proteoglycan and, to a lesser extent, collagen. The elastic fibers thicken and fragment; there is a reduction in the capillary network, which contributes to gradual atrophy of the skin and which may be partly responsible for the decreased inflammation and rate of healing with injury seen in elderly skin. Finally, the size and number of fibroblasts are reduced.[1]

Subcutaneous Fat

The underlying subcutaneous fat also thins with age. It cannot adequately carry out its role of protecting the internal structures from trauma and cold. Many elderly people frequently feel cold due in part to this loss of protection.[1]

Appendages

One of the first and most noticeable changes during aging is hair loss. Two common processes lead to hair loss: androgenic alopecia and involutional alopecia. Androgenic alopecia is dependent on genetics and male sex hormones and usually has an onset before age 40 years. Hair loss is noted primarily on the vertex and frontal areas of the scalp as terminal hairs turn into vellus hairs.[2] Involutional alopecia is a phenomenon of aging, with narrowing of hair shaft diameters, decreasing anagen phase and growth rate, and fewer active follicles. Unlike androgenic alopecia, involutional alopecia is not limited to the scalp but involves all body hair.

Graying of hair is considered synonymous with aging. By age 50 years, approximately half of all body hairs are gray. This is due to loss of melanocytes and melanocytic function in the hair bulb.[2]

The rate of growth of the nail plates also diminishes with age. Some nails become thin and brittle, while others, especially the toenails, become thick and dystrophic. Longitudinal ridging is common.[1]

Sebaceous glands do not decrease in size with age but actually undergo hypertrophy on the back and face in many elderly people. Their function, however, does diminish, which adds to the problem of dry skin in the elderly. Eccrine and apocrine glands do diminish in number with aging, and they are less able to respond to appropriate stimuli. This reduced perspiring capacity makes the elderly person more susceptible to hyperthermia.[1]

Changes in Aging Skin from Physical Elements

Since the skin is exposed to all the physical elements in the environment, it is continually damaged and changed by these forces. It is difficult to distinguish the changes of intrinsic aging from those caused by the environment. Many of the skin changes assumed to be due to intrinsic aging actually are from exposure to physical elements. Therefore, protecting skin from the environment can prevent many undesirable effects previously thought to be unavoidable.

Sun Exposure

The most damaging physical element to the skin is the sun. The term *dermatoheliosis* is used to describe all of the findings that occur in photoaged skin. Ultraviolet B light (wavelengths 290 to 320 nm) is most responsible for chronic damage from the sun, and ultraviolet A light (320 to 400 nm) less so. A large percentage of ultraviolet light could easily be blocked by clothing and commercially available sunscreens, preventing harm to the skin.[3]

The degree of photoaging varies not only with solar exposure but also with the individual. The photoabsorbing melanin pigment system is protective against the sun's effect, so a fair-skinned person is far more susceptible to sun damage than someone with greater pigmentation. Of course, the areas of heavier sun exposure, the face and arms, sustain more damage.

The epidermis is thinned by chronic sun exposure, and atypical keratinocytes become more prevalent. Some melanocytes are destroyed by excessive ultraviolet light, leading to spotty hypopigmentation, while, in nearby areas, melanocytes may be stimulated by solar energy to cause hyperpigmentation.

The dermis is markedly changed after years of sun exposure. Its fibrillar nature is replaced by irregular homogeneous clumps of connective tissue, a process called elastosis. Elastosis is probably due to the production of defective collagen and elastin by sun-damaged fibroblasts. These dermal changes are partly responsible for the sagging and wrinkling of aging skin. The elastotic dermis provides inadequate structural support for blood vessels, leading to ectasia and thin vessel walls.[4]

Solar Elastosis

The first change of solar elastosis is wrinkling. How this occurs is not entirely clear. Wrinkling does not occur in some of the most photoexposed areas, like the nose and ears, so it may be confined to skin that is elastic. Not all wrinkling is sun induced; some wrinkle lines run in families and can be considered genetic. The most common areas for wrinkles are the periorbital (crow's feet) and perioral areas, the cheeks, and the forehead (Fig. 29.1). The skin also will show yellowing and a rough texture with solar elastosis.[4]

Cutis Rhomboidalis Nuchae

This condition is most common in men after years of sun exposure.[5] Deep furrows on the back of the neck form a rhomboid pattern. The skin is thick and yellow or red.

Nodular Elastoidosis with Cysts and Comedones (Favre-Racouchot Syndrome)

Numerous comedones and cysts develop primarily in the periorbital and temporal areas.[5] The comedones have a dark central plug, are filled with keratinous debris, and are commonly called blackheads (Fig. 29.2).

Colloid Millium

This is caused by a degenerative change in the dermis from years of overexposure to sunlight.[5] The dermis contains globules of homogeneous, eosinophilic material termed colloid. Clinically, yellow papules approximately 2 mm in diameter form on the face and the back of the hands.

Stellate Pseudoscars

These are white, atrophic scars found commonly on the forearms after years of sun exposure.[5] They have irregular, stellate shapes and form after minor trauma. The origin probably is poor repair in a dermis with solar elastosis.

Senile Purpura (Bateman's Purpura)

Senile purpura refers to the red to purple patches that form over the forearms and back of the hands in elderly people (Fig. 29.3).[5] The thin dermis of aged skin does not provide adequate support for the cutaneous blood vessels. Therefore, even trivial shearing trauma to the skin can cause the vessels to rupture and form purpuric lesions, which may persist for weeks.

Heat

Chronic exposure to heat also can damage the skin. Elderly people who are sensitive to the cold frequently warm themselves by a fire, space heater, or with an electric blanket. This can lead to a condition known as erytherma ab igne (Fig. 29.4).[6] The area chronically exposed to heat develops a reticulated brown pigmentation. Keratotic lesions may form in this area and rarely have developed into squamous cell carcinomas. The condition is most common on the lower extremities.

Cold

Winter weather, with its cold temperatures, low humidity, and wind, is poorly tolerated by aging skin. With the decrease in eccrine and sebaceous gland function, the skin becomes dry and pruritic. Due to the loss of subcutaneous fat and a reduced vascular supply to the extremities, the elderly also are more prone to frostbite.

Inflammatory Dermatoses in Aging Skin

Xerosis and Eczema Craquelé

An almost universal problem among the elderly is xerosis, which usually is worse during the winter with the low humidity of heated rooms.[7] The exact etiology is unclear, but a decrease in sebaceous and eccrine gland function, as well as an increase in transepidermal water loss, may play a role. The skin is dry and scaly and may be very pruritic. Often called asteototic eczema, xerosis is most common on the legs, back, and arms. The skin may become inflamed with erythema, lichenification, and fissuring, a condition which is referred to as eczema craquelé (Fig. 29.5).

This problem usually is transient and clears with the warm weather. During the winter months, the patient should decrease the frequency of bathing, avoid hot bath water, and limit the use of soap. This will help prevent further drying of the skin. A topical emollient, preferably an ointment, should be used daily to hydrate the skin. If inflammation is present, low-dose topical corticosteroid ointment, such as 1% to 2.5% hydrocortisone, may be used twice daily. Due to the thin nature of elderly skin, potent topical corticosteroids should be avoided. For persistent associated pruritus, a low-dose oral antihistamine at bedtime is useful.

Nummular Eczema

A condition related to xerosis is nummular eczema.[8] It appears as coin-shaped patches with erythema, scaling, and sometimes vesiculations, most commonly on the limbs of people with dry skin (Fig. 29.6). Treatment with emollients and low-dose topical corticosteroids may be of help.

Lichen Simplex Chronicus

This is a localized area of chronic eczema with extreme pruritus.[9] Areas commonly involved include the dorsum of the feet, the back of the neck, and the wrists. Pruritus is thought to be the initiating problem, and the chronic scratching leads to the skin changes. The skin is thickened, the skin markings are enhanced, and the plaque may show erythema and excoriations. The patient must try to resist scratching; potent topical corticosteroids are often necessary.

Pruritus

Many elderly people suffer from chronic pruritus without any obvious skin disorder. This can be extremely bothersome. Patients may be unable to sleep and may severely excoriate their skin. The condition can be localized or generalized. The physician must carefully look for an underlying skin disease that could be causing the eruption. Due to the muted inflammatory response in elderly people, many skin conditions, including scabies, urticaria, and eczema, are difficult to detect. Systemic disease,[10] including renal failure, liver disease, cancer, thyrotoxicosis, and diabetes, may also present as or cause pruritus. Frequently, no etiology is uncovered and the patient must be treated symptomatically. Emollients and topical antipruritic agents, such as 0.5% menthol and 0.5% phenol, may provide some relief. The use of sedatives and antihistamines may be helpful, but excessive drowsiness and paradoxical restlessness are concerns in elderly patients.

Angular Cheilitis

Frequently, elderly people develop inflammation at the corners of the mouth, which is called angular cheilitis or perlèche (Fig. 29.7).[11] This condition is characterized by erythema and painful fissures. It is most common in the edentulous patient. The skin of the cheek loses support due to the loss of teeth and the normal aging process, thereby causing overlaps at the angles of the mouth. Saliva is trapped in this area, leading to maceration and candida infections. Properly fitting dentures may eliminate the problem by restoring the normal cheek contour. Topical antifungal agents can help resolve the secondary *Candida* infection, and low-dose topical corticosteroids will decrease the inflammation.

Seborrheic Dermatitis

Seborrheic dermatitis is a chronic eczematous disorder of the scalp, face, chest, and intertriginous areas that affects over 20% of the elderly population.[12] It is characterized by erythema and greasy scales. The eruption usually starts in the scalp and often is mistaken for dandruff. It then progresses to the eyebrows and paranasal area. In its most severe form, the disorder can become generalized and develop into an erythroderma. The cause of seborrheic dermatitis is unknown. *Pityrosporum*, a yeast that is part of the normal flora of the skin, is found in increased numbers in the greasy scales and may be involved in the pathogenesis. Usually, seborrheic dermatitis can be easily brought under control, but there is no cure. One of the dandruff shampoos, either selenium sulfide or tar based, frequently can clear the scalp. Hydrocortisone 1% cream may be required to treat the skin of the face. In view of the possible role of *Pityrosporum*, topical antifungal agents may be useful.[13]

Psoriasis

This condition usually has its onset during young adult life but is common and can be disabling in the elderly population. Approximately 2% of the population is affected. Psoriasis is characterized by sharply de-

marcated, erythematous plaques with silvery scales. It is most common on the extensor surfaces, especially knees and elbows, and frequently involves the scalp. Areas of trauma and chronic irritation often develop psoriasis. Psoriasis can generalize into an erythroderma or may be pustular. Approximately 7% of psoriatic patients will have an associated arthritis usually of the distal phalanges. Psoriasis is a disease of rapid epidermal cell growth and inflammation, but despite extensive investigation its cause remains unknown. Localized areas of psoriasis usually can be treated with topical corticosteroids, tar preparations, anthralin, and ultraviolet light. For more extensive or generalized disease, oral psoralen and ultraviolet light (PUVA), methotrexate, or the oral retinoid etretinate may be necessary. Recently, cyclosporine has shown promise. There is no cure for this condition.[14]

Pityriasis Rubra Pilaris

This is a rare condition that may be acquired or inherited.[15] The most common form is acquired. Onset is rapid, commonly in the 5th decade of life. It begins in the scalp and on the face and then proceeds downward to involve the whole body. This condition resembles psoriasis but has a characteristic orange color, marked follicular involvement, and hyperkeratosis of the palms and soles. The disease usually lasts only 1 to 3 years. Topical medications usually are ineffective. Oral etretinate has been used with some benefit.

Contact Dermatitis

Often older persons treat their dry and pruritic skin with a variety of topical medications. These may contain various antibiotics, anesthetics, preservatives, and keratolytics that can lead to contact allergic and irritant dermatoses. Plants, nickel, and rubber additives frequently cause contact dermatitis in the general population and may also affect the elderly.[16] Although aging skin is thin and fragile, it has a depressed inflammatory response. As a result, contact dermatitis may be relatively mild. Clinically, the involved skin is erythematous and swollen, with vesicles and crusting. With chronic exposure, the eruption becomes lichenified and scaly. The most important intervention is to discover the responsible agent and prevent further contact. Topical corticosteroids hasten healing.

Drug Eruptions

Because of the increased likelihood of polypharmacy in elderly patients, this age group has many more drug-induced eruptions than the general population.

Some of the drugs that commonly cause skin eruptions are diuretics, antibiotics, psychotropics, and nonsteroidal antiinflammatory agents.[17] Almost 50% of the eruptions are maculopapular, about 25% urticarial. All types of drug eruptions have been observed in the elderly, including fixed drug eruptions, phototoxic reactions, erythema multiforme, toxic epidermal necrolysis, lupus-like syndromes, and lichenoid drug eruptions.

Bullous Pemphigoid

This is a blistering disease found almost exclusively in elderly persons; it is rare before the age of 60 years. Large, tense bullae filled with clear serum form on normal and urticarial skin (Fig. 29.8). Lesions predominate in the flexural aspects of the limbs and abdomen. Approximately 25% of patients will have oral lesions. The eruption frequently is extensive and impressive in appearance, but the general health of the patient usually is good.

The diagnosis of bullous pemphigoid is made by means of skin biopsy. Routine light microscopy of lesional skin shows a subepidermal blister. Immunoflourescence of perilesional skin demonstrates linear deposits of immunoglubulin G and C3 along the basement membrane.[18] Its exact etiology is unknown, but the condition is thought to be due to the formation of an autoimmune antibody directed against the epidermal basement membrane. There is no explanation for why this antibody forms.

Bullous pemphoid usually runs a benign course with eventual remission. Relapses do occur, and debilitated patients have died from this condition. Systemic corticosteroids (prednisone, 60 mg/d) usually brings the disease under control and is considered the standard therapy. The dosage should be slowly tapered to avoid a relapse. An immunosuppressant agent, usually azathioprine, can be used to help the tapering.

Pemphigus vulgaris should be considered in the differential diagnosis of bullous pemphigoid. Usually this condition involves middle-aged people, is characterized by flaccid and fragile bullae, and is fatal unless high-dose systemic corticosteroids are used. In pemphigus vulgaris, the blister and immune deposits are found at skin biopsy to be intraepidermal, making it easy to distinguish from bullous pemphigoid.[18]

Anogenital Disease in Aging Skin

Pruritus Ani

Persistent pruritus of the perianal area is a common and troublesome problem in the elderly. Fecal contamination and moisture chronically irritate the skin, leading to pruritus and even eczematous changes. Cutaneous infections and hemorrhoids may be the cause of pruritus ani in some cases. To treat this condition, the patient should be carefully educated in proper hygiene.[19] Fecal evacuation should be limited to once daily if possible and the area cleaned gently. Hydrocortisone cream may help alleviate the pruritus and irritation. When used in a cautious, temporary fashion, potent topical corticosteroids may be helpful in difficult cases.

Senile Vulvar Atrophy

This condition is quite common in postmenopausal women.[5] Clinically, the vaginal mucosa is dry and there is atrophy of the labia majora, labia minora, and clitoris. The dryness may lead to pruritus, scratching, and eventual lichenification. A topical emollient can provide some relief (see Chapter 23).

Lichen Sclerosus et Atrophicus, Balanitis Xerotica Obliterans

Lichen sclerosus et atrophicus occurs primarily in women at menopause but can also affect prepubital girls.[20] It most commonly involves the vulva and anus, forming the characteristic "hourglass" appearance. The condition consists of ivory-white, atrophic papules and plaques with a violaceous rim. The most common complaint is pruritus, but some people also are bothered by soreness and dyspareunia. In approximately 50% of patients, leukoplakia will form, and 5% eventually will develop squamous cell carcinoma. Therapy includes the frequent application of bland emollients and the occasional use of a mild topical corticosteroid to control the pruritus. In severe cases, topical 2% testosterone propionate has been used with some success. Unfortunately, this medication can lead to the side effects of systemic testosterone excess. The patient also must be carefully followed up to identify any developing carcinomas.

The male counterpart of lichen sclerosus et atrophicus is balanitis xerotica obliterans. It consists of white atrophic plaques on the glans and prepuce (Fig. 29.9). Phimosis and urethral stricture may develop.[21]

Angiokeratomas of Fordyce

This is a common lesion in men over age 50 years. Numerous red-purple lesions with minimal hyperkeratosis are found on the scrotum (Fig. 29.10).[22] The lesions are benign and asymptomatic, so removal is not necessary.

Infections in Aging Skin

Herpes Zoster

This is a vesicular dermatomal disease due to the varicella virus.[23] Primary infection leads to chicken pox and usually occurs in childhood. Herpes zoster (shingles) is caused by the reactivation of the latent virus in the dorsal root ganglia. Although most people with this condition are in good health, patients with neoplastic disease or on immunosuppressant drugs are at higher risk. Zoster is common and may be severe in the elderly population (see Chapter 25).

The disease begins as pain and paresthesia in the involved dermatome. Clusters of vesicles on an erythematous base then erupt in the same area (Fig. 29.11). The condition can affect any nerve, but the ophthalmic division of the trigeminal nerve and the thoracic nerves are the most common. The rash usually involves only one dermatome and is typically unilateral, rarely crossing the midline.

The most common complication is postherpetic neuralgia, lasting over 1 year in half the patients above age 60 years. Involvement of the corneal branch of the ophthalmic division of the trigeminal nerve can lead to keratitis and iritis. In an immunosuppressed patient, the virus can disseminate and be life threatening.

During the acute phase of infection, the patient may require narcotic analgesics for pain relief and Burow's solution to help dry the vesicles. Some physicians advocate the use of oral corticosteroids (prednisone, 60 mg/d) for 2 weeks in patients over age 50 years, to decrease the risk of postheraptic neuralgia. The use of intravenous acyclovir can halt the progression of herpes zoster and may be useful in immunosuppressed patients.[24] The varicella virus is less sensitive to acyclovir than the herpes simplex virus, and a higher dose is needed (10 mg/kg/8 h, given intravenously). If eye involvement occurs, an ophthalmologist should be consulted.

Dermatophytes and *Candida*

Dermatophyte infection of the toenail plate, called tinea unguium or onychomycosis,[25] is a common and persistent problem in elderly men. The involved nail becomes thick and yellow with subungual debris. An associated chronic tinea pedis with mild erythema and scales often is found. Similar nail changes can be due to aging without any fungal infection. Before treatment is initiated, a confirmed diagnosis should be made by demonstrating hyphae on a microscopic preparation or culturing dermatophytes from the subungual debris. Therapy frequently is disappointing. One topical antifungal cream, ciclopirox olamine, has been used with modest improvement. Oral griseofulvin (500 mg/d) sometimes can clear the toenail, but 1 to 2 years of therapy often is required, and recurrences are common.

The elderly also are susceptible to *Candida* and dermatophyte infections in the moist areas of the groin, axilla, and submammary region. These are especially common in obese persons during the summer months. Candidiasis causes a shiny erythematous rash with pustules and satellite lesions. The eruption of a dermatophyte infection is annular and sharply margined, with a raised and scaly edge. Treatment includes keeping the area dry and applying a topical antifungal agent twice a day.

Benign and Malignant Skin Tumors in Aging Skin

One of the most common concerns of an elderly patient is the many different growths that appear on the skin with aging. The physician frequently will be questioned about which lesions are or may become malignant. Also, many of these lesions are unsightly to the patient, and their removal will be requested.

Seborrheic Keratosis

This is a common epidermal growth found in almost every elderly patient.[26] They begin to appear in the 4th decade and may occur anywhere on the body. The size ranges from 2 mm to 4 cm, and the color varies from tan to black. These rough-surfaced lesions are sharply marginated and appear "stuck on" the skin (Fig. 29.12). An occasional lesion may resemble a malignant melanoma, and a biopsy is then required. A variant form common in the elderly consists of white, keratotic plaques on the extremities, called stucco keratosis. Seborrheic keratosis may become irritated and unsightly. If the patient desires removal, the least damaging procedure should be used. Curettage and liquid nitrogen cryosurgery are two simple techniques that work well.

Skin Tags (Acrochordons)

Skin tags are benign lesions frequently found on the obese elderly patient, especially around the neck and flexural areas. They are pedunculated, pink to brown papules. Removal can be easily performed by means of scissor excision or light electrodesiccation if they are irritated or cosmetically unacceptable to the patient.

Sebaceous Hyperplasia

These lesions are slow growing, benign papules found mostly on the face after age 50 years.[27] They are yellow, dome-shaped, and may have a central umbilication. Sebaceous hyperplasia has been mistaken for a basal cell carcinoma, and a biopsy is sometimes necessary. Light electrodesiccation can remove any unwanted lesions.

Cherry Angiomas

These benign lesions, also known as senile angiomas, are found on the trunk of almost every person over age 30 years. They become more numerous and larger with age. The typical lesion is 1 to 4 mm in size, dome shaped, and cherry red (Fig. 29.13). Removal is not necessary, but electrodesiccation, cryosurgery, and shave excision all have been used successfully.

Venous Lakes

These blue to black lesions are found primarily on the lips, face, and ears of elderly patients. They are due to dilated venous channels in elastotic skin. Treatment with shave excision and electrodesiccation usually is successful. Occasionally, the venous lakes may be mistaken for melanomas.

Spider Veins

A common complaint of older women is dilated, star-shaped, blue veins on the feet and legs. They represent a cosmetic problem and are due to elevated venous pressure over a lifetime. The preferred treatment, sclerotherapy, involves injecting the lumen of the vein with 20% hypertonic saline.[28]

Actinic Keratosis

Actinic or solar keratoses are common, premalignant lesions found on sun-exposed skin in fair-skinned middle-aged to elderly people.[29] The lesions usually are due to accumulated damage to the skin from the ultraviolet rays of the sun. Chronic heat exposure and arsenic ingestion can lead to similar lesions. A typical lesion is pink with dry, rough adherent scales. They often are easier to feel than to see. The most commonly involved areas include the face and the back of the hands. A severely sun-damaged patient may have numerous lesions.

A small percentage of actinic keratoses transform into squamous cell carcinomas, so these lesions should be removed. Individual lesions can be easily treated with electrodesiccation, cryosurgery, or excision. For multiple small lesions, a course of 5% fluorouracil cream may be useful. The medication is applied twice daily for approximately 3 weeks, and the patient should be warned that the treated area becomes inflamed. Topical tretinoin also may be useful.

Basal Cell Carcinoma

Basal cell carcinoma is the most common of all human malignancies. The lesions are locally invasive but rarely if ever metastasize. They usually occur on sun-exposed areas of older, fair-skinned individuals. Ultraviolet radiation is thought to be the primary cause, although some lesions form on sun-protected areas.

There are several different morphologic forms of basal cell carcinoma. The most common is the nodular ulcerative lesion. It appears as a pearly, translucent nodule with rolled borders and telangiectasias (Fig. 29.14). The lesions may ulcerate or become pigmented. Another type, the superficial basal cell carcinoma, is a persistent, erythematous plaque on the torso that can easily be mistaken for eczema. The morpheaform basal cell carcinoma is the rarest, presenting as a pale, indurated plaque with poorly defined borders.

These lesions are locally destructive and disfiguring, so definitive treatment should be initiated promptly. The goal is to eradicate the cancer with a good cosmetic result.[30] Scalpel excision, electrodesiccation and curettage, cryosurgery, and ionizing radiation all have been used successfully. The choice of therapy depends on the patient's age and the size and location of the lesion. The procedure with the highest cure rate is Mohs' microscopically controlled surgery, but it is time consuming and requires special equipment and training to perform. It is primarily used for large or recurrent basal cell carcinomas.

Bowen's Disease

Bowen's disease is actually an intraepidermal squamous cell carcinoma in situ. The lesion appears as a sharply marginated erythematous plaque with scales that slowly enlarge over years (Fig. 29.15).[29] With time it can develop into an invasive squamous cell carcinoma. Typical Bowen's disease can easily be mistaken for eczema or psoriasis. Therefore, any dermatitis that is consistently resistant to therapy should be submitted to biopsy to rule out this cancer. Adequate therapy requires destruction of the entire lesion. As with basal cell carcinomas, scalpel excision, electrodesiccation and curettage, cryosurgery, and ionizing radiation all have been used successfully.

A variant of Bowen's disease, erythroplasia of

Queyrat, occurs on the glans penis in uncircumsised men. The lesion is a red, velvety plaque with sharp borders. It must be recognized immediately because metastatic disease may occur early.

Squamous Cell Carcinoma

Squamous cell carcinoma of the skin is another common cancer in elderly persons. It usually arises on sun-damaged skin or from an actinic keratosis in fair-skinned patients. Most lesions are only locally destructive and rarely spread, but those that arise on the lips, in Bowen's disease, or from a chronic skin ulcer tend to be more invasive and can metastasize early.[29] The initial lesion may be a firm, erythematous nodule with a scaly surface. If not treated, it may become a large ulcerated tumor fixed to the underlying structures (Fig. 29.16). Treatment involves the complete removal of the lesion, usually by scalpel excision or Mohs' surgery. Electrodesiccation with curettage, cryosurgery, and ionizing radiation may also be used.[30]

Keratoacanthoma

This is a rapidly enlarging skin tumor that resembles a squamous cell carcinoma but usually runs a benign course.[31] The lesion is a firm, dome-shaped nodule with a central keratotic plug, found primarily on sun-exposed skin (Fig. 29.17). It may grow to over 1 cm in only 6 weeks but may spontaneously heal over the next 2 months, leaving a scar. Even with a skin biopsy it may be difficult to distinguish a keratoacanthoma from a squamous cell carcinoma. Therefore, removal with scalpel excision or electrodesiccation with curettage is recommended.

Solar Lentigos (Senile Lentigos)

These are well-circumscribed macules found on sun-exposed skin in almost all white persons over age 60 years. The lesions are uniformly tan to dark brown in color and range in size from 1 mm to greater than 2 cm. They are due to a benign proliferation of melanocytes in the epidermis. These lentigos are benign but may be removed with a light liquid nitrogen freeze if the patient finds them displeasing. Topical tretinoin decreases the pigmentation as well.

Lentigo Maligna and Lentigo Maligna Melanoma

Lentigo maligna begins as a tan macule that slowly darkens and enlarges over many years. It is found almost exclusively on sun-exposed skin in elderly patients. Various shades of brown to jet black occur in the same lesion. It consists of an intraepidermal proliferation of atypical melanocytes.[32] This lesion should be removed completely by scalpel excision or freezing with liquid nitrogen.

If the lesion is not treated, nodules may appear, indicating evolution to lentigo maligna melanoma (Fig. 29.18). At this point, the atypical melanocytes have penetrated through the basement membrane of the epidermis.[32] The lesion usually is larger than 3 cm and is almost always located on the face or neck. The entire lesion should be removed and the deepest area of invasion measured under the microscope. The prognosis of the disease is best determined by the depth of penetration into the dermis.[33] Lesions that are less than 1 mm thick are almost always cured by surgical excision with a 1 cm margin of normal skin. Thick lesions, over 4 mm in depth, frequently metastasize and are associated with less than a 50% 5-year survival. Wider excision and lymph node dissection often is recommended for thick lesions. Unfortunately, metastatic melanoma has been very resistant to chemotherapy, radiation therapy, and immunotherapy.

Paget's Disease

The two forms of Paget's disease are mammary[34] and extramammary.[35] It is an intraepidermal carcinoma of glandular origin with onset after age 50 years. The mammary form presents as a sharply-marginated, eczematous plaque on the areola and nipple. As it is associated with an intraductal carcinoma of the breast, mastectomy is recommended. Extramammary disease usually is found in the groin and has the same clinical appearance as on the nipple. An associated malignancy in an underlying organ or adnexal structure is frequently but not always found. Treatment of extramammary disease includes surgical excision of the lesion and a search for an associated malignancy. Either form of Paget's disease can easily be mistaken for eczema, so any treatment-resistant dermatitis of the nipple or groin should be biopsied.

Kaposi's Sarcoma

The classic form of this vascular malignancy is largely restricted to elderly men of Eastern European or Jewish descent.[36] Multiple dermal plaques and nodules are found on the lower legs (Fig. 29.19). The lesions are red to purple in color and may become large tumors that ulcerate. Metastatic disease may occur as the condition progresses. In this form of Kaposi's sarcoma, the spread is slow and many elderly patients will die of an unrelated cause. Although there is no cure for this malignancy, it is radiosensitive and local cutaneous disease responds to radiation therapy.

Kaposi's sarcoma also occurs in two other patient populations. It is an endemic disease in Africa and it frequently occurs in patients with the acquired immunodeficiency syndrome (AIDS). These patient are young, have more extensive disease, and have a poorer prognosis than those with the classic form.

Angiosarcoma

This is a rare and fatal vascular malignancy of the elderly. Dusky, erythematous plaques and nodules are found on the scalp and face.[37] Angiosarcoma metastasizes early and treatment usually is unsuccessful.

Cutaneous Metastases

Most malignant tumors can cause cutaneous metastases. Approximately 4% of internal malignancies eventually will involve the skin.[38] The most common sites of the primary tumor are the breasts, gastrointestinal tract, lung, and kidney. Cutaneous metastases usually are multiple and a manifestation of extensive disease. Rarely, they may be the presenting sign of an internal malignancy. There is no classic appearance to these lesions. They often are pink, intradermal nodules with a firm consistency (Fig. 29.20). These lesions are found predominately on the scalp and trunk.

Ulcerations in Aging Skin

Stasis Dermatitis and Venous Ulceration

Stasis dermatitis is due to venous hypertension in the lower legs. Predisposing factors include a history of thrombophlebitis, obesity, or multiple pregnancies and a positive family history. Initially, the patient complains of ankle edema and aching in the limb. The skin around the medial malleolus becomes brown and eczematous, with enlarged, blue veins. The conditions usually will respond to low-dose topical corticosteroids and an elastic bandage to reduce the edema.

Venous ulcerations[39] may occur spontaneously or from a superficial injury. They usually are located on the medial aspect of the ankle. The initial ulcer is small and shallow, but it can become quite large. It has a red base with an irregular border. Secondary bacterial infections are common, but they are frequently not clinically significant. With long-standing disease, the skin becomes fibrotic and calcifications can occur in the subcutaneous tissues. The treatment of venous ulcers is difficult and recurrences are common. Relieving the ankle edema by elevating the feet and wearing elastic bandages may help to promote healing. The use of an occlusive dressing (eg, Duoderm) has been effective in some cases with ulcerations.

Arterial Ulceration

This condition is due primarily to atherosclerosis of the limb vessels leading to ischemia of the skin.[39] Arterial ulcers have distinguishing features from venous ulcers. They are located primarily on the toes and pretibial area. Even small ulcers are very painful, especially at night. The lesions have a punched-out appearance with a gray to black base. Due to the decreased blood supply, the surrounding skin is cold and atrophic. Local treatment for arterial ulcers includes keeping the area clean and dressed. Healing is slow, and reconstructive vascular surgery often is needed.

One variant of this condition is the hypertensive ulcer. It predominantly affects women over age 50 years with essential hypertension.[39] This extremely painful ulcer usually is located on the lateral aspect of the lower leg. The initial lesion is a red plaque that becomes purpuric and ulcerates. Controlling the hypertension helps to promote healing.

Diabetic Ulceration

Diabetes mellitus has many pronounced effects on the vasculature. It can cause a microangiopathy of the arterioles, venules, and capillaries. The proliferation of endothelial cells and thickening of the basement membrane in the small vessels lead to a decreased lumen and blood flow. In addition, atherosclerosis of both large and medium-sized arteries is more common with diabetes.

With this diminished blood flow, the patients are prone to arterial ulcerations, frequently in the toes.[39] Since both large and small blood vessels are involved, healing is very difficult. Also, diabetics have a lower resistance to bacterial diseases and cutaneous infections can be a serious complication.

Elderly diabetics may develop a symmetric distal neuropathy and lose sensation in their feet. Because they are unaware of chronic friction, pressure, or trauma to their feet, ulcers may form. The ulcers are painless, penetrate deeply into the soft tissue, and are surrounded by hyperkeratotic skin.[40] To heal these lesions, the surrounding hyperkeratotic skin must be débrided, and any chronic rubbing or pressure to the area must be eliminated. Further ulcerations may be prevented by instructing these patients in proper foot care. They must never go barefoot, and they should avoid trauma to the feet and inspect their feet daily. Shoes must fit perfectly, and special orthotic shoes may be necessary to distribute weight evenly and prevent friction (see Chapter 18).

Nutritional Deficiences and Aging Skin

Many elderly people suffer from malnutrition. Often they live alone or on a fixed income and are unable to prepare or afford an adequate diet.[41] Also, they may suffer from chronic diseases that diminish the appetite. Therefore, they may develop protein and vitamin deficiencies. The skin, composed of rapidly proliferating tissue, is one of the first tissues affected by a nutritional deficiency.

With inadequate protein intake, the skin becomes fragile and heals slowly; the hair and nails become thin and brittle. Certain vitamin deficiencies lead to characteristic cutaneous changes. Vitamin A deficiency causes follicular hyperkeratosis and xerosis. Patients lacking vitamin B complex develop cheilitis and dermatitis (pellagra). A vitamin C deficiency leads to perifollicular hemorrhage with coiled hairs (scurvy).

Cosmetic Treatment of Aging Skin

Our society puts a strong emphasis on appearance. One of the hardest aspects of aging for people is the loss of physical attractiveness. When people maintain an attractive appearance throughout life, they have a better mental outlook and are perceived more favorably by others.

Cosmetic use in elderly women has been found to improve significantly their appearance and their perception of themselves. Elderly patients seeking advice on the use of cosmetics should not be discouraged.

Whether someone has severe sun-damaged skin or simple wrinkling and roughness, he or she may seek treatment for the reversal of these changes. Until recently, the only options for patients were various moisturizing creams with unfounded promises of healing properties or plastic surgery. Recently, a topical medication, tretinoin (all-*trans*-retinoic acid) has demonstrated efficacy in the improvement of sun-damaged skin. Decreased fine and coarse wrinkling, increased smoothness of skin, and even fading hyperpigmentation and lentigenes can be achieved by using 0.1% tretinoin cream daily.[42] This medication also has been effective for nodular elastosis.

For more severe damage, various procedures have been developed to repair the skin. Collagen injection may diminish the wrinkles of the forehead and nasolabial folds. Chemical peels and dermabrasion can remove superficial wrinkles and areas of hyperpigmentation from the face. Trichloroacetic acid is the safest method of inducing a chemical peel but does not penetrate deeply and therefore is the least effective; phenol has a more pronounced effect but has a risk of producing cardiac arrhythmias when applied. With dermabrasion, some people will develop hypertrophic scarring. If the major problem is sagging skin, a face-lift is the procedure of choice.

References

1. Fenske NA, Lober CW. Structural and functional changes of normal aging skin. *J Am Acad Dermatol* 1986;15:571–585.
2. Rook A, Dawber R. *Diseases of the Hair and Scalp.* Boston, Mass: Blackwell Scientific Publication Inc; 1982.
3. Kligman LH. Photoaging: manifestations, prevention and treatment. *Dermatol Clin* 1986;4:517–528.
4. Gilchrest BA. *Skin and Aging Processes.* Boca Raton, Fla: CRC Press Inc, 1984.
5. Ogawa CM. Degenerative skin disorders: toll of age and sun. *Geriatrics* 1975;30:65–69.
6. Shahrad P, Marks R. The wages of warmth: changes in erythema ab igne. *Br J Dermatol* 1977;97:179–186.
7. Sneddon IB. Winter ailments of skin. *Practitioner* 1968;201:886–891.
8. Hellgren L, Mobacken H. Nummular eczema: clinical and statistical data. *Acta Derm Venereol* 1969;49:189–196.
9. Schaffer B, Beerman H. Lichen simplex chronicus and its variants. *Arch Dermatol* 1951;64:340–351.
10. Lyell A. The itching patient: a review of the causes of pruritus. *Scott Med J* 1972;17:334–347.
11. Schoenfeld RJ, Schoenfeld FL. Angular cheilitis. *Cutis* 1977;19:213–216.
12. Young AW, Jr. Seborrhea in the geriatric patient: incidence, implication, management. *Geriatrics* 1969;24:144–150.
13. Farr PM, Shuster S. Treatment of seborrheic dermatitis with topical keotconazole. *Lancet* 1984;2:1271–1272.
14. Roenigk HH Jr, Maibach HI. *Psoriasis.* New York, NY: Marcel Dekker Inc; 1985.
15. Gross DA, Landau JW, Newcomer VD. Pityriasis rubra pilaris. *Arch Dermatol* 1969;99:710–716.
16. Fisher AA. *Contact Dermatitis,* 3rd ed. Philadelphia, Pa: Lea & Febiger; 1986.
17. Arndt KA, Jick H. Rates of cutaneous reactions to drugs: a report from the Boston Collaborative Drug Surveillance Program. *JAMA* 1976;235:918–923.
18. Lever WF. Pemphigus and pemphigoid. *J Am Acad Dermatol* 1979;1:2–31.
19. Alexander-Williams J. Pruritus ani. *Br Med J* 1983;287:159–160.
20. Barker LP, Gross P. Lichen sclerosus et atrophicus of the female genitalia. *Arch Dermatol* 1962;85:362–373.
21. Khezri AA, Dounis A, Dunn M. Balanitis xerotica obliterans. *Br J Urol* 1979;51:229–231.

22. Imperial R, Helwig EB. Angiokeratoma of the scrotum (Fordyce type). *J Urol* 1967;98:379–387.

23. Burgoon CF, Burgoon JS, Baldridge GD. The natural history of herpes zoster. *JAMA* 1957;164:265–269.

24. Balfour HH Jr, Bean B, Laskin OL, et al. Acyclovir halts progression of herpes zoster in immunocompromised patients. *N Engl J Med* 1983;308:1448–1453.

25. Walshe MM, English MP. fungi in nails. *Br J Dermatol* 1966;78:198–207.

26. Mehregan AH, Rahbari H. Benign epithelial tumors of the skin, I: epidermal tumors. *Cutis* 1977;19:43–48.

27. Mehregan AH, Rahbari H. Benign epithelial tumors of the skin, II: benign sebaceous tumors. *Cutis* 1977;19:317–320.

28. Bodian EL. Techniques of sclerotherapy for sunburst venous blemishes. *J Dermatol Surg Oncol* 1985;11:696–704.

29. Brownstein MH, Rabinowitz AD. The precursors of cutaneous squamous cell carcinoma. *Int J Dermatol* 1979;18:1–16.

30. Albright SD III. Treatment of skin cancer using multiple modalities. *J Am Acad Dermatol* 1982;7:143–171.

31. Schwartz RA. The keratoacanthoma: a review. *J Surg Oncol* 1979;12:305–317.

32. Clark WH Jr, Mihm MC Jr. Lentigo maligna and lentigo maligna melanoma. *Am J Pathol* 1969;55:39–67.

33. Rigel DS, Rogers GS, Friedman RJ. Prognosis of malignant melanoma. *Dermatol Clin* 1985;3:309–314.

34. Ashikari R, Park K, Huvos AG, et al. Paget's disease of the breast. *Cancer* 1970;26:680–685.

35. Lee SC, Roth LM, Ehrlich C, et al. Extramammary Paget's disease of the vulva: a clinicopathologic study of 13 cases. *Cancer* 1977;39:2540–2549.

36. Reynolds WA, Winkelmann RK, Soule EH. Kaposi's sarcoma: a clinicopathologic study with particular reference to its relationship to the reticuloendothelial system. *Medicine* 1965;44:419–443.

37. Mehregan AH, Usndek HE. Malignant angioendothelioma. *Arch Dermatol* 1976;112:1565–1567.

38. Reingold IM. Cutaneous metastases from internal carcinoma. *Cancer* 1966;19:162–168.

39. Leu HJ. Differential diagnosis of chronic leg ulcers. *Angiology* 1963;14:288–296.

40. Kelly PJ, Coventry MB. Neutropic ulcers of the feet: review of 47 cases. *JAMA* 1958;168:388–393.

41. Gambert SR, Gaunsing AR. Protein-calorie malnutrition in the elderly. *Am Geriatr Soc* 1980;28:272–275.

42. Weiss JS, Ellis CN, Headington JT, et al. Topical tretinoin improves photoaged skin: a double-blind, vehicle-controlled study *JAMA* 1988;259:527–532.

30

Ophthalmology

L. F. Rich

To an elderly person, vision is perhaps even more important than it is to a younger individual. As aging proceeds and the acuity of other senses becomes blunted, the need for adequate visual orientation increases. Yet, advancing years take their toll on the visual system; ocular disease, visual loss, and blindness itself are far more common in elderly persons. The incidence of potentially blinding eye diseases increases dramatically after the age of 40 years and astronomically after the age of 65 years. The need for frequent eye examinations increases proportionately.

The ocular system evolves throughout life, and certain aging changes are expected and are normal. The distinction between normal aging changes and disease states often is difficult. Nevertheless, the physician must recognize that significant visual loss is not necessarily a part of aging, and satisfactory vision may remain throughout an individual's life. An awareness of the subtle onset of many ophthalmic diseases may aid in recognizing, treating, and preventing visual disorders in a patient and help to maintain an elderly individual's contact with the environment.

In elderly persons, as with emaciated, younger individuals, the fat cushion behind the globe of the eye atrophies and produces a recession of the eye into its orbit. This may be exacerbated when the patient assumes a supine position. The skin of the eyelids becomes wrinkled, which in combination with atrophy of orbital fat, produces a deepening of the upper eyelid sulcus. The eyelids become lax and thinner, and they may droop. Upper eyelid skin folds may become so flaccid as to obstruct the superior or temporal visual fields.[1]

The lower eyelid loosens similarly and may actually fall away from the globe, in which case it is definitely abnormal. A more subtle change occurs when the inner puncta no longer lie against the globe, and tear drainage is impaired. In these cases, the tears spill over the eyelid margin onto the cheeks (epiphora), compelling the patient to wipe the lower eyelids frequently. If the patient wipes away tears with a laterally directed motion, a greater stretching of the eyelid occurs, and the puncta are pulled further away from the globe. Whenever eyelid laxity is encountered, the physician should encourage the patient to blot the tears medially toward the inner canthus to push the lower eyelid inward, thus preventing a worsening of the problem.

In some elderly individuals, the blink rate is diminished, particularly in conditions such as Parkinson's disease. Blinking serves two major purposes: (1) it distributes the tear film across the globe, providing nourishment to the ocular surface; and (2) it is a vital part of the pumping mechanism in tear drainage. Looseness of the eyelids, malposition of the puncta, alterations of blink frequency, or habits of excessive squeezing of the eyelids interfere with these functions and can lead to true disease states.

The most common abnormality of the tear film is a deficiency of the aqueous layer. Physiologically, a diminution of the aqueous component of tears occurs with advancing years. Postmenopausal females are particularly prone to this disorder, which implicates a role of hormonal changes in dryness of the eyes. In milder states, decreased tear production may merely dull the luster of the cornea, causing the commonly observed "loss of gleam" in the eye of an elderly person. In moderate dryness states, the patient may experience a burning sensation, a gritty feeling of the eyes, or a vague ocular discomfort. If dryness is the cause, the symptoms worsen the longer the eyes remain open and are typically more pronounced during the evening hours. In more severe cases, a true keratitis sicca results. Ocular dryness is generally managed by frequently applying artificial tears.

The conjunctiva, the thin membrane covering of the anterior portion of the globe (Fig. 30.1), loses its elasticity with age and becomes yellowed due to fat deposition. Large collections of fatty tissue and hyalinization of the conjunctiva in the interpalpebral fissure are more common in individuals who have lived or worked outdoors most of their lives. These are actinic changes and, when localized to the conjunctiva, are termed *pingueculae;* a pterygium is an overgrowth of conjunctivalike scar tissue beyond the corneoscleral junction (limbus) onto the cornea.

The cornea is the main refracting element of the eye, and changes in its structure influence visual function. Gerontoxon, or arcus senilis, is a peripheral corneal lipid deposition. In its earlier stages, this condition may be noted on examination only when magnification is used. Typically, it is more pronounced superiorly and inferiorly and progresses to a complete ring years later. There is a characteristically clear zone of cor-

nea, known as the lucid interval, between the lipid deposition and the limbus.[2] The condition is bilateral and symmetric, except when there is a severe, unilateral carotid vascular disease, in which case there is a less prominent arcus senilis on the side with the more compromised blood flow. An obvious arcus should be considered abnormal in an individual younger than 35 years of age and should lead the physician to evaluate the patient's serum triglyceride and cholesterol levels.[2] Arcus senilis can be confused with more severe disorders, such as peripheral corneal thinning and certain ulcerative states; however, these are often accompanied by pain or changes in vision.

The corneal endothelium, the innermost monolayer of corneal cells, is most responsible for the maintenance of corneal clarity. Normally, the population density of this cell layer diminishes with age,[3] but if trauma occurs, additional endothelial cells die, and the cornea may eventually decompensate and lose transparency.

The sclera often becomes the repository for various fats and pigments. These depositions can produce yellowish or grayish discoloration of the globe. If the deposition is not uniform, a mottled appearance may result.[1] This must be differentiated from scleral thinning, which is an abnormal condition not associated with aging that gives the globe a characteristically blue tinge. Typically, the rigidity of the sclera increases with age, producing a profound impact on the measurement of intraocular pressure.[3,4]

Pressure inside the eye must exceed that of the

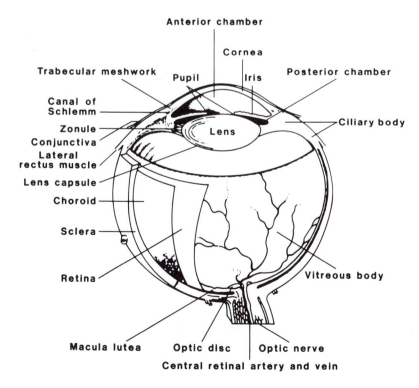

Fig. 30.1. Internal structures of normal human eye. Nasal aspect of eye is on reader's right.

atmosphere to prevent collapse of the globe. Normal values of intraocular pressure are between 10 and 22 mm Hg, but variations (1 to 2 mm Hg) occur with heartbeats and respirations. Wider swings (2 to 4 mm Hg) occur as diurnal variations.[4]

Intraocular pressure is determined by the rate of aqueous humor formation in the ciliary body and by aqueous humor outflow, which occurs primarily through the trabecular meshwork into the canal of Schlemm (Fig. 30.1). With increasing age, the rate of aqueous humor formation decreases slightly, but the resistance to outflow of fluid from the eye increases. Thus, intraocular pressure rises slightly with advancing age but as a general rule is remarkably stable.[5]

The depth of the anterior chamber diminishes with age as the lens increases in thickness.[6] Increasing lens thickness does not cause an elevation in intraocular pressure unless the lens has changed rapidly and dramatically, displacing the iris against the trabecular meshwork. Similarly, a tumor inside the eyes does not grow fast enough to increase intraocular pressure unless it directly invades the aqueous outflow pathways. A sudden hemorrhage into the eye or into a tumor may alter the pressure.

The lens of the eye is a unique structure with regard to aging. In embryonic life, the lens placode invaginates from the surface ectoderm to form the lens vesicle in which the apexes of the cells point inward, and their bases are externalized. Unlike other cells of ectodermal origin, such as hair and nail cells, lens fibers derived from these epithelial cells cannot be sloughed off because of this unique orientation.[3] Rather, they are compacted centrally as the lens continues to grow throughout life with successive annulation of new lens fibers. A dense nucleus of older fibers surrounded by a cortical layer of new fibers results.

Although it is living, the lens is avascular; its nourishment is derived from the surrounding aqueous humor. Transient changes in a person's health may alter the clarity of growing lens fibers. In this way, isolated opacities result, and if the cataractogenic effect subsides, transparent lens fibers will subsequently be laid down, with the opaque "island" becoming a permanent record of the disturbance.

The density of the lens nucleus increases with age due to a loss of water, compression of older fibers, and a conversion of lower weight crystalline proteins into higher weight, insoluble albuminoid proteins. This results in a higher lens weight and decreased transparency with increased age.

The lens and its capsule, although not composed of elastin, are in fact elastic; this allows the lens to change shape when accommodating for near vision.

With advancing age, the lens becomes less elastic due to an increased density of its nucleus and cortex and a diminished elasticity of the capsule. When the ciliary body muscle contracts in an older individual, the lens is less able to increase convexity, and powers of accommodation are subsequently diminished. Thus, the amplitude of accommodation, which is the amount that the eye can alter its refraction, slowly decreases until it is essentially nil in late middle age (Fig. 30.2).[7] As a person ages, the nearest point to which that person can focus gradually recedes. If clear vision is to be maintained, converging lenses in the form of reading eyeglasses or bifocals are necessary. This is the result of normal aging changes that slowly but invariably occur in every human; the condition is called presbyopia.

The uvea comprises three structures: the iris, ciliary body, and choroid (Fig. 30.1). The iris controls the size of the pupillary aperture, the average diameter of which gradually increases up to the 15th year of age but decreases thereafter until the minimal average pupillary diameter is reached in the sixth decade.[1] The aged iris thins and rigidifies,[6] the stroma atrophies, and the posterior pigment layer degenerates with advancing age.

The ciliary body, which has both secretory and muscular functions, thickens gradually with age due to connective tissue accumulation.[8] The epithelial cells of the ciliary process, which are responsible for secreting aqueous humor, become attenuated with age, and the production of aqueous humor concomitantly diminishes.[3,5]

The choroid is the most posterior portion of the uveal system. Its principal functions are to nourish the outer retina while providing a pathway for vessels that supply the anterior portion of the eye. Bruch's membrane, which is the innermost elastic layer of the choroid lying directly beneath the retina, exhibits the most dramatic changes of all choroidal tissues. Beginning in young adult life, accumulations of granular and

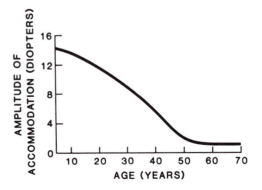

Fig. 30.2. Amplitude of accommodation vs age.

filamentous material are found on Bruch's membrane. These changes are more prominent in the macula and near the optic nerve and may lead to drusen, which are collections of amorphous granular material between Bruch's membrane and the retina (Fig. 30.3).[3]*

The vitreous humor is a semisolid gel that supports the retina and fills the posterior cavity of the eye. The solid components of the vitreous humor undergo gradual shrinkage with age, leaving the posterior portion of the vitreous cavity filled with liquid vitreous humor. This frequently results in a separation of the solid vitreous humor from the macular and/or optic disc, which is called a *posterior vitreous detachment*. Visual symptoms, such as seeing flashes of light, may follow, particularly during movements, and these must be distinguished from early retinal detachments.[9] The distinction, therefore, between a "normal" vitreous detachment (a more physiologic process) and a retinal detachment (a clearly pathologic process) is not always clear from symptoms alone.

Aging changes in the retina are more likely to be seen as functional aberrations than as gross anatomic alterations. Anatomic changes do occur nevertheless. Loss of the normal pigment xanthophyll in the macular area accompanies a reduction of central acuity to the 20/25 level in the eighth decade.[9] Earlier, there is a loss of the foveal light reflex on examination by ophthalmoscopy. A significant percentage of the adult population will exhibit senile, peripheral retinal degenerations, which seldom impair visual function or progress to actual retinal detachment.

As a rule, retinal arterioles develop sclerotic changes with aging, which are manifest on ophthalmoscopy, both as a narrowing of the visible blood column and an increased visibility of the arteriolar wall light reflex (Figs. 30.4 and 30.5). Unless the underlying venous column is compressed, these changes are not necessarily pathologic and are more indicative of advanced age.[9]

"Dark adaptation," the increase in the ability to see light that occurs after being in the dark for a few minutes, occurs more slowly in higher age groups. Furthermore, the visually evoked potential, which involves cortical activity, changes significantly with older age groups. This suggests a significant increase in the time needed by these subjects for cognitive processing.[10] Color perception may be altered with advancing age by a variety of mechanisms. As the lens becomes more yellow with age, short wavelength light is filtered, producing a greater difficulty in detecting violet and blue light, which is compounded by alterations in macular pigmentation.[1]

---

* Figures 30.3 to 30.8 appear in the four-color insert.

Pathologic Conditions in the Aged Eye

Visual Loss in Elderly Persons—Magnitude of the Problem

Visual impairment and blindness produce a tremendous impact on our society, both socially and economically. In the general population, nearly 11.5 million persons in the United States—1 of every 19—have some degree of visual impairment. Nearly 500,000 Americans, a prevalence of 225 of every 100,000 persons, are legally blind.[11] Legal blindness includes persons whose corrected visual acuity in the better eye is 20/200 or poorer, or is restricted to less than 20° in its widest diameter. The cost of professional care, including hospitalization, surgery, office visits and professional treatments, rehabilitation benefits, and support for visually handicapped persons, exceeds $5 billion each year in this nation alone.[11]

Statistics on the prevalence of blindness have a particular significance for the geriatrician. Over 50% of all blind persons in the United States are 65 years of age or older. The prevalence of blindness rises sharply with age to 3,000 of every 100,000 persons 85 years of age or older. For those persons 65 years of age or older, the leading causes of blindness are glaucoma, macular degeneration, senile cataracts, and diabetic retinopathy. New cases of legal blindness in the elderly age group are primarily due to macular degeneration.[11]

Visually impaired persons are those who have some trouble seeing with one or both eyes even when they are wearing eyeglasses or corrective lenses, but they do not fit the definition of legal blindness. Of the more than 11 million Americans in this category, 43% are 65 years of age or older. Cataracts and glaucoma are the leading causes of new cases of visual impairment.[11]

Glaucoma

Glaucoma is a progressive eye disease, resulting from excessive pressure within the eye. It is the leading cause of blindness in the United States for persons of all ages. Over 2 million Americans (approximately 2% of the population) have glaucoma; 3% of persons older than 65 years of age have this disease.[11]

Glaucoma causes visual loss by damaging the optic nerve and the retinal nerve cells due to excessive pressure within the eye. Frequently, there are no symptoms, so glaucoma escapes detection unless regular eye examinations and pressure measurements are performed. Chronically elevated intraocular pressure first destroys the peripheral retinal nerve fibers; therefore, the initial symptoms might be decreased side vision or an inability to see in the dark. Central vision is typically spared until the end stage of the disease. Although glaucoma-induced visual loss cannot be restored, treatment can generally prevent a progression of the disease and, in some cases, may permanently eliminate the excessive pressure.

The diagnosis of glaucoma is based on three characteristic clinical findings: (1) increased intraocular pressure, (2) atrophy and cupping of the optic nerve head (Fig. 30.6) and (3) visual field defects. Elevations of intraocular pressure alone, without the accompanying changes in the nerve head or visual field, may not mandate treatment although they require close observation. In "low-tension glaucoma," the intraocular pressure is not elevated, but the optic disc nevertheless undergoes gliosis, which is characteristic of glaucoma. In these rare cases, even intraocular pressures in the "normal" range lead to optic disc and nerve damage. Thus, the ophthalmologist does not treat intraocular pressure as an isolated phenomenon but aims to prevent optic nerve injury.

Clinically, glaucoma behaves as a pressure-induced, chronic optic neuropathy. Glaucoma is classified as an open-angle or angle-closure type. Of all glaucomas, 95% are the open-angle variety, with angle-closure glaucoma accounting for most of the remainder (congenital glaucoma accounts for less than 1% of all cases). The cause(s) of primary open-angle glaucoma have not been identified, although the trabecular meshwork is known to be the site of the blockage. In open-angle glaucoma, the aqueous humor has free access from the ciliary body (where it is formed) through the posterior chamber, the pupil, into the anterior chamber, and to the trabecular meshwork (Fig. 30.1).[12] Angle-closure glaucoma, on the other hand, involves anatomic, intermittent obstruction of the trabecular meshwork region by the root of the iris. This occurs in individuals who have an anatomically shallow anterior chamber. When the pupil becomes partially dilated in people with this condition, the aqueous humor flow through the pupil becomes relatively blocked (relative pupillary block). This causes the pressure to rise in the posterior chamber, driving the iris against the cornea, closing the angle, and blocking aqueous humor outflow. These individuals typically have sudden elevations of intraocular pressure when the pupil is dilated, such as with emotional stress, or when mydriatic eye drops are given. Rapid, marked elevations of intraocular pressure result; the patient will experience acute pain, a clouding of vision, and (not uncommonly) headache and nausea.

It is important to realize that the vast majority of glaucomas, the open-angle variety, do not produce acute elevations of intraocular pressure with pain. Therefore, patients are not aware of their condition, and the disease can be detected only if frequent ocular examinations are performed.

Once a diagnosis of glaucoma has been made, therapy is aimed at the underlying pathophysiologic condition. In the vast majority of cases, this involves the use of topical pharmaceutical agents.

There are several classes of drugs used in the treatment of glaucoma.[13] Miotics, such as pilocarpine and carbachol, constrict the pupil and stimulate the longitudinal muscle fibers of the ciliary body, thus opening the trabecular meshwork pores. Miotics, therefore, decrease resistance to the outflow of aqueous humor and, in the case of angle-closure glaucoma, prevent the iris root from mechanically blocking the trabecular meshwork. There are a variety of parasympathomimetic drugs that are useful for this purpose, and they usually must be taken for the remainder of a person's life. They have undesirable side effects, such as altered visual acuity due to induced myopia, headaches on initiating treatment, and dimming of vision from the smaller pupil. Longer-acting parasympathomimetic drugs, such as the anticholinesterases, cause less fluctuation in vision after eye drops are used. However, they have the disadvantage of being highly toxic if accidentally taken internally.[14]

Another approach to controlling intraocular pressure with drugs is to diminish inflow, ie, lower the rate of aqueous humor production.[13] Levoepinephrine, in 1% or 2% concentrations, diminishes intraocular pressure when applied as topical eye drops primarily by decreasing aqueous humor production through its vasoactive effects. Its side effects include eye pain, headaches, and conjunctival redness. Adrenochrome deposits may occur in the cornea and conjunctiva with prolonged use. β-Adrenergic blocking agents, such as timolol maleate, have been proved to be safe and effective in lowering intraocular pressure by decreasing aqueous humor formation when applied topically.[14] These drugs do not cause miosis and must be instilled only twice daily in the affected eye. As with systemically administered β-blockers, these drugs are to be avoided or used cautiously in individuals with a history of asthma, bradycardia, or congestive heart failure.

Systemic medications are used when topical medications alone are ineffective or contraindicated. Carbonic anhydrase inhibitors lower the production of aqueous humor by interfering with the enzymatic equilibrium between carbonic acid and carbon dioxide. They are effective agents for reducing intraocular pressure, but side effects, such as paresthesias, anorexia, drowsiness, renal lithiasis, and blood dyscrasias, are not uncommon, and confusion or depression may occur in elderly patients.[13]

Agents that increase serum osmolality withdraw fluid from the eye and lower intraocular pressure. This phenomenon occurs in diabetic hyperosmolar states. Osmotically active agents may be used to decrease intraocular pressure and volume for a short period of time, eg, to break an attack of angle-closure glaucoma, or before some forms of intraocular surgery when a lower pressure is desired. The osmotic agents most commonly used are glycerol and isosorbide, which may be given orally. Mannitol, the alcohol of the sugar mannose, must be given intravenously as a 20% solution.[14]

Surgical therapy for glaucoma is indicated when pharmacologic agents alone are insufficient in maintaining intraocular pressure at normal levels, or if there is a progression of glaucomatous field loss or optic nerve damage with maximal medical therapy. For patients who exhibit poor compliance in the use of their medications (as often occurs in confused, elderly individuals), surgery may also become necessary.

Conventional glaucoma surgical procedures are designed to produce a fistula between the anterior chamber and the subconjunctival space, forming an alternative pathway for the aqueous humor to exit from the eye.[12] Successful maintenance of this opening is the limiting factor. A significant number of patients will scar the opening closed, rendering them glaucomatous once again.

In some cases, the ophthalmologist may be able to control intraocular pressure in many patients with glaucoma by using laser treatment on the trabecular meshwork, termed *laser trabeculoplasty*. This procedure is much less complicated for the patient, because it does not require hospitialization.

Macular Degeneration

The macula is the central portion of the retina that surrounds the fovea centralis and is the area necessary for clear central vision. It is located between the upper and lower temporal arcade of the vessels and extends temporally from the optic disc approximately 2 disc diameters. The photoreceptor population is markedly skewed in this region with a high concentration of cones, necessary for color vision, and very few rods, making this the area responsible for high-resolution visual acuity.[3] A small lesion that would not affect vision, if located peripherally, may lead to a severe loss of visual acuity when present in the macula.

Anatomically, retinal vessels diminish in caliber as the fovea centralis is approached. Nourishment for the macula is derived principally from the underlying

choroidal vasculature.[3] This is at least partially responsible for the unique involvement of the central retina in a variety of degeneration conditions termed *macular degeneration.*

In general, degenerations of the macula are easily seen with an ophthalmoscope (Fig. 30.7). However, the ophthalmoscopic appearance cannot be correlated with the level of visual acuity, for many conditions in this area that destroy vision are microscopic. In recent years, a great deal has been learned about the causes of senile macular degeneration by using fluorescein angiography. This technique permits an evaluation of the retinal and choroidal vasculature, including areas of vessel leakage, regions of hypovascularization, and abnormalities of the pigment epithelium or Bruch's membrane.

Several therapeutic modalities are now available for treating macular degeneration. For example, some forms of macular degeneration can be improved with laser photocoagulation, and certain inflammatory conditions of the macula and central retina can be treated pharmacologically.[15,16] Patients in whom laser and medical therapy is of no value may derive useful vision from low-vision aids.

Macular degeneration is the second leading cause of blindness; the majority of patients who experience this degeneration are 65 years of age or older.[11] Unlike glaucoma, the symptoms of macular degeneration are readily noticeable to patients as a loss of central acuity. With the continuing aging of the population, the proportion of blindness due to this disorder likely will increase in the future.

Cataracts

The term cataract is misunderstood by many people, including some physicians. Any opacity of the lens, whether it interferes with vision or not, is a cataract by definition. In the United States, 50% of the population older than 40 years of age has some form of a cataract, but cataracts are responsible for only 1 of every 12 cases of legal blindness.[11] The most common type of cataract is a senile cataract, which typically progresses slowly (Fig. 30.8). Cataracts can occur in conjunction with other medical disorders or can result from physical, chemical, or radiation injury. Many diseases, such as diabetes mellitus, hasten the development of cataracts. Some forms of cataracts are iatrogenic; corticosteroid-induced lens changes are the most notorious.

There is no effective nonsurgical treatment of cataracts at this time. Certain types of cataracts can be prevented, or their progression can be arrested; however, existing cataracts do not regress. Those due to galactosemia, diabetes mellitus, hypoparathyroidism, or the ingestion of toxic drugs can be prevented, or their progression can be halted or slowed by controlling the underlying disease.

Some patients with cataracts will see better when the pupil is dilated. Vision will not return to normal with mydriatic eye drops, but their use may permit the postponement of cataract extraction or allow the patient to function at a more normal level until surgery is indicated.

With modern microsurgical techniques, removal of cataracts is highly successful. Indeed, cataract extraction is one of the most commonly performed surgical procedures in the United States; over 330,000 cases are performed each year, with the vast majority being done for elderly individuals.[11] Although 75% of all persons older than 60 years of age probably have cataracts, only 15% will experience a significant visual loss, and fewer than 15% will need surgery.[11]

Cataract surgery offers improvement of vision in 95% of cases. A common misconception, perhaps arising from surgical techniques of the past, is that a cataract must be "ripe" before it can be removed. At present, the decision to operate depends more on the degree to which the cataract influences the patient's life-style; some patients may require a lens extraction with a visual acuity of 20/60, whereas others may not need surgery until visual acuity is 20/200 or less.

Visual loss due to cataracts is caused by the opacification of the lens, which interferes with the transmission of light through the eye on its way to the retina. However, the lens contributes refractive power to the eye, and when the opacified lens is removed, the refractive error must be corrected by artificial means. At present, there are four ways of correcting aphakia (the postoperative condition of an eye with its lens removed): spectacles (eyeglasses), contact lenses, intraocular lenses, and refractive corneal surgery. Each has its own indications and complications. For example, if a cataract has been present and is removed from only one eye (producing monocular aphakia), eyeglasses cannot be used, because the severe magnification that is induced results in a marked disparity in the size of the image presented to the refractively corrected aphakic eye compared with that entering the uninvolved phakic eye. Only by placing the refractive correction onto or into the eye is this induced magnification minimized, thus permitting cerebral fusion of the images. Even when cataracts have been removed from both eyes, a refractive correction with aphakic spectacles is abnormal. Not only is magnification induced, making objects appear closer than they really are, but distortion also results. Straight lines, such as doorways and walls, appear to be bowed. This produces the so-called pincushion effect. Furthermore, a midperipheral ring-shaped visual field defect is pro-

duced by these spectacles, and objects moving from the peripheral visual field into the magnified central field appear to jump or dart into view: the "jack-in-the-box" phenomenon. Because of the characteristics of aphakic spectacles, patients corrected in this manner have difficulty adjusting to their eyeglasses, particularly when they are walking or moving about. In elderly people, who may be less adaptable than younger individuals, this adjustment period is trying.

Many of the problems in the correction of aphakia are minimized or eliminated by contact lenses. By placing the optical correction closer to the eye, the magnification is far less than it would be with the same correction via eye glasses. Whereas an aphakic spectacle lens magnifies as much as 20% to 30%, a contact lens at the same diopter power magnifies only 7% or 8%. Furthermore, there is little or no distortion or visual field limitation induced by aphakic contact lenses. Contact lenses do have their drawbacks, however; they often are irritating to the eyes, and many patients are only able to wear them for a portion of the day. Spectacles, then, must be used as a supplement if functional vision is to be enjoyed for the entire day. Many elderly persons experience difficulty in handling contact lenses, particularly when they are aphakic and cannot see the tiny devices with their uncorrected vision. The need for such handling is decreased with soft contact lenses for continuous (extended) wear, which the patient may leave on the eye for weeks or months. These patients must return to the ophthalmologist's office at regular intervals for skilled removal, cleaning, and replacement of the lens on the eye. The use of extended-wear soft contact lenses is more risky than daily wear. Blood vessels may invade the normally avascular cornea, and abrasions or infected ulcers may develop. Furthermore, extended-wear contact lenses are not indicated in patients with extremely dry eyes, severe glaucoma, or greater than moderate levels of corneal astigmatism.

A rapidly changing and increasingly accepted mode of aphakic correction is the use of intraocular lenses (pseudophakos). The theoretical advantages of intraocular lenses are enormous. The refractive correction is placed at or near the physiologic lens plane inside the eye, and magnification from refractive correction following cataract extraction is negligible. Patients also experience a recovery of vision almost immediately after surgery, although most patients require some form of minor adjustment in the form of eyeglasses. This type of aphakic correction produces a more natural type of vision than contact lenses or aphakic spectacles. An intraocular lens is inadvisable in certain situations: high myopia, glaucoma, corneal endothelial dystrophies, diabetic retinopathy, or retinal detachment.

New methods of correcting aphakia, collectively termed *refractive keratoplasty,* are being studied in many medical centers throughout the world. With these techniques, the corneal contour is surgically altered to correct the refractive error in aphakia. To date, the use of these procedures is limited and is most widely used for those patients in whom the other three modalities are contraindicated or unsuccessful.[17]

Diabetic Retinopathy

A threat to every person with diabetes mellitus is the possibility of developing diabetic retinopathy. This disease affects the blood vessels of the eye and accounts for 1 of every 15 cases of blindness in the United States. Diabetic retinopathy ranks third, behind glaucoma and macular degeneration, as a cause of new cases of blindness.[11] Those persons who are most at risk for developing diabetic retinopathy are patients who have had diabetes for over 10 years.

Visual loss due to diabetic retinopathy is often related initially to vascular changes in and around the macula. Microaneurysms lead to hemorrhages and exudates, and related vascular abnormalities may produce a leakage of serous fluid or blood.[8] When one or more of these phenomena occur in the macular area, visual acuity deteriorates. With fluorescein angiography and laser photocoagulation, these areas often can be detected and treated, which restores the vision.[15] In advanced cases of diabetic retinopathy, neovascularization occurs in, over, or beneath the retina and is called *proliferative retinopathy.* This also is treatable with photocoagulation therapy. For reasons that are incompletely understood, panretinal photocoagulation (in which the chorioretinal layers anterior to the equator of the eye are ablated by photocoagulation) often preserves the central vision as proliferative neovascularization involutes postsurgically.

Corneal Disease

The cornea, like the lens and vitreous humor, must remain transparent if light is to reach the retina. Corneal disorders cause visual loss less frequently than the previously mentioned ocular diseases, but are often correctable with therapy.

Herpetic keratitis is the most common cause of cornea-induced blindness in this nation.[11] Repeated bouts of infection with herpesvirus may lead to opacification of the cornea with subsequent visual loss. Several pharmacologic and surgical means of treating herpes simplex keratitis are now available. Antiviral drugs shorten the course of herpes keratitis but do not prevent recurrences.

Disorders of the corneal endothelium are not uncommon causes of corneal-induced blindness in elderly persons. Progressive, primary endothelial cell loss (Fuchs' corneal dystrophy) and endothelial damage following cataract surgery may lead to corneal edema and blisters of the corneal epithelium. These blisters, or vesicles, may coalesce and form bullae that rupture and expose bare nerve endings, which produces severe pain. This pain may be intermittent in its early stages, but it eventually becomes chronic. The patient may become withdrawn due to pain and photophobia.

Corneal scars and edematous or damaged corneas can, in many cases, be treated successfully with corneal transplantation. Visual acuity is often restored to near-normal levels when a clear graft is obtained and an optical correction is prescribed.

Healing of corneal grafts is a very slow process, since the cornea is avascular and cells must migrate relatively long distances into the area of the wound. Following corneal transplantation, 6 to 12 months of healing must transpire before functional vision can be obtained with eyeglasses or contact lenses. Yet, corneal transplantations are performed in individuals in the 8th, 9th, or even 10th decade of life, with subsequent improvement in the quality of life. Corneal transplant surgery is presently no more stressful for an individual than the removal of cataracts. Long periods of bed rest and hospitalization are not necessary, and excellent general health is not a prerequisite to corneal surgery.

Ocular Infections

The use of antimicrobial drugs in eye infections is guided by the physician's general knowledge. An awareness of ocular microbiology is helpful and sometimes essential, because certain microorganisms invade ocular tissues preferentially; selected eye structures may be more prone to infection with a specific microorganism. For example, by virtue of its avascularity, the cornea is an immunologically unique structure.

Obviously, the first requirement of treating ocular infection is to diagnose the cause. Although an external ocular infection produces a redness of the eye, there may be other causes for this symptom (such as acute glaucoma, iritis, etc). Second, the selection of an appropriate antimicrobial agent depends on a correct identification of the offending organism and a knowledge of those drugs to which it is sensitive. Finally, the toxic effect of drugs is particularly important in ophthalmology, because many highly effective antimicrobial agents cannot be used topically due to their ocular side effects.

Topical antibiotics are used prophylactically before surgery more frequently in ophthalmology than in other surgical specialities. The rationale is that sterilization of the eye preoperatively is highly desirable; a minute inoculum of bacteria that might not cause an infection in a skin incision may produce devastating consequences when present in the eye.

Antiviral drugs are effective in decreasing the duration of herpes simplex keratitis, and they offer prophylaxis against reactivation of viral disease when topical corticosteroids are used for ocular inflammation. They are not without their complications, however, and a thorough knowledge of their side effects and contraindications is essential before use.[18]

Antifungal drugs often are extremely toxic to ocular tissues. Treatment of intraocular fungal infections is often disappointing, for the drugs are so toxic that the concentrations necessary to inhibit the microorganism frequently destroy ocular tissues. Newer antifungal agents, such as natamycin (pimaracin), flucytosine, and ketoconazole, show promise by virtue of their safer therapeutic indexes.

Ocular Inflammation

A variety of anti-inflammatory agents are useful in treating ocular disease or trauma. The site of inflammation, as well as the underlying cause, must be kept in mind when using such drugs. For example, inflammations of the eyelids or ocular surface are best treated with agents that penetrate the globe poorly. This minimizes the intraocular side effects and concentrates the drug where it is most needed. With infectious processes, it is always best first to attack the microorganism and use anti-inflammatory agents only when the infection is controlled and/or the inflammatory process itself is a threat to sight. The use of corticosteroids in ocular reactions should be limited to those situations in which the inflammation is severe enough to threaten a permanent structural change. Mild intraocular inflammation may require corticosteroid therapy, whereas moderately severe external inflammations may not require such treatment. Corticosteroids are the most frequently used ocular anti-inflammatory agents. There are multiple corticosteroid preparations available for ophthalmic use, and the physician must select an agent or mode of therapy appropriate to the condition. The patient's general health status influences this selection process.[14]

Corticosteroids may be given topically in the form of eye drops or ointments, as a periocular injection, or systemically. Systemic side effects are not usually produced by topical corticosteroids, even if use is prolonged. Periocular injections of steroids are reserved for severe inflammatory processes in which systemic administration is contraindicated, or when maximal intraocular concentration is required and topical or systemic administrations are insufficient. These injections are useful for concentrating the drug in a given area of the ocular system.[14] They may be given in soluble forms, in which case they are present for a short time, or in the depot variety, which prolongs their action.

The major contraindication to the use of corticosteroids is a lack of a specific indication for their need; these drugs should never be given as a placebo or as "shotgun" therapy. Just as systemic corticosteroids reduce the resistance of the body to infection, the same effect is noted locally in the eye with topical administration.

Glaucoma may be induced by topical, periocular, or systemic corticosteroid use, particularly after prolonged treatment. A glaucomatous response to corticosteroid use is hereditarily determined and found in one third of the population.[14]

The degree of intraocular pressure elevation following corticosteroid use depends on the potency of the steroid and the frequency and duration of its use. Researchers have sought to separate the anti-inflammatory activity from the pressure-elevating properties of corticosteroids. Fluorometholone allegedly retains both anti-inflammatory potency and significant intraocular penetration, but it is said not to elevate intraocular pressure as the most potent agents do.[14]

Anticholinergic preparations are of value in the treatment of anterior uveitis (iritis). Atropine is an effective drug that acts to reduce the pain of iritis, helps to prevent adhesions of the iris to adjacent structures, and reduces the permeability of inflamed vessels, which decreases exudation of protein and inflammatory cells.[14] The duration of action of atropine may be as long as 14 days. Other anticholinergic preparations with shorter action have been developed for topical use. All anticholinergic drugs produce a paresis of accommodation, dilate the pupil, and can have systemic side effects, such as dryness of the mouth, fever, delirium, and tachycardia.

Drugs that interfere with prostaglandins have great theoretic implications in ophthalmic use. Their anti-inflammatory activity in the treatment of ocular disease is being investigated. The role of prostaglandins in glaucoma therapy has yet to be established.[13]

Adnexal Problems

If the eyelid falls away from the globe so that the eye is incompletely covered, tear distribution is compromised, and localized dryness may occur. In some cases, excessive reflex tearing from chronic exposure develops. In other cases, dryness leads to keratinization of the ocular surface. Laxity of the lower eyelid that produces malposition is termed *ectropion* and is usually correctable by surgery.

Senile entropion is a condition in which the eyelid margin is turned inward onto the globe and the eyelashes irritate the eye. The spastic variety of senile entropion is caused by an overaction of the orbicularis oculi muscle that is associated with weakness of its antagonists. This allows the eyelid to turn inward. The atonic type of entropion is associated with a loss of tone of several eyelid muscles and may occur alone or in combination with the spastic variety. Entropion is frequently intermittent in its early stages. Asking a patient to squeeze the eyelids forcibly may reveal the tendency toward infolding. Temporary relief of the condition may be accomplished by taping the lower eyelid, but a permanent cure requires surgical intervention.

Incomplete eyelid closure may also result from a senile laxity of the eyelids. Thyroid disorders or seventh cranial nerve malfunction may cause or complicate the situation. If the underlying cause is temporary, the eye may be maintained on artificial teardrops and ointment lubricants, combined with taping the eyelids shut until the underlying cause is corrected. In more permanent disorders, such as endocrine exophthalmos, a partial or total surgical closure of the eyelids (tarsorrhaphy) may be necessary.

An annoying problem to many elderly individuals is epiphora, which is an excessive tearing of the eye that spills over the eyelid margin onto the cheeks. This may be caused, paradoxically, by ocular dryness. In this situation, the baseline secretion of tears is inadequate, dry spots develop on the cornea producing an irritation, and reflex tearing occurs in copious amounts. Treatment in this situation is aimed at tear supplementation to prevent the development of dry spots.

Adequate tear drainage is prevented, and epiphora results if the tear drainage system is blocked either through (1) a closure or malposition of the lacrimal puncta of the inner canthus or (2) an obstruction of the lacrimal canaliculi or lacrimal duct system.[12] These conditions are usually treated by surgical means, but they may be effectively managed with minor manipulations of the lacrimal drainage system, such as probing or dilation of the lacrimal passages.

Neurosensory Blindness

Ischemia or atrophy of the optic nerve accounts for approximately 5% of the cases of blindness in people older than 65 years of age.[11] Ischemia of the optic nerve may produce a slight edema of the disc that is associated with an altitudinal (superior) field defect.

Temporal (giant cell) arteritis (see Chapter 16) may lead to a sudden visual loss through optic nerve ischemia. An immediate diagnosis is urgent and must not await the results of laboratory tests. Treatment should begin as soon as possible with high doses of systemic corticosteroids if vision is to be preserved.

Other forms of optic nerve disease, such as optic neuritis, may be idiopathic and associated with multiple sclerosis or lead poisoning. Intracranial mass lesions or vasculitides other than temporal arteritis may cause neurologic deficits, including optic atrophy.

Low-Vision Aids

Patients with subnormal vision and many legally blind individuals may be helped with telescopic lenses, magnifiers, or specially devised optical and electronic devices that are now available.[19] Although the number of patients who can learn to use these devices may be small, a low-vision aid evaluation is often worthwhile. Older patients, who may be less adaptable than younger individuals, frequently find that they are able to use nothing more than simple magnifying lenses. A patient should have reasonable expectations, an understanding of the underlying condition, and a high degree of motivation for success with low-vision aids. Low-vision aids merely allow patients to maximize the use of their remaining vision.

Physicians should reassure macular degeneration patients that although central vision is lost, their condition will not lead to total blindness, and that they may be able to experience a better life if they can learn to use one of these aids. Hence, it is important for the geriatrician to understand the distinctions between, as well as the causes of, visual impairment, legal blindness, and total blindness.

References

1. Weale RA. *The Aging Eye.* London, England: Bartholomew Press for Harper & Row Publishers Inc; 1963.
2. Grayson M. *Diseases of the Cornea.* St Louis, Mo: CV Mosby Co; 1979.
3. Hogan MJ, Alvarado JA, Weddell JE. *Histology of the Human Eye: An Atlas and Textbook.* Philadelphia, Pa: WB Saunders CO; 1971.
4. Moses RA. *Adler's Physiology of the Eye: Clinical Applications.* 5th ed. St Louis, Mo: CV Mosby Co; 1980.
5. Brubaker RF, Nagataki S, Townsend DJ, et al. The effect of age on aqueous humor formation in man. *Ophthalmology* 1981;88(suppl 3):238–288.
6. Berens C. Aging changes in the eye and adnexa. *Arch Ophthalmol* 1943;29:171–209.

7. Duane A. Subnormal accommodation. *Arch Ophthalmol* 1925;54:568.

8. Hogan M, Zimmerman L. *Ophthalmic Pathology: An Atlas and Textbook*. 2nd ed. Philadelphia, Pa: WB Saunders Co; 1962.

9. Keeney AH, Keeney VT. A guide to examining the aging eye. *Geriatrics* 1980;35:81–91.

10. Beck EC, Swanson C, Dustman RE. Long latency components of the visually evoked potential in man: effects of aging. *Exp Aging Res* 1980;6(suppl 6):523–545.

11. National Society to Prevent Blindness. *Vision Problems in the United States: A Statistical Analysis*. New York, NY: National Society to Prevent Blindness; 1980.

12. Newell FW. *Ophthalmology: Principles and Concepts*. 4th ed. St Louis, Mo: CV Mosby Co; 1978.

13. Samples RJ. Pharmacologic management of glaucoma. *Ration Drug Ther* 1987;21:1–7.

14. Lamberts DW, Potter DE, eds. *Clinical Ophthalmic Pharmacology*. Boston, Mass: Little Brown & Co Inc; 1987.

15. Bressler NM, Bressler SB, Fine SL. Age-related macular degeneration. *Surv Ophthalmol* 1988;32:375–413.

16. Yannuzzi LA. A perspective on treatment of aphakic cystoid macular edema. *Surv Ophthalmol* 1984;28:540–553.

17. Lass JH, Stocker EG, Fritz ME, et al. Epikeratoplasty: the surgical correction of aphakia, myopia and keratoconus. *Ophthalmology* 1987;94:912–923.

18. Kaufman HE, Varnell ED, Centifanto-Fitzgerald, et al. Virus chemotherapy: antiviral drugs and interferon. *Antiviral Res* 1984;4:333–338.

19. Woo GC, ed. *Low Vision Principles and Application: Proceedings of the International Symposium on Low Vision*. New York, NY: Springer-Verlag NY Inc; 1986.

31

Otology

Ernest Mhoon

Harris[1] reports that hearing impairment is the second most common medical problem affecting the geriatric age group, second only to arthritis. Moreover, the most common cause of hearing loss in the adult population is presbycusis,[2] hearing loss attributed to aging. Once a diagnosis of presbycusis or other disorder is established, a program of aural rehabilitation can be initiated. Dizziness and imbalance are very common complaints among older persons but are often difficult to diagnose and manage, because balance is subserved by a complex interrelationship between the vestibular, visual, and somatosensory systems along with their central nervous system connections and pathways. Furthermore, each system is subject to the degenerative processes of aging. This chapter will focus on those problems affecting the elderly patient relative to the field of otology: the auditory system, clinical audiology, and the vestibular system.

The Auditory System

The effects of aging on the auditory and vestibular systems result in a gradual diminution of function that is largely bilaterally symmetric. This symmetry of the dysfunction is often helpful in ruling out a large number of disorders that primarily present unilaterally: neoplasms of the cerbellopontine angle, vascular occlusion, hemorrhage, viral illness, and posttraumatic injuries to the skull base and temporal bone.

The auditory system is very important in maintaining social interactions through communication, especially when an individual has spent the greater part of his or her life with relatively normal hearing. Hearing impairment may result in a significant decrease in the ability of the patient to interact effectively with friends, relatives, and other members of society.[3-5] For the elderly patient, family members and friends are often the first to notice the problem and recommend that the patient seek assistance. Failure to obtain help may lead to feelings of isolation and psychological disturbances.[6-9] Physicians who regularly treat elderly patients should be keenly aware of the significance and frequency of hearing loss among these patients and be knowledgeable of the diagnostic and therapeutic measures that are currently available.

Although hearing loss is the most common complaint associated with disorders of the ear, other complaints, such as tinnitus, itching, discharge, and pain, frequently are cited. As is true with other organ systems, there is no substitute for beginning an otologic workup with a thorough history and physical examination. Afterward, appropriate audiologic and other diagnostic studies can be selected and administered.

External Ear

The external auditory canal extends from the caudal cartilage and tragus of the auricle laterally to the tympanic membrane medially (Fig. 31.1). The skin of the lateral one half to one third of the canal is similar to skin located elsewhere on the body. It has well-

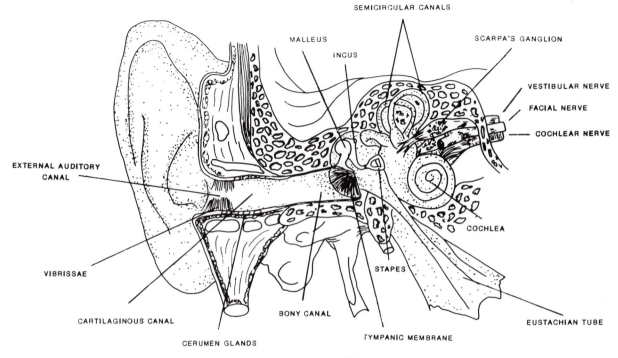

Fig. 31.1. Diagram of the ear.

developed dermal and subcutaneous layers with many hair follicles as well as sebaceous and cerumen glands. It has a thickness of approximately 0.5 to 1 mm, but the medial one half to two thirds of the canal has a thickness of only 0.2 mm and is firmly attached to the underlying periosteum.[10] Because the lateral part of the canal is supported by cartilage, it is often referred to as the cartilaginous canal. Similarly, the medial part of the canal is supported by bone and is thus called the bony canal.

Two of the most common complaints relative to the external auditory canal among elderly patients are cerumen impactions and itching. Cerumen impactions in older persons usually are the result of several factors. Cerumen glands, which are modified apocrine sweat glands, decrease in number and activity, causing an overall reduction in moisture. Dry cerumen predisposes the patient to impactions, in that the normal transport of cerumen from the cartilaginous canal to the external meatus is impaired. These impactions are more frequent in older men because the cerumen becomes entangled in large, laterally placed vibrissae (hairs), which are a secondary sex characteristic.[11] The vibrissae become more prominent in the 3rd and 4th decades and appear on the tragus, antitragus, and helix as well as in the external canal. Complete occlusion of the canal may cause a conductive hearing loss in the range of 15 to 30 dB (Table 31.1). There is no correlation between the amount or color of cerumen and the age of the patient.[11] Cerumen impac-

tions may be prevented by the regular use of agents that readily soften wax. When the wax is soft, normal transport mechanisms usually are effective in clearing it. Patients may use household agents such as mineral oil, cooking oil, or glycerin to achieve the same effect achieved with commercial agents such as carbamide peroxide 6.5% and triethanolamine polypeptide oleate. Gentle irrigation of the canal with water heated to 37°C often will result in a successful disimpaction without causing dizziness through caloric stimulation of the vestibular system. If the patient has a history of a tympanic membrane perforation or chronic ear disease, irrigations are contraindicated. If the patient has a history of recurrent otitis externa ("swimmer's ear"), the canal should be rinsed after irrigation with three to four drops of a solution that will return the external canal to its baseline pH of 5 to 5.5. This discourages the growth of organisms that commonly infect the external ear canal. Solutions commonly used

Table 31.1. Hearing threshold scale.

Degree of loss	Pure-tone average, dB*	Speech equivalent
Normal	<25	Whisper
Mild	26–40	Soft voice
Moderate	41–60	Normal speech
Severe	61–90	Loud speech
Profound	>81	Shouting

* 500, 1000, 2000 Hz

for this purpose include half-strength white vinegar solution or commercially prepared solutions that contain weak acids such as acetic and boric acids. Antibiotic-containing ear drops usually are unnecessary.

Itching of the external canal is also a common complaint among elderly persons. The sensation of itching can be related to dryness of the skin, which undergoes senile changes in the cartilaginous portion of the external auditory canal. The itching is often worsened by the patient's efforts to remove the dry cerumen and epithelial debris with cotton-tipped applicators, hairpins, or other similar objects. Atrophy of the epithelium and underlying sebaceous and cerumen glands results in decreased hydration of the skin[12] and an increased susceptibility to damage from trauma and irritation caused by strong soaps and shampoos. Once the itch develops, it is often maintained by an itch-scratch-itch cycle.[13] This symptom can usually be successfully managed if patients avoid traumatizing the ear canal and using irritating substances. The itch may be controlled by the use of steroid-based creams or solutions, and dryness can be avoided with the use of skin moisturizers.

Other disorders that may affect the external auditory canal include foreign bodies, infections, dermatoses, tumors, and congenital anomalies (Table 31.2). Interestingly, the aging changes associated with the external auditory canal are not associated with a higher incidence of infections.[13] Malignant otitis externa is commonly found in elderly diabetic patients but may affect children as well.[14] It is caused by a *Pseudomonas* osteitis of the bony canal. The major predisposing factor of this disease is immunoincompetence rather than aging.

The skin overlying the pinna and cartilaginous portion of the canal is susceptible to many forms of dermatologic change. As the pinna is often exposed to sunlight, skin changes related to actinic radiation are often found. Common benign neoplasms of the external canal include osteomas and exostoses. Neither of these are particularly associated with aging. Common malignant neoplasms include basal cell carcinomas, which are most often found on the pinna, squamous cell carcinomas, which usually begin in the external auditory canal and progress both medially and laterally, and ceruminomas, which include adenoid cystic carcinoma and adenocarcinoma. Fortunately, malignancies involving the ear are relatively rare, but the median ages for all types of tumors range from the 5th to the 6th decade.[15] Malignancy should be seriously considered in all patients with complaints of a chronic aural discharge associated with constant pain. Most patients with chronic otorrhea do not complain of otalgia. Any patient with an otologic symptom associated with facial nerve weakness or paralysis also should be evaluated for malignancy.

Table 31.2. Causes of hearing loss in elderly persons.

Conductive	Sensorineural
A. External ear canal	A. Sensory disorders (cochlear)
Cerumen impactions	Presbycusis
Foreign bodies	Hereditary or congenital
Cotton	abnormalities
Tissue paper	Vascular insufficiency
Otitis externa	Acoustic trauma
Bacterial	Ototoxicity
Fungal	Meniere's disease
Dermatitis	Infection
Benign tumors	Viral
Osteomas	Bacterial (syphilis,
Exostoses	meningitis)
Malignant tumors	Metabolic or hormonal
Squamous cell	disorders
carcinoma	Diabetes mellitus
Adenoid cystic	Hypothyroidism
carcinoma	Autoimmune or
Adenocarcinoma	granulomatous
Congenital anomalies	diseases
Atresia	Cogan's syndrome
Stenosis	Sarcoidosis
	Head Trauma
B. Middle ear	B. Neural disorders (retrocochlear)
Otitis media	Presbycusis
serous	Brainstem ischemia or
acute	infarction
chronic	Neoplasms
Tympanic membrane	Acoustic neuroma
perforation	Meningioma
Traumatic	Metastatic tumors
Inflammatory	Demyelinating disease
Cholesteatoma	
Congenital	
Acquired	
Head trauma	
Ossicular	
disruption	
Otosclerosis	
Congenital defects	
Ossicular fixation	
or malformation	
Eustachian tube	
anomalies	
Neoplasms	
Glomus tumors	
Squamous cell	
carcinoma	

Middle Ear

The middle ear encompasses the medial surface of the tympanic membrane, the ossicular chain, eustachian tube, and air spaces of the tympanic cavity, mastoid, and petrous apex (Fig. 31.1). Disorders of the middle ear often result in an impairment of sound conduction between the tympanic membrane and inner ear. Hearing loss that results from an abnormality of the mechanical transmission of sound, as found in external canal and middle-ear abnormalities, is termed conductive. Hearing loss associated with an abnormality of the sensory and/or neural structures of the inner ear is termed sensorineural. Some of the more common problems affecting the middle ear include serous otitis media (otitis media with effusion), acute and chronic otitis media, tympanic membrane perforation, cholesteatoma, otosclerosis, traumatic injuries, congenital defects, and neoplasms (Table 31.2). All of these problems may be found among geriatric patients but are not found with any greater frequency than in the general population, with the exception of malignant neoplasms, as previously discussed in the section on external canal disorders.

The middle ear undergoes changes with aging. Many histologic studies have demonstrated changes in the ossicular joints, incudomalleal and incudostapedial, which are synovial diarthrodial joints (Fig. 31.2). Etholm and Belal[16] reported that some of the earliest changes in the middle-ear joints are fibrillation, fraying, and vacuolation in the articular cartilages. Hyalinization of the joint capsule, thinning and calcification of the articular cartilage, and narrowing of the joint space followed the early changes. The most severe changes included diffuse calcification of the joint capsule and articular cartilages and fusion or obliteration of the joint space. Ears from individuals ranging in age from infancy to 96 years were studied. No persons less than 1 year of age showed abnormalities in the middle-ear joints. All temporal bones from individuals over 70 years of age showed moderate to severe arthritic changes in the joints. No differences were present between males and females. Interestingly, in the same group of patients, audiometric studies showed no correlation between the severity of middle-ear joint involvement and conductive hearing loss. A previous study by Elpern et al[17] demonstrated that experimental fixation of the middle-ear joints and human temporal bones had no effect on sound transmission. Subsequent studies have also been unable to show a significant difference in hearing among individuals with arthritis of the ossicular joints and those without.[3,18,19]

Inner Ear

The inner ear includes the sensorineural auditory and vestibular systems (Fig. 31.1). Disorders affecting the inner ear may involve either system independently or in combination. Hearing loss resulting from inner-ear disease is of the sensorineural type. A sensorineural loss can be further subdivided into a sensory loss and a neural loss. A sensory or cochlear loss is usually the result of an abnormality within the cochlea or organ of Corti, and a neural or retrocochlear loss results from the dysfunction of neural structures that are medial to the cochlea: peripheral nerve fibers, ganglion cells, auditory nerve, and/or central pathways[20] (Fig. 31.3). Factors that commonly cause sensorineural hearing loss include presbycusis, congenital and hereditary influences, vascular insufficiency, autoimmune or granulomatous diseases, neoplasms, acoustic trauma, ototoxicity, Meniere's disease, infection, metabolic and hormonal disorders, demyelinating disease, and head trauma (Table 31.2). Among this list, presbycusis is by far the most common cause of sensorineural hearing loss in elderly persons. Another frequent cause of hearing loss in the geriatric population is ototoxicity, a diagnosis that often is overlooked. Several drugs used in the treatment of arthritis, such as salicylates and ibuprofen, may be ototoxic in sensitive patients. Other important ototoxic drugs are quinine, ethacrynic acid, furosemide, and aminoglycoside antibiotics[21] (Table 31.3). A careful history and physical examination along with an audiogram is often all that is needed to make a firm diagnosis in a patient with sensorineural hearing loss.

Presbycusis

Hearing loss associated with aging was first described by Zwaardemaker[22] in 1891, and the term *presbycusis* has been in use since 1897 to denote this phenomenon[8], which is that of a slowly progressive, bilaterally symmetric decrease in hearing primarily affecting high

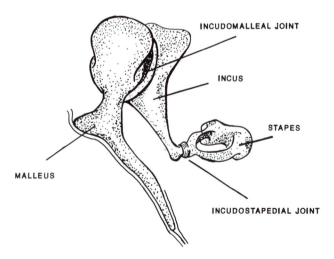

Fig. 31.2. Schematic representation of the ossicular chain, illustrating the relative positions of the incudomalleal and incudostapedial joints.

INCUDOMALLEAL JOINT

INCUS

STAPES

MALLEUS

INCUDOSTAPEDIAL JOINT

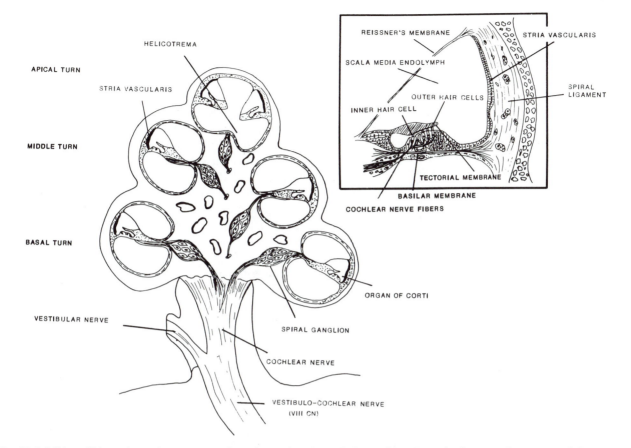

Fig. 31.3. Midmodiolar schematic representation of a section through the cochlea. Inset depicts an enlargement of the organ of Corti within the scala media (adapted from Honrubia and Goodhill[20]).

tones and associated with the aging process. The results of numerous studies worldwide have shown that most persons over the age of 40 years have some degree of progressive hearing loss.[13,23] The loss tends to be greater in frequencies above 2,000 Hz[24] (Fig. 31.4). Many attempts have been made to define the etiologic factors contributing to the development of presbycusis. Factors that have been widely studied include diet, nutrition, cholesterol levels, blood pressure, metabolism, arteriosclerosis, exercise, genetic factors, noise, and emotional stress. In 1962, Rosen et al[25] tested the hearing of the Mabaans, a Sudanese tribe that lives in a relatively silent environment. The tribe's members exercised daily, maintained a diet that was low in cholesterol, and did not smoke. When their hearing results were compared with those of age-matched control subjects from industrialized areas of the United States, their thresholds were significantly better from 500 to 6,000 Hz. At first glance, the results of this study suggest that a noise-free environment, low-cholesterol diet, exercise, and lack of smoking may lead to better hearing in old age. Unfortunately, similar studies on other populations have not been able to duplicate these results. For example, Royster and

Thomas[26] studied a population of over 10,000 subjects and discovered that black men had significantly better hearing thresholds than age-matched white men. At 25 years of age the difference was only 5 dB, but at 60 years of age the difference was 20 dB. Furthermore, the hearing thresholds of black men exposed to industrial noise were lower than those of age-matched white men who had no history of industrial noise exposure. Both the study by Rosen et al and the one by Royster and Thomas suggest that genetic predisposition plays an important role in the development of presbycusis.

Many investigators have studied the histopathologic correlates of presbycusis in human temporal bones. Crowe et al[27] in 1934 and Saxen[28] in 1937 described two types of histologic changes associated with presbycusis, one involving the cochlear epithelial tissues and the other involving the spiral ganglion (Fig. 31.3).[20]

Schuknecht[29] in 1964 described at least four types of presbycusis, including those described by Crowe et al and Saxon. *Sensory presbycusis* involves the atrophy of the organ of Corti in the basal end of the cochlea. It usually begins in middle age and is characterized by an abrupt high-tone hearing loss. It is slowly progressive

Table 31.3*. Ototoxic drugs.

Aminoglycoside antibiotics	Antiprotozoal drugs
Amikacin	Chloroquine
Gentamicin	Quinine
Kanamycin	Loop Diuretics
Neomycin	Bumetanide
Netilmicin	Ethacrynic acid
Streptomycin	Furosemide
Tobramycin	Topical aural preparations
Other Antibiotics	Antibiotics (polymyxin B,
Ampicillin	neomycin,
Chloramphenicol	chloramphenicol,
Erythromycin	erythromycin, tetracycline)
Polymyxin B	Antiseptics
Ristocetin	Chromic acid
Vancomycin	Formaldehyde (in absorbable
Viomycin	gelatin sponges)
Anticancer drugs	Chlorhexidine
Cisplatin	Local anesthetics
Cyclophosphamide	Framycetin
Bleomycin	Miscellaneous
Antiinflammatory drugs	Arsenicals
(nonsteroidal)	Quinidine
Fenoprofen	Thalidomide
Ibuprofen	
Indomethacin	
Naproxen	
Phenylbutazone	
Salicylates	
Sulindac	

* Adapted from Sevy.[21]

but does not involve those areas of the cochlea that subserve the speech frequencies. The supporting cells of the organ of Corti are the first to degenerate. Neural degeneration follows.

Neural presbycusis, originally described by Schuknecht as neural atrophy, develops as a loss of cochlear neurons predominantly occurring in the basal end but often involving the entire cochlea. The audiogram has a typical downward slope in the high frequencies. The most significant clinical manifestation of neural presbycusis is that of a loss of speech discrimination that appears to be much worse than that expected for the pure-tone thresholds, which are often reasonably good. This can be explained by the relative sparing of the organ of Corti, which better subserves pure-tone hearing. When the number of neural connections decrease beyond a certain limit, the ability to understand speech also decreases. Neural presbycusis may begin at any age.

Strial presbycusis is characterized audiometrically by a relatively flat pure-tone response with excellent speech discrimination. The hearing loss is slowly progressive, with a pure-tone average that falls below 50 dB. Cochlear atrophy is primarily seen in the stria vascularis and is usually located in the middle and apical turns. The relative lack of degeneration of the cochlear neurons is believed to be responsible for the excellent speech discrimination associated with moderate hearing losses.

Cochlear conductive presbycusis begins in middle

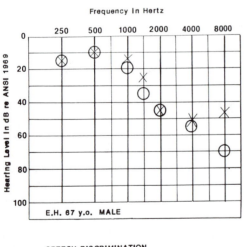

SPEECH DISCRIMINATION

RIGHT EAR: 60%/40dBSL
LEFT EAR: 68%/40dBSL

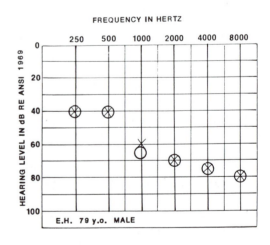

SPEECH DISCRIMINATION

RIGHT EAR: 24%/30dBSL
LEFT EAR: 36%/30dBSL

SPEECH DISCRIMINATION IN SOUND FIELD

UNAIDED: 48%/55dBSL
AIDED: 84%/55dBSL

Fig. 31.4. Audiograms of a presbycusic patient that were taken 12 years apart, at 67 and 79 years of age. The patient refused a hearing aid initially but consented to a hearing aid evaluation 12 years later. Because of his poor speech discrimination scores (24% in the right ear and 36% in the left ear), he was at first considered a poor candidate for a hearing aid; however, during his hearing aid evaluation in sound field, his aided speech discrimination score was noted to be much better than the unaided score, 84% and 48%, respectively. Consequently, he received substantial benefit from amplification.

age and has an audiometric pattern characterized by a descending straight line. Unlike neural and strial presbycusis, speech discrimination and the degree of pure-tone hearing loss are directly related. An interesting histopathologic feature of this type of hearing loss is that the degenerative changes are inadequate to explain the loss. The diagnosis is therefore largely based on the history and clinical findings.

Although many ears can be placed into one of these four categories of presbycusis, many have more than one type of degenerative change occurring simultaneously. Thus, in the final analysis, the diagnosis of presbycusis depends on the presence of a slowly progressive, bilaterally symmetric, sensorineural hearing loss that begins in middle to older age, the etiology of which is undetermined.

Statistics compiled by the US Public Health Service[30] and Department of Health, Education, and Welfare[31] have indicated that approximately 25% of individuals between 65 and 74 years of age and nearly 50% of those aged 75 years or older experience problems with hearing. As there are more than 25 million people in the United States over 65 years of age,[32] hearing loss in this population is a problem deserving of careful attention and consideration.

Concepts in Clinical Audiology

The evaluation of a patient with impaired hearing is incomplete unless a thorough otologic and audiologic examination has been performed. The otologic evaluation is performed by an otologist or otolaryngologist and includes a history and physical examination and all studies needed to arrive at a diagnosis. The audiologic evaluation is performed by an audiologist who has received a master's or doctorate degree in the field of audiology. In some states, patients may receive a hearing aid without undergoing an otologic examination by signing a waiver following audiometric testing. Although most audiologists refer patients for otologic clearance before fitting them with a hearing aid, a few, most of whom are associated with hearing aid dealerships, do not. Fortunately, most patients who are fitted with a hearing aid without undergoing an otologic examination do not have treatable otologic illnesses. Nonetheless, just because an elderly patient has a hearing loss is no reason to assume that the cause is presbycusis until a thorough evaluation has been completed. Clearly, the patient benefits most when the physician and the audiologist work together. When it is determined that the patient's hearing loss is not amenable to medical or surgical intervention, only then can effective audiologic rehabilitative services be initiated: assistive listening devices, hearing aids, speech reading, educational programs, guidance, and counseling.

Audiologic Evaluation

A pure-tone audiogram that shows both air and bone conduction gives information on the relative degree of hearing loss, the configuration (descending, flat, or ascending), and the type of loss (conductive or sensorineural). Before it is decided that a patient is a candidate for a hearing aid, speech audiometry is performed. As previously discussed in the section on presbycusis, the ability to discriminate speech varies widely among patients with presbycusis. Those classified as having "neural presbycusis" have poor speech discrimination scores, whereas those with "strial presbycusis" have high scores, even when the pure-tone average of the patient with "neural presbycusis" is higher than the pure-tone average of the patient with "strial presbycusis." Thus, recommendations for amplification cannot be based on pure-tone averages alone.

The assessment of a patient's ability to discriminate speech begins with a presentation of monosyllabic words that are presented at a comfortable listening level, usually around 40 dB above pure-tone thresholds.[33] Patients who demonstrate an improvement in speech discrimination with increased amplification are usually good candidates for hearing aids. Patients who experience a decrease in speech discrimination with increasing intensity exhibit a phenomenon termed "rollover," which is indicative of a retrocochlear abnormality that may be caused by lesions of the eighth nerve, brain stem, or cortex.[34,35]

Another test of speech is that of the speech reception threshold, which measures a patient's ability to hear two-syllable words presented in the speech frequency ranges (500, 1,000, and 2,000Hz).[33] If the results of this test do not closely match the pure-tone thresholds, a nonorganic or functional hearing loss must then be ruled out.

More sophisticated audiologic techniques which are often used in site-of-lesion testing include impedance audiometry (including tympanometry) and auditory brain-stem response testing.[36] Impedance audiometry may provide information on tympanic membrane compliance, middle-ear pressures, size of the external canal and middle-ear cavities, eustachian tube function, and acoustic reflexes. Although each subtest measures some aspect of middle-ear function, acoustic reflex testing also measures the integrity of the peripheral and central pathways of the reflex arc and is helpful in the investigation of central lesions, such as acoustic neuromas and other brain-stem lesions that may cause an absence or decay of the acoustic reflex during intense auditory stimulation of the involved ear (70 dB to 90 dB above threshold). The auditory brain-stem response is useful for threshold testing in infants, children, and adults who are unable to be tested accurately with behavioral audiometry. It is also a highly sensitive test for the detection of small acoustic neuromas or other cerebellopontine angle masses and lesions of the brain stem that may affect nerve conduction. Tumors of the eighth nerve may cause prolonged latencies of wave forms I through V, poor wave-form morphology, or complete absence of wave forms.

The tests presented here represent only a few of the tests available to the audiologist but are among those most commonly used in an audiologic evaluation.

Audiologic Rehabilitation

Upon completion of the otologic and audiologic evaluations, an aural rehabilitation program can begin. Over the past 10 to 20 years, substantial technologic advances have occurred in the devices used to aid the hearing impaired. These advances are evident in the improvement of conventional hearing aids, the introduction of surgically implantable hearing aids, and the development of cochlear implant devices. As each patient has specific characteristics with regard to the degree of pure-tone hearing loss, the ability to understand speech, noise tolerance, manual dexterity for the manipulation of small controls and component parts, cognition, and overall life-style, the type of listening device or rehabilitative program must be custom-designed to suit the individual's specific needs. Furthermore, patients with presbycusis often have psychosocial problems that make audiologic rehabilitation more difficult. Often, elderly patients associate hearing aids with aging and are not willing to accept them for that reason. Unfortunately, it is difficult to change these attitudes as they are generally shared by the society at large. Nevertheless, thorough guidance, counseling, and education can go a long way in helping patients adjust to amplification. Family members and friends may assist in this adjustment but may require a certain amount of counseling and education themselves before they can become helpful in the rehabilitative process.

Many devices other than hearing aids can be helpful to the hearing-impaired patient in certain environmental settings. Assistive listening devices or systems[37] can be used both for large group settings—as in churches, restaurants, auditoriums, and conference rooms—and for personal use in or out of the home. The most common such device is an FM system whereby a microphone is attached to an amplifier-

transmitter and is placed close to the sound source to improve signal-to-noise ratio. The microphone often is clipped to a speaker's lapel, attached to a television set by a plug, or placed on a lectern or table. An individual with a clothing microphone and a pocket amplifier-transmitter can be heard by a person with a receiver anywhere in the house or yard. The devices may be used with or without hearing aids. Other devices are based on AM transmissions, direct wire transmission, electromagnetic loop induction, and infrared systems that transmit speech and music using infrared light as a carrier medium. They are most often used for television viewing.

The use of the telephone is often problematic for hearing-impaired patients. The average telephone system has a frequency response between 300 to 3,000 Hz and is prone to significant distortion or noise during transmission.[37] Understandably, persons with hearing losses involving those frequencies may have difficulty using the telephone. To assist the hearing impaired, two types of telephone amplification devices have been developed: a device that increases the volume and one with a magnetic induction that couples with the circuitry in certain hearing aids. Neither of these devices improves signal-to-noise ratio, reduces distortion, or extends the frequency response.

Recent studies have shown that failure to diagnose and manage hearing problems early in their course may result in significant sensory deprivation.[38,39] With this in mind, some otologists recommend routinely screening patients over age 50 years for pure-tone sensitivity as part of the general physical examination.[38] However, when testing elderly patients, it must be remembered that presbycusis is only one cause of hearing impairment and may coexist with other causes. Usually a good history and physical examination is adequate to screen for hearing loss, but if there is any doubt, formal testing should be initiated.

Hearing Aids

Before a hearing aid is prescribed, the physician and audiologist must make certain that the patient has realistic expectations regarding the benefits and limitations of its use. Unless these patients are informed about the circumstances under which amplification will and will not be of help, they may reject the use of amplification after a relatively limited trial period. Corrado[40] reports that 20% of hearing aids administered in his practice are not used within 6 months of being supplied. Brooks[41] reported that only 25% of a group of hearing-impaired persons considered hearing aids as a treatment choice. The remainder of the patients were expecting medical or surgical treatment or were forced to have a hearing evaluation by family or friends. With proper counseling and orientation, even the poorest candidates for hearing aids may find unsuspected benefits from the use of amplification (Fig. 31.4). In a survey on the rejection of hearing aids by geriatric patients, Franks and Beckman[42] found that of 35 possible scale responses, the major reasons for the nonuse of hearing aids included cost, calling attention to the handicap, dealer practices, concern about the nature of the amplified sound, difficulty in manipulating hearing aid controls, and not knowing where to obtain a hearing aid. Kapteyn[43] in 1977 found that satisfaction with hearing aid use related more strongly to motivation, personal adjustment, and family support than to the ability to understand speech or the fit of the hearing aid.

Following otologic clearance, a hearing aid evaluation is the next step. This evaluation primarily consists of audiometric testing to determine the intensity levels at which sound is most comfortable and at which it is uncomfortable. In a sound field environment, the patient is first tested without a hearing aid and again with a variety of hearing aids that have been selected to match the patient's hearing deficit. The aid or aids that produce the best responses on prescribed tests are recommended. A 30-day trial period is usually given to allow for acclimation, adjustments, and counseling before the final purchase is made. Other rehabilitative services that may be needed include classes in speech reading and instructions on the use of assistive listening devices in and outside of the home.

Technologic improvements in hearing aids are accelerating rapidly. Not only are the aids smaller and more unobtrusive, they have higher fidelity and are more frequency specific, and many have noise-suppression units that allow for better speech discrimination in noise, a feature that is most helpful for the presbycusic patient. There are three basic categories of hearing aids: body-type aids, which are larger and easier to adjust; in-the-ear aids, which are smaller and thus more cosmetic in appearance and are easier to insert into the ear; and behind-the-ear aids, which are the more conventional-appearing aids with the electronic parts located behind the ear. Because the controls on the behind-the-ear aids are somewhat larger, they are easier to operate. The hearing aid mold may be open or closed depending on the frequency needs of the patient or on whether or not a chronic aural discharge is present. A mold that completely occludes the external canal may predispose the patient to cerumen impactions, otitis externa, or an exacerbation of preexisting chronic otitis media in patients with tympanic membrane perforations or mastoid cavities. Poorly fitting molds may result in the "squeal" of

auditory feedback when the fit is inadequate or ulceration of the meatus and auricular cartilages when the fit is too tight. In-the-ear aids are often contraindicated in patients with a chronic aural discharge. However, these patients may use a bone-conduction hearing aid, which is worn like a headset behind the ears, or a surgically implanted bone-conduction aid, which has been recently developed and may be used under a variety of circumstances. Other alternatives to conventional hearing aids include bone-conduction aids that stimulate the ossicular chain directly and are thus more effective than conventional air-conduction aids or other types of bone-conduction aids in providing auditory stimulation to patients with moderately severe sensorineural or conductive hearing losses. Patients who are unable to perceive auditory stimulation from conventional amplification in either ear may be candidates for cochlear implant devices that produce auditory responses by stimulating the eighth nerve through electrodes that are placed into or near the cochlea.

Successful hearing aid use in elderly persons with hearing impairment depends on a carefully prescribed program of audiologic rehabilitation. The education, guidance, and counseling that make up an important part of the rehabilitative services should not be limited to the patient but should be expanded to include those family members, friends, and professionals who have a direct impact on the patient's psychosocial well being. Matkin and Hodgson[44] formulated the following guidelines to improve communication with elderly persons who are hearing impaired:

1. The speaker should make certain to get the person's attention before speaking.
2. The speaker's face should be visible to the listener and well lighted (not backlit), and the speaker should avoid eating, smoking, or covering the mouth while talking.
3. The speaker should speak toward the better or aided ear at a distance of approximately 2 to 3 ft and make an attempt to reduce unnecessary background noise.
4. Speech should be slow and clear with more pauses than usual. If the listener is not wearing a hearing aid, the speaker should speak loudly but avoid shouting.
5. If the listener fails to understand a word or sentence, the speaker should paraphrase rather than repeat.
6. Before proceeding to a new topic, the speaker should alert the listener to sudden changes in the subject of the conversation.

Other helpful hints include making certain that one is in the same room with a hearing-impaired person when communicating. Radio and television sets should be turned down or off during periods of conversation. When possible, the presbycusic patient should select activities and forms of entertainment that are associated with low background noises. Observing these pointers in association with an effective aural rehabilitation program can greatly enhance communication with the hearing-impaired patient.

The Vestibular System

Disorders of the vestibular system among elderly patients are so common that if the related symptoms are not severe or incapacitating, they are often ignored by both the patient and physician. An enormous amount of time and expense can be involved in a complete vestibular workup, and the returns may be minimal. This tends to discourage some physicians who are unfamiliar with balance disorders from pursuing vestibular symptoms enthusiastically. Dizziness may be related to a variety of factors that may directly or indirectly affect the vestibular, visual, or soma-

tosensory systems, alone or in combination, and this contributes to the complexity of the problem (Figs. 31.5[45] and 31.6[20]). The dizzy patient is therefore approached as having a multisensory disorder rather than a simple inner-ear disturbance.

A good history and physical examination is essential in the initial evaluation of dizziness. These can usually differentiate between central, peripheral, and systemic causes of dizziness (Table 31.4). Patients often find it difficult to describe the symptom precisely and often require the assistance of the examining physician to find the word that best describes the sensation. Dizziness is a general term that is used to describe various sensations of disequilibrium related to varying degrees of spatial disorientation in both the internal and external environment. Included in this definition are sensations of light-headedness, fainting, imbalance, unsteadiness, swaying, giddiness, swimming in the head, tilting, staggering, falling, and rocking, to name a few. Vertigo, however, is a term that is used to describe misperceptions of motion, most notably sensations of spinning, whirling, and falling. Vertigo is also usually associated with autonomic nervous sys-

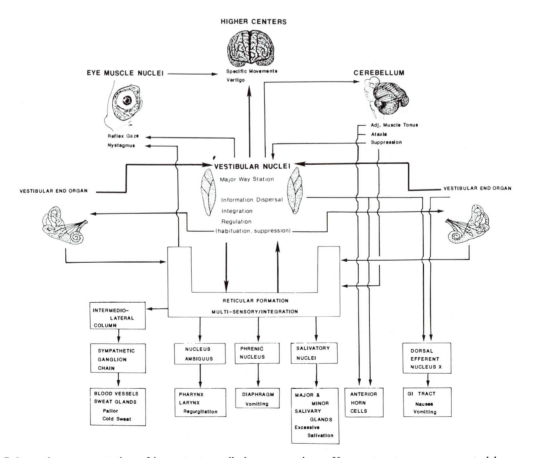

Fig. 31.5. Schematic representation of important vestibular connections. Known tracts are represented by arrows. Under normal conditions the vestibular system is primarily somatosensory (upper half of schema), but under abnormal conditions it initiates considerable motor activity (lower half of schema) (adapted from McCabe, BF[45]).

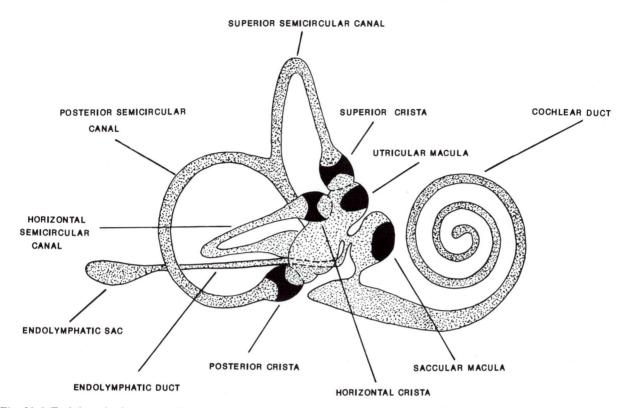

Fig. 31.6. Endolymphatic system of the labyrinth illustrating the relative positions of the cristae of the semicircular canals and the maculae of the utricle and saccule (Adapted from Honrubia and Goodhill[20]).

tem responses such as nausea, vomiting, diaphoresis, and pallor. Central vestibular disorders are usually related to mild symptoms of dizziness, whereas peripheral vestibular disorders are most often associated with severe symptoms of vertigo. Systemic factors may cause dizziness or vertigo, depending on which component of the balance system is most affected.

On physical examination, the dizzy patient often will be found to have spontaneous nystagmus, gaze nystagmus, and/or positional nystagmus. Nystagmus induced by peripheral vestibular changes has a latency of 3 to 45 seconds, is fatigable, diminishes on repetition of a provocative maneuver, is direction-fixed, and is associated with symptoms of vertigo when present. Centrally induced nystagmus has no latency, does not fatigue, may change direction, and may be asymptomatic or associated with relatively mild forms of dizziness or vertigo. Patients with a normal Romberg

Table 31.4. Causes of dizziness in elderly persons.

Peripheral	Central	Systemic
Motion sickness	Brain-stem ischemia or infarction	Vascular insufficiency
Benign paroxysmal positional vertigo	Cerebellopontine angle tumors 　Acoustic neuroma 　Meningioma 　Metastatic tumors	Infections 　Syphilis 　Viral syndromes 　Bacterial sepsis
Benign positional vertigo		
Vestibulotoxic drugs	Vascular anomalies 　Arteriovenous malformations 　Vascular loops	Autoimmune or granulomatous diseases
Vestibular neuronitis or labyrinthitis		Metabolic or hormonal disorders
Meniere's disease	Demyelinating disease	Drug effects
Posttraumatic vertigo	Seizure disorders	
Perilymph fistula	Psychogenic disorders	
Otosclerosis		

and abnormal tandem Romberg test are likely to have a peripheral vestibular disorder, which if unilateral will cause them to fall toward the side of the lesion. In addition to a thorough head and neck examination, neurologic and general medical examinations are often needed to complete the evaluation.

Additional testing may include audiologic testing, auditory brain-stem response testing, electronystagmography, magnetic resonance imaging of the internal auditory canals with gadolinium enhancement, an electrocardiogram, a complete blood cell count, sedimentation rate, serum chemistry profile, urinalysis, thyroid function test, serology for syphilis, and electroencephalography. Rarely are all of these studies needed to make a diagnosis.

Common causes of peripheral vestibular disorders among elderly persons include motion sickness, benign paroxysmal positional vertigo, which can be successfully treated with vestibular habituation exercises, drug-induced vertigo, which is usually diagnosed by means of a carefully taken drug history (Table 31.5),[21] and the disequilibrium of aging. Belal and Glorig[46] reported that of 740 patients over 65 years of age with complaints of dizziness, 79% were found to have the disequilibrium of aging that they called "presbyastasis." However, histopathologic evidence for presbyastasis is lacking when compared with its counterpart in the auditory system, presbycusis. Other causes of peripheral vestibular dysfunction include benign positional vertigo, vestibular neuronitis, Meniere's disease, posttraumatic vertigo, perilymph fistula, and otosclerosis (Table 31.4).

Table 31.5. Drugs that may cause vertigo and/or dizziness.

Analgesics	Antihypertensive drugs
Butorphanol	Atenolol
Hydromorphone	Clonidine
Meperidine	Guanethidine
Morphine	Hydralazine
Pentazocine	Methyldopa
Propoxyphene	Metoprolol
Anesthetics	Nitroprusside
Ketamine	Phenoxybenzamine
Methoxyflurane	Phentolamine
Antiarrhythmic drugs	Prazosin
Amiodarone	Antiinflammatory drugs
Bretylium	(non-steroidal)
Encainide	Allopurinol
Lidocaine	Diflunisal
Procainamide	Fenoprofen
Propranolol	Gold
Quinidine	Ibuprofen
Tocainide	Ketoprofen
Anticancer drugs	Indomethacin
Cisplatin	Naproxen

Anticancer drugs (cont)	Antiinflammatory drugs (cont)
Cyclophosphamide	Phenylbutazone
Fluorouracil	Salicylates
Anticonvulsants	Sulindac
Carbamazepine	Tolmetin
Clonazepam	Antimicrobial drugs
Ethosuximide	Aminoglycosides
Phensuximide	Colistin
Phenytoin	Cycloserine
Primidone	Griseofulvin
Antihistamines	Erythromycin
Cimetidine	Ethambutol
Diphenhydramine	Isoniazid
Tripelennamine	Minocycline
Antimuscarinic drugs	Nalidixic acid
Atropine	Nitrofurantoin
Scopolamine	Paromomycin
Antiprotozoal and	Polymyxin
Antihelminthic drugs	Rifampin
Chloroquine	Spectinomycin
Metronidazole	Sulfonamides
Oxamniquine	Trimethoprim
Pentamidine	Vancomycin
Pyrantel Pamoate	Vidarabine
Quinacrine	Drugs used for
Quinine	psychiatric
Thiabendazole	disorders
Appetite depressants	Benzodiazepines
Fenfluramine	Ethchlorvynol
Mazindol	Lithium
CNS Active drugs	Meprobamate
Amantadine	Monoamine-oxidase
Baclofen	inhibitors
Barbiturates	Phenothiazines
Dantrolene	Tricyclic
Disulfiram	antidepressants
Ethyl alcohol	Hormones and hormone
Methylphenidate	antagonists
Diuretics	Bromocriptine
Acetazolamide	Estrogens
Bumetanide	Insulins
Ethacrynic acid	Oral hypoglycemic
Furosemide	agents
	Progesterone-estrogen
	combinations
	Parasympatholytic
	drugs
	Dicyclomine
	Sympathomimetics
	Amphetamine
	Epinephrine
	Isoproterenol
	Vasodilators and
	antianginal drugs
	Isoxuprine
	Nitroglycerin
	Nylidrin

* Adapted from Sevy.[21]

Some of the central causes of vertigo include infarcts and brain-stem ischemia, cerebellopontine angle tumors such as acoustic neuromas, metastatic tumors, vascular anomalies, demyelinating diseases, seizure disorders, and psychogenic disorders (Table 31.4). Drop attacks are often related to central phenomena, but some may be related to a disturbance of the otolith organs in the peripheral vestibular system, Tumarkin's otolithic crisis.[47] Peripherally induced drop attacks are unassociated with a change in mental alertness, whereas centrally induced drop attacks, such as those of vascular or central nervous system origin, are often associated with an aura, "blackout," visual disturbance, state of confusion, or brief loss of memory.

Systemic causes of dizziness are extensive and include vascular and cardiac problems, infectious disease states, autoimmune and granulomatous diseases, metabolic abnormalities such as diabetes and hypothyroidism, and drug-induced effects (Table 31.4).

The treatment of peripheral vestibular disorders is primarily directed toward the alleviation of symptoms. In cases of acute vestibular neuronitis and benign paroxysmal positional vertigo, patients usually respond well to a program of vestibular habituation exercises.[48] The exercises are based on the habituation of the vestibular system by repetitive stimulation through maneuvers that cause vertigo. Mathog and Peppard[49] demonstrated that recovery from vestibular injury in cats is enhanced by exercise. Vertigo that results from an indirect insult on the vestibular system from diseases affecting other organ systems is usually controlled by the successful treatment of the underlying disease process. Unfortunately, many cases of vertigo are associated with an ill-defined etiology, and treatment is thus directed toward relief of the symptoms. The most widely used method in the control of vestibular symptoms is that of vestibulosuppression with various drugs and drug combinations from a variety of categories. The most commonly used drugs for the treatment of dizziness in general include meclizine, diazepam, promethazine, dimenhydrinate, scopolamine, oxazepam, chlorpromazine, and perphenazine. Medication choices are often based on patient tolerance, efficacy of response, and safety of long-term use. Patients with Meniere's disease are often treated with diuretics and/or vasodilators in addition to vestibular suppressants. Unfortunately, almost all of the drugs used to treat vertigo produce side effects that are particularly disturbing to the elderly patient. Some of these side effects include drowsiness, jitteriness, insomnia, blurred vision, and xerostomia, which may cause or exacerbate dysphagia. Most cases are managed fairly well with medical therapy, but some require surgery before relief is obtained.

Surgery for uncontrolled vertigo is divided into two categories: procedures that spare cochlear function and those that do not. Those procedures that preserve hearing include vestibular nerve section, singular nerve section, vascular loop decompressions, and operations on the endolymphatic sac for Meniere-type disorders, the efficacy of which is controversial. If the patient's hearing is not serviceable, the entire labyrinth, including cochlear function, may be destroyed by either a transmastoid or transcanal technique. Most patients are severely vertiginous for the first several days following vestibular ablative surgery, but this condition gradually tapers as vestibular compensation, which is mediated through the cerebellum, occurs over the next several weeks or months. Vestibular compensation is usually prolonged in the elderly patient.

Histopathology of the Aging Labyrinth

The labyrinth undergoes degenerative changes similar to those found in the aging cochlea. There is a loss of sensory epithelium, hair cells, peripheral nerve fibers, and ganglia. However, because of the complex anatomic arrangement of the sensory and neural structures of the peripheral vestibular sense organs, the evaluation and quantification of degenerative changes are difficult when compared to the cochlea.

As in the cochlea, hair cell loss is a prominent feature of degenerative change associated with aging in the labyrinth. A loss of up to 40% of the sensory epithelium of the cristae in the semicircular canals and 20% of the maculae of the otolith organs has been found in humans.[50] Another common finding believed to be associated with aging is the presence of epithelial cysts within the cristae and occasionally in the maculae.[51] Intracellular vesicles also are often found within the supporting cells.[50] According to Bergstrom,[52] a reduction in the number of peripheral neural fibers begins to occur after the age of 40 years. The loss is greatest among the thick myelinated fibers of the cristae. It has also been reported that after 50 years of age, the number of cell bodies in Scarpa's ganglion is reduced.[53]

Another change that has been found to occur after 50 years of age is a degeneration of otoconia of the saccule.[54] Interestingly, the otoconia of the utricle are only minimally affected. This tends to support several observations that have indicated that the phylogenetically younger pars inferior, which is composed of the cochlea and saccule, is more sensitive to the degenerative changes of aging than the older pars superior, which consists of the utricle and semicircular canals.[55,56] Schuknecht[57] proposed that deposits located around the cupula of the posterior semicircular canal were dislodged otoconia and were probably responsible for the symptoms and findings related to benign paroxysmal positional vertigo or cupulolithiasis, a controversial term which describes his histopathologic findings. Benign paroxysmal positional vertigo is believed to be the result of trauma in younger patients and degenerative processes associated with aging in older patients. Because the ampulla of the posterior semicircular canal is located in the most dependent part of the vestibule, dislodged otoconia or products of degeneration are likely to settle there and cause symptoms (Fig. 31.6). The best supporting evidence for this theory comes from the observation that denervation of the ampulla of the posterior semicircular canal through singular nerve section results in a cure of symptoms.[58] However, patients with symptoms related to this disorder often experience spontaneous resolution within 1 year of onset. Those with symptoms persisting beyond 1 year may become candidates for surgery.

As we continue to learn more about auditory and vestibular anatomy and function through basic and clinical research, more information regarding how aging affects these functions will follow. Moreover, a thorough understanding of the underlying mechanisms can lead to the development of more effective methods of diagnosis and treatment.

References

1. Harris CS. *Fact Book on Aging: A Profile of America's Older Population.* Washington, DC: National Council on the Aging; 1978.
2. Naunton RF. Presbycusis. In: Paparella MM, Shumrick D, eds. *Otolaryngology.* Philadelphia, Pa: WB Saunders Co; 1973;2:368–376.
3. Klotz RE, Kilbane M. Hearing in an aging population, preliminary report. *N Engl J Med* 1962;266:277–280.
4. McShane DP, Dayal VS. Hearing impairment: diagnostic and therapeutic measures. *Geriatr Med* 1986;2:32–36.
5. Salomon G. Hearing problems and the elderly. *Dan Med Bull* 1986;33(suppl 3):1–22.
6. Eastwood MR, Corbin SL, et al. Acquired hearing loss and psychiatric illness: an estimate of prevalence and co-morbidity in a geriatric setting. *Br J Psychiatry* 1985;147:552–556.
7. Jones DA, Victor CR, Vetter NJ. Hearing difficulty and its psychological implications for the elderly. *J Epidemiol Community Health* 1984;38:75–78.
8. Mader S. Hearing impairment in elderly persons. *J Am Geriatr Soc* 1984;32:548–553.
9. Ulhmann RF, Larson EB, Koepsell TD. Hearing impairment and cognitive decline in senile dementia of the Alzheimer type. *J Am Geriatr Soc* 1986;34:207–210.
10. Senturia BH, Marcus MD, Lucente FE. *Diseases of the External Ear.* 2nd ed. New York, NY: Grune & Stratton; 1980:4–6.
11. Perry ET. *The Human Ear Canal.* Springfield, Ill: Charles C Thomas Publishers; 1957:57–70.
12. Waisman M. A clinical look at the aging skin. *Postgrad Med* 1979;66:87–94.
13. Anderson RG, Meyerhoff WL. Otologic manifestations of aging. *Otolaryngol Clin North Am* 1982;15:353–370.
14. Horn KL, Gherini S. Malignant external otitis in children. *Am J Otol* 1981;2:402–404.
15. Dehna LP, Chen KTK. Primary tumors of the external and middle ear. *Arch Otolaryngol Head Neck Surg* 1980;106:13–19.
16. Etholm B, Belal A. Senile changes in the middle ear joints. *Ann Otol Rhinol Laryngol* 1974;83:49–54.
17. Elpern BS, Greisen D, Anderson HC. Experimental studies on sound transmission in the human ear. *Acta Otolaryngol* 1965;60:223–230.
18. Melrose J, Welsh OL, Luterman DM. Auditory responses in selected elderly men. *J Gerontol* 1963;18:267–270.
19. Sataloff J, Vassallo L, Menduke H. Presbycusis: air and bone conduction thresholds. *Laryngoscope* 1965;75:889–901.
20. Honrubia V, and Goodhill V. Clinical anatomy and physiology of the peripheral ear. In: Goodhill V, (Ed). *Ear Diseases, Deafness and Dizziness.* Hagerstown, Md: Harper & Row Publishers Inc; 1979;4–63.
21. Sevy RW. Drugs as a cause of dizziness and vertigo. In: Finestone AS, (Ed). *Evaluation and Clinical Management of Dizziness and Vertigo.* Boston, Ma: John Wright PSG Inc; 1982;105–113.
22. Zwaardemaker H. Der Verlust an hochen Toenen mit Zunehmendem Alfer: ein neues Gesetz. *Arch Ohrenheilk* 1891;32:53–56.
23. Goodhill V. *Ear Diseases, Deafness and Dizziness.* Hagerstown, Md: Harper & Row Publishers Inc; 1979.
24. Glorig A, Davis H. Age, noise and hearing loss. *Ann Otol Rhinol Laryngol* 1961;70:556–571.
25. Rosen S, Bergman M, Plester D, et al. Presbycusic study of a relatively noise-free population in Sudan. *Ann Otol Rhinol Laryngol* 1962;71:727–743.
26. Royster LH, Thomas WG. Age effect hearing levels for a white nonindustrial noise exposed population (NINEP) and their use in evaluating industrial hearing conservation programs. *Ann Ind Hyg Assoc J* 1979;40:504–511.
27. Crowe SJ, Guild SR, Polvogt LM. Observations on the pathology of high tone deafness. *Bull Johns Hopkins Hosp* 1934;54:315–379.
28. Saxen A. Pathologie und Klinik der Altersschwerhuerigkeit. *Acta Otolaryngol* 1937;(suppl 23):1–85.
29. Schuknecht HF. Further observations on the pathology of presbycusis. *Arch Otolaryngol Head Neck Surg* 1964;80:369–382.
30. *Hearing Status and Ear Examination: Findings Among Adults, United States 1960–1962.* Washington, DC: Health Services and Mental Health Administration. Public Health Service publication 1000. Series 11, No. 32.
31. *Prevalence of Selected Impairments: United States,*

1971. Rockville, Md: 1975. US Dept of Health, Education, and Welfare publication (HRA) 75-1527.

32. *1980 Census of Population*. Washington, DC: Bureau of the Census; 1981. Bureau of the Census publication PC80-51-1.

33. Martin F. *Introduction to Audiology*. Englewood Cliffs, NJ: Prentice-Hall International Inc; 1975.

34. Gang R. The effects of age on the diagnostic utility of the rollover phenomenon. *J Speech Hear Disord* 1976;41:63–69.

35. Jerger J, Jerger S. Psychoacoustic comparison of cochlear and VIIIth nerve disorders. *J Speech Hear Res* 1967;10:659–688.

36. Hosford-Dunn H. Auditory function tests. In: Cummings WC, Fredrickson JM, Harker LA, et al, eds. *Otolaryngology–Head and Neck Surgery*. St Louis, Mo: CV Mosby Co; 1986;4:2779–2817.

37. Harper-Barduch P, Harker A. Advances for the hearing impaired. In: Cummings WC, Fredrickson JM, Harker LA, et al, eds. *Otolaryngology–Head and Neck Surgery*. St Louis, Mo: CV Mosby Co; 1986;4:3247–3277.

38. Miller MH. Restoring hearing to the older patient: the physician's role. *Geriatrics* 1986;41:75–88.

39. Silman S, Geltand SA, Silverman CA. Late-onset auditory deprivation: effects of monaural vs binaural hearing aids. *J Acoust Soc Am* 1984;76:1357–1362.

40. Corrado OJ. Hearing aids. *Br Med J* 1988;296:33–35.

41. Brooks D: Hearing aid use and the effects of counseling. *Aust J Audiol* 1979;1:1–6.

42. Franks JR, Beckmann NJ: Rejection of hearing aids: attitudes of a geriatric sample. *Ear Hear* 1985;6:161–166.

43. Kapteyn T. Satisfaction with fitted hearing aids, II: an investigation into the influence of psychosocial factors. *Scand Audiol* 1977;6:171–177.

44. Matkin ND, Hodgson WR. Amplification and the elderly patient. *Otolaryngol Clin North Am* 1982;15:371–386.

45. McCabe BF. Vestibular physiology: its clinical application in understanding the dizzy patient. In: Paparella MM and Shumrick DA, (Eds). *Otolaryngology*. Philadelphia, Pa: WB Saunders Co; 1973;318–328.

46. Belal A, Glorig A. Dysequilibrium of ageing (presbyastasis). *J Laryngol Otol* 1986;100:1037–1041.

47. Black FO, Effron MZ, Burns DS. Diagnosis and management of drop attacks of vestibular origin: Tumarkin's otolithic crisis. *Otolaryngol Head Neck Surg* 1982;90:256–262.

48. Norré ME, Beckers A. Benign paroxysmal positional vertigo in the elderly: treatment by habituation exercises. *J Am Geriatr Soc* 1988;36:425–429.

49. Mathog RH, Peppard SB. Exercise and recovery from vestibular injury. *Am J Otolaryngol* 1982;3:397–407.

50. Engstrom H, Ades HW, Engstrom D, et al. Structural changes in the vestibular epithelia in elderly monkeys and humans. *Adv Otorhinolaryngol* 1977;22:93–110.

51. Rosenthal U. Epithelial cysts in the human vestibular apparatus. *J. Laryngol Otol* 1974;88:105–112.

52. Bergstrom B. Morphology of the vestibular nerve, II: the number of myelinated vestibular nerve fibers in men at various ages. *Acta Otolaryngol* 1973;76:173–179.

53. Richter E. Counts of neurons in Scarpa's ganglion from human temporal bones. In: Lim DJ, ed. *Abstracts of the Second Midwinter Research Meeting* of the *Association for Research in Otolaryngology;* January 22–24, 1979; St Petersburg Beach, Fl. Abstract 38.

54. Ross MD, Peacor D, Johnson L, et al. Observations on normal and degenerating human otoconia. *Ann Otol Rhinol Laryngol* 1976;85:310–326.

55. Babin RW, Harker LA. The vestibular system in the elderly. *Otolaryngol Clin North Am* 1982;15:387–393.

56. Johnsson LG. Sensory and neural degeneration with aging, as seen in micro-dissections of the human inner ear. *Ann Otol Rhinol Laryngol* 1972;81:179–193.

57. Schuknecht HF. *Pathology of the Ear*. Cambridge, Mass: Harvard University Press; 1974.

58. Gacek RR. Transection of the ampullary nerve for relief of benign paroxysmal positional vertigo. *Ann Otol Rhinol Laryngol* 1974;80:596–605.

32

Oral Disease

Robert S. Felder

Edentulism, once a hallmark of aging, is declining. Data from national surveys (1957–1983) indicate that edentulism among 65- to 74-year-old persons decreased from 55.4% to 34.1%.[1-3] This trend is expected to continue as the younger, dentally aware, population ages.

Along with the benefits associated with tooth retention, dentate elderly persons may expect increased dental problems—decay, gingivitis, and periodontitis—and their caregivers will be faced with complex oral care procedures. Dental surveys have noted needs among dentate elderly persons as comparable with or greater than younger cohorts,[4,5] challenging the youth-orientated concepts depicted in dentrifice advertising.

In addition to tooth-related diseases, oral lesions and denture problems are common in elderly persons.[6,7] Despite the prevalence of these oral problems, elderly persons are poor utilizers of dental services.

Although almost one third of elderly persons reported dental visits within 12 months, 44% had not seen a dentist in 5 or more years.[8] Significantly, the majority of these infrequent dental utilizers were edentulous; 74% of edentulous elderly persons interviewed had not been to a dentist in 5 or more years.

Since these patients, who are irregular users of dental services, receive regular medical care, it is important for physicians to perform thorough oral examinations and to distinguish normal aging changes from oral disease.

Significance of Oral Disease

Diseases of the oral cavity can be prevented or treated with routine dental visits and patient cooperation. If neglected, however, insidious, progressive oral diseases become increasingly difficult and expensive to treat; small lesions become crowns, requiring root canal treatment, or become unsalvable, requiring extraction. Extracted teeth decrease the patient's ability to chew, and replacements often are poor substitutes; complete maxillary and mandibular dentures have only 17% to 20% the biting force of natural teeth.[9]

Deteriorating oral health can lead to systemic problems. There is the obvious, though difficult to document, effect on nutrition,[10] as well as an association with asphyxiation secondary to incomplete mastication.[11] Most orofacial infections are odontogenic in origin. Complications include maxillary sinusitis, osteomyelitis, Ludwig's angina, and cavernous sinus thrombosis.[12-14]

Hematogenous spread of oral flora has been documented in odontogenic infections, during dental procedures, and during eating or toothbrushing.[15,16] These bacteremias have been implicated in bacterial endocarditis,[17] infections of prosthetic cardiac valves[18] and hip prostheses,[19] and brain abscesses.[20,21] Because bacteremias are more likely in the presence of gingivitis and periodontitis,[22,23] as well as in odontogenic infections,[12] it is particularly important for people susceptible to endocarditis to maintain oral health (see Chapter 11).

Infections in elderly persons often present as an alteration in mental functioning.[24] Considering that even mild periodontal infections expose approximately 20 cm^2 of connective tissue to the complex bacterial flora of the oral cavity,[25] infections of the oral cavity may very likely cause changes in mental functioning as well. In addition, fevers of unknown origin have occasionally been attributed to dental causes.[26]

The oral cavity contributes to appearance: a good dental condition fosters self-confidence and improved self-image.[27,28] With elderly persons at an increased risk for depression and social isolation, edentulism, poorly fitting dentures, teeth in disrepair, and halitosis affect socialization. A healthy mouth also is important for communication, both for clear enunciation and to provide necessary information during lipreading.

Oral Structures: Aging and Disease

Teeth

Elderly people, especially the oldest age groups, had very different dental experiences than young people do today. They were not exposed to preventive dental techniques (annual checkups, fluoridated dentifrices/water supplies), and they did not benefit from modern dental knowledge (eg, many teeth were extracted because of arthritis and other systemic problems) or improved dental techniques (eg, local anesthesia, high-speed handpieces, root canal therapy). They sought dental services only when they were in pain and were treated by extractions.

Although tooth loss clearly increases with age, sufficient numbers of very old individuals with complete, or nearly complete, dentitions exist to dispel the notion that tooth loss is inevitable. The predominant cause of tooth loss in elderly persons is thought to be periodontal disease, a disease of the supporting tissues. However, recent longitudinal data suggest that dental decay continues to be a major cause of tooth loss in elderly persons.[29]

Among elderly persons with teeth, there is a high prevalence of decay.[4,30] While this may be due to decreased dental utilization and reflect a long-term process, a recent longitudinal study reported that elderly persons are at an increased risk for new decay as well, finding newly decayed lesions at 36-month follow-up in 78% of a random sample of community-dwelling elderly persons.[31]

Patterns of decay change with age. Root surface lesions, which are common only in older age groups, must be preceded by gingival recession.[31,32] Recession and root decay, though associated with elderly persons, actually seem to be due to declining oral care and not aging per se.[33] Age-related changes reliably observed in teeth include increased wear, discoloration, and the gradual constriction of pulp chambers and root canals.

Supporting Tissues

Periodontal disease (periodontitis) is an insidious, painless disease common in adults. Most tooth loss after the age of 40 years is attributed to this disease. Periodontitis can present as inflamed, bleeding gingiva, gingival recession, mobile teeth, and halitosis. Like decay, periodontal disease is associated with dental plaque that accumulates on teeth, in gingival pockets (under the gingiva along the tooth root), and in calculus (the calcified deposits often noted on teeth and in gingival pockets). As the disease progresses, the supporting structures of the teeth—the periodontal ligaments and the alveolar bone—are destroyed, eventually causing tooth mobility and ultimately resulting in tooth loss. The disease is irreversible. In addition to the decreased function associated with periodontitis, it causes a break in the body's physical defenses, exposing the blood stream to a complex bacterial flora.

Alveolar Ridges

Alveolar ridges in edentulous people are needed to support dentures, or in the absence of dentures, to aid in mastication. Edentulous ridges should appear healthy, covered with firm attached gingiva, without evidence of edematous or redundant tissue. Alveolar ridges resorb with time, often quite rapidly, significantly interfering with masticatory function. Resorption has been attributed to normal aging, denture use, trauma, and certain metabolic processes[34] (eg, osteoporosis has been linked with rapid ridge resorption[35]).

Dentures are designed to distribute the forces of mastication over the largest possible surface area. As alveolar ridges change, these forces become concentrated, resulting in rapid focal resorption. Although denture age per se is not a good indicator of denture problems, one study noted that 40% of dentures that were 5 years old, and 80% of dentures 11 years old, needed replacement.[36] Therefore, to protect the health of the oral tissues, as well as to preserve denture function, dentures must be examined, refitted, and replaced periodically.

Oral Mucosa

The oral cavity is lined by a stratified squamous epithelium that functions as a barrier between the internal and external environments. This provides protection against entry of noxious substances and organisms, as well as decreasing mechanical damage. The masticatory mucosa of the gingiva and hard palate is keratinized, has a dense lamina propria, and serves to withstand the forces of functional trauma. The lining mucosa of the cheek, soft palate, floor of the mouth, and ventral tongue surface is nonkeratinized with increased elastic fibers within a less dense lamina propria. It serves to permit movement and extension.

Often, the oral mucosa in elderly persons appears to be thin, smooth, and dry, with a satinlike, edematous appearance and loss of elasticity and stippling. A study of 70-year-old persons found only 23% with healthy oral mucosae. Edentulous patients had the lowest rate of healthy mucosal tissues: 6% for men and 10% for women.[37] Much of the observed clinical variation seems to be due to the effects of systemic disease or medications, rather than age, on the oral cavity.[38]

Oral lesions are common in elderly individuals. A prevalence study of over 23,000 white Americans, with an average age of 56 years, discovered oral lesions in 10.3%; leukoplakia was the most common lesion reported.[39] The study noted the prevalence of squamous cell carcinoma to be 2.4/1,000 males, 1.1/1,000 overall.[39] Oral mucosal lesions were found in 23% of community-dwelling elderly persons, the majority of whom were denture wearers.[6]

Some of these lesions are due to medication side effects (Table 32.1). Oral lesions temporally associated with new medication use, or increased medication dose, often fall into this category.

Oral cancer increases with age. It is estimated that of the 985,000 new cases of all cancers (excluding skin) diagnosed during 1988 in the United States, approximately 30,200 (3.1%) will be oral cancer, and approximately 9,000 deaths will result.[40] Oral cancers are more common in men and increase dramatically with age (Fig. 32.1).

Oral lesions should arouse suspicion of oral cancer in the presence of risk factors (Table 32.2), or if the lesion is erythematous, leukoplakic, ulcerated, erosive, or fixed. The vast majority of oral cancers occur in three areas: the floor of the mouth, the soft palate–anterior pillar–retromolar complex, and the ventro-lateral portion of the tongue.[41]

A biopsy and/or dental consultation is indicated to evaluate any undiagnosed lesion present in the oral cavity for more than 2 weeks. The dye toluidine blue, a metachromatic nuclear stain, has been shown to be useful in differentiating between innocuous oral le-

Table 32.1. Oral manifestations of drug therapy*

Condition	Examples
Xerostomia	All medications that either stimulate sympathetic activity or depress parasympathetic activity
Sialorrhea	Neostigmine
Gingival hyperplasia	Phenytoin
Candidiasis	Corticosteroids
Mucositis/glossitis	Cytotoxic drugs (5-fluorouracil)
Salivary gland problems	Methyldopa
Petechiae/bleeding gums	Warfarin sodium
General oral lesions	Gold compounds
Lichenoid lesions	Methyldopa
Erythema multiforme	Sulphonamides
Lupus erythematosus	Hydralazine
Tardive dyskinesias	Neuroleptic drugs
Taste changes,	ACE† inhibitors (eg, captopril)
Pigmentation	Tetracycline
Facial neuritis	Nitrofurantoin

*Adapted from Felder et al.[81]
†ACE indicates angiotensin converting enzyme.

sions and cancerous ones and in detecting lesions at very early stages.[42,43]

Salivary Glands

The major salivary glands (parotid, submandibular, and sublingual) should be palpated during oral exami-

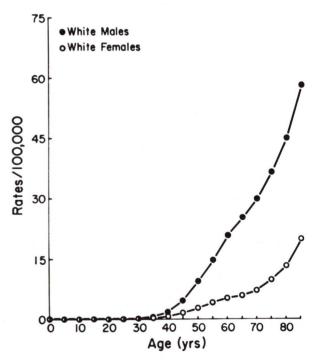

Fig. 32.1. Incidence of oral cavity cancers by age (adapted from McKay et al[80]).

Table 32.2. Risk factors associated with oral cancer

Risk Factor	Association
Gender	Male: female ratio, 2.1 : 1
Age	Rare below the age of 40 years; increases dramatically thereafter
Tobacco	Overwhelming evidence linking tobacco (including smokeless) with oral cancer
Alcohol	Overwhelming evidence linking alcohol with oral cancer, also strong evidence showing that alcohol and tobacco act synergistically
Oral status	One study reported that when controlling for tobacco and alcohol, a poor dentition increased the odds of developing oral cancer by factor of 3[82]
Diet	Certain dietary deficiencies are associated with oral cancer (vitamins A, C, and E, and beta carotenes), though the effect is small compared with tobacco and alcohol
Sunlight	Implicated, though not well proved, in cases in lower lip cancers
Systemic	Immunosuppression, syphilis, Plummer-Vinson syndrome

nations. Wharton's ducts, emptying into the anterior floor of the mouth, and Stensen's ducts, located in the cheeks approximately opposite the maxillary second molars, should be examined for evidence of infection or blockage. By "milking" the parotid or submandibular glands, they can be observed for the expression and character of saliva and the presence of pus or stones.

Salivary gland swelling can be due to sialolithiasis (calculus forming in a duct), sialadenitis (nonspecific inflammation of the salivary glands), epidemic parotitis (mumps), Sjögren's syndrome, sarcoidosis, or neoplasms.

Salivary gland disorders have significant dental effects due to changes in the quality and quantity of saliva. Saliva, in addition to its role in food digestion, lubricates the oral mucosa, decreasing abrasion and facilitating speech and swallowing. Xerostomatic patients have difficulty with eating; food adheres to oral structures and cannot be formed into a bolus for swallowing. Taste is also altered. Saliva protects teeth by cleansing, buffering, and providing antibacterial activity, as well as by remineralizing small lesions in enamel surfaces.[44] Xerostomatic patients also have difficulty with denture retention, because they lack the adhesive (wetting) properties of saliva.

Xerostomia can cause dramatically rapid carious destruction of the teeth. Xerostomatic patients are also at increased risk for chronic recurrent sialadenitis, *Candida albicans* infections, and a painful or burning mouth.

Although dry mouth is a frequent complaint of elderly persons, generally this does not correspond well to measured declines in major salivary gland secretion. However, complaints of dry mouth associated with eating (difficulty with swallowing food, needing liquid to aid in swallowing dry food) are good indications of compromised salivary function.[45] In extreme cases, a diagnosis of xerostomia is straightforward: a dry, erythematous oral mucosa to which tongue blades often adhere during the oral examination.

The current literature reports that clinically detectable xerostomia in aged individuals is not due to aging.[46] Often, this xerostomia is due to medications that either stimulate sympathetic activity or depress parasympathetic activity; a recent review cited 375 medications with xerostomatic effects.[47] Studies of salivary flow rates in medicated subjects noted reduced rates, in general, with increased drug use[48] and, in particular, with tricyclic antidepressants, neuroleptic medications, and hypotensive agents.[49] If the underlying cause for xerostomia cannot be treated, symptomatic approaches to management must be implemented. In addition to intensive oral care to protect the teeth, which should include increased use of fluorides (rinses, gels), saliva substitues are available and are effective. Medications to stimulate flow, ie, pilocarpine, have been effective in some cases.[50]

Changes in Oral Function With Age

The ability to perform the complex, coordinated movements associated with speech, swallowing, and mastication seems to decline with normal aging. Along with general declines in muscle size, numbers of motor fibers, and sensory abilities,[51] studies have reported decreased lip competency, decreased masticatory functions, and alteration in tongue function.[51,52] Changes in swallowing abilities were not seen in these studies. Among frail elderly persons, these changes can significantly affect nutrition, communication, and deglutition.

Oral-facial dyskinesias, ie, involuntary movements of the face, lips, tongue, and jaw, have been associated with a spontaneous onset, psychiatric disorders, tardive dyskinesia, senile dyskinesias, and poorly fitting dentures or edentulism.[53–56] Dyskinesias due to dental problems can usually be eliminated with treatment. Tardive dyskinesia, a severely debilitating oral-facial dyskinesia, is associated with long-term neuroleptic medication use (see Chapter 33). Tardive dyskinesia significantly interferes with mastication, communication, and the ability to use removable oral prostheses.[55]

Facial Pain in Elderly Persons

The temporomandibular joint (TMJ) is a gliding, hingelike connection between the glenoid fossa of the temporal bone and the condylar process of the mandible. It has been implicated in a variety of facial pain disorders that may originate either in the joint or in related structures.

Temporomandibular joint dysfunction can be difficult to diagnose; one study reported that, on average, patients with TMJ problems presenting to a California facial pain center had been seen by seven health professionals (physicians, dentists, psychologists, and others) without a proper diagnosis.[57] Temporomandibular joint disorders are found with equal frequency among men and women in their third to fifth decades, although women outnumber men among those actively seeking treatment for the disorder.[58] Because many of the joint disorders are a result of structural changes of the TMJ, one would expect an increased frequency of TMJ problems in elderly persons. However, few patients older than 60 years of age present with complaints attributable to TMJ problems.[59] Studies of TMJ problems among community-dwelling elderly persons, while showing a decline with age, suggest it is more prevalent than treatment-seeking behavior indicates.[59,60] Prevalence does not seem to vary between dentate and edentulous individuals.[61]

The TMJs should be palpated, bilaterally, just anterior to the external auditory meatus. Pain or crepitus that is noted while the patient opens and closes the mouth, or when moving the jaw from side to side, may indicate joint or muscle dysfunction. Auscultation may reveal abnormal joint sounds (popping, clicking) as well. Restricted maximum opening may indicate TMJ disorders. Average adult maximal opening, measured between the tips of the incisors, ranges from 40 to 55 mm.

Some longitudinal studies suggest that TMJ disorders follow a general pattern: from joint noises alone, to joint noise and pain, to joint remodeling, and to cessation of symptoms.[62,63] However, great variability has been reported, with various symptoms lasting from 1 month to 46 years.

Burning Mouth

Patients often have vague complaints of burning mouth (stomatopyrosis), or generalized mouth/tongue pain (mucusitis/glossitis). This disorder, most often presenting in postmenopausal women, has been associated with a variety of causes, including denture problems, infections, xerostomia, systemic disorders (anemias, vitamin deficiencies, hormonal changes, immunologic abnormalities), and psychologic disorders.[64–68]

Although the evidence for psychologic disorders as a component of burning mouth is usually anecdotal, psychiatric assessment performed in one study noted that 44% of patients with idiopathic burning mouth had mixed anxiety and depressive symptoms compared with 16% of cases of burning mouth with identifiable causes.[68]

Prostheses

Missing teeth can significantly disrupt masticatory function. Edentulous areas often are occluded by adjacent teeth that tilt or drift and by opposing teeth that supererupt into the vacant space. In addition to disrupting function, this process jeopardizes the health of the surrounding teeth and makes future restoration of the area more difficult and expensive.

Replacement teeth can be either fixed or removable. Fixed bridges attach replacement teeth to crowns made for adjacent natural teeth, and these are cemented into place. Removable dentures are plastic or porcelain teeth attached to an acrylic and/or metal base; they can replace any or all of the teeth. These are removed after meals for cleaning.

Denture problems are common. One study suggested that over one third of elderly denture wearers need prosthodontic treatment.[7] Removable prostheses should be inspected for damage, general hygiene, and identification. Dentures should be stable and retentive. Patients should be questioned as to the fit of their dentures, and this should be confirmed clinically. Dentures should be labeled, especially among institutionalized patients, with the patient's name or other identifying information. This can be done simply with a marking pen and clear varnish, or with a commercially available marking kit.

Diet orders for edentulous patients need to be individualized. There is much variability in function among denture wearers and among edentulous people without dentures. The routine placement of edentulous patients on soft diets does them a disservice, and it may jeopardize their nutrition by the reduced intake of food in this unappetizing form.

Dentures, like teeth, need daily oral care; they should be rinsed and brushed after every meal. Dentures should be soaked overnight in plain water or some freshening preparation. The oral tissues, including the tongue, should be brushed with a soft toothbrush and rinsed with water.

Some patients find that they cannot sleep without their dentures; some just cannot get used to it, others develop orofacial muscle or joint pain, and still others find it socially unacceptable. These patients must maintain the health of their tissue by removing their dentures and brushing their oral tissues periodically.

Oral Care Among Institutionalized Residents

Institutionalized residents are at risk for the rapid destruction of their teeth due to a variety of factors. Medication use among institutionalized residents is much higher than in other groups. Many medications have oral side effects, especially xerostomia; others have a high sugar content, eg, phenytoin suspension. Medications also can mask symptoms of oral disease (eg, pain medications) or the patient's ability to discuss them (eg, psychotropics). Many patients receive multiple snacks to improve caloric intake, without increased attention to oral care.

The resident's ability for adequate self-care is often compromised by depression, physical problems, and mental changes. Regular, adequate assistance in oral care often is difficult to obtain in institutions.

Access to dental care is often a problem as well. While some dentists and dental hygienists provide ongoing treatment at long-term care facilities, most require that the patient be brought to the dentist's office. Studies have shown that the average nursing home patient has not seen a dentist for about 5 years.[69,70]

Oral care can be improved by emphasizing its importance to long-term care staff and by consultation with other disciplines. Occupational therapists can determine the best method for the resident to use a toothbrush. Simple adaptations, such as changing grips on toothbrushes, or supplying hemiplegic patients with suction denture brushes, can make the difference between adequate and inadequate care. Dentists and dental hygienists can recommend specific brushes, including double-headed brushes[71] or electric toothbrushes, and can assess the patient's ability to brush with these adaptations.

Chemotherapeutic methods of oral care, such as fluoridated dentrifices, fluoride rinses, and some of the plaque-reduction rinses (eg, chlorhexidine), are useful adjuncts to oral care[72,73] and should be considered in dentate institutionalized patients.

Dental Treatment of Compromised Elderly Patients

All conditions that lower a patient's ability to handle stress need to be considered during dental treatment. This can range from a history of cerebrovascular accidents to long-term steroid use. Routine dental care in the presence of cardiac disease has a good safety record. Studies of cardiac changes during dental treatment on healthy[74,75] and cardiac patients[76,77] show only slight increases in cardiac output (due to either an increased heart rate or increased stroke volume—

blood pressure changes vary). Hypertensive patients should be treated cautiously; patients with diastolic pressures greater than 115 mm Hg should not receive dental treatment until under better control. Recent myocardial infarctions (within 6 months) or unstable angina are also considered to place dental patients at increased risk.[78] Routine dental treatment should be also be deferred in these cases.

Particularly anxious patients, especially those with medical risks associated with stress, may need antianxiety medication before treatment. Geriatric doses of short-acting benzodiazepines (oxazepam, lorazepam, alprazolam) or choral hydrate usually are helpful. Also, nitrous oxide, available in many dental offices, and a drug that the dentist is skilled at using, is often an excellent choice with elderly patients.

Antibiotic prophylaxis often is necessary in the treatment of geriatric patients. It has been recommended for various cardiac conditions (see Chapter 11), as well as for joint prostheses,[19,79] although the basis for the latter is less firm.

Summary

Oral health among elderly individuals has implications beyond the oral cavity. Quality of life must be considered: an attractive, functional oral cavity is important to people of all ages. Oral health enhances the taste and enjoyment of food. Broken-down teeth, poorly fitting dentures, and oral pain will significantly influence which foods can be managed, decreasing choices and much of the pleasure associated with eating. With extreme age or disability, such pleasures may be paramount.

References

1. Burnham CE. Edentulous persons, United States, 1971. *Vital Health Stat 10* 1974;89:1–30.
2. Kelly JE, Harvey CR. Basic dental examination findings of persons 1–74 years. *Vital Health Stat 11* 1979;214:1–33.
3. Ishmail AI, Burt BA, Hendershot GE, et al. Findings from the dental care supplement of the National Health Interview Survey, 1963. *J Am Dent Assoc* 1987;114:617–621.
4. Hughs JT, Rosier RG, Ramsey DL. *Natural History of Dental Diseases in North Carolina 1976–1977.* Durham, NC: Carolina Academic Press; 1982.
5. National Institutes of Health. *Oral Health of United States Adults—National Findings: The National Survey of Oral Health in US Employed Adults and Seniors: 1985–1986.* Washington, DC: National Institutes of Health NIH publication 87-2868; 1987.
6. Hand JS, Whitehill JM. The prevalence of oral mucosal lesions in an elderly population. *J Am Dent Assoc* 1986;112:73–76.

7. Hunt RJ, Srisilapanan P, Beck JD. Denture-related problems and prosthodontic treatment needs in the elderly. *Gerodontics* 1985;1:226–230.

8. Current estimates from the National Health Interview Survey: United States, 1980. *Vital Health Stat 10* 1981;139:28–31.

9. Haroldsson T, Carlsson GE, Ingervall B. Bite force and oral function in patients with complete dentures. *J Oral Rehabil* 1979;6:41.

10. Hartsook E. Food selection, dietary adequacy and related dental problems of patients with dental prostheses. *J Prosthet Dent* 1974;32:32–40.

11. Mittleman RE, Wetli CV. The fatal café coronary: foreign-body airway obstruction. *JAMA* 1982;247:1285–1288.

12. Chow AW, Roser SM, Brady FA. Orofacial odontogenic infections. *Ann Intern Med* 1978;88:392–402.

13. Goteiner D, Sonis ST, Faciano R. Cavernous sinus thrombosis and brain abscess initiated and maintained by periodontally involved teeth. *J Oral Med* 1982;37:80–83.

14. Fielding AF, Matise JL, Cross S, et al. Cavernous sinus thrombosis: report of a case. *J Am Dent Assoc* 1983;106:342–345.

15. De Leo AA, Schoenkneckt FD, Anderson MW, et al. The incidence of bacteremia following oral prophylaxis on pediatric patients. *Oral Surg Oral Med Oral Pathol* 1974;37:36–45.

16. Balth AL, Schaffer C, Hammer MC, et al. Bacteremia following dental cleaning in patients with and without penicillin prophylaxis. *Am Heart J* 1982;104:1335–1339.

17. Shulman At, Amren DP, Bisno AL, et al. Prevention of bacterial endocarditis: a statement for health professionals by the committee on rheumatic fever and infective endocarditis of the Council on Cardiovascular Disease in the Young. *Circulation* 1984;70:1123A–1127A.

18. Baumgartner JC, Plack WF. Dental treatment and management of a patient with a prosthetic heart valve. *J Am Dent Assoc* 1982;104:181–184.

19. Jacobson JJ, Matthews LS. Bacteria isolated from late prosthetic joint infections: dental treatment and chemoprophylaxis. *Oral Surg Oral Med Oral Pathol* 1987;63:122–126.

20. Aldous JA, Powell GL, Stensaas SS. Brain abscess of odontogenic origin: report of a case. *J Am Dent Assoc* 1987;115:861–863.

21. Ingham HR, High AS, Kalbag RM, et al. Abscesses of the frontal lobe of the brain secondary to covert dental sepsis. *Lancet* 1978;2:497–499.

22. Okell CC, Elliott SD. Bacteraemia and oral sepsis. *Lancet* 1935;2:869–872.

23. McEntegart MG, Poterfield JS. Bacteraemia following dental extractions. *Lancet* 1949;2:596–598.

24. Garibaldi RA. Infections in the elderly. *Am J Med* 1986;81(suppl 1A):53–58.

25. Bennett JS, Creamer HR. Oral diseases. In: Cassel CK, Walsh JR, eds. *Geriatric Medicine.* New York, NY: Springer-Verlag NY Inc; 1984:545.

26. Shinoda T, Mizutani H, Kaneda T, et al. Fever of unknown origin caused by dental infection. *Oral Surg Oral Med Oral Pathol* 1987;64:175–178.

27. Albino JE, Tedesco LA, Conny DJ. Patient perceptions of dental-facial esthetics: shared concerns in orthodontics and prosthetics. *J Prosthet Dent* 1984;52:9–13.

28. Ofstehage J. The social and psychological importance of dental-facial attractiveness in the elderly. *Geriatr Dent Update Newsletter* 1987;1:31–33.

29. Beck J. Trends in oral disease and health. *Gerodontology* 1988;7:21–25.

30. Hand JS, Hunt RJ, Beck JD. Incidence of coronal and root caries in an older adult population. *J Public Health Dent* 1988;48:14–19.

31. Hand JS, Hunt RJ. Coronal and root caries in older adults: 36 month incidence. *J Dent Res* 1988;67:176. Abstract.

32. Wallace MC, Retief DH, Bradley EL. Prevalence of root caries in a population of older adults. *Gerodontics* 1988;4:84–89.

33. Vehkulahti MM, Paunio IK. Occurrence of root caries in relation to dental health behavior. *J Dent Res* 1988;67:911–914.

34. Atwood DA. The problem of reduction of residual ridges. In: Winkler S, ed. *Essentials of Complete Denture Prosthodontics.* 2nd ed. Philadelphia, Pa: WB Saunders Co; 1980:22–38.

35. Engstrom H, Libanati C, Schultz ES, et al. Spinal density and dentition in osteoporotic patients. Presented at the American Association of Dental Research, October, 1985.

36. Hoad-Reddick G, Grant AA, Griffiths C. The search for an indicator of need for denture replacement in an edentulous elderly population. *Gerodontics* 1987;3:223–226.

37. Osterberg T, Ohman A, Heyden G, et al. The condition of the oral mucosa at age 70: a population study. *Geriodontology* 1985;4:71–75.

38. Mackenzie IC, Holm-Pedersen P, Karring T. Age changes in the oral mucous membranes and periodontium. In: Holm-Pedersen P, Loe H, eds. *Geriatric Dentistry.* Copenhagen, Denmark: Munksgaard, International Publishers Ltd; 1986:102–113.

39. Bouquot JE. Common oral lesions found during a mass screening examination. *J Am Dent Assoc* 1986;112:50–57.

40. Silverberg E, Lubera JA. Cancer Statistics, 1988. *CA* 1988;38:14–15.

41. Mashberg A. Anatomical site and size of 222 early asymptomatic oral squamous cell carcinomas, II: a continuing prospective study of oral cancer. *Cancer* 1976;37:2149–2157.

42. Mashberg A. Final evaluation of tolonium chloride rinse for screening of high-risk patients with asymptomatic squamous carcinoma. *J Am Dent Assoc* 1983;106:319–323.

43. Moyer GN, Taybos GM, Pelleu GB. Toluidine blue rinse: potential for benign lesions in early detection of oral neoplasms. *J Oral Med* 1986;41:111–113.

44. Baum BJ. Salivary gland function during aging. *Gerodontics* 1986;2:61–64.

45. Fox PC, Busch KA, Baum BJ. Subjective reports of xerostomia and objective measures of salivary gland performance. *J Am Dent Assoc* 1987;115:581–584.

46. Heft MW, Baum BJ. Unstimulated and stimulated parotid salivary flow rate in individuals of different ages. *J Dent Res* 1984;63:1182–1185.

47. Sreebny LM, Secwartz SS. A reference guide to drugs and dry mouth. *Gerontology* 1986;5:75–99.

48. Osterberg T, Landahl S, Hedegard B. Salivary flow, saliva, pH and buffering capacity in 70-year-old men and women. *J Oral Rehabil* 1984;11:157–170.

49. Parvinen T, Parvinen I, Larmas M. Stimulated salivary flow rate, pH and lactobacillus and yeast concentrations in medicated persons. *Scand J Dent Res* 1984;92:179–187.

50. Fox PC, van der Ven PF, Baum BJ, et al. Pilocarpine for the treatment of xerostomia associated with salivary gland dysfunction. *Oral Surg Oral Med Oral Pathol* 1986;61:243–245.

51. Baum BJ, Bodner L. Aging and oral motor function: evidence for altered performance among older persons. *J Dent Res* 1983;62:2–6.

52. Feldman RS, Kapur KK, Aalman JE, et al. Aging and mastication: changes in performance and in the swallowing threshold with natural dentition. *J Am Geriatr Soc* 1980;28:97–103.

53. Koller WC. Idiopathic oral-facial dyskinesia. In: Jankovic J, Tolosa E, eds. *Advances in Neurology*. New York, NY: Raven Press; 1988, vol 49: *Facial Dyskinesias*. pp 177–183.

54. Sutcher HD, Underwood RG, Beatty RV, et al. Orofacial dyskinesia: a dental dimension. *JAMA* 1971; 216:1459–1461.

55. Sutcher HD, Beatty RA, Underwood RG. Orofacial dyskinesia: effective prosthetic therapy. *J Prosthet Dent* 1973;30:252–262.

56. Klawans HL, Tanner CM, Goetz CG. Epidemiology and pathophysiology of tardive dyskinesias. In: Jankovic J, Tolosa E, eds. *Advances in Neurology*. New York, NY: Raven Press; 1988, vol 49: *Facial Dyskinesias*, pp 185–197.

57. Tanaka TT. A rational approach to the differential diagnosis of arthritic disorders. *J Prosthet Dent* 1986;56:727–731.

58. Greene CS, Marbach JJ. Epidemiologic studies of mandibular dysfunction: a critical review. *J Prosthet Dent* 1982;48:184–190.

59. Clark GT, Mulligan R. A review of the prevalence of temporomandibular dysfunction. *Gerodontology* 1984; 3:231–236.

60. Heft MW. Prevalence of TMJ signs and symptoms in the elderly. *Gerodontology* 1984;3:125–130.

61. Sakurai DK, San Biacomo T, Arbree NS, et al. A survey of temporomandibular joint dysfunction in completely edentulous patients. *J Prosthet Dent* 1988;59:81–85.

62. Rasmussen OC. Description of population and progress of symptoms in a longitudinal study of temporomandibular arthropathy. *Scand J Dent Res* 1981;89:196–203.

63. Brooke RI, Leeds LDS, Grainger RM. Long-term prognosis for the clicking jaw. *Oral Surg Oral Med Oral Pathol* 1988;65:668–670.

64. Zegarelli DJ. Burning mouth: an analysis of 57 patients. *Oral Surg Oral Med Pathol* 1984;58:34–38.

65. Basker RM, Sturdee DW, Davenport JC. Patients with burning mouths: a clinical investigation of causative factors, including the climacteric and diabetes. *Br Dent J* 1978;145:9–16.

66. Grushka M. Clinical features of burning mouth syndrome. *Oral Surg Oral Med Oral Pathol* 1987;63:30–36.

67. van der Ploeg HM, Wal van der N, Eijkman HM, et al. Psychological aspects of patients with burning mouth syndrome. *Oral Surg Oral Med Oral Pathol* 1987; 63:664–668.

68. Browning S, Hislop S, Scully C, et al. The association between burning mouth syndrome and psychosocial disorders. *Oral Surg Oral Med Oral Pathol* 1987;64:171–174.

69. Bagramian RA, Heller RP. Dental health assessment of a population of nursing home residents. *J Gerontol* 1977;32:168–174.

70. Emprey G, Kiyak A, Milgrom P. Oral health in nursing homes. *Spec Care Dent* 1983;3:65–67.

71. Gibson MT, Joyston-Bechal S, Smales FC. Clinical evaluation of plaque removal with a double-headed toothbrush. *J Clin Periodontol* 1988;15:94–98.

72. Swango PA. The use of topical fluorides to prevent dental caries in adults: a review of the literature. *J Am Dent Assoc* 1983;107:447–450.

73. Fardal O, Turnbull RS. A review of the literature on use of chlorhexidine in dentistry. *J Am Dent Assoc* 1986;112:863–869.

74. Chernow B, Balestrieri F, Ferguson CD, et al. Local dental anesthesia with epinephrine: minimal effects on the sympathetic nervous system or on hemodynamic variables. *Arch Intern Med* 1983;143:2141–2143.

75. Abraham-Inpijn L, Borgmeiger-Hoelen A, Gortzak RA. Changes in blood pressure, heart rate, and electrocardiogram during dental treatment with use of local anesthesia. *J Am Dent Assoc* 1988;116:531–536.

76. Hirota Y, Sugiyama K, Joh S, et al. An echocardiographic study of patients with cardiovascular disease during dental treatment using local anesthesia. *J Oral Maxillofac Surg* 1986;44:116–121.

77. Cintron G, Medina R, Reyes AA, et al. Cardiovascular effects and safety of dental anesthesia and dental interventions in patients with recent uncomplicated myocardial infarction. *Arch Intern Med* 1986;146:2203–2204.

78. Little JW, Falace DA. *Dental Management of the Medically Compromised Patient*. 2nd ed. St Louis, Mo: CV Mosby Co; 1984.

79. Jacobsen PL, Murray W. Prophylactic coverage of dental patients with artificial joints: a retrospective analysis of thirty-three infections in hip prostheses. *Oral Surg Oral Med Oral Pathol* 1980;50:130–133.

80. McKay FW, Hanson MR, Miller RW. *Cancer Mortality in the United States, 1950–1977*. National Cancer Institute Monograph 59, 1982. National Institutes of Health NIH publication 82-2435.

81. Felder RS, Millar SB, Henry RH. Manifestations of drug therapy. *Spec Care Dent* 1988;8:119–124.

82. Graham S, Cayal H, Rohrer T, et al. Dentition, diet, tobacco, and alcohol in the epidemiology of oral cancer. *JNCI* 1977;59:1611–1618.

33

Dementia

Jeffrey L. Cummings and Lissy F. Jarvik

Elderly people may manifest a variety of behavioral syndromes produced by brain dysfunction. They may show evidence of multiple deficits in the delirious and dementia syndromes or single deficits in amnestic and aphasic disorders. In addition, brain lesions may cause "productive" behavioral syndromes, such as anxiety, delusions, hallucinations, depression, mania, and personality alterations. Furthermore, these disorders are not mutually exclusive: delirium may be superimposed on dementia and is frequently accompanied by anxiety, delusions, and/or manic behavior; demented patients may manifest personality alterations, delusions, or mood changes in addition to their intellectual deficits; personality alterations often develop in patients with amnesia; and patients with aphasia may exhibit delusions or mood changes that result from their underlying disease.

Behavioral changes are among the most common presentations of illness in elderly persons and can herald the presence of a psychiatric disorder, neurologic disease, physical illness, or any combination of these. The differential diagnosis, so critical to appropriate management, can be particularly difficult in persons who often have a coexisting illness or take multiple medications and whose symptom presentation, metabolism, and performance on psychodiagnostic instruments differ from that of younger adults.

Dementia is the most common organic mental syndrome that occurs in elderly individuals. It affects 2% to 3% of 60-year-old persons and becomes increasingly common among old old individuals. Dementia is a clinical syndrome in which the potential causes include psychiatric, neurologic, systemic, and toxicologic disorders. It may be reversible or irreversible; even dementias with no available curative interventions frequently can be substantially ameliorated by appropriate clinical management. In this chapter, the definition, causes, evaluation, and treatment of dementia are presented. Behavioral syndromes of elderly individuals that must be distinguished from dementia are briefly described before the dementing disorders are discussed.

Delirium

Delirium is characterized by a reduced ability to maintain or shift attention appropriately, disorganized thinking, a reduced level of consciousness, perceptual disturbances, increased or decreased psychomotor activity, disturbances of the sleep-wake cycle, disorientation to time, place or person, and memory impairment.[1] In contrast to dementia, delirium generally has an abrupt onset and is of a relatively short duration (days to weeks); delirium also exhibits a greater impairment of arousal and more fluctuation in the level of consciousness than dementia.

In its clinical presentation, delirium is often manifested by an incoherent verbal output and frequent erratic changes in the stream of thought. Illusions, hallucinations, delusions, and signs of autonomic dysfunction are common. Errors in writing and mistakes on the Digit Span Tests are two sensitive indicators of the presence of a confusional state, but delirious patients may fail any test that requires a sustained effort, including tasks that assess comprehension, calculation, abstraction, and construction.[2] Delirious patients may draw attention to themselves through agitation and hyperactivity, or they may be outwardly calm and quiet with a minimum of overt signs; fluctuations in the level of arousal are characteristic.

Elderly (and very young) patients are particularly vulnerable to the development of delirium in the course of a medical illness. The condition is four times more common among those patients aged older than 40 years than among younger patients, and it is most frequent in those patients aged older than 70 years. Patients aged older than 75 years may have incidence rates approximately twice as high as those for patients between the ages of 65 and 75 years. Approximately one third to one half of aged patients will have a delirious episode during the course of a hospitalization for medical or surgical care.[3] Factors that predispose to the development of delirium include advanced age, combinations of medications, sensory impairment, chronic illness, structural brain disease, drug or alcohol abuse, sleep deprivation, and social isolation or unfamiliar surroundings. Delirium is more likely to develop in patients with a preexisting intellectual compromise associated with a dementing illness than in those patients with a normal premorbid cognitive status.[3] Early diagnosis and treatment of delirium are important because most patients can recover with appropriate treatment. However, advanced age and longer duration of illness worsen the prognosis, and mortality rates range from 15% to 30% among elderly persons with delirium.[4]

Virtually any acute disorder of cerebral function can produce a confusional state. Lipowski[3] recognized four classes of diseases associated with delirious states: (1) primary cerebral diseases, such as central nervous system (CNS) infections, brain tumors, and stroke; (2) systemic illnesses that secondarily affect brain function, including cardiac disease, pulmonary failure, hepatic dysfunction, uremia, deficiency states, anemia, endocrine disturbances, systemic infections, and inflammatory diseases; (3) intoxication with exogenous substances, including alcohol, illicit drugs, prescribed medications, and industrial toxins; and (4) withdrawal from dependency-producing agents, such as alcohol, barbiturates, and benzodiazepines.

Medications, drugs, and alcohol are particularly important causal factors in delirium; an excess or combination of many of these substances can cause delirium directly in the course of intoxication and secondarily during withdrawal. Geriatric patients with age-related alterations in pharmacokinetics are at special risk because the usual therapeutic dosages of medication may result in toxic drug levels.

Delirium usually is indicative of diffuse brain dysfunction, but occasionally focal lesions produce identical clinical syndromes. In such cases, the lesion is most likely in the posterior medial aspects of the left occipital lobe or in the superior posterior lateral aspects of the right parietal region.

Amnestic Syndromes

Amnesia is characterized by an impairment of memory. It is not accompanied by an impairment in judgment or abstract thinking, personality change, or other disturbance of higher cortical function.[1] Amnestic patients are not demented and are able to abstract, calculate, name, and copy normally; their attention and concentration are also normal, and their recall of remote material beyond the period of their retrograde amnesia is intact. Amnesia cannot be diagnosed in a delirious patient. Amnesia typically consists of an anterograde amnestic period that begins at the time of the precipitating event and during which learning new material is difficult or impossible, as well as a period of retrograde amnesia that extends from minutes to years backward from the time of onset of the amnesia. For that period, the patient has difficulty in recalling previously learned information. Recollection of remote information, such as childhood events, early family memories, and occupational history, is unimpaired.

Conditions that produce amnesia affect the medial hemispheric limbic circuitry and include hippocampal injury from trauma, stroke, anoxia, hypoglycemia, or infection; fornix lesions, such as trauma and neoplasms; hypothalamic-diencephalic diseases, including the Wernicke-Korsakoff syndrome (secondary to thiamine deficiency) and thalamic neoplasms; and electroconvulsive therapy.[5] Dementia is distinguished from monosymptomatic neuropsychiatric syndromes, such as aphasia and amnesia, by the simultaneous occurrence of deficits that involve several cognitive functions.

Organic Delusional Syndrome

Organic delusional syndrome is characterized by the predominance of delusions in the presence of a specific organic factor.[1] The delusions may be of any type (eg, persecutory, somatic) and may range from well organized and elaborate to crude and simple.[1] They comprise incorrect but unequivocally endorsed beliefs in the threat of harm, theft, or infidelity.[6] The most common cause of organic delusional syndrome is pharmacologic toxicity. Any one or a combination of a variety of drugs (eg, amphetamines, cocaine, marijuana) may be responsible, but cerebral lesions (eg, stroke, trauma), complex partial seizures, systemic illnesses, vitamin deficiency states, endocrinopathies, collagen-vascular disorders, and degenerative neurologic diseases (eg, Huntington's disease) also may produce an organic delusional syndrome. Medications, such as anticonvulsants, analgesics, and cancer chemotherapeutic agents, also have been implicated in the development of delusions.[7]

Organic Hallucinosis

Prominent or persistent hallucinations in the presence of a specific organic factor and not attributable to delirium are the criteria for a diagnosis of organic hallucinosis.[1] Hallucinations may be visual, auditory, tactile, olfactory, or gustatory in nature. Visual hallucinations are the most common and occur with particular frequency in delirium. Auditory hallucinations may accompany organic delusional syndromes. Causes are similar to those that produce the organic delusional syndrome; drugs (eg, LSD, mescaline, psilocybin, phencyclidine), alcohol, cerebral lesions, and sensory changes all have been associated with this syndrome.

Organic Mood Syndromes

The diagnosis of organic mood syndrome applies when there is a prominent and persistent depressed, elevated, or expansive mood, due to a specific organic factor.[1] Numerous causes have been adduced for organic mood syndrome, including medications, structural lesions of the brain, endocrinologic disorders, and viruses.[8,9] Depression syndromes are common following stroke and in the extrapyramidal disorders, whereas mania is infrequent in organic diseases but may occur in deliria or with local lesions that involve the thalamus and adjacent structures of the right hemisphere.[7]

Organic Anxiety Syndromes

Organic anxiety syndrome is characterized by the occurrence in the setting of brain dysfunction of the following symptoms on either an ongoing basis or in discrete attacks: intense feelings of fear or discomfort; dyspnea; dizziness; palpitations; trembling; sweating; choking; nausea or abdominal distress; depersonalization or derealization; paresthesias; hot flashes or chills; chest pain or discomfort; and fear of dying,

going crazy, or losing control.[1] Organic anxiety syndrome occurs with thyroid and adrenal disturbances, hypoglycemia, stimulant use, withdrawal syndromes, epilepsy, parkinsonism, pulmonary and cardiac disease, multiple sclerosis, inflammatory disorders, and infections.

Organic Personality Syndrome

Organic personality syndrome refers to a persistent personality disturbance due to a specific organic factor. It may be lifelong or represent a change or accentuation of a previously characteristic trait, including affective lability, aggression out of proportion to any provocative stimulus, impaired social judgment, apathy or indifference, or suspiciousness or paranoid ideation produced by a brain disorder. Such personality alterations occur with traumatic brain injuries, CNS neoplasms, dementia syndromes, multiple sclerosis, the extrapyramidal disorders, stroke, epilepsy, and long-term use of psychoactive substances.[1,10]

Aphasic Syndromes

Aphasia refers to a language disturbance secondary to brain damage.[9] Loss of the ability to name items and to write normally occurs in nearly all forms of aphasia. If the brain lesion is located anteriorly in the left hemisphere, the spontaneous speech of the patient will be nonfluent with few words, little paraphasia, and relative preservation of comprehension (eg, Broca's aphasia); posterior lesions produce syndromes characterized primarily by fluent output with many words, preserved speech melody, frequent paraphasia, and poor comprehension (eg, Wernicke's aphasia); and lesions large enough to encompass both anterior and posterior left hemispheric regions produce nonfluent disorders with impairments in all linguistic abilities (eg, global aphasia). Dementia is distinguishable from aphasia by the simultaneous occurrence of deficits that involve several cognitive functions.

Age-Associated Memory Impairment

The organic mental disorders must be distinguished from alterations in memory function that may accompany the normal aging process. Age-associated memory impairment, or benign senescent forgetfulness, designates a process observed in normal elderly individuals that is characterized by poor recall of specific items, such as names of people, street addresses, or rarely used vocabulary items.[11] The memory loss is variable, and the items are frequently recalled a few minutes or hours later. Age-associated memory impairment, is not incapacitating, nor does it portend the emergence of a dementing illness; individuals are able to continue to lead their lives in an unimpaired manner despite the inconvenience. The deficits of age-associated memory impairment appear to be a consequence of the reduced speed and efficiency with which the eye, ear, and brain process information. Although the early stages of dementia often are difficult to distinguish from aging changes, serial neuropsychologic assessment over time will help to make the distinction.

Dementia

Dementia is a clinical syndrome characterized by acquired persistent disturbances in multiple areas of neuropsychologic function.[12] Its onset is less abrupt, and dementia lasts longer than delirium and exhibits less impairment of arousal and less fluctuation in the level of consciousness. Dementia is distinguished from mental retardation by its late occurrence and the corresponding decline from a higher level of intellectual functioning. Dementia is distinguished from monosymptomatic neuropsychologic syndromes, such as aphasia and amnesia, by the simultaneous occurrence of deficits that involve several cognitive functions. While the syndrome must have been present for several months or more to be labeled as a dementia, the decline in intellectual ability is not necessarily irreversible, and appropriate diagnosis and treatment may produce improvement in cognitive functions. Dementing illnesses become increasingly common in old age but should not be regarded as an expected component of the normal aging process. Regardless of the patient's age, a thorough search for the cause of dementia is warranted.

The American Psychiatric Association *Diagnostic and Statistical Manual, 3rd Edition, Revised (DSM-III-R),*[1] provides the following diagnostic criteria for dementia:

A. Impairment in short- and long-term memory.
B. At least one of the following:
  1. impairment of abstract thinking, as indicated by difficulty in defining words and concepts or the relationships between objects;
  2. impaired judgment, as indicated by inability to make reasonable plans to deal with problems and issues;
  3. other disturbances of higher cortical function such as language disorder, inability to carry out motor activities despite intact comprehension and motor function, failure to recognize or identify objects

despite intact sensory function and "constructional difficulty", e.g. inability to copy three-dimensional figures, assemble blocks or arrange sticks in specific designs.
  4. personality changes.
C. The disturbance in the two preceding categories significantly interferes with work or usual social activities or relationships with others.

Dementia may result from degenerative, vascular, traumatic, neoplastic, infectious, hydrocephalic, toxic-metabolic, or depressive disorders (Table 33.1). In most cases, the character of the mental status alterations will indicate the appropriate differential diagnosis and suggest the necessary laboratory evaluations.

Primary Dementias

Dementia of the Alzheimer Type. The most prevalent of the primary dementias is known as Alzheimer's disease or dementia of the Alzheimer type (DAT); it is estimated to affect 3% to 5% of individuals aged older than 65 years, increasing to about 20% after the age of 80 years.[13] First described in 1907 by Alois Alzheimer, a German psychiatrist and neuropathologist, the disease was reported in a 51-year-old woman and, until the 1960s, was considered to be a cause of presenile dementia (onset before the age of 65 years). The typical Alzheimer-type brain lesions, neurofibrillary tangles and neuritic plaques, however, also are found in the brains of patients whose dementia has its onset in old age. Neuropathologically, the age at onset does not constitute a reliable distinguishing feature, and it is now believed that there is only one type of Alzheimer's disease, and that it occurs with a markedly increased frequency late in life. Women may be affected by DAT somewhat more commonly than men. Together, senile and presenile DAT are estimated to account for approximately 50% of progressive dementias.[14]

Genetic Aspects. In a few families, the disease manifests a pattern consistent with autosomal dominant inheritance (affecting 50% of all offspring who survive the risk period), and evidence suggests that a gene for familial DAT is located on chromosome 21—a finding of great interest, since Alzheimer-like changes eventually develop in the brains of virtually all individuals with Down's syndrome (due primarily to an extra chromosome 21). In other families, however, the inheritance pattern is obscure, and data from twin studies point to the importance of both genetic and nongenetic variables in DAT.[15,16]

Other Causal Hypotheses. In addition to a genetic factor, other hypothesized causes for DAT include a deficiency in the enzymes that mediate acetylcholine

Table 33.1. Conditions reported to produce dementia syndromes.

Condition
Primary dementing illnesses
Alzheimer's disease
Pick's disease
Huntington's disease
Parkinson's disease
Progressive supranuclear palsy
Parkinson-dementia complex of Guam
Spinocerebellar degenerations
Idiopathic basal ganglia calcification
Striatonigral degeneration
Metachromatic leukodystrophy
Adrenoleukodystrophy
Cerebrotendinous xanthomatosis
Secondary dementing illnesses
Vascular dementias
Thrombotic disorders
Atherosclerosis
Arteriosclerosis (including lacunar state and Binswanger's disease)
Fibromuscular dysplasia and other rare syndromes
Embolic disorders
Hemorrhagic conditions
Inflammatory vascular conditions
Systemic lupus erythematosus
Temporal arteritis
Behçet's syndrome
Trauma
Posttraumatic encephalopathy
Dementia pugilistica
Intracranial conditions
Brain tumors
Primary, metastatic
Brain abscesses
Subdural hematoma
Hydrocephalus
Communicating (normal-pressure hydrocephalus)
Noncommunicating
Multiple sclerosis
Marchiafava-Bignami disease
Metabolic and endocrine disturbances
Hypothyroidism and hyperthyroidism
Hypoadrenalism and hyperadrenalism
Hypopituitarism
Hypoparathyroidism and hyperparathyroidism
Hypoglycemia and hyperglycemia
Hepatic encephalopathy
Nonwilsonian hepatocerebral degeneration
Wilson's disease
Uremic encephalopathy
Dialysis dementia
Hyperlipidemia
Porphyria
Anemia (severe)
Anoxic and postanoxic dementias
Cardiac disease
Pulmonary insufficiency

Table 33.1. Continued

Condition
Chronic electrolyte disturbances
Remote effects of systemic cancer
Deficiency states
Vitamin B_{12}
Folate
Pellagra (vitamin B_6)
Infections
Acquired immunodeficiency syndrome
Fungal meningoencephalitis
Parasitic meningoencephalitis
Tuberculous meningoencephalitis
Syphilitic meningoencephalitis
Postencephalitic dementia
Jakob-Creutzfeldt disease
Gerstmann-Straussler syndrome
Kuru
Whipple's disease
Progressive multifocal leukoencephalopathy
Intoxications
Alcohol
Prescription medications
Antihypertensives
Adrenocorticosteroids
Nonsteroidal anti-inflammatory agents
Antidepressant agents
Lithium
Neuroleptic agents
Anticholinergic agents
Barbiturates
Benzodiazepines and other sedative-hypnotics
Anticonvulsants
Digitalis preparations
Antiarrhythmics
Opiate drugs
Gastrointestinal agents
Polydrug abuse
Aluminum
Heavy metals (arsenic, lead, mercury, manganese, thallium)
Organic solvents
Carbon monoxide
Psychiatric disorders
Depression
Mania
Schizophrenia

metabolism, a microtubular defect, an impaired philothermal response, an abnormal brain protein, infectious agents (eg, "slow viruses"), head injury, abnormal blood flow to the brain, chronic leakage of the blood-brain barrier, environmental toxins (eg, aluminum, other minerals, heavy metals, pesticides, and other chemicals), neurotoxic plants, nutritional deficiencies, alcohol, and drugs. Fundamental cell biology in patients with DAT is being studied, and there are numerous reports of abnormalities in non-neural tissues, including skin fibroblasts, lymphocytes, red blood cells, and platelets, as well as polymorphonuclear leukocytes.[17] Abnormalities also may occur in calcium and oxidative metabolism, membranes, and messenger RNA. It is possible that there are several causes of DAT and that a combination of different mechanisms is responsible for the disease in each individual. As postulated many years ago, the manifestation of symptoms may indicate that cumulative damage has exceeded a threshold of vulnerability.[18] It is important to note that there is, as yet, no confirmed infectious agent for DAT, despite numerous attempts to identify one.

Diagnosis and Clinical Course. The *DSM-III-R* criteria for primary degenerative dementia of the Alzheimer type require that a diagnosis of dementia be made first.[1] Beyond that, DAT is characterized by an insidious onset with a generally progressive deteriorating course. The diagnosis of DAT requires exclusion of all other known specific causes of dementia by history and by results of physical examinations and laboratory tests. There is, at present, no biologic or neuropsychologic marker for DAT, and as mentioned above, the definitive diagnosis can be made only from a combination of clinical and histopathologic findings. The accuracy of the clinical diagnosis of DAT has improved in recent years due to more precise specification of criteria and the advent of neuroimaging. Careful application of current diagnostic criteria is reported to predict correctly the pathologic diagnosis in 85% to 90% of cases.[19,20] That rate, however, applies to major research centers, not to primary care facilities. Since research studies are conducted by experts in DAT who tend to exclude all but the most ''pure'' cases from their protocols, it is unlikely that such diagnostic accuracy prevails in a clinical practice setting. Nevertheless, diagnostic progress has been made. To increase the fidelity between the clinical and pathologic diagnosis of DAT, the clinical diagnosis has been stratified into definite, probable, or possible DAT,[19] with cerebral biopsy or autopsy required for the diagnosis of definite DAT (Table 33.2).

On examination, patients with DAT exhibit abnormalities in both remote and recent memory; in all but the earliest stages of the illness, they are disoriented for time and have difficulty in learning new information. In the linguistic domain, impairments of naming usually appear first; as the disease progresses, anomia is followed by loss of the ability to understand spoken language, and in the final stages, patients exhibit palilalia or become mute. Constructional skills are lost early in the clinical course, and patients have difficulty with copying progressively simpler drawings as the

Table 33.2. Criteria for the diagnosis of definite, probable, and possible DAT.*

DAT	Criteria
Definite	Meets clinical criteria for probable DAT and has histopathologic evidence of DAT obtained from biopsy or autopsy specimens.
Probable	Dementia with progressive worsening in 2 or more areas of intellectual function (including memory) established by clinical examination results, documented by a mental status questionnaire, and confirmed by neuropsychologic testing results. There is no delirium; onset is between the ages of 40 and 90 years; there is no alternative systemic or brain disease present that could account for the intellectual decline. The diagnosis of probable DAT is supported by evidence of progressive aphasia, apraxia, or agnosia; by impaired activities of daily living; by a positive family history of a similar disorder, particularly if confirmed pathologically; by normal findings on lumbar puncture; by normal patterns or nonspecific changes on the electroencephalogram; and by cerebral atrophy on a computed tomographic scan of the head.
Possible	There are variations from the classic course of DAT in onset, presentation, or course in the absence of any alternative explanation for the deficits; a second systemic illness or brain disorder is present but is thought not to be the cause of the dementia syndrome; or there is slow progression in only 1 area of neuropsychologic function.

* Adapted from McKhann et al.[19] DAT indicates dementia of the Alzheimer type.

disease advances. Abstraction, calculation, and judgment also are compromised. Persecutory delusions commonly appear during the course of the illness, and depressive symptoms may occur. Changes in personality are seen in virtually every patient. Indifference, dependence, and passivity are the most common alterations; shouting, lewd behavior, and violence occasionally are observed. Oddly, social integrity, or at least its appearance, often is maintained well into the course of the illness. In contrast to the marked intellectual and behavioral changes, somatosensory, auditory, visual, endocrine, and autonomic functions are relatively preserved; motor function generally remains intact until the final phases of the illness, when ambulation is lost, incontinence supervenes, and dysphagia makes the patient vulnerable to aspiration pneumonia.[12,21]

The course of DAT typically involves three stages: mild, moderate, and severe. Mild DAT is characterized by minor changes in memory and language; one neuropsychologic ability may be disproportionately affected. In moderately advanced DAT, many behavioral domains are involved, and the classic clinical syndrome is identifiable. In the severe form of DAT, all intellectual abilities are markedly impaired, and motor dysfunction emerges. Death often is caused by aspiration pneumonia, urinary tract infection, sepsis from decubitus, or a concomitant medical illness.[12,22]

While there are no pathognomonic laboratory findings in DAT, the laboratory evaluation is important to exclude other conditions that may be responsible for or may be exacerbating the dementia.[23] Specific findings on certain tests, although not diagnostic alone, may contribute to the differential diagnosis. The National Institutes of Health Consensus Statement on the Differential Diagnosis of Dementing Disorders[23] cautions against too much reliance on laboratory findings; it stresses that ordering laboratory tests beyond those routinely recommended should be guided by the patient's history and the findings of the physical and mental examinations. It further notes that the clinician must walk a tightrope between overtesting and undertesting in elderly demented patients, with discomfort, inconvenience, excess costs, and the likelihood of false positives on one side, balanced on the other by missed diagnoses of treatable disorders.

It should be noted that an electroencephalogram (EEG) usually is normal when DAT begins, slowing progressively as the disease advances. Computed tomographic (CT) scans often reveal nonspecific cerebral cortical atrophy with dilatation of the ventricles and enlargement of the cerebral sulci.

Autopsy Findings. Histopathologic changes in DAT include diffuse cortical atrophy and diminished total brain weights, neuronal loss, gliosis, intraneuronal neurofibrillary tangles and granulovacuolar degeneration, neuritic plaques, and amyloid angiopathy,[12,24] especially in the hippocampus and cortex. These changes are not distributed evenly throughout the cortex, but preferentially affect the medial temporal regions and the lateral temporal-parietal-occipital junction areas bilaterally.[25] There is also atrophy and plaque and tangle formation in the nucleus basalis of Meynert (the principal source of cholinergic innervation of the cerebral cortex) and a corresponding deficit in acetylcholine and related cholinergic system enzymes in the cortex.[26]

The quantitative criteria for a tissue diagnosis of DAT vary according to the age of the patient and whether or not a clinical diagnosis of DAT was made during the patient's life.[27]

The importance of a neuropathologic examination of patients with clinically diagnosed DAT cannot be stressed too highly; it is essential to confirm the diagnosis. An autopsy should be performed by a pathologist who is knowledgeable about DAT who will provide the required counts of plaques and tangles (that are present but fewer in the brains of nondemented older patients). Since the clinical diagnosis of DAT may mistakenly be made when the dementia is due to an infectious agent (such as in acquired immunodeficiency syndrome [AIDS] dementia or Jakob-Creutzfeldt disease), pathologists and others who come in contact with a patient's tissues need to exercise prudent caution; however, refusal to handle tissues under appropriate safeguards is unacceptable.

As noted above, the accuracy of the clinical diagnosis for unselected groups of patients remains unknown; autopsy confirmation, therefore, is still of major importance, especially for family members who are concerned about genetic risk.

Pick's Disease. The rare dementia that bears his name was first described by Pick in 1892. The cause of Pick's disease is not known; one estimate places its prevalence in the United States at 20 to 100 times lower than that of DAT.[12] Pedigree studies indicate an autosomal dominant mode of inheritance in some families and a recessive mode in others; further study of large families is needed to determine the mode of transmission and genetic defect of Pick's disease.

Pick's disease resembles DAT in age at onset and duration. Like DAT, it has a prominent aphasia with fluent output, anomia, and impaired comprehension, as well as a slowly progressive course and lack of focal neurologic signs. These similarities may confuse the diagnosis. Pick's disease can, however, often be distinguished from DAT by the retention of memory, by visuospatial and arithmetic skills in the early and middle stages of the illness, and by the more flamboyant personality changes early in the course.[12] Patients with Pick's disease may exhibit elements of the Klüver-Bucy syndrome (ie, hypersexuality, dietary changes, placidity, agnosia, hypermetamorphosis, hyperorality) early in the disease process. A CT scan and magnetic resonance imaging (MRI) may reveal focal lobar atrophy of the temporal or frontal lobes, and EEG studies may demonstrate focal slowing in the temporal or frontal regions.

Diagnostic confirmation of Pick's disease currently requires an autopsy. A postmortem examination shows focal atrophy in the temporal and/or frontal regions with widened sulci and knife-edged gyri in the involved regions. Microscopically, there is neuron loss and gliosis of the cortex and the subcortical white matter. Inflated cells and cells with Pick bodies may be identified in the medial temporal or inferior frontal areas.[28]

Dementia With Extrapyramidal Disorders. Dementia commonly occurs in Parkinson's and Huntington's diseases, as well as in rarer extrapyramidal syndromes, eg, progressive supranuclear palsy, striatonigral degeneration, spinocerebellar degenerations, and a variety of other system atrophies. The dementia syndrome that occurs in these diseases has clinical features that distinguish it from the dementia of DAT or Pick's disease. The descriptive terms *cortical* and *subcortical* are used by some investigators to separate the two presentations of dementia, and a comparison of the distinguishing features is presented in Table 33.3. The cardinal clinical characteristics of subcortical dementias are as follows: slowing of cognition or bradyphrenia; a memory impairment that involves prominent recall deficits with relative preservation of recognition abilities; cognitive dilapidation with decline of executive functions, abstraction, and judgment; and alterations in mood and personality.[12,29] Aphasic symptoms and more profound memory disturbances that affect both recall and recognition are evident in DAT and reflect cortical dysfunction. The subcortical dementias usually occur in diseases with prominent motor symptoms, whereas cortical dementias typically exhibit motor system involvement only late in the clinical course. Not all dementias can be categorized in this manner; multi-infarct dementia (MID) or dementias due to infection, for example, may

Table 33.3. Distinguishing features of cortical and subcortical dementia syndromes.

Clinical characteristic	Cortical dementia	Subcortical dementia
Language	Aphasia	Minimal abnormalities
Memory	Poor encoding, impaired recall and recognition	Poor recall, intact recognition
Abstraction	Severely impaired	Impaired on most difficult tasks
Personality	Indifferent, dependent	Labile, withdrawn
Mood	Severe depression uncommon	Severe depression common
Motor function	Normal until late	Abnormal early
Principal site of pathologic condition	Hippocampus and association cortex	Basal ganglia, thalamus, brain stem
Diseases	Alzheimer's disease, Pick's disease	Parkinson's disease, Huntington's disease, progressive supranuclear palsy

exhibit a mixture of "cortical" and "subcortical" symptoms.

Parkinson's Disease. The reported prevalence of Parkinson's disease varies between 100/100,000 and 150/100,000. It is a disease primarily of those patients in late middle age and older with a mean age of onset from 58 to 62 years; 80% of parkinsonian patients are aged from 60 to 79 years.[30] The prevalence of dementia in Parkinson's disease is controversial; reports have ranged from 8% to 80%.[31] Parkinson's disease produces the clinical tetrad of resting tremor, limb rigidity, bradykinesia, and loss of righting reflexes. The intellectual deficits are most evident in those patients who are older, who have had the disease for a longer period of time, and who have marked akinesia. Mental status may improve with levodopa therapy, but usually declines as the disease advances. Pathologically, there is cell loss and gliosis in the substantia nigra, and a portion of the remaining neurons contain Lewy bodies. There is a marked deficiency of dopamine in Parkinson's disease, with variable losses of norepinephrine, serotonin, acetylcholine, and selected neuromodulators. In the brains of some patients with Parkinson's disease, the classic lesions of DAT also have been found.[31,32] Brain implants are being investigated as a means of ameliorating the symptoms, but findings are preliminary.[33]

Huntington's Disease. The classic presentation of Huntington's disease includes dementia, and in some patients, the dementia may precede the characteristic movement disorder. The disease most commonly begins in the fourth or fifth decade of life, but in approximately 20% of patients, the onset is after the age of 50 years.[34] Huntington's disease is an autosomal dominant disorder that is transmitted by a parent to 50% of the offspring. The Huntington's disease gene has now been localized to chromosome 4.[35] The disease may have a course that spans 10 to 20 years and is marked by choreiform movements of the limbs, trunk, neck, and face, as well as a dementia syndrome with features indicative of subcortical dysfunction (eg, early cognitive changes include the loss of the ability to plan and organize, while the memory loss and language difficulties typically seen in DAT usually are absent or delayed). While neuroleptic agents may ameliorate the chorea, there is, as yet, no treatment available for the dementia syndrome. Neuropathologically, there is degeneration of the small cells of the caudate and putamen, and the caudate nucleus becomes markedly atrophic as the disease advances; γ-aminobutyric acid is preferentially depleted from the involved areas.

Other Extrapyramidal Disorders. Progressive supranuclear palsy, striatonigral degeneration, Wilson's disease, spinocerebellar degenerations, and other movement disorders exhibit various combinations of parkinsonism, ataxia, chorea, and ophthalmoplegia; most disorders manifest a dementia syndrome in the late phases of the illness. The parkinsonism dementia complex of Guam is a dementing illness that occurs in Guam, Papua, New Guinea, and Japan. It combines factors of Parkinson's disease, DAT, and amyotrophic lateral sclerosis.

Secondary Dementias

Vascular Dementia Syndromes. Scientists have been seeking a connection between dementia and cerebral vascular disease since the days when arteriosclerosis was offered as an explanation for senility. Today, it is generally acknowledged that dementia associated with vascular changes is second in prevalence only to DAT, accounting for from 8% to 29% of all dementias. It is widely attributed to multiple infarctions of the brain with relatively little contribution from hypoperfusion of viable tissue.[36] The criteria for MID[1] and vascular dementia[1,36] include the presence of dementia with a stepwise deteriorating course, a "patchy" or uneven distribution of cognitive deficits, focal neurologic signs and symptoms, and evidence from the history, physical examination, or laboratory tests of cerebral or systemic vascular disease presumed to be the cause of the dementia. Other characteristic features include emotional lability, dysarthria and dysphagia, transient depression, episodes of clouded consciousness, and nocturnal confusion. A definitive diagnosis is possible by examining brain tissue.

In an effort to distinguish MID and DAT, the Hachinski Ischemia Scale quantifies 13 diagnostic items; a high score points to MID and a low score to DAT.[36] Review of the literature, however, suggests that caution is needed in applying these scores and a Modified Ischemia Scale has been published.[37] It must be noted that the Ischemia Scale is not a means of identifying dementia but assists in distinguishing MID from other forms of dementia, *after the diagnosis of dementia has been made.*

Treatment of vascular dementia has not been well studied; control of hypertension is the major concern, and treatment with platelet anti-aggregation agents is recommended for most patients.

Classification of the vascular dementia syndromes is still in its infancy, but several vascular dementias are recognized, each determined by the cause of the vascular disease, the size of the vessel affected, and the region of the brain infarcted.[12,38] Emboli and atherosclerosis of large vessels result in multiple large-vessel occlusions with wedge-shaped infarctions that involve the cerebral cortex and produce motor, sen-sory, and visual field defects, as well as aphasia, apraxia, amnesia, agnosia, and other instrumental deficits. Small vessels are disproportionately affected by sustained hypertension that leads to fibrinoid necrosis of vessel walls with gradual occlusion and eventual infarction of perfused tissues. This process is most marked in arterioles, and the resulting ischemic injury usually affects the deep structures of the brain supplied by the penetrating branches of the larger cerebral vessels. The dementia syndrome associated with lesions of the deep nuclear structures has features of the subcortical dementia with prominent signs of frontal lobe dysfunction.[39]

To complicate the picture further, both the neurofibrillary tangles and the neuritic plaques of DAT and the multiple areas of cerebral infarction of MID sometimes are found together in the same brain; this "mixed" DAT and MID may be present in 10% to 20% of patients with dementia.[14]

There are a few specifically named vascular dementia syndromes. When brain lesions found at autopsy result from occlusion of the lenticulostriate and thalamoperforant branches, the infarctions occur in the basal ganglia, thalamus, and internal capsule, and the disorder is known as the *lacunar state*. If the longer vessels that penetrate through the cortex to supply the hemispheric white matter are the primary site of involvement, the lesions will be most intense in the periventricular regions, and the syndrome is known as Binswanger's disease. The lacunar state and Binswanger's disease commonly occur together.[39,40] Cerebral anoxia has been proposed as a causal factor in cognitive impairment by a number of investigators who have attempted to account for the dementia that sometimes accompanies primary cardiac illness or advanced pulmonary disease, but the issue remains in dispute.

Drug-Induced Dementia. The high frequency of systemic illnesses in elderly patients leads to treatment with a panoply of pharmaceutical agents, both prescribed and self-chosen. Although elderly persons represent about 12% of the population, they consume approximately 30% of all prescribed medications. In addition, up to 70% of elderly persons regularly use over-the-counter preparations, particularly analgesics.[41] Hence, drug-drug and drug-disease interactions are common. Decreased serum protein concentrations, diminished renal and hepatic blood flow, and increased target organ and brain sensitivity to drug actions all predispose elderly persons to toxic complications of drug use. The actual prevalence of drug-induced dementia among elderly patients is unknown; nevertheless, it is sufficiently high that drugs are considered to be a leading cause of secondary dementia.

Although any drug potentially can cause cognitive or behavioral changes, some medications are associated with dementia syndromes more often than others; these include psychotropic, anticholinergic, and antihypertensive agents, anticonvulsants, and cardiac drugs.[11] The possibility of a drug-related complication may be signaled in the geriatric patient by fatigue, falls, depression, delusions, syncope, postural hypotension, hallucinations, hypovolemia, hypokalemia, confusion, or the new onset of incontinence. The presence of cognitive impairment calls for a careful inventory of both prescribed and nonprescribed medications; a period during which all medications are discontinued (to the extent that the patient's health is not endangered) is recommended, with close observation for up to several weeks (depending on the half-life of the drug). Many clinicians report dramatic improvement of dementia symptoms when following these recommendations. If discontinuing a drug is contraindicated, assessment of the contribution of the medication(s) to the treatment of a dementia syndrome may be attempted by other methods, such as determining blood levels or substituting another drug with a similar efficacy but different mode of action.

Alcohol-Induced Dementia. Long-term use of alcohol produces a dementia syndrome with prominent apathy and frontal lobe dysfunction, apparently independent of head trauma, malnutrition, or hepatic failure.[42,43] Alcohol-related dementia may partially remit if abstinence can be maintained for several months.[43] (See also "Amnestic Syndromes" section above.)

Toxic Encephalopathies (Other Than Drugs). Heavy metals (lead, arsenic, mercury, manganese) are unusual causes of dementia in elderly persons. Industrial agents, pesticides, and other chemicals, as well as neurotoxic plants, all have been suspected in the etiology of dementia, although direct causal relationships have not been established. The most persistent interest has been focused on aluminum, and active research continues to delineate the role of this particular metal in dementia.[44]

Infectious Causes of Dementia

AIDS Dementia. Acquired immunodeficiency syndrome is caused by the human immunodeficiency virus (HIV) that attacks cells of the immune system and leaves the patient defenseless against disease, notably infections and tumors. Bisexual and homosexual men, intravenous drug users, and individuals who require multiple blood transfusions are at highest risk for the disease in the United States. Patients with AIDS are doubly at risk for dementia—both from the AIDS virus itself and from opportunistic brain infections. Dementia is evident in approximately one third of patients when the diagnosis of AIDS is made, and it is present in nearly all patients when the terminal stage of the illness is reached. Acquired immunodeficiency syndrome dementia is now the most common of the dementias caused by infection.[45]

The AIDS dementia complex has subcortical features, including apathy, impaired concentration and memory, indifference, and poor motivation. However, AIDS symptoms can produce many neuropsychiatric disorders, including abrupt or insidious changes in cognition, mood, and behavior, that may lead to diagnostic confusion—especially in older persons in whom the possibility of AIDS may not be considered. Temporary improvement in intellectual function after treatment with the drug zidovudine has been reported.[46]

Neuropathologically, HIV infection produces diffuse demyelination of the hemispheric white matter, perivascular inflammation, and invasion of the deep structures by multinucleated macrophages; neurons and oligodendrocytes are relatively unaffected.

Jakob-Creutzfeldt Disease. An uncommon cause of progressive dementia is Jakob-Creutzfeldt disease, which is the result of infection of the brain by an unconventional or "slow" virus; the estimated frequency is 1 case per 1 million population. Several families with an autosomal dominant pattern of inheritance have been described, and in one report, about 10% of the families had at least one other affected family member. Because of the infectious nature of Jakob-Creutzfeldt disease, contact with the patient must be taken into account when interpreting familial occurrence.

Jakob-Creutzfeldt disease may be confused with DAT on initial presentation, but its duration usually is weeks or months rather than years—although occasional cases of long duration have been reported. The rapid course, early involvement of multiple neurologic systems, and a characteristic EEG pattern—periodic bursts of polyspike and wave activity—often enable the clinician to make the correct diagnosis.[47] Onset most often occurs between the ages of 50 and 60 years, but is reported to range from 21 to 79 years. In one study, 39% of the patients with Jakob-Creutzfeldt disease had only one presenting symptom; the three most common of these were severe asthenia, weight loss, and sleep disturbance. Myoclonus frequently is present in Jakob-Creutzfeldt disease, but it also may occur late in the course of DAT. Rarely, patients with DAT exhibit periodic sharp waves on EEGs and myoclonus that closely mimic Jakob-Creutzfeldt disease.

Neuropathologic examination reveals prominent fibrous astrocytes and spongiform changes that involve the cerebral cortex. Jakob-Creutzfeldt disease is an infectious disorder, and transmission by stereotactic instruments, as well as corneal grafts, has been reported.[48]

Gerstmann-Straussler Syndrome. First described by Gerstmann in 1928, the Gerstmann-Straussler syndrome is a form of cerebellar ataxia with dementia that develops slowly and is characterized at autopsy by a large number of unusual amyloid plaques that are distributed throughout the brain; degenerative changes in white matter are common, and the brain tissue may be "spongy." In addition to dementia, there are cerebellar and pyramidal signs (extensor plantar responses). Both sporadic and familial (autosomal dominant) cases have been reported, and a transmissible virus was isolated from patients with Gerstmann-Straussler syndrome whose brains showed spongiform changes. Some investigators have concluded that this syndrome is a virus-induced spongiform encephalopathy similar to Jakob-Creutzfeldt disease.

General Paresis. Delirium is more commonly produced by generalized infections with sepsis than is dementia, but the localized effects on the brain of CNS infections may produce chronic cognitive impairment. Syphilis, though rare, is now increasing in incidence; it may produce dementia through direct spirochetal invasion of the brain in general paresis, through inflammation and increased pressure in chronic meningitis, or through vascular mechanisms in meningovascular syphilis.[12] Laboratory evaluation for lues and examination of the spinal fluid are essential. Antimicrobial therapy will halt the progress of the dementia and may lead to a partial recovery of intellectual function.

Chronic Meningitis. Chronic meningitis may present with a dementia syndrome that is accompanied by cranial nerve palsies and evidence of a raised intracranial pressure. The meningitis may be bacterial (tuberculosis, Whipple's disease), parasitic (malaria, cysticercosis, toxoplasmosis), or fungal (eg, *Cryptococcus, Histoplasma, Candida, Coccidioides, Aspergillus*) in origin.[49] Diagnosis is made through examination of the cerebrospinal fluid, and treatment is determined by the specific causal agent identified.

Noninfectious Systemic Illnesses (Including Neoplasms) Causing Dementia. Elderly persons may develop a wide variety of systemic illnesses, many of which are capable of altering brain function and producing a dementia syndrome. Only 13% of nursing home residents are without at least one chronic illness, and 50% have two or more chronic illnesses. Thus, systemic illness must be considered in the differential diagnosis of dementia in elderly persons. The diagnosis depends on the results of the physical examination and appropriate laboratory tests. Among the systemic

illnesses that may produce dementia are cardiac disease, pulmonary failure, uremia, hepatic encephalopathy, and systemic infections.[49] Endocrine disturbances, including thyroid diseases, parathyroid dysfunction, and adrenal disorders, also are potential causes of dementia syndromes. Vitamin B_{12} and folate deficiency states are rare causes of intellectual decline. Inflammatory disorders, such as temporal arteritis and other forms of vasculitis, are unusual causes of dementia in elderly patients. These conditions may cause dementia syndromes or may exacerbate intellectual deterioration when they occur in individuals with preexisting dementing illnesses.

Neoplasms become increasingly common with advancing age and must be considered in the differential diagnosis of dementia. Brain tumors may cause mental status changes through direct invasion of brain tissue, as in the case of intrinsic and metastatic lesions, or through compression of the brain from extracerebral masses, such as meningiomas. Neoplasms that affect the frontal lobes are particularly likely to present with dementia; most tumors produce focal neurologic signs and increased intracranial pressure, as well as intellectual changes.

Traumatic Dementias

Traumatic brain injury is a cause of dementia in old persons, as well as in young persons. Brain dysfunction with intellectual compromise may result from direct contusion of the brain or shearing injuries that affect primarily white-matter tracts. Intracerebral hematomas, posttraumatic obstructive hydrocephalus, and subdural and extradural hematomas also may complicate head injuries and produce a dementia syndrome.[12] Subdural hematomas may develop in elderly persons after relatively minor closed-head injuries, and a rapidly progressive confusional state with focal neurologic findings should lead to a search for intracranial bleeding. Dementia that occurs in boxers, who sustain repeated blows to the head, has been termed *dementia pugilistica*.[50] The exact mechanism is not known. Neuroimaging often is helpful in identifying the underlying pathologic condition of most dementias due to trauma.

Hydrocephalus

Enlarged ventricles may result from a loss of tissue (hydrocephalus ex vacuo) or from failure to absorb cerebrospinal fluid. The latter is known as obstructive hydrocephalus and may be either communicating or noncommunicating. In communicating obstructive hydrocephalus, there is a free flow between the ventricular system and the subarachnoid space, but the fluid is prevented from being absorbed through the pacchionian granulations into the superior sagittal sinus. This condition also is known as normal-pressure hydrocephalus because the cerebrospinal fluid pressure is not elevated; it often is idiopathic, but may follow trauma, meningitis, encephalitis, subarachnoid hemorrhage, stroke, or neoplasia. Noncommunicating obstructive hydrocephalus results from occlusion of the ventricular system preventing the flow of cerebrospinal fluid either through the ventricular system or between the ventricles and the subarachnoid space. The cause is usually a neoplasm, cyst, or late manifesting congenital abnormality, such as aqueductal stenosis. Cerebrospinal fluid pressure is usually elevated in this form of hydrocephalus.

Diagnosis of the type of hydrocephalus is pursued by identifying enlarged ventricles on a CT scan or by MRI and by determining the pattern of cerebrospinal fluid flow with radionuclide cisternography. In hydrocephalus ex vacuo, the tracer substance enters the ventricles and then flows normally over the convexities of the brain; in obstructive communicating hydrocephalus, the tracer usually enters the ventricles but is prevented from flowing over the convexities and is not visualized in the midsagittal region; and in obstructive noncommunicating hydrocephalus, the tracer does not enter the enlarged ventricular system.

Communicating obstructive hydrocephalus has been treated by redirecting the cerebrospinal fluid through a ventriculoperitoneal shunt from the intracranial cavity to the serosal surfaces of the abdominal cavity. The results of surgical intervention have been inconsistent, but some patients have shown unquestioned improvement. The best predictor of response, according to one review that encompassed 62 patients, was the presence of the complete triad of dementia, gait disturbance, and urinary incontinence.[51] In general, patients with significant gait disturbance, minimal cognitive impairment, and little or no cortical atrophy shown on CT scans appear to profit most from surgical intervention. Even among selected patients, it seems that only slightly more than one half have shown improvement. The risk-benefit ratio of surgical intervention has to be weighed carefully since complications, such as subdural hematoma and infection, are common. Noncommunicating hydrocephalus may require shunting in addition to treatment of the obstructing process.

The behavioral changes of hydrocephalus are attributed to frontal lobe damage that results from the enlargement of the anterior horns of the lateral ventricles and compression of the surrounding areas, while the gait, reflex, and bladder changes can be explained by the stretching and subsequent malfunction of the motor fibers to the lower limbs and the bladder,

both of which lie closely adjacent to the ventricular margin.

Depression

The interactions between dementia and depression are complex. Patients with DAT, vascular dementias, and dementias associated with extrapyramidal syndromes may show mood changes. Frontal lobe syndromes with significant apathy may mimic a depressive syndrome and so may pseudobulbar palsy with prominent weeping. Depression may develop in demented patients, particularly early in the illnesses.

In elderly depressed patients, "vegetative" symptoms, such as sleep disturbance, constipation, and weight loss, are very common; sadness, a history of previous episodes of mood disorder, abrupt onset, and rapid progression of symptoms also point to depression. Feelings of guilt and low self-esteem are less prominent among older compared with younger depressed patients.

The dementia syndrome of depression has been called *pseudodementia*, but the term is misleading because the symptoms of dementia are real. Thus, major depressive illness may produce intellectual, memory, and behavioral impairment that is indistinguishable from a dementia due to degenerative brain disease—except that it may revert to normal with appropriate antidepressant treatment. The proportion of depressed patients who exhibit this syndrome has been estimated at 10% to 15%. While neuropsychologic evaluation may be helpful in arriving at the correct diagnosis,[52] the difficulties in distinguishing a dementia syndrome due to depression from that caused by progressive brain disease are numerous, and the issue is further complicated by the fact that depression and dementia may coexist. Therapeutic trials of electroconvulsive therapy or antidepressants may be required to resolve the issue, although only a positive treatment outcome is of value. Depressions in elderly patients may fail to respond to treatment even when there is no doubt of the diagnosis of uncomplicated major depressive disorder and dementia is absent.

Once the diagnosis of a depressive disorder has been made, a number of standardized observer- and self-rating measures may be employed for recording quantitative changes in depression severity. Among those commonly used are the Hamilton Rating Scale for Depression[53] and the Zung Self-Rating Depression Scale.[54] Despite its emphasis on somatic complaints, the Hamilton depression scale has continued to prove its value as a measure of treatment response in depressed elderly patients.

Neuropsychiatric Assessment

The basic elements of the geriatric neuropsychiatric assessment are the history; mental status, neurologic, and physical examinations; and laboratory tests. If these are not diagnostic, additional specialized examinations are indicated.

History

The most important part of the diagnostic assessment is the neuropsychiatric history. Obtaining a thorough anamnesis can be time-consuming, especially when multiple informants must be consulted, as is necessary with patients with dementia. Previous medical records should be examined and, when possible, information obtained from community health workers, such as nurses and social workers, should be reviewed. The history should precisely document the signs and symptoms, as well as details concerning their onset. A medical history, including specific diseases, injuries, operations, hospitalizations, psychiatric disorders, alcohol and substance use, nutrition, and exposure to environmental toxins, is fundamental.

A complete drug history, including past and present use of medications (both prescribed and nonprescribed), is critical, and patients or other informants should be asked about the use of over-the-counter medications (including laxatives, analgesics, antacids, sedatives, decongestants, eye or nose drops, skin ointments, vitamins, nutritional supplements, and pills or chewing gum used in diets or to stop smoking). Having drugs brought in for inspection is often valuable. A careful social history also is important, particularly with regard to events that have affected the patient's emotional state.

When a patient has symptoms of dementia, obtaining a family history is crucial; it should include detailed information about similar illness in other family members, including grandparents, aunts and uncles, as well as parents, siblings, and children. More than one informed source should be contacted when possible. This is also an excellent opportunity to introduce family members to the concept of autopsy-confirmed diagnoses. In the rare case in which an autosomal dominant transmission is suggested by family history, more specific recommendations and counseling may be appropriate.

A history of psychopathology, coupled with a relatively rapid onset of symptoms, should alert the clinician to investigate closely underlying psychiatric disturbances. The dementia syndrome of depression, for example, usually has a more precise onset in time or in reaction to a life event than other dementias, as well as a more rapid development of symptoms. A family history of depressive disorder further increases the likelihood of that diagnosis.

Mental Status Examination

The Mental Status Examination is the clinical means by which changes of normal aging are distinguished from pathologic intellectual and behavioral alterations. Although one might expect that the increased study of the dementing illnesses during the last decade would lead to widespread familiarity with the Mental Status Examination and testing, a study of physicians' awareness of dementing disorders[55] found that of 50 general internists and family physicians interviewed, only 42% included mental status testing among the diagnostic procedures used in a dementia workup, and only 12% mentioned the use of any formal testing procedure.

Areas to be assessed in the Mental Status Examination include the level of consciousness, attention, orientation, short- and long-term memory, language ability (including naming, repeating, understanding, reading, and writing), visuospatial skills, abstraction, calculation, affect, continuity and content of thought, insight, and judgment. Many of these functions can be evaluated during the interview by close attention to verbal and nonverbal communication. It is important to remember that the patient with declining intellectual abilities is often embarrassed by the impairment, and special care should be taken to preserve dignity, respect the desire to appear competent, and avoid the discouragement of ''failing'' a test.

The most sensitive measure of attention is the Digit Span Test, in which the clinician reads single digits aloud at a rate of one per second, and the patient is asked to repeat the sequence from memory and in the same or reverse order of presentation. Individuals with intact attention can repeat a minimum of five digits forward and four backward. When testing language, it is important to include observations regarding the characteristics of spontaneous speech, assessment of auditory comprehension by asking the patient to follow spoken commands, and exploration of naming abilities by asking the patient to name common and uncommon objects. Memory evaluation includes tests of recall of both recent and remote information. Recent memory is often tested by asking the patient to learn a short list of words for later recall. Remote memory is assessed by inquiring about personal and political events of the past. Visuospatial skills can be evaluated by having the patient copy figures, such as a circle, a cross, and a cube. Abstraction skills are assessed by having the patient interpret common proverbs; calculation by asking the patient to perform additions, subtractions, multiplications, and divisions; and orientation by inquiring about the three spheres, ie, time, place, and person. The presence of neuropsychiatric disturbances (eg, delusions, hallucinations, mood abnormalities, anxiety, personality changes) is determined by careful probing and, at times, by obtaining corroborating information from others.

More quantitative information regarding the patient's mental state can be obtained by the use of brief rating scales; while they are not diagnostic, they often can help in assessing the relative severity of the cognitive changes, document the impairment, and (especially in serial examinations) follow the course of the disease. No instrument can be substituted for the clinician in establishing a diagnosis of dementia. Instruments are used to document the clinician's findings and to add a quantitative dimension to the assessment.

The commonly used structured scales fall primarily into two categories—mental status screening examinations and measures of severity (or sometimes "stages") of the disease, usually based on both cognitive and behavioral symptoms. In the first group, the Mini-Mental State Examination (Table 33.4[56]) is a widely used instrument that can be administered in a relatively short time (5 to 15 minutes), provides a numerical score, and has been well documented in terms of replicable results and interrater reliability. It also has been correlated with the Blessed Dementia Scale, ie, the instrument used in the landmark studies that linked the clinical and pathologic changes of DAT.[57] Among the limitations of the Mini-Mental State Examination are the fact that it does not distinguish delirium from dementia and that it is insufficiently sensitive to early symptoms of dementia or those produced by dysfunction of subcortical structures. The Mental Status Questionnaire[58] is another scale that is used widely throughout the United States; it takes only 5 to 10 minutes to perform and, based on the answers to 10 questions, yields a numeric score that estimates the degree of brain dysfunction. A recently developed tool, the Neurobehavior Cognitive Status Examination,[59] provides a more diagnostic profile of intellectual dysfunction, giving scores for each neuropsychologic domain assessed. Another frequently used bedside instrument is the Short Portable Mental Status Questionnaire.[60] One of the newest scales, the Cambridge Mental Disorders of the Elderly Examination,[61] is designed to assist in the early diagnosis of dementia in elderly persons.

Among the group of rating scales for dementia designed to measure severity or place the impairment in a staging system, the Blessed Dementia Scale,[57] quantifies changes in cognition, as well as performance of daily activities, habits, personality, interests, and drive, based on information provided not only by the patient but also by a person in close contact with the patient. Blessed and associates reported that scores for the Blessed Dementia Scale correlate significantly with mean counts of senile plaques from postmortem examinations. The Clinical Dementia Rating (CDR) Scale[62] was designed as a global measure of dementia, based on behavioral and cognitive performance and relying on an extensive structured interview of knowledgeable informants, as well as the patient. The six separately rated categories are memory, orientation, judgment and problem solving, home and hobbies, community affairs, and personal care, with memory the most important category. Patients are rated in relation to both their cognitive ability and their past performance, with scores ranging from CDR-0 (healthy) to CDR-3 (severe dementia). It has shown good interrater reliability and is being validated by autopsy findings. The Global Deterioration Scale[63] sorts symptoms into seven stages of a continuum, from normal to completely demented, and correlates behavioral, mood, and other symptoms with scores on standard memory and mental status tests.

More detailed information regarding intellectual deficits in the various diseases can be obtained through the use of neuropsychologic testing (See Chapter 5). Like rating scales, neuropsychologic investigations provide information that is useful in the characterization and long-term follow-up of patients, but the test results are not diagnostically specific.

Physical Examination

A thorough physical and neurologic examination is crucial when evaluating a patient for dementia. As described above, manifold causes may produce cognitive impairment in a geriatric patient (Table 33.1). Concomitant physical illness can add to the severity of dementia, and patients with stroke, epilepsy, sensory impairment, or pulmonary, hepatic, renal, or cardiovascular disease need particularly careful evaluations due to the potential complications of drug-drug, drug-disease, and disease-disease interactions. In older patients, an additional concern in both the history and physical examination is the possible presence of undiagnosed conditions other than those related to dementia. Underreporting of symptoms and the overuse of medications are common in cognitively impaired patients. In one study,[64] congestive heart failure, urinary tract infections, skin diseases, arthritis, anemia, and chronic lung disease were some of the previously undiagnosed conditions found among outpatients who were referred for evaluation of cognitive impairment.

Table 33.4. Mini-mental state examination.*

I. Orientation (Maximum score 10) Ask "What is today's date?" Then ask specifically for parts omitted; eg, "Can you also tell me what season it is?"	Date (eg, January 21) ....1 ___ Year............................2 ___ Month........................3 ___ Day (eg, Monday) ....4 ___ Season ....5 ___
Ask "Can you tell me the name of this hospital?" "What floor are we on?" "What town (or city) are we in?" "What county are we in?" "What state are we in?"	Hospital ....6 ___ Floor ....7 ___ Town/City ....8 ___ County ....9 ___ State ....10 ___
II. Registration (Maximum score 3) Ask the subject if you may test his/her memory. Then say "ball," "flag," "tree" clearly and slowly, about one second for each. After you have said all 3 words, ask subject to repeat them. This first repetition determines the score (0–3) but keep saying them (up to 6 trials) until the subject can repeat all 3 words. If (s)he does not eventually learn all three, recall cannot be meaningfully tested	"ball" ....11 ___ "flag" ....12 ___ "tree" ....13 ___ Record number of trials: _____
III. Attention and calculation (Maximum score 5) Ask the subject to begin at 100 and count backward by 7. Stop after 5 subtractions (93, 86, 79, 72, 65). Score one point for each correct number.	"93" ....14 ___ "86" ....15 ___ "79" ....16 ___ "72" ....17 ___ "65" ....18 ___ OR

If the subject cannot or will not perform this task, ask him/her to spell the word "world" backwards (D, L, R, O, W). The score is one point for each correctly placed letter, eg, DLROW = 5, DLORW = 3. Record how the subject spelled "world" backwards: _____
                    D L R O W
	Number of correctly-placed
	   letters ....14 ___

IV. Recall (Maximum score 3) Ask the subject to recall the three words you previously asked him/her to remember (learned in Registration)	"ball" ....19 ___ "flag" ....20 ___ "tree" ....21 ___
V. Language (Maximum score 9) Naming: Show the subject a wrist watch and ask "What is this?" Repeat for pencil. Score one point for each item named correctly	Watch..........................22 ___ Pencil ....23 ___
Repetition: Ask the subject to repeat, "No ifs, ands, or buts." Score one point for correct repetition	Repetition ....24 ___
3-Stage Command: Give the subject a piece of blank paper and say, "Take the paper in your right hand, fold it in half and put it on the floor." Score one point for each action performed correctly	Takes in right hand ....25 ___ Folds in half ....26 ___ Puts on floor ....27 ___
Reading: On a blank piece of paper, print the sentence "Close your eyes." in letters large enough for the subject to see clearly. Ask subject to read it and do what it says. Score correct only if (s)he actually closes his/her eyes	Closes eyes ....28 ___
Writing: Give the subject a blank piece of paper and ask him/her to write a sentence. It is to be written spontaneously. It must contain a subject and verb and make sense. Correct grammar and punctuation are not necessary	Writes sentence..............29 ___
Copying: On a clean piece of paper, draw intersecting pentagons, each side about 1 inch, and ask subject to copy it exactly as it is. All 10 angles must be present and two must intersect to score 1 point. Tremor and rotation are ignored Eg,	Draws pentagons ....30 ___

Score: Add number of correct responses. In section III include items 14–18 or item 19, not both. (Maximum total score 30)

Total score _____

Rate subject's level of consciousness: _____ (a) coma, (b) stupor, (c) drowsy, (d) alert

* Reprinted with permission from Folstein MF. et al. Mini-mental state: A practical method of grading the cognitive state of the patient for the clinician. *J Psychiatr Res* 12:189, 1975.

Medication intoxication was found to be the most common cause for reversible dementia (6 of 15 patients). Depressive disorders, too, may aggravate dementia, and complications due to drug side effects and drug interactions are common.

Laboratory Evaluation

The absence of pathognomonic laboratory findings in many dementias prohibits a purely laboratory approach to the diagnosis of dementia. Laboratory analyses, appropriate to specific dementias, have been noted above. Some tests should be done routinely to search for causes of dementia or to identify abnormalities that may be exaggerating the effects of intellectual deficits; these include the complete blood cell count, electrolyte panel, screening metabolic panel, thyroid function tests, vitamin B_{12} and folate levels, tests for syphilis and HIV antibodies, urinalysis, electrocardiogram, and chest x-ray.[23] Discontinuing all medications that are not absolutely necessary may reveal a drug-related dementia. These laboratory tests, together with the history and mental and physical examinations, will reveal the presence of most readily reversible metabolic, endocrine, deficiency, and infectious states, whether causative or complicating. When these tests do not identify a reversible cause for the dementia, other studies may be appropriate. In the elderly patient, there are hazards of overtesting and undertesting to consider, and undue weight should not be placed on isolated laboratory findings unless they are consistent with clinical information.

Electroencephalography is appropriate when there is altered or fluctuating consciousness, when seizures are suspected, when the cause of the dementia is uncertain, or when the presentation is unusual. Topographic mapping of the resting state EEG may be useful in identifying focal lesions. Event-related potentials may show normal early components and nonspecific increases in the latency of the P300 element.

The routine need for a neuroimaging procedure in the investigation of dementia is controversial. They are costly, and it has been suggested that the presence of a reversible intracranial pathologic condition is predictable by findings in the clinical examination, allowing neuroimaging tests to be used selectively. Prospective studies, however, demonstrate that clinical guidelines to predict adequately the existence of an intracranial pathologic condition have not yet been constructed[65]; moreover, the purpose of the complete evaluation of dementia is not focused exclusively on the detection of reversible conditions. Accurate diagnosis also aids in providing patients and family with prognostic information, supports genetic counseling

when hereditary disease is present, and may help in the choice of treatment (such as choosing to treat a patient with platelet anti-aggregation agents in cases where the presence of vascular disease as a cause of dementia, or in addition to DAT, is difficult to establish on clinical grounds). For these reasons, a CT scan or MRI should be considered as a part of the dementia evaluation if no reversible cause has been detected for the dementia, or if the dementia persists despite apparently appropriate treatment. Specifically, a CT scan of the brain (without contrast enhancement) is appropriate when there is a history of a mass, in the presence of focal neurologic signs, and in dementia of brief duration. Magnetic resonance imaging is more sensitive than CT scanning for detection of small infarcts, most mass lesions, and atrophy of the brain stem and other subcortical structures.[66] Single-photon emission computed tomography (SPECT) may reveal a diminished cerebral blood flow in the parietal lobes bilaterally in DAT[67,68]; positron emission tomography (PET) with a fluorodeoxyglucose label can demonstrate decreased metabolic activity in both parietal lobes in the early stages of DAT, and combined bilateral parietal and bilateral frontal hypometabolism in the later stages.[69] The value of PET and SPECT for predicting Huntington's or Alzheimer's disease in individuals at risk is currently being investigated.

Follow-Up Assessment

Because of its progressive course, the diagnosis of dementia requires repeated evaluations. Several measures that sample different domains of mental functioning are superior to any single one in carrying out longitudinal investigations. Serial assessments add to knowledge about the course of the disease, and abrupt changes or the absence of decline over prolonged intervals should signal the clinician that the diagnosis needs to be reconsidered. A suggested checklist for periodic reassessment (intervals of 6 months to a year) is presented in Table 33.5.

Caregiver needs, too, are likely to change, and reassessments of the caregiver's medical and psychologic status, as well as social support needs, are important (Table 33.5). The physician's relationship with the family, fostered during periodic visits, is a valuable source of support to patients and caregivers.

Treatment of Dementia

Etiology-Specific Treatments

Specific treatments, when available, were included in the appropriate sections above. For dementias such

Table 33.5. Periodic review: checklist for patients with dementia.*

Medical and psychiatric condition	Caregiver needs
Medications	Social supports
Coexistent medical illnesses	Respite services
Neurologic changes	Support group
Nutrition, anorexia	Financial aid
Dental conditions	Psychologic issues
Foot problems	Evidence of depression
Sleep disturbances	Evidence of other psychopathology
Incontinence	Abuse by the patient
Depression	Abuse of the patient
Agitation, restlessness, irritable behavior	Medical issues
Inappropriate affect	Symptoms of physical illness?
Suspiciousness, paranoid thoughts	Use of drugs? alcohol?
Hostility, verbal and physical threats	Sleep disturbance?
Sexual problems, disinhibitions	Health habits?
Care needs of patient	Legal
Activity and functional status	Property
What is daily schedule?	Durable power of attorney
Problems with wandering or getting lost	Arrangements for decisions regarding medical treatment; durable power of attorney for health care, living will
Activities of daily living	
Instrumental activities of daily living	
Problems with transportation, driving	
Drug or alcohol use or abuse	
Supervision of medications	
Management of finances	
Social skills	
Social activities	
Personal relationships	
Reaction to visitors	
Reaction to environmental change	
Social supports	
Living arrangements	
Housing	
Financial resources	
Human resources	
Available family	
Available friends	
Counseling	
In-home services	

* Adapted from Winograd.[76]

as DAT, where there is, as yet, no treatment to halt or reverse the cognitive decline, treatment is symptomatic.

Symptomatic Treatments. The major areas for symptomatic treatment are depression, anxiety, paranoid and other delusions, agitation, assaultive and other disruptive behaviors, wandering, insomnia, incontinence, infection, hydration, nutrition, and skin care. Regardless of the symptom presentation, the first principle of treatment is to listen and respond to the patient's concerns, a task often rendered particularly difficult by the patient's communication problems. Even early in the dementia, the concerns of the patient often are not those of the physician; for example, patients may be less concerned about the loss of intellectual function than about how to provide for the family's financial security or how to ensure that no heroic measures will be taken when they themselves are no longer able to prevent them. One study[70] of the ways in which psychiatric disorders are overlooked during medical evaluations found that certain physician behaviors tended to suppress expression by patients of the verbal and vocal cues that are so important in alerting the physician to the presence of a psychiatric illness. The authors suggested that lack of eye contact during the initial portion of the interview, failure to clarify the patient's complaint, and asking closed questions about physical symptoms contribute to discouraging the patient from revealing psychologic symptoms. These findings should be borne in mind when interviewing a patient with cognitive impairment not only during the process of diagnosis, but also throughout treatment. The second principle that guides treatment of the patient with dementia is to seek a cause other than the dementia to explain a behavioral symptom.

Delusions and Paranoid States. Delusions are common in many dementia syndromes. Approximately 50% of patients with DAT and an equal number of those with vascular dementia, as well as patients with Huntington's disease, traumatic brain injuries, neoplasms, infections, and toxic-metabolic encephalopathies manifest delusions in the course of their illness.[6] The delusional content often is persecutory, and many patients have maladaptive and disruptive behaviors that are motivated by their delusional beliefs. It is wise to check on the delusional content, however, before assuming that a patient's accusations of theft or abuse are indeed delusional, and not grounded in reality. Open-minded, active listening, supplemented by psychotherapeutic intervention, may ameliorate the symptoms. If not, small doses of neuroleptic (antipsychotic) agents may lead to a remission of symptoms, allowing patients to remain at home for longer periods of time or to avoid restraints in institutional settings. Potential side effects of these agents include sedation, hypotension, and a variety of motor system disturbances, such as parkinsonism, akathisia, and tardive dyskinesia (Table 33.6); patients should therefore be carefully monitored for adverse drug effects. Low-potency agents, such as thioridazine, are more likely to produce postural hypotension; high-potency drugs, such as haloperidol or fluphenazine hydrochloride, are less sedating and cause little hypotension but have a greater tendency to cause motor system abnormalities.[71] The anticholinergic properties of neuroleptics may exacerbate cognitive deficits in demented patients.

Agitation and Combativeness. For symptoms of anxiety, restlessness, irritation, and fearfulness, the first line of treatment is, again, to listen and try to uncover the circumstances that provoke and maintain the patient's behavior. Common underlying causes include tension, depression or feelings of loss, concomitant physical illness, pain, or side effects of medication. Benzodiazepines should be used cautiously to treat anxiety in demented patients; they may produce paradoxic agitation, depression, incontinence, confusion, instability, and further impairment of cognition. Benzodiazepines with a long half-life (eg, diazepam) or an active metabolite with a long half-life (eg, flurazepam) should be avoided.[72] Violent behaviors, such as pushing, threatening, and striking, also may occur, and if precipitating factors cannot be identified and handled successfully, neuroleptics may control the symptoms. Again, starting doses should be low and increased very gradually. If the patient is dangerous to self or others, restraints may be needed. Agitated behaviors should be distinguished from the more benign hyperactivity that is exhibited by many patients with dementia, particularly those with DAT, that requires no treatment.

Pacing, Wandering, and Similar Behavioral Disturbances. Pacing, wandering, constant picking (carphologia), and continuous talking are among the behaviors that are most frustrating for caregivers and generally resistant to treatment; yet, carefully controlled research is notable for its absence. Drugs are rarely effective; allowing the patient as much freedom

as possible in a safe contained environment generally is more satisfactory.[73] When behavioral disturbances are intolerably disruptive, medications are usually prescribed.[72] Restraints are a last resort; they may cause more agitation in the patient, and their use is very disturbing to caregivers. Nevertheless, the patient's safety may require occasional use of restraints, for example, if the patient must be left alone for a short time. A geriatric chair (padded, with a high back and a waist-level tray) often is less disturbing than the usual restraints.[71]

Insomnia. In patients with dementia, sleep disturbance usually is more severe than that considered to be characteristic of normal aging and is often accompanied by nighttime wandering, a major challenge to caregivers. As with other problem behaviors, there may be an underlying cause; ascertaining and treating that cause is the first priority, whether it is physical illness, pain (eg, nocturnal leg muscle cramps), change in the environment, medication toxicity, anxiety, or depression. If no underlying cause is identified, simple practical interventions can be tried, including a darkened room, night-lights, and familiar surroundings. Rationing daytime sleep without depriving the patient of needed rest, as well as moderate physical exercise (eg, walking or swimming) are helpful, as are avoiding nighttime fluids and diuretics, and having the patient empty the bladder just before going to bed. For most patients, behavioral and environmental interventions can improve sleep; when the problem of sleep disturbance requires additional treatment, medication may be useful. Warm milk (containing tryptophan) has the least side effects; if that is not effective, chloral hydrate or short-acting benzodiazepines may be tried. Long-acting sedatives, in general, are to be avoided because they easily produce oversedation and may further impair cognitive function.

Depression. Depression may aggravate the intellectual deficits of dementia and may itself be a cause of dementia in elderly patients (see above). There are few data that bear on the treatment of depression in the demented patient, and psychotherapeutic interventions are often ignored. Yet, early in the course of dementia, supportive psychotherapy may be of considerable value. Drugs are the mainstay of treatment, despite the fact that nearly all antidepressants have significant and potentially deleterious anticholinergic actions (see chapter 36). Trazodone is an exception, but its therapeutic efficacy in demented patients is yet to be established. In the patient with delusions or hallucinations, current or past, antidepressants frequently have to be combined with neuroleptic treatment. Even in depressed patients who are not demented, antidepressant drugs produce remission in only about half of the patients, and most antidepressants have prominent side effects. On the whole, the differ-

Table 33.6. Some side effects of neuroleptic drugs commonly prescribed to manage behavioral symptoms in elderly demented patients.*

Drug	Sedation	Postural hypotension	Anticholinergic	Parkinsonian
Chlorpromazine	+++	+++	++	+
Thioridazine	+++	++	++	+
Haloperidol	+	+	+	+++
Perphenazine	+	+	+	++

* Three plus signs indicate most severe; one plus sign, least severe.

ent classes of antidepressants have similar efficacy; therefore, the choice of medication is usually made on the basis of side effect profiles. The antidepressant agents that are reputed to have the fewest side effects in elderly patients are nortriptyline, desipramine, trazodone, and doxepin.[41] Electroconvulsive therapy should be considered in patients who are intolerant of or unresponsive to other treatments of their mood disorder.

Incontinence. Urinary and fecal incontinence occur in the later stages of dementia and require medical assessment. Memory aids, exercise, attention to habit timing, changes in diet, and modifying drug regimens all are helpful in controlling incontinence, alleviating the distress of the patient and family, and helping to postpone nursing home placement.

Concomitant Illness. "Excess disability" refers to the aggravation of the cognitive and behavioral symptoms of dementia exhibited by patients with dementia who have a concomitant physical or mental disorder. As mentioned earlier, for example, cognition and behavior may improve with antidepressant treatment or with treatment of paranoid disorders, urinary tract infection, chronic respiratory infection, immobility, sensory deprivation, and other disorders. Demented patients are vulnerable to a variety of medical illnesses, particularly in the late stages of the disease. Incontinence predisposes to urinary tract infections, and dysphagia frequently leads to aspiration pneumonia. Agitation and lack of cooperation may cause dehydration or nutritional deprivation. When immobility supervenes, decubitus ulcerations may occur if the patient is not turned and shifted frequently. Any abrupt change in the behavior of a demented patient may be the clue to the occurrence of one of these conditions and should lead to a search for an occult medical disorder. In advanced stages of dementia, the family, with physician counsel and ideally based on the patient's previously expressed wishes, may decide not to treat a complicating medical illness, allowing it to become the terminal event of the dementia.

Experimental Treatments. Numerous drugs have been tried throughout the years to treat dementia, including cerebral vasodilators, anticoagulants, psychostimulants, neuropeptides, neurotransmitters, neuroleptics, antidepressants, hyperbaric oxygen, carbonic anhydrase inhibitors, nootropics, lipofuscin reducers, aluminum chelators, and procaine hydrochloride. None has been successful, although there have been flurries of encouragement from time to time. As mentioned above, zidovudine has been reported to cause a temporary improvement in the cognitive function of patients with AIDS. A multicenter controlled study of tetrahydroaminoacridine in patients with DAT currently is attempting to replicate preliminary reports[74] that tetrahydroaminoacridine can improve the level of cognitive functioning in patients with DAT.

Participation in experimental treatment programs is a positive action that we can offer the patient and the family, although special attention must be paid to the ethical issues and the protection of human subjects.

Caregivers

Family members provide most of the care for demented patients, and a major role of the clinician is to educate them, as well as assist them in obtaining appropriate support. Attention to the caregivers' psychologic, social, and legal needs is crucial. The burden experienced by caregivers is the primary determinant of how long the patient will be able to remain at home and how well the family adjusts to the long-term and ever-increasing needs of the patient.[75] The sense of burden experienced by the primary caregiver may be ameliorated by encouraging participation of other family members and the use of alternate care, such as day-care and respite care centers. Psychologic support for caregivers may be obtained through referral to disease-related lay organizations (eg, Alzheimer's Association); in some cases, psychotherapy or pharmacotherapy may be needed. Legal counsel regarding guardianship (or other means of taking responsibility for the patient), estate management, and testamentary procedures is frequently required.

Conclusion

The aged individual is vulnerable to a panoply of clinical syndromes produced by brain dysfunction. Of these, dementia is among the most common. Dementia refers to a syndrome of acquired persistent intellectual impairment with deficits in several intellectual and behavioral domains. Dementia may result from degenerative, vascular, infectious, neoplastic, traumatic, toxic, metabolic, or psychiatric disorders. A thorough evaluation is required to identify factors responsible for or contributing to the intellectual deterioration. Specific interventions are available for some dementias, symptomatic treatments for all. The needs of caregivers, as well as patients, should be monitored by the clinician.

Acknowledgment

This work was supported in part by the Veterans Administration. The opinions expressed herein are those of the authors and not necessarily those of the Veterans Administration.

References

1. American Psychiatric Association. *Diagnostic and Statistical Manual of Mental Disorders*. 3rd ed, *Revised (DSM-III R)*. Washington, DC: American Psychiatric Association; 1987.

2. Chedru F, Geschwind N. Disorders of higher cortical function in acute confusional states. *Cortex* 1972;8:395–411.

3. Lipowski ZJ. Delirium (acute confusional states). *JAMA* 1987;258:1789–1792.

4. Rabins PV, Folstein MF. Delirium and dementia: diagnostic criteria and fatality rates. *Br J Psychiatry* 1982;140:149–153.

5. Small GW. Dementia and amnestic syndromes. In: Karasu TB, et al, eds. *Treatment of Psychiatric Disorders: A Task Force Report of the American Psychiatric Association*. Washington, DC: American Psychiatric Press Inc. In press.

6. Cummings JL, Miller B, Hill MA, et al. Neuropsychiatric aspects of multi-infarct dementia and dementia of the Alzheimer type. *Arch Neurol* 1987;44:389–393.

7. Cummings JL. Organic delusions: phenomenology, anatomical correlations, and review. *Br J Psychiatry* 1985;146:184–197.

8. Spar JE. Organic mood syndrome. In: Karasu TB, et al, eds. *Treatment of Psychiatric Disorders: A Task Force Report of the American Psychiatric Association*. Washington, DC: American Psychiatric Press Inc. In press.

9. Cummings JL. *Clinical Neuropsychiatry*. New York, NY: Grune & Stratton; 1985.

10. Spar JE. Organic personality syndrome. In: Karasu TB, et al, eds. *Treatment of Psychiatric Disorders: A Task Force Report of the American Psychiatric Association*. Washington, DC: American Psychiatric Press Inc. In press.

11. Larrabee GT, Levin HS, High WM. Senescent forgetfulness: a quantitative study. *Dev Neuropsychol* 186;2:373–385.

12. Cummings JL, Benson DF. *Dementia: A Clinical Approach*. Stoneham, Mass: Buttersworths; 1983.

13. Ineichen B. Measure the rising tide: how many dementia cases will there be by 2001? *Br J Psychiatry* 1987;150:193–200.

14. Tomlinson BE, Blessed G, Roth M. Observations on the brains of demented old people. *J Neurol Sci* 1970;11:205–224.

15. Kallmann FJ. *Heredity in Health and Mental Disorder*. New York, NY: WW Norton & Co Inc; 1953.

16. Nee LE, Eldridge R, Sunderland T, et al. Dementia of the Alzheimer type: clinical and family study of 22 twin pairs. *Neurology* 1987;37:359–363.

17. Jarvik LF, Matsuyama SS, Kessler JO, et al. Philothermal response of polymorphonuclear leukocytes in dementia of the Alzheimer type. *Neurobiol Aging* 1982;3:93–99.

18. Roth M, Tomlinson BE, Blessed G. The relationship between quantitative measures of dementia and of degenerative changes in the cerebral grey matter of elderly subjects. *Proc R Soc Med* 1967;60:254–258.

19. McKhann G, Drachman D, Folstein M, et al. Clinical diagnosis of Alzheimer's disease: report of the NINCDS-ADRDA Work Group under the auspices of the Department of Health and Human Services Task Force on Alzheimer's Disease. *Neurology* 1984;34:939–944.

20. Tierney MC, Fisher RH, Lewis AJ, et al. The NINCDS-ADRDA Work Group criteria for the clinical diagnosis of probable Alzheimer's disease: a clinicopathologic study of 57 cases. *Neurology* 1988;38:359–364.

21. Mayeux R, Stern Y, Spanton S. Heterogeneity in dementia of the Alzheimer type: evidence of subgroups. *Neurology* 1985;35:453–461.

22. Chandra V, Bharucha NE, Schoenberg BS. Conditions associated with Alzheimer's disease at death: case-control study. *Neurology* 1986;36:209–211.

23. NIH (National Institutes of Health), Consensus Development Conference Statement. *Differential Diagnosis of Dementing Diseases. JAMA* 1987;258:3411–3416.

24. Katzman R. Alzheimer's disease. *N Engl J Med* 1986;314:964–973.

25. Brun A, Gustafson L. Distribution of cerebral degeneration in Alzheimer's disease. *Arch Psychiatr Nervenk* 1976;223:15–33.

26. Whitehouse PJ, Price DL, Clark AW, et al. Alzheimer's disease and senile dementia: loss of neurons in the basal forebrain. *Science* 1982;215:1237–1239.

27. Khachaturian ZS. Diagnosis of Alzheimer's disease. *Arch Neurol* 1985;42:1097–1105.

28. Wechsler AF, Verity M, Rosenchein S, et al. Pick's disease. *Arch Neurol* 1982;39:287–290.

29. Albert ML, Feldman RG, Willis AG. The 'subcortical dementia' of progressive supranuclear palsy. *J Neurol Neurosurg Psychiatry* 1974;37:121–130.

30. Martilla RJ. Epidemiology. In: Koller WC, ed. *Handbook of Parkinson's Disease*. New York, NY: Marcel Dekker Inc; 1987.

31. Cummings JL. Intellectual impairment in Parkinson's disease: clinical, biochemical, and pathologic correlates. *J Geriatr Psychiatr Neurol* 1988;1:24–36.

32. Boller F. Alzheimer's disease and Parkinson's disease: clinical and pathological associations. In: Reisberg B, ed. *Alzheimer's Disease: The Standard Reference*. New York, NY: The Free Press; 1983.

33. Lewin R. Dramatic results with brain grafts. *Science* 1987;237:245–247.

34. Hayden MR. *Huntington's Chorea*. New York, NY: Springer-Verlag NY Inc; 1981.

35. Gusella JF, Wexler NS, Conneally PM et al. A polymorphic DNA marker genetically linked to Huntington's disease. *Nature* 1983;306:234–238.

36. Hachinski VC, Iliff LD, Zilhka E, et al. Cerebral blood flow in dementia. *Arch Neurol* 1975;32:632–637.

37. Rosen WG, Terry RD, Fuld PA, et al. Pathological verification of ischemic score in differentiation of dementias. *Ann Neurol* 1980;7:486–488.

38. Erkinjuntti T. Types of multi-infarct dementia. *Acta Neurol Scand* 1987;75:391–399.

39. Ishii N, Nishahara Y, Imamura T. Why do frontal lobe symptoms predominate in vascular dementia with lacunes? *Neurology* 1986;36:340–345.

40. Roman GC. Senile dementia of the Binswanger type. *JAMA* 1987;258:1782–1788.

41. Thompson TL II, Moran MG, Nies AS. Psychotropic drug use in the elderly. *N Engl J Med* 1983;308:134–138, 194–199.

42. Cutting J. The relationship between Korsakov's syndrome and 'alcoholic dementia.' *Br J Psychiatry* 1978;132:240–251.

43. Ron MA. Brain damage in chronic alcoholism: a neuropathological, neuroradiological, and psychological review. *Psychol Med* 1977;7:103–112.

44. McLachlan C. Aluminum and Alzheimer's disease. *Neurobiol Aging* 1986;7:525–532.

45. Price RW, Brew B, Sidtis J, et al. The brain in AIDS: central nervous system HIV-1 infection and AIDS dementia complex. *Science* 1987;239:586–592.

46. Yarchoan R, Brouwers P, Spitzer AR, et al. Response of human-immunodeficiency-virus-associated neurological disease to 3′-azido-3′-deoxythymidine. *Lancet* 1987; 1:132–135.

47. Brown P, Cathala F, Castaigne P, et al. Creutzfeldt-Jakob disease: clinical analysis of a consecutive series of 230 neuropathologically verified cases. *Ann Neurol* 1986; 20:597–602.

48. Gajdusek DC. Unconventional viruses and the origin and disappearances of kuru. *Science* 1977;197:943–960.

49. Mahler ME, Cummings JL. Treatable dementias. *West J Med* 1987;146:705–712.

50. Corsellis JAN. Posttraumatic dementia. In: Katzman R, Terry RD, Bick KL, eds. *Aging: Alzheimer's Disease: Senile Dementia and Related Disorders*. New York, NY: Raven Press; 1973:7.

51. Black PM. Idiopathic normal-pressure hydrocephalus: results of shunting in 62 patients. *J Neurosurg* 1980; 52:371–377.

52. LaRue A, D'Elia LF, Clark EO, et al. Clinical tests of memory in dementia, depression, and healthy aging. *Psychology Aging* 1986;1:69–77.

53. Hamilton M. A rating scale for depression. *J Neurol Neurosurg Psychiatry* 1967;23:56–62.

54. Zung WWK. A self-rating depression scale. *Arch Gen Psychiatry* 1965;12:63–70.

55. Rubin SM, Glasser ML, Werckle MA. The examination of physician's awareness of dementing disorders. *J Am Geriatr Soc* 1987;35:1051–1058.

56. Folstein MF, Folstein SE, McHugh PR. 'Mini-Mental State': a practical method for grading the cognitive state of patients for the clinician. *J Psychiatr Res* 1975;12:189–198.

57. Blessed G, Tomlinson BE, Roth M. The association between quantitative measures of dementia and of senile change in the cerebral grey matter of elderly subjects. *Br J Psychiatry* 1968;114:797–811.

58. Kahn RL. Psychological aspects of aging. In: Rossman I, ed. *Clinical Geriatrics*. Philadelphia, Pa: JB Lippincott; 1971.

59. Schwamm LH, Van Dyke C, Kiernan RJ, et al. The neurobehavior cognitive status examination: comparison with the Cognitive Capacity Screening Examination and the Mini-Mental State Examination in a neurosurgical population. *Ann Intern Med* 1987;107:486–491.

60. Pfeiffer E. A short portable mental status questionnaire for the assessment of organic brain deficit in elderly patients. *J Am Geriatr Soc* 1975;23:433–441.

61. Roth M, Tym E, Mountjoy CQ, et al. CAMDEX: a standardized instrument for the diagnosis of mental disorders in the elderly with special reference to the early detection of dementia. *Br J Psychiatry* 1986;149:698–709.

62. Hughes CP, Berg L, Danzinger WL, et al. A new clinical scale for the staging of dementia. *Br J Psychiatry* 1982;140:566–572.

63. Reisberg B, Ferris SH, DeLeon MJ, et al. The global deterioration scale for assessment of primary degenerative dementia. *Am J Psychiatry* 1982;139:1136–1139.

64. Larson EB, Reifler BV, Featherstone HJ, et al. Dementia in elderly outpatients: a prospective study. *Ann Intern Med* 1984;100:417–423.

65. Martin DC, Miller J, Kapoor W, et al. Clinical prediction rules for computed tomographic scanning in senile dementia. *Arch Intern Med* 1987;147:77–80.

66. Garber HJ, Weilburg JB, Buonanno FS, et al. Use of magnetic resonance imaging in psychiatry. *Am J Psychiatry* 1988;145:164–171.

67. Jagust WJ, Budinger TF, Reed BR. The diagnosis of dementia with single photon emission computed tomography. *Arch Neurol* 1987;44:258–262.

68. Johnson KA, Mueller ST, Walshe TM, et al. Cerebral perfusion imaging in Alzheimer's disease. *Arch Neurol* 1987;44:165–168.

69. Foster NL, Chase TN, Mansi L, et al. Cortical abnormalities in Alzheimer's disease. *Ann Neurol* 1984;16:649–654.

70. Davenport S, Goldberg D, Millar T. How psychiatric disorders are missed during medical consultations. *Lancet* 1987;2:439–441.

71. Jarvik LF, Trader DW. Treatment of behavioral and mood changes. In: Aronson M, ed. *Understanding Alzheimer's Disease*. New York, NY: Charles Scribner's Sons; 1988:128–145.

72. Winograd CH, Jarvik LF. Physician management of the demented patient. *J Am Geriatr Soc* 1986;34:295–308.

73. Burnside I. Nursing care. In: Jarvik LF, Winograd CH, eds. *Treatments for the Alzheimer Patient: The Long Haul*. New York, NY: Springer Publishing Co Inc; 1988.

74. Summers WK, Majovski LV, Marsh GM, et al. Oral tetrahydroaminoacridine in long-term treatment of senile dementia, Alzheimer type. *N Engl J Med* 1986;315:1241–1245.

75. Zarit SH, Reever KE, Bach-Peterson J. Relatives of the impaired elderly: correlates of feelings of burden. *Gerontologist* 1980;20:649–655.

76. Winograd CH. The physician and the Alzheimer patient. In: Jarvik LF, Winograd CH, eds. *Treatments for the Alzheimer Patient: The Long Haul*. New York, NY: Springer Publishing Co Inc; 1988.

34

Cerebrovascular Disease and Stroke

Louis Caplan

Stroke is a problem of major importance in the geriatric age group. In 1984, one-half million Americans had a stroke, more than 150,000 died of stroke, and there was a prevalence of 2 million stroke survivors. A great majority of strokes occur in individuals older than 65 years of age. During 1980, death rates from stroke for men and women aged 65 to 69 years were more than five times higher than for individuals aged 50 to 54 years. And for individuals older than 85 years of age, the stroke death rate was over 50 times higher than for individuals in their 50s[1]. In nearly all age groups, men have more strokes and more stroke deaths than women.

More impressive than the numbers, are the qualitative aspects of morbidity after stroke. Quality of life depends so much on having preserved brain function. The two worst robbers of dignity in the last decades of life are dementia and stroke. Many stroke victims have an impaired ability to see, think, walk, feel, communicate, speak, read, write, and recall. Yet, there is reason for hope. The incidence of stroke is dramatically declining as is the stroke mortality rate.[2] New advances in technology, especially in neuroimaging and ultrasound, now make it possible to pinpoint the location and degree of brain damage from stroke and to detect the location and severity of disease within the larger extracranial and intracranial arteries. These advances should facilitate stroke prevention, treatment, and recovery.

Stroke is a heterogeneous category of disease. There are two major large categories, hemorrhage and ischemia, which cause drastically opposite problems—too much blood in hemorrhage and insufficient blood supply in ischemia. These large categories can be further subdivided in a clinically useful way (Fig. 34.1). Hemorrhage causes brain injury by increasing intracranial pressure, creating local pressure on focal brain regions, disconnecting vital nerve pathways, and irritating blood vessels to cause vasoconstriction and subsequent brain ischemia. Ischemia causes damage by depriving brain tissue of vital nutrients: ischemia can be generalized when there is cardiac pump failure or circulatory collapse, but is most often focal when a supplying artery is obstructed by local atherostenosis, thrombosis, or an embolus. Treatment depends on the location and severity of the vascular lesion, the presence and degree of brain damage, and the presence of coexistent neurological and medical problems. This chapter will emphasize age-related differences in stroke patterns and treatment of elderly persons.

Hemorrhagic Stroke

Within the large category of hemorrhagic stroke are two quite different syndromes, subarachnoid hemorrhage (SAH) and intracerebral hemorrhage (ICH); each syndrome has quite different causes, clinical findings and problems, and treatment. Subarachnoid hemorrhage is due to leakage of blood at the surface of the brain into the cerebrospinal fluid (CSF) spaces around it. It is most often due to the rupture of an artery on the surface, especially an aneurysm. Less

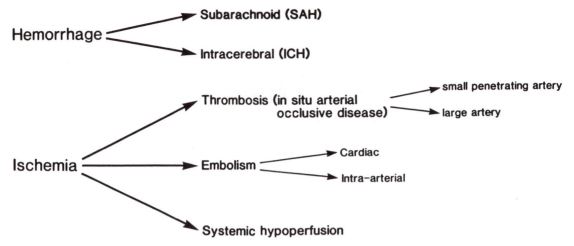

Fig. 34.1. Two major categories of stroke.

often, vascular malformations or abnormal or traumatized arteries bleed. Blood is quickly distributed throughout the subarachnoid space. When bleeding is massive, the patient usually does not survive the initial bleeding. In survivors, the major goal of medical care is to prevent subsequent hemorrhage (the abnormal or damaged artery, once it leaks, has a high rate of rebleeding) and to deal with the following complications of having blood under pressure in the subarachnoid space: increased intracranial pressure, increased systolic blood pressure, cardiac changes, hydrocephalus, and constriction of arteries bathed by the blood.[3] In contrast, ICH is caused by leakage of smaller arteries or arterioles directly into the brain parenchyma. Most often, this is due to hypertension, but vascular malformations and abnormal arteries (eg, those infiltrated with amyloid) can bleed into the brain substance as can aneurysms on occasion. Massive hemorrhages cause death quickly. In most patients, the brain substance limits and contains the hemorrhage, and rebleeding is much less common compared with SAH. The aims of treatment are to limit the size of the hematoma, minimize damage to the local regions of the brain, and prevent death from increased intracranial pressure.[4] Bleeding diatheses can cause either SAH or ICH.

Subarachnoid Hemorrhage

Subarachnoid hemorrhage accounts for about 8% to 10% of strokes. In many physicians' minds, SAH is considered a young person's disease; these physicians probably recall instances of a tragic outcome from aneurysmal SAH in individuals in their 20s or 30s. Actually, SAH is common in elderly persons, and the age-specific annual incidence of SAH increases with advancing age to the oldest age group studied.[5] The average age of patients with SAH in the Framingham study was 63 years,[6] and the median age of patients with SAH in Rochester, Minn, was 58 years.[5] Women predominate over men; the rates in Rochester, Minn, were 12.2/100,000 for women and 7.6/100,000 per year for men.[5] The incidence of SAH, unlike that of other stroke types, has not changed appreciably during the past three decades, and virtually all stroke registries and data banks find that SAH accounts for about 1 stroke in 10.

The majority of patients with SAH harbor saccular aneurysms as the cause of bleeding. In necropsy studies, between 6% and 10% of patients in each decade have cerebral aneurysms at postmortem examination.[7] Saccular aneurysms form at the bifurcation of large arteries and are probably caused by a combination of congenital and degenerative changes in arteries. Hemodynamic stresses at arterial bifurcations and hypertension lead to degenerative changes in the internal elastic lamina, weakening of the arterial wall, and aneurysmal outpouching. The most common sites for aneurysm formation are at the internal carotid (ICA)–posterior communicating artery junction, the anterior cerebral (ACA)–anterior communicating artery junction, and the bifurcation of the middle cerebral artery (MCA) within the anterior circulation. Posterior circulation aneurysms are less common; when present, the most common sites are at the bifurcation of the basilar artery and the vertebral artery–posterior inferior cerebellar artery junction. Most aneurysms probably remain asymptomatic until they bleed, but some larger aneurysms distort and compress adjacent nerves, brain tissues, or meningeal structures, causing headache and cranial nerve or parenchymatous dysfunction.

When aneurysms rupture, they leak blood into the CSF under arterial pressure. Patients invariably describe a sudden onset of severe headache, often "the worst headache of my life." The sudden increase in intracranial pressure often causes an immediate cessation of activity, loss of ability to make new memories, and vomiting. There usually is some alteration in alertness, ranging from deep coma in massive bleedings to sleepiness or restlessness with agitation in smaller bleedings. Unless bleeding also occurs directly into the brain (called *meningocerebral hemorrhage*), patients usually do not have severe focal neurological signs, such as hemiplegia or hemianopia. Blood around the aneurysm or layered within the cisterns around the brain often irritates local structures, causing minor focal abnormalities. Posterior communicating artery aneurysms may cause a third nerve palsy; MCA aneurysms cause slight aphasia, minor contralateral weakness, or sensory abnormalities; and anterior communicating artery aneurysms often cause bilateral leg weakness and bilateral Babinski's signs.

Arteriovenous malformations (AVMs) also can leak onto the surface and cause SAH, but more often bleed into brain parenchyma. Bleeding from AVMs is usually less brisk than from aneurysms, and symptoms may evolve more slowly. Most AVMs become symptomatic during the first four decades of life by causing headache, seizures, or bleeding. Arteriovenous malformations are a much less common cause of bleeding in elderly persons. Investigation of geriatric patients with SAH yields a higher percentage of individuals in whom neither aneurysms nor AVMs can be identified in contrast to patients younger than 60 years of age, in whom these lesions are invariably found. Hypertension sometimes causes leakage of surface arteries. Unrecognized head trauma, amyloid angiopathy, and bleeding diatheses, especially administration of anticoagulants, cause more episodes of SAH in elderly persons than among younger patients.

Computed tomography (CT) is a very important investigation tool for patients with SAH and is, at present, far superior to magnetic resonance imaging (MRI). CT scan can show the presence of blood in the subarachnoid space and thus confirm the diagnosis. The distribution of the blood can suggest the likely aneurysmal site; the amount of blood and its thickness and distribution can also help to predict the likelihood of delayed cerebral ischemia developing.[8] A contrast-enhanced CT scan can occasionally opacify the aneurysm, allowing its identification.[9] Smaller hemorrhages and SAH, occurring longer than 48 hours before the scan, can be missed by CT. Lumbar puncture still is a very important test in patients whose symptoms are suggestive of SAH.[10] All patients with SAH have blood in the CSF when tapped within 48 hours. Some patients have a small "warning leak" before massive aneurysmal rupture. These small hem-

orrhages are often missed by CT and will be detected only by lumbar puncture. No patient with a serious suspicion of SAH should leave the emergency room without a lumbar puncture, unless they are to be admitted to the hospital for further study. If SAH is confirmed, hematological studies for a bleeding diathesis should be performed. If the patient's condition does not preclude treatment, angiography to detect an aneurysm or AVM should be pursued when surgical treatment becomes feasible.

Aneurysmal SAH is a disease in which surgical treatment is preferred whenever possible. The incidence rate of further bleeding is so high, and the morbidity and mortality of subsequent bleedings are so devastating, that surgical obliteration of the aneurysm is warranted whenever possible. The physicians and surgeons attempt to get the patient into the best possible condition for surgery, trying to anticipate further aneurysmal leakage. During the period of preparation for surgery, delayed cerebral ischemia can develop. Delayed ischemia is due to a reaction in the basal arteries that are surrounded by blood.[11] These vessels constrict and appear as narrowed thin threads on cerebral angiograms. Treatment of delayed ischemia usually consists of volume expansion and attempts to decrease intracranial pressure. Calcium channel blockers are being investigated to see if these agents will prevent or decrease vasoconstriction and so prevent delayed ischemia. Hydrocephalus is another complication of SAH and occasionally necessitates placement of a ventricular drain. Cardiac arrhythmias and hyponatremia are important medical complications of SAH that require early recognition and treatment.

Intracerebral Hemorrhage

Intracerebral hemorrhage accounts for about 8% of strokes, but their frequency is declining. The average age for patients with ICH was 64 years in the Framingham study.[6] Contrary to common belief, ICH increases in frequency with age and is quite common in patients in their 70s and 80s. The most common cause of ICH is hypertension. Hypertension causes degenerative changes in small penetrating cerebral and brain-stem arteries and arterioles that can lead to microaneurysm formation and rupture. Acute increases in blood pressure can also cause rupture of these small penetrating arteries.[12] Arteriovenous malformations are a common cause of ICH in young adults but are an unusual source of hemorrhage after the sixth decade. Amyloid angiopathy, anticoagulant-related hemorrhages, and trauma are very important causes of ICH in elderly persons.

In most cases of ICH, the bleeding is under arteriolar or capillary pressure and is not as brisk as in aneurysmal SAH, explaining why the clinical symptoms and signs evolve more gradually. The first symptoms are related to the local brain region where the bleeding is located. Bleeding into the internal capsule causes weakness or numbness of the contralateral limbs, while bleeding into the left temporal lobe might cause speech abnormalities as the first symptom. Continued bleeding causes the hematoma to enlarge. The pressure that develops within the hematoma exerts pressure on surrounding capillaries, causing them, in turn, to break.[13] The hematoma gradually enlarges during a period of a few minutes, up to an hour or more. As the ICH grows, tissue pressure also increases locally and acts to contain the bleeding. The enlarging ICH causes a gradual increase in the focal symptoms over a period of minutes. Patients will describe minor weakness in an arm, evolving to hemiplegia during a 5- to 15-minute span. The enlarging hematoma, if it becomes sizable, causes pressure shifts and increases intracranial pressure, causing headache, vomiting, and a decreased level of consciousness. The clinical findings of gradually increasing focal neurological signs with a decreasing level of alertness during a period of minutes is virtually diagnostic of ICH. In some elderly patients, cerebral atrophy may provide considerable room inside the cranium, so that small or medium hemorrhages may not cause headache or alterations in alertness. In the Harvard Stroke Registry series, about one half of patients with ICH did not complain of a prominent headache.[14] Hypertensive ICH favors regions that contain penetrating arteries, especially the putamen, caudate nucleus, cerebral white matter, thalamus, pons, and cerebellum. Table 34.1 lists the frequency of hemorrhages at various sites and the usual accompanying clinical findings.

Bleeding diatheses, especially the use of anticoagulants, are an important cause of ICH in the geriatric age group. Patients may not mention that they are taking warfarin. Sometimes, the warfarin has been prescribed because of transient cerebral ischemia, so that the unwary physician falsely attributes the focal neurological signs to recurrent ischemia. Anticoagulant hemorrhages often begin slowly and evolve more gradually than hypertensive hemorrhages.[15] They commonly affect the cerebellum or cerebral white matter and have a higher mortality than other causes of ICH. Sometimes, the anticoagulant has been given to prevent a cerebral embolism from prosthetic heart valves or other cardiogenic sources. When the hemorrhage is small and the threat of embolism is high, the treating physician may be tempted to watch the patient without reversing the hypoprothrombinemia with aquamephyton (vitamin K). This is a bad mistake.

Anticoagulant-related ICH must be treated quickly and aggressively to prevent a disastrous outcome.

Amyloid angiopathy is another frequent cause of ICH in elderly persons. This disorder affects small arteries and arterioles in the meninges and cerebral white and gray matter. These arteries are thickened by an acellular hyaline material that stains positively with periodic–acid Schiff stains and has an apple-green birefringence with a polarized Congo red stain.[16] The arterial lesions are not common in the brain stem or basal ganglia. Most ICHs due to amyloid angiopathy are in the subcortical white matter. Hemorrhages can be multiple and frequently patients are demented due to an accumulation of disability caused by the hemorrhages and frequently coexistent Alzheimer's disease.

Computed tomography is a nearly ideal diagnostic tool for patients with ICH. During the acute period, blood within the brain parenchyma is readily recognized and easily separated from ischemic lesions. Computed tomography defines the location, size, and shape of the hemorrhage; dissection and drainage of the lesion into the ventricles or onto the brain surface; edema and shift of brain tissue; and the presence of accompanying subarachnoid blood and hydrocephalus.[9] Magnetic resonance imaging also shows hemorrhages well, but experience is needed to differentiate ICH from ischemia; MRI is especially useful for showing occult vascular malformations. Angiography and lumbar puncture are ordinarily not needed unless an aneurysm is suspected because of the clinical symptoms or location of the blood.

Treatment usually consists of control of the causal factors when possible. Correction of bleeding abnormalities and reduction of blood pressure in hypertensive individuals are the two most important methods of treatment. Small hematomas usually resolve by themselves without a problem; large hematomas, greater than 4 cm, are usually fatal, and the patient is irreversibly damaged by the time of arrival at a medical facility. Medium hematomas near the cerebral surface can be drained if they are causing progressive focal neurological signs or decreasing levels of alertness.

Ischemic Stroke

Ischemia accounts for approximately 80% of strokes. There are four major subcategories of ischemic stroke: (1) lacunes due to disease of small penetrating cerebral arteries; (2) atherostenosis of large extracranial and intracranial arteries, causing ischemia by intra-arterial embolism and reduced flow distal to the obstructing lesion; (3) hypoperfusion due to cardiac factors or hypovolemia; and (4) cerebral embolism of cardiac origin. In the geriatric age group, cardiogenic embo-

Table 34.1. Neurological findings in patients with ICH at common sites.*

Locale	Frequency, %	Motor weakness	Sensory loss	Hemianopia	Pupils	Eye movements	Other
Caudate	7	Hemiparesis, + −	−	−	Normal	Normal or transient conjugate gaze palsy, contralateral	Confusion
Putamen, small	35	Hemiparesis, + +	+	−	Normal	−	
Putamen, large		Hemiparesis, + + + +	+ +	+ +	+ − ipsilateral fixed, dilated	Conjugate gaze palsy, contralateral	L: aphasia; R: L-side neglect, constructional apraxia
Thalamus	15	Hemiparesis, +	+ + +	+ −	Small, nonreactive	Eyes down, or down and in; vertical gaze palsy; conjugate palsy, ipsilateral or contralateral; pseudo–6th nerve palsy	Confusion, L: aphasia
Lobar	25						
Frontal		Hemiparesis, + −	−	−	Normal	−	Abulic,
Parietal		Hemiparesis, +	+ + +	+ +	Normal	−	L: aphasia, R:L-side construction
Temporal		−	−	+ +	Normal	−	L: aphasia
Occipital		− or transient	− or transient	+ + + +	Normal	−	−
Pontine	8						
Median, large		Quadraparesis + + + +	+ −	−	Small reaction	Bilateral horizontal conjugate gaze palsy, bobbing	Hyperventilation
Lateral tegmental		− or transient	Contra-lateral, hemisen-sory + + +	−	ipsilateral, small reaction	1½ syndrome	Limb ataxia
Cerebellar	10	−	−	−	Small reaction	Ipsilateral 6th nerve palsy or ipsilateral conjugate gaze palsy	Gait ataxia

*ICH indicates intracerebral hemorrhage; plus sign, present; minus sign; not present; L, left-sided lesion; and R, right-sided lesion.

lism and lacunae account for a disproportionate number of strokes compared with ischemic strokes in younger patients. Except for systemic hypoperfusion that starts abruptly, the signatures of ischemic stroke are transient ischemic attacks (TIAs) and a stepwise, fluctuating, or progressive clinical course.

Cerebral Embolism of Cardiac Origin

Until very recently, cardiogenic embolism was considered to be rare. Prior classifications required the presence of a known cardiac source, a sudden maximal-at-onset neurological deficit, and peripheral systemic embolism. Myocardial infarction and rheumatic mitral stenosis with atrial fibrillation were the only accepted cardiac embolic sources. Newer cardiac-testing technology, including echocardiography, ambulatory rhythm monitoring, and radionuclide imaging, have now uncovered many more potential cardiac embolic sources. Furthermore, ultrasonography and digital angiography have often made it possible to exclude large artery pathological conditions, thus making cardiogenic embolism a more likely explanation for cerebral cortical infarction in a given patient.

Cerebral embolism accounts for at least 30% of ischemic strokes.[17] A variety of different cardiac sources of embolism are now well established and include various valvular lesions, myocardial diseases (especially ischemia), rhythm disturbances, and cardiac tumors. These are outlined in Table 34.2. The two most important sources probably are ischemic heart disease and arrhythmias, each of which is more prevalent with advancing age. Coronary artery disease is a frequent cause of clot formation on the endocardial surface of the heart. Echocardiographic studies of patients with myocardial infarction and angina pectoris often reveal hypokinetic zones, regions of old myocardial damage, ventricular aneurysms, and poor ejection function. Mural thrombi are found less often. Atrial fibrillation is now a very well-established cause of cerebral embolism. The incidence of atrial fibrillation increases with advancing age during each decade. As many as 5% of all individuals older than 70 years of age have atrial fibrillation, and atrial fibrillation has been estimated to be responsible for as many as 25% of

Table 34.2. 12F2C—Cardiac sources of emboli.

Cardiac source
Ischemic heart disease
Mural thrombi
Ventricular aneurysms
Hypokinetic zones
Atrial infarcts
Myocardial infarcts
Arrhythmias
Atrial fibrillation
Sick sinus syndrome
Valvular heart disease
Rheumatic mitral and aortic stenosis
Bicuspid aortic valve
Mitral valve prolapse
Mitral annular calcification
Nonbacterial thrombotic endocarditis
Bacterial and fungal endocarditis
Myocardiopathies
Cardiomyopathy
Myocarditis
Amyloidosis
Sarcoidosis
Endocardial fibroelastosis
Atrial aneurysms
Intracardiac lesions or defects
Myxomas and other cardiac tumors
Ball valve thrombi
Atrial septal defects ⎫ "Paradoxical embolism"
Patent foramen ovale ⎭

strokes in individuals between 75 and 84 years of age.[18]

Sinoatrial pacemaker disturbances (the so-called sick sinus syndrome)[19] also is an important cause of cerebral embolism, and the disorder is more common in older patients. In one series of 100 patients with sick sinus syndrome, 16 had systemic embolism, among which 13 were to the brain.[19] Patients with sick sinus syndrome, in addition to periods of sinus bradycardia and sinus arrests, have attacks of atrial fibrillation and atrial fibrillation-flutter. Poor atrial function leads to stagnation of blood in the atria and subsequent embolization, especially if the atria regain contractility. This series of events probably is common in patients with atrial fibrillation and enlarged atria.[18]

In most patients, cerebral emboli produce symptoms abrupty, but not always maximal at outset, and not always during physical activity as was formerly thought. Progression of symptoms during the first 24 to 48 hours occurs in some patients and is due to distal passage of emboli that then block distal arteries.[20] Systemic embolism is common, but its recognition is infrequent, approximately 2% in the Harvard Stroke Registry and Michael Reese Registry cases of cerebral embolism.[21] Most emboli in the anterior circulation go to middle cerebral artery branches, causing surface infarcts. About 20% of emboli go to the posterior circulation, usually causing cerebellar or posterior cerebral artery territory infarction. Recurrent infarction in different vascular territories is especially suggestive of cardiogenic embolism.

Investigation of patients for cerebral embolism should involve cardiac testing to establish a possible cardiogenic source, neuroimaging tests to define the areas of infarction, and exclusion of other potential causes of ischemia, such as large artery ischemic disease and coagulopathies. Computed tomography or MRI is often the first test performed. Wedge-shaped, superficial cortical, or cortical and subcortical infarcts in the territory of the MCAs and posterior cerebral arteries (PCAs), especially when multiple and bilateral, are supportive of a diagnosis of a cardioembolic mechanism. If the CT scan shows only lacunar infarcts, cardiogenic embolism becomes very unlikely. Echocardiography is a particularly useful test, especially in groups of patients who do not have strong risk factors for atherosclerosis (young people, women, and those with hypertension, diabetes, hyperlipidemia, a history of coronary or peripheral vascular disease, or smoking) or who have known heart disease. Echocardiography, however, misses many cardioembolic lesions because of an image-resolution problem. A 1- to 2-mm thrombus can block an intracerebral artery, leading to devastating neurological damage, and yet be below the resolution capacity of the present technology. Furthermore, mural atrial and ventricular thrombosis is a dynamic disorder, with clots being formed that dissolve or embolize. When a clot has left its "nest" in the heart and flown the coop, it will no longer be present and so will not be detectable by cardiac imaging.[22] The use of Doppler devices after intravenous injection of air bubbles during echocardiography improves the detection of cardiac septal defects that could lead to cerebral embolism.[23] Rhythm monitoring also is important. Angiography, especially if done soon after symptoms develop, can show the embolism, as well as provide evidence for or against coexistent artery disease.[17]

Treatment will depend on the nature of the cardiac source, the likelihood of a further embolism, and the medical and neurological state of the patient. Cardiac thrombi are usually red clots that form in stagnant regions of the atria or ventricles. Warfarin and heparin have theoretical advantages over platelet antiaggregates for prevention of further thrombi and embolization. During the acute period of cerebral ischemia, if the infarct is very large or hemorrhagic and if the patient is hypertensive, acute heparinization, especially by bolus injection, carries a substantial risk of bleeding into the infarct. If the risk of further embolization is low, I would advise waiting to treat the patient with anticoagulants. When anticoagulants are used prophylactically to prevent embolization, keeping the prothrombin time at 16 to 19 seconds, $1\frac{1}{2}$ times control, usually is effective and is less hazardous than more intense anticoagulation.

Lacunar Infarction

Lacunes are small, deep infarcts caused by degenerative changes within small penetrating arteries to the internal capsule, basal ganglia, cerebral white matter, thalamus, and pons. Hypertension is the most important cause of lipohyalinosis, the most common mechanism of disease within the media of these microscopic arteries. Sometimes, microatheroma originating at the orifice of these pentrating arteries leads to occlusion.[24] Lacunar infarcts are the most common vascular lesions found within the brain at necropsy. In various series and registries, they account for about 25% or more of ischemic strokes.

Symptoms may begin abruptly or evolve gradually during hours to days. Transient ischemic attacks precede the development of a persistent deficit in about 30% of cases. The neurological symptoms depend on the region of ischemia. The most common clinical presentations are as follows: (1) "pure motor stroke" due to ischemia to the pons or internal capsule—weakness of the face, arm, and leg on one side of the body without sensory, visual, cognitive, or behavioral abnormalities; (2) pure sensory stroke due to infarction in the lateral part of the thalamus or posterior limb of the internal capsule—numbness and/or paresthesia of the face, arm, leg, and trunk on one side of the body without paralysis, visual, cognitive, or behavioral abnormalities; and (3) "ataxic hemiparesis" due to infarction in the internal capsule or pons—a mixture of cerebellar-type incoordination and weakness on one side of the body without other major findings.[24] Some patients have a combination of motor and sensory abnormalities, and some patients with lacunar infarcts in the caudate nucleus, thalamus, or cerebral white matter may have prominent cognitive and/or behavioral abnormalities. Since lacunes are small lesions, headache, vomiting, and a decrease in the level of consciousness are not found.

The diagnosis of lacunar infarction is based on the presence of risk factors, the nature of the clinical signs and symptoms, and the results of neuroimaging tests. Most often, patients with lacunar infarction have hypertension or a history of hypertension or antihypertensive treatment. Diabetes also is common and probably predisposes to microatheroma. The absence of any history of either hypertension or diabetes should weigh against the diagnosis of lacunar infarction. The presence of prominent headache, vomiting, or a decreased level of alertness also makes lacunar infarction unlikely. The clinical symptoms and signs should be compatible with a small, deep lesion. Aphasia, hemianopia, and signs of solely tegmental brain-stem disease are strong evidence against lacunar disease. Computed tomography or MRI should show a small, deep infarct or be normal. A surface infarct or a large, deep infarct in the territory that would account for the symptoms excludes the diagnosis of lacunar infarction. The electroencephalogram (EEG) is usually not very much affected by a small lacunar infarct, so that lateralized EEG abnormalities also argue against the diagnosis of lacunar disease. In some cases, the clinical and neuroimaging tests are equivocal and do not establish a lacunar cause. In these patients, a search for other ischemic causes, such as coagulopathy, an embolism of cardiac origin, and large artery ischemic disease, is warranted.

The arterial lesions that cause lacunes predominantly affect the media of the small arteries. They are not subintimal nor is arterial thrombosis prominent. Agents that affect platelet aggregation and standard anticoagulants, such as heparain or warfarin, have little hypothetical reason to be effective. In fact, when anticoagulants have been used in small anecdotal series of patients with lacunar infarction, they have been proved to be ineffective. Treatment consists primarily of risk factor control, especially treatment of hypertension and/or diabetes.

Large Artery Occlusive Disease

Atherostenosis is a generalized process. Most often, the disease affects the extracranial large arteries in the neck, especially the origin of the ICA from the common carotid artery and the vertebral artery origin from the subclavian artery. Other, albeit less common, sites for atherostenosis are the ICA within the bony siphon and the proximal portion of the MCA within the anterior circulation, as well as the intracranial portion of the vertebral artery and the basilar artery in the posterior circulation. There are prominent racial and sex differences in the prevalence and distribution of atherostenosis.[25] Men and white patients have lesions that predominantly affect the origins of the ICA and vertebral artery extracranially, while women, black patients, and individuals of Chinese or Japanese origin have predominantly intracranial disease. Extracranial artery disease correlates with hypertension, hyperlipidemia, and the presence of coexistent coronary and peripheral arterial occlusive disease.

Atherostenosis causes brain infarction by decreasing blood flow and by acting as a source of intra-arterial embolism. The rough, craggy surfaces of arterial plaques serve as a nidus for aggregation and adhesion of platelet clumps and for superimposed thrombosis. Narrowing of the arterial lumen promotes thrombosis. Intra-arterial emboli can be composed of plaque material, including calcium, cholesterol crystals, red clots, or fibrin-platelet aggregates. Once a severe degree of stenosis is reached (about 70%), hemodynamic changes and turbulence with uneven flow develop. Ulceration, cracking of plaques, superimposed thrombus, and hemorrhage into plaques develop as a complication of the altered flow dynamics. The plaque grows; the lumen is progressively compromised, and the potential for intra-arterial embolism increases. Thrombosis of the small residual lumen is frequently the culminating event that precipitates symptoms, although occlusion often occurs without symptoms.[26,27] Initially, recently formed clots are loosely adherent to the arterial wall and can readily propagate or break off and embolize. Gradually, during the first 2 to 3 weeks after occlusion, the thrombus becomes more organized and adherent to the arterial wall, making embolization less likely. The thrombus decreases blood flow distally in the involved arterial bed, causing ischemia. Decreased blood flow and local accumulation of metabolites and other factors, such as lactic acid, prostacyclins, and leukotrienes, promote vasodilatation and development of collateral circulation that protect against ischemia. During the first 2 to 3 weeks after occlusion of a large artery, the situation often is unstable while a clot is organizing and collateral circulation is becoming established.

Treatment during these few weeks is therefore most important for limiting the extent of ischemic damage.

The most important clinical symptoms are headache and TIAs or persisting small stroke deficits. Headache is probably due to dilatation of collateral arteries and may precede or accompany the neurological symptoms. Transient ischemic attacks often are multiple, brief, and not stereotyped episodes of ischemia.[28] Specific symptoms will depend on the artery affected.[29]

Anterior Circulation

ICA in the Neck

This is the most common site for atherostenosis in the cerebrovascular bed. Lesions begin on the posterior wall of the ICA opposite the flow divider between the ICA and the external carotid artery. A high-pitched, focal, and long bruit may be audible if the lumen becomes compromised. The ICA supplies the ophthalmic artery as its first branch. Small emboli or reduced flow to the ophthalmic artery causes attacks of transient monocular blindness called *amaurosis fugax*. These are usually described as a shade or curtain descending from above or the side generally obscuring vision in the eye ipsilateral to the ICA lesion. Attacks usually last seconds to minutes and rarely cause lasting visual deficits. Small cholesterol emboli or fibrin-platelet plugs occasionally can be seen in the fundus oculi during or after an attack of amaurosis.[30] Hemispheric ischemia causes attacks of numbness and/or weakness of the face, arm, or leg contralateral to the ICA lesion and aphasia or behavioral symptoms, depending on the hemisphere affected. The arm is the most commonly affected part.[27] Usually, hemispheric attacks are not stereotypical. An arm might be affected during one attack, the leg in another, and the arm and leg in a third. The presence of both ipsilateral transient monocular blindness and contralateral limb symptoms due to hemispheric ischemia is virtually diagnostic of ICA disease.[31] In patients with ICA origin disease, TIAs are more common than strokes.

ICA Within the Siphon

Atherostenosis of the ICA in the neck above the first few centimeters of the artery is unusual. However, within the osseous canal, the artery sometimes becomes stenosed and calcified. This can involve the portion of the artery before the ophthalmic artery branch or more distally until the artery pierces the dura mater to become intracranial in its supraclinoid segment. When the artery is stenosed before the ophthalmic artery branch, transient monocular blindness can occur. The prognosis for patients with ICA siphon disease is not as good as for patients with ICA origin disease.[32] Strokes are more common than TIAs.[29] Symptoms and signs probably affect the anterior cerebral artery territory more often than in patients with ICA origin disease.

MCA

Atherostenosis of the MCA usually affects the proximal horizontal portion of the main-stem vessel or its proximal superior division branch. Women, diabetic patients, black persons, and individuals of Japanese or Chinese origin have a predilection for MCA disease.[25] Patients with MCA disease frequently do not have coronary or peripheral vascular disease or hyperlipidemia. The most common symptoms are aphasia "confusion" and face and hand weakness. Most patients with MCA disease do develop a stroke, but the size of the stroke usually is more limited than in patients with ICA disease. A common area of involvement is the deep territory supplied by the lenticulostriate arteries. These lesions are bigger than lacunae but are deep and best called striatocapsular infarcts.[29,33,34] The evolution of symptoms and signs often is longer than in patients with ICA disease,[33] and there is an increased incidence of bilateral MCA disease.

Other anterior circulation arteries are affected less often. *Anterior cerebral artery* (ACA) territory infarction is most often caused by propagation or embolization of a clot from the ICA.[29,35] Leg weakness and numbness are the most common findings. The *anterior choroidal artery* can be blocked by microatheroma, causing a deep infarct in the globus pallidus, posterior limb of the internal capsule, optic tract, and lateral geniculate body. Contralateral hemiparesis, hemianopia, and variable hemisensory symptoms result.[29,36]

Posterior Circulation

Subclavian Artery

The subclavian artery can be the site of atherostenosis, usually before its vertebral artery branch. Disease occurs more often on the left. Most often, subclavian artery disease is asymptomatic and is detected by noninvasive testing of patients with peripheral vascular or carotid artery disease. Some patients have coldness, fatigue, or cramping of the ischemic arm, especially after exercise. Brain ischemia is less common and, when present, is often due to coexistent carotid artery stenosis. Dizziness, staggering, diplopia, and visual blurring can occur in attacks and are due to diminished anterograde vertebral artery flow. Strokes in the posterior circulation are rare.[37,38] In many patients with subclavian artery stenosis, noninvasive testing[39] or angiography does document retrograde flow down the ipsilateral vertebral artery to supply the ischemic arm, the so-called subclavian steal syndrome.

Vertebral Artery in the Neck

Plaques can extend from the subclavian artery into the orifice of the vertebral artery, or can affect the first few centimeters of the nuchal vertebral artery. Vertebral artery origin lesions often coexist with ICA origin disease and also correlate with coronary and peripheral vascular occlusive disease. The symptoms of vertebral artery disease in the neck are identical to those found with subclavian artery disease except, of course, for the lack of ischemic arm symptoms. Transient ischemic attacks are common, but strokes are much less common.[40] When strokes occur, they are usually due to intra-arterial embolism to intracranial arteries within the posterior circulation.[38] Collateral circulation develops quickly after vertebral artery occlusion in the neck, usually deriving from branches of the subclavian artery, thyrocervical trunk, and external carotid artery.

Vertebral Artery Intracranial Segment (IVA)

Atherostenosis of the vertebral artery in the neck is unusual at any site above the most proximal portion of the artery, although the distal extracranial vertebral artery is vulnerable to injury and can be torn or spontaneously dissect after minor trauma or neck turning. The IVA is a relatively frequent site of disease. The most common symptoms are those of lateral medullary dysfunction or cerebellar infarction.[38] The IVA supplies the medulla and posterior inferior portion of the cerebellum and ends usually at the pontomedullary junction where the two IVAs join to form the basilar artery. Clots, formed within the IVA, can propagate into the basilar artery or embolize to the more distal intracranial basilar artery or the posterior cerebral arteries and their branches.[38]

Basilar Artery

The basilar artery is another frequent area of atherostenosis. Disease often affects the most proximal portion of the basilar artery but also frequently involves the middle and distal segments.[41] The basilar artery supplies the pons and ends at the pontomesencephalic junction. The most common symptoms are motor and oculomotor. Bilateral or alternating hemiplegia, diplopia, and ophthalmoplegia are common. Surprising is the fact that some patients survive quite well after basilar artery occlusion with little or no deficit.[42] In these patients, collateral circulation has formed from the circumferential cerebellar arteries and from the ICA posterior communicating, PCA pathway. Severe stenosis or occlusion of both IVAs is tolerated less well because of the paucity of available collateral circulation to supply the lower brain stem.[39]

PCAs

Atherostenosis of the PCAs also has a predilection for black persons and individuals of Oriental origin. Ischemia to the occipital and temporal lobes supplied by the PCAs causes hemianopia; hemisensory loss, amnesia, alexia, and anomia occur but less commonly and depend on the location and extent of the ischemia. Most infarcts within the PCA territory are due to embolism arising either from the heart or from the proximal part of the vertebrobasilar arterial system.[38,43,44] Patients with stenosis of the PCA origin may have TIAs that consist mostly of dysfunction in the contralateral hemianopic visual field.[45]

Diagnosis and Treatment

A veritable revolution in technology has now made it possible for clinicians to localize and quantitate the severity of disease within the arterial bed and to study the resulting brain damage. Neuroimaging tests, CT, and MRI are very important in localizing the arterial territory of the ischemia. Certain patterns of infarction correlate well with disease at various loci in the extracranial and intracranial arterial bed.[29] Some patients with transient or even persisting but reversible ischemia have normal CT scans that indicate that the ischemic insult has probably not led to irreversible brain damage. On the other hand, some patients with TIAs have lesions in appropriate loci for their symptoms on CT and MRI.[28] Once the arterial territory has been clarified by clinical symptoms and signs and neuroimaging tests, a variety of noninvasive ultrasound tests often can yield information about the offending arterial lesion. B-mode ultrasound and Doppler (pulsed or continuous wave), especially when combined in a duplex system, can usually accurately quantitate the presence and severity of disease in the nuchal ICA,[27] vertebral arteries, and subclavian arteries. Transcranial Doppler ultrasound can give accurate information about flow in the intracranial ICA, ophthalmic, ACAs, MCA, and PCAs, as well as the IVA and basilar arteries.[46] Angiography is still frequently needed to define further the arterial pathological condition and can be performed safely in most large centers with large numbers of cases and neuroradiologists and neurologists supervising the cases.[47] Although digital subtraction angiography can be done on an outpatient basis, lack of detail, complications, and lack of good intracranial opacification limit the usefulness of this relatively new procedure.

When the patient has had multiple TIAs in the same vascular territory, cardiogenic embolism is quite unlikely, and cardiac testing is important only to evaluate coexistent coronary artery disease. However, if there has been only a single stroke or TIA, the clinician may not be able to tell if the cause was cardiac or a proximal large artery lesion, so that cardiac evaluation for an embolic source would be very important and would complement ultrasound and angiography of the cardiovascular bed. Coagulopathies are becoming increasingly recognized as patients are being tested more often and more thoroughly. Hypercoagulability alone may explain multiple vascular occlusions or may complicate atherosclerotic disease. Complete blood cell counts, platelet counts, inspection of a stained blood smear, and prothrombin time should be routinely performed in all stroke patients. In young patients, those without vascular risk factors or known cardiac disease, and in patients with systemic symptoms, a full coagulation battery, including partial thromboplastin time, measurement of levels of antithrombin III, protein C, and protein S, testing for lupus anticoagulant and anticardiolipin antibodies, and measurement of serum complement, should also be requested.

Treatment of patients with ischemic disease should depend on: (1) the nature, location, and severity of the occlusive vascular lesion; (2) the mechanism of ischemia—low flow, embolism, or vasoconstriction; (3) the presence of hematological abnormalities; (4) the presence and severity of persisting brain ischemia and infarction; and (5) the presence of coexisting arterial and/or neurological disease.[48] Treatment should *not* be chosen simply because of the time course of the symptoms.[28] I follow rather simple schema for treatment. If the problem is inadequate distal flow, then measures to augment flow should be pursued (Table 34.3). In occlusive lesions, thrombosis and propagation of clots and embolization of material account for much of the problem. I try to distinguish between

Table 34.3. Augmentation of blood flow.

Augmentation
Surgical
Endarterectomy
Bypass
Angioplasty—(by invasive radiological methods)
Medical
Fibrinolysis and clot lysis
Raising blood pressure
Augmenting blood volume
Avoiding hypotension
Decreasing intracranial pressure if raised

situations in which white clots (fibrin-platelet clumps) and red clots (fibrin-dependent thrombi) are more likely to form. White clots are most common in irregular regions of rapid blood flow. Platelets tend to adhere to plaques and can be broken off into the arterial stream or form the nidus for superimposed thrombin deposition. Plaque disease in nonstenosing lesions is the optimal environment for white clots. On the other hand, red clots form more readily in slow-moving stagnant regions, such as dilated cardiac atria, ventricular aneurysms, and tightly stenotic large arteries. Theoretically, agents that decrease platelet aggregation and agglutination, such as aspirin, ibuprofen, or sulfinpyrazone, would be most effective in preventing white clots, while heparin and warfarin would be most effective against red clots. I also distinguish between situations that require short-term treatment but with low long-term risk, eg, acute thrombosis of a large artery, and situations, such as tight stenosis of a large artery, in which the risk of stroke is more prolonged. Short-term therapy is more appropriate for the former and long-term treatment for the latter. Guidelines for management of large artery lesions are outlined in Table 34.4.

Systemic Hypoperfusion

Because the brain is very vulnerable to any decrease in its blood, oxygen, or fuel supply, patients with hypotension, hypoxia, or cardiac pump failure often present to emergency rooms because of cerebral dysfunction. The most common causes of this global brain hypoperfusion are cardiac arrest and severe arrhythmias. Less often, acute hypovolemia caused by acute gastrointestinal bleeding, pulmonary embolism, and severe postural hypotension can be responsible. The symptoms are usually light-headedness, dizziness, difficulty in concentrating, confusion, and decreased alertness or delirium. The neurological symptoms are always accompanied by pallor and changes in pulse and blood pressure. Tragically, prolonged cerebral hypoperfusion often causes irreversible brain damage, but the heart dysfunction can be reversed. New technology can prolong the existence of these brainless souls at great personal, family, and community expense and loss.

The clinical findings are invariably related to bilateral cerebral dysfunction. Brain areas in the so-called border-zones between arterial territories are preferentially affected. Cortical blindness, amnesia, and arm weakness and numbness are the most prevalent symptoms. Computed tomography and MRI may show ischemia in the areas between the ACA and MCA anteriorly and between the MCA and PCA posteriorly. Sometimes, the brain-stem nuclei and cerebellum are involved preferentially or in addition to the cerebral lesions.[48] Treatment consists of rapid correction of the underlying cause of the hypoperfusion.

Stroke Prevention

The preceding remarks relate to the cause of stroke and their treatment. Once brain damage has occurred, the efforts of the treating physician are limited. Much better, of course, would be to prevent the stroke in the first place. Each patient who has a stroke or TIA has risk factors that caused these symptoms and that are likely to lead to further cerebrovascular symptoms in the future. Often lost sight of, in the urgency of acute evaluation and treatment of the patient with stroke, is the importance of controlling these risk factors to prevent further progression of vascular damage. Also, physicians and educators must begin to teach the general public the need for modifying correctable risk factors as early in life as possible.[50]

Hypertension

Hypertension is probably the single, most important risk factor. Even systolic hypertension is detrimental to the vascular endothelium and can lead to degenerative vascular changes and accelerate the process of atherostenosis. Some racial groups, especially black persons and persons of Japanese and Chinese origin, have a particularly high incidence of hypertension. Patients with a family history of hypertension are also quite likely to become hypertensive sometime in the

Table 34.4. Guidelines for treatment of patients with large-artery disease.*

Condition	Rx	Dose control	Duration
Nonstenosing plaques	Aspirin	300 mg QD	Long term
Tight stenosis Surgically accessible and nondisabling deficit	Endarterectomy	. . .	. . .
Inaccessible or nonsurgical candidate	Warfarin	PT 1.5 × control	Long term
Thrombosis of large artery	Heparin	aPTT 1.5-2.5 × baseline	Short term (3–6 wk)
	Warfarin	PT, 1.5 × control	

*RX indicates treatment; QD, every day; PT, prothrombin time; and aPTT, activated, partial thromboplastin time.

second or third decade of life. Frequent surveillance and testing, particularly in high-risk groups, and aggressive treatment as early as possible are very important. Undoubtedly, more effective control of hypertension has contributed to the decline in stroke incidence and mortality (see Chapter 13).

Smoking

Data are accumulating at a rapid rate showing cigarette smoking to be extremely detrimental to blood vessels. It has long been known that peripheral vascular and coronary artery disease are accelerated by smoking. New convincing and conclusive data link smoking to premature cerebrovascular occlusive disease.

Cardiac Disease

Heart diseases of all types are highly correlated with cerebrovascular damage. Cardiogenic embolism, hypoperfusion, and coexisting atherosclerotic disease are the most frequent explanations. Early recognition and treatment of cardiac disease is important in stroke prevention.

Hyperlipidemia

Evidence that links abnormalities of cholesterol and triglycerides to stroke is less persuasive than the data that link these abnormalities to cardiac disease. Undoubtedly, hypercholesterolemia, especially a reduced high-density lipoprotein/low-density lipoprotein ratio, contributes to the formation of atherostenosis at the origins of the carotid and vertebral arteries in the neck. Dietary advice early in life and treatment of hyperlipidemia as early in life as possible may reduce the likelihood of cerebrovascular atherostenosis later in life.

Oral Contraceptives

Although the topic is controversial, birth control pills unquestionably increase the probability of stroke in young women, especially those who also smoke or have migraine headaches.

Family History

Perhaps the sagest advice is to choose your parents well. Individuals whose parents have had premature vascular disease also have a high incidence of coronary and peripheral vascular disease. A recent informal study of schoolchildren, conducted under the auspices of the American Heart Association, showed that screening of children who had a family history of heart disease uncovered a number of risk factors that could be treated. Screening of children of parents with known vascular risk factors or vascular disease might be very effective in preventing stroke and heart disease in later life.

Complications and Rehabilitation

Brain injury, disability, bed rest, and coexisting medical disease explain the high rate of complications that affect stroke patients. The most important cerebral complications are progressive ischemia, transtentorial herniation, and seizures. Thrombosis in dependent leg veins, sometimes resulting in pulmonary embolism, also is common. Dysphagia, aspiration, and hypoventilation all contribute to the frequency of pneumonia. Contractures, bed sores, and pressure-induced neuropathies result from immobility and poor nursing care. Knowledge of these possible complications is the first step toward prevention and treatment.

Recovery from stroke is complex. Some ischemic lesions are reversible. Although some brain regions may be irreversibly injured and connecting pathways interrupted, other pathways and regions may be able to assume new functions formerly subserved by the damaged area. Adaptation to the clinical deficit often is possible despite lack of neurological improvement.

Rehabilitation hopes to activate new brain regions by training and helps to educate and train the individual and family to overcome and adapt to the deficit. To be effective, rehabilitation should be started early and should be directed to the particular neurological deficits and the whole individual. Often, particular problems, such as arm weakness, are emphasized, but the trees sometimes obscure the forest. The aim of rehabilitation is *not* to increase arm function, but to allow the stroke patient to regain former life functions as much as possible. Sometimes, this can occur even though the arm does not improve much. Overattention to the arm and intense frequent exercise and therapy can delay the patient's reentry into life in a more global sense (see Chapter 12).

Dementia Due to Cerebrovascular Disease

Senility and decline in intellectual function in the geriatric age group have often been blamed on "hardening of the arteries" in common parlance. Actually, most individuals who develop dementia have brain degeneration due to Alzheimer's disease, a condition that has no vascular basis. There are some patients, probably less than 10% of the geriatric population with dementia, who do have so-called multi-infarct dementia, the common term for dementia caused by cerebrovascular pathological conditions. Others have a mixture of Alzheimer's disease and strokes.

Patients with vascular dementia usually (1) have a high incidence of risk factors for stroke, such as hypertension, smoking, diabetes, etc; (2) have a high frequency of accompanying coronary and peripheral vascular disease; (3) have a history of strokes or sudden onset of neurological signs and symptoms; and (4) have prominent motor, sensory, and visual abnormalities that exceed or parallel their intellectual deficits. The key regions needed for effective function as an organism, ie, movement, sensation, vision, and speech, are directly in the center of supply of the major cerebral arteries. Occlusion of arteries rarely damages the associative cortex without concomitant injury to regions that control elementary neurological function. Weakness, hyperreflexia, pseudobulbar dysarthria and dysphagia, and hemianopia are common findings. The dementia is characterized by focal deficits in cognitive function, such as aphasia or amnesia, and a high frequency of frontal lobe deficits. Neuroimaging tests invariably identify multifocal regions of brain damage (See Chapter 33).

Multi-infarct dementia is a broad term that can be conveniently divided into two large groups[51]: large-artery pathological conditions and microangiopathies. The large-artery group includes patients with multiple cardiogenic emboli, multiple occlusions of extracranial and/or intracranial arteries, and multiple old ICHs. All of these patients have a history of stroke, often severe and usually multiple. Computed tomography shows multiple surface infarcts or old, healed hemorrhage cavities. The microangiopathy group includes patients with multiple lacunar infarcts and patients who have lacunae and wider areas of white-matter damage called *subcortical arteriosclerotic encephalopathy (Binswanger's disease)*.[52] In Binswanger's disease, either chronic hypertensive encephalopathy with edema formation and gliosis or tandem damage to white matter due to widespread arteriolar sclerosis leads to chronic white-matter loss and scarring. Magnetic resonance imaging can help make this diagnosis.[53] Treatment will depend on the nature of the causative vascular disease.

References

1. Wolf PA, Kannel WB, McGee D. Epidemiology of strokes in north America. In: Barrett HJ, Mohr JP, Stein BM, et al, eds. *Stroke, Pathophysiology, Diagnosis, and Management.* New York, NY: Churchill Livingstone Inc; 1986:19–29.

2. Anderson GL, Whisnant JP. A comparison of trends in mortality from stroke in the United States and Rochester, Minnesota. *Stroke* 1982;13:804–809.

3. Caplan LR, Stein RW. *Subarachnoid Hemorrhage in Stroke: A Clinical Approach.* Stoneham, Mass: Butterworths; 1986:231–260.

4. Caplan LR, Stein RW. *Intracerebral Hemorrhage in Stroke: A Clinical Approach.* Stoneham, Mass: Butterworths; 1986:261–292.

5. Phillips LH, Whisnant JP, O'Fallon M, et al. The unchanging pattern of subarachnoid hemorrhage in a community. *Neurology* 1980;30:1034–1040.

6. Sacco RL, Wolf PA, Bharucha N, et al. Subarachnoid hemorrhage: natural history, prognosis and precursive factors in the Framingham study. *Neurology* 1984;34:847–854.

7. Parkarinen S. Incidence, etiology, and prognosis of primary subarachnoid hemorrhage: a study based on 589 cases diagnosed in a defined urban population during a defined period. *Acta Neurol Scan* 1967;43(suppl 29):1–128.

8. Fisher CM, Kistler JP, Davis JM. Relation of cerebral vasospasm to subarachnoid hemorrhage visualized by computed tomographic scanning. *Neurosurgery* 1980;6:1–9.

9. Caplan LR. Computed tomography and stroke. In: McDowell F, Caplan LR, eds. *Cerebrovascular Survey Report for the National Institute of Neurological and Communicative Disorders and Stroke.* 1985:61–74.

10. Caplan LR, Flamm ES, Mohr JP, et al. Lumbar puncture and stroke. *Stroke* 1987;18:540A–544A.

11. Heros RC, Zervas NT, Varsos V. Cerebral vasospasm after subarachnoid hemorrhage: an update. *Ann Neurol* 1983;14:599–608.

12. Caplan LR. Intracerebral hemorrhage revisited. *Neurology* 1988;38:624–627.

13. Fisher CM. Pathological observations in hypertensive cerebral hemorrhages. *J Neuropathol Exp Neurol* 1971;30:536–550.

14. Caplan LR, Mohr JP. Intracerebral hemorrhage: an update. *Geriatrics* 1978;33:42–52.

15. Kase C, Robinson K, Stein R, et al. Anticoagulant-related intracerebral hemorrhage. *Neurology* 1985;35:943–948.

16. Gilbert J, Vinters H. Cerebral amyloid angiopathy: incidence and complications. *Stroke* 1983;14:915–923, 923–928.

17. Mohr JP, Caplan LR, Melski J, et al. The Harvard Cooperative Stroke Registry: a prospective registry. *Neurology]* 1978;29:754–762.

18. Caplan LR, D'Cruz I, Hier DB, et al. Atrial size, atrial fibrillation, and stroke. *Ann Neurol* 1986;19:158–161.

19. Fairfax AJ, Lambert CD, Leatham A. Systemic embolism in chronic sinoatrial disorder. *N Engl J Med* 1976;295:190–193.

20. Fisher CM, Perlman A. The nonsudden onset of cerebral embolism. *Neurology* 1967;17:1025–1032.

21. Caplan LR, Hier DB, D'Cruz I. Cerebral embolism in the Michael Reese Stroke Registry. *Stroke* 1983;14:530–536.

22. DeWitt LD, Pessin MS, Pandian NG, et al. Benign disappearance of ventricular thrombus after embolic stroke. *Stroke* 1988;19:393–396.

23. Lechat P, Mas JL, Lascault G, et al. Prevalence of patent foramen ovale in patients with stroke. *N Engl J Med* 1988;318:1148–1152.
24. Mohr JP. Lacunes. *Stroke* 1982;13:3–11.
25. Caplan LR, Gorelick PB, Hier DB. Race, sex, and occlusive vascular disease: a review. *Stroke* 1986; 17:648–655.
26. Chambers BR, Norris JW. Outcome in patients with asymptomatic neck bruits. *N Engl J Med* 1986;315:860–865.
27. Caplan LR, Pessin MS. Symptomatic carotid artery disease and carotid endarterectomy. *Annu Rev Med* 1988;39:273–299.
28. Caplan LR. TIAs: we need to return to the question "What's wrong with Mr. Jones?" *Neurology* 1988; 38:799–793.
29. Caplan LR. Cerebrovascular disease: large artery occlusive disease. In: Appel S. *Current Neurology*. Chicago, Ill: Year Book Medical Publishers Inc; 1988;3:179–226.
30. Fisher CM. Observations of the fundus oculi in transient monocular blindness. *Neurology* 1959;9:333–347.
31. Pessin MS, Duncan G, Mohr J, et al. Clinical and angiographic features of carotid transient ischemic attacks. *N Engl J Med* 1977;296:358–362.
32. Marzewski D, Furlan A, St Louis P, et al. Intracranial internal carotid artery stenosis: long term prognosis. *Stroke* 1982;13:821–824.
33. Caplan LR, Babikian V, Helgason C, et al. Occlusive disease of the middle cerebral artery. *Neurology* 1985;35:975–982.
34. Bladin P, Berkovic S. Striatocapsular infarction: large infarcts in the lenticulostriate arterial territory. *Neurology* 1984;34:1423–1430.
35. Gacs G, Fox A, Barnett HJM, et al. Occurrence and mechanisms of occlusion of the anterior cerebral artery. *Stroke* 1983;14:952–959.
36. Helgason C, Caplan LR, Goodwin J, et al. Anterior choroidal territory infarction: case reports and review. *Arch Neurol* 1986;43:681–686.
37. Hennerici M, Kleman C, Rautenberg W. The subclavian steal phenomenon: a common vascular disorder with rare neurologic deficits. *Neurology* 1988;38:669–673.
38. Caplan LR. Vertebrobasilar occlusive disease. In: Barnett HJ, Mohr J, Stein B, eds. *Stroke: Pathophysiology, Diagnosis and Management*. New York: Churchill Livingstone Inc; 1985:549–620.
39. Caplan LR. Bilateral distal vertebral artery occlusion. *Neurology* 1983;33:552–558.
40. Moufarrij N, Little J, Furlan A, et al. Vertebral artery stenosis: long term follow-up. *Stroke* 1984;15:260–263.
41. Pessin MS, Caplan LR. Basilar artery stenosis—middle and distal segments. *Neurology* 1987;37:1742–1746.
42. Caplan LR. Occlusion of the vertebral or basilar artery. *Stroke* 1979;10:277–282.
43. Castaigne P, L'hermitte F, Gautier J, et al. Arterial occlusions in the vertebral-basilar system. *Brain* 1973;96:133–154.
44. Pessin MS, Lathi E, Cohen MB, et al. Clinical features and mechanisms of occipital infarction in the posterior cerebral artery territory. *Ann Neurol* 1987;21:290–299.
45. Pessin MS, Kwan E, DeWitt LD, et al. Posterior cerebral artery stenosis. *Ann Neurol* 1987;21:85–89.
46. DeWitt LD, Wechsler L. Transcranial Doppler. *Stroke* 1987;22:31–36.
47. Caplan LR, Wolpert SM. Conventional cerebral angiography: occlusive cerebrovascular disease. In: Wood JH, ed. *Cerebral Blood Flow: Physiologic and Clinical Aspects*. New York, NY: McGraw-Hill International Book Co; 1987;23:356–384.
48. Caplan LR, Stein RW. *Treatment in Stroke: A Clinical Approach*. Stoneham, Mass: Butterworths; 1986:85–104.
49. Caplan LR. Neurology of the acute cardiac. In: Donoso E, Cohen S, eds. *Critical Cardiac Care*. New York, NY: Stratton International Medical Books; 1979:183–197.
50. Wolf P, Dyken M, Barnett HJM, et al. Risk factors in stroke. *Stroke* 1984;15:1105–1111.
51. Caplan LR. Chronic vascular dementia. In: Jones HR, ed. *Primary Care: Cerebrovascular Disorders*. Philadelphia, Pa: WB Saunders Co; 1979:843–848.
52. Caplan LR, Schoeme W. Subcortical arteriosclerotic encephalopathy (Binswager's disease): clinical features. *Neurology* 1978;28:1206–1217.
53. Caplan LR. Binswager disease: current opinion in neurology and neurosurgery. *Gowers Academic J* 1988; 1:57–62.

35

Abnormalities of Posture and Movement

John G. Nutt

Alterations of posture and gait commonly accompany aging and are indicators of the health and biologic age of an individual. They also may be disabling, by decreasing confidence, restricting mobility, and causing injuries. Posture and gait may be compromised by cardiovascular, arthritic, and orthopedic disorders, but are most commonly impaired by neurologic dysfunction. The neurologic disturbances that produce postural and gait abnormalities can be categorized under three headings: (1) afferent or sensory dysfunction, (2) efferent or motor dysfunction, and (3) central or integrative dysfunction.

Humans depend primarily on three sensory modalities for orienting themselves in space: proprioceptive, vestibular, and visual. The sensory input is redundant, and posture and gait are generally normal in the absence of one or even two of the sensory modalities. However, if all are compromised, or if there is erroneous or conflicting input (such as in acute vestibular disease or the initial use of bifocals), postural and gait disturbances may result. The more common sensory causes of postural difficulties, the accompanying signs, and the characteristic gaits are summarized in Table 35.1.

Disturbances in the efferent or motor system are manifested by weakness and alterations in muscle tone. Primary muscle disease (dystrophy, myopathy, or myositis) preferentially affects proximal muscles symmetrically. Weakness of the muscles of the pelvic girdle produces exaggerated lumbar lordosis, waddling gait, and particular difficulties in rising from chairs and negotiating stairs. Motor neuropathies commonly affect distal musculature, but they also may involve proximal muscles (most dramatically seen in diabetic amyotrophy or radiculoplexopathy). Both muscle and peripheral nerve disorders are associated with normal or decreased muscle tone. Weakness on the basis of corticospinal tract damage is associated with hyperactive reflexes, Babinski's signs, and increased ("spastic") tone. The salient features of these motor abnormalities and the associated gait disturbances are summarized in Table 35.2.

The integration of sensory input and organization of appropriate motor output for postural responses and ambulation use the frontal lobes, basal ganglia, cerebellum, and vestibular nuclei. Diseases that affect these structures may produce characteristic postural and gait disturbances, as well as involuntary movements, alterations in muscle tone, and disruption of voluntary and automatic motor acts. In addition, there are gait abnormalities in elderly persons, often termed *senile gaits*, that cannot be readily explained by afferent or efferent abnormalities or by any of the classic "central" gait disorders. Central gait disorders are summarized in Table 35.3. Spastic, ataxic, and senile gaits are considered below; parkinsonian, marche à petits pas, and apractic gaits are discussed in the section on parkinsonism.

Gait

Spastic Gaits

The hemiparetic gait with unilateral spasticity is easily recognized: the circumduction of the leg, reduced arm

Table 35.1. Sensory abnormalities producing postural and gait disturbances.

Modality	Lesion	Signs	Gait
Proprioceptive	Peripheral nerves	Loss of position sensation, stocking glove sensory loss, decreased or absent DTRs,* Romberg's sign	Ataxic
	Spinal posterior columns	Loss of position sensation, other signs of spinal cord dysfunction	Ataxic
Vestibular	Peripheral: labyrinth and vestibular nerve	Nystagmus, hearing deficits, past pointing	Weaving "drunken"
	Central: vestibular nuclei and pathways	Nystagmus, past pointing, cerebellar and other cranial nerve signs	Weaving or ataxic
Visual	Lens, vitreous, retina, extraocular muscles	Altered visual acuity, diplopia, or deficient downgaze	Tentative, uncertain

*DTRs indicates deep tendon reflexes.

swing, flexed posture of the arm, and extended leg are characteristic. On examination, the presence of the ipsilateral weakness, hyperreflexia, and hypertonus confirms the diagnosis. Hemiparkinsonism can produce diagnostic confusion if it is not accompanied by tremor, because parkinsonism commonly starts with unilateral hypertonus, an absent arm swing, and foot-dragging. Reflexes may sometimes be brisker on the affected side. Hemiparkinsonism can be differentiated from hemiparesis by a careful evaluation of tone (plastic rigidity vs the velocity-sensitive spastic "catch") and the presence of other subtle parkinsonian signs (masked facies, soft voice, and mild contralateral rigidity).[1]

Paraparesis with bilateral leg spasticity produces a gait characterized by (1) bilateral circumduction; (2) short steps; (3) narrow base; and, if severe, (4) scissoring. The bilaterally brisk reflexes, Babinski's signs, and hypertonus are diagnostic. A coexisting, mild peripheral neuropathy may dampen ankle jerks and mislead the clinician.

Spasticity is caused by chronic metabolic (eg, vitamin B_{12} deficiency), degenerative (eg, amyotrophic lateral sclerosis), and structural (eg, cervical spon-

dylosis) lesions disrupting the corticospinal tracts anywhere from the cortex to the spinal cord. If the cause is not historically obvious, this problem is best evaluated in conjunction with a neurologic consultant.

Therapeutic efforts should be directed to bracing, ambulation aids, and gait training. Antispasticity agents, such as baclofen, diazepam, and dantrolene sodium, generally produce weakness and disequilibrium at doses that reduce spasticity and, consequently, are of little assistance in the potentially ambulatory patient; however, they may be worthwhile in treating patients confined to wheelchairs and beds whose care is compromised by spasticity or flexor spasms.

Ataxic Gait

Cerebellar ataxia is characterized by a wide-based stance and irregularity of the amplitude and timing of steps, particularly on turns. An unsteady, weaving gait without a wide base may be seen with acute vestibular lesions (peripheral or central), midline cerebellar lesions, and sedative-hypnotic intoxication. It is important to recognize that gait ataxia need not be ac-

Table 35.2. Motor abnormalities producing postural and gait disturbances.

Lesion	Signs*	Gait
Muscle	Proximal weakness, normal DTRs	Waddling
Distal motor nerve	Distal weakness, decreased DTRs	Slapping, footdrop steppage
Proximal motor nerve or roots	Patchy weakness, proximal and distal	Waddling and/or slapping
Corticospinal tracts	Distal greater than proximal weakness, increased DTRs, increased tone, Babinski's sign	Circumduction, "spastic"

*DTRs indicates deep tendon reflexes.

Table 35.3. Central or integrative dysfunction producing postural and gait disturbances.

Lesion	Signs	Gait
Corticospinal tracts	Weakness, increased DTRs,* and tone	"Spastic," stiff legged, circumduction
Frontal lobes	Dementia, perseveration, hand and foot grasp reflexes	"Apractic"
Deep white and gray matter	Corticospinal tract signs, pseudobulbar palsy, history of "strokes"	Marche á petits pas
Basal ganglia	Tremor, rigidity, bradykinesia	Parkinsonian
	Choreic movements of face, trunk, limbs	Dancing or choreic
Cerebellum	Limb dysmetria, intention tremor	Ataxic
Brain stem, midline cerebellum, thalamus	Cranial nerve signs, severe imbalance	Unable without assistance
Multiple central and peripheral sites	Absence of other significant central or peripheral disturbances to explain gait disorder	"Senile" or "cautious"

*DTRs indicates deep tendon reflexes.

companied by abnormalities of other coordination tests, such as the finger-to-nose or heel-to-shin tests.

Treatable causes of ataxia in the geriatric population include thiamine or vitamin B_{12} deficiency, hypothyroidism, sedative-hypnotic intoxication, and the Arnold-Chiari malformation.[2] Other than the recognition of these remediable entities, treatment consists of ensuring safe living quarters and providing for mobility with a walker or wheelchair.

Senile Gaits

"Senile" gait is not a diagnosis but a label for the unsteady gait of older persons that cannot be attributed to orthopedic causes or the other neurologic causes detailed in Tables 35.1 through 35.3.[3] Most commonly, this takes the form of a shortened stride, a normal or minimally widened base, and "en bloc" turning. These changes may be nonspecific, for they can be observed in younger individuals who are uncertain of their footing when, for example, walking on a slippery or swaying surface. Indeed, most of the elderly patients with this gait pattern have objective and subjective imbalance. These patients do not have difficulty in initiating walking and do not freeze. Their gait may improve if allowed to hold another person's arm, a fact that may be falsely interpreted as evidence that the gait is "functional." However, the offered arm may contribute significantly to postural stability and, by this means, improve gait. This gait may be more accurately termed a *cautious gait pattern*, an appropriate response to instability that may arise from musculoskeletal or peripheral and central nervous system dysfunction.

A related pattern that may have a more functional basis is the "post fall syndrome." This typically occurs in elderly women who fall, or have closely averted a fall, and subsequently cannot walk without assistance, despite no objective signs of neurologic or orthopedic dysfunction sufficient to explain an inability to walk. This appears to be a psychologic response or acute anxiety about falling and often responds to intensive gait retraining.

There are several hypotheses to explain senile gaits.[3] One attributes senile gait to normal-pressure hydrocephalus.[4] The evidence supporting this is an increased ventricular span on computed tomography (CT scan) in patients with gait disturbance compared with a geriatric population with no gait disturbance and an improvement in gait following removal of cerebrospinal fluid (CSF) by lumbar puncture. However, in many of these patients, there is also sulcal enlargement, indicating generalized cerebral atrophy rather than isolated hydrocephalus.[5] The criteria for making a diagnosis of normal-pressure hydrocephalus remain problematic, and in most clinicians' experience, normal-pressure hydrocephalus is an uncommon cause of gait disturbance. Furthermore, ventricular shunting for normal-pressure hydrocephalus is associated with significant morbidity and mortality.[6,7]

A second hypothesis is that multiple, minor neurologic deficits result in the gait and postural instability. There is a progressive loss of Betz cells, Purkinje cells, dopaminergic neurons, and spinal motor neurons with aging.[8] Furthermore, there are age-related alterations in sensation, motor power, monosynaptic reflexes, vestibular reflexes, and control of body sway.[8–10] No single abnormality is sufficient to destabilize posture and disrupt gait, but the combination of these minor deficits may do so.

Pharmacologic intervention is of no benefit and often is detrimental in these patients. Antiparkinsonian agents do not help, and sedatives, antivertiginous drugs, and antihypertensives (occasionally) exacerbate the imbalance. Treatment of contributing musculoskeletal disorders is worthwhile.[11] Gait training is of limited benefit. However, ambulatory aids and teaching the patient to make wide turns and to use caution in confined spaces, such as closets and bathrooms, may avoid falls. The living quarters should be evaluated for loose rugs, obstructions, handrails, and lighting to minimize accidents.

Parkinsonism

Epidemiology

Parkinson's disease is exceedingly common in the geriatric population; estimates are that 1 in 100 individuals who are older than 60 years of age are parkinsonian.[12] The incidence continues to increase with age. The sexes are affected equally.

Pathology

Parkinsonism is caused by a disruption of dopaminergic neurotransmission. Processes that destroy the pigmented dopaminergic neurons of the substantia nigra, disrupt the synthesis, storage, and release of dopamine, alter the postsynaptic dopamine receptors, or damage the postsynaptic striatal neurons can produce clinical parkinsonism. The most common form of parkinsonism in the geriatric population is idiopathic Parkinson's disease, which is characterized by the loss of pigmented neurons in the substantia nigra and locus ceruleus. Eosinophilic inclusion bodies, termed *Lewy bodies*, are present in the remaining pigmented neurons of these structures, as well as in the neurons of the nucleus basalis, the dorsal nucleus of the vagus, and the autonomic ganglia.[13] The loss of cortical and nucleus basalis neurons and the presence of neurofibrillary tangles in cortical neurons in demented parkinsonian patients raise a question of the relationship between Alzheimer's disease and Parkinson's disease.[14,15]

Clinical Features

Four groups of signs characterize parkinsonism. The first is tremor. Classically, a 4- to 6-Hz tremor is present when the limb is supported or suspended (ie, arm resting in lap or hanging by the side) and is abolished by complete relaxation (such as during sleep) or by voluntary movement of the limb. The tremor generally begins insidiously in one hand, then spreads to the ipsilateral foot, subsequently to the contralateral limbs, and perhaps to the tongue and jaw. In addition to the resting tremor, many patients have a faster 6- to 9-Hz postural tremor. The presence of tremor is neither sufficient nor required for a diagnosis of parkinsonism. The diagnosis of parkinsonism in patients with tremor alone, and no bradykinesia or rigidity, is hazardous and generally reflects a confusion with essential tremor. Conversely, although it is a common presenting sign, tremor may never develop in the course of Parkinson's disease.

The second cardinal feature of parkinsonism is rigidity. The rigidity is "plastic" or "lead pipe" and is perceived as a constant or ratchety (cogwheeling) resistance to passive movement of a joint. Rigidity often is detected first in the nuchal musculature. All muscles may eventually be affected, but the distribution of rigidity need not be symmetric. Rigidity must be differentiated from spasticity and gegenhalten (paratonia). In spasticity, the resistance to passive joint movement tends to be greater the faster the limb is moved and to increase initially, and then melt away. In gegenhalten or paratonia, there is variable resistance because the patient cannot relax the limb and moves it either against or with the examiner. The later tone abnormality is common in dementing illnesses. Although it is teleologically attractive to attribute many of the bradykinetic and postural parkinsonian features to the rigidity, there is poor correlation between the severity of rigidity and other parkinsonian signs.

The third feature is bradykinesia, which encompasses the slowness and impreciseness of voluntary movements and the loss of automatic or associated movements. Voluntary movements may be visibly slowed. Repetitive dexterous movements become irregular in tempo and amplitude, leading to scratchy, small handwriting (micrographia), difficulty with hand tools (especially screwdrivers) and eating utensils, and problems with dressing and grooming. The blink rate is decreased, facial expression is fixed, and the voice is soft and monotonous. Speech, however, is sometimes hurried—a festination of sound production that is reminiscent of the festinating gait. A reduced frequency of unconscious swallowing is responsible for drooling. The normal fidgety movements, readjustments of sitting or standing posture, crossing and uncrossing of the legs while sitting, and the arm swing while walking are reduced or absent.

The final feature comprises static and kinetic postural abnormalities. Characteristically, the parkinsonian patient assumes a flexed posture (simian posture) with flexion of the knees, trunk, elbows, wrists, and metacarpophalangeal joints. Fixed spinal deformities (scoliosis) may develop. When standing or sitting, the trunk may unconsciously drift to the side or back. Inadequate defensive postural responses to perturbations of equilibrium lead to propulsion, retropulsion, and falls.

The mental status of parkinsonian patients is classically thought to be normal. James Parkinson, in the original description of "paralysis agitans," stated that "the senses are left intact." However, it has become increasingly clear that dementia is more common in patients with parkinsonism than in an age-matched control group.[16] Although the prevalence of this complication is debated, recent estimates are that about 15% to 20% of parkinsonian patients have dementia.[17] An anatomic basis for this is suggested by the observations of cortical and nucleus basalis cell loss, senile plaques, tangles, and granulovacuolar degeneration, suggesting a relationship to Alzheimer's disease.[14,15]

The dementia associated with parkinsonism does not have unique features that allow a clear separation from other dementias, although focal deficits (aphasia, agnosia, and apraxias) occur less frequently than in Alzheimer's disease. It is important not to confuse the slow responses and dysarthria that are common in parkinsonism with true dementia. In addition to the functional difficulties produced by dementia, drug therapy is often complicated by the condition; many of the antiparkinsonian medications increase confusion and precipitate hallucinations or frank psychosis in these patients.

Differential Diagnosis

The clinician is faced with two diagnostic branch points in evaluating a hypokinetic motor disorder. First, does the patient have parkinsonism at all? Disorders that may superficially resemble parkinsonism include hypothyroidism and depression with psychomotor retardation.

Disorders that are more difficult to separate from parkinsonism are those with gait disturbances resembling that of parkinsonism. These include gaits that have been termed *marche à petits pas* or *gait apraxia* and that are associated with vascular disease,[18] frontal lobe disease,[19] and hydrocephalus.[20] These gaits are characterized by short shuffling steps, often a widened base, difficulty in initiating gait, and freezing and are accompanied by postural instability. Features of this gait that differ from a parkinsonian gait are the variably widened base and the retention of the arm swing. Other features of parkinsonism (particularly tremor and bradykinesia) are generally absent, and other evidence of vascular disease (history of hypertension,

"small strokes," pseudobulbar palsy, and corticospinal tract signs) and frontal lobe dysfunction (dementia, motor perseveration, and grasp reflexes) are present. Essential tremor, discussed later in this chapter, also must be differentiated from parkinsonism.

Second, if the patient does have parkinsonism, is it the common, idiopathic form of the syndrome, is it secondary to an identifiable cause,[21] or is it part of another neurologic entity?[22-24] Table 35.4 summarizes some of the secondary causes of parkinsonism, and Table 35.5 gives the system degenerations that may have parkinsonism as a major component of the clinical picture. The differentiation between the various parkinsonian syndromes has prognostic significance; only idiopathic Parkinson's disease responds reliably to levodopa. In other forms of parkinsonism, levodopa is less beneficial and commonly produces confusion, hallucinations, or psychosis without benefiting the parkinsonism. Because drug induced parkinsonism is reversible over days to months following withdrawal of the offending drug, it is important to consider this cause. The dopamine antagonists used to treat gastrointestinal diseases (antiemetics and gastric motility stimulants) are commonly overlooked causes of parkinsonism.

Despite the many causes of parkinsonism, the idiopathic form is by far the most common. The practiced geriatrician can confidently make this diagnosis based on the individual's history and examination. If the history or examination suggests another cause or a more widespread neurologic dysfunction, then a neurologic consultation should be obtained.

Table 35.4. Secondary parkinsonism.*

Cause	Features differentiating from IPD
Major tranquilizers	History of neuroleptic usage
Antihypertensives	History of reserpine, α-methyldopa, or some calcium-channel blockers usage
Gastrointestinal drugs	History of use of dopamine antagonists (as antiemetics, promoters of gastric emptying, or in drug combinations)
Encephalitis	History, pupillary and extraocular abnormalities, oculogyric crises, other neurologic signs
Head trauma	History, other neurologic signs
Toxins	History of carbon monoxide, carbon disulfide, cyanide, manganese, mercury, methanol, or MPTP exposure
Hydrocephalus	CT scan

*IPD indicates idiopathic Parkinson's disease; MPTP, 1-methyl-4-phenyl-1,2,3,6-tetrahydropyridine; and CT, computed tomographic.

Table 35.5. Neurologic syndromes in which parkinsonism may be a prominent feature.

Disorder	Features differentiating
Multiple-system atrophy (Shy-Drager, olivopontocerebellar degeneration, striatonigral degeneration)	Autonomic dysfunction (particularly orthostatic hypotension), corticospinal and cerebellar signs
Progressive supranuclear palsy	Paresis of voluntary vertical gaze (particularly downgaze), pseudobulbar palsy, marked postural instability with relatively preserved locomotion
Alzheimer's disease	Early and prominent dementia preceding motor abnormalities, other focal cortical signs
Creutzfeldt-Jakob disease	Rapidly progressing illness with dementia, cerebellar signs, upper and lower motor neuron signs, and myoclonus
Rigid Huntington's disease	Family history of Huntington's disease

Treatment of Parkinsonism

The therapy for Parkinson's disease may be considered under three headings: Who? When? What?

Who

Approximately 85% of patients with idiopathic Parkinson's disease will respond, to some extent, to levodopa or to levodopa plus carbidopa (Sinemet). The response is generally minimal in other parkinsonian syndromes; these latter patients often experience adverse psychiatric effects with this drug. It still may be elected to try levodopa in these patients, but it should be done cautiously, and the drug should be withdrawn if no obvious benefit accrues.

When

The efficacy of levodopa wanes with continued therapy. Psychiatric side effects and a fluctuating response to the drug ("on-off phenomenon") commonly develop with prolonged use and may limit the usefulness of the drug.[25] There is concern that long-term levodopa administration itself may be responsible for the development of these problems. Therefore, many neurologists choose to wait until the parkinsonian symptoms become a significant hindrance to the patient's life-style before starting levodopa therapy.[26]

What

The secondary or subsidiary antiparkinsonian agents (anticholinergics, amantadine, and diphenhydramine) offer mild to moderate relief of parkinsonian symptoms and are often employed as initial or adjunct therapy. All these drugs have anticholinergic actions, and they are particularly useful in patients with sialorrhea or tremor. However, the anticholinergic side effects must be carefully considered in a geriatric population, because the drugs may exacerbate angle-closure glaucoma, cause urinary retention in patients with prostatic hypertrophy, aggravate constipation, and produce psychiatric and cognitive difficulties. If some preparation of levodopa is added later, it is worthwhile to try to discontinue anticholinergics, as their combination with levodopa is generally no more effective than levodopa alone; in this way, the side effects of the anticholinergics may be avoided. Abrupt cessation of anticholinergics will, sometimes, markedly exacerbate parkinsonism, and therefore, these drugs should be gradually withdrawn.

Levodopa is generally prescribed in combination with the peripheral decarboxylase inhibitor carbidopa (the combination is marketed as Sinemet—with carbidopa to levodopa ratios of 10:100 mg, 25:100 mg, and 25:250 mg) to lessen the peripheral side effects of levodopa, nausea, and cardiac arrhythmias. The drug is best started at low doses (one half or one 25:100-mg tablet three times per day), then slowly increased during the ensuing weeks to a dose giving a satisfactory response without side effects (usually in the range of 300 to 900 mg of levodopa administered daily in three to six doses). The most common causes for apparent therapeutic failure are as follows: (1) a rapid increase in drug dosage, leading to unacceptable nausea or other side effects; (2) a failure to increase the dose until a benefit accrues or side effects prohibit further increases; (3) a therapeutic response judged from the effects on tremor, the symptom most resistant to levodopa; and (4) the patient does not have idiopathic parkinsonism.

The dopamine agonists, bromocriptine and pergolide, generally are not first-line antiparkinsonian drugs and are reserved for patients whose response to levodopa is limited by rapid swings between being underdosed and overdosed ("on-off" and "wearing-off" phenomena) and/or by dyskinesia. However, they are increasingly being added to levodopa early in treatment to reduce the need for higher doses of levodopa and to avert dyskinesia and the fluctuating response. Orthostatic hypotension and psychiatric side effects can be prominent with dopamine agonists. They should be used with caution in patients with postural hypotension, dementia, or psychiatric illness.

Abnormal Involuntary Movements

Tremor

Tremor is categorized by the activity that maximizes the tremor. A rest tremor is that tremor most evident when the limb is inactive, lying in the lap or hanging at the side. A postural or action tremor is most evident when an antigravity posture is being maintained, often most dramatically as the patient holds a tea cup. Kinetic or intention tremor is a rhythmic movement present in a limb as it approaches a goal, and it is characteristic of cerebellar dysfunction.

The majority of tremors occurring in the geriatric population is due to three entities: parkinsonism, benign essential tremor, and metabolic/toxic tremor.

Parkinsonian rest tremor is considered above. Mention has been made of the fact that these patients may have a postural tremor alone or in combination with a rest tremor.

Benign essential tremor primarily is a postural tremor, but it also may be present at rest and with intention. Onset occurs from early adulthood to senescence. It commonly affects the upper extremities, head, and voice, but only rarely the legs. The amplitude may vary from barely noticeable to very wide. The tremor is aggravated by emotional tension and fatigue. A family history of tremor is generally obtained. A most characteristic feature is the amelioration of the tremor by alcohol: a fact that most patients discover for themselves and sometimes employ therapeutically. Findings from the neurologic examination are unremarkable except for the tremor, and specifically, there is no rigidity or other evidence of parkinsonism and no evidence of cerebellar disease. The handwriting is large and irregular (tremorous), rather than small as in parkinsonism.[27]

Propranolol in doses of 20 to 320 mg/d often is effective for this disorder. It reduces the amplitude, but does not abolish the tremor. The drug must be given with caution in patients with congestive heart failure, asthma, and insulin-dependent diabetes. The selective β_1 antagonists have been used successfully to treat tremor in patients with bronchospasm. Primidone (Mysoline) also is effective, although the sedative effects may be prominent in elderly persons. Introduction at 25 mg at bedtime with gradual escalation of the single bedtime dose reduces this problem.[27]

A variety of toxic and metabolic insults accentuate the normal physiologic tremor to produce an irregular postural tremor, which may be associated with asterixis (see Table 35.6).

Choreoathetosis

Choreiform movements are "spontaneous" or "involuntary" brief muscle contractions (jerks) that produce simple movements, such as flexion or extension of a finger, and/or complex semipurposeful movements, such as raising the hand to the face. These choreic movements may occur when the limb is at rest or may be superimposed on voluntary movements. Facial, respiratory, truncal, and limb muscles may be involved. The temporal and spatial pattern generally is irregular; this helps to differentiate the movements from tics, which are stereotyped. Athetosis is similar to chorea except that the movements are slower and often blend one into another, which leads to a sinuous or writhing quality rather than the jerky movements of chorea. The distinction between the two often is difficult and has no pathologic significance.

The more common causes of choreoathetosis are listed in Table 35.7. The disorder most frequently encountered by the geriatrician is tardive dyskinesia (discussed in Chapter 33, Dementia). Meige's syndrome, described below, is often confused with tardive dyskinesia.

Myoclonus

Myoclonic movements are exceedingly brief, shock-like contractions of muscle that may lead to almost undetectable movement or produce large excursions of the limb or trunk. They are irregular in timing and distribution. Some forms are induced by touch, noise, or intentional movements. Myoclonic movements must be differentiated from tics (which are repetitive stereotyped movements), from chorea (which is less

Table 35.6. Common metabolic and toxic causes of tremor.

Cause
Hyperthyroidism
Uremia
Liver failure
Alcohol withdrawal
Lithium
Tricyclic antidepressants
Caffeine, theophylline
Isoproterenol
Valproate sodium
Steroids

Table 35.7. Choreoathetosis in the geriatric population.*

Cause	Features
Drug induced	
Neuroleptics	History of drug use,
Reserpine	predominantly affects
Levodopa	face, lips, and tongue
Other psychoactive drugs	
Metabolic	
Hyperthyroidism	Abnormal thyroid function test results
Hypocalcemia	Low serum calcium level
Miscellaneous	Abnormal liver function test results
Vascular	
Contralateral Subthalamic or Striatal stroke	Sudden onset of hemichorea or hemiballismus
Vasculitis	ANA, elevated ESR, angiographic evidence of vasculitis
Polycythemia	Increased RBC mass
Infectious	
Encephalitis (acute and as a sequela)	CSF pleocytosis (acute phase)
Creutzfeldt-Jacob disease	Dementia, other neurologic signs, abnormal EEG
AIDS	HIV antibody positive

*ANA indicates positive antinuclear antibody; ESR, erythrocyte sedimentation rate; RBC, red blood cell; CSF, cerebrospinal fluid; EEG, electroencephalogram; AIDS, acquired immunodeficiency syndrome; and HIV, human immunodeficiency virus.

Table 35.8. Commonly encountered causes of myoclonus.

Cause
Metabolic
Hypoxic encephalopathy
Uremic encephalopathy
Hepatic encephalopathy
Other, including drug intoxication
Infectious
Acute viral encephalitis
Creutzfeldt-Jakob disease
Idiopathic seizure disorders
Benign
Sleep jerks (nocturnal myoclonus)
Hiccups

shocklike), from asterixis (which is caused by brief electromyogram silence and loss of muscle tone), and from irregular tremor. Myoclonus may arise from disorders of the spinal cord, brain stem, and cerebral hemispheres; it is, thus, variably associated with cortical electroencephalogram abnormalities. Myoclonus may be benign, as exemplified by the "sleep jerks" that most people experience as they fall asleep or by hiccups. However, myoclonus often is an accompaniment of idiopathic epilepsy, central nervous system infections, Creutzfeldt-Jakob disease, and metabolic disorders, particularly hypoxic encephalopathy[28] (see Table 35.8).

Dystonia

Dystonic movements are characterized by slow, protracted muscle contractions that produce abnormal postures of limbs and axial structures. The dystonic contractures often are bizarre, commonly are exacerbated by emotion and stress, and only may appear during certain motor acts. These features commonly lead to the erroneous diagnosis of a functional or hysterical disorder. Another feature that confuses the diagnosis of dystonia is that many patients with dystonia will have a postural tremor or other "jerky" movements.

A classification of dystonia is presented in Table 35.9. Generalized dystonia is uncommon in the geriatric population; however, the focal dystonias occur in this age group, and Meige's syndrome is almost exclusively an illness of elderly persons.

Meige's syndrome is named after a French neurologist who described "midline spasms" manifest by a forceful, involuntary closure of the eyelids (blepharospasm), involuntary opening of the jaw, and tongue protrusion. A variety of other manifestations are now recognized, including retraction of the corners of the mouth, contraction of the platysma, jaw clenching, lip pursing, and torticollis. Any of these movements may be the only manifestation of the syndrome, and particularly, blepharospasm is often a solitary sign. Meige's syndrome is only of cosmetic importance to many patients, but in some, the blepharospasm sufficiently interferes with vision to prevent driving, reading, or watching television. The oromandibular involvement may produce dysarthria and dysphagia.[29] The entity most commonly confused with Meige's syndrome is tardive dyskinesia. The blepharospasm and prolonged jaw opening or tongue protrusion are not classic for tardive dyskinesia, but certainly may occur in that disorder. The history of neuroleptic use and the appearance of the movements while patients are receiving neuroleptics or shortly after their withdrawal are the sine qua non for tardive dyskinesia. Spontaneous oral and facial dyskinesias occur in elderly persons, especially those who are edentulous; they do not appear to be part of Meige's syndrome or related to neuroleptic use, but the frequency is controversial.[30] These are rarely of more than cosmetic significance.

The onset of Meige's syndrome occurs commonly in the sixth and seventh decades, and females are more commonly affected than males. The course is, in general, slowly progressive with long periods of stability. Although other facial and cervical muscles may eventually become involved, it is distinctly rare for the dystonia to spread to the limbs or trunk. Other focal dystonic syndromes include dystonia restricted to the larynx (spasmodic dysphonia),[31] to the cervical musculature (torticollis),[32] or to the upper limb during specific skilled tasks (writer's cramp and other occupational cramps).[33] Some patients will have two or more of these focal dystonic syndromes.

Drug therapy of focal dystonias is of limited efficacy. Some patients respond to anticholinergics, benzodiazepines, or neuroleptics.[29] The treatment of choice for blepharospasm is now injection of botulinum toxin into the orbicularis oculi, and injection into other sites is under investigation for treatment of other focal dystonias.[34] Blepharospasm also may be treated surgically by destruction of the fibers of the facial nerve that innervate the orbicularis oculi, or by myectomy of the affected muscles, but with resultant facial weakness.

Tics

Tics are repetitive, stereotyped movements that generally involve the face, respiratory musculature (leading to snorts, grunts, and calls), neck, and shoulder. The movements can be voluntarily reproduced and, likewise, suppressed. The patient consciously experiences a need to make a movement.[35] The nervous twitch of the periorbital musculature is the most common tic; this, as well as other tics, are often accepted as "mannerisms" and not brought to the

physician's attention. Generally, tics are benign and not indicative of central nervous system disease, although they may be a sequela of encephalitis. Geriatricians should be aware that Gilles de la Tourette's syndrome, characterized by multiple tics and involuntary vocalizations with onset in childhood,[35] continues through life and, thus, may be encountered in older age groups.

A disorder that may be confused with tics or blepharospasm and occurs almost exclusively in older age groups is hemifacial spasm.[36] It is characterized by rapid clonic contractions of the facial musculature, usually unilateral, that cannot be willfully suppressed and that may be exacerbated by anxiety and fatigue. This disorder appears to result from a lesion about the facial nerve exit zone from the pons, and it may be produced by tumor, demyelination, or blood vessels impinging on the nerve. This may respond to carbamazepine (Tegretol) or to surgical placement of a sponge between the nerve and any adjacent vessels.[37]

References

1. Gilbert GJ. A pseudohemiparetic form of Parkinson's disease. *Lancet* 1976;2:442–443.
2. Friede RL, Rosessmann V. Chronic tonsillar herniation. *Acta Neuropathol (Berl)* 1976;34:219–235.
3. Sabin TD. Biologic aspects of falls and mobility limitations in the elderly. *J Am Geriatr Soc* 1982;30:51–58.
4. Fisher CM. Hydrocephalus as a cause of disturbances of gait in the elderly. *Neurology* 1982;32:1358–1363.
5. Koller WC, Wilson RS, Glatt SL, et al. Senile gait: correlation with computed tomographic scans. *Ann Neurol* 1983;13:343–344.
6. Hughes CP, Siegel BA, Coxe WS, et al. Adult idiopathic communicating hydrocephalus with and without shunting. *J Neurol Neurosurg Psychiatry* 1978;41:961–971.
7. Black PM. Idiopathic normal-pressure hydrocephalus: results of shunting in 62 patients. *J Neurosurg* 1980;52:371–377.
8. Jenkyn LR, Reeves AG. Neurologic signs in uncomplicated aging (senescence). *Semin Neurol* 1981;1:21–30.
9. Woollacott MH, Shumway-Cook A, Nashner L. Postural reflexes and aging. In: Mortimer LA, Pirozzolo G, Maletta F, eds. *The Aging Motor System*. New York, NY: Praeger Publishers; 1982;98–119.
10. Sheldon JH. The effect of age on the control of sway. *Gerontology* 1963;5:129–138.
11. Steinberg FU. Gait disorders in old age. *Geriatrics* 1966;21:134–143.
12. Kurland LT. Epidemiology: incidence, geographic distribution and genetic considerations. In: Fields WS, ed. *Pathogenesis and Treatment of Parkinsonism*. Springfield, Ill: Charles C Thomas Publisher; 1958:5–49.
13. Alvord EC. The pathology of parkinsonism. In: Minekler J, ed. *Pathology of the Nervous System*. New York, NY: McGraw-Hill International Book Co; 1968:1152–1161.
14. Boller F, Mizutani T, Roessman U, et al. Parkinson

Table 35.9. Dystonia.

Classification	Features
Generalized	
Torsion dystonia (dystonia musculorum deformans)	Widespread axial and limb musculature involvement
Focal	
Meige's syndrome, blepharospasm, oromandibular dystonia	See text
Spasmodic dysphonia	Strained, forced voice, breathy voice
Torticollis	Involuntary rotation, flexion, or extension of neck
Writer's cramp and writer's tremor	Appearance of a dystonic posture or tremor with attempted writing

disease dementia and Alzheimer disease: clinicopathological correlations. *Ann Neurol* 1980;7:329–335.

15. Hakim AM, Mathieson G. Dementia in Parkinson disease: a neuropathologic study. *Neurology* 1979;29:1209–1214.

16. Loranger AW, Goodel H, McDowell FH. Intellectual impairment in Parkinson's syndrome. *Brain* 1972;95:405–412.

17. Brown RG, Marsden CD. Neuropsychology and cognitive function in Parkinson's disease: an overview. In: Marsden CD, Fahn S, eds. *Movement Disorders*. 2nd ed. Stoneham, Mass: Butterworths; 1987:99–123.

18. Critchley M. Arteriosclerotic parkinsonism. *Brain* 1929;52:23–83.

19. Meyer JS, Barron DW. Apraxia of gait: a clinicophysiological study. *Brain* 1960;83:261–284.

20. Estanol BV. Gait apraxia in communicating hydrocephalus. *J Neurol Neurosurg Psychiatry* 1981;44:305–308.

21. Rail D, Scholtz C, Swash M. Post-encephalatic parkinsonism: current experience. *J Neurol Neurosurg Psychiatry* 1981;44:670–676.

22. Bannister R, Oppenheimer DR. Degenerative diseases of the nervous system associated with autonomic failure. *Brain* 1972;95:457–474.

23. Steele JC. Progressive supranuclear palsy. *Brain* 1972;95:693–704.

24. Pearce J. The extrapyramidal disorder of Alzheimer's disease. *Eur Neurol* 1974;12:94–103.

25. Marsden CD, Parkes JD. Success and problems of long-term levodopa therapy in Parkinson's disease. *Lancet* 1977;1:345–349.

26. Fahn S, Calne DB. Considerations in the management of parkinsonism. *Neurology* 1978;28:5–7.

27. Larsen TA, Calne DB. Essential tremor. *Clin Neuropharmacol* 1983;6:185–206.

28. Swanson PD, Luttrell CN, Magladery JW. Myoclonus: a report of 67 cases and a review of the literature. *Medicine (Baltimore)* 1962;41:339–356.

29. Jankovic J, Ford J. Blepharospasm and orofacial-cervical dystonia: clinical and pharmacological findings in 100 patients. *Ann Neurol* 1983;3:402–411.

30. Kane JM, Weinhold P, Kinon B, et al. Prevalence of abnormal involuntary movements ('spontaneous dyskinesias') in the normal elderly. *Psychopharmacology (Berlin)* 1982;77:105–108.

31. Aminoff MJ, Dedo HH, Izdebski K. Clinical aspects of spasmodic dysphonia. *J Neurol Neurosurg Psychiatry* 1978;41:361–365.

32. Patterson RM, Little SC. Spasmodic torticollis. *J Nerv Ment Dis* 1943;98:571–599.

33. Sheehy MP, Marsden CD. Writers' cramp: a focal dystonia. *Brain* 1982;105:461–480.

34. Jankovic J, Orman J. Botulinum A toxin for cranial-cervical dystonia: a double-blind, placebo-controlled study. *Neurology* 1987;37:616–623.

35. Jankovic J. The neurology of tics. In: Marsden CD, Fahn S, eds. *Movement Disorders*. (2nd ed. Stoneham, Mass: Butterworths; 1973:383–405.

36. Ehni G, Wollman HW. Hemifacial spasm. *Arch Neurol Psychiatry* 1945;53:205–211.

37. Jannetta PJ, Abbasy M, Maroon JC, et al. Etiology and definitive microsurgical treatment of hemifacial spasm. *J Neurosurg* 1977;47:321–328.

Depression and Other Affective Disorders

Harold G. Koenig and Dan G. Blazer II

Depression, the prototype affective disorder, is a common and pervasive syndrome that includes some of the most painful emotional experiences that humans can endure. The intense suffering during a depressive episode can drain life of meaning, desire, excitement, and pleasure. Depressed elders may perceive their past to have been wasted, their present without meaning, and their future without hope. Some prefer and may choose death as an alternative. Poets and clinicians, since ancient times, have noted symptoms of depression to be common among older persons. Age is accompanied by loss and challenges adaptive capacity; yet, most older adults do not suffer from depression and report higher life satisfaction than younger adults.[1] Nevertheless, many elders do suffer from loneliness, discouragement, and feelings of worthlessness and uselessness, having lost hope in the future and believing that they are destined to endure this painful existence for the rest of their lives. Because older adults often see their personal physician for relief from such symptoms, a solid understanding by clinicians of the principles of diagnosis and management of affective disorders is essential.

Epidemiology

Psychiatric symptoms are frequently encountered by clinicians who treat older adults. Problems with sleep, hypochondriacal complaints, cognitive impairment, and depressive symptoms are among the difficulties often reported to clinicians. While depressive symptoms are prevalent among older persons, depressive disorders appear to be less frequent in later life than at other stages of the life cycle. The prevalence of depressive symptoms among older persons varies, depending on the type of population studied, with rates higher for hospitalized and institutionalized elderly patients compared with those persons dwelling in the community. Significant depressive symptoms, determined by self-rated checklists, are present in about one fifth of healthy, community-dwelling populations.[2] Among older persons hospitalized with medical illness, the rate of significant depressive symptoms averages about 38%.[3,4] The severity of medical illness and a history of psychiatric illness are strong correlates of depressive symptoms.

Current prevalence data for major depression and other depressive disorders in relatively healthy community-dwelling adults have been derived from the Epidemiologic Catchment Area (ECA) surveys.[5,6] The 1-year prevalence for major depression among 5500 persons aged 65 years and older was only 1.0% (<one half the prevalence for younger adults), and the prevalence among women was three times that in men. Dysthymias (chronic milder depressions or depressive neuroses) were more common (1.8%). Adjustment disorders and mixed depression-anxiety disorders available from one site were diagnosed in 5.2% of elders, and dysphoria (mild depression) was present in 18.7%.[7] Bipolar disorder was rare.

Among medically ill hospitalized patients, the rates for major depression have been much higher than those found in the community, ranging from 12% to

45%.[8,9] In a study that used standardized methods for diagnosing depressive disorders, 11.5% of 130 male patients aged 70 years and older had a major depression, 2.5% had a dysthymia, 3.1% had an adjustment reaction, 1.6% had an organic affective disorder, and 15.3% had a dysphoria.[8] The severity of medical illness was the factor most strongly associated with depression. For medical outpatients, little information exists concerning the prevalence of depressive disorders, although the rates for major depression appear to be less than those found among inpatients. Borson and colleagues[10] found 24% of their sample of 404 elderly medical outpatients with clinically significant depressive symptoms, estimating the prevalence of major depression to be about 10%. A recent study that screened for depressive disorders among medical outpatients of all ages found 6.2% with major depression by using the Diagnostic Interview Schedule.[11] For elderly patients residing in nursing homes, the rates of depressive disorders approximate those of medical inpatients. In a study of 958 older adults living in congregate housing and nursing homes, 11.3% met criteria for having a major depressive disorder, and 21.3% met criteria for minor depressions.[12] Kafonek et al[13] found a somewhat lower prevalence for depression in their sample of 70 nursing home patients, with 21% (N=15) having major depression, dysthymia, or adjustment disorder. All patients in the latter study were examined by psychiatrists. In conclusion, the rates for serious depressive disorders are highest among older persons who are hospitalized with medical illness or among those persons who reside in nursing home settings.

Etiology

The etiology of depressive symptoms in an older adult usually is multifactorial. Biological and psychosocial factors interact to predispose and later precipitate the onset of the depressive syndrome. These factors, along with the depressive behavior and cognitions of the older adult, fuel the course of the syndrome through time.

Genetic and Biological Factors

Family studies and molecular genetics suggest that both major depression and bipolar disorders are, at least, partly inheritable, although the contribution by genetic factors in later life is less than for early-onset disorders. The risk of depression for immediate relatives of index cases with onset after the age of 50 years is only one half to one third that of relatives of patients with early-onset disorder (age, <50).[14]

The activity and metabolism of neurotransmitters with aging may also affect late-life depression. In an autopsy study of biogenic amines in the hindbrains of 55 normal persons of various ages, Robinson et al[15] found that levels of both norepinephrine and serotonin decreased, while levels of 5-hydroxyindoleacetic acid and monoamine oxidase (MAO) increased with age. Given the role of these neurotransmitters in mood disorders, such aging changes might predispose older adults to dysphoric states.

Investigators have found an increase in the 24-hour excretion of cortisol in depressed patients, suggesting a relationship between changes in the hypothalamic-pituitary-adrenal (HPA) axis and depression. Both growth hormone and thyroid stimulating hormone demonstrate blunted responses in normal and depressed older persons.

A disruption of biological circadian rhythms also may be associated with depressive disorders and is manifested by an altered sleep-wake cycle, a disturbed cyclic neuroendocrine release pattern, and a change in diurnal variation in mood.[16] There is a known alteration in the sleep cycle with aging, with a gradual reduction in total sleep time and sleep continuity. It is unclear to what extent this predisposes the older adult to depression.

Despite changes in neurotransmitters and neuroendocrine substances with aging, the lower prevalence of major depression and bipolar disorders in late life suggest that biological predisposition may not be as potent among elderly persons when compared with persons in mid-life.

Psychosocial Factors

A loss commonly precedes a depressive disorder. Depletion of financial reserves, failure of health, loss of independence, death or relocation of family or friends, forced retirement, or loss of a social role may act alone or synergistically to threaten the elder's ability to cope. Studying the role of sociodemographic factors in the development of depressive *symptoms* in more than 1200 persons aged 55 years and older, Pfifer and Murrell[17] found that health and social support played both independent and interactive roles in the genesis of these symptoms in 66 individuals at 6 months of follow-up. An especially high-risk condition was a weak social support system in a person with poor physical health. Social support may relate to depression by contributing to the onset, affecting the outcome, or being adversely affected by depression. The latter possibility was tested by Blazer[18] in a random sample of 331 community residents whose social support and affective state were assessed at the baseline and again 30 months later. Social support was associated with major depression at the baseline. At follow-up, the depressed persons were more likely to exhibit improvement in social support. Therefore, depressive symptoms do not necessarily impair the support available to the older adult.

Symptoms

Symptoms of depression may be divided into two major groups: (1) vegetative or biological and (2) psychological. Vegetative symptoms include insomnia, loss of appetite and/or weight, fatigue, concentration difficulties, constipation, loss of sexual interest, and severe psychomotor agitation or retardation. Psychological symptoms include depressed mood, guilt and self-reproach, feelings of worthlessness, loss of interest, and suicidal ideation. The number, severity, time course, and combination of these symptoms determines which of the specific depressive disorders is present. Depressions characterized by prominent vegetative symptoms are thought to be more biologically driven and, therefore, more likely to respond to biological interactions, such as antidepressant therapy or electroconvulsive therapy (ECT).

Depressions may vary in their presentation, and include agitated, retarded, apathetic, or hypochondriacal varieties. The agitated type is characterized by restlessness, anxiety, an inability to relax, and a need to be moving all the time; hostility or aggressiveness may also occur. Patients with retarded depressions present with psychomotor retardation and complaints of fatigue, and they may actually appear to be slowed up in their physical movements or speech. Apathetic, depressed persons show little personal initiative, are socially withdrawn, and have little interest in their surroundings. A hypochondriacal presentation may have multiple complaints of dizziness, abdominal complaints, ringing of the ears, vague aches and pains, headaches, and sensory changes, such as tingling of the extremities. These varying presentations may have implications concerning the type of antidepressant therapy. Many conditions can mask the presence of depression, including alcoholism, drug abuse, any type of change in behavior, paranoia, schizophrenia, and dementia. These will be discussed further in a later section.

Prognosis

An increase in all-cause mortality for depressed older persons has been reported and may be attributed to decreased social support, poor nutrition from loss of appetite, possible adverse effects of depression on the immune system, increased carelessness, and loss of motivation for self-care. Research findings in this regard, however, are not certain. While several studies have demonstrated a higher mortality rate for depressed persons than nondepressed persons, variables other than age were seldom controlled in these analyses. The ECA surveys conducted in North Carolina examined the 2-year mortality among 1600 persons aged 60 years and older, controlling for age, activities of daily living, sex, and cognitive impairment.[19] Neither depressive symptoms nor the diagnosis of major depression contributed significantly to the prediction of mortality. Murphy et al,[20] however, reported increased mortality rates for depressed elderly men referred to inpatient and outpatient psychiatric facilities. Thus, the relationship between depression and mortality in late life remains unresolved.

The natural history of major depression follows a pattern of remission and relapse. Recurrent episodes usually have similar symptoms and last about the same time. The duration of a particular episode of major depression, regardless of age, averages 9 months, although the variation around this mean is appreciable. Some severe depressions last only a few days, whereas others may last for years. Antidepressants will induce a remission in approximately 60% to 70% of cases. The dexamethasone suppression test (DST) may assist clinicians in predicting recovery; the return of suppression of cortisol, after an original nonsuppressed state, may precede clinical improvement and herald a positive response to therapy.[21] A single DST may be less useful for long-term follow-up, but serial tests may have predictive value.

Older persons with depression have, in general, a poor prognosis. In later life, relapses occur frequently, at times coalescing to produce a chronic depressive state. Post,[22] following up 92 depressed older persons for 3 years, reported that only 26% (N = 24) had a complete recovery from their index episode; half of the remaining patients had further attacks with good recoveries, and the other half were either continuously ill or had recurrent attacks superimposed on a chronic depressive state. Murphy[23] following up 124 patients with a primary diagnosis of depression during a 1-year period, reported that 35% recovered completely, while 29% remained ill throughout the period of observation, and 14% died. Recently, in a study of middle-aged and older adults with major depression, Blazer et al[24] reported that 48% of older adults vs 46% of middle-aged adults had not recovered from the index episode of depression by 1 to 2 years of follow-up; 27% of elders vs 45% of middle-aged adults recovered from the index episode but had recurrent episodes. However, 25% of older adults recovered completely with no recurrences compared with only 9% for the middle-aged group. For the group as a whole, older patients had more depressive symptoms (Center for Epidemiologic Studies-

Depression Scale, >15) at follow-up (59%) than did middle-aged persons (43%), suggesting that the elder group was more likely to suffer from residual symptoms.

Factors that have been found to predict long-term recovery from depressive disorder include the amount and quality of social support, as well as certain personality traits. Following up 104 inpatients with major depression for a period of 1 to 2 years, George et al[25] reported that those inpatients who perceived their social support network as adequate were 2.3 times more likely to have recovered than those inpatients who reported inadequate support in the midst of a depressive episode. More than half of this sample was aged 60 years or older. Social support remained a strong and significant predictor of recovery even after age, sex, and baseline Center for Epidemiologic Studies-Depression Scale score (CES-D) were controlled. Personality pathological conditions may also impair outcomes from major depression.

Little is known concerning the outcome of bipolar disorders in older persons. There is some information to suggest that early-onset bipolar disorder may "burn out" with time. Shulman and Post[26] found that few of their sample of elderly persons with bipolar disorder had the early-onset variety. If bipolar disorder does reemerge in late life, then episodes may cluster in the same manner observered with the early-onset type.

Suicide

Persons aged 65 years and older commit suicide at a higher rate than any other age group in the United States. While making up only 11% of the population, they commit 17% of all suicides, and suicide ranks in the top 10 causes of death in the older than 65 years age group. Even these rates of suicide in elderly persons probably are an underestimate, given the suspected high rate of underreporting in this population. Older persons are more likely to have chronic medical conditions that require powerful life-sustaining medications for control, and either excess ingestion or willed noncompliance could easily cause a death, which might be interpreted as a side effect of therapy or progression of disease.

In 1980, older white males committed suicide at a rate of 46/100,000 nearly double the rate of the next highest group (young white males, 27/100,000) (Table 36.1).[27] Concomitant physical illness, especially in men living alone with little social support, may result in even higher risk. While suicide attempts are less frequent in older adults (0.3% vs 1.2%), the ratio of suicide attempts to completed suicide drops from 20:1 in younger adults to 4:1 in persons aged 65 years and older, suggesting that when older persons attempt

Table 36.1. Death rates per 100,000 from suicide for 1980 by age, sex, and race.*

Age, sex, and race	Death rate
White males	
18–24 y	26.53
25–44 y	24.51
65–74 y	32.84
75–84 y	45.52
White females	
18–24 y	7.70
25–44 y	8.23
65–74 y	7.20
75–84 y	5.67
Nonwhite males	
18–24 y	17.00
25–44 y	16.94
65–74 y	11.42
75–84 y	11.17
Nonwhite females	
18–24 y	3.26
25–44 y	4.70
65–74 y	2.16
75–84 y	2.57

*Source: Tabulations of US Mortality Files from Blazer et al[27].

suicide, they mean business.[28] The increase in suicide in the oldest of old persons, those aged 85 years and older, is particularly worrisome in that this is the most rapidly growing segment of the population.

Clinical Picture

Phenomenology

Depression in later life can be perceived in three ways, each of which has clinical relevance. First, depression can be seen as a single entity in which the severity varies along a continuum. Today, however, most investigators and clinicians view depression as a series of discrete disorders, each fulfilling certain diagnostic criteria as specified in the recently revised *Diagnostic and Statistical Manual of Mental Disorders* (*DMS-III-R*). Categorization has important therapeutic implications, in that biological and psychosocial interventions today are more efficacious for some affective disorders than for others.

The third and final way in which depression may be perceived is from a functional approach. The clinical significance of depressive symptoms is determined by the degree to which a patient's function, particularly social functioning, is impaired. This approach is often of even greater relevance to the family, for whom the patient's isolation and disinterest in surroundings may be more troublesome than disturbed appetite and sleep pattern or suicidal ideation, which are of more immediate interest to the clinician. Thus, careful follow-up of social and physical functioning is important, in addition to the monitoring of clinical symptoms.

Since most modern investigators and clinicians approach depression from the categorical perspective, this is the approach taken in the present chapter. The following affective disorders are discussed here:

Depressive disorders
  Major depression (single episode vs recurrent)
  Major depression with melancholia (endogenous)
  Major depression with psychotic features
  Seasonal affective disorder
  Dysthymia (depressive neurosis)
  Depressive disorder not otherwise specified (dysphoria)
  Adjustment disorder with depressed mood
  Organic affective disorder
  Bereavement (uncomplicated)
Bipolar disorders
  Bipolar disorder (mixed, manic, depressed)

To illustrate the range of depressive symptoms across these diagnostic categories, several case examples are presented.

Case Examples

Case 1

Major Depression

A 73-year-old white woman came to see her physician with complaints of a 3-month history of severe constipation, feeling tired all the time, and trouble with sleeping. She took no medication, except for a stool softener, and her medical history was unremarkable, except for occasional urinary incontinence with coughing or sneezing. A widow of 10 years, she had been living independently in her own home and was active in her church and community until about 9 months ago, when she had contracted influenza. Getting up out of bed one morning, she slipped on a rug and landed on her right hip, resulting in an intertrochanteric fracture. The consequent hospitalization, surgery, and prolonged convalescence placed a serious strain on her financial reserves, forcing her to sell her house and move into an apartment. During this time, a close neighbor and friend of hers was found to have widespread metastatic colon cancer, requiring her hospitalization and eventual placement in a nursing home for terminal care. The patient had been upset over the loss of this lifelong friend.

During the 6 months preceding evaluation, she had become increasingly irritable and spent more time alone in her apartment. She stopped attending church and withdrew from volunteer work at the local senior center because of health reasons and squabbles with other members. An avid reader earlier in life, her failing vision made this activity difficult. Lately, watching television or listening to her favorite radio programs had also become less interesting.

Questioning by her physician also revealed that her appetite was poor and that she had lost about 4.5 kg in the past 6 weeks. Food just did not taste like it used to, and she did not like to bother with cooking just for herself. On direct inquiry, she admitted to feeling like a burden on her daughters, and she felt especially bad because she had so often failed them in the past. For the patient, the future seemed to be bleak. While she had not contemplated suicide, she often thought that she would be better off dead. After her sister-in-law died, her older brother had taken his life several years before. She herself had experienced periods of depression in the past, particularly when her children were small and after her husband had died. She now complained of feeling drained, knew that there must be something physically wrong with her, and was hoping that her physician would find out what it was or at least prescribe something to relieve her symptoms.

Physical examination findings were unremarkable, except for pain and restricted motion in her right hip and poor vision. Laboratory evaluation included mammography, an electrocardiogram, and thyroid function studies, which disclosed unremarkable findings. A diagnosis of major depression was made, therapy was started with 25 mg of desipramine daily, and a follow-up appointment was made for 2 weeks, with clear instructions that she should call the physician if things should worsen, particularly if any thoughts of suicide should emerge.

Somatic complaints, such as constipation, fatigue, appetite disturbance, and insomnia, are common in later life. Both normal aging and the effects of disease may predispose to such problems, in the absence of depression. These, of course, must first be ruled out by a comprehensive medical and neurological evaluation. The presence of increased irritability, worthlessness, guilt, hopelessness, social withdrawal, thoughts about death, and a history of problems with depression, however, suggest the presence of a major depression. This is particularly true in light of major losses and changes in this patient's social environment, deteriorating health, and financial difficulties.

Case 2

Adjustment Disorder With Depressed Mood

A 70-year-old man was followed up in a medical outpatient clinic for stable angina and moderately severe congestive heart failure. In the past 2 years, he had experienced two myocardial infarctions and had recently been admitted for heart failure, which was now under fair control with diuretics and vasodilators. He complained to his physician that he was having trouble doing the things he used to do because of shortness of breath and fatigue. He had always been a handyman around the house and loved to plant a big garden every year. Lately, his wife had taken over many of the chores that he used to do, and his garden had become overrun with weeds. During the past year, he had begun to feel pretty useless and now spent a lot of time watching television and feeling sorry for himself. Also, he felt discouraged about the results of a coronary bypass operation a year ago that had promised him better function and relief of symptoms. The patient had experienced brief spells of depression following each of his heart attacks and after bypass surgery, but never severe enough to warrant therapy.

On careful questioning, the patient said that he was still hopeful and was not to the point of giving up. He appeared to interact fairly well with his physician and brightened up when talking about his family. He still enjoyed watching sports programs and was an avid baseball fan. While he looked forward to visits from his grandchildren, large family get-togethers seemed to wear him out. He also complained that his appetite was not like it used to be, in large part due to the low-sodium diet that made food almost tasteless. He had not lost any weight, however, and did not appear to be fluid overloaded at the time of the examination. His sleep was fair, but interrupted with nocturia and occasional orthopnea. The patient did think a lot about his illness, which was hard to get off his mind because of the limiting nature of his symptoms. When asked if he still thought life was worth living, he immediately said that it was, given the alternative.

This patient has an adjustment disorder with depressed mood. His still-hopeful attitude, continued interest in his environment and family, and failure to exhibit significant vegetative signs argue against a severe depression. Since he has not suffered a major depression, he would be unlikely to benefit from antidepressants or intensive psychotherapy. Supportive counseling and cognitive or behavioral therapy might be particularly effective in helping him to develop interests within his current abilities, to avoid isolating himself from others, and to maintain a positive attitude. Of concern during the examination is the physician's assurance that this patient's medical condition is optimally managed and that his depressive symptoms are not secondary to reversible illness or to drugs that could be discontinued or altered.

Case 3

Major Depression and Medical Illness

A 77-year-old man lived with his wife in a small home into which they had recently moved. Less than 6 months ago, they sold their ranch in the country and moved into the city to be nearer to stores and the local hospital. This patient, with a 75 pack-year history of smoking and a long history of alcoholism, had emphysema, hypertension, and poorly controlled congestive heart failure. Once an active man and fore-man of a large crew of construction workers, he now could walk only to the mailbox before becoming short of breath and exhausted. He had also recently complained of difficulty with emptying his bladder due to problems with his prostate gland.

One afternoon, the patient was admitted through the emergency room to his local hospital with a diagnosis of biventricular heart failure. On questioning by the physician, he admitted to allowing his heart medication to run out and now had not taken his digoxin for approximately 3 weeks. He had also cut back on his diuretics about a week ago because of distressing nocturia. On examination, he was gruff and irritable, complaining that all he wanted was to be left alone. A chest examination revealed rales halfway up both posterior lung fields, an S₃, distended neck veins, and marked swelling of both extremities to his knees. X-ray films and other laboratory studies were consistent with an exacerbation of congestive heart failure, probably due to medication noncompliance. An electrocardiogram showed a bifascicular block, but no acute changes.

His wife noted that for the past 2 months his appetite had been poor. Because of fluid retention from his illness, it was unclear whether he had experienced a net loss or gain of weight. She noted that he recently seemed to be more irritable when approached and preferred to be left alone. His sleep was poor and frequently interrupted by nocturia and periods of dyspnea. The patient complained that his nerves ''were shot,'' and he needed something to calm him down and help him sleep. He had stopped reading the news because of difficulties with concentration, but had never experienced any psychiatric problems previously, and no one in his family had been treated for depression or other mental problems. When asked specifically about how he felt about himself, the patient growled that he could not do any of the things he used to enjoy, felt like he was no good to anyone anymore, could no longer care for his family, and was now simply a burden on everyone around him. When asked about thoughts of taking his life, he admitted to feeling tempted at times to swerve into oncoming traffic.

This patient is a man with multiple medical problems that presented with a major depression, which might have gone undetected without the information provided by his wife and his own acknowledgement of feelings of worthlessness and suicidal thoughts (illicited only by the physician's direct questioning). Insomnia could have been attributed to his illness (heart failure or prostatism) or the effects of medications (diuretics). Loss of appetite could be explained away by liver congestion due to right-sided heart failure. Loss of energy and fatigue are common physiological accompaniments of heart failure, and memory problems might be attributed to early dementia. The use of long-acting minor tranquilizers to control anxiety can further impair cognition and actually worsen an ongoing depression. Because of his chronic illness, age older than 75 years, and history of alcoholism, this patient is in a high-risk group for suicide. His noncompliance, in fact, may represent an occult suicide attempt and herald more direct efforts in the future.

Treatment of this patient's depression will be a challenge. Antidepressants may be dangerous in the setting of bladder outlet obstruction, severe heart failure, bifascicular block, and multiple drugs predisposing to orthostasis.

Differential Diagnosis

Difficulties with Diagnosis

Most older persons experience episodes of depressed mood, loss of interest, fatigue, or discouragement that last from hours to days to weeks; yet, these episodes are not severe enough to warrant a diagnosis of major depression or even one of the other affective disorders. These episodes require no more treatment than an encouraging and supportive word from a friend or a good night's rest. On the other hand, elders may find themselves locked into a depressive syndrome that does require some planned outside intervention for its resolution. In a longitudinal study of normal aging, Gianturco and Busse[29] demonstrated that 70% of community-dwelling older men experienced some degree of depression throughout the 17-year span of the study. Differentiating clinically significant depressive disorders from minor mood fluctuations, or from other psychiatric or medical conditions that mimic depression, is not always easy.

It now has been well established that older persons commonly seek help for mental health problems from their general medical provider rather than from mental health specialists. In the ECA study, participants aged 65 to 74 years were five times more likely to see their medical provider for mental health concerns than they were to see mental health professionals.[30] Among persons aged 75 years and older, all mental health visits were made to medical providers and none to mental health specialists.

At the same time, however, it also has been well established that primary care physicians commonly either miss the diagnosis of depression in older persons or do not manage it effectively. German et al[31] examined detection and management rates for depression in medical outpatients aged 65 years and older compared with those under age 65. Detection rates were poor in both groups, but were slightly lower among older patients (35% vs 41%). Similarly, adequate management of recognized depressive disorders was present in a lower percentage of older patients (46%) compared with younger patients (57%). Detection rates of major depression among hospitalized older patients with medical illness are also poor. One study found that only 20% of male patients older than 70 years of age with major depression were detected.[32] Self-rated depression scales have been sought to assist clinicians in this regard. A number of such instruments have been used among elderly, medically ill patients, but only the Geriatric Depression Scale, a brief, easily administered self-rating scale developed specifically for use among older persons, has been validated in medical outpatients[33] and medical inpatients.[34]

Diagnostic Evaluation

A patient's history should focus on the length of the current episode, any history of previous episodes, a history of drug or alcohol abuse, therapies tried in the past and the response to them, and an assessment of the degree to which the patient is suffering, particularly with respect to suicidal thoughts. If possible, confirmation of responses by the patient should be obtained from a relative or caretaker. In the physical examination, attention should be directed toward such neurological findings as lateralization, frontal release signs, cogwheeling, or tremor, muscle tone, and slowed reflexes.

Laboratory Workup

Thyroid function studies, along with a complete blood cell count, are sometimes informative. Vitamin B_{12} deficiency may present with depressive symptoms, as well as dementia, even in the face of a normal vitamin B_{12} serum level or hemogram. The quest for a biological marker for depression has been an intense one. A number of tests purport varying sensitivities and specificities for depressive illness. Several tests are thought to be particularly sensitive for detecting depressions that are biologically driven (such as major depression with melancholia). The first is the DST, based on the long-known hyperactivity of the HPA axis in depression. The test is performed by administering 1 mg of dexamethasone at 11 PM and drawing serum cortisol levels at 8 AM, 4 PM, and 11PM on the following day; if any one of the three cortisol levels excedes 5 mg/L, the test is considered to be positive.

In 1981, Carroll et al[31] introduced the DST as a possible diagnostic aid for endogenous depression or major depression with melancholia. In that study, the test was 50% sensitive and more than 90% specific for endogenous depression. Since then, the specificity of the test has been challenged by other investigators, who have found a positive DST in persons with other psychiatric disorders and a variety of nonpsychiatric conditions. Rosenblaum et al,[36] administering the DST to a large sample of adults of all ages, found that nearly twice as many persons aged 65 years and older were nonsuppressors as those persons younger than 65 years (18% vs 9%, respectively), implying that older persons were more susceptible to alterations in the HPA axis.[36] The DST has been reported to have a sensitivity of 73% for major depression among hospitalized depressed elderly patients.[4] Others have found it useful in distinguishing depressed from nondepressed patients with early Alzheimer's disease.[37] In general, however, the prevalence of nonsuppression in nondepressed persons increases with age.

Sleep electroencephalographic (EEG) patterns may be another marker for identifying patients with depressive disorder.[38] Patients with endogenous depression have a number of EEG changes that include a general disruption of the usual sleep pattern, reduced slow-wave sleep (stages 3 and 4), a shortened rapid eye movement (REM) latency (time before onset of REM sleep after falling asleep), and an increased REM density (number of eye movements per time period in REM). However, many of these changes in the sleep EEG patterns can be normal accompaniments of aging (Chapter 43).

Most recently, platelet-tritiated, imipramine-binding density has been heralded as a biological marker for depression. The density of platelet-tritiated, imipramine-binding sites is lower in patients with major depression than in nondepressed subjects. This finding is particularly notable among older individuals and is not present in patients with Alzheimer's disease or schizophrenia.[39] In summary, there are no validated biological markers, at present, that are specific for depressive illness.

Major Depression

Major depression is characterized by a depressed mood that is experienced most of the day, nearly every day during at least a 2-week period. Instead of a depressed mood, the individual may exhibit a marked loss of interest or pleasure in all, or almost all, activities most of the day, nearly every day during the same time period. Along with either of those two symptoms, the experience of any four of the following eight symptoms nearly every day during the 2-week period qualifies a person for the diagnosis of major depression: (1) weight loss (>5% of body weight in a month) or a loss of appetite, (2) insomnia or hypersomnia, (3) psychomotor agitation or retardation, (4) fatigue or a loss of energy, (5) feelings of worthlessness or guilt, (6) diminished concentration, (7) thoughts of suicide, or (8) loss of interest (including decreased sexual interest). To qualify for major depression, this mood disturbance cannot be a result of an organic factor or be associated with normal bereavement. No mood-incongruent delusions, hallucinations, or other psychiatric disorder can be present.

Melancholic or endogenous depression is a severe form of major depression that is characterized by three or more of the following six symptoms: (1) vegetative symptoms, (2) psychomotor change, (3) guilt, (4) anhedonia, (5) distinct quality of mood, and (6) lack of reactivity. This biologically driven entity varies little in its presentation in old and young persons.[40] It is severe, incapacitating, and carries an unusually high risk for suicide; yet, it is often responsive to appropriate doses of antidepressant medication or to electroconvulsive therapy. Although cases of major depression with melancholia can be diagnosed easily in the clinical setting, many older persons with this disorder still remain unidentified. Families, in frustration, may come simply to ignore the patient or attribute the behavior to aging or dementia. While patients may not volunteer their depressive symptoms, they will seldom deny them when asked.

Psychotic depression is characterized by the presence of delusions concerning persecution, the presence of a terminal illness, or of nothingness (mood-congruent). The focus is often on the abdomen. Hallucinations and guilt are uncommon. This disorder is of special concern among elderly persons. When severe endogenous depression occurs for the first time in persons aged older than 60 years, it is more likely to be accompanied by delusions than when it occurs in younger persons.[5] This variety of depression may be particularly responsive to electroconvulsive therapy, rather than antidepressants.

Seasonal affective disorder occurs when a patient with major depression has a history of at least 2 consecutive years when a depressive episode occurs in the fall or winter, resolves as spring or summer appears, and is not due to any other psychiatric cause. This rapidly cycling depression is becoming increasingly recognized.

Other Affective Disorders

Dysthymic disorders (depressive neuroses) are more frequent among elderly patients than major depression.[6] These are chronic depressions of less severe intensity than major depression that last for 2 years or more. Underlying personality factors may be predisposing. Dysthymia in late life is likely to result from a loss of self-esteem due to the older person's inability to supply needs and drives or to defend against threats or insecurity. Cultural factors may also contribute to dysthymia in late life, such as habit patterns that emphasize activity and productivity. With retirement and cessation of childcare responsibilities, recognition and self-esteem are often lost and not easily regained through substitution of other activites.

An adjustment disorder with a depressed mood occurs when there is a maladaptive reaction to an identifiable stressor. The relationship between the symptoms of a depressed mood and a stressful event is clear. Examples of such stressors may include retirement, marital problems, financial difficulties, social role adjustment, change of residence, or physical illness. An adjustment disorder may be designated when symptoms of depression occur concurrently with a physical illness and are out of proportion to that expected from the severity of the illness or the disruption of life caused by it. Reactive depressions may become more frequent with aging and are associated with bereavement or losses of other kinds.

An organic affective syndrome occurs when there is a disturbance of mood that resembles a major depressive episode, but has a specific organic agent as its origin. Medications are a prime example (Table 36.2). Withdrawal of these agents may result in a dramatic improvement. Symptoms associated with medication-induced depressions include mild cognitive impairment, fearfulness, anxiety, irritability, and excessive

Table 36.2. Medications frequently implicated in organic affective disorders.

Medication
CNS drugs*
Benzodiazepines
Alcohol
Tricyclic antidepressants
Levodopa
Amantadine
Major tranquilizers
Stimulants (rebound)
Antihypertensives
β-blockers
Clonidine
Reserpine
Methyldopa
Prazosin
Guanethidine
Chemotherapeutic drugs
Vincristine
L-asparaginase
Interferon
Steroids
Prednisone
Estrogen preparations
Anticonvulsants
Procarbazine
Others
Cimetidine
Digitalis

*CNS indicates central nervous system.

somatic concerns. Likewise, a metabolic disorder (Table 36.3) or other physical illness (Table 36.4) may be either the primary culprit or interact with psychological causes to induce depression.

A depressive disorder not otherwise specified (ie, atypical depression) may present as a dysthymic disorder, but with intermittent periods of a normal mood lasting more than a few months (disqualifying the dysthymia diagnosis), as a brief episode of depression that does not last long enough to fulfill criteria for major affective disorder and is not reactive to a psychosocial stress, or as an episode that does not meet the criteria for any specific mood disorder (encompassing both atypical depressions and dysphorias). Dysphoria may be used to describe persons whose level of a depressed mood is appropriate for their circumstances. For instance, older adults with a severe chronic medical illness that compromises their function and physical well-being appropriately may experience some degree of depression, yet remain hopeful and not develop vegetative symptoms or negative thought patterns.

Bereavement or grieving cannot be classified as a psychiatric disorder since it is a universal human experience. Bereaved persons may be preoccupied with thoughts of their loved one, may experience guilt over small commissions or omissions concerning the deceased, and may become irritable and hostile. Restlessness may be prominent, and an inability to initiate or maintain normal activities commonly occurs. While the symptom complex may closely resemble major depression, the older adult recognizes these symptoms as normal to the situation, and there is no serious interference with the ability to function. Despite increased bereavement in later life, little evidence suggests that community-dwelling older adults experience severe or continuing dysphoria secondary to this condition. The ECA study found low rates of bereavement or grieving among persons aged older than 65 years.[5] Because loss of a spouse in later life represents an expected event, this condition may be better tolerated.

Problems can result from strong denial of the loss

Table 36.3. Metabolic and nutritional disorders that may manifest as organic affective syndromes.

Disorder
Hypokalemia or hyperkalemia
Hyponatremia or hypernatremia
Hypocalcemia or hypercalcemia
Hypoglycemia or hyperglycemia
Hypomagnesemia
Metabolic acidosis or alkalosis
Hypoxemia
Uremia
Vitamin deficiencies (B vitamins, folic acid)

Table 36.4. Physical illnesses associated with depression.

Illness
End-stage renal disease (dialysis)
Cardiovascular disease
Postmyocardial infarction
Postcoronary artery bypass surgery
Cardiomyopathy (congestive or other)
Endocrine disorders
Thyroid (hyperthyroidism and hypothyroidism, autoimmune thyroiditis)
Parathyroid (hyperparathyroidism and hypoparathyroidism)
Adrenal (Cushing's and Addison's diseases)
Disorders of insulin secretion
Hypopituitarism
Neurologic diseases
Parkinson's disease
Stroke
Alzheimer's disease
Subdural hematoma
Amyotrophic lateral sclerosis
Temporal lobe epilepsy
Multiple sclerosis
Normal-pressure hydrocephalus
Cancer
Brain tumors (primary or secondary)
Leukemia
Pancreatic cancer
Lung cancer (oat cell)
Bone metastases with hypercalcemia
Hepatic failure with encephalopathy
Anemia
Infections (particularly viral)
Chronic pain

(delayed grief). In this case, grieving may become excessive in degree. Common symptoms of pathological grief are overactivity (without a sense of loss), psychosomatic illness, hostility toward family members, and a marked loss of the ability to interact socially.

In bipolar disorder, at least three of the classic manic symptoms are required for a diagnosis of a manic episode: overactivity, pressured speech, decreased sleep (without a need for sleep), overspending, and grandiosity. Mood may be elevated, irritable, labile, or a mixture with depressive symptoms. Patients in later life with bipolar disorder often exhibit a mixture of manic and depressive symptoms. The manic elderly patient may present atypically, with a depressed mood denying any manic symptoms, and is less likely to experience euphoria. Irritability, hostility, and resentment are common when grandiose

plans are not realized. Differentiating an agitated depression from a manic episode may be difficult. Manic delirium is a special case, where cognitive functioning is markedly altered and may include hallucinations. First-time manic episodes after the age of 60 years may often occur in the setting of head injury or stroke.

Cyclothymic disorder is the bipolar equivalent of dysthymic disorder, but includes the cycling between hypomanic and minor depressive states, without marked impairment, during at least a 2-year period. A "bipolar disorder not otherwise specified" is the *DSM-III-R* equivalent of a "depressive disorder not otherwise specified," in that the former is any disorder with manic or hypomanic features that does not fulfill the criteria for any other bipolar disorder.

Normal Aging

A depressed mood also has been attributed by some investigators to changes that occur with normal aging. Biological changes with aging may predispose older adults to depressive symptoms. They may spend more time lying in bed trying unsuccessfully to sleep and, therefore, complain of poor sleep. The REM sleep latency, a marker for depression, gradually decreases with aging, and depth and quality of sleep may thus be altered (Chapter 43). Decreased activity due to disease or disability may make older persons feel more lethargic. Decreased appetite, due to poor dentition or altered taste perception, may also reduce the energy level.

Results of longitudinal studies, however, have not supported this supposition. As noted earlier, severe depression in late life is significantly less common than it is at any other stage of the life cycle. Well-being and adjustment were found to remain constant during a 4-year longitudinal study of an elderly cohort.[41]

Other Psychiatric Disorders

Psychiatric conditions with depressive symptoms may be confused with depression. These include the organic mental disorders (Chapter 33), paranoid disorders (Chapter 37), sleep disorders (Chapter 43), hypochondriasis, alcoholism, and schizophrenia.

Hypochondriasis is both a symptom of depression and a separate disorder itself. The essential features are an unrealistic interpretation of physical signs or sensations as abnormal and a preoccupation with the imagined physical illness underlying these sensations. Between 60% and 70% of depressed persons in one study were found to have hypochondriacal symptoms.[42] When hypochondriacal complaints appear in later life for the first time, there is a high likelihood that either depression or an undetected physical illness is present. Hypochondriasis as a disorder is usually distinguishable from depression by (1) the length of the episode (hypochondriasis persisting for years), (2) the degree of suffering by the patient (more among depressed patients), (3) and the waxing and waning course of symptoms in depression, which by nature is cyclical. Differentiating the older adult with hypochondriasis or a generalized anxiety disorder from the one who is depressed has therapeutic implications; the former usually does not tolerate antidepressants because of real or imagined side effects.

Alcoholism, while less frequent in older than in younger persons, still occurs in about 5% to 8% of persons aged older than 60 years.[43] A heavy alcohol intake may cause both physical and psychological symptoms that mimic depression. Conversely, many alcoholics drink to relieve the pain of depression that recurs when they become sober.

The sudden appearance of a psychosis in later life, with paranoid or delusional thinking, may herald the onset of a major depression. Differentiating depression from late-life schizophrenia may be difficult, but the latter is not associated with profound depression. Late-life schizophrenia seldom begins suddenly. Rather, it is characterized by gradual withdrawal, bizarre complaints, and paranoia.

Depression in the Setting of Medical Illness

The spectrum of depressive disorders described can occur in older persons with a medical illness. The mental strain associated with progressive disability and dependence, chronic pain, unpleasant side effects from drugs, alterations in diet and life-style, financial insecurity, and feelings of guilt from being a burden on family members can result in dysphoric mood states ranging from mild dissatisfaction with life to major depression. In general, depressive disorders associated with a physical illness tend to be less severe although this is not always the case.

The relationship between a medical illness and depression is a complex one. Organic symptoms associated with severe congestive heart failure, end-stage chronic obstructive pulmonary disease, or metastatic cancer include fatigue, restlessness, poor appetite, and sleeplessness; these symptoms are sometimes impossible to differentiate from psychological symptoms originating from a depression. A high prevalence of depression has been reported in older patients with a severe medical illness.[8] The response of depressive symptoms to treatment of the underlying medical illness may provide a clue to their origin. Dysphoria, loss of interest, or feelings of worthlessness that persist despite reversal of physical disease suggest a functional diagnosis.

Specific Medical Conditions

Hyperthyroidism (apathetic) and hypothyroidism are both commonly associated with depression; yet, changes of normal aging and the altered presentation of thyroid disorders in elderly patients may hinder a correct diagnosis. A depressed affect may be a normal accompaniment of hypothyroidism, along with psychomotor retardation, cognitive changes, and constipation. Treatment of the underlying thyroid disorder should reverse symptoms and signs of depression.

Occult cancer, presenting with weight loss and fatigue, may likewise be confused with depression and vice versa. In fact, several investigators have found higher rates of cancer in persons suffering from depression.[44] Alterations in the immune system with aging and depression may increase the individual's susceptibility to neoplasia. On the other hand, metabolic factors released from tumors might underlie depressive symptoms (cancer of the pancreas).

Stroke, particularly left hemispheric lesions, have been associated with high rates of depression in older populations.[45] The finding that lesions in the brain may cause specific depressive syndromes supports the hypothesis that localized areas of brain dysfunction, rather than a generalized neurochemical abnormality, may be responsible for certain depressive states.

Chronic pain syndromes frequently give rise to symptoms that mimic depression, and depressed patients may be unusually sensitive to pain. Depression rating scales often cannot distinguish persons with chronic pain from those persons with depression.

Parkinson's disease and depression frequently coexist; yet, if either of these conditions is present alone, the other may be difficult to rule out. Older patients with Parkinson's disease may have a flat affect, appear to be socially withdrawn, feel helpless and hopeless, and experience anger and frustration over their disability. Levodopa may cause disorientation, paranoia, and aggressiveness. The progression of disease may also mimic depression as psychomotor retardation worsens. Consequently, the degree of depressed affect may be overestimated in such patients, resulting in intervention inappropriately directed toward depression rather than Parkinson's disease.

Management

The treatment of depression in later life may be divided into four major components: (1) individual psychotherapy, (2) pharmacotherapy, (3) ECT, and

(4) family therapy. Individual and family psychotherapy are purported to be equal in their ability to relieve symptoms, particularly in nonendogenous depression.

Psychotherapy

Given the high prevalence of known and occult medical illness in later life, the tolerance of biological interventions may lessen with increased age. Side effects of powerful psychoactive drugs are common and may predispose the older person to falling or convey other unpleasant side effects. Psychotherapy, on the other hand, circumvents the dangers of physiological instability and susceptibility. Increased attention is being directed toward refining both cognitive and behavioral therapies for depression in later life, therapies that may be particularly applicable to the frail older patient with medical illness.

Cognitive-behavioral therapy is designed specifically for depression.[46] Interpersonal psychotherapy uses the methods of cognitive-behavioral therapy to improve interpersonal relationships of depressed individuals and, thus, improve their social functioning.[47] The cognitive-behavioral approach is useful among older persons because it is time limited and directive. Approximately 10 to 25 sessions are usually required for good results. Few medical interventions for chronic, disabling, and potentially life-threatening illnesses require less expenditure of health care resources. The effectiveness of cognitive-behavioral strategies has been studied in elderly patients, and improvements have been documented in this population.[48]

The cognitive-behavioral approach has, as its goals, to change behavior and restructure modes of thinking. Behavioral interventions may include a weekly activity schedule, mastery and pleasure logs, and graded assignments. Cognitive methods include attempts to change negative-thinking patterns and automatic thoughts. Cognitive restructuring is accomplished by the reality testing of negative cognitions, examining distorted cognitions, and coming up with new ways of thinking about self and life. Depressed patients overgeneralize and think in terms of black or white (good or bad) without considering shades or degrees. Depressed patients regard themselves and their futures from a negative perspective. They believe that the defect is in themselves and that they are inadequate, ineffective, worthless, helpless, and hopeless. Depressed elders may convince themselves that they will never get better and are doomed to suffer for the rest of their lives with no possibility for relief. The symptoms of depression, then, result from these negative cognitions that generate internal distress and dissipate energy.

Adjustment disorders seldom require intensive psychotherapy, drugs, or other biological therapies. Often, all that is required are simple counseling and time that involve active listening, warm understanding, suggestions on different ways of viewing and solving problems, and provision of steady support in the context of a strong physician patient relationship.

Pharmacotherapy

When patients' distress from depression is great and significantly interferes with their functioning, pharmacological therapy should be considered. Depressions that are severe and associated with melancholic or endogenous symptoms (insomnia, loss of weight and appetite, constipation, and loss of pleasure and interest) are more likely to be driven biologically and are thought to be more responsive to pharmacological therapy. However, drugs also may be effective to varying degrees in depressive episodes without melancholic symptoms.

The three major classes of medications used to treat affective disorders are (1) tricyclic and newer antidepressants, (2) MAO inhibitors, and (3) lithium carbonate (or other medications to prevent a recurrence of affective episodes). Tricyclic antidepressants remain the drugs of choice for depression in later life. Heterocyclic antidepressants (sometimes called "second-generation" antidepressants) include trazodone, maprotiline, and amoxapine. More recently, bupropion, fluoxetine, and sertaline have appeared. Preferred medications are those that, while effective, have as few side effects as possible, particularly orthostatic hypotension and anticholinergic effects (Table 36.5).

Tricyclic and Second-Generation Antidepressants

Nortriptyline, desipramine, and doxepin are popular drugs for treating older adults with endogenous depressions. Lower doses than those for younger adults are preferred, since high blood levels may occur in older adults even at reduced dosages.[49] Doses of 25 to 50 mg of nortriptyline or desipramine at bedtime is often adequate to relieve symptoms. If higher doses are required, a divided dosage during the day may decrease the likelihood of orthostatic hypotension. If side effects are prohibitive or no response is seen after 3 to 4 weeks of treatment, trazodone may be tried. This drug's virtual lack of anticholinergic side effects makes it an attractive alternative for use in elderly patients. Cases of priapism have been associated with its use in elderly men. Despite the absence of anticho-

Table 36.5. Recommended doses, reported side-effects, and therapeutic blood levels of antidepressants in older persons.*

Drug	Dose (initial-maintenance), mg	Therapeutic serum level, ng/dl	Relative sedation	Relative anticholinergic	Postural hypotension
Tricyclics and heterocyclics					
Doxepin	25–100	>100	+++	+++	+++
Nortriptyline	10–100	50–150	++	++	++
Desipramine	25–100	>125	+	+	++
Trazodone	50–200	NA	+++	0	+
Fluoxetine	20	NA	0	+	?
MAO inhibitors					
Phenelzine	15–45	>80% inhibition of MAO	+	++	+++
Lithium carbonate	150–300	0.4–0.7 mmol/L	++	0	?
Stimulants					
Methylphenidate	5–10	NA	0	0	?

*NA indicates not applicable; three plus signs, strong; two plus signs, moderate; one plus sign, weak; zero, none; MAO, monoamine oxidase; and question mark, unknown.

linergic effects, trazodone can lead to significant drowsiness, a symptom that is not well tolerated by elderly patients. When doses exceeding 100 mg/d of a tricyclic antidepressant or 200 mg/d of trazodone are not sufficient to control depression in an older patient, the drug should be discontinued.

Certain features of a depressive episode may suggest the use of one antidepressant over another. The patient with agitation, restlessness, or insomnia may respond better to either doxepin or trazodone; both of these drugs tend to have sedation as a prominent side effect. Both trazodone and doxepin have been studied in medically ill older patients, and improvements in mood and function have been noted.[50,51] On the other hand, when psychomotor retardation, fatigue, and listlessness are prominent, desipramine may be more appropriate because it is less sedating and has a low incidence of anticholinergic side effects. Nortriptyline is intermediate in both sedative and anticholinergic side effects, has been demonstrated to be effective in older medically ill patients, and has little effect on cardiac output in patients with congestive heart failure.[52,53]

Before starting therapy with an antidepressant, the older patient should undergo a thorough history and physical examination to detect contraindications to these drugs. Special care should be employed to elicit any history of closed-angle glaucoma, difficulty with urination, severe dizziness with standing, seizure disorder, severe hypertension, recent myocardial infarction, or unstable angina. The physical examination should include measurement of orthostatic blood pressure changes and examination of the heart for murmurs and gallops, the abdomen for liver enlargement, and the prostate gland. Baseline liver and kidney

function test results should also be obtained because tricyclic antidepressants are metabolized in the liver and excreted in the urine.

An electrocardiogram should be obtained before starting therapy with antidepressants. If bifascicular block, second-degree heart block, or prolongation of the QT interval are present, antidepressants should not be started unless the patient is under careful observation in the hospital. Patients with atrial fibrillation may experience an acceleration in heart rate due to anticholinergic side effects that enhance conduction through the atrioventricular (AV) node. Simple first-degree AV block or bundle-branch block does not increase the risk of cardiac complications. A follow-up electrocardiogram, after the start of treatment, is essential in all patients with heart disease. The dose should be decreased or the drug should be stopped if there is a marked prolongation of the PR, QT, or QRS durations or if AV block worsens or ventricular arrhythmias increase. Use of tricyclic antidepressants concurrently with quinidine, procainamide hydrochloride (Pronestyl), or other type 1 antiarrhythmics may produce additive cardiac effects.

Assuring compliance is an important part of pharmacological therapy. The depressed older person may commonly forget to take medicine or lack the motivation to comply; hence, involvement of a concerned family member can increase the chance of success. Compliance will also depend on physicians providing patients and their families with information about the benefits to be expected, their time course, and possible side effects. While improvement in sleep may be noted almost immediately, 3 to 4 weeks at a therapeutic blood level may be required before mood changes occur. Some investigators, however, have found that of the older patients who are going to respond, more than two thirds do so by the end of the first week of treatment.[54] Patients should be informed of side effects, such as dizziness with sudden standing, difficulty with urination, dry mouth, and constipation. These effects are often experienced soon after starting the drug therapy, but may gradually improve throughout a couple weeks of therapy. When there is concern over the patient's suicidal potential, no more than 1 g of a tricyclic antidepressant should be dispensed at any one time. Once a response is achieved, antidepressants should be continued for 6 to 9 months and then gradually tapered. Patients who experience more than one relapse within 2 years of the initial episode may require long-term maintenance therapy.

Other Antidepressants

Monoamine oxidase inhibitors are an alternative to tricyclic antidepressants. Three caveats are in order. First, if a patient develops intolerance to side effects with a tricyclic antidepressant, it is unlikely that he or she will better tolerate an MAO inhibitor. Second, if the patient is seriously depressed and there is a risk of suicide, management can require the emergent use of electroconvulsive therapy. However, ECT cannot be safely performed until 10 days to 2 weeks after discontinuation of the MAO inhibitor. Dietary modifications are required to prevent a hypertensive crisis. Foods high in tyramine content are to be avoided: certain cheeses, canned meat or fish, wines, chocolate, and others. The older adult, who lives alone, has marginal financial reserves, and seldom cooks, may subsist on inexpensive canned foods that contain ingredients to be avoided. If an MAO inhibitor is used, blood levels of MAO activity before and during treatment should be measured to ensure that adequate inhibition (ie, 80%) is accomplished.

Lithium carbonate may be useful in preventing the recurrence of unipolar depression, although its efficacy in this regard is not as well proved as for bipolar disorder. Some investigators have suggested that lithium carbonate be used either alone or in combination with tricyclic antidepressants in the short-term treatment of depression. The usefulness of the latter combination is based on the assumption that lithium carbonate may sensitize postsynaptic adrenergic receptors and, thus, enhance the effects of tricyclic antidepressants. Other agents, such as carbamazapine, may be prescribed if lithium carbonate fails to control recurrences. Use of lithium carbonate by nonpsychiatric physicians in the treatment of depression is not recommended.

Alprazolam, a benzodiazepine, has been reported to have antidepressant, as well as antianxiety, effects. At doses of 2 to 4 mg/d, the antidepressant effects of this drug have been reported to equal those of imipramine. Nevertheless, alprazolam has a strong tendency toward habituation, and it may be difficult to get patients to discontinue this drug once it has been started. No studies have examined its efficacy in treating depression in later life. Benzodiazepines in general, however, should not be used to treat depression. They can induce excessive sedation and may even worsen the depressive state.[55,56]

Low-dose stimulants, such as methylphenidate, 5 mg every morning, may enhance the mood of an apathetic older adult. At such a dose, side effects are rare, and abuse or addiction is seldom encountered. Stimulants have been used to treat depression in medically ill older patients.[57]

The treatment of acute manic episodes is best accomplished with lithium carbonate; supplementation with phenothiazines, such as haloperidol or thioridazine, may be necessary. In rare circumstances, a manic episode will respond only to electroconvulsive therapy.

Major depression with dementia probably should be treated with antidepressant medication. The starting dose should be low (eg, 10 mg of nortriptyline), increasing slowly to a maximum of 75 mg/d. Anticholinergic effects can worsen dementia and may precipitate an acute delirium.

ECT

For severe, major depressive illness that is persistent and refractory to psychotherapy and pharmacotherapy, ECT can be a most effective treatment. Electroconvulsive therapy is primarily effective in major depression with melancholia and in major depression with psychotic features, especially when associated with agitation or withdrawal. Despite its effectiveness, ECT should be performed only after other methods of treatment have been tried and have failed. In cases where the patient becomes suicidal or attempts to starve to death, ECT may be the treatment of choice.

For an adequate therapeutic response, treatments are usually given 3 times per week for a total of 6 to 15 times. A marked improvement usually is noted after one of the treatments. Following this improvement, two or three further treatments are usually given. The overall success rate for ECT in drug nonresponders is about 80%, a rate that is not significantly decreased in the elderly patients. In the absence of prophylactic drug therapy, the relapse rate 1 year following ECT exceeds 50%. Maintenance ECT (weekly or monthly) may reduce these relapse rates, but the use of tricyclic antidepressants or lithium carbonate usually is effective in decreasing the relapse rate to around 20% in the year following ECT.

Family and Social Therapies

There are two reasons for including the family in therapy. First, family dysfunction may be contributing to the genesis and maintenance of depression in the patient. Second, support from the family is essential to a successful outcome. First, the clinician should focus on whoever is going to be in contact with the older person in the home. Next, the overall atmosphere among that group of people identified as family should be evaluated. Interactions between the older patient and other family members should be observed, as should interactions between family members themselves. How do they regard psychiatric therapy? What are the chances that a family member will undermine efforts to shape new behaviors and attitudes in the patient? The clinician should try to assess the level of support and tolerance within the family, as well as what other stressors exist.

After permission has been obtained from the patient to allow the interaction with the family, the clinician should inform them about the nature of the depressive disorder and the risks associated with it. In particular, families should be prepared for the possibility of a suicide attempt. They should be instructed to remove instruments that might facilitate such an attempt, especially when the patient has mentioned a likely method. A schedule of constant observation of, or frequent checks on, the patient may have to be arranged. A telephone number should be provided to relatives that will assure them an immediate response from the health care team should a suicide attempt occur. The family can also assist the clinician in monitoring the patient for signs of improvement or worsening. Methods of dealing with overly dependent elders should be taught to family members to prevent burnout and relieve guilt.

Family members must be told that many of the behaviors exhibited by the patient at this time (apathy, crying, hostility, criticism) are part of the illness of depression, and that many of these symptoms will abate once the depression resolves. They should be warned to brace themselves for expressions of anger or rejection by the patient. The family should be encouraged to maintain their warmth and support toward the patient and to engage the patient in outside activities with them as much as possible. Where family tensions exist, it may be helpful to see the patient and family together and observe their interaction. Family therapy also may resolve ongoing conflicts, which may account for recurrent depression.

A determined effort may be needed to counteract the depressed person's natural tendency to withdraw from others. Social support is an important predictor of recovery from depression in later life.[25] Friendships outside the immediate family are important in this regard. A number of voluntary social organizations, such as churches, senior centers, special support groups, and various clubs and associations, may be important sources of social contact for older persons. Organizations that provide meaningful volunteer work in the community may do much to help older persons develop new relationships and direct their minds to activities outside of themselves. Shepherds' Centers provide an innovative model in this regard. These privately funded groups are organized and operated by older adults themselves who volunteer their time and talents to help more disabled elderly persons in the community.[58]

Treatment of Depression in Medically Ill Patients

The population of older adults at highest risk for the development of significant depressive disorders comprises medically ill patients, particularly those who are hospitalized with a severe illness. Prevalence rates for major depression are 3 to 10 times more common in medically ill patients than in healthy community-dwelling elderly persons. Treatment of depressive disorders in older medically ill patients is difficult. Of five studies that examined the efficacy of antidepressants in the treatment of depression among medically ill older patients, two have demonstrated a benefit over placebo.[53,54] Inadequate dosing, the uncertainty of the diagnosis, and the failure to include individuals with severe medical illness limit the conclusions of these positive studies. However, the serious side effects experienced by medical patients receiving these drugs are well known. In one study, 80% to 90% of hospitalized medical patients older than age 70 years with major depression had relative or absolute contraindications to the use of antidepressants.[32]

Psychotherapy, a mode of treatment associated with little morbidity, may be more optimal in this setting, particularly for less severe depressions that are reactive to physical illness and chronic disability. Supportive counseling, cognitive therapy, or interpersonal psychotherapy can be effective and avoid side effects of conventional biological treatments. Cognitive therapies might be especially effective in maintaining self-esteem and motivation toward recovery by dispelling negative thought patterns and replacing them with more realistic, hopeful, and forward-looking cognitions. Few studies, however, have systematically examined the efficacy of psychotherapy in this setting. Electroconvulsive therapy is effective and safe for the treatment of severe and biologically driven depressions of the melancholic or endogenous variety, particularly where suicidal ideation, starvation, or serious noncompliance are a problem. Treatment complications with ECT increase with age and the severity of medical illness, and prolonged remission from depressive symptoms with ECT has been difficult to effect.

Management of Grief

First, the physician must distinguish normal from pathological grieving. Normally grieving elders may have all the symptoms of depression; yet, they may not require conventional therapy for depression. When uncomplicated bereavement is taking place, the physician's most important task is to be available, to show interest, and to encourage the patient to express feelings and ask questions. An effort should be made to free patient from any unnecessary guilt or responsibility by assuring the patient that he or she had done everything possible for the deceased, and by allowing the expression of any doubts that the patient may have in this area. A follow-up telephone call or a scheduled visit to the office 1 month after death can be helpful to both the family and the physician.

Grief work is a necessary component of a healthy adjustment to a loss, and the patient should be encouraged to take time for this. Failure to complete the work of grieving may result in disordered grieving characterized by either long-term mourning (an abnormal extension of the period of grieving marked by disorganization and failure to restructure life) or inhibited mourning (the prolonged absence of grieving, with subsequent hypochondriasis, generalized dissatisfaction with life, and difficulty in connecting with one's feelings). Disordered mourning may require both intensive psychotherapy and antidepressants for its resolution.

Management of the Suicidal Patient

Clinicians should sensitively inquire about suicidal thoughts among any older patients who appear to be depressed or who abuse alcohol. The interest and concern shown by the physician often are reassuring, allowing the patient to release these thoughts to another person. Such inquiry will not increase the likelihood of suicide. Gentle exploration for suicidal thoughts may begin by the following series of questions. "Do you ever feel so discouraged about the way things are that you wonder whether life is really worth living?" If the response is yes, then inquire, "Have you felt that way recently?" If again affirmative, then ask, "Have you felt low enough recently to think about taking your life?" If yes, then ask, "Have you thought about how you might do it, and do you have the means (gun, medication, etc) to carry out the job?" Affirmative responses to the latter questions indicate a serious enough level of intent to warrant some sort of interventive action. Such action may be particularly appropriate when a combination of any of the following risk factors is present: age older than 65 years, male sex, presence of painful or disabling illness, living alone, history of suicide attempts, or family history of suicide.

Specific interventions include a psychiatric consultation, establishment of a contract with the patient, communication with relatives concerning careful monitoring of the patient, and removal of the means by which suicide might be accomplished. Treatment of depression, if present, should be started, and the patient should be hospitalized, if necessary. Great care should be expressed in dispensing antidepressant medication, for these drugs themselves often become the instrument of suicide.

Acknowledgment

This work was supported in part by grant MH40159, Clinical Research Center for Psychopathology in the Elderly (CRC/PE), at Duke University Medical Center, Durham, NC.

References

1. Koenig HG. Depression and dysphoria among the elderly: dispelling a myth. *J Fam Pract* 1986;23:383–385.
2. Blazer DG. *Depression in Late Life*. St Louis, Mo: VC Mosby Co; 1982:113.
3. Cavanaugh S. The prevalence of emotional and cognitive dysfunction in a general medical population: using the MMSE, GHQ, and BDI. *Gen Hosp Psychiatry* 1983;5: 15–24.
4. Magni G, Diego DL, Schifano F. Depression in geriatric and adult medical inpatients. *J Clin Psychol* 1985;41: 337–344.
5. Myers JK, Weissman MM, Tischler GL, et al. Six-month prevalence of psychiatric disorders in three communities. *Arch Gen Psychiatry* 1984;41:959–967.
6. Weissman MM, Leaf PF, Tischler GL, et al. Affective disorders in five United States communities. *Psychol Med* 1988;18:141–153.
7. Blazer DG, Hughes DC, George LK. The epidemiology of depression in an elderly community population. *Gerontologist* 1987;27:281–287.
8. Koenig HG, Meador KG, Cohen HJ, et al. Depression in elderly men hospitalized with medical illness. *Arch Intern Med* 1988;148:1929–1936.
9. Kitchell MA, Barnes RF, Veith RC, et al. Screening for depression in hospitalized geriatric medical patients. *J Am Geriatr Soc* 1982;30:174–144.

10. Borson S, Barnes RA, Kukull WA, et al. Symptomatic depression in elderly medical outpatients, I: prevalence, demography, and health services utilization. *J Am Geriatr Soc* 1986;34:341–347.
11. Schulberg HC, McClelland M, Gooding W. Six-month outcomes for medical patients with major depressive disorders. *J Gen Intern Med* 1987;2:312–317.
12. Parmalee PA, Katz IR, Lawton MP. Depression among institutionalized aged: Assessment and prevalence estimation. Presented at the Gerontological Society of America annual meeting, 1987; Washington, DC.
13. Kafonek S, Ettinger W, Roca R, et al. Dementia, depression, and functional status in a long-term care facility. *In:* Proceedings of the AGS/AFAR Annual Meeting; May 1987; Kafonek S, Ettinger WH, Roca R, Kittner S, Taylor N, German PS. Instruments for screening for depression and dernentia in a long term care facility. JAGS 1989;37:29–34.
14. Hopkinson G. A genetic study of affective illness in patients over 50. *Br J Psychiatry* 1964;110:244–254.
15. Robinson DS, Davies JM, Nies A, et al. Relation of sex and aging to monoamine oxidase activity of human plasma and platelets. *Arch Gen Psychiatry* 1971;24:536–541.
16. Vogel GW, Vogel F, McAbee RS, et al. Improvement of depression by REM sleep deprivation: new findings and a theory. *Arch Gen Psychiatry* 1980;37:247–253.
17. Pfifer JF, Murrell SA. Etiologic factors in the onset of depressive symptoms in older adults. *J Abnorm Psychol* 1986;95:282–291.
18. Blazer DG. Impact of late-life depression on the social network. *Am J Psychiatry* 1983;140:162–166.
19. Fredman L, Schoenbach VJ, Kaplan BH, et al. The association between depressive symptoms and mortality among older participants in the Epidemiologic Catchment Area-Piedmont Health Survey, 1986.
20. Murphy E, Smith R, Lundesay J, et al. Increased mortality rates in late-life depression. *Br J Psychiatry* 1988;152:347–353.
21. Schweitzer I, Maguire KP, Gee AH, et al. Prediction of outcome in depressed patients by weekly monitoring with the dexamethasone suppression text. *Br J Psychiatry* 1987;151:780–783.
22. Post F. The management and nature of depressive illness in late life: a follow-through study. *Br J Psychiatry* 1972;121:393–404.
23. Murphy E. The prognosis of depression in old age. *Br J Psychiatry* 1983;142:111–119.
24. Blazer D, Fowler N, Hughes D. Follow-up of hospitalized depressed patients: an age comparison.
25. George LK, Blazer DG, Hughes DC, et al. Social support and the outcome of major depression. 1989;154:478–485.
26. Shulman K, Post F. Bipolar affective disorder in old age. *Br J Psychiatry* 1980;136:26–32.
27. Blazer DG, Bachar JR, Manton KG. Suicide in late life: review and commentary. *J Am Geriatr Soc* 1986;34:519–525.
28. Parkin D, Stengal E. Incidence of suicide attempts in an urban community. *Br Med J Clin Res* 1965;2:133–134.
29. Gianturco DT, Busse EW. Psychiatric problems encoun-
tered during a long-term study of normal ageing volunteers. In: Issacs AD, Post F, eds. *Studies in Geriatric Psychiatry* New York, NY: John Wiley & Sons Inc; 1978:1–16.
30. German PS, Shapiro S, Skinner EA. Mental health of the elderly: use of health and mental health services. *J Am Geriatr Soc* 1985;33:246–252.
31. German PS, Shapiro S, Skinner EA, et al. Detection and management of mental health problems of older patients by primary care providers. *JAMA* 1987;257:489–493.
32. Koenig HG, Meador KG, Cohen HJ, et al. Detection and treatment of major depression in older medically ill hospitalized patients. *Intl J Psychiatry Med* 1988;18:17–31.
33. Norris JT, Gallagher D, Wilson A, et al. Assessment of depression in geriatric medical outpatients: the validity of two screening measures. *J Am Geriatr Soc* 1987;35:989–995.
34. Koenig HG, Meador KG, Cohen HJ, et al. Self-rated depression scales and screening for major depression in the older hospitalized patient with medical illness. *J Am Geriatr Soc* 1988;36:699–706.
35. Carroll BJ, Feinberg M, Greden JF, et al. A specific laboratory test for the diagnosis of melancholia: standardization, validity, and clinical utility. *Arch Gen Psychiatry* 1981;38:15–22.
36. Rosenbaum AH, Schatzberg AF, MacLaughlin MS, et al. The DST in normal control subjects: a comparison of two assays and the effects of age. *Am J Psychiatry* 1984;141:1550–1555.
37. Jenike MA, Albert MS. The dexamethasone suppression test in patients with presenile and senile dementia of the Alzheimer's type. *J Am Geriatr Soc* 1984;32:441–444.
38. Kupfer DJ, Foster FG, Coble P, et al. The application of EEG sleep for the differential diagnosis of affective disorders. *Am J Psychiatry* 1978;135:69–74.
39. Knight DL, Krishnan KRRR, Blazer DG, et al. Tritiated imipramine binding to platelets is markedly reduced in elderly depressed patients. *Soc Neurosci Abstr* 1986;12:1251.
40. Blazer DG, Bachar JR, Hughes DC. Major depression with melancholia: a comparison of middle-aged and elderly adults. *J Am Geriatr Soc* 1987;35:927–932.
41. Palmore E, Kivett V. Change in life satisfaction: a longitudinal study of persons age 46–70. *J Gerontol* 1977;32:311–316.
42. de Alarcon R. Hypochondriasis and depression in the aged. *Gerontology* 1964;6:266–277.
43. Shoenborn CA, Cohen BH. *Trends in Smoking, Alcohol Consumption, and Other Health Practices Among US Adults, 1977 and 1983.* (1986.) US Dept of Health and Human Services publication (PHS) 86-1250.
44. Whitlock FA, Siskind M. Depression and cancer: a follow-up study. *Psychol Med* 1979;9:747–752.
45. Robinson RG, Szetela B. Mood change following left hemisphere brain injury. *Ann Neurol* 1981;9:447–453.
46. Beck AT, Rush AJ, Shaw BF, et al. *Cognitive Therapy of Depression.* New York, NY: Guilford Press; 1979.
47. Klerman GL, Weissman MM, Rounsaville BJ, et al. *Interpersonal Psychotherapy of Depression.* New York, NY: Basic Books Inc. Publishers; 1984.

48. Gallagher D, Thompson LW. Differential effectiveness of psychotherapies for the treatment of major depressive disorder in older adult patients. *Psychother Theory Res Pract* 1982;19:42–49.

49. Nies A, Robinson DS, Friedman MJ, et al. Relationship between age and tricyclic antidepressant pharmacokinetics and plasma levels. *Am J Psychiatry* 1977; 134:790–793.

50. Reding MJ, Orto LA, Winter SW et al. Antidepressant therapy after stroke: a double-blind trial. *Arch Neurol* 1986;43:763–768.

51. Lakshmanan M, Mion LC, Frengley JD. Effective low dose tricyclic antidepressant treatment for depressed geriatric rehabilitation patients. *J Am Geriatr Soc* 1986;34:421–426.

52. Lipsey JR, Robinson RG, Pearlson GD. Nortriptyline treatment of post-stroke depression: a double-blind study. *Lancet* 1984;1:297–300.

53. Roose SP, Glassman AH, Giardina, EGV, et al. Nortriptyline in depressed patients with left ventricular impairment. *JAMA* 1986;256:3253–3257.

54. Jarvik LF, Mintz J, Steuer J, et al. Treating geriatric depression: a 26-week interim analysis. *J Am Geriatr Soc* 1982;30:713–717.

55. Tyrer P, Murphy S. The place of benzodiazepines in psychiatric practice. *Br J Psychiatry* 1987;151:719–723.

56. Greenblatt DJ, Shader RI, Abernathy DR. Current status of benzodiazepines: clinical use of benzodiazepines. *N Engl J Med* 1983;309:410–405.

57. Katon W, Raskind M. Treatment of depression in the medically ill elderly with methylphenidate. *Am J Psychiatry* 1980;137:963–965.

58. Koenig HG. Shepherds' Centers: elderly people helping themselves. *J Am Geriatr Soc* 1986;34:73–74.

Anxiety, Paranoia, and Personality Disorders

Richard C. U'Ren

The five disorders discussed here—anxiety, phobia, obsessive-compulsive disorder, hypochondriasis, and conversion disorder—were once known collectively as the *neuroses.* The term *neurosis* is now out of fashion in American psychiatry, however, and the first three of the above disorders are now considered to be *anxiety disorders,* while the last two are *somatoform disorders.* Physical symptoms without a demonstrable organic basis that are linked with psychological factors or conflicts characterize somatoform disorders.[1(p255)]

Panic and obsessive-compulsive disorders are rare in elderly persons. Phobias, however, are not. Phobic disorders are the most common psychiatric disorders in women aged older than 65 years and are second only to cognitive disorders in men aged older than 65 years. Yet, despite the relatively high frequency of phobias in older men and women, the overall prevalence of anxiety disorders (including phobias) is lower in elderly persons than it is in younger individuals, thus belying a common perception that aging is associated with an increase in neurotic behavior.[2]

The occurrence of these disorders in old age, whether arising for the first time after the age of 60 years or representing merely a worsening of a lifelong affliction, is always caused by a combination of personal predisposition, life experience, and stress. Common stresses in old age include a decrease in strength and stamina, physical illness, isolation, loneliness, lack of money, loss of independence, loss of a spouse, relocation, and retirement. Anxiety symptoms are usually indicative of situations that are unsettling to elderly patients.[3]

These five disorders rarely present as pure types. Elderly patients may present, for example, with a mixture of anxiety, obsessiveness, and hypochondriasis. Furthermore, depression commonly accompanies anxiety disorders and exacerbates the symptoms.

Patients older than 65 years of age who suffer from either anxiety of somatoform disorders can be roughly divided into those whose symptoms developed much earlier in life and those whose symptoms have developed after 65 years of age. The two groups differ from each other in significant ways. Individuals with late-onset disorder report more feelings of loneliness, have more trouble in caring for themselves, and have fewer hobbies than either patients with long-standing neurotic symptoms or normal older people. Individuals with late-onset anxiety disorders also have more actual physical illness than either normal elderly persons or patients with long-standing anxiety disorders. This finding underscores the importance of searching for an unrecognized medical illness when anxiety disorders appear for the first time in late life.[4]

Little is known about the long-term course of anxiety and somatoform disorders when they begin early in life. In one review, 40% of such patients showed a definite improvement as they got older, and another 30% showed a slight improvement with age; the intensity of the symptoms of these disorders also may diminish with the passage of time.[5]

Anxiety

Symptoms of anxiety, especially feelings of tension and apprehension, are common in old age. The threatened or actual loss of economic or personal security, dependency, pain, and failing health all can create a state of anxiety. The Reverend Sidney Smith once observed "The evil in old age is that as your time has come, you think every little illness is the beginning of the end. When a man expects to be arrested, every knock at the door is an alarm."[6] An underlying medical cause always should be sought when episodes of anxiety occur for the first time in old age, since physical illness is the most common precipitant of anxiety in this age group. Table 37.1 lists the major organic causes of anxiety in old age.[7,8]

Common symptoms of anxiety are nervousness, tension, restless sleep, apprehensiveness, and fear of impending doom, as well as a variety of somatic complaints: dyspnea, palpitations, chest pain, hyperventilation, dizziness, light-headedness, headaches, sweating, trembling, diarrhea, urinary frequency, and abdominal pain. When distinct and discrete episodes of these symptoms occur, the condition is called a *panic disorder* and further qualified by the presence or absence of agoraphobia, a fear of being in places or situations from which escape would be impossible or embarrassing, or a fear of being in a place or situation in which help would not be available should a panic attack occur. Panic disorder is uncommon in elderly persons.[2] If the symptoms of anxiety are chronic and continuous, the condition is referred to as a *generalized anxiety disorder.*

Anxiety also can be a prominent feature of other psychiatric syndromes, including delirium, dementia, and, particularly, depression. The anxiety that occurs with delirium is associated with a sudden change in alertness and awareness. Anxiety associated with dementia occurs early in the illness, when the patient is aware of memory loss, and later in the course of the disease whenever threats to routine and security occur. Anxiety symptoms with agitation and restlessness are especially prominent in major depressive episodes. Other symptoms of depression—low mood, loss of energy and interest, and sleep and appetite disturbances—make this diagnosis likely.

The management of anxiety depends on the type and etiology. A careful history, a physical examination, and a laboratory investigation that are relevant to the particular symptoms of the patient are imperative, particularly when the anxiety is of a recent onset. A careful pharmacological history also is imperative. Discontinuation of benzodiazepines, neuroleptics, and even tricyclic antidepressants may cause anxiety and withdrawal symptoms.

Anxiety associated with delirium or depression usually disappears when the underlying illness is treated. The anxiety that occurs with dementia diminishes when the disease progresses (and insight is lost) or when measures are taken that diminish threats to security, eg, when provisions are made so that a demented person is not left alone at home.

When generalized anxiety symptoms seem to be more sociogenic and psychogenic, a physician should pay careful attention to a patient's history to understand the issues that underlie the symptoms. Simply listening to a patient's worries may be therapeutic. Giving the condition a name ("From your symptoms, it sounds to me that you are having anxiety symptoms") and making practical suggestions about ways to deal with the situation responsible for the symptoms may be helpful. If a great deal of stress has caused the symptoms, a physician should encourage a patient to talk to friends or relatives about his or her feelings. Regular, but limited, appointments during the time of stress also are advisable.

Benzodiazepines have become widely known and publicized as the treatment of choice for anxiety states. However, there are many reasons to be cautious about prescribing them for older patients despite their usefulness in generalized anxiety, panic disorder, agoraphobia, and social phobia.[9-11] Side effects that are especially unwelcome in elderly persons include dizziness, ataxia, sedation, insomnia, depression, disinhibition, and memory impairment and amnesia that resembles dementia. These drugs are capable of pro-

Table 37.1. Organic disorders associated with anxiety.*

Organic disorder
Cardiopulmonary
Coronary insufficiency
Cardiac arrhythmias
Mitral valve prolapse
Recurrent pulmonary emboli
Endocrine
Hypoglycemia
Hyperthyroidism
Hypoparathyroidism
Pheochromocytoma
Cushing's syndrome
Neurologic
Early primary degenerative dementia (senile dementia)
Transient ischemic attacks and major strokes
Epilepsy
Toxic metabolic
Medications/drugs (caffeine, thyroid preparations, barbiturates, steroids, psychostimulants, propranolol, vasodilators)
Withdrawal states (from benzodiazepines, alcohol, barbiturates, neuroleptics, tricyclic antidepressants)
Other
Chronic pulmonary disease
Chronic pain from any source
Anemia

* Data from references 7 and 8.

ducing physical dependence and have been associated with relapse, rebound, and withdrawal symptoms.[12,13] Even single nighttime doses of benzodiazepine may produce delirium.[14] A history of benzodiazepine use may put patients at greater risk for developing more severe withdrawal symptoms if benzodiazepines are subsequently prescribed and withdrawn.[15] Older patients often are reluctant to stop taking them once started, and this class of drugs contributes to the growing problem of adverse drug reactions in elderly persons.[16]

Given these risks, the benzodiazepines probably should be used only when anxiety symptoms are intense and disruptive. Drugs with a shorter half-life, such as oxazepam, 10 mg two or three times each day, are favored and should not be prescribed for longer than 2 or 3 weeks. Alprazolam, 0.25 mg three times each day, also is a popular drug but one that should also be used cautiously.

Panic disorders (formerly called *acute anxiety*) usually require the use of medication, psychotherapy, and, if agoraphobia is present, behavioral exposure techniques, which makes referral to a psychiatrist advisable. Tricyclic antidepressants (imipramine), monoamine oxidase inhibors (phenelzine), and benzodiazepines (alprazolam) are equally effective in treating panic episodes,[17] but tricyclic antidepressants are usually the first choice because of the dietary restrictions necessary with phenelzine and the risk of dependence and withdrawal with alprazolam.

Treatment can be started for the occasional older person who suffers from panic disorder with either imipramine (Tofranil) or desipramine (Norpramin). The patient's blood pressure should be taken in both the sitting and standing positions and recorded; an electrocardiogram also should be requested, since tricyclic antidepressants can affect cardiac conductivity. The benefits and possible side effects of treatment should be outlined. The patient is then instructed to take a single 10-mg dose of, for example, desipramine the next morning and call the physician's office if any untoward effects occur. Some patients are extremely sensitive to tricyclic antidepressants and experience a temporary stimulant effect from the drug, principally jitteriness and more anxiety, which actually may predict a positive response to the medication in the long run. If such a reaction occurs, the patient should be instructed to crush the 10-mg tablet and take a small proportion of the remainder, eg, 3 to 5 mg. Alternatively, the brief use of a β-adrenergic blocking agent or a benzodiazepine should be considered.

In most cases, however, the patient will tolerate the drug, and the medication should then be increased by 10 mg/d, taken in two divided doses, until the symptoms disappear or side effects intervene. Blood pressure should be taken at each office visit, and a systolic drop of 20 mm Hg or more on arising from a sitting position should be cause for concern. Some patients will report that their panic symptoms are blocked by small to moderate doses of the tricyclic antidepressant, eg, 20 to 50 mg, while others will require several weeks' treatment with doses ranging from 100 to 150 mg and sometimes higher. Serum tricyclic antidepressant levels can be useful at this point in helping the physician decide whether to increase the dose yet more or consider recommending a switch to a different medication. If tricyclic antidepressant treatment is successful, patients continue to receive the medication until they are free of panic episodes for 6 months; the medication is then tapered gradually during a period of several weeks. A few patients, however, will require constant maintenance medication.[18]

Phobias

Phobias are of three types: agoraphobia, social phobia, and simple phobia. Most have their beginnings in earlier life (rarely later than the fourth decade), but occasionally a phobia will appear for the first time in later life, particularly agoraphobia associated with panic disorder.

Agoraphobia is anxiety about, and avoidance of, places that are perceived as possible entrapments. Standing in a crowd or in a line, driving over a bridge or a freeway, traveling, or shopping in a store all are common agoraphobic situations.

A social phobia is a fear that one will be exposed to scrutiny by others and that something humiliating or embarrassing will result. Public speaking is the most common, but fears of choking while eating in front of others or fears of having one's hand tremble when working in front of others also are frequent. Simple phobia is a persistent fear of a discrete object (such as a cat) or of a situation (driving, heights, dentists' offices, closed spaces, air travel, etc). Simple phobias are common in all age groups, but they are rarely incapacitating, so treatment for them is rarely sought.[1(p244)]

The management of phobias has become so specialized that physicians are best advised to refer such patients for treatment. The most effective behavioral approach to agoraphobia, for example, uses exposure to the phobic stimulus.[10] Imipramine, when used in doses above 150 mg/d (and probably lower doses for elderly patients), can enhance the effects of exposure.[19,20] With social phobias, monoamine oxidase inhibitors, exposure to the feared situation, and cognitive restructuring techniques have all been useful.[21,22]

Physicians can best help in the management of

phobic disorders by ensuring that no underlying medical disorder goes undetected and by recognizing the presence of major depression. A depression will exacerbate phobias, and adequate treatment of the mood disorder often will alleviate the phobic symptoms.

Obsessive-compulsive Disorder

Severe obsessive states rarely begin in old age. Obsessive symptoms, however (repetitive, irrational, unwanted thoughts), are not uncommon and are often associated with a depression. Individuals who have suffered from an obsessive-compulsive disorder earlier in life may experience a serious worsening of their condition in old age, especially if depression intervenes. The treatment of late-onset obsessional symptoms usually is the treatment of a clinical depression.

Hypochondriasis

Hypochondriasis is a preoccupation with the fear of having or the belief that one has a serious physical disease. Symptoms that trigger hypochondriacal fears are remarkably diverse and include palpitations, chest or abdominal pains, dyspnea, dyspepsia, diarrhea, constipation, and headaches. The degree of concern can be remarkable, and a patient's persistent "organ recital" can be taxing. The onset of hypochondriasis at any age may be precipitated by a combination of factors: a stressful event that connotes loss or threat including an actual physical illness; experiences earlier in life that taught the individual to use somatic symptoms as idioms of distress or exposed him to physical illness or pain; and a perception of the sick role as a means to obtain attention and support or to avoid demands and obligations.[23] Hypochondriasis is usually a language of distress. Its meaning, however, is highly idiosyncratic, though hypochondriacal fears often reflect cultural and societal themes that have become highly personalized, eg, fear of inability to control events, fear of risks in life, or fear of decline with aging.[24]

There are chronic hypochondriacs (patients who have had their symptoms for a long time) and hypochondriacs whose symptoms have developed later in life. Individuals with long-standing hypochondriacal symptoms differ little from normal older people, except that they have more persistent physical complaints. In contrast, late-onset hypochondriacs more often have an actual physical illness and experience more loneliness and difficulty with self-care than normal elderly persons or chronic hypochondriacs.[4]

As a rule, it is wise to assume that all late-onset hypochondriacs have a depression or a serious (and sometimes undiscovered) physical illness until proved otherwise. Somatic symptoms often are associated with major and minor depressions. Mood and energy disturbances, sleep and appetite problems, or feelings of hopelessness and low self-esteem point to the diagnosis. Hypochondriacal complaints are associated with an increased risk of suicide in depressed older patients.[25] Serious cardiovascular disease, undetected cancer, and early cerebral degeneration are examples of physical illness that may underlie late-onset hypochondriasis.

In a number of instances, however, late-onset hypochondriasis will not portend a serious emotional or physical illness, but will instead serve as a signal of conflict or insecurity produced by the same stressors that cause anxiety. The same techniques that a physician uses to alleviate anxiety (careful listening, advice, reassurance) can be useful.

The management of chronic hypochondriacs can be difficult but rewarding, not only because proper management can prevent a patient from undergoing unnecessary diagnostic and surgical procedures, but also because symptoms may abate if physicians are persistent, patient, and try to understand the meaning of the symptoms. The principles of management include the following items[26]:

1. A thorough initial medical assessment.
2. If no disease is found, the patient should be told so unambiguously. But the patient should also be told the symptoms are "real" in the sense that they are real experiences to the patient, ie, you believe they are having such experiences.
3. Evaluation of psychological state with particular attention to the possibility of depression.
4. Avoid confrontation ("Your symptoms have no physical basis," "Your symptoms are in your head"), since this will only spur the patient on to prove the existence and reality of the symptoms.
5. Schedule regular but limited appointments. This shows interest in the patient and helps with continuity of care.
6. Inquire about (and discuss if possible) aspects of the patient's life that may be associated with the symptoms, eg, recent threats, fears, insecurities, living circumstances, relationship problems, and so on. Family members should also be interviewed for clues to understanding.

This kind of program, while not dramatic, serves to provide hypochondriacal patients with support and consistency. The goals are to reeducate a patient in such a way that somatic concerns can be dealt with on a regular basis and to understand the meaning of the symptoms. The plan also frees patients from having to prove constantly to their physicans that their symptoms are real.

Conversion Disorder

Conversion disorders, also called *hysterical neurosis, conversion type,* present as paralysis, blindness, hyperesthesias, ataxias, or hysterical dissociative states (fugues, wandering, or memory loss) and almost never begin in old age. If they do, they are usually a sign of depression or of a rapidly developing organic disease. As an example, three older patients whose conditions were diagnosed as either a dissociative state or a conversion reaction were found, on follow-up examination, to be suffering from cerebral metastases from bronchogenic carcinomas (two cases) or from cerebral embolus (one case), probably following a myocardial infarction.[27(pp578,579)] In the first two cases, the psychiatric illness manifested itself several months before neurological signs became apparent. As one author has said, "It is best to assert dogmatically that primary hysterical illness does not begin in old age."[4]

Paranoid Disorders

The word *paranoia* refers to experiences in which an individual falsely, or to an exaggerated extent, believes himself or herself to be the object of attention of others. These beliefs usually are persecutory in nature; patients believe that others are conspiring against or harassing them.

Paranoid symptoms are common in elderly persons.[28] Their diagnostic significance varies greatly. Table 37.2 shows the conditions in which paranoid symptoms occur.[29–31]

Clinical Considerations

The sudden onset of a paranoid delusion should always suggest the possibility of delirium caused by a physical illness or drugs. A misinterpretation of sounds and actions, ideas of reference, and persecutory delusions are common in delirium, but they fluctuate in intensity and usually are poorly organized. Persecutory symptoms are common in demented patients, who deny their forgetfulness, misplace objects, and accuse others of stealing their clothing and jewelry. A wide assortment of pharmacological agents may precipitate paranoid symptoms and states that usually—but not invariably—are associated with delirium.

Table 37.2. Conditions in which paranoid symptoms occur in elderly persons.*

Condition
Organic conditions
Delirium (any cause)
Dementia (any cause)
Auditory and visual impairment (any cause)
Stroke
Hypothyroidism and hypoparathyroidism
Head injury
Temporal lobe epilepsy
Multiple sclerosis
Vitamin B^{12} deficiency and pernicious anemia
Syphilis
Brain tumors
Drugs
Corticotropin (ACTH†) and cortisone
Levodopa
Psychotropics (eg, imipramine, benzhexol monoamine oxidase inhibitors)
Phenytoin
Psychostimulants
Alcohol
Barbiturates
Bromides
Withdrawal from alcohol, minor tranquilizers, barbiturates, and hypnotics
Paranoid symptoms associated with other psychiatric conditions
Mood disorders (depression, mania)
Paranoid personality disorders
Functional paranoid states
Acute paranoid states secondary to any major procedure in hospital
Psychological stress (eg, bereavement, loneliness, isolation)
Paraphrenia (late-onset schizophrenia)
Schizophrenics who have grown old
Monosymptomatic hypochondriacal delusions (eg, parasitosis)

* Data from references 29–31.
† ACTH indicates adrenocorticotropic hormone.

The majority of deaf older people are not paranoid, but there is evidence to show that a hearing loss predisposes one to paranoia.[32] Persecutory feelings and auditory hallucinations of noises, music, and voices are common. Poor vision and blindness can be associated with visual illusions and hallucinations.[33]

Paranoid symptoms commonly occur in both depression and mania. In the course of a severe depressive episode, patients may accuse others of talking about them, plotting against them, withholding medications, trying to poison them, and so on. Delusions of poverty and somatic delusions also occur. Paranoia often is prominent in mania. In fact, delusions of persecution may be the presenting feature of mania, along with irritability and sometimes even auditory hallucinations. Overactivity and overtalkativeness with circumstantiality and repetitiveness, along with (in most instances) a history of manic or depressive episodes, should enable a physician to make the diagnosis.

Acute paranoid reactions may occur in response to great stress among predisposed individuals, and they are not uncommon on medical and surgical wards where a wide range of stressors are operative, including sensory deprivation, immobility, apprehension, exhaustion, unfamiliar surroundings, major medical or surgical procedures, electrolyte imbalance, and drugs.

Most schizophrenics seen in old age are those persons whose illness began earlier in life. Many of them have a history of long periods of hospitalization throughout their lives and show a combination of residual schizophrenic defects, institutional deficits, and (in many cases) tardive dyskinesia. Schizophrenia may appear for the first time in later life, however, and is then called *late-onset schizophrenia* or *paraphrenia*.[34] Paraphrenia differs from early-onset schizophrenia in that patients' personalities and affects are well preserved and do not deteriorate; also, thought disorder is rare. Most paraphrenics present with hallucinations and delusions, but about 20% of them present with delusions alone.

Paraphrenic patients typically are female, solitary, and eccentric. There often is a history of a hearing loss, of long-standing interpersonal difficulties (such as failure to marry, early divorce without remarriage, or a late and troubled marriage), and of a paranoid or schizoid type of personality.[27(p582)] In most cases, there is no history of a previous breakdown—a contrast to depressed elderly persons, many of whom have had depressive episodes before 65 years of age.

A paraphrenic illness usually starts with an accentuation of previous personality traits, such as increased suspiciousness, withdrawal, and depression. Irritability, hypochondriasis, insomnia, weakness, and anxiety may be prominent. Suspiciousness is usually directed at neighbors or young people in the neighborhood, who are accused of stealing mail, pounding on the house at night, shining headlights into the windows, or (in one case) putting lint into the clothes dryer. Paraphrenics also may believe that their neighbors are talking about them critically. Frequent telephone calls to the police, in which an individual complains of harassment by the neighbors, may finally exhaust the officers' patience, and the individual is brought to the hospital for psychiatric evaluation.

The illness may remain at this phase, or the delusions may become more firmly held and extensive, so that a patient may believe that a conspiracy of people exists who are out to do him or her harm. Relatives or neighbors are often implicated. Patients may believe that they are being spied on, that their house is being broken into in their absence and things are being stolen, that poisonous gas is being wafted through the house, that their water is poisoned, or that they are being attacked by x-ray guns from outside (one woman explained the presence of seborrheic keratoses on the back of her hands in that way). In most cases, auditory hallucinations that often develop suddenly also are prominent. They consist of "threatening, demanding, commanding, accusing, or cajoling" voices and nonverbal noises.[27(p583)] Voices that talk about the patient, comment on his or her activities, or repeat and anticipate a patient's thoughts, feelings, and sensations are not uncommon and may be unusually vivid, as are beliefs that other people are controlling the patient's thoughts, feelings, and even movements.

Unfortunately, there is no way of discriminating, on the basis of clinical characteristics alone, between paraphrenia and organically caused paranoid states in elderly patients. Medical and neurological evaluation of seemingly "functional" paraphrenic patients often reveals occult neurological disorders,[35,36] and as many as a third of patients whose conditions are initially diagnosed as paraphrenia may progress to dementia within 3 years.[37,38] The need to evaluate medically older patients presenting with paranoid or other delusional symptoms is evident.

Other forms of delusional syndromes exist but are rare.[39] Two of them, however—delusional jealousy and monosymptomatic hypochondriacal delusions—are occasionally seen in older patients. In delusional or pathological jealousy, one partner in a marriage believes the spouse has been—or is being—unfaithful. The syndrome occurs more often in men than women and is usually a discrete syndrome, although it can be seen in association with several psychiatric conditions (late-onset schizophrenia, depression, alcoholism) and medical diseases, including Alzheimer's disease and other degenerative conditions, neoplasms, syphilis, and endocrine dysfunction. Patients who show pathological jealousy deserve close attention, not only because their jealousy disrupts their marriage, but also because they may be dangerous. Once medical and psychiatric evaluation has been completed, a course of phenothiazines, eg, perphenazine 2 to 4 mg at night, should be tried, although some patients are notoriously resistant to treatment. Once physical violence occurs, separation of the partners may be mandatory; frequently, in such patients, the only effective treatment is geographical.[40]

Monosymptomatic hypochondriacal delusion, also

called *somatic delusional syndrome,* usually takes one of two forms in older people: a delusion of parasitosis or a delusion that one is emitting a foul smell. In the former case the patient usually presents to a dermatologist, complaining of itching, tickling, or prickling sensations on or under the skin that are ascribed to an infestation by insects, such as lice, fleas, beetles, or bees.

Other unusual preoccupations with bodily parts or functions (eg, the delusion that one's bowels are blocked or a sensation of a persistent burning feeling in the perineal area) usually are associated with major depression and are alleviated once the depression is treated. Patients with monosymptomatic hypochondriacal delusions may show little or no depressive symptoms; however, the condition is chronic and difficult to treat. The neuroleptic pimozide represents a promising treatment for a certain proportion of patients who suffer from parasitosis.[41]

Management of Paranoid Disorders

The treatment of paranoid symptoms that are secondary to organic conditions or pharmacological agents is the treatment of the underlying illness or withdrawal of the drug. However, if persecutory symptoms are disruptive and a patient is overly fearful, agitated, or belligerent, then haloperidol may be prescribed orally in doses of 0.5 to 5 mg once per day. Paranoid symptoms that accompany dementia may be treated in the same fashion or with perphenazine, 2 to 4 mg at bedtime. Attempts to distract the patient and to provide a highly structured environment also may be useful and, in some cases, may make psychopharmacology unnecessary.

Paranoid symptoms associated with mood disorder often require the addition of neuroleptics to the antidepressant regimen, but most patients should be referred to a psychiatrist, as should patients with paraphrenia. The treatment of paraphrenia is a combination of drug therapy and social intervention. The correction of hearing or visual deficits is imperative, of course, and relocation sometimes is necessary.

The outcome of therapy for paraphrenia (which, untreated, is a chronic illness) is surprisingly good, provided that patients continue to receive the medication. Post[42] found that, of 71 patients with this condition, 61% had a complete remission of symptoms with treatment, while another 31% had a social recovery but with residual symptoms, such as mild delusions. Only 8% of these paraphrenics failed to respond at all to treatment.[42] Neuroleptic agents used to control symptoms include haloperidol (1 to 6 mg/d taken orally), perphenazine (8 to 24 mg/d), and thioridazine (50 mg/d to begin with, increasing to a total dose of 150 to 200 mg/d in divided doses after several weeks).[43,44] The maintenance dose of medication that is needed to control the symptoms is about one quarter of the dose that is needed to suppress the symptoms. Only in occasional cases are intramuscular depot injections of fluphenazine (Prolixin) necessary.

Personality Disorders

When long-standing personality traits are exaggerated and are associated with rigidity, inflexibility, a pattern of difficulty in getting along with other people, isolation, and personal distress, they are referred to as *personality disorders.* The major personality disorders that are seen in old age are well depicted by their descriptive adjectives in Table 37.3.[1(pp335–358) 45,46]

While most personality disorders tend to increase an individual's vulnerability to the stresses of advancing age, there are exceptions. Schizoid personalities, for example, may fare relatively well in old age because their lack of personal relationships leaves them untouched by the deaths that cause grief to other people. Many dependent personalities also cope well with old age because their lifelong wish to be taken care of is finally fulfilled. Patients with paranoid personalities, who are often at odds with others, frequently engage in struggles that, however unpleasant, give meaning to life and leave them little time for the usual anxieties that go with aging.[4]

Patients present themselves to physicians with symptoms, not with personality disorders, but a patient's personality colors every clinical presentation. The physical and emotional stresses of advancing age cause preexisting personality traits to be exaggerated. Old age is a stern personality test: the ordeals to which an aging personality is put reveal clearly its strengths and vulnerabilites.

Patients with paranoid and compulsive personalities are apt to cause the most trouble for the staff on a geriatric medical ward. These patients cause frustration and irritation for the staff because their need to gain control over others increases with insecurity. Compulsive individuals may become more fastidious and demanding, while paranoid patients become more mistrustful, negativistic, and oppositional.

The management of personality disorders by physicians can be facilitated by first recognizing and treating any associated physical illness, depression, or sensory deficits, all of which exacerbate troublesome personality traits. Second, a physician should make an effort to dampen the feelings of irritation and frustration that difficult patients arouse, to react not with anger and threats, but by trying to understand the situation through the patient's eyes. This means spending some

Table 37.3. Personality disorders and response to age-related stress.*

Type of disorder	Traits	Response to age-related stress
Paranoid	Suspicious; mistrustful, rigid; lack of warmth; critical, argumentative	Increased suspiciousness, paranoid symptoms, reclusiveness
Compulsive	Perfectionistic; excessive devotion to work; personal stiffness, formality; preoccupation with rules, procedures, and details; insistence on conformity and control	Pervasive anxiety, major depression, hypochondriasis, paranoid symptoms
Narcissistic	Need for constant attention and admiration, grandiose, lack of empathy, manipulative	Depression, suicide, drug or alcohol abuse
Dependent	Lack of confidence, passivity, wants others to assume responsibility, subordinates needs, unwillingness to make demands	Depression
Schizoid	Lack of social involvement; lack of warmth; aloofness; indifference to criticism, praise, and feelings; reserved, withdrawn, and seclusive	Reclusiveness
Histrionic	Lively, dramatic, and colorful; exaggerates feelings, thoughts, and reactions; excitable, egocentric, and vain	Depression, hypochondriasis, exaggeration of physical illnesses

Table 37.3. Continued

Type of disorder	Traits	Response to age-related stress
Passive-aggressive	Resentment of demands manifested by procrastination, obstructionism, and stubbornness, and inefficiency	Increased aggressiveness at first, helpless dependency, regression

* Data from references 1 (pp 335–358), 45, and 46.

time alone with a patient, sitting and talking, and getting to know him or her. When becoming tense in the presence of an irritating patient, the physician may find it useful (instead of expressing anger) to relax the shoulder muscles and say to the patient, "Tell me more."

For patients with paranoid personalities especially—who are mistrustful, prickly, independent, and controlling—a hospital routine, which demands dependency, as well as frequent intrusions, is threatening and annoying. After gaining an understanding of the patient's feelings, it is often advisable to assign one member of the treatment team—the person who gets along best with the patient—to serve as a liaison between the patient and medical personnel. Procedures and their rationales should be explained patiently. Allowing a patient to decide when he or she wants to undergo a certain procedure, which thereby increases a sense of control, is worthwhile. Only a couple of people should go into a patient's room at any time, since a cluster of people may be viewed as overwhelming and more threatening. The same guidelines that are useful in the management of paranoid personalities (correction of associated physical and psychiatric problems, avoidance of overreactions on the part of physicians, and a willingness to spend extra time with a patient and to understand his or her feelings) are, in fact, useful with all personality disorders; in most cases, they can be managed satisfactorily by an understanding physician. A psychiatric consultation will be warranted, of course, when these guidelines do not work.

Behavior Disorders

The term *behavior disorders* refers to antisocial acts that are not the result of mental illness and do not obviously rise from a patient's previous personality. In many cases, however, a careful history reveals that behavior disorders are consistent with earlier personality defects that have merely become more obvious with advancing age. Hoarding, miserliness, stubbornness, extreme dependency, set and irritating habits, social disinhibition (eg, tactless outspokenness, sexual offenses), milder forms of aggressiveness, apathy, and an occasional case of urinary incontinence constitute the list.

Urinary incontinence is not inevitably a manifestation of infection, local neuromechanical defects, or dementia. Sometimes it represents an older dependent patient's way of showing resentment and anger.

Sexual misbehavior, which is actually more common earlier in life than after 65 years of age, has been falsely attributed in older males to early dementia. It is, in fact, a relatively rare problem in older males and most often occurs in individuals who are becoming impotent. There rarely is a history of previous psychiatric or legal problems. It is believed that children are selected for sexual activities that range from exhibitionism to masturbation (but rarely intercourse) because older males feel unable to attract females and because children tend to be submissive. Sexual offenses, once they have brought satisfaction, tend to recur despite threats and actual punishment if a patient is not provided with supervision and support.[44] A psychiatric consultation is advisable, and if sexual urges persist despite other measures, diethylstilbestrol (1 to 3 mg/d) can be helpful.

The senile squalor syndrome, also termed the *Diogenes syndrome,* after the reclusive Greek Cynic philosopher who ended up living in an earthenware jar, describes withdrawn older people who live in socially unacceptable disorder and filth. About 40% of them turn out to be schizophrenic; however, the majority are not psychiatrically ill or demented, although the prevalence of alcoholism in this group may be higher than previously reported.[47] Many of these older people have never married, and some have shared their isolated existence with a sibling. They tend to be quarrelsome, independent, and domineering and to reject help. If forced to enter a hospital, they usually resume their old way of life on discharge.

Most behavior disorders, as with personality disorders, must be accepted. However, the correction of associated physical and psychiatric conditions and attempts to understand the feelings (eg, powerlessness, resentment, anger, frustration) that lie behind troublesome behaviors always should be undertaken and may be useful in at least ameliorating the more troublesome problems.

Violent and aggressive behavior occurs among older people and often is associated with a major psychiatric illness. In a survey of 220 consecutive admissions to a geriatric unit in a state hospital, it was found that 18 (8.1%) of the patients—called *violent*—had used guns or knives in their assaults on others. Another 121 patients, referred to as *aggressive,* constituted 63% of all patients, and these patients had either threatened or had actually struck another person but had not used weapons.

In this survey, the violent and aggressive groups differed from each other. In the violent group, almost one third of the patients' conditions were diagnosed as paraphrenia. Atypical organic states (eg, associated with normal-pressure hydrocephalus or brain tumors) and the manic phase of bipolar affective illness each accounted for another 17% of the cases. In contrast, one third of the aggressive patients were demented, and another 28% were long-standing schizophrenics. Paraphrenia was the least common diagnosis in the aggressive group, in contrast to the violent group in whom paraphrenia was the most common diagnosis.[48]

While one must be cautious about generalizing these findings to geriatric patients in the community, it seems that dangerous and violent behavior is more likely to occur in older patients with paraphrenia, who direct their violence toward their imagined prosecutors, than in patients with any other psychiatric disorders, eg, dementia, who are more likely to be aggressive than violent.

References

1. *Diagnostic and Statistical Manual of Mental Disorders,* revised. 3rd ed. Washington, DC: American Psychiatric Association: 1987.
2. Myers JK, Weissman MM, Tischler GL, et al. Six-month prevalence of psychiatric disorders in three communities. *Arch Gen Psychiatry* 1984;41:959–967.
3. Simon A. The neuroses, personality disorders, alcoholism, drug use and misuse, and crime in the aged. In: Birren JE, Sloane RB, eds. *Handbook of Mental Health and Aging.* Englewood Cliffs, NJ: Prentice-Hall International Inc; 1980:653–670.
4. Bergmann K. Neurosis and personality disorder in old age. In: Isaacs AD, Post F, eds. *Studies in Geriatric Psychiatry.* New York, NY: John Wiley & Sons Inc; 1978:41–75.
5. Mueller C. Cited by: Brocklehurst JC, ed. *Textbook of Geriatric Medicine and Gerontology.* ed 2. New York, NY: Churchill Livingstone Inc; 1978:188.
6. Pearson H. *The Smith of Smiths.* New York, NY: Harper & Row Publishers Inc; 1934:314.
7. Hall RCW. Anxiety. In: Hall RCW, ed. *Psychiatric Presentations of Medical Illness: Somatopsychic Disorders.* Jamaica, NY: Spectrum Publications Inc; 1980: 13–35.
8. Dietch JT. Diagnosis of organic anxiety disorders. *Psychosomatics* 1981;22:661–669.
9. Elie R, Lamontagne Y. Alprazolam and diazepam in the treatment of generalized anxiety. *J Clin Psychopharmacol* 1984;4:125–129.

500   Richard C. U'Ren

10. Roy-Byrne PP, Katon W. An update on treatment of the anxiety disorders. *Hosp Community Psychiatry* 1987; 38:835–843.

11. Reich J, Yates W. A pilot study of treatment of social phobia with alprazolam. *Am J Psychiatry* 1988;145: 590–594.

12. Juergens SM, Morse RM. Alprazolam dependence in seven patients. *Am J Psychiatry* 1988;145:625–627.

13. Pecknold J, Swinson RP, Kuch K, et al. Alprazolam in panic disorder and agoraphobia: results from a multicenter trial, III: discontinuation effects. *Arch Gen Psychiatry* 1988;45:429–436.

14. Patterson J. Triazolam syndrome in the elderly. *South Med J* 1987;80:1425–1426.

15. Rickels K, Schwiezer E, Csaralosi I, et al. Long-term treatment of anxiety and risk of withdrawal: prospective comparison of clorazepate and buspirone. *Arch Gen Psychiatry* 1988;45:444–450.

16. Need we poison the elderly so often? *Lancet* 1988;2:20–22. Editoral.

17. Sheehan DV. The relative efficiency of phenelzine, imipramine, and placebo in the treatment of panic disorder. Presented at the annual meeting of the American Psychiatric Association; May 5–11, 1984; Los Angeles, Calif.

18. Klein DF, Gittelman R, Quitkin F, et al. *Diagnosis and Drug Treatment of Psychiatric Disorders: Adults and Children*. 2nd ed. Baltimore, Md: Williams & Wilkins; 1979:560–565.

19. Marissakalian M, Michelson L, Dealy RS. Pharmacological treatment of agoraphobia: imipramine versus imipramine with programmed practice. *Br J Psychiatry* 1983;143:348–355.

20. Telch MJ, Agras WS, Taylor CB, et al. Combined pharmacological and behavioral treatment for agoraphobia. *Behav Res Ther* 1985;23:325–355.

21. Liebowitz M. Cited by Roy-Byrne pp, Katon W. An update on treatment of the anxiety disorders. *Hosp Community Psychiatry* 1987;38:835–843.

22. Heimberg RG, Becker RE, Goldfinger KT, et al. Treatment of social phobia by exposure, cognitive restructuring and homework assignments. *J Nerv Ment Dis* 1985;173:236–245.

23. Lipowski ZJ. Somatization: a concept and its clinical application. *Am J Psychiatry* 1988;145:1358–1368.

24. Kleinman A. *The Illness Narratives*. New York, NY: Basic Books; 1988:194–208.

25. Stengel E. *Suicide and Attempted Suicide*. London, England: Penguin Books Ltd; 1964:61.

26. Busse EW, Blazer D. Disorders related to biological functioning. In: Busse EW, Blazer D, eds. *Handbook of Geriatric Psychiatry*. New York, NY: Van Nostrand Reinhold Co; 1980:390–414.

27. Slater E, Roth M. *Clinical Psychiatry*. 3rd ed. Baltimore, Md: Williams & Wilkins; 1969.

28. Christenson R, Blazer D. Epidemiology of persecutory ideation in the elderly population in the community. *Am J Psychiatry* 1984;141:1088–1091.

29. Manschreck TC, Petri M. The paranoid syndrome. *Lancet* 1978;2:251–253.

30. Cumming JL. Organic delusions: phenomenology, correlations, and review. *Br J Psychiatry* 1985;146:184–197.

31. Bridge TP, Wyatt RJ. Paraphrenia: paranoid states of late life, I: European research. *J Am Geriatr Soc* 1980;28:193–200.

32. Cooper AF, Garside RF, Kay DWK. A comparison of deaf and non-deaf patients with paranoid and affective psychoses. *Br J Psychiatry* 1976;129:297–302.

33. Barrios G, Brook P. Visual hallucinations and sensory delusions in the elderly. *Br J Psychiatry* 1984;144: 662–664.

34. Roth M. The natural history of mental disorder in old age. *J Ment Sci* 1955;101:281–301.

35. Leuchter AF, Spar TE. The late-onset psychoses. *J Nerv Ment Dis* 1985;173:488–494.

36. Miller BL, Bensen DF, Cummings JL, et al. Late-life paraphrenia: an organic delusional syndrome. *J Clin Psychiatry* 1986;47:204–207.

37. Holden NL. Late paraphrenia or the paraphrenias? *Br J Psychiatry* 1987;150:635–639.

38. Craig TJ, Bregman Z. Late onset schizophrenia-like illness. *J Am Geriatr Soc* 1988;36:104–107.

39. Cummings JL. Organic psychosis. *Psychosomatics* 1988;29:16–26.

40. Gelder M, Gath D, Mayou R. *Oxford Textbook of Psychiatry*. New York, NY: Oxford University Press Inc; 1983:282–286.

41. Munro A. Paranoia revisited. *Br J Psychiatry* 1982; 141:344–349.

42. Post F. The functional psychosis. In: Isaacs AD, Post F, eds. *Studies in Geriatric Psychiatry*. New York, NY: John Wiley & Sons Inc; 1978:77–94.

43. Varner RB, Gaitz CM. Schizophrenic and paranoid disorders in the aged. *Psychiatr Clin North Am* 1982;5:107–118.

44. Post F. Psychiatric disorders. In: Brocklehurst JC, ed. *Textbook of Geriatric Medicine and Gerontology*. New York, NY: Churchill Livingstone Inc; 1978:185–200.

45. Straker M. Adjustment disorders and personality disorders in the aged. *Psychiatr Clin North Am* 1982;5: 121–129.

46. Verwoerdt A. Anxiety, dissociative and personality disorders in the elderly. In: Busse ED, Blazer D, eds. *Handbook of Geriatric Psychiatry*. New York, NY: Van Nostrand Reinhold Co; 1980:368–380.

47. Kafetz KK, Cox M. Alcohol excess and the senile squalor syndrome. *J Am Geriatr Soc* 1982;30:706.

48. Petrie WM, Lawson EC, Hollender MH. Violence in geriatric patients. *JAMA* 1982;248:443–444.

Voiding Dysfunction and Urinary Incontinence

Neil M. Resnick

Urinary incontinence affects 15% to 30% of community-dwelling elderly persons,[1,2] one third of older individuals in acute care settings,[3,4] and roughly half of institutionalized elderly patients.[5] Its burden is substantial and must be measured in medical, psychosocial, and economic terms.[6] Medically, individuals are predisposed to perineal rashes, pressure sores, urinary tract infections, urosepsis, falls, and fractures. Another unappreciated complication is recurrent lower-limb cellulitis. This occurs when incontinent individuals' shoes are chronically soaked by urine, become hardened, and abrade the feet; it is especially apt to occur in individuals with impaired peripheral sensation.

The psychosocial concomitants of incontinence also are significant. Individuals are frequently embarrassed, isolated, stigmatized, depressed, and regressed; they are also predisposed to institutionalization, although the extent remains undefined.[2,7] Economically, the costs of incontinence are startling. In America, more than $8 billion was devoted to incontinence in 1984.[8] This figure exceeds the annual amount devoted to dialysis and coronary artery bypass surgery combined![6]

Despite its considerable prevalence, morbidity, and expense, however, incontinence remains a largely neglected problem. Only the minority of incontinent individuals consult a health care provider; sadly, when they do, the physician who initiates even the most rudimentary evaluation is the exception.[6] This is unfortunate, because incontinence is no more a part of normal aging than is chest pain; like chest pain, it is a symptom of a variety of underlying conditions. Moreover, several studies have documented that, regardless of the context in which it is found, incontinence is a highly treatable and even curable disorder.[3,6,9–16]

This chapter will review the basics of urinary incontinence in elderly persons. This will entail a brief review of the anatomy and physiology of the lower urinary tract, an examination of the impact that normal aging has on the system, a theoretical consideration of what can go wrong, and a review of what does go wrong. This knowledge will be used to formulate a targeted clinical evaluation of the incontinent individual and to propose a logical diagnostic and therapeutic approach.[17]

Lower Urinary Tract Anatomy and Physiology

Details of the anatomy and physiology of normal micturition remain controversial and have been reviewed elsewhere.[18] For the present purposes, however, we can simplify both. The lower urinary tract includes the urethral outlet and a muscular storage and contractile portion known as the detrusor. The proximal portion of the urethra comprises a sphincter (internal urethral sphincter), which is located in the region of the bladder neck, is predominantly smooth muscle, and is autonomically innervated. A few centimeters distal to this is the external sphincter, which is composed of striated muscle and lies primarily in the mural portion of the urethra, at the level of the urogenital diaphragm.

The innervation of the lower urinary tract is derived from three sources: (1) the parasympathetic nervous system (S2-4), (2) the sympathetic nervous system (T-10–L-2), and (3) the somatic (voluntary) nervous system (S2-4). The parasympathetic nervous system innervates the detrusor; increased cholinergic activity increases the force and frequency of detrusor contraction, while reduced activity has the opposite effect. The sympathetic nervous system innervates both the bladder and the urethra, with its effect determined by local receptors. Although adrenergic receptors are sparse in the bladder body, those normally present are β-receptors; their stimulation relaxes the bladder. Receptors at the base of the bladder and in the proximal portion of the urethra, on the other hand, are α-receptors; their stimulation contracts the internal sphincter. Thus, activation of the sympathetic nervous system facilitates storage of urine in a coordinated manner. The somatic nervous system innervates the urogenital diaphragm and the external sphincter, although the external sphincter probably receives other innervation as well.[18] The central nervous system integrates control of the urinary tract. The pontine micturition center mediates synchronous sphincter relaxation and detrusor contraction, while higher centers in the frontal lobe, basal ganglia, and cerebellum (among others) exert inhibitory and facilitatory effects.

Storage of urine is mediated by detrusor relaxation and closure of the sphincters. Detrusor relaxation is accomplished by central nervous system inhibition of parasympathetic tone, while sphincter closure is mediated by a reflex increase in α-adrenergic and somatic activity. Voiding occurs when detrusor contraction, mediated by the parasympathetic nervous system, is coordinated with sphincter relaxation.

Impact of Age on Continence

Normal aging affects the lower urinary tract in a variety of ways, but incontinence is not one of them. Although there is still a dearth of data (and no longitudinal studies), several points emerge from cross-sectional studies. Bladder capacity, the ability to postpone voiding, bladder compliance, and urinary flow rate probably decline in both sexes, while maximum urethral closure pressure and urethral length probably decline in women.[16] The prevalence of uninhibited contractions probably increases with age, but there are few studies of younger individuals available for comparison.[16,19] Postvoiding residual volume (PVR) may increase, but probably to no more than 25 to 50 mL.[16] Another important age-related change is an alteration in the pattern of fluid excretion. Younger individuals excrete the bulk of their daily ingested fluid before bedtime, but many healthy elderly persons excrete the bulk of theirs during the night. This is true even for those persons without peripheral venous insufficiency, renal disease, heart failure, or prostatism. Thus, one to two episodes of nocturia per night may be normal, especially if the pattern is long-standing and unchanged, and other conditions have been excluded.[16] Finally, virtually all men experience an age-related increase in prostatic size.

None of these age-related changes causes incontinence, since each has been documented in studies of either asymptomatic or continent individuals. Nonetheless, each predisposes to incontinence. This predisposition, coupled with the increased likelihood that an older person will be subjected to an additional pathologic, physiologic, or pharmacologic insult, underlies the higher incidence of incontinence in elderly persons. The corollary is equally important. The new onset or exacerbation of incontinence in an older person is likely to be due to a precipitant outside the lower urinary tract that is amenable to medical intervention. Treatment of the precipitant alone may be sufficient to restore continence. These principles provide a rationale for dividing the causes of incontinence in elderly persons into categories of transient and established incontinence.

Causes of Incontinence

Transient Incontinence

Transient incontinence is common in elderly persons, affecting up to one third of community-dwelling incontinent individuals and up to one half of hospitalized incontinent patients.[16] The causes can be recalled easily using the mnemonic "DIAPPERS" (misspelled with an extra "P") as follows[20]:

> *D*elirium/confusional state
> *I*nfection—urinary (symptomatic)
> *A*trophic urethritis/vaginitis
> *P*harmaceuticals
> *P*sychologic, especially depression
> *E*ndocrine (hypercalcemia, hyperglycemia)
> *R*estricted mobility
> *S*tool impaction

In the setting of *delirium,* incontinence is merely an associated symptom that will abate once the underlying cause of confusion is identified and treated. The patient needs medical rather than bladder management.

Asymptomatic *urinary tract infection* causes transient incontinence when dysuria and urgency defeat the older person's ability to reach the toilet. On the other hand, asymptomatic infection, which is more common in elderly persons, is usually not a cause of incontinence.[16,21]

Atrophic vaginitis only occasionally causes transient incontinence, but it commonly contributes.[22] It can present as urethral "scalding," dysuria, dyspareunia, urinary urgency, or urge or stress urinary incontinence. In demented individuals, vaginitis may present as agitation. The symptoms are readily responsive to treatment with a low dose of estrogen, administered either orally (0.3 mg of conjugated estrogen per day) or topically. The optimal route is unclear. Orally administered, estrogen has adverse hepatic-mediated effects but beneficial effects on blood lipids[23] and costs less than 10 cents per day. Applied intravaginally, estrogen is considerably more expensive and inconvenient; additionally, levels attained are equivalent to orally administered estrogen, and the hepatic effect is not eliminated. More recently, estrogen has been given transcutaneously, but studies of its impact on atrophic vaginitis are not yet available. The transcutaneous route seems to be promising, however, because it requires application only twice weekly, and preliminary data suggest that it may have beneficial effects on lipids without adverse hepatic effects.[24] Whichever route is chosen, symptoms respond in a few days to 6 weeks, although the intracellular biochemical response may take much longer.[25] While the duration of therapy has not been well established, my colleagues and I administer a low dose of estrogen on a daily basis for 1 to 2 months and then start to taper it. Eventually, most patients can probably be weaned to a dose given as infrequently as two to four times per month; after 6 months, estrogen can be discontinued entirely in some patients, although recrudescence is common. Since the estrogen dose is low and given briefly, its carcinogenic effect is likely slight, if present at all. In fact, the only adverse effect that we have seen is mild and irregular vaginal bleeding in a small percentage of patients. However, if long-term treatment with estrogen is required, a progestin should probably be added if the patient still has a uterus (see Chapter 22). In addition, because estrogen-responsive breast cancer is common in older women, mammography should probably be performed before starting hormone therapy. Of note, the dose of estrogen employed for treatment of atrophic vaginitis is substantially lower than the dose required to prevent bone loss.

Pharmaceuticals are one of the most common causes of voiding dysfunction (Table 38.1). Long-acting sedative hypnotics, such as diazepam and flurazepam, have longer half-lives in elderly patients and thus may accumulate, inducing confusion and secondary incontinence.[16] Another sedative used by patients is alcohol, which both induces a diuresis and clouds the sensorium. "Loop" diuretics induce a brisk diuresis, which may overwhelm bladder capacity and result in incontinence. Vincristine can cause a partially reversible neuropathy associated with urinary retention.[26]

Drugs with anticholinergic properties are in common use. Older patients often take several nonprescribed preparations for conditions such as insomnia, coryza, pruritus, and vertigo. Because three quarters of elderly patients use nonprescription agents,[27] and because many do not regard them as "medicines" worth mentioning to their physicians, it is worth inquiring about such drugs directly. If the agents have anticholinergic effects, urinary retention and overflow incontinence may result.

Adrenergic agents also affect the lower urinary tract. Because the proximal urethra contains primarily α-adrenoceptors, its tone can be decreased by α-antagonists and increased by α-agonists. α-Antagonists are contained in many antihypertensive medications. When taken by an older women, whose urethra has shortened and weakened with age, these drugs may precipitate stress incontinence.[28] On the other hand, nonprescribed preparations containing α-agonists (such as decongestants) may provoke acute retention in a man with otherwise asymptomatic prostatic enlargement—especially if the preparation additionally

Table 38.1. Common medications that can cause incontinence.*

Medication
Sedative hypnotics
Flurazepam
Diazepam
Ethyl alcohol
Diuretics
Furosemide
Ethacrynic acid
Bumetanide
Anticholinergic agents
Antipsychotic agents
Antidepressants
Drugs for Parkinson's disease (trihexyphenidyl and benztropine mesylate, not levodopa)
Disopyramide
Antispasmodic agents
Antihistamines
Opiates
Adrenergic agents
Sympathomimetics
Sympatholytics

* Adapted from Resnick.[20]

contains an antihistamine (anticholinergic). It is apparent that many nonprescription cold remedies are effectively, albeit inadvertently, formulated to cause lower urinary tract dysfunction in older men. In fact, a not uncommon cause of urinary retention occurs when an older man medicates himself with a multicomponent "cold" capsule, long-acting nose drops, and a hypnotic (usually an antihistamine).[16] How commonly this scenario results in an unnecessary or premature prostatectomy is unknown.

Calcium channel blockers reduce smooth-muscle contractility throughout the body, and the bladder is no exception; they not infrequently induce urinary retention which is occasionally significant.[16]

Psychological causes of incontinence have not been well studied in elderly persons, but are probably much less common than in younger individuals. Intervention is properly directed at the psychologic disturbance, usually depression or lifelong neurosis. However, once the psychologic disturbance has been treated, persistent incontinence warrants further evaluation. *Endocrine* causes of incontinence include those conditions that both cloud the sensorium and induce a diuresis, primarily hypercalcemia and hyperglycemia. Diabetes insipidus also may cause incontinence, albeit rarely.

Restricted mobility commonly contributes to incontinence in elderly persons. It can result from arthritis, hip deformity, poor eyesight, inability to ambulate, fear of falling, a stroke,[29] or simply being restrained in a bed or a chair. A careful search will often identify correctable causes. If not, a urinal or bedside commode may still improve or resolve the incontinence.

Stool impaction has been implicated as a cause of urinary incontinence in up to 10% of patients referred to incontinence clinics;[16] the mechanism may involve stimulation of opioid receptors.[30] Patients usually present with either urge or overflow incontinence and typically have associated fecal incontinence as well. Disimpaction restores continence.

These eight reversible causes of incontinence should be assiduously sought in every elderly patient. In our series of hospitalized patients, when these causes were identified, continence was regained by most of those who became incontinent in the context of acute illness.[3] Regardless of their frequency, however, their identification is important in all settings because they are easily treatable.

A case presentation may illustrate these points more effectively.[31] An 80-year-old man was referred for evaluation of urinary incontinence. He had been healthy until a year ago, when he noted progressive generalized stiffness and trouble with walking. He then fell and was hospitalized for a hip fracture, and subsequently, pneumonia and confusion developed.

The confusion was treated with haloperidol, and the pneumonia was treated with antibiotics. He was noted to be newly incontinent, and this persisted even after the pneumonia cleared. A urologist thought the prostate was palpably enlarged and suggested a prostatectomy, but the family refused. Awaiting placement in a nursing home, the patient continued to receive haloperidol. A physical examination revealed confusion, congestive heart failure, parkinsonism, a distended bladder, an enlarged prostate gland, and fecal impaction.

The etiology of his incontinence was multifactorial. During the prior year, Parkinson's disease had developed that limited his mobility, was the cause of his fall, and was exacerbated by haloperidol. The anticholinergic effect of haloperidol also contributed to fecal impaction and urinary retention. Congestive heart failure, as well as the discomfort of urinary retention and fecal impaction and the anticholinergic effect of haloperidol, all led to his becoming confused. Obviously, the role played by his prostate could not yet be determined, especially since the size of the prostate as palpated rectally correlates poorly with the presence of outlet obstruction.[16,32] Therefore, he was treated with disimpaction and diuresis, haloperidol therapy was discontinued, the bladder was drained, physical therapy was started, and fiber was added to his diet. Levodopa/carbidopa (Sinemet) therapy was started, because moderately severe Parkinson's disease had preceded treatment with haloperidol. Within 2 weeks, parkinsonian stigmata subsided, bowel movements became regular, exercise tolerance increased, ambulation improved, and incontinence resolved; the postvoid residual was 10 mL, and a prostatectomy was deferred. He remained dry and asymptomatic a year later.

Established Incontinence

Lower Urinary Tract Causes

If leakage persists after transient causes of incontinence have been addressed, the lower urinary tract causes of established incontinence must be considered. These are due to dysfunction of the bladder, the outlet, or both.

The lower urinary tract can malfunction in only four ways. Two involve the bladder, and two involve the outlet. The bladder either contracts when it should not (detrusor overactivity) or fails to contract when or as well as it should (detrusor underactivity); alternatively, outlet resistance is high when it should be low (obstruction) or low when it should be high (outlet incompetence). Since incontinence in older individuals is frequently due to a cause other than the classic types of "neurogenic bladder,"[33] it is probably better to think of the causes of incontinence in terms of the four pathophysiologic mechanisms just mentioned and to realize that each mechanism has a set of "neurogenic" as well as "nonneurogenic" causes (Table 38.2). This section provides an overview of the four basic mechanisms and their causes; a later section provides more clinical details and treatment strategies for each.

Detrusor overactivity, the most common cause of geriatric incontinence,[16,33] is a condition in which the bladder contracts precipitantly, usually emptying itself completely. Recently, however, detrusor overactivity has been found to exist as two physiologic subsets—one in which contractile function is preserved and one in which it is impaired. The latter condition has been

Table 38.2. Lower urinary tract causes of established incontinence.*

Urodynamic diagnosis	Some neurogenic causes	Some nonneurogenic causes
Detrusor overactivity	Stroke, Parkinson's disease, Alzheimer's disease	Urethral obstruction/incompetence, cystitis, bladder carcinoma, bladder stone
Detrusor under-activity	Disk compression, plexopathy, surgical damage (eg, anterior/posterior resection), autonomic neuropathy (eg, diabetes mellitus, alcoholism, vitamin B_{12} deficiency)	Chronic outlet obstruction, or idiopathic (common in women)
Outlet incompetence	Surgical lesion (rare), lower motor neuron lesion (rare)	Urethral hypermobility (type 1 and 2 SUI),† sphincter damage (type 3 SUI),† post-prostatectomy
Outlet obstruction	Spinal cord lesion with detrusor-sphincter dyssynergia	Prostatic enlargement, urethral stricture, large cystourethrocele

* Adapted from Resnick and Yalla.[6]
† SUI denotes stress urinary incontinence.

termed *detrusor hyperactivity with impaired contractility* (DHIC),[34] and is discussed below under the "Cystometry" subsection.

Detrusor overactivity presents clinically as urge incontinence. It may result from damage to the central nervous system inhibitory centers due to a stroke, Alzheimer's disease, or Parkinson's disease. Alternatively, the cause may be in the urinary tract itself, where a source of irritation—such as cystitis (interstitial, radiation, or chemotherapy-induced), a bladder tumor, or a stone—overwhelms the brain's ability to inhibit bladder contraction. Two other important local causes are outlet obstruction and outlet incompetence, both of which may lead to secondary detrusor overactivity.[35,36]

Traditionally, detrusor overactivity has been thought to be the primary cause of incontinence in demented patients. While this is true, it is also the most common cause in nondemented patients, and a recent study found no definite association between cognitive status and detrusor overactivity.[33] Thus, it is no longer tenable to ascribe incontinence in demented individuals merely to detrusor overactivity; other etiologies must also be considered.[16]

Detrusor underactivity, the least common cause of geriatric incontinence, may result from mechanical injury to the nerves supplying the bladder (eg, disk compression, tumor involvement) or from the autonomic neuropathy of diabetes, pernicious anemia, Parkinson's disease, alcoholism, Guillain-Barré syndrome, or tabes dorsalis. Alternatively, the detrusor may be replaced by fibrosis and connective tissue, as occurs in men with chronic outlet obstruction, so that even when the obstruction is removed, the bladder fails to empty normally. Detrusor replacement by fibrosis also may occur in women, but the cause is unknown.

Outlet incompetence is the second most common cause of incontinence in older women,[16,33] and is most often due to pelvic floor laxity. This results in "urethral hypermobility" and allows the proximal portion of the urethra and bladder neck to "herniate" through the urogenital diaphragm when abdominal pressure increases. Such herniation results in unequal transmission of abdominal pressure to the bladder and urethra and consequent stress incontinence (Fig. 38.1). A less common cause of stress incontinence is "sphincter incompetence," in which the sphincter is so weak that merely the hydrostatic weight of a full bladder overcomes outlet resistance. This condition is known as *type 3 stress incontinence.*[37] In elderly persons, it generally results from repeated operative trauma or diabetes, but occasionally no precipitant is identified.

Outlet obstruction is the final lower urinary tract cause of incontinence and the second most common

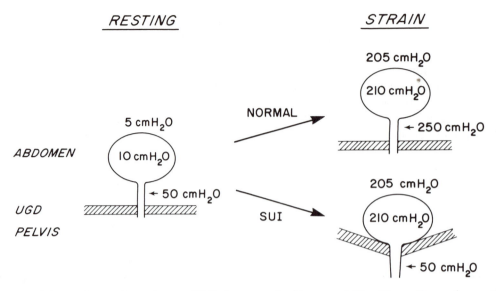

Fig. 38.1. Pathophysiology of stress incontinence (SUI) due to urethral hypermobility. Normally, resting urethral pressure is greater than bladder pressure; with a stress maneuver (such as coughing, straining, laughing, or bending over), the increase in abdominal pressure is transmitted equally to the bladder and the outlet, and the individual remains dry. In the woman with urethral hypermobility, however, the proximal urethra "herniates" through the urogenital diaphragm (UGD) into the pelvis with a stress maneuver. Since abdominal pressure is no longer transmitted equally, instantaneous leakage occurs (from Rowe and Besdine[74]).

cause in older men.[16,33] If due to neurologic disease, it is invariably associated with a spinal cord lesion. In this situation, pathways are interrupted to the pontine micturition center, where outlet relaxation is coordinated with bladder contraction. Then, rather than relaxing when the bladder contracts, the outlet contracts simultaneously, leading to severe outlet obstruction, a "Christmas tree bladder," hydronephrosis, and renal failure—a condition termed *detrusor-sphincter dyssynergia*. Alternatively, and much more commonly, obstruction results from prostatic enlargement, carcinoma, or urethral stricture in men; anatomic obstruction is uncommon in women in the absence of a large cystocele, which can prolapse and kink the urethra if the patient strains to void.

Clinically, it is useful to rearrange these four basic pathophysiologic mechanisms into two categories: (1) disorders of storage (detrusor overactivity or outlet incompetence), in which the bladder empties at inappropriate times; and (2) disorders of evacuation (detrusor underactivity or outlet obstruction), in which the bladder empties incompletely, leading to progressive urine accumulation and overflow. In the first category, the bladder is normal in size; in the second it is distended.

Functional Incontinence

Of course, factors other than lower urinary tract dysfunction can contribute to established incontinence in elderly persons, since continence is also affected by environmental demands, mentation, mobility, manual dexterity, and motivation. These factors are important to keep in mind because small improvements in each can result in a marked amelioration of both incontinence and functional status. In fact, once one has excluded serious lesions of the urinary tract, attention to these factors will often obviate the need for further investigations.

Diagnostic Approach

The diagnostic approach has three purposes: (1) to determine the cause of the incontinence, (2) to detect a related urinary tract pathologic condition (Table 38.3),

Table 38.3. Serious conditions that may present as incontinence.*

Condition
Lesions of the brain and spinal cord
Carcinoma of the bladder or prostate
Bladder stones
Hydronephrosis
Decreased bladder compliance
Detrusor-sphincter dyssynergia

* Adapted from Resnick.[17]

and (3) to evaluate comprehensively the patient, the environment, and the available resources. The extent of the evaluation must be tailored to the individual and tempered by the realization that not all detected conditions can be cured (eg, invasive bladder carcinoma), that optimal diagnostic and treatment strategies remain to be determined, that simple interventions may be effective even in the absence of a diagnosis,[12,17,38] and that, for many elderly persons, diagnostic tests are themselves often interventions. Fortunately, however, the diagnostic approach outlined below is relatively noninvasive, accurate, and easily tolerated, and it will detect most underlying pathologic conditions (Tables 38.3 and 38.4).

History

The first step is to characterize the voiding pattern and determine if symptoms of abnormal voiding are present, such as straining to void or a sense of incomplete emptying. However, one must be careful in eliciting these symptoms because many patients strain at the end of voiding to empty the last few drops. On the other hand, many patients have been straining for so long that they fail to acknowledge it. Thus, additional observations by the physician and family members are extremely useful.

One then elicits a detailed description of the incontinence, focusing on its onset, frequency, severity, pattern, precipitants, palliating features, and associated symptoms and conditions. It is also helpful to know if the patient leaks at night. Generally, individuals with detrusor overactivity gush intermittently both day and night, while those with pure stress incontinence are usually dry at night because they are in the supine position and not straining. However, individuals with type 3 stress incontinence, especially those who also have a poorly compliant bladder, may leak only at night if they allow their bladder to fill to a volume greater than their weakened outlet can withstand. These individuals may admit to postural-related dribbling as well, leaking continually while they are sitting or standing.

Prostatism is another symptom complex that is worth additional comment. Regardless of whether the patient has "irritative" or "obstructive" symptoms, the physician can be misled easily. Several investigators have found that about one third of patients referred for a prostatectomy are not obstructed.[39,40] Usually, the problem is an overactive detrusor, which, if unaccompanied by outlet obstruction, may be exacerbated by operative intervention.[41] Thus, symptoms are a clue to the diagnosis of obstruction, but alone are insufficiently specific to confirm it.

Table 38.4. Clinical evaluation of the incontinent patient.*

Evaluation
History
Type (urge, reflex, stress, overflow, or mixed)
Frequency, severity, duration
Pattern (diurnal, nocturnal, or both; also, eg, after taking medications)
Associated symptoms (straining to void, incomplete emptying, dysuria)
Alteration in bowel habit/sexual function
Other relevant factors (cancer, diabetes, acute illness, neurologic disease, pelvic or lower urinary tract surgery [especially abdomininoperineal resection and radical hysterectomy, which can cause decreased detrusor compliance])
Medications, including nonprescription agents
Functional assessment
Physical examination
Identify other medical conditions (eg, congestive heart failure, peripheral edema)
Test for stress-induced leakage when bladder is full
Observe/listen to void
Palpate for bladder distention after voiding
Pelvic examination (atrophic vaginitis or urethritis, pelvic muscle laxity, pelvic mass)
Rectal examination (resting tone and voluntary control of anal sphincter, prostate nodules, fecal impaction)
Neurologic examination (mental status and elemental examination, including sacral reflexes and perineal sensation)
Initial investigation
Voiding/incontinence chart
Metabolic survey (serum levels of electrolytes, calcium, glucose, and creatinine)
Measurement of postvoiding residual volume
Urinalysis and culture
Renal ultrasound†
Urine cytologic study†
Uroflowmetry†
Cystoscopy?†

* Adapted from Resnick and Yalla[6] and Resnick.[17]
† See text.

Voiding Record

One of the most helpful components of the history is the voiding record kept by the patient or caregiver. Recorded for a 48- to 72-hour period, these charts note the time of each void at 2-hour intervals. Many incontinence records have been proposed; a sample of ours is shown in Table 38.5.

To record the volume voided at home, an individual can use a measuring cup, coffee can, pickle jar, or other large container. Information regarding the volume voided provides an index of functional bladder capacity and, together with the pattern of voiding and leakage, can be helpful in pointing to the cause of the

Table 38.5. Sample voiding/incontinence record.*

Time	Wet/dry	How wet? (mild, moderate, severe)	Volume voided, oz	Comment
8	Wet	Severe	1	On way to bathroom
10	Dry	. . .	4	Voided before going out
noon	Dry	. . .	. . .	
2	Wet	Moderate	5	Abrupt urge—could not get to bathroom in time

* The chart is completed for 24 to 72 hours, recording the information every 2 hours. Voiding habits should not be changed; the patient should not be told to void every 2 hours while obtaining these baseline data. The physician should review the record with the patient, as part of the clinical evaluation (see text) (modified from Resnick[20]).

leakage. For example, incontinence that occurs only between 8 AM and noon may be caused by a morning diuretic. If a chairfast man with congestive heart failure wets himself frequently at night but remains dry during a 4-hour daytime nap in his wheelchair, the problem is probably not prostatic enlargement but rather the postural diuresis associated with heart failure.[20] A patient may also void frequently because of polyuria due to a metabolic abnormality. One woman's chart showed a single episode of leakage each day, always at 1 AM. Closer questioning revealed her regular use of a "nightcap" to induce sleep.

The information gathered from the history and voiding record permits a symptomatic characterization of the incontinence as *urge,* in which precipitant leakage of a large volume is preceded by a brief warning of seconds to minutes; *reflex,* in which precipitant leakage is not preceded by a warning; *stress,* in which leakage occurs coincident with, and only in association with, increases in abdominal pressure; *overflow,* in which continual dribbling occurs; and *mixed,* which is usually a combination of urge and stress.[42] Each of these types correlates fairly well with the following pathophysiologic mechanisms already mentioned: urge and reflex with detrusor overactivity, stress with an incompetent outlet, overflow with outlet obstruction or detrusor underactivity, and mixed with both an overactive detrusor and an incompetent outlet.

Targeted Physical Examination

The examination should check for signs of neurologic disease—such as delirium, dementia, stroke, Parkinson's disease, cord compression, and neuropathy (autonomic of peripheral)—as well as for functional impairment and general medical illnesses, such as heart failure and peripheral edema. Additionally, one should check for spinal column deformities or dimples suggestive of dysraphism, for bladder distention (pointing to an evacuation disorder), and for stress leakage. Stress incontinence is assessed by asking the patient, whose bladder should be full, to assume a position as close to upright as possible, to relax, spread her legs, and cough. The diagnosis of stress incontinence can be missed if any of these maneuvers is omitted. If leakage occurs, it also is important to note whether it occurs coincident with the stress maneuver or is delayed for more than 5 to 10 seconds. If delayed, such leakage suggests detrusor overactivity (triggered by coughing) rather than outlet incompetence.

The rectal examination checks for fecal impaction and masses. The size of the prostate is less important to assess because, as determined by palpation, it correlates poorly with the presence or absence of outlet obstruction.[20,32] The remainder of the rectal examination actually is a detailed neurourologic examination, since the same sacral roots (S2-4) innervate both the external urethral and the anal sphincters. With the finger in the rectum, one assesses motor innervation by asking the patient to contract and relax the anal sphincter. Because abdominal straining may mimic sphincter contraction, it is useful to place one's hand on the patient's abdomen to check for this. Many neurologically unimpaired elderly patients are unable to contract their sphincters, but, if they can, it is strong evidence against a cord lesion. One can assess motor innervation further by testing the anal wink (S4-5) and bulbocavernosus reflexes (S2-4). In an older person, however, the absence of these reflexes is not necessarily pathologic, nor does their presence exclude an underactive detrusor (due to diabetic neuropathy, for example). Finally, the afferent supply is assessed by testing the perineal sensation.

In women, one should check for pelvic muscle laxity (cystocele, rectocele, enterocele, uterine prolapse). After removing one blade of the vaginal speculum (or using a "tongue blade"), one checks for laxity by sequentially applying the remaining blade to the anterior and posterior vaginal walls and asking the patient to cough. If bulging of the anterior wall is detected with the posterior wall is stabilized, a cystocele is present; conversely, if bulging of the posterior wall is detected, a rectocele or enterocele is present. While the extent of pelvic floor laxity may be underestimated if one checks the patient in only the supine position, the presence of laxity can usually be determined in any position. It is important to realize, however, that the presence or absence of pelvic floor laxity reveals little about the cause of an individual's leakage. Detrusor overactivity may exist in addition to a cystocele, and stress incontinence may exist in the absence of a cystocele. Thus, knowledge of pelvic muscle strength is useful primarily in informing the surgeon's choice of operation. The one exception to this statement occurs in the woman with a large cystocele: descent of the cystocele may kink the urethra and cause obstruction.

Atrophic vaginitis also must be sought. It is characterized by mucosal friability, petechiae, telangiectasia, and vaginal erosions;[22] loss of rugal folds and the presence of a thin, shiny-appearing musoca are signs of vaginal atrophy rather than atrophic vaginitis. The bimanual examination excludes pelvic masses.

Two other tests should be mentioned. The first is the Q-tip test, in which a lubricated, sterile Q-tip is inserted into the urethra, and the patient is asked to strain abdominally. The change in the Q-tip angle is measured and used as a measure of pelvic floor laxity. As pointed out earlier, however, checking for pelvic floor laxity is of little value in determining the cause of a patient's leakage, and hence, the utility of this test is limited. The second test is the Bonney (or Marshall) test. If one detects stress leakage that occurs coincident with abdominal straining, the Bonney test checks to see if such leakage can be prevented by stabilizing (not occluding) the bladder base and thereby preventing its herniation through the urogenital diaphragm. This is accomplished by placing a finger in each lateral vaginal fornix and asking the patient to cough again. Urethral hypermobility is considered present if leakage is prevented. However, the value of this test is limited in elderly patients, because vaginal stenosis is common and may lead to a false-positive result by precluding accurate finger placement; if one's fingers are not placed far enough laterally, rather than stabilizing the bladder outlet, they may occlude it and prevent leakage even in a patient with detrusor instability. Furthermore, even if the test is correctly performed, a false-positive result may occur if the first episode of leakage was due to a cough-induced detrusor contraction, which, having emptied the bladder, does not recur during the Bonney test. A final caveat: one should not check for stress leakage if the patient suddenly feels a strong urge to void, since the urge may be due to an uninhibited contraction. If the contraction is accompanied by physiologic sphincter relaxation and if the patient then coughs, she will leak

instantaneously, prompting the physician to misdiagnose a detrusor abnormality as outlet incompetence. Finally, if stress testing provokes delayed leakage of a large amount, suggestive of detrusor overactivity, the patient should be asked to interrupt the stream. If she is able to do so, this probably bodes well for bladder retraining.

The examination concludes when the patient voids and is catheterized for a PVR. Adding the PVR to the voided volume provides an estimate of total bladder capacity and a crude assessment of bladder proprioception. A PVR above 50 to 100 mL suggests either bladder weakness or outlet obstruction, but smaller values do not exclude either diagnosis, especially if the patient has strained to void. Thus, it is important to observe or listen to the voided stream. If straining is observed, one must ask the patient whether this is typical and take that information into account when interpreting the PVR. Of note, relying on the ease of catheterization to establish the presence of obstruction can be misleading, since difficult catheter passage can be caused by urethral tortuosity, a "false passage," or a catheter-induced spasm of the distal sphincter, while easy passage can be seen in severely obstructed patients.[43]

Laboratory Investigation[17]

In addition to a urinalysis, urine culture, and PVR determination, one should measure the serum urea nitrogen and creatinine levels. If the voiding record suggests polyuria, serum concentrations of glucose and calcium should be measured as well. In a man whose PVR exceeds 150 to 200 mL, renal sonography should be performed to exclude hydronephrosis. In any patient with sterile hematuria, or in a patient at high risk for bladder carcinoma (eg, a male smoker), a urine cytologic study should be obtained. The role of cystoscopy remains to be determined; the roles of uroflowmetry and radiography are discussed below.

Although the literature is replete with statements and uncontrolled studies asserting that "the bladder is an unreliable witness" and that the clinical evaluation is an unreliable guide to the cause of incontinence, our experience differs. In a prospective and blinded study, we found that the clinical evaluation correctly predicted the urodynamically determined cause of leakage in more than 90% of cases.[44] The discrepancy between our experience and that of others may arise because we do not rely on any single symptom or sign. Rather, we dissect each symptom for its full diagnostic significance, and we integrate information from the history with that from the voiding record, physical examination, the observed void, and the PVR determination. Furthermore, even in nursing home patients, an algorithmic approach—relying only on information obtainable at bedside by a nurse—has yielded the correct diagnosis in 83% of cases and correctly guided treatment in 93%.[45] Therefore, although the specificity of a given symptom may be low, we believe that an informed, carefully performed, and comprehensive clinical evaluation can determine the cause of incontinence most of the time.

Urodynamic Testing

If the cause of the patient's incontinence still cannot be determined, urodynamic evaluation is the next step to consider. Although "beside testing" has long been advocated,[46–48] its marginal utility is unknown for the 10% to 20% of patients whose diagnosis eludes clinical evaluation. Urodynamic testing is probably warranted when diagnostic uncertainty may affect therapy, when empiric therapy has failed and other approaches would be tried, and when surgical intervention is contemplated.[6,33]

"Urodynamics" consists of a battery of tests. It is difficult to know in advance what to include in the battery; therefore, only someone conversant with the pathophysiology of incontinence should perform the evaluation. Generally, the evaluation includes simultaneous measurement of bladder, urethral, and rectal pressures during the filling and emptying phases of the micturition cycle. Optimally, the study is fluoroscopically monitored, and periurethral electromyography (EMG) may occasionally be required. Some of the more commonly used tests will be described below.

Cystometry

CMG evaluates bladder proprioception, compliance, capacity, and stability (re detrusor overactivity). It assesses only the bladder—not the outlet—and only during filling, not voiding. Therefore, it yields only one fourth of the information needed to establish a diagnosis. It is performed by inserting a catheter into the bladder, filling it with gas or fluid, and plotting the bladder's pressure response to increasing volume. Artifacts are common, especially when investigating elderly patients, but they can be minimized by having the test performed by a knowledgeable person (preferably a physician), by infusing fluid rather than gas, by using moderate infusion rates rather than rapid ones (<100 mL/min), by using fluoroscopy, and by measuring abdominal and bladder pressures simultaneously to differentiate rises in bladder pressure from rises in abdominal pressure.

Uninhibited contractions are phasic bladder contractions and are usually seen easily. They may be missed, however, especially in patients in whom detrusor hyperactivity coexists with detrusor weakness (DHIC).[34] In these patients, detrusor contraction pressure may rise only 2 to 6 cm H_2O. Because DHIC is the most common cause of incontinence in nursing home patients,[33] and because it is easily missed, it can be a great mimic, masquerading variously as "reflex urethral instability," stress incontinence, and outlet obstruction.[33] For instance, if the low-pressure uninhibited contraction is missed cystometrically, physiologic relaxation of the urethral sphincter may be misdiagnosed as "urethral instability." If the low-pressure contraction coincides with a stress maneuver, coincident leakage may be misdiagnosed as stress incontinence. Because the symptoms, flow rate, and PVR of DHIC are all similar to those seen in prostatism, a man with DHIC might easily be misdiagnosed as obstructed. The first two mistakes can be avoided by fluoroscopically monitoring the urodynamic evaluation, since visual evidence of a bladder contraction will be seen to coincide with leakage. DHIC can be distinguished from obstruction by the use of pressure/flow studies and *micturitional urethral pressure profilometry* (MUPP), as described below. If these tools are unavailable, however, the distinction can be difficult. My colleagues and I are currently devising ways to simplify the diagnosis of DHIC, examining the importance of the distinction, and exploring whether DHIC will exacerbate or simplify our ability to treat detrusor hyperreflexia.

Urethral Profilometry (During Filling and Voiding)

There are two types of profilometry, depending on whether urethral pressure is measured during bladder filling or contraction. The first is called *urethral closure pressure profilometry* (UCPP), and the second is known as MUPP. Both are performed by inserting a catheter into the bladder, slowly withdrawing it through the urethra and plotting urethral pressure at each point.[49] By using this trace, UCPP measures the urethral anatomic length, functional length, maximum urethral pressure, maximum urethral closure pressure (urethral pressure minus bladder pressure), and the length and height of the prostatic area (in males). Although there is a correlation between the presence of stress incontinence and both the strength of the sphincter and the length of the urethra, continent and incontinent values overlap considerably, reducing the utility of these measurements for the individual patient. Similarly, values obtained for prostatic length and area are of limited value. Nonetheless, UCPP is occasionally useful to test the bulbocavernosus reflex, and for fluid bridge testing; the latter is an extremely sensitive test for stress incontinence.[50,51] Additionally, UCPP will help to differentiate stress incontinence due to urethral sphincter weakness from that due to urethral hypermobility; in the former, the urethral pressure is low, while in the latter, it is normal.[35]

Urethral profilmetry is also used to exclude detrusor-sphincter dyssynergia. Generally, only the distal urethral sphincter is evaluated; normally it should relax just before, or coincident with, detrusor contraction. The response of the smooth-muscle sphincter is more complex and is reviewed elsewhere.[52]

The MUPP is useful for evaluating men.[53] It is performed by simultaneously measuring pressure in the bladder and along the urethra as the patient voids. Its interpretation is based on the principle that urethral pressure proximal to the membranous urethra normally equals bladder pressure during voiding. In the setting of a urethral obstruction, however, the pressure distal to the obstruction is lower than bladder pressure. If an obstruction is detected, fluoroscopy will usually localize the site. The MUPP is more accurate than cystoscopy for determining the presence of an obstruction and judging its severity.

Uroflowmetry

Uroflowmetry is often used in males to screen for obstruction. The flow rate depends not only on the presence of an outlet obstruction, however, but also on the strength of detrusor contraction. To interpret the test, one must know the voided volume, the residual volume, whether the void was augmented by abdominal straining, the peak and mean flow rates, and the configuration of the accompanying trace. Interrupted and oscillatory patterns are suggestive of abdominal straining, bladder weakness, or outlet obstruction. Although age-related norms have been devised to facilitate interpretation of the test, the studies on which they are based have been flawed and included few patients older than 70 years.[16] Moreover, while its sensitivity may increase with age, the specificity of uroflowmetry almost certainly declines. Thus, the utility of isolated uroflowmetry in elderly males remains undefined. One can, however, derive some information from it. In the older man with symptoms of prostatism, a normal flow rate and a low PVR probably exclude a clinically significant obstruction. On the other hand, when performed in conjunction with a full urodynamic evaluation, uroflowmetry is helpful in assessing detrusor contractility and detecting obstruction.

EMG[54]

Electromyography evaluates the distal urethral sphincter by determining the integrity of its inner-

vation, testing its response to reflex stimuli (such as bladder filling [guarding reflex] and bulbocavernosus stimulation), and characterizing its behavior during voiding. A variety of techniques are available for EMG, depending on whether one employs surface or needle electrodes, records the response of single or multiple nerve fibers, and evaluates the nerve supply to the urethral sphincter or the pelvic floor musculature (through vaginal, anal, or perineal probes). The most accurate technique is to insert a needle electrode directly into the distal urethral sphincter. Although most elderly patients can tolerate this, the results can be difficult to interpret (eg, are a few polyphasic potentials in a 90-year-old patient really abnormal?), the equipment is expensive, and if urodynamic testing is performed as already detailed, EMG adds little. If fluoroscopically monitored, multichannel urodynamic capability is not available, however, EMG is useful. Unfortunately, in these situations, only surface or anal EMG is usually performed. Because these techniques are fraught with artifacts, they should be interpreted with caution.

Radiographic Evaluations

Optimally, the radiographic and urodynamic evaluations are performed simultaneously, allowing the correlation of visual and manometric information. If this is not feasible, substantial information can still be gleaned from cystography. A full evaluation includes posterior-anterior and oblique (or lateral) views of the bladder at rest and during straining and voiding. These films check for bladder trabeculation, diverticula, masses, bladder neck competence, and ureteral reflux. Although the urethrovesical angle and axis also are generally measured, their reliability and relevance are controversial.[55] The voiding films allow one to check for outlet obstruction. The PVR also can be assessed radiographically, but there are pitfalls. Elderly patients are frequently rushed through busy radiography departments and may feel too inhibited to void to completion; the radiologist, who may have been absent during the examination, may then erroneously conclude that the residual volume is elevated. Conversely, a low volume does not exclude a weak bladder if the patient augmented voiding by straining. Therefore, the radiographer should be viewed as a partner in the evaluation rather than being asked to read films blindly after the examination is completed.

The precise role of urodynamic testing in the evaluation of the incontinent elderly individual remains to be determined. Although it pinpoints pathologic abnormalities, it may not identify which of the abnormalities actually causes the patient's incontinence unless it is performed by a trained urodynamicist and incorporated into the overall clinical evaluation.[33]

Whatever its role, however, urodynamic evaluation of elderly patients is reproducible, safe, and feasible to perform, even in frail and debilitated individuals. In our series of more than 100 consecutively evaluated nursing home patients, whose mean age was 89 years and all of whom received prophylactic antibiotics, we induced only three cases of asymptomatic bacteriuria; no cases of urosepsis, pyelonephritis, endocarditis, or cardiac ischemia were observed. All but two patients were able to complete the examination at one sitting, and the original diagnosis was confirmed in all 30 cases in which the examination was repeated. It must be emphasized, however, that an extra person was employed whose sole job was to explain the procedure and comfort the patient during the test. Several modifications in the urodynamic suite were made as well.[56]

Therapy

Like the diagnostic approach, treatment must be individualized, because factors outside the lower urinary tract also are important. For instance, although both may have detrusor overactivity that can be managed successfully, a severely demented and bedridden patient will be treated differently from one who is ambulatory and cognitively intact. Thus, this section will suggest several treatments for each condition and try to provide some guidance for their use. It assumes that serious underlying conditions and transient causes of incontinence have already been excluded.

Detrusor Overactivity

Detrusor overactivity is characterized by frequent but periodic voiding; the patient is generally dry in between. Leakage is moderate to large in volume, nocturnal frequency and incontinence are common, sacral sensation and reflexes are preserved, voluntary control of the anal sphincter is intact, and the PVR is generally low. A residual volume in excess of 50 mL in a patient with detrusor overactivity suggests outlet obstruction (although the residual volume may be nil in early obstruction), DHIC, or pooling of urine in a cystocele. This also is found in patients with Parkinson's disease or spinal cord injury.[34]

Initial management involves identification and treatment of reversible causes. Suspicion of a spinal cord disorder (an appropriate history and/or the finding of a dermatomal sensory "level") warrants a complete neurourologic evaluation. Sterile hematuria, if present, must be evaluated to exclude a bladder stone, carcinoma in situ, or carcinoma. Uroflowmetry, if available, can exclude important outlet obstruction, as described above.

It cannot be overemphasized that obstruction and stress incontinence may cause secondary detrusor overactivity that will remit with correction of the outlet abnormality.[35,36] Failure to evaluate the outlet may not only cause the patient harm (eg, prescribing an anticholinergic agent to an obstructed patient), but will also lead to overlooking easily correctable incontinence. Obstruction and stress incontinence are common in elderly persons, even frail and cognitively impaired individuals.[33] With recent medical and surgical advances, treatment of outlet abnormalities is now feasible even for these patients.[16,33] Thus, evaluation of the outlet is critically important.

Unfortunately, many of the causes of detrusor overactivity are not amenable to specific therapy, or a cause may not be found. Treatment must then be symptomatic. Simple measures, such as providing a bedside commode or urinal, are often successful. Toileting regimens, based on the analysis of the voiding record, also are beneficial, even in patients with advanced cognitive impairment.[57,58,58a] For the demented patient, the technique known as prompted voiding is used. One uses the voiding record to predict when leakage is likely to occur, asks the patient if he or she needs to void, and escorts the patient to the bathroom in advance. Positive reinforcement is employed, while negative reinforcement is avoided. A randomized, controlled study, conducted in two nursing homes, found a 50% decrease in incontinence within the first day of using the technique in this manner, a decrease that persisted as long as it was utilized.[12] In nondemented patients, techniques such as behavior modification permit the voiding interval to be lengthened progressively. For instance, if the incontinence chart reveals that the patient is wet every 3 hours, one asks the patient to void every 2 hours. Once the patient remains dry for 3 consecutive days using this regimen, the interval is lengthened by a half hour, and the process is repeated. One need not ask patients to void at night; once they are dry during the day, they are generally dry at night as well. Biofeedback may be added to this regimen, but its marginal benefit is unclear.

The voiding record can be helpful in other ways. For instance, as noted above, patterns of fluid excretion alter with age. If incontinence is worse at night and the chart discloses a nocturnal diuresis, incontinence can be ameliorated by altering the pattern of fluid intake or judiciously prescribing a rapidly-acting diuretic at dinner time; nocturnal use of an antidiuretic agent has proved to be less effective.[16,59] If nocturnal diuresis is due to peripheral edema in the absence of heart failure, a pressure-gradient stocking may avert fluid accumulation and the resultant nocturnal leakage. Another example is the patient with DHIC whose voiding record and PVR reveal that uninhibited contractions are provoked only at high volumes. By voiding every few hours during the day he or she may remain dry, but nocturnal leakage will persist, since functional bladder capacity is low. However, catheterization just before bedtime will remove the residual urine, thereby increasing bladder capacity, and restoring both continence and sleep. Significantly, in each of these cases, pharmacologic suppression of detrusor contractions can be avoided.

Pharmacologic intervention can be added, but there is a dearth of data regarding efficacy and toxicity in this population, and comparative or controlled trails are rare.[16] Smooth-muscle relaxants, such as flavoxate (300 to 800 mg/d) and calcium channel blockers, have been used, as have anticholinergic agents, such as propantheline (15 to 120 mg/d). Oxybutynin (5 to 20 mg/d), combining both smooth-muscle relaxant and anticholinergic properties, and imipramine (50 to 150 mg/d), in which the mechanism of action is more complex, are also frequently successful. All these drugs are given in divided doses. The decision regarding which drug to employ is often based on factors unrelated to bladder function.[6,16] In the incontinent patient with dementia or the patient taking other anticholinergic agents, propantheline is best avoided. In the patient with associated hypertension, angina pectoris, or abnormalities of cardiac diastolic relaxation, a calcium channel blocking agent may be preferred. Orthostatic hypotension often precludes the use of imipramine and nifedipine and should be watched for if these agents are used. Occasionally, combining low doses of two agents with complementary actions, such as oxybutynin and imipramine, will maximize benefits, and minimize side effects. Medications with a rapid onset of action, such as oxybutynin, can be employed prophylactically if incontinence occurs at predictable times. But regardless of which medication is used, since urinary retention may develop, the PVR and common indexes of renal function (serum urea nitrogen and creatinine levels and urine output) should be monitored, especially in DHIC where the detrusor is already weak. On the other hand, inducing urinary retention and using intermittent catheterization may be a viable approach for patients whose incontinence defies other remedies (such as those with DHIC) and for whom intermittent catheterization is feasible. Other remedies for urge incontinence, including electrical stimulation, bladder distention, and selective nerve blocks, are less widely used, although some are successful in selected situations.

Adjunctive measures, such as pads and special undergarments, are invaluable if incontinence proves to be refractory, and a wide variety of these are now available, allowing the recommendation to be tailored to the individual's problem. For instance, for bedridden individuals, a launderable bed pad may be preferable,[60] while for those with a stroke, a diaper or pant that can be opened by using the good hand may be preferred. For ambulatory patients with large gushes of incontinence, a wood pulp–containing product is generally preferable to those containing a polymer gel, since the polymer gel generally cannot absorb the large amount and rapid flow that these individuals produce, while the woodpulp product can easily be doubled up if necessary. Optimal products for men and women also differ because of the location of the "target zone." Finally, one must know whether the patient has fecal incontinence as well, to choose the most appropriate product.[9,60]

Condom catheters are helpful for men, although they are associated with skin breakdown and, often, a decreased motivation to become dry. A satisfactory external-collecting device has not yet been devised for women, especially for elderly women in whom the problem is further complicated by the high prevalence of atrophic vaginitis and vaginal stenosis. Indwelling urethral catheters are not recommended for this condition because they usually exacerbate detrusor overactivity. If they must be used (eg, to allow healing of a pressure sore in a patient with refractory detrusor overactivity), a small cathether with a small balloon is preferable to minimize irritability and consequent leakage around the catheter. Such leakage almost invariably results from bladder "spasm," not a catheter that is too small. Increasing the size of the cathether and balloon only aggravates the problem and, over time, may result in progressive urethral erosion and sphincter incompetence. If "bladder spasm" persists, agents such as oxybutynin can be employed. Especially in elderly persons, alternative agents with more potent anticholinergic side effects (eg, belladonna suppositories) should be avoided.

Stress Incontinence

Involuntary leakage that occurs only during stress is common in elderly women, but uncommon in men unless the sphincter has been damaged by surgery. The definition excludes overflow incontinence, which, although exacerbated by stress, occurs at other times as well and is associated with bladder distention. Typical stress incontinence is characterized by daytime loss of small to moderate amounts of urine, infrequent nocturnal incontinence, and a low PVR (in the absence of urine pooling in a large cystocele). The sine qua non of the diagnosis is leakage that, in the absence of bladder distention, occurs coincident with the stress maneuver. The usual cause is "urethral hypermobility" due to pelvic floor laxity (Fig. 38.1), but other conditions must be considered. These include intrinsic "sphincter incompetence" (type 3 stress incontinence), stress-induced detrusor overactivity, and urethral instability.[35,37,61,62]

Sphincter incompetence (type 3 stress incontinence) was described above. One should realize that the term stress incontinence is in this case a misnomer, because, if the weight of urine in the bladder exceeds the ability of the weakened sphincter to retain it, leakage can occur even when the patient sits quietly, a helpful diagnostic point.

Stress-induced detrusor instability is merely an uninhibited bladder contraction triggered by stress maneuvers. These uninhibited contractions occur at other times as well, giving rise to urgency, frequency, nocturia, urge incontinence, and nocturnal incontinence. The key point is to assess the integrity of the outlet as described earlier. If it is competent, then the problem is detrusor-mediated and should be treated as detrusor overactivity. If the outlet is incompetent, then the patient has either stress incontinence or mixed incontinence (see below) and should be treated as such.

Urethral instability occurs when the sphincter abruptly and paradoxically relaxes in the absence of a detrusor contraction. In our experience this condition is rare in elderly persons. In fact, it may be less common than believed in younger individuals as well, since most investigators have failed to use fluoroscopic monitoring. This omission may lead one to miss an uninhibited contraction (DHIC) and mistakenly identify the accompanying physiologic sphincter relaxation as a pathologic sphincter abnormality.[33,34]

The most common cause of stress incontinence, however, is urethral hypermobility, which is improved by weight loss if the patient is obese, by therapy for precipitating conditions (such as coughing or atrophic vaginitis), and occasionally by insertion of a pessary.[63] Pelvic floor muscle exercises are time honored and frequently effective.[16,57,64] The patient is instructed to sit on the toilet and begin voiding. Once voiding has started, she is asked to interrupt the stream by contracting the sphincter for as long as possible. Initially, most elderly women are able to do so for no more than a second or two, but after a few weeks, many women can prolong the duration of the contraction. Once she recognizes which muscle to contract, she can do the exercises at any time and during any activity. The optimal regimen remains to be determined. My associates and I advise patients to increase the duration of muscle contraction to about 10 seconds, to contract

the muscle as many as 25 times per set, and to complete three to four sets per day. When the patient is able to comply, the exercises are extremely efficacious. However, many older women are unable or unmotivated to follow this regimen. If so, we contact them more frequently or add biofeedback, if available.[64a] If not contraindicated by other medical conditions, treatment with an α-adrenergic agonist, such as phenylpropanolamine (50 to 100 mg/d in divided doses) may be added and is often beneficial for women, especially when administered with estrogen. In fact, these two agents work for women with sphincter incompetence as well. Phenylpropanolamine is inexpensive, available without a prescription, and contained in many "diet pills." However, the physician should prescribe the dose and guide the choice of preparation, since some capsules contain additional agents, such as chlorpheniramine, in doses that can be troublesome for elderly patients. Imipramine, with beneficial effects on the bladder and the outlet, is a reasonable alternative for patients with evidence of both stress and urge incontinence if postural hypotension has been excluded.

If these methods fail, further evaluation of the lower urinary tract may be warranted. If urethral hypermobility is confirmed, surgical correction may be performed and is successful in the majority of selected elderly patients.[16,64b,64c] If sphincter incompetence is diagnosed instead, it too can be corrected, but a different surgical approach is often required, morbidity is higher, and precipitation of chronic urinary retention is more likely than with correction of urethral hypermobility.[16,62] Other treatments for sphincter incompetence include periurethral injection of polytef (Teflon) or collagen and insertion of an artificial sphincter, all of which are effective in selected cases.[16]

If all other interventions fail, prostheses, such as condom catheters or penile clamps, may be useful for men, but most such prostheses require substantial cognitive capacity and manual dexterity, and are often poorly tolerated. An alternative product for men is a penile sheath, such as the McGuire prosthesis (similar to an athletic supporter) or the self-adhesive sheath produced by several manufacturers; especially desirable are those lined with a polymer gel or cellulose. Unfortunately, no similar satisfactory prostheses are available for elderly women. As discussed above, pads and undergarments are employed as adjunctive measures, but in these cases, thin, superabsorbent polymer gel pads are frequently successful because the gel can more readily absorb the smaller amount of leakage. Some products (eg, Tranquility) consist of pads that can actually be flushed down the toilet, which is convenient for ambulatory women. Electrical stimulation is promising, whether applied rectally or vaginally, but is still investigational.[16]

Outlet Obstruction

Outlet obstruction is the cause of incontinence in up to 5% of elderly women.[16,33] As noted earlier, the cause is usually a large cystocele that distorts or kinks the urethra during voiding.[43] Other causes of obstruction include bladder stones and bladder neck obstruction, which are rare, and distal urethral stenosis, which may afflict as many as 2% of 3% of incontinent women.[33] If a large cystocele is the problem, surgical correction is usually required and should include an outlet suspension if urethral hypermobility also is present. Prior urodynamic evaluation is helpful as well: if bladder neck incompetence or low urethral closure pressure (<20 cm H_2O) is observed, a different surgical approach may be required to avoid converting incontinence due to obstruction into incontinence due to sphincteric incompetence. Bladder neck obstruction also is corrected easily, using local anesthesia, and is thus feasible for even the most frail elderly patients. Distal urethral stenosis can be dilated and treated with estrogen. If meatal stenosis is present, more extensive intervention may be necessary; alternatively, dilation can be repeated at fairly frequent intervals. It should be noted that many women who undergo dilation do not have urethral stenosis but rather an underactive detrusor; for these women, dilation usually is not helpful and may be harmful.

In men, the cause of obstruction usually is a stricture, carcinoma, or prostate enlargement. As noted above, neither the size of the prostate nor a past history of prostatectomy correlates well with obstruction, since estimates of prostate size are unreliable,[32] and following a prostatectomy the patient may have a bladder neck contracture or stricture. Although a prostatectomy is optimal and feasible for most elderly patients,[65] newer approaches (eg, bladder neck incision with bilateral prostatotomy)[16,66] have made surgical decompression possible for even the most frail individuals. These procedures, as well as a TURP in some instances,[67] can be done with the patient under local anesthesia and can be completed in less than 30 minutes of operating time. Unlike the TURP and open resections, these newer procedures do not fully resolve the problem, but in frail elderly individuals recrudescence of obstruction 2 to 3 years later may not be an issue.

Another new approach to the obstructed individual involves administration of α-adrenergic antagonists, such as prazosin or phenoxybenzamine. Numerous double-blind placebo-controlled trials have documented the symptomatic efficacy of these agents, and in some trials, the PVR, outlet resistance, and urinary flow rate have improved as well.[68] Phenoxybenzamine in adequate doses (5 to 20 mg/d) is probably superior to prazosin (1 to 2 mg two to four times a day), but concern about its carcinogenic potential in mice has militated against its use. Neither agent is a panacea for outlet obstruction. Rather, each allows the physician to treat the problem symptomatically until more definitive therapy is necessary and feasible.

Underactive Detrusor

Incontinence due to an underactive detrusor is associated with a large PVR and overflow incontinence. Leakage of small amounts of urine occurs frequently throughout the day and night. The patient may also notice hesitancy, a diminished and interrupted flow, a need to strain to void, and a sense of incomplete emptying. If the problem is neurologically mediated, perineal sensation, sacral reflexes, and control of the anal sphincter are frequently impaired. Before this entity can be diagnosed, one must first exclude outlet obstruction.

Management of detrusor underactivity is directed at reducing the residual volume, eliminating hydronephrosis (if present), and preventing urosepsis. The first step is to use indwelling or intermittent catheterization to decompress the bladder for up to a month (at least 7 to 14 days), while reversing potential contributors to impaired detrusor function (fecal impaction and medications). If this does not restore bladder function, once obstruction has been excluded, augmented voiding techniques (such as double voiding and implementation of the Credé's or Valsalva's maneuver) may help if the patient is able to initiate a detrusor contraction. An α-blocker, such as prazosin, may further facilitate emptying by reducing outlet resistance. Bethanechol (40 to 200 mg/d in divided doses) is occasionally useful in a patient whose bladder contracts poorly because of treatment with anticholinergic agents that cannot be discontinued (eg, neuroleptic agents). In other patients, bethanechol may decrease the PVR if sphincter function and local innervation are normal, but evidence for its efficacy is equivocal,[69,70] and residual volume should be monitored to assess its effect.

On the other hand, if after decompression the detrusor is acontractile, these interventions are apt to be fruitless, and the patient should be treated with intermittent catheterization or an indwelling urethral catheter. Intermittent self-catheterization is preferable and requires only clean, rather than sterile, catheter insertion. The individual can purchase two or three of these catheters inexpensively. One or two catheters are used during the day, and another is kept at home. Men can carry their catheter in a coat pocket, and women can carry theirs in a purse (the catheter used for females is only a few inches long). The catheters are cleaned daily, allowed to air dry at night, sterilized periodically, and may be reused repeatedly. Prophylaxis against urinary tract infection is probably warranted if the individual gets more than an occasional infection or has an abnormal heart valve. Intermittent catheterization is painless, safe, inexpensive, and effective, and it allows individuals to carry on with their usual daily activities.

Unfortunately, despite the benefits and proven feasibility of intermittent catheterization, most elderly individuals choose indwelling catheterization instead. Complications of long-term indwelling catheterization include bladder and urethral erosions, bladder stones, and bladder cancer, as well as urosepsis. There is still no consensus regarding the optimal composition of the catheter or the best time to change it, but several points should be mentioned. First, asymptomatic bacteriuria is ubiquitous in patients undergoing long-term catheterization.[71,72] It is pointless to treat these asymptomatic infections, since all one does is replace one organism with a more virulent one; symptomatic infections, on the other hand, should be treated. Second, recent studies have revealed that organisms that colonize catheter encrustations may be unrelated to the organisms that cause a given bladder infection.[73] For this reason, before treating a symptomatic infection, one should pull the old catheter and obtain a culture from a newly inserted one. Third, methenamine mandelate (mandelamine) for treatment of the patient undergoing long-term catheterization is useless, both theoretically and in practice. Methenamine is inert unless activated, a process that takes at least 60 to 90 minutes in acidic urine. Because urine in the catheterized patient remains in the bladder for only a few minutes, methenamine will do nothing to sterilize it.

When indicated, indwelling catheters can be extremely effective, but their use should be restricted. They are indicated in the acutely ill patient to monitor fluid balance, in the patient with a nonhealing pressure sore, and in the patient with overflow incontinence refractory to other measures. Even in long-term care facilities, they probably should not be used in more than 1% or 2% of patients.[16]

Mixed Incontinence

Especially in elderly persons, more than one type of incontinence may be present. For example, urge incontinence may develop in a woman with a history of stress incontinence. Such mixed incontinence differs from stress-induced detrusor overactivity; in the latter, only detrusor overactivity is present, whereas in the former, both detrusor overactivity and impaired outlet integrity are present. Urodynamic evaluation is frequently helpful in such cases because it can help the physician to decide which is the predominant lesion and to target therapy more effectively.

Conclusion

Incontinence is a common, morbid, and costly condition that has been neglected too long. While the approach to it can be time consuming, it can also challenge one's diagnostic and therapeutic skills, and its successful treatment can be tremendously gratifying to patient, caregiver, and clinician.

The approach to the incontinent elderly patient should be stepped. Transient causes and a serious underlying pathologic condition should be excluded, and contributing factors should be identified and pursued. If incontinence persists, the clinician must weigh the risks and benefits of empiric therapy against those of further investigation. While urodynamic investigation will probably be necessary in only the minority of cases, it can be done safely when it is indicated, and it can be extremely helpful if conducted by an experienced urodynamicist. In summary, if the clinician is prepared to devote patience, skill, and compassion to the problem, most incontinent patients can be helped.

Acknowledgments

Supported in part by grants from the National Institute on Aging and The Medical Foundation.

References

1. Resnick NM, Wetle TT, Scherr P, et al. Urinary incontinence in community-dwelling elderly: prevalence and correlates. In: Proceedings of the 16th annual meeting of the International Continence Society, In: 1986; Boston, Mass.

2. Herzog AR, Diokno AC, Fultz NH. Urinary incontinence: medical and psychosocial aspects. *Annu Rev Geriatr Gerontol* In press.

3. Resnick NM, Paillard M. Natural history of nosocomial incontinence. In: Proceedings of the 14th annual meeting of the International Continence Society; In: 1984; Innsbruck, Austria.

4. Sier H, Ouslander J, Orzeck S. Urinary incontinence among geriatric patients in an acute-care hospital. *JAMA* 1987;257:1767–1771.

5. Ouslander JG, Kane RL, Abrass IB. Urinary incontinence in elderly nursing home patients. *JAMA* 1982;248:1194–1198.

6. Resnick NM, Yalla SV. Management of urinary incontinence in the elderly. *N Engl J Med* 1985;313:800–805.

7. Ory MG, Wyman JF, Yu L. Psychosocial factors in urinary incontinence. *Clin Geriatr Med* 1986;2:657–671.

8. Hu T. The economic impact of urinary incontinence. *Clin Geriatr Med* 1986;2:673–687.

9. Willington FL. Problems in urinary incontinence in the aged. *Gerontology* 1969;11:330–365.

10. Yarnell JWG, St Leger AS. The prevalence, severity, and factors associated with urinary incontinence in a random sample of the elderly. *Age Ageing* 1979;8:81–85.

11. Fossberg E, Sander S, Beisland HO. Urinary incontinence in the elderly: a pilot study. *Scand J Urol Nephrol Suppl* 1981;60:51–53.

12. Schnelle JF, Traughber B, Morgan DB, et al. Management of geriatric incontinence in nursing homes. *J Appl Behav Anal* 1983;16:235–241.

13. Castleden CM, Duffin HM, Asher MJ, et al. Factors influencing outcome in elderly patients with urinary incontience and detrusor instability. *Age Ageing* 1985;14:303–307.

14. Overstall PW, Rounce K, Palmer JH. Experience with an incontinence clinic. *J Am Geriatr Soc* 1980;28:535–538.

15. Pannill FC III, Williams TF, Davis R. Evaluation and treatment of urinary incontinence in long-term care. *J Am Geriatr Soc* 1988;36:902–910.

16. Resnick NM. Voiding dysfunction in the elderly. In: Yalla SV, McGuire EJ, Elbadawi A, et al, eds. *Neurology and Urodynamics: Principles and Practice.* New York, NY: Macmillan Publishing Co, Inc; 1988:303–330.

17. Resnick NM. The initial approach to the incontinent patient. *J Am Geriatr Soc* 1989, in press.

18. Torrens M, Morrison JFB, eds. *The Physiology of the Lower Urinary Tract.* New York, NY: Springer-Verlag NY Inc; 1987.

19. Diokno AC, Brown MB, Brock BM, et al. Clinical and cystomertric characteristics of continent and incontinent noninstitutionalized elderly. *J Urol* 1988;140: 567–571.

20. Resnick NM. Urinary incontinence in the elderly. *Med Grand Rounds* 1984;3:281–290.

21. Boscia JA, Kobasa WD, Abrutyn E, et al. Lack of association between bacteriuria and symptoms in the elderly. *Am J Med* 1986;81:979–982.

22. Robinson JM. Evaluation of methods for assessment of bladder and urethral function. In: Brocklehurst JC, ed. *Urology in the Elderly.* New York, NY: Churchill Livingstone Inc; 1984:19–54.

23. Chetkowski RJ, Meldrum DR, Steingold KA, et al. Biologic effects of transdermal estradiol. *N Engl J Med* 1986;314:1615–1620.

24. Jensen J, Riis BJ, Strom V, et al. Long-term effects of percutaneous estrogens and oral progesterone on serum lipoproteins in postmenopausal women. *Am J Obstet Gynecol* 1987;156:66–71.

25. Semmens JP, Tsai CC, Semmens EC, et al. Effects of estrogen therapy on vaginal physiology during menopause. *Obstet Gynecol* 1985;66:15–18.

26. Wheeler JS, Siroky MB, Bell R, et al. Vincristine-induced bladder neuropathy. *J Urol* 1983;130:342–343.

27. Goldsmith MF. Research on aging burgeons as more Americans grow older. *JAMA* 1985;253:1369–1405.

28. Matthew TH, McEwen J, Rohan A. Urinary incontinence secondary to prazosin. *Med J Aust* 1988;148:305–306.

29. Brocklehurst JC, Andrews K, Richards B, et al. Incidence and correlates of incontinence in stroke patients. *J Am Geriatr Soc* 1985;33:540–542.

30. Hellstrom PM, Sjoqvist A. Involvement of opioid and nicotinic receptors in rectal and anal reflex inhibition of urinary bladder motility in cats. *Acta Physiol Scand* 1988;133:559–562.

31. Resnick NM, Yalla SV. Aging and its effect on the bladder. *Semin Urol* 1987;5:82–86.

32. Meyhoff HH, Ingemann L, Nordling J, et al. Accuracy in preoperative estimation of prostatic size. *Scand J Urol Nephrol* 1981;15:45–51.

33. Resnick NM, Yalla SV, Laurino E. The pathophysiology and clinical correlates of established urinary incontinence in frail elderly. *N Engl J Med* 1989;320:1–7.

34. Resnick NM, Yalla SV. Detrusor hyperactivity with impaired contractile function: an unrecognized but common cause of incontinence in elderly patients. *JAMA* 1987;257:3076–3081.

35. McGuire EJ, Savastano JA. Stress incontinence and detrusor instability/urge incontinence. *Neurourol Urodynam* 1985;4:313–316.

36. Abrams P. Detrusor instability and bladder outlet obstruction. *Neurourol Urodynam* 1985;4:317–328.

37. McGruire EJ, Lytton B, Pepe V, et al. Stress urinary incontinence. *Obstet Gynecol* 1976;47:255–264.

38. Tobin GW, Brocklehurst JC. The management of urinary incontinence in local authority residential homes for the elderly. *Age Ageing* 1986;15:292–298.

39. Eastwood HDH. Urodynamic studies in the management of urinary incontinence in the elderly. *Age Ageing* 1979;8:41–48.

40. Abrams PH, Feneley RCL. The significance of the symptoms associated with bladder outflow obstruction. *Urol Int* 1978;33:171–174.

41. Abrams PH. Prostatism and prostatectomy: the role of urine flow rate measurement in the preoperative assessment for operation. *J Urol* 1977;117:70–71.

42. Hald T, Bates P, Bradley WE. The standardisation of terminology of lower urinary tract function. International Continence Society; 1984; Pp. 1–34 Glasgow, Scotland.

43. Klarskov P, Andersen JT, Asmussen CF. Symptoms and signs predictive of the voiding pattern after acute urinary retention in men. *Scand J Urol Nephrol* 1987;21:23–28.

44. Resnick NM, Yalla SV. The baldder is a 'reliable witness': a prospective, blinded study. *J Urol* 1989;141 (4/2):575A.

45. Resnick NM, Yalla SV, Laurino E, et al. Evaluation of a clinical algorithm to identify the cause of incontinence in the elderly. *J Urol* 1986;135:168 Abstract.

46. Stamey TA. Endoscopic suspension of the vesical neck for urinary incontinence in females. *Ann Surg* 1980;192:465–471.

47. Sutherst JR, Brown MC. Comparison of single and multichannel cystometry in diagnosing bladder instability. *Br Med Clin Res* 1984;288:1720–1722.

48. Ouslander J, Leach G, Abelson S. et al. Simple versus multichannel cystometry in the evaluation of bladder function in an incontinent geriatric population. *J Urol* 1988;140:1482-1486.

49. Schmidt RR, Witherow R, Tanagho E. Recording urethral pressure profile. comparison of methods and clinical implications. *Urology* 1977;10:390–397.

50. Sutherst JR, Brown, MC. Detection of urethral incompetence in women using the fluid bridge test. *Br J Urol* 1980;52:138–142.

51. Yalla SV, Finn D, DeFelippo N. Fluid bridge test in the evaluation of male urinary continence. *J Urol* 1982;128:1241–1245.

52. Resnick NM, Yalla, SV. Initiation of voiding in human subjects: the temporal relationship and nature of urethral sphincter responses. Submitted.

53. Yalla SV, Resnick NM. Vesicourethral static pressure profile during voiding: methodology and clinical utility. *World J Urol* 1984;2:196–202.

54. Blaivas JG, Sphincter electromyography. *Neurourol Urodynam* 1983;2:269–288.

55. Fantl JA, Beachley MC, Bosch HA, et al. Bead-chain cystourethrogram: an evaluation. *Obstet Gynecol* 1981;58:237–240.

56. Resnick NM, Yalla SV, Laurino, E. Feasibility, safety, and reproducibility of urodynamics in the elderly. *J Urol* 1987;137(4/2):189A.

57. Hadley E. Bladder training and related therapies for urinary incontinence in elderly people. *JAMA* 1986;256:372–379.

58. Burgio KL, Burgio, LD. Behavior therapies for urinary incontinence in the elderly. *Clin Geriat Med* 1986; 2(4):809–827.

58a. Schnelle JF. Treatment of urinary incontinence in nursing home patients by prompted voiding. *J Amer Geriatr Soc,* in press.

59. Pedersen PA, Johansen PB. Prophylactic treatment of adult nocturia with bumetanide. *Brit J Urol* 1988;62:145–147.

60. Brink CA, Wells TJ. Environmental support for incontinence: toilets, toilet supplements, and external equipment. *Clin Geriat Med* 1986;2(4):829–840.

61. McGuire EJ. Reflex urethral instability. *Br J Urol* 1978;50:200–204.

62. Blaivas JG, Olsson CA. Stress incontinence: classification and surgical approach *J Urol* 1988;139:727–731.

63. Bhatia NN, Bergman A, Gunning JE. Urodynamic effects of a vaginal pessary in women with stress urinary incontinence. *Am J Obstet Gynecol* 1983;147:876–884.

64. Wells TJ. Pelvic floor exercises. *J Am Geriat Soc,* in press.

64a. Burgio KL, Engel BT. Biofeedback-assisted behavioral training for elderly men and women. *J Amer Geriatr Soc,* in press.

64b. Raz S. Vaginal surgery for stress incontinence. *J Am Geriatr Soc;* in press.

64c. Stanton SL. Suprapubic approaches for stress incontinence in women. *J Am Geriatr Soc;* in press.

65. Mebust WK, Holtgrewe HL, Cockett ATK., et al. Transurethral prostatectomy: immediate and postoperative complications. A cooperative study of 13 participating institutions evaluating 3,885 patients. *J Urol* 1989;141:243–47.

66. Orandi A. Transurethral incision of prostate (TUIP): 646 cases in 15 years—a chronological appraisal. *Br J Urol* 1985;57:703–707.

67. Sinha B, Haikel G, Lange PH, et al. Transurethral resection of the prostate with local anesthesia in 100 patients. *J Urol* 1986;135:719–721.

68. Caine M. The present role of alpha-adrenergic blockers in the treatment of benign prostatic hypertrophy. *J Urol* 1986;136:1–4.

69. Downie JW. Bethanechol chloride in urology—a discussion of issues. *Neurourol Urodynam* 1984;3:211–222.

70. Finkbeiner A. Is bethanechol chloride clinically effective in promoting bladder emptying? A literature review. *J Urol* 1985;134:443–444.

71. Warren JW, Muncie HL, Bergquist EJ, et al. Sequelae and management of urinary infection in the patient requiring chronic catheterization. *J Urol* 1981;125:1–8.

72. Warren JW. Urine collection devices for use in adults with urinary incontinence. *J Am Geriat Soc,* 1989; in press.

73. Grahn D, Norman DC, While ML, et al. Validity of urinary catheter specimen for diagnosis of urinary tract infection in the elderly. *Arch Int Med* 1985;145:1858–1860.

74. Rowe JW, Besdine RW, eds. *Geriatric Medicine,* ed 2. Boston, MA: Little Brown & Co; 1988.

39

Pressure Sores

Thomas G. Cooney and James B. Reuler

A pressure sore is one of those common clinical problems to which many physicians have been exposed, but about which few possess any knowledge. In part, this is due to the facts that these festering wounds often occur in patients who are deemed "undesirable,"[1] that their management is frustrating and fatiguing for both physician and patient, and that the topic is viewed as intellectually unattractive by health care providers. This lack of interest has led to inadequate attention to prevention, the institution of ineffective therapeutic measures, increases in health care expenditures, and adverse impacts on patient morbidity and mortality. In this chapter, we will review the salient features of the pathophysiology and management of pressure sores, highlighting issues that are particularly germane to the geriatric population.

The term *decubitus ulcer,* which is derived from the Latin word *decub,* meaning *lying down,* frequently is used to describe this problem. This is a misnomer, however, because many of these lesions develop while a patient is in a sitting position. Therefore, the term *pressure sore* is preferred because it is more accurate and emphasizes the underlying pathophysiology.

Epidemiology

At the turn of this century, pressure sores most often were seen in young persons afflicted with a variety of debilitating diseases, which included tuberculosis, osteomyelitis, and chronic renal disease.[2] At present, the groups that account for the vast majority of pressure sores include those persons with spinal cord injuries, those persons with chronic neurologic diseases (such as cerebrovascular disease and multiple sclerosis), and elderly persons.[3] In the first group, 25% to 85% of all afflicted patients develop pressure sores that account for 50% of admissions to specialized cord injury centers and for 7% to 8% of all related deaths.

A survey from Glasgow, Scotland, that involved more than 10,000 patients revealed that 8.8% of both the hospitalized and home care groups had at least one pressure sore, and that those persons aged 70 years and older accounted for 70% of all patients with pressure sores (the proportion of the total population of the area older than 70 years of age was 8.4%).[4] More recently, a survey from Baltimore, Md, identified a point prevalence of pressure sores of 4.7% in hospitalized patients.[5] Of all elderly patients admitted to a hospital, 10% to 25% will develop pressure sores, usually within the first 2 weeks. The following factors have been implicated in the high prevalence rate of pressure sores in elderly persons: fractures with attendant immobility, incontinence, hypoalbuminemia, and impaired cognition.[3,5]

Notably, development of pressure sores among hospitalized elderly patients is associated with a fourfold increase in the mortality rate and, in failure of the sore to heal, a sixfold increase. Pressure sore–associated sepsis carries a 50% mortality rate in elderly patients.

Health care costs of patients with or at risk for pressure sores are increased substantially over those of other hospitalized patients. In the 1984 Baltimore study, the mean charges for patients with sores was

$37,000; for those patients at risk for pressure sores, it was $28,000. For all other patients, the mean charges were $7,000.[5]

Pathophysiology

Of the many factors that contribute to the development of pressure sores, four appear to be critical: pressure, shearing forces, friction, and moisture.[6] Of these factors, pressure, which is the force exerted on a unit area, is the most important; however, the precise mechanism by which pressure produces tissue necrosis remains clinically controversial.

Pressure

Experimental work reveals that, in skin, the capillary arteriolar limb pressure is 32 mm Hg, the midcapillary pressure is 20 mm Hg, and the venous limb pressure is 12 mm Hg.[7] A 70-kg male lying in the supine position with evenly distributed pressure would have an average pressure exerted, at any given point, of 5.7 mm Hg. Unfortunately, pressure is not equally distributed, but is concentrated in focal areas, generally over bony prominences (Fig 39.1).[8] Increased pressure over these areas leads to a wide, three-dimensional pressure gradient.

Within the tissues, a negative interstitial fluid pressure exists that is balanced by a positive solid tissue pressure, which results in a total tissue pressure of 0 mm Hg. On application of external pressure, interstitial fluid pressure increases, and when pressure in the venous limb is exceeded, a marked increase in total tissue pressure results. This leads to an increased capillary arteriolar pressure, filtration of fluid from capillaries, edema, and autolysis.

The occlusion of lymphatic vessels is another consequence of these pressure gradients. An impairment of the active contractility of lymphatic vessels, combined with changes in the blood microvascular system, leads to an accumulation of anaerobic metabolic waste products and, ultimately, tissue necrosis.[9]

Early investigative work by Dinsdale[10] showed that a pressure of 70 mm Hg, applied for more than 2 hours, produced irreversible tissue damage. However, if pressure was intermittently relieved, a minimal change was seen, even to pressures of 240 mm Hg. Kosiak[11] confirmed these findings, but noted that if pressure was alternated every 5 minutes, few changes were seen. No difference was noted between animals with injured and uninjured spinal cords, thus negating the existence of the hypothesized neurotropic factor that was believed

to be responsible for the increased incidence of pressure sores in cord-injured patients. These studies suggest that the critical period of pressure application is less than 2 hours, after which time irreversible changes occur.

Studies of pressure measurements under the buttocks of a person sitting in a wheelchair demonstrated that pressures were greatest (up to 500 mm Hg) under and just lateral to the ischial tuberosities. Pressures at these points remained higher than 150 mm Hg despite the addition of 5 cm of foam padding to the chair. All other points of measurement were greater than the capillary arteriolar pressure.

More recently, the traditional ischemic cause of pressure sores has been questioned. By using a swine model, Daniel et al[12] showed that initial pathologic changes occur in muscle and subsequently progress toward the skin with increasing pressure and/or duration. Muscle damage occurred at a high pressure of short duration (500 mm Hg, 4 hours), whereas skin destruction required a high pressure of long duration (800 mm Hg, 8 hours) and was not evident after 15 hours at 200 mm Hg. This information suggests that normal tissue is much more resistant to a pressure-induced ischemia than earlier studies would suggest, and that the pressure-duration threshold for the development of pressure sores is lowered significantly by changes in soft-tissue coverage.

Shearing Forces

Tangential pressures, or shearing forces, are caused by the sliding of adjacent surfaces of laminar elements that provides a progressive relative displacement. At high levels of shear pressure, approximating 100 g/cm^2, the normal pressure that is necessary to produce vascular occlusion is 50% of the pressure required when shear forces are absent.[13] Clinically, these forces are in play when the head of the bed is raised, which causes the torso to slide down, or when a patient slides forward in a wheelchair, transmitting pressure to the sacrum and deep fascia. At the same time, the posterior sacral skin is fixed secondary to friction with the bed or wheelchair, and shearing forces in the deep part of the superficial fascia lead to the stretching and angulation of vessels, thus causing a thrombosis and undermining of the dermis. The most vulnerable vessels are the posterior branches of the lateral sacral arteries and the superficial branches of the superior gluteal artery; these branches pass through the posterior sacral foramen to perforate the muscles and deep fascia. In addition, subcutaneous fat, which lacks tensile strength and is particularly susceptible to mechanical forces, accentuates the shearing phenomenon.

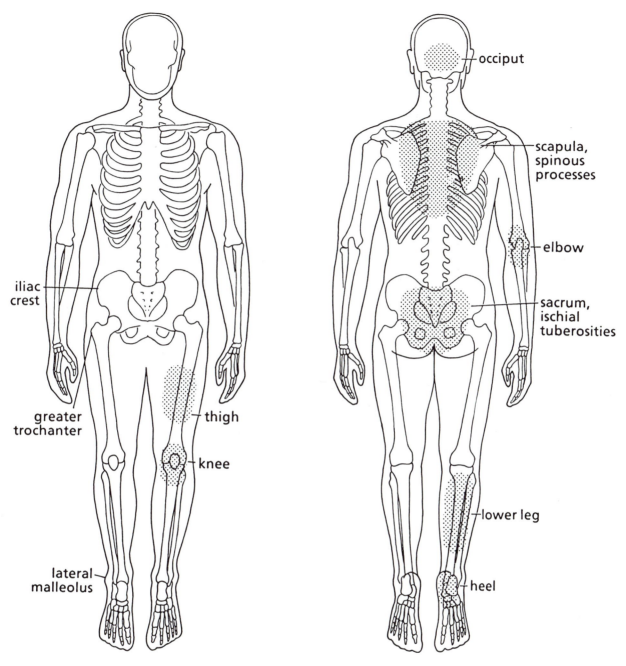

Fig. 39.1. Common locations of pressure sores.

Friction

Friction, which is the force created when two surfaces in contact move across each other, is exemplified when a patient is dragged across the bed sheets. The impact of friction is to remove the outer protective stratum corneum, thus accelerating the onset of ulceration. Age-related changes in the skin (see chapter 29 entitled "Dermatology"), including epidermal atrophy, a decreased turnover rate of cells in the stratum corneum, stiffening of dermal collagen, and a decrease in dermal blood vessels, all may combine to amplify the effects of friction and, therefore, increase the risk of pressure sore development in elderly persons.

Moisture

The final critical causative factor is moisture, which is caused by fecal or urinary soilage or perspiration; it substantially increases the risk of pressure sore formation.

Clinical Evaluation

More than 90% of all pressure sores are located in the lower part of the body, with the majority found in the sacral and coccygeal areas and over the ischial tuberosities and greater trochanters (Fig 39.1).[14] In an individual patient, however, the location of a pressure sore is dependent on a combination of factors that are both intrinsic (immobility, incontinence, malnutrition) and extrinsic (support surfaces, positioning, humidity) to the patient.

Of the many classifications of pressure sores to be found in the available literature, the classification devised by Shea[15] is most clinically applicable (Fig 39.2). A stage 1 sore involves an acute inflammatory response in all layers, with an irregular ill-defined area of soft-tissue swelling, induration, and heat. This resembles an abrasion, is confined to the epidermis, and is reversible. A stage 2 ulceration includes an inflammatory and fibroblastic response that extends through the dermis to the subcutaneous fat and also is reversible. A stage 3 ulcer is essentially a full-thickness skin defect that extends into the subcutaneous fat with extensive undermining. A stage 4 lesion includes penetration into the deep fascia with involvement of muscle and bone.

A physical examination is essential, particularly for early identification. Early in its development, a pressure sore is irregular in shape contrasted with chronic sores, which tend to have regular edges with a thick fibrous ring under the surface. Due to the pressure gradient phenomenon, a small defect at the surface may overlay a large undermining lesion, highlighting the necessity of palpation of the ulceration. On occasion, bimanual palpation of an ischial ulcer may reveal an extension to the rectum.

Given the usual locations and clinical settings, little concern generally is given to a differential diagnosis of these wounds. Occasionally, however, an incipient pressure sore may be mistaken for an early ischial-rectal abscess. Vasculitis may present as a pressure sore, most notably in a bedridden patient afflicted with rheumatoid arthritis. The presence of pustular lesions at the surface may suggest a deep mycotic infection, and the finding of verrucous margins should raise the suspicion of a malignant neoplasm. When these latter diagnoses are entertained, obtaining a biopsy specimen of the area is advisable.

Complications of pressure sores are multiple and can be associated with significant morbidity and mortality (Table 39.1). Infectious complications occur most frequently and are among the most common infections that occur in residents of nursing homes. Because of the loss of the epidermal barrier and the frequent contamination with urine and feces, pressure sores are colonized routinely with a wide variety of organisms. Cultures of these polymicrobial wounds are poorly predictive of the specific organism that causes the infection and should not be used to guide therapy.

Sepsis is a life-threatening complication of infected pressure sores and should be considered seriously in

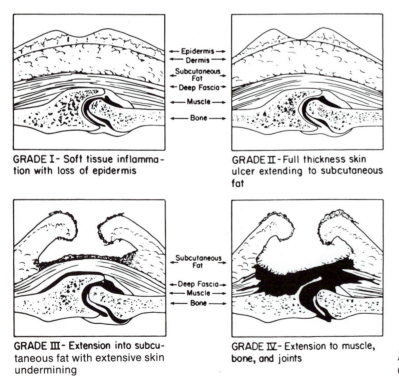

GRADE I - Soft tissue inflammation with loss of epidermis

GRADE II - Full thickness skin ulcer extending to subcutaneous fat

GRADE III - Extension into subcutaneous fat with extensive skin undermining

GRADE IV - Extension to muscle, bone, and joints

Fig. 39.2. Clinical stages of pressure sores. (from Cooney and Reuler[48]).

Table 39.1. Pressure sores: complications.

Complication
Sepsis
Osteomyelitis
Pyarthroses
Joint disarticulation
Extension to deep organs
Heterotopic calcifications
Tetanus
Amyloidosis

the differential diagnosis of febrile patients afflicted with pressure sores. In one series of 21 patients with pressure sore–associated sepsis, 10 of 21 died, 8 of 21 developed osteomyelitis, and 18 of 21 developed extensive tissue necrosis.[16] All patients older than 60 years of age (7 of 7) died. Anaerobic bacteria, particularly *Bacteroides fragilis*, *Peptococcus* and *Peptostreptococcus,* enteric gram-negative organisms, including *Proteus mirabilis* and *Escherichia coli,* and *Staphylococcus aureus* were the most common bacteria recovered from blood cultures. Importantly, the bacteremia was polymicrobial in half of the patients.

There are sparse data on the effectiveness of various antibiotics in the treatment of infected pressure sores. First- and second-generation cephalosporins have not been shown to penetrate into pressure sores; clindamycin and gentamicin have been shown to achieve therapeutic tissue levels in surgically resected pressure sores. In patients whose symptoms are suggestive of sepsis from an infected pressure sore, a combination of clindamycin and an antipseudomonal aminoglycoside is indicated as initial therapy, pending isolation of the causative organisms.[16,17] The role of third-generation cephalosporins and the newer quinolone class of antimicrobials is undefined.

Early surgical débridement of infected pressure sores with secondary sepsis is necessary to improve the chances of survival. Despite appropriate antimicrobial agents, bacteremia can be persistent and may be terminated only after surgical débridement.

Extension to a bone frequently is encountered, which may lead to osteomyelitis, pyarthroses, and joint disarticulation. In addition to bone, pressure sores may extend to any of the deeper structures, including the bowel and bladder. These deep, indolent infections may cause formation of heterotopic calcifications or may increase the susceptibility to tetanus.[18] Studies suggesting that most older adults have not been appropriately immunized against tetanus, and the high mortality rate, make an awareness of this complication particularly important.[19] The administration of tetanus toxoid should be considered in any patient with a deep pressure sore and inadequate documentation of immunization status.

The diagnosis of osteomyelitis underlying higher grade pressure sores is problematic. Differentiation of osteomyelitis from soft-tissue infection is difficult due to the inability of most available tests to distinguish between these two conditions.[20,21] Plain radiographs are neither sensitive nor specific. False positives are a particular problem due to pressure-related bony changes. Radionuclide bone scanning is more sensitive than plain radiographs (range, 64% to 100%) but is nonspecific (range, 30% to 57%). Gallium scans have similar sensitivities and specificities. Computed tomography is useful for defining the extent of soft-tissue involvement and for detecting abscesses, but its role in facilitating the diagnosis of osteomyelitis is less well defined. There is a wide range of sensitivities (10% to 50%) in reported studies, although the specificity is high (90%). Bone cultures (from bone biopsy specimens) are very sensitive and represent the only means for identifying definitively the infecting organism(s), although positive blood cultures are highly suggestive. Unfortunately, bone cultures are not specific. The "gold standard" for the diagnosis of osteomyelitis is abnormal histologic findings on a bone biopsy specimen, obtained either via a needle biopsy or through surgical resection.

Patients with high-grade (3 or 4) pressure sores, non-healing pressure sores, pressure sore–associated spesis, unexplained elevated white blood cell counts (15,000/mm^3), or an elevated erythrocyte sedimentation rate ($\geq$120 mm/hr) should be suspected of having underlying osteomyelitis.[20,21] Although various combinations of tests may offer improved sensitivity and specificity over single tests,[21] no combination offers the diagnostic accuracy or usefulness of a bone biopsy specimen with culture. Complications of a bone biopsy, in experienced hands, are low; they include pain and fracture. Infection and bleeding are rare.[20]

When there is clinical uncertainty about the size or extent of a pressure sore, particularly one with undermined margins and sinus tracts, sinography may be indicated. This study not only will demonstrate the internal size of the cavity, but it may reveal an extension to the joint space or other structures.[22,23] A computed tomographic scan usually is reserved for complicated lesions that are greater than 5 cm, particularly when a soft-tissue or pelvic abscess is suspected; it is most useful in the ischial, sacral, and trochanteric sites due to the generous amounts of subcutaneous fat present.

Systemic amyloidosis, which was a frequently reported complication of spinal cord injury found in the older available literature, may be a consequence of these chronic, suppurative wounds.

Table 39.2. Pressure sores: risk score.

General physical condition	Mental status	Activity	Mobility	Incontinence
4. Good	4. Alert	4. Ambulant	4. Full	4. Not
3. Fair	3. Apathetic	3. Walks with help	3. Slightly limited	3. Occasional
2. Poor	2. Confused	2. Chair-bound	2. Very limited	2. Usually: urinary
1. Very bad	1. Stupor	1. Confined to bed	1. Immobile	1. Urinary and fecal

Prevention

The dictum, "an ounce of prevention is worth a pound of cure," is particularly germane to the management of pressure sores. Due to the morbidity that is associated with these lesions and the limited resources, it is crucial that patients who are at risk are identified, so that preventive measures may be selectively (but intensively) employed. Numerous prediction rules designed to identify patients at risk have been described. Unfortunately, few have been validated properly. The Norton scale, or a modification thereof, appears to be one clinically applicable and sensitive assessment tool.[3] This system assesses five variables (physical condition, mental condition, activity, mobility, and incontinence), may be scored by nursing personnel, and possesses good interrater reliability (Table 39.2). An almost linear relationship exists between the initial score and the incidence rate of pressure sores; the lower the score, the higher the incidence rate. In the original study, 48% of all patients with an initial score of 12 or less developed a pressure sore, whereas those with scores of 18 to 20 had an incidence rate of only 5%.[3] Of all the sores, 70% developed within the first 2 weeks of hospitalization. Although each individual component was associated to a high degree with the development of early sores, incontinence was the single best indicator of risk. One study that used a discriminant function analysis, as applied to the Norton score, suggested that ratings of activity and mobility alone may be as reliable as using all five factors.[24]

Another instrument (Table 39.3) uses absolute and relative criteria to generate a risk score. In the validation study, the instrument had a sensitivity of 88% and specificity of 89% when a score of 3 or greater was used as an indicator of risk.[25]

Finally, epidemiologic surveys of hospitalized patients have established that hypoalbuminemia, fecal incontinence, and fractures are independently and significantly associated with pressure sores.[5] Unfortunately, these factors have not been developed into a prediction rule.

In preventing pressure sores in patients at risk, quality nursing care is crucial. To minimize friction, particulate matter (eg, food) should be removed from the bed, sheets should be loose so that movement is not restricted, and patients should be lifted, not dragged. The skin should be patted dry, not rubbed, and the surface should not be kept too dry or too moist.

Spasticity may interfere with proper positioning and increase the risk of friction. Therapeutic alternatives include medications, such as diazepam, baclofen, and dantrolene sodium; rarely, intrathecal injections or neurosurgical ablation may be indicated.

The head of the bed should not be raised to greater than an angle of 30° and an upright position should be maintained while the individual is sitting in a wheelchair to minimize shearing forces. When it is necessary to tilt the bed, the use of a firm footboard will reduce slippage. Sheepskin pads are useful in this regard due to their shear resistance properties.[26]

Moisture control depends on timely skin care, prevention of soilage, and maintenance of a low-humidity interface. The evaluation and management of urinary incontinence, which is a frequently encountered problem in elderly persons, is extremely important.[27] Surgically created fecal diversion has been used for fecal incontinence but represents an extreme remedy. Again, because of its high capacity to absorb water vapor, sheepskin provides an excellent contact surface.

The most important preventive measure is the relief of pressure itself.[3,28] Rotation of the patient is the simplest mechanism to accomplish this goal. Given the previously cited experimental data, rotation should be performed at roughly 2-hour intervals. Bridging, by using six or more soft pillows placed at strategic loca-

Table 39.3. Pressure sores: risk criteria.*

Absolute criteria (score 2)	Relative criteria (score 1)
Unconsciousness	Age (≥70 y)
Dehydration	Restricted mobility
Paralysis	Incontinence
	Emaciation
	Redness over bony prominence

* Score of 3 or greater identifies a patient at risk (adapted from Andersen et al[25]).

tions, also may provide pressure relief.[29] The use of "donuts" is to be avoided, however, due to the resulting undesirable stress distribution and vessel occlusion.

With good nursing care, it is possible to prevent most pressure sores without the use of special equipment. In some instances, however, alternate support surfaces may be useful adjuncts, although the clinical efficacy and cost-effectiveness of, and indications for, these specialized support surfaces for the prevention of pressure sores have not been established. Pressure-relief devices include fluid-support systems,[30] in which the body floats and evenly distributes weight over the surface that is in contact with the fluid medium; air-support systems,[31] which provide a form of levitation; and air-fluidized beds, in which warm, pressurized air is forced through ceramic beads covered by a closely woven polyester sheet. Alternating pressure mattresses and mud beds also are included in this category of systems.[32] One of these alternatives should be available for the handling of special problems, particularly a patient with multiple sores who cannot be positioned adequately to unload pressure from the at-risk sites. It must be cautioned that an inordinate reliance on gadgetry, much of which may malfunction, often diverts attention from good positioning. No substitute exists for vigilance in nursing care.

In the geriatric population, in contrast to the cord-injury group, a wheelchair is a less significant, but still important, source of pressure ulceration. This issue, however, remains a major problem that confronts rehabilitation engineers. None of the available cushions are as effective as an intermittent, complete unloading of pressure, although appropriate seating, combined with flat support boards and thick polyurethane foam cushions, may reduce the risk.[33]

Management

Once present, the management of a pressure sore is similar to that of other wounds; the primary goal is a promotion of wound healing.[6] General medical care should begin with assessing nutritional status, given the prevalence of protein-calorie malnutrition in hospitalized geriatric patients and its deleterious effect on wound healing.[34] A correction may require enteral or intravenous hyperalimentation to reverse protein catabolism and promote wound healing.[34] A higher intake of protein nitrogen has been shown to be a highly significant predictor of wound healing.[35] Correction of edema and anemia, control of hyperglycemia, and improvement in oxygenation and tissue perfusion, all may contribute to more rapid wound healing. Insufficient information exists to recommend routine vitamin C or

zinc supplementation, as some authors have advocated.[36,37]

The majority of pressure sores are superficial and will heal by secondary intention. The objectives of the management plan include the relief of pressure, wound débridement, and the promotion of healing. Rarely in elderly persons, in contrast to the younger patient with a spinal cord injury, will excision and closure of defects be necessary.

The relief of pressure is the most critical factor in the healing of pressure sores. Without effective pressure relief, other interventions to enhance healing are likely to be fruitless. Indeed, the efficacy of numerous agents alleged to accelerate wound healing are more likely due to unintended improvements in pressure relief than in the intrinsic activity of the actual agent.[38] Methods for relief of pressure have been discussed in the section on prevention. Special support surfaces such as air-fluidized beds may be indicated in patients with particularly large sores (>7.8 cm^2),[35] or patients with multiple sores who are difficult to position.

The goals of wound débridement are to remove devitalized tissue that, if allowed to remain, promotes infection, delays granulation, and impedes healing. Devitalized tissue may be removed through wound cleansing and wound débridement. Numerous agents, including soaps, astringents, disinfectants, and topical antibiotics, are available for wound cleansing. Most of these agents suffer significant limitations, including skin irritation, interference with wound healing (toxicity to the regenerating epithelial layer), systemic absorption (iodide), and contact sensitization (antibiotic creams).[39]

Wound débridement may be mechanical, chemical, or surgical. Mechanical débridement is accomplished with wet-to-"dry" dressings,[40] by using fine mesh gauze soaked in normal saline solution and loosely packed in the wound, with removal every 3 to 4 hours. To prevent pain and reduce the damage to granulation and epithelial tissue, saline solution may be applied to loosen the contact layer of gauze if it is adherent to the wound. A number of agents have been developed to provide chemical débridement (collagenase, sutilains, fibrinolysin, streptokinase, and trypsin-papain).[41,42] None have been adequately studied to establish their clinical usefulness. Dextranomer is a novel agent that acts through the capillary action of beads, by absorbing wound debris.[43] It may be useful in more purulent wounds, but it has not been shown to be superior to less expensive methods (ie, wet-to-dry dressings). Once a wound has been débrided adequately and there is evidence of new granulation tissue, care should be taken not to use any agents or techniques that will damage or inhibit the growth of this tissue.

Surgical débridement is most useful in higher stage

pressure sores (stage 3 and 4) and is mandatory in patients with pressure sore–associated sepsis.[16] At any stage, the presence of a thick eschar usually will require surgical débridement.

Clinicians have long sought agents and methods to promote wound healing. Innumerable topical agents have been advocated, including sugar, insulin, antacids, and karaya gum. There are no adequate clinical trials that substantiate their efficacy. Some agents may actually inhibit cell growth, and hence, great caution should be used in the decision to place any topical agent on a pressure sore. Hyperbaric oxygen has been used on a limited basis, but its cost-effectiveness has not been established.[44] Wound dressings have been investigated for the ability to promote wound healing. The most promising agents are an adhesive hydrocolloid occlusive dressing (Duoderm) and a polyurethane film dressing (Op-Site). One advantage of these dressings is that they can be left in place for several days, reducing consumption of valuable nursing time. Unfortunately, this may have a deleterious effect on efforts at pressure relief. They may also protect the wound from contamination by fecal and urinary soilage. Limited trials suggest that these dressings are most useful in lower stage pressure sores (stage 2) and are not superior to wet-to-dry dressings in higher stage sores.[45,46]

Stage 1 pressure sores are managed with simple cleansings, dressings, and pressure relief. The management of stage 2 sores is similar, although special dressings (Duoderm, Op-Site) may be indicated occasionally. Stage 3 and 4 wounds require aggressive mechanical and, often, surgical débridement, pressure relief, careful attention to nutritional repletion, and identification and treatment of any underlying infection (eg, osteomyelitis). Although these wounds are routinely colonized with multiple organisms, systemic antibiotics are not indicated unless there is evidence of sepsis, cellulitis/fasciitis, or osteomyelitis.

The exact role of surgery, which has been defined extensively in younger patients with spinal cord injuries, remains problematic in elderly persons because of the poor prognosis of many patients in long-term care facilities and the increased risk of recurrence. Surgical objectives include the excision of ulcerated areas, resection of bony prominences that may delay healing and cause a recurrence of the ulcer if left in place, resurfacing of the defect, formation of large flaps, and the obtainment of additional padding by using muscle flaps. Many surgical techniques have been employed to accomplish these goals.[47]

References

1. Papper S. The undesirable patient. *J Chronic Dis* 1970;22:777–779.

2. Shaw TC. On so-called bed-sores in the insane. *St Bartholemew's Hosp Rep* 1872;8:130–133.

3. Norton D, McLaren R, Exton-Smith AN. *An Investigation of Geriatric Nursing Problems in Hospital (1962, Reissued)*. New York, NY: Churchill Livingstone Inc; 1975:194–236.

4. Barbenel JC, Jordan MM, Nicol SM, et al. Incidence of pressure-sores in the greater Glasgow health board area. *Lancet* 1977;2:548–550.

5. Allman RM, Laprade CA, Noel LB, et al. Pressure sores among hospitalized patients. *Ann Intern Med* 1986;105:337–342.

6. Reuler JB, Cooney TG. The pressure sore: pathophysiology and principles of management. *Ann Intern Med* 1981;94:661–666.

7. Kosiak M, Kubicek WG, Olon M, et al. Evaluation of pressure as a factor in the production of ischial ulcers. *Arch Phys Med Rehabil* 1958;39:623–629.

8. Lindan O, Greenway RM, Piazza JM. Pressure distribution on the surface of the human body, I: evaluation in lying and sitting positions using a "bed of springs and nails." *Arch Phys Med Rehabil* 1965;46:378–385.

9. Krouskop TA, Reddy NP, Spencer WA, et al. Mechanisms of decubitus ulcer formation: an hypothesis. *Med Hypotheses* 1978;4:37–39.

10. Dinsdale SM. Decubitus ulcers: role of pressure and friction in causation. *Arch Phys Med Rehabil* 1974;55:147–152.

11. Kosiak M. Etiology of decubitus ulcers. *Arch Phys Med Rehabil* 1961;42:19–29.

12. Daniel RK, Priest DL, Wheatley DC. Etiologic factors in pressure sores: an experimental model. *Arch Phys Med Rehabil* 1981;62:492–498.

13. Bennett L, Kavner D, Lee BK, et al. Shear vs pressure as causative factors in skin blood flow occlusion. *Arch Phys Med Rehabil* 1979;60:309–314.

14. Vasconez LO, Jurkiewicz MJ, Schneider WJ. Pressure sores. *Curr Probl Surg* 1977;14:1–62.

15. Shea JD. Pressure sores: classification and management. *Clin Orthop* 1975;112:89–100.

16. Galpin JE, Chow AW, Bayer AS, et al. Sepsis associated with decubitus ulcers. *Am J Med* 1976;61:346–350.

17. Rissing JP, Crowder JG, Dunfee T, et al. Bacteroides bacteremia from decubitus ulcers. *South Med J* 1974;67:1179–1182.

18. LaForce FM, Young LS, Bennett JV. Tetanus in the United States (1965–1966): epidemiologic and clinical features. *N Engl J Med* 1969;280:569–574.

19. Crossley K, Irvine P, Warren JB, et al. Tetanus and diphtheria immunity in urban Minnesota adults. *JAMA* 1979;242:2298–2300.

20. Sugarman B. Pressure sores and underlying infection. *Arch Intern Med* 1987;147:553–555.

21. Lewis Jr VL, Bailey MH, Pulawski G, et al. The diagnosis of osteomyelitis in patients with pressure sores. *Plast Reconstr Surg* 1988;81:229–232.

22. Hendrix RW, Calenoff L, Lederman RB, et al. Radiology of pressure sores. *Radiology* 1981;138:351–356.

23. Putnam T, Calenoff L, Betts HB, et al. Sinography in management of decubitus ulcers. *Arch Phys Med Rehabil* 1978;59:243–245.

24. Goldstone LA, Roberts BV. A preliminary discriminant function analysis of elderly orthopaedic patients who will or will not contract a pressure sore. *Int J Nurs Stud* 1980;17:17–23.

25. Andersen KE, Jensen O, Kvorning SA, et al. Prevention of pressure sores by identifying patients at risk. *Br Med J Clin Res* 1982;284:1370–1371.

26. Denne WA. An objective assessment of the sheepskins used for decubitus sore prophylaxis. *Rheumatol Rehabil* 1979;18:23–29.

27. Staskin DR, Nehra A, Ouslander JG. Urinary incontinence in the elderly. *Hosp Pract Off* 1988;23:133–140.

28. Anonymous. Sore afflicted. *Lancet* 1981;2:21–22.

29. Stewart P, Wharton GW. Bridging: an effective and practical method of preventive skin care for the immobilized person. *South Med J* 1976;69:1469–1473.

30. Weinstein JD, Davidson BA. Fluid support in the prevention and treatment of decubitus ulcers. *Am J Phys Med Rehabil* 1966;45:283–290.

31. Scales JT, Lunn HF, Jeneid PA, et al. The prevention and treatment of pressure sores using air-support systems. *Paraplegia* 1974;12:118–131.

32. Reswick JB, Rogers JE. Experience at Rancho Los Amigos Hospital with devices and techniques to prevent pressure sores. In: Kenedi RM, Cowden JM, Scales JT, eds. *Bedsore Biomechanics.* Baltimore, Md: University Park Press; 1976:301–310.

33. Lim R, Sirett R, Conine T, et al. Clinical trial of foam cushions in the prevention of decubitus ulcers in elderly patients. *J Rehabil Res Dev* 1988;25:19–26.

34. Cashman MD. Geriatric malnutrition: recognition and correction. *Postgrad Med* 1982;71:185–194.

35. Allman RM, Walker JM, Hart MK, et al. Air fluidized beds or conventional therapy for pressure sores. *Ann Intern Med* 1987;107:641–648.

36. Taylor TV, Rimmer S, Day B, et al. Ascorbic acid supplementation in the treatment of pressure sores. *Lancet* 1974;2:544–546.

37. Hallbook T, Lanner E. Serum-zinc and healing of venous leg ulcers. *Lancet* 1972;2:780–782.

38. Fernie GR, Dornan J. The problems of clinical trials with new systems for preventing or healing decubiti. In: Kenedi RM, Cowden JM, Scales JT, eds. *Bedsore Biomechanics.* Baltimore, Md: University Park Press; 1976: 315–320.

39. Longe RL. Current concepts in clinical therapeutics: pressure sores. *Clin Pharm* 1986;5:669–681.

40. Kucan JO, Robson MC, Heggers JP, et al. Comparison of silver sulfadiazine, povidone-iodine and physiologic saline in the treatment of chronic pressure ulcers. *J Am Geriatr Soc* 1981;29:232–235.

41. Constantian MB, Jackson HS. Biology and care of the pressure wound. In: Constantian MB, ed. *Pressure Ulcers: Principles and Techniques of Management.* Boston, Mass: Little Brown & Co Inc; 1980:69–100.

42. Lee LK, Ambrus JL. Collagenase therapy for decubitus ulcers. *Geriatrics* 1975;30:91–98.

43. Floden CH, Wikstrom K. Controlled clinical trial with dextranomer (Debrisan™) on venous leg ulcers. *Curr Ther Res* 1978;24:753–760.

44. Rosenthal AM, Schurman A. Hyperbaric treatment of pressure sores. *Arch Phys Med Rehabil* 1971;52:413–415.

45. Gorse GT, Messner RL. Improved pressure sore healing with hydrocolloid dressings. *Arch Dermatol* 1987; 123:766–771.

46. Sebern MD. Pressure ulcer management in home health care: efficacy and cost effectiveness of moisture vapor permeable dressing. *Arch Phys Med Rehabil* 1986; 67:726–729.

47. Constantian MB, Jackson HS. The ischial ulcer. In: Constantian MB, ed. *Pressure Ulcers: Principles and Techniques of Management.* Boston, Mass: Little Brown & Co Inc; 1980:215–246.

48. Cooney TG, Reuler JB. Pressure sores. *West J Med* 1984;140:622–624.

40

Falls

Mary E. Tinetti

Until the 1940s, falls and fall-related injuries were considered accidents, that is "acts of God," random or chance events without observable or understandable explanations.[1] However, beginning with the early studies by Droller, Sheldon, and Fine, falls have increasingly been recognized as predictable, and potentially preventable, health problems worthy of careful investigation.[2-4] As evidenced by their association with other functional problems, such as incontinence, and by a high mortality rate not due to injury, falls by the very frail elderly may simply be markers for deterioration. However, falls by elderly persons other than the very frail appear to result from either single specific causes or, more often, from the accumulated effect of multiple identifiable risk factors.

Prevalence and Morbidity

About one-third of community elderly persons over age 65 fall each year.[5-7] The number increases to 50% by age 80. The majority of fallers have multiple episodes. The average reported annual incidence of falling among nursing home residents is 1,600 falls per 1,000 beds.[8] More than half of ambulatory nursing home residents fall each year.

Falls are a major health concern, not only because of frequency, but because of associated morbidity. An accident, of which falls constitute the majority, is the sixth leading cause of death over age 65.[9] Fall-related injuries are reported as an underlying cause of 9,500 deaths each year in persons over age 65.

Nonfatal injuries include fractures and serious soft tissue trauma. An estimated 5% of falls by community and institutionalized elderly result in a fracture; less than 1% in a hip fracture.[10] The most common fall-related fractures are those of the humerus, wrist, pelvis, and ankle, as well as the hip.[11] An additional 5% of falls result in serious soft tissue injuries requiring medical attention.[10] These injuries include hemarthoses, joint dislocations, sprains, and hematomas. Subdural hematomas and cervical fractures are devastating but rare.

The mortality rate, acute and long term health care costs, and effect of hip fractures on a person's functioning have been well studied and are discussed elsewhere. The health care costs and lasting effect on function of other fractures and serious soft tissue injuries have not yet been described. However, it is likely that these other injuries result in decreased function, both directly from the physical effect of the injury as well as indirectly from self-imposed activity restrictions that result from fear of further injury. It is not yet known whether there are subgroups of fallers at increased risk of injury. Risk appears to result from impaired protective responses of the faller and force of impact of the fall. Some evidence suggests that healthier, more active fallers have a higher incidence of injury per fall than frailer fallers, perhaps because of greater force of impact.

Self-imposed activity restriction because of fear, while as yet not well studied, is well known to care providers, family members, and to elderly persons themselves. In a recent community study, one of four fallers reported avoiding activities because of fear. In addition, family members and care providers often discourage activity following falls because of concern for injury. This concern often results in a decision to seek institutionalization. Falls are mentioned as one reason in 40% of nursing home admissions.[10]

Fall Etiology

Between 1 and 5% of falls by community elderly result from such overwhelming intrinsic events as syncope, seizure, or stroke.[7] An additional 3 to 5% of falls result from overwhelming environmental hazards, such as being hit by a car or being pushed.[7] Specific diseases such as Parkinson's disease, strokes, normal pressure hydrocephalus, and cervical spondylosis, are responsible for a small, but unknown, percent of falls by elderly persons. The manifestations, diagnostic evaluation, and treatment of these diseases are discussed elsewhere and are beyond the scope of this chapter.[12]

The majority of falls by elderly persons are likely to be multifactorial, that is, they result not from a single intrinsic or environmental cause, but from the accumulated effect of multiple etiologies. These multifactorial falls do not represent a homogeneous entity. Investigators have attempted to deal with this heterogeneity by classifying falls or by developing fall models. Methods of classification have included separating falls into those that are predominantly intrinsically or environmentally caused—by mechanism of fall such as slip, trip, or drop attack—and by those with a major presumed cause, such as orthopedic, cardiovascular, or postural hypotension.[8] Development of a clinically useful classification system is an ongoing research effort.

The epidemiologic model of host, activity, and environmental factors perhaps best explains the multifactorial etiology of most falls. Under this model, there is a reciprocal relationship among host, activity, and environmental factors. The importance of these three categories of factors varies in individual falls.

A related method for explaining fall etiology that is clinically useful is to consider both predisposing as well as situational factors. Predisposing risk factors are those intrinsic characteristics of the individual that chronically impair stability. Situational factors are those host, activity, and environmental factors present at the time of the fall. The individual factors that have been associated with falling can be placed in one of these two categories. The predisposing and situational risk factors for both community and institutionalized elderly are described below and summarized in Table 1.

Predisposing Risk Factors

Stability depends on the intricate functioning of sensory, central integrative, and musculoskeletal effect or components. The predisposition to falling results from accumulated disabilities and diseases affecting these components superimposed on age-related changes.[13]

Sensory impairments involving visual, auditory, vestibular, and proprioceptive modalities increase risk of falling.[10] Impairment of both visual acuity and perception have been associated with falling. Perception, a visual function involved in spatial orientation, has been shown to be especially relevant to postural stability and falling.[14]

An age-related decline in vestibular function has been suggested as an explanation for increased postural sway, as well as dizziness and perhaps falling in elderly persons.[15] In addition, vestibular function can be compromised by medications, including aminoglycosides, aspirin, furosemide, and Quinidine, as well as by trauma and infections. Elderly persons with vestibular problems will complain of worsening stability in the dark because of increased reliance on visual input.

Proprioceptive abnormalities may result from peripheral neuropathies or posterior column disease, as well as from cervical disorders such as spondylosis. Predisposing factors for cervical spondylosis include past whiplash injuries and cervical arthritis.[16] Patients with proprioceptive problems complain of worsening difficulties in the dark or on uneven ground. They may complain of true vertigo. Their gait often improves with even minimal support.

The central nervous system channels inputs from the sensory modalities to the appropriate efferent components of the musculoskeletal system. Given the multiple connections and their complexity, essentially any central nervous system disorder can contribute to instability and falling. Specific diseases such as Parkinson's disease, normal pressure hydrocephalus, and stroke are associated with falling. Also, some investigators postulate that specific pathologic changes, perhaps in the frontal cortex where the locomotor control is located, may result in an essential gait disorder.[17] In addition, patients with impaired mental status or dementia have consistently been found to have an increased incidence of falling.

Any disability within the musculoskeletal system including muscles, joints, and bones will impair stability and increase risk of falling. Arthritis, myopathies, and hemiparesis are all associated with falling. Hip, knee, and ankle weakness have all been found significant in previous investigations.[8,18] Reciprocal flexion and extension of lower extremity muscles appears essential to postural stability. Ankle dorsiflexion weakness may explain the tendency of some elderly patients to fall backward with even minimal displacement. Foot disabilities such as callouses, bunions, and deformed nails may provide incorrect proprioceptive information.

Systemic diseases may contribute to instability by impairing sensory, neurologic, or musculoskeletal functioning or by causing decreased cerebral blood flow, fatigue, or confusion. Further, the medications prescribed to treat these diseases may contribute to instability and falling.

Postural Hypotension

Postural hypotension, diagnosed remote from the fall, has been associated with falling in nursing homes, but not community falls.[7,19] The lack of blood pressure and heart rate measurements at the time of falls is one impediment to determining the role of postural hypotension in community falls. In addition, the prevalence of orthostatic hypotension, defined as a drop of 20 mm Hg, or more than 10%, in systolic blood pressure, is probably lower than the 15 to 20% previously thought.[20] Postural hypotension, like falling, often is multifactorial.[21] Contributing factors include age-related autonomic changes, decreased baroreceptor sensitivity, decreased renin-angiotension response to upright position, and decreased venous lymphatic return. The effects of diseases, such as diabetes or Parkinson's disease, and medications, such as antidepressants, antihypertensives, and diuretics, are further contributing factors. Postural hypotension should be considered if the fall occurred while going from a lying or sitting to standing position, during exertion, or soon after a meal—a condition referred to as postprandial hypotension. The patient may complain of lightheadedness, blurred vision, or other types of dizziness including vertigo.

Medications may result in instability through multiple mechanisms, including impaired cognitive functioning, postural hypotension, dehydration, fatigue, or electrolyte disturbance. Centrally acting medications, including hypnotics, tranquilizers and antidepressants, have repeatedly been associated with an increased risk of falls and injuries.[5,7,10,22] Other drugs such as diuretics, antiarrhythmics, and anticonvulsants may contribute as well.

Situational Factors

Syncope, seizures, and strokes are obvious direct causes of falling. However, other acute illnesses, such as pneumonias or urinary tract infections, also may precipitate falls, probably by temporarily impairing stability.[7,19] Indeed, falling is a well-recognized non-specific presentation for acute illness in elderly patients.

The role of physical activity in falling is complex. On the one hand, increased physical activity results in improved muscle strength, coordination, and flexibility. On the other hand, controlling for the effect of other risk factors, more active elderly individuals have a higher risk of falling, probably because of increased opportunity.[7] The majority of falls by both community and institutionalized elderly persons occur during usual, relatively nonhazardous activities, such as walking, changing positions, or performing basic activities of daily living. Only a small percent of falls occur during clearly hazardous activities, such as climbing on chairs or ladders, or participating in sports.

While overwhelming environmental hazards, such as being pushed or being hit by a car, account for few falls, environmental factors probably contribute to the majority of falls by institutionalized and community elderly. The precise role of environmental factors is difficult to ascertain because studies lack control data on nonfallers or fallers at times other than their fall. Over 70% of falls by community elderly occur at home.[7] About 10% occur on stairs, with descending being more hazardous than ascending. The most commonly mentioned environmental hazards include tripping over objects, slippery floors, poor lighting, and carrying heavy objects, as well as ice and snow. Slippery or improperly fitting shoes are other potential hazards. Finally, patterns on floors and walls, depending on their quality, may either distort or improve visual perception.[23]

Environmental factors are felt to be less important among institutionalized, than community, elderly persons. The greater frailty and larger numbers of disabilities predispose institutionalized elderly to fall under situations where more functional persons would not. Also, institutions are safer environments than the community, since many hazards are removed. Further, institutionalized elderly persons have fewer opportunities to engage in such hazardous activities as climbing on ladders or walking on ice. However, even among institutionalized elderly persons, environmental contributors do exist. Examples include ill-fitting shoes, untied shoelaces, long pants, or slippery floors.[8] Furniture may be hazardous as well. Beds that are too high or too low, bedrails that can be climbed over, and chairs that are too low or soft may be dangerous.[8] Walking aids are an underappreciated fall hazard. Canes and footrests can be tripped over, walkers may be an added weight displacing an individual backward. Restraints, used to prevent falls and injury, also can contribute to falls. Many patients are able to remove the restraints. In addition, restrained patients may take their wheelchairs or chairs over with them in a fall.

Evaluation and Prevention

The goal of evaluation and prevention is to minimize risk of falling without compromising mobility or functional independence, a difficult task at times. Perhaps a better goal would be to prevent fall-related injuries. However, no method exists at present to identify fallers or falls at risk for injury.

The first step in prevention is to identify possible contributing factors. The following components of the evaluation provide complementary information: 1) thorough risk assessment; 2) balance and gait evaluation; and 3) a review of previous fall situations.

The risk assessment involves a careful evaluation aimed at identifying all predisposing risk factors. This evaluation is similar to that recommended by the Canadian Task Force on the Periodic Health Examination for elderly patients.[24] Because elderly patients may deny or may not be aware of their disabilities, the assessment needs to be initiated by care providers. It is important to bear in mind that the multiple disabilities and diseases suffered by individual patients may render the signs and symptoms of specific processes obscure, vague, or nonspecific. For example, nonvestibular disorders may present with vertigo, although patients with vestibular dysfunction may complain of only vague dizziness. Therefore, a thorough, careful assessment in all patients is needed. The governing concept in fall assessment is that it may be possible to decrease risk by eliminating as many contributing factors as possible.[7,19] Based on individual assessments, combinations of medical, surgical, rehabilitative, and environmental interventions should be considered as outlined in Table 1.

Balance and gait represent the end product of the accumulated effects of disease, age-related changes, and disabilities on sensory, neurologic, and musculoskeletal functions. Therefore, a careful assessment of an individual's balance and gait is an essential component of the fall evaluation. There is mounting evidence that this assessment will identify community and nursing home patients at increased risk of falling. The assessment should reproduce the position changes and gait maneuvers used during daily activities.[7,10,13,19,25] In addition to identifying persons at risk for falling, and, perhaps, the situations under which falls are likely to occur, the assessment can be used to determine rehabilitative and environmental interventions that may decrease risk. For example, if a patient has difficulty getting up from a chair, the combination of strengthening exercises, transfer training under physical therapy, and the use of high firm chairs with arms should be recommended. The use of balance and gait assessment to guide choice of interventions is discussed elsewhere.[26]

While computerized, precise methods of balance and gait analysis are available, these techniques are not feasible for widespread clinical use. Simple, yet reliable methods for observing patients' balance and gait are available for use in clinical practice. The "Get up and Go" test and the Performance-oriented Assessment of Mobility both involve observing the patient get up from a chair, perform several common maneuvers such as reaching up, turning, and bending over, walk at a usual and rapid pace, and return to sit in the chair.[26,28] The examiner watches for instability or difficulty with performing each maneuver. Components of a simple balance and gait assessment are included in Table 2. Again, based on these observations, combinations of medical, rehabilitative, and environmental interventions can be recommended.

The third component of the fall evaluation is a careful review of recent fall situations. In determining possible intrinsic host factors, the clinician should obtain information on premonitions, feelings of light headedness, vertigo or unsteadiness, recent medications or alcohol consumption, or symptoms of acute illness, postural hypotension, or dysrhythmias. A precise description of activity at the time of the fall is important as well. Was the patient standing still; performing a simple activity of daily living such as getting dressed; walking, and if so, on what type of surface; getting up or sitting down from a lying or sitting position; going up or down stairs or curbs, and so on. If the fall occurred during routine and relatively nonhazardous activities, the goal is to improve the safety and effectiveness of the maneuver through balance and gait training and environmental safety assessments. If the fall occurred while performing more hazardous activities, such as climbing on chairs or ladders, substitution of safer activities or avoidance should be recommended.

Environmental details include obstacles in immediate area of the fall, volume and intensity of lighting, floor or ground surface, objects being carried, footwear including fit, height of heel and type of sole, and walking aid used at time of fall.[8,29] A home safety evaluation as well as careful review of specific fall situations may reveal remediable environmental hazards. While common sense dictates eliminating obvious hazards such as tripping hazards, experimental data are not yet available on the efficacy of environmental assessment and adaptation. It is well known that compliance is poor and that careful education, specific recommendations, and close follow up are necessary components of environmental safety programs.

Situations relevant specifically to nursing home residents include presence of side rails if fall occurred while getting into or out of bed, inappropriate use of walking aids such as walkers or wheelchairs, and presence and appropriate application of vest, belt, and

Table 40.1. Predisposing and situational factors associated with risk of falling.

Predisposing factors with contribution to falling	Possible interventions
Sensory	
Vision—acuity, perception,	Medical—refraction; cataract extraction
Impaired hazard recognition; distorted environmental signals; spatial disorientation	Rehabilitative—balance and gait training
	Environmental—good lighting; home safety assessment; architectural design that minimizes distortions and illusions
Hearing	Medical—cerumen removal; audiologic evaluation with hearing aid if appropriate
Spatial disorientation	Rehabilitative—training in hearing aid use
	Environmental—decrease background noise
Vestibular dysfunction	Medical—avoid vestibulotoxic drugs; surgical ablation
Spatial disorientation at rest; impaired visual fixation	Rehabilitative—habituation exercises
	Environmental—good lighting (increased reliance on visual input); architectural design that minimizes distortions and illusions
Proprioceptive-cervical disorders; peripheral neuropathy	Medical—diagnose and treat specific disease (e.g., spondylosis, B_{12} deficiency)
Spatial disorientation during position changes or while walking on uneven surfaces or in dark	Rehabilitative—balance exercises; correct walking aid
	Environmental—good lighting (increased reliance on visual input); good footwear; home safety assessment
Central neurologic	
Central nervous system diseases	Medical—diagnose and treat specific diseases (e.g., Parkinson's, normal pressure hydrocephalus)
Impaired problem-solving, strength, sensation, balance, gait, tone, or coordination	Rehabilitative—physical therapy; balance and gait training; correct walking aid
	Environmental—home safety assessment; appropriate adaptations (e.g., high, firm chairs, raised toilet seats, grab bars in bathroom)
Dementia	Medical—avoid sedating or centrally acting drugs
Impaired problem-solving	Rehabilitative—supervised exercise and ambulation
	Environmental—safe, structured, supervised environment
Musculoskeletal	
Arthritides	Medical—diagnose and treat specific diseases
Impaired gait, muscle strength	Rehabilitative—balance and gait training; muscle strengthening exercises; back exercises; correct walking aid; correct-foot wear; good foot care (nails, bunions)
Ankle	
Impaired postural stability	
Feet	Environmental—home safety assessment; appropriate adaptations
Impaired proprioception	
Back	
Impaired ability to regain stability	
Other	
Postural hypotension	Medical—diagnose and treat specific diseases; avoid offending drugs; rehydrate
Impaired cerebral blood flow	
Depression	Rehabilitative—tilt table if severe; reconditioning if component of decondition; graded pressure stockings
? accident-proneness	
? poor concentration	Environmental—elevate head of bed
Medications especially sedatives, phenothiazines, antidepressants	?-antidepressants associated with increased risk of falling
Impaired alertness; postural hypotension; instability	Medical—lowest effective effective dose of essential medications; readjust and discontinue when possible

Situational factors	Possible interventions
Acute host factors	
Acute illness; new or increased medications	Medical—diagnose and treat specific diseases; start medications low and increase slowly
Transiently impaired alertness; postural hypotension; fatigue	Environmental—increase supervision during illnesses or with new medication
Displacing activity	Rehabilitative—recommend avoiding only clearly hazardous and unnecessary activities (e.g., climbing on chairs); balance and gait training
Increased opportunity to fall	

Table 40.1. Continued

Situational factors	Possible interventions

Environmental—hazards
  Slipping or tripping hazards (e.g., loose rugs, wet floors, ice, small objects)
  Stairs, lighting, and furniture
	Environmental—home safety assessment with appropriate adaptive or structural changes (See Reference 7)

other restraints. Restraints, while used to prevent falls, can be a contributor to falls if applied incorrectly, or when used on very active individuals. Active nursing home residents often are able to remove the restraints or fall with the restraints in place. Therefore, restraints should not replace careful supervision and attention to the fall-preventive measures described above.

Summary

Falling is a common event for both nursing home residents and community-living elderly persons. These falls may result in morbidity ranging from self-imposed activity restriction because of fear to serious injury or death. There is no way at present to distinguish those fallers at risk for serious morbidity. Therefore, all fallers are assumed to be at risk for morbidity.

A small percent of falls result from a single, overwhelming, intrinsic event such as syncope, from the effects of a single disease process such as Parkinson's disease, or from overwhelming environmental hazards. The majority of falls are multifactorial resulting from various combinations of intrinsic, activity-related, and environmental factors.

Although results from controlled trials are not yet

Table 40.2. Position changes, balance maneuvers, and gait components included in performance-oriented mobility assessment.

Position change or balance maneuver	Observation
	Potential fall risk if patient:
Getting up from chair*	Does not get up with single movement; pushes up with arms or moves forward in chair first; unsteady on first standing
Sitting down in chair	Plops in chair; does not land in center
Withstanding nudge on sternum (examiner pushes lightly on sternum 3 times)	Moves feet; grabs object for support; feet not touching side by side
Eyes closed	Same as above (tests patient's reliance on visual input for balance)
Neck turning	Moves feet; grabs object for support; feet not touching side by side; complains of vertigo, dizziness, or unsteadiness
Reaching up	Unable to reach up to full shoulder flexion standing on tiptoes; unsteady; grabs object for support
Bending over	Unable to bend over to pick up small object (eg, pen) from floor; grabs object to pull up on; requires multiple attempts to arise
Gait component or maneuver†	
Initiation	Hesitates; stumbles; grabs object for support
Step height (raising feet with stepping)	Does not clear floor consistently (scrapes or shuffles); raises foot too high (more than two inches)
Step continuity	After first few steps, does not consistently begin raising one foot as other foot touches floor
Step symmetry	Step length not equal (pathologic side usually has longer step length-problem may be in hip, knee, ankle, or surrounding muscles)
Path deviation	Does not walk in straight line; weaves side to side
Turning	Stops before initiating turn, staggers; sways; grabs object for support

* Use hard, armless chair.
† Patient walks down hallway at "usual pace," turns and comes back using usual walking aid. Examiner observes single component of gait at a time (analogous to heart examination). (Reproduced from reference 27 with permission.)

available, it is likely that careful assessment and targeted interventions may decrease risk of falling in community and institutionalized elderly persons. The assessment consists of identifying the presence and severity of the diseases and disabilities listed in Table 1, careful observation of balance and gait as in Table 2, and review of previous fall situations.

Based on an individual's assessment, targeted interventions should be recommended. These interventions need to be considered within the context of overall health and functioning. Most frequently, a combination of medical, rehabilitative, and environmental manipulations will be appropriate.

Most frequently, the goal of fall prevention will be to minimize risk without compromising functioning and mobility. However, as with all geriatric patients, the goals and priorities may be different for individual patients. Most importantly, falls should not be considered random, unavoidable, or inevitable consequences of aging.

References

1. Hogue CC. Epidemiology of injury in older age. In: *Second Conference on the Epidemiology of Aging.* 1980; NIH publication No. 80–969. pp. 127–138.
2. Droller H. Falls among elderly people living at home. *Geriatrics* 1955;May:293–344.
3. Sheldon JH. On the natural history of falls in old age. *Br Med J* 1960;2:1685–1690.
4. Fine W. An analysis of 277 falls in hospital. *Gerontol Clin* 1959;1:292–300.
5. Campbell AJ, Reinken J, Allan BC, et al. Falls in old age: A study of frequency, and related clinical factors. *Age Ageing* 1981;10:264–270.
6. Prudham D, Evans JG. Factors associated with falls in the elderly: A community study. *Age Ageing* 1981; 10:141–146.
7. Tinetti ME, Speechley M, Ginter SF. Predisposing and situational risk factors for falls in community elderly (submitted).
8. Rubenstein LZ, Robbins AS, Schulman BL, et al. Falls and instability in the elderly. *J Am Geriatr Soc* 1988;36:266–278.
9. Baker SP, Harvey AH. Fall injuries in the elderly. *Clin Geriatr Med* 1985:1:501–508.
10. Kennedy TE, Coppard LC, eds. The prevention of falls in later life. *Danish Medical Bulletin.* Supplement 4, 1987.
11. Melton LJ, Riggs BL. Risk factors for injury after a fall. *Clin Geriatr Med* 1985;525–536.
12. Tinetti ME: Instability and falling in the elderly. *Seminars in Neurology* (accepted).
13. Wolfson LI, Whipple RH, Amerman PM, et al. Gait and balance in the elderly: Two functional capacities that link sensory and motor ability to falls. *Clin Geriatr Med* 1985;1:649–659.
14. Tobis JS, Reinsch S, Swanson JM, Byrd M, Scharf T. Visual perception dominance of fallers among community-dwelling adults. *J Am Geriatr Soc* 1985;33:330–333.
15. Hazel JWP. Vestibular problems of balance. *Age Ageing* 1979;8:258–260.
16. Wykce B. Cervical articular contributions to posture and gait: Their relations to senile disequilibrium. *Age Ageing* 1979;8:251–258.
17. Koller WC, Glatt SL, Fox JH. Senile gait: A distinct clinical entity. *Clin Geriatr Med* 1985;1:661–669.
18. Whipple RH, Wolfson LI, Amerman PM. The relationship of knee and ankle weakness to falls in nursing home residents: An isokinetic study. *J Am Geriatr Soc* 1987;35:13–20.
19. Tinetti ME, Williams TF, Mayewski R. Fall risk index for elderly patients based on number of chronic disabilities. *Am J Med* 1986;429–34.
20. Mader SL, Josephson KR, Rubenstein LZ. Low prevalence of postural hypotension among community-dwelling elderly. *JAMA* 1987;258:1511–1514.
21. Lipsitz LA. Syncope in the elderly. *Ann Int Med* 1983;99:92–105.
22. Ray WA, Griffin MR, Schaffner W, et al. Psychotropic drug use and the risk of hip fracture. *N Engl J Med* 1987;316:363–369.
23. Owens DH. Maintaining posture and avoiding tripping. *Clin Geriatr Med* 1985;1:581–599.
24. Canadian Task Force on the Periodic Health Examination: The periodic health examination. *Can Med Assoc J* 1979;121:1193–1254.
25. Wild D, Nayak USL, Isaacs B. Characteristics of old people who fell at home. *J Clin Exper Gerontol* 1980;2:271–287.
26. Tinetti ME. Performance-oriented assessment of mobility problems in elderly patients. *J Am Geriatr Soc* 1986;34:119–126.
27. Tinetti ME, Ginter SF. Identifying mobility dysfunctions in elderly patients. *JAMA* 1988;259:1190–1193.
28. Mathias S, Nayak USL, Isaacs B. The "Get up and Go" test: A simple clinical test of balance in old people. *Arch Phys Med Rehabil* 1986;67:387–389.
29. Tideiksaar R. Preventing falls: Home hazard checklists to help older patients protect themselves. *Geriatrics* 1986;41:26–28.

41

Nutrition

Cynthia T. Henderson

As the number of older adults in the United States and industrialized world increases along with increasing health care expenditures, the need for guidance on health promotion and maintenance for these individuals also grows. While promotion of good nutrition, exercise, and healthy habits is routinely advanced, there is a considerable gap between empiric advice and the scientific data to support specific recommendations. More research is needed to define the needs of elderly persons at different decades of life. The impact of chronic illness, medications, and alterations in functional ability on nutritional needs, nutritional status, and dietary prescriptions is not clearly defined in the older individual. Among healthy elderly individuals, the variation in dietary needs and nutritional status as a function of the type and degree of physical exercise needs clarification. Furthermore, such research must delineate clinical approaches to nutritional problems in elders as a function of the setting in which they primarily are seen for medical evaluation. For example, studies are needed of elders in long-term care facilities that not only stratify them according to level of care and activity, but also examine the effects of intercurrent illness and dietary intake on nutrient needs and clinical outcomes.

The effect of nutrition on the aging process in humans is unclear. Current theories of aging include some hypotheses tested in animals that have nutritional implications, but are not confirmed in humans. Of particular relevance in this regard is the free radical theory of aging, supported by the results of studies in which dietary antioxidants increase life expectancy and re-

duce the incidence of various cancers in mice. Dietary manipulation also affects life expectancy in animals, with restriction of fat, calories, and easily oxidized amino acids in rats after weaning resulting in increased longevity.[1,2] Although the relevance of these observations to humans has not been conclusively proved and studies would be difficult, circumstantial evidence does exist to support these hypotheses. A review of mortality records from World War II revealed a decrease in mortality and morbidity due to atherosclerosis and heart disease in the Nordic countries; this decrease has been attributed to the food restrictions imposed by the conflict.[3] This observation and the results of numerous animal studies suggest that in humans, life expectancy and morbidity can be decreased to some extent by dietary manipulation, including avoidance of excessive fat and carbohydrate consumption and increased consumption of foods with natural antioxidants (vitamin E, selenium, and beta carotene). What remains to be seen is the effect in humans of dietary manipulation at later points in the life cycle.

Effect of Age on Nutrient Requirements and Intake

Nutritional needs are the amounts of those essential nutrients necessary for health and normal growth. These needs vary with age, sex, and body weight and are influenced by such factors as illness, physical activity, and drugs. These daily requirements are expressed as recommended dietary allowances (RDAs), which are the amounts of essential nutrients needed to meet the needs of 95% of all healthy persons. The RDAs are broad limits and were intended to be applied to populations over time, not to serve as a rigid frame into which all individuals should fit. The RDAs do not, for example, take into account interindividual variability in nutrient requirements, nor do they account for the effect of age after 70, 80, or 90 years. In fact, the highest age category specifically addressed is "51 years and over."[4] The lack of information on the effects of chronic illness and changes in physical activity over time also is not addressed by the RDAs. These omissions reflect our incomplete knowledge of the issues and provide fertile, though difficult, ground for study. Thus, when an individual's intake of a nutrient is below the RDA, the diet is not necessarily inadequate for that nutrient in that individual. However, in those elderly persons who consume less than two thirds of the RDA, the risk of nutrient deficiency and resultant illness increases with increasing duration of low-nutrient intake. In many studies of dietary intake, 67% of the RDA is taken as a reference standard.

Table 41.1 details some of the food sources, signs of deficiency, and RDAs for the nutrients described below. In addition, recommended intakes, derived from a variety of sources, are listed for several common clinical situations, including bedridden patients, those patients with sepsis or other forms of catabolism, and patients with decubitus ulcers.[5-8]

Energy

Energy needs are determined by the basal metabolic rate (BMR) and the energy needed for activity, and these energy needs are influenced by age, height, weight, sex, and the proportion of metabolically active tissue, particularly bone and muscle. With increasing age, there is, in general, a decline in lean body mass and an increase in total body fat. Diminished muscle mass accounts for the greatest decline in energy production, and it parallels the decreasing physical activity. Energy intake and requirements decrease with increasing age. Basal energy needs are decreased by 10% for individuals aged from 51 through 75 years, and by 20% in those persons aged older than 75 years, as compared with energy allowances for young persons.[7] Deductions also are made to account for reduced activity, and women require less energy than men (Table 41.1). The level of physical activity is a major influence on energy requirements, which has definite implications for the small but growing subset of today's physically active, aging athletes. The 70- to 80-year-old marathon runners and weight lifters who continue a high level of physical

activity have less change in body composition.[9] Although the elderly athlete has received considerable publicity, the majority of older adults do not participate in sports or regular exercise. A National Center for Health Statistics survey, conducted in 1975, revealed that only 9.9% of all persons aged older than 65 years regularly engaged in exercise or any sports activity. Of these, 16% of men and only 5.2% of women participated in sports regularly; the remainder cited walking as their regular exercise. No doubt these numbers have increased in the past decade as the benefits of exercise continue to be widely publicized and as our aging society includes more former athletes who continue to exercise (See Chapter 42).

Physical activity may be significantly limited by obesity or chronic musculoskeletal, cardiac, pulmonary, neurologic, or vascular disease. Fear of injury or exacerbation of symptoms may further inhibit physical activity. From the ages of 65 through 74 years, arthritis of the knees afflicts 25% of women and 14% of men; 11% of these individuals report limitation of physical activity. In individuals with osteoarthritis and obesity, the resulting reduction in caloric expenditure may create a vicious cycle of worsening obesity and arthritis, especially in the knees and hips.

Among institutionalized elderly persons, physical activity often is markedly limited, with a reduction in caloric needs. This population is heterogeneous, however, and activity levels may vary depending on such factors as institutional facilities, programs for rehabilitation and exercise, wandering or pacing, and intercurrent illness. The growing number of wheelchair athletes warrants study in this regard. Patients with sepsis or injuries require additional calories (Table 41.1).

Energy is supplied primarily by the metabolism of carbohydrate and fat. Fiber and protein are lesser energy sources. The average American diet provides 45% to 70% of total daily calories as carbohydrate, 38% to 42% as fat, and 10% to 12% as protein.

Fat

There is now widespread agreement that the amount of fat in the diet should be reduced to 30% or less of total daily caloric intake.[10] This reflects the increasing epidemiologic evidence for the role of dietary fat in the development of atherosclerosis, as well as various cancers.[10,11] However, the effect of reducing dietary fat in elderly persons on the risk of these diseases is unclear.

At least 10% of calories must be provided as fat to assure intake of fat-soluble vitamins and essential fatty

Table 41.1. Food sources, recommended intakes, and signs of deficiency: selected nutrients.*

Nutrient	Common food sources	Signs of deficiency	Men 51-74	Men 75+	Women 51-74	Women 75+	Bedridden	Pressure sores	Sepsis
Calories (kcal), protein (g)	Carbohydrates, fats, meats, fish, eggs, legumes	Anorexia, apathy, irritability, flaking dermatitis, depigmentation, parotid gland enlargement, bradycardia, hypotension, respiratory depression, edema, transverse lines on nails, hepatomegaly, anemia	2,400 56	2,050	1,800 44	1,600	BMR+0%-20%, 0.8 g/kg	BMR+10%-20%, 1.0-2 g/kg	BRM+10%-25%, 0.8 g/kg+30%-100%
Vitamin A (μg of retinol)	Yellow-orange vegetables (beta-carotene equivalents) carrots, liver, fish, fish liver oils	Follicular hyperkeratosis, night blindness, decreased recovery after glare, photophobia, xerosis, senile macular degeneration, poor wound healing	1,000		800		RDA		3,333
Vitamin D (μg)	Fish, milk, egg yolks	Bone tenderness, muscle weakness	5		5		RDA		10
Vitamin E (mg of α-tocopherol)	Vegetable and seed oils, wheat germ, nuts, egg yolks	Cerebellar degeneration, peripheral neuropathy	10		8		RDA		10-15
Ascorbic acid (mg)	Citrus fruits, berries, tomato, cabbage, greens, melons	Perifollicular petechiae, bruising, bleeding gums, poor wound healing	60		60		RDA		75-1,000
Thiamine (mg)	Seeds, nuts, wheat germ, legumes, lean meat, enriched cereals, potatoes	Confusion, edema, muscle tenderness, peripheral neuropathy	1.2		1.0		RDA		0.5-1.0/ 1,000 kcal
Riboflavin (mg)	Milk, eggs, nuts, seeds, organ meats, green leafy vegetables, enriched cereals, bread	Flaking dermatitis, scrotal dermatitis, photophobia, blurring, glossitis, cheilosis, angular stomatitis, tongue atrophy	1.4		1.2		RDA		1.4
Niacin (mg)	Meats, nuts, legumes, fish, milk	Flaking dermatitis, hyperpigmentation, diarrhea, dementia, glossitis, tongue fissuring, tongue atrophy	16		13		RDA		15-20
Pyridoxine (mg)	Liver, wheat germ, nuts, beans, avocados, bananas, pork, oatmeal	Peripheral neuropathy/paresthesias, loss of reflexes, wrist/foot drop	2.2		2.0		RDA		2.2
Folate (μg)	Green leafy vegetables	Glossitis, macrocytic anemia, decreased thiamine absorption	400		400		RDA		400
Vitamin B$_{12}$ (μg)	Liver, meats	Megaloblastic anemia, glossitis, loss of position and vibratory sense, dementia	3.0		3.0		RDA		4.0
Calcium (mg)	Milk, dairy products, tofu, bones	Tetany, muscle weakness, osteoporosis, osteomalacia	800		800		RDA		800–1,200
Phosphorus (mg)	Present in nearly all foods	Hemolysis, cardiac arrhythmias, weakness, anorexia, malaise, bone pain	800		800		RDA		800
Magnesium (mg)	Nuts, beans, fish	Weakness, tremors, seizures, behavioral disturbances	350		300		RDA		350
Iron (mg)	Meat	Microcytic anemia, koilonychia (nail spooning), tongue atrophy	10		10		RDA		10
Zinc (mg)	Meat, seafood	Flaking dermatitis, hypogeusia, poor wound healing	15		15		RDA		Up to 60 (in divided doses)

* RDAs indicates recommended daily allowances; BMR; basal metabolic rate.
Adapted from reference 44 with permission.

acids. There is no evidence that older individuals require more or less fat than younger persons.

Carbohydrate

There is no minimum dietary requirement for carbohydrates. The major issue in carbohydrate intake in elderly individuals is the development of glucose intolerance with increasing age. This may be further exacerbated by the onset of acute illness. The use of complex carbohydrates instead of simple sugars improves glucose tolerance and may avoid mislabeling and overtreatment of elderly persons with glucose intolerance.

Fiber

Dietary fiber is not a single entity; rather, it comprises multiple components of plants that are resistant to human digestion. Each component has different physiochemical properties and physiologic effects. The three major fractions of dietary fiber are as follows: structural polysaccharides (cellulose, hemicellulose, and some pectins); structural nonpolysaccharides (predominantly lignin); and nonstructural polysaccharides (gums and mucilages secreted by cells, and polysaccharides from algae and seaweed, such as carrageenan and agar). Particulate, water-insoluble fiber is comprised mainly of lignin, which is resistant to degradation in the human small and large intestine. Lignin content is high in wheat bran, carrots and other root vegetables, and fruits with edible seeds, such as strawberries. Diets high in wheat bran increase stool bulk and have been used effectively in the treatment of constipation. In one study conducted at a 300-bed nursing home, the addition of bran to breakfast cereals of residents decreased laxative costs by $44,000/y.[12] Oat bran has been shown to be effective in lowering total cholesterol and low-density lipoprotein levels in hypercholesterolemia.[13] Water-soluble components of dietary fiber, including gums (found in oatmeal and legumes), pectins (from strawberries, citrus, and apples), and psyllium, have been shown to lower the peak blood glucose response and the serum cholesterol level.[14,15] While there is no RDA for fiber, the National Cancer Institute has recommended a daily intake of 25 to 35 g, which can be achieved by bran supplementation and inclusion of five servings of fruit and/or vegetables in the daily diet. Other proposed benefits of dietary fiber include reductions in the incidence of cholelithiasis, improvement in irritable bowel syndrome and colonic diverticulosis (common problems among elderly persons), and possibly improved weight reduction.

Protein

Breakdown and synthesis rates of protein are decreased in aging humans. There is also a redistribution of protein synthesis sites, with a relative decline in the contribution of skeletal muscle accompanied by an increase in the proportion of whole-body protein contributed by the visceral organs.[16]

There are conflicting reports in the literature regarding whether protein and certain amino-acid needs increase in aging persons. The findings from the studies are difficult to interpret due to a lack of comparability in methodology and subjects. The recommended protein allowance of 0.8 g/kg/d has been considered adequate for healthy elderly persons by some investigators, while others have concluded this level to be inadequate for long-term nitrogen balance. In general, at least 12% to 14% of daily caloric intake should be in the form of protein.[16] In elderly persons with chronic illnesses, very little information is available, particularly for those persons in long-term care settings. Recently, one group of investigators performed nitrogen balance studies on female nursing home residents with chronic illnesses in whom pressure sores were prone to develop. During the 6 months of study, many of the women required 1 g or more of protein per kilogram per day to remain in positive nitrogen balance.[6] Elders who experience acute illnesses with sepsis, trauma, burns, and postoperative states require increased dietary protein just as do their younger counterparts.[8] Those elders with pressure sores in whom balance studies are not performed should receive at least 1 g/kg/d, depending on renal function.

One important unresolved issue is the role of dietary protein in the decline of renal function with age. The prevalence of renal insufficiency and renal failure rises as a function of age. However, there is evidence that aging per se does not necessarily cause a decline in renal function.[17] Furthermore, although dietary protein restriction is useful as a means of slowing the rate of glomerular function decline if started early in the course of renal disease, protein intake does not appear to alter the glomerular filtration rate in otherwise healthy elderly persons.[18]

At this time, it appears to be prudent to recommend 0.8 to 1.0 g/kg/d of protein intake to elderly persons, with any reductions below this level based on the presence of demonstrated renal disease.

Vitamins

Fat-soluble Vitamins

Vitamin A deficiency is seldom encountered in community-living elderly persons, and most elders studied appear to consume at least 67% of the RDA for vitamin A. On the other hand, elderly individuals commonly use vitamin supplements that may contain 100% of the RDA for vitamin A and may be at increased risk of hypervitaminosis A. In elderly persons, alterations in mental status, headaches, gait disturbance, liver dysfunction, and other symptoms may not be attributed to retinol overdosage. There is no evidence that older persons' requirement for vitamin A is different from their younger counterparts.

Vitamin D is much more likely to be deficient in geriatric patients, especially those who are homebound or institutionalized, but community-living elderly persons who take vitamin supplements actually may consume well over the RDA for vitamin D. A number of factors contribute to low vitamin D levels in aging persons, including a decreased intake and exposure to sunlight, a reduced intestinal absorption by up to 40% in elderly vs younger persons, a decreased hepatic synthesis of 25OH-vitamin D, an impaired renal conversion of 25OH-D to 1,25OH-D, and increased metabolic requirements.[19,20] Serum 25OH-D levels can be moderately increased by sunlight exposure for 30 minutes daily.[21] Another factor in long-term care patients is the common use of phenytoin and phenobarbital. The prevalence of anticonvulsant-related metabolic bone disease in long-term care patients is not known, but low serum 25OH-D, calcium, and phosphate levels and high alkaline phosphatase levels are commonly seen, and bone disease may go unrecognized.[22] Efforts should be made to taper and discontinue anticonvulsants whenever feasible.

Supplementation of vitamin D should be cautious. The risk of hypervitaminosis D is not insignificant, and it may result in metastatic soft-tissue calcification, with renal dysfunction and, ironically, bone resorption.

Vitamin E supplementation has received considerable publicity due to claims of its antiaging properties and benefit in vascular disease, claims that have not been scientifically proved. However, such a role has not been demonstrated in elderly individuals. The role of vitamin E in the retardation of the aging processes, presumably due to its antioxidant properties, is yet to be demonstrated in humans, although many older individuals take vitamin E supplements in the belief that aging may be slowed. Deficiency of vitamin E in adults is seen in individuals with malabsorption that causes steatorrhea and abetalipoproteinemia. Given the extreme rarity of clinical vitamin E deficiency in developed countries, supplementation beyond the current RDA for adults aged older than 51 years probably is of no benefit. Unlike vitamins A and D, however, toxicity due to vitamin E does not appear to be a significant clinical problem.

Vitamin K deficiency due to dietary inadequacy is extremely uncommon. Prolonged sulfa or other antibiotic therapy may kill vitamin K–producing colonic bacteria, producing deficiency, as may chronic fat malabsorption due to pancreatic disease.

Laxative abuse, which is common among elderly individuals, may lead to excessive losses of fat-soluble vitamins due to rapid intestinal transit.

Water-soluble Vitamins

Thiamine is essential to energy metabolism, and requirements are linked to energy intake. The enrichment of breads, cereals, and other products with thiamine has decreased the incidence of clinical deficiency among free-living populations in the United States. However, because of the reduced absorption of thiamine by alcohol, elderly alcoholics are at increased risk of deficiency. The difficulty of obtaining an accurate history of alcohol abuse in elders, coupled with the potential for altered mental status and memory impairment, requires a high index of suspicion among health care providers. Population studies (National Health and Nutrition Examination Survey, NHANES) measuring urinary thiamine have shown a low prevalence of thiamine deficiency among free-living individuals aged 65 through 74 years. However, 10% of black men examined had low urinary excretion of thiamine. Elderly patients with chronic illnesses, especially those in long-term care facilities, are likely to be at higher risk for thiamine deficiency, since total-energy intake, and thus dietary thiamine, is often reduced in institutionalized persons. An increase in postoperative confusion has been noted in elderly patients undergoing hip surgery, and a concomitant low-thiamine status was observed.[23] For elderly persons, even at caloric intakes below 2,000 kcal/d, the recommended thiamine intake is 1.0 mg/d.

Riboflavin needs are, like thiamine, related to energy intake. Most studies have shown riboflavin intakes to be adequate in the general population. However, earlier data from the NHANES I study (1971–1974) showed that a greater proportion of elderly blacks had lower urinary excretion of riboflavin than did elderly whites. Minor degrees of deficiency may produce marked behavioral changes.

Niacin deficiency, in its severe form, causes the classic symptoms and signs of pellagra—diarrhea, dementia, and dermatitis. Niacin requirements also are related to total-energy intake. Because tryptophan is converted to niacin, intake of this amino acid influences niacin needs, and 60 mg of tryptophan is equivalent to 1 mg of niacin. Animal protein is a better source of tryptophan than vegetable protein. There is no evidence that elderly persons have increased or decreased niacin needs.[4]

Pyridoxine (vitamin B$_6$) deficiency, as with other B-complex vitamins, presents as behavioral abnormalities and appears to be common in elderly persons. Up to 30% of elderly nursing home patients, studied in New Jersey and Maryland, had low levels of serum vitamin B$_6$, with corresponding low dietary intakes.[24] Pyridoxine needs are related to the protein content of the diet, and cooking may significantly alter bioavailability. It does not appear that elderly persons require increased intake of pyridoxine, unless protein intake is low.

Folic acid deficiency has been demonstrated in several biochemical studies of elderly persons. Low levels of serum folate were seen in 6% of those persons aged 65 to 74 years who took part in the NHANES I. In a study of low-income persons, up to 60% had low red blood cell folate levels (a more sensitive indicator, reflecting recent intake), as compared with 5% to 10% of all elderly subjects living at home.[25] Folate deficiency, which can antagonize dietary thiamine absorption, has been found in 13% to 20% of elderly nursing home and hospitalized patients.[26] Folate absorption is reduced in the presence of antacids, which are commonly used by elderly persons.

Cobalamin levels recently have been shown to be low or low normal in the absence of typical macrocythemia or anemia in some persons with neurologic abnormalities.[27] Although the average American diet provides 5 to 15 μg of vitamin B$_{12}$ per day, many elderly persons with low cobalamin levels have poor absorption of the vitamin from food. As a result, they may have low or low normal levels of cobalamin in the face of a normal Schilling test (the Schilling test uses free vitamin B$_{12}$). The prevalence of low normal serum vitamin B$_{12}$ levels in the elderly population as a whole, as compared with those with cognitive impairment, behavioral changes, and/or peripheral neuropathy, is not known. However, serum vitamin B$_{12}$ levels should be obtained when these signs or symptoms are present and when a low normal cobalamin level and normal Schilling test are obtained, a food Schilling test should be performed, if available. Cobalamin assays may yield falsely low vitamin B$_{12}$ levels in the presence of megadoses (> 2 g/d) of ascorbic acid. In the event a food Schilling test cannot be performed, cobalamin supplementation should be provided, and the patient should be monitored for serum and neurologic response. Some practitioners may opt simply to supplement cobalamin on the basis of a low or low normal serum level, monitoring clinical response and serum level, without performing a Schilling test. Although this approach has not been subjected to large clinical studies, it may be more cost effective.

Ascorbic acid supplementation is widely practiced among elderly persons. In one study of 304 elderly men and women, more than 56% of the subjects regularly took vitamin C supplements. In this population, less than 2% of the subjects were considered at risk for ascorbic acid deficiency, and, as in other studies, women more often took supplements than men.[28] Low plasma levels of vitamin C have been documented more often in the institutionalized elderly population, attributed to decreased dietary intake. These levels can be increased to normal with supplementation at intakes as low as 50 mg/d.[29] Ascorbic acid may affect neutrophil function, wound healing, and drug metabolism. Therefore, adequate levels in long-term care patients are crucial.

Ascorbic acid has been positively correlated with increased high-density lipoprotein levels, without an increase in the total cholesterol level. This effect appears to be significant in persons aged 60 to 69 years, mild in the 70 to 79-year-old group, and negligible in those persons aged older than 80 years.[30] Double-blind, randomized, placebo-controlled trials are needed over a wide age range to confirm these observations and to establish the magnitude of vitamin C intake necessary to affect the incidence of atherosclerotic disease.

Minerals

Calcium absorption declines in efficiency with advancing age, and the role of calcium in osteoporosis has received increasing attention of late. Although many studies have shown calcium intake to be deficient in elderly persons, other factors affect calcium balance and bone health. Among some populations, particularly blacks, calcium intakes often are well below the RDA; yet, the prevalence of osteoporosis and related hip fractures is lowest among black persons, which may reflect nonnutritional factors, such as increased bone density. Alterations in calcium balance in older adults may be due to a variety of factors, including the changes previously mentioned in vitamin D metabolism. Reduced estrogen production has been clearly implicated in the pathogenesis of osteoporosis in postmenopausal women, and estrogen replacement, combined with calcium supplementation, can slow the progression of bone loss if started early after menopause.[5] Improvements in bone density have been shown in elderly women with osteoporosis who received supplemental calcium without estrogen replacement. In elderly osteoporotic men, the addition of milk to increase calcium intake from 800 to 1,200 mg daily reduced the percentage of those with negative calcium balance from 41% to 13%.[31] The National Institutes of Health Consensus Conference on Osteoporosis recommended a calcium intake of 1,000 to 1,500 mg/d for females (See Chapter 15).[5]

Other factors that may affect calcium balance include dietary fiber, protein, and phosphorus. The increasing use of high-fiber diets in elderly and other persons with constipation has led to concern over the possibility that some unrefined cereals may interfere with absorption of calcium and other minerals. Elderly persons with marginal calcium intakes may be at increased risk of negative calcium balance as a result.

Physical activity clearly is an important factor in bone mineralization and calcium balance. Immobilization increases bone loss and diminishes absorption of dietary calcium, in addition to causing increased calciuria. A program of physical exercise slows bone loss and promotes utilization of dietary calcium.

Phosphorus is plentiful in most foods, and dietary deficiency is not a problem. Phosphorus levels are most likely to decrease when there is refeeding after prolonged periods of starvation. With the introduction of large amounts of carbohydrates for metabolism, phosphorus is consumed as adenosine triphosphate, and severe hypophosphatemia may result. The decreased cardiovascular reserve and skeletal muscle depletion, induced by malnutrition and starvation, leave the elderly person at high risk of sudden cardiac death in the presence of severe hypophosphatemia. Phosphorus depletion also may result from long-term use of antacids, such as aluminum hydroxide.

Plasma inorganic phosphate levels, normally 2.5 to 4.4 mg/dL in adults, decline with advancing age in men. On the other hand, plasma phosphate levels increase in postmenopausal women, and a positive correlation has been reported between plasma phosphate level and bone resorption in postmenopausal and elderly women.[32]

Magnesium is essential to normal neuromuscular function. Deficiency of this mineral causes weakness, depression, and behavioral changes. Low magnesium levels have been associated with a decreased myocardial tolerance to ischemia, hypertension, and sudden death.[33]

Zinc deficiency has been associated with a loss of taste acuity, skin changes, impaired wound healing, and depressed immune function in humans.[34] Meats are a particularly good source of zinc, and among elderly persons who consume less meat because of low incomes, poor dentition, or other reasons, the risk of zinc deficiency may be increased. Data from the NHANES II study revealed that 3% of those persons aged 65 to 74 years had subnormal serum zinc levels; this figure reached 16% among low-income blacks.[35] Acute illness and surgical conditions often result in increased utilization of zinc. Coupled with a decreased intake during these periods, patients are at an increased risk of zinc deficiency, which may result in hypogeusia, which is correctable with zinc supplementation. Other

groups of elderly persons who may be at particular risk of zinc deficiency include those with alcoholism and malabsorption. While serum zinc levels are a commonly used measure, serum zinc may not be a very sensitive indicator of zinc nutriture. More recent studies indicate that cellular levels of zinc are better correlated with mild zinc deficiency.[34] There is evidence that the plasma response to an oral dose of zinc is lower in older adults, and zinc uptake by old cells in cell culture is lower than that of younger cells.[36]

Iron nutriture actually improves with advancing age. The NHANES I study found that the prevalence of iron deficiency, as measured by low transferrin saturation, decreased from 7.2% in men aged 45 to 54 years, to 4.2% in those aged 65 to 74 years. Among women, iron deficiency was found in 9.5% of those aged 45 to 54 years, and in 6.8% of those between the ages of 65 and 74 years. As with other nutrients, the prevalence of deficiency was greater among blacks, particularly black women, with 9.5% of those aged 65 to 74 years iron deficient.[37] Normally, in the face of iron deficiency, the intestinal absorption of iron increases. However, even when iron intake is low, serum ferritin and bone marrow iron stores increase with age (see Chapter 26). The prevalence of hypochlorhydria or achlorhydria among elderly persons may increase the risk of impaired absorption, as hydrochloric acid is needed to reduce ferric iron to the ferrous form for optimal absorption. Other factors that interfere with iron absorption include antacids (commonly used in elderly persons), phytates, tannic acid in tea, and salts of calcium and phosphates. The bioavailability of dietary iron also depends on the form in which it is consumed. Heme iron constitutes 40% of the iron in meat, and it is more readily available for absorption (20%) than non–heme iron, of which 5% or less is absorbed. Iron deficiency due solely to an inadequate dietary intake does not appear to be a major cause of anemia in elderly persons, and it does not appear that iron requirements exceed the current RDA. Iron deficiency in elderly individuals is more likely a reflection of bleeding, most often from a gastrointestinal source, and should be evaluated. When iron supplementation is used, particularly if there is evidence of hypochlorhydria or achlorhydria, the supplement will be better absorbed in the presence of ascorbic acid.

Selenium has received increasing attention because of its relationship with vitamin E and intracellular antioxidant functions. In addition, selenium deficiency has been demonstrated as a cause of cardiomyopathy and skeletal muscle dysfunction, establishing its place as an essential nutrient for humans. Individuals who are maintained for prolonged periods on total parenteral nutrition, as well as with enteral tube feedings, are at particular risk for selenium deficiency.[38] There is no information available on the prevalence or sequelae of selenium deficiency in long-term tube-fed elderly patients.

Chromium, which acts as a cofactor of insulin, is essential to normal carbohydrate and lipid metabolism. It is also a cofactor in nucleic acid metabolism and may play a role in the regulation of gene expression. Patients who are maintained on prolonged total parenteral nutrition are most at risk for deficiency. Improved glucose tolerance following chromium supplementation in human subjects has been documented. However, in healthy elderly persons, chromium intakes below the RDA did not appear to be harmful in one study.[39] A relationship between chromium and ischemic heart disease has been suggested, but not proved.

Nutritional Evaluation

The goals of nutritional evaluation are to determine the risk for significant undernutrition, identify likely nutrient deficiencies, assess somatic nutrient reserves, and determine the severity of nutritional deficits. This information, coupled with ongoing reevaluation, should lead to an appropriate nutritional prescription.

The assessment of nutritional status in the elderly person includes a careful history and physical examination, which are aimed at eliciting clues to possible risk factors for undernutrition, and a determination of the patient's functional capacity for nutrient intake. Some important risk factors are listed in Table 41.2, and others are described below.

History

Symptoms, such as nausea, vomiting, abdominal pain, flatulence, diarrhea, or constipation, can limit dietary intake. Diarrhea also may result in significant losses of fluid, potassium, magnesium, and zinc. Oral discomfort due to ill-fitting dentures or poor dentition may compromise the amount and variety of foods consumed. Anorexia, commonly occurring during the course of various chronic illnesses, may be a result of malnutrition itself.

Polypharmacy may cause anorexia, increased losses of specific nutrients, altered nutrient utilization, and decreased nutrient absorption. Nutrient interactions with drugs may alter drug bioavailability. Some important drug-nutrient interactions are listed in Table 41.3.

Alterations in taste and smell may result from a range of causes, including viral infections, toxic exposures, drugs, and intracranial disease. Aging per se appears to produce some decline in taste and smell acuity.

Eating-feeding and swallowing disorders occur frequently in elderly persons with strokes, dementia, and

Table 41.2. Risk factors for malnutrition in geriatric patients.

Risk factor
Altered taste and smell
Anorexia
Chronic illness
Deglutition disorders
Altered mental states
Gastrointestinal disorders
Recent surgery
Recent hospitalization
Alcoholism
Need for tube feeding
Decubitus ulcers
Physical incapacity
Previously homebound
Poverty
Cultural diet restrictions
Loss of control over food choices
Depression
Unattractive surroundings
Distraction at meals
Inappropriate food timing and food temperature
Need for assisted feeding
Elder abuse

Adapted from the Illinois Department of Aging Report.

degenerative neurologic diseases. The prevalence of deglutition and eating disorders was found to be 46% in one study of 2,500 patients in 28 nursing homes.[40] The need for assisted feeding may place some elders at nutritional risk. Hand-feeding may be considered demeaning and may evoke resistance in a previously independent individual, with a resultant decline in intake; persistently low intakes with weight loss often result in the need for enteral tube feeding.

Enteral tube feeding per se may be associated with deficiencies of certain nutrients. These include essential fatty acid deficiency, with scaly dermatitis, seen in

Table 41.3. Drug-nutrient interactions.

Drug	Nutrient(s) affected
Antipsychotics	Protein/calorie; produce disinterest in food
Digitalis glycosides	Protein/calorie; anorexia
Laxatives (mineral oil)	Vitamins A, D, E, and K malabsorption
Diuretics	Loss of potassium, magnesium, and zinc
Isoniazid	Vitamin B_6
Phenytoin and phenobarbital	Altered vitamin D metabolism
Salicylates	Iron loss due to gastrointestinal bleeding
Corticosteroids	Calcium absorption inhibited

patients on long-term elemental diets (which are low in essential fatty acids) and in some patients not on elemental diets.[8] Serum carnitine levels are low in long-term tube-fed patients.[38] Beta carotene, which has been under increasing scrutiny for its possible anticarcinogenic properties, is undetectable in most enteral formulas, and tube-fed patients rapidly become hypocarotenemic.[41] The long-term consequences of chronically low serum beta carotene and carnitine levels are unclear. Selenium deficiency, which has been observed in unsupplemented patients who are receiving long-term tube feeding or long-term total parenteral nutrition, may cause muscle cramps and cardiomyopathy. Dietary prescriptions that are inadequate to meet the patient's energy and protein needs during and after recurrent acute illness may further compromise nutritional status. On the other hand, a common practice, unsupported by hard clinical data, is routinely to provide additional daily multivitamins to patients who are receiving tube feeding. This practice has not been shown to be beneficial and may have as yet unrecognized adverse effects. If the patient is receiving the amount of formula recommended by the manufacturer, then the RDA for essential nutrients will be provided by the formula. Since most routinely used multivitamin supplements contain up to 100% of the RDA for most fat- and water-soluble vitamins, the potential for vitamin A and D toxicity exists. The effects of long-term oversupplementation of patients who are receiving tube feeding are unclear and need further study.

Altered mental status and depressed consciousness are commonly observed in acutely ill elderly people, and their capacity for oral intake often is significantly reduced. Tube feeding is frequently used during these periods. In patients with fluctuating levels of consciousness, oral intake may be inadequate to meet nutrient needs, with resultant nutritional compromise.

Social isolation, depression, and bereavement increase the risk of undernutrition in elderly persons. Depression is underdiagnosed among elders and may be precipitated by significant life changes, including new onset of illness, institutionalization, and loss of loved ones and friends. A loss of the sense of control over living situations may have implications for the health of older adults and may be reflected in a decreased dietary intake.[42] In nursing home patients, the loss of control over food choices, meal timing, and meal frequency particulary is problematic and may lead to disinterest in food. Loss of mobility further limits food choices, and decreased nutrient intakes have been shown in homebound elderly persons.

Elder abuse is frequently unrecognized by health professionals, and it may have serious nutritional and medical complications. A recent study by the Illinois Department on Aging revealed that of 641 reported cases, 11% of abused elders had been denied food and/ or medical care.[43] Those elderly persons who are most dependent are at greatest risk, especially when their needs outweigh the resources of their caregiver (See Chapter 49).

The *eating environment* has an impact on dietary intake, particularly in nursing homes and hospitals. Such factors as uncomfortable room temperature, noisy, unattractive surroundings, and inappropriate timing, temperature, and portion sizes of food served can affect meal intake.

Dietary restrictions may pose a risk for undernutrition if food choices are dramatically limited. Diabetics, those patients with liver and renal disease, and patients on modified consistency diets may find prescribed diets unpalatable, with diminished intake.

Poverty clearly limits access to adequate amounts and varieties of food. The prevalence of multiple chronic illnesses in elders on fixed incomes, requiring polypharmacy, may force patients to choose between food and medication, resulting in both undernutrition and undertreatment.

Physical Examination

Physical signs of malnutrition may be difficult to discern in the aging person. Sparse, thinning hair, dry skin, and loss of muscle mass all may accompany normal aging. They also are commonly seen with protein-calorie malnutrition, as well as with zinc and vitamin A deficiency. In patients who are fed through nasogastric tubes in the institutional setting, mouth breathing is common, with drying and cracking of oral mucous membranes that can be mistaken for the cheilosis and stomatitis seen in B-complex vitamin deficiency (Table 41.1).[44]

Anthropometric measures that are used to assess nutritional status include height, weight, skin-fold thickness (to evaluate body fat stores), and arm muscle circumference or arm muscle area (AMA) (to estimate somatic protein reserves). These measures all are affected by aging, especially height.

Height is used as a reference point for evaluating weight and for determining the creatinine-height index as an indicator of lean body mass. However, height may be difficult to measure accurately in older individuals. Height decreases by 1.2 cm/20 y to 4.2 cm/20 y as a result of vertebral bone loss, kyphosis, and osteoporosis. Accurate measurement is particularly difficult in those individuals who are unable to stand, are bedridden, are amputees, or have extremity contractures. Alternative measures, such as recumbent length, knee height, arm span, and total arm length, may be useful, but each has limitations. In clinical practice, height often is not measured directly, and the practitioner simply asks the patient his or her height. This is probably the most inaccurate means of determining stature, and it may be misleading due to patients' memory deficits and failure to account for loss of height with aging.

Weight should be regularly monitored, and changes should prompt further evaluation. Hydration status and the presence or absence of edema should be noted at the time of weighing. Generally, weight increases during middle age, up to the ages of 40 to 50 years, reaches a plateau and remains stable up to about the age of 70 years, and then declines. It is difficult to compare a very old person's weight to a standard table, especially among those aged older than 80 years, because most standard tables used to determine "ideal body weight" were not developed by using reference groups this age or above. The argument has been advanced that mild obesity may actually have a protective effect in old age.[45] A recent study of the nutritional status of a group of residents in a teaching nursing home showed a positive relationship with change in the level of function: activities of daily living increased with weight gain and decreased with weight loss, independent of acute changes in medical status.[46]

Weight loss should be considered significant if it exceeds 1% to 2% loss in 1 week, 5% loss in 1 month, 7.5% in 3 months, or 10% loss in 6 months. More important than the absolute percentage of loss is the weight trend. One study of geriatric nursing home patients found a decreased 4-year survival among those who had lost 4.5 kg or more during a 2-year period.[47] In the long-term care setting, weight loss should prompt the nursing staff to notify the physician, and nursing home policies should so state.

Skin-fold thickness and AMA or arm muscle circumference are used in nutritional practice to estimate body fat and somatic protein stores, respectively. The reliability of these measures is affected by the loss of elasticity and altered compressibility of normally aging skin. Skin-fold thickness most often is measured over the midpoint of the triceps. There also appear to be gender differences in the predictive capacity of skin fold thickness for body fat stores. Subscapular and suprailiac measures may be more reliable predictors of body fat in men, while triceps skin-fold thickness (TSF) may better correlate with body fat in women.

Arm muscle area or arm muscle circumference is calculated based on the midarm circumference (MAC) and the TSF. The MAC is measured at the midpoint between the olecranon process of the elbow and the acromion process of the shoulder. In severely malnourished geriatric patients with very low AMA, the 90-day mortality may reach 50%.[48]

Unfortunately, skin-fold and arm muscle measurements have not been widely used in ambulatory clinical geriatric practice or in the long-term care setting. Such measures are more likely to be used in hospital-based situations where there is a nutrition support team or where it is a routine part of the dietitian's practice. These measures are especially limited, because they do not predict early malnutrition. Among long-term care patients and those in other settings who may have contractions, paralysis, or other postural abnormalities, these measures may be very difficult to obtain due to problems in properly positioning the patient.

Functional Nutritional Assessment

Functional assessment of nutrient intake capacity should be an integral part of nutritional evaluation. Just as the hallmarks of geriatric medical practice are the assessment of function and the use of an interdisciplinary team approach, similar elements should characterize the nutritional assessment of elderly persons.

Sensory perception should be assessed, to determine the degree, if any, of impairment of sight, taste, and smell and the effect on nutrient intake. Taste and smell can be evaluated by the physician or dietition, by using common household substances, such as coffee, sugar, and salt.

A *mental status evaluation* can include questioning about food preferences and dietary recall. This may enable simultaneous evaluation of recent recall and the dietary history.

Dentition, if poor, can pose a significant risk to the nutritional status of elderly persons. An estimated 50% of Americans aged older than 60 years and 75% of those aged older than 75 years have lost more than half of their teeth. As a result, they may eat a less challenging diet, decreasing their intake of fresh fruits and vegetables and other sources of fiber. An unknown number of dentures are lost during transfer of long-term care patients to and from acute care hospitals, and Medicare does not pay for dentures.

Swallowing abnormalities should be sought in patients with strokes, degenerative neurologic disorders, and head and neck malignant neoplasms. Recent onset of a refusal to swallow may herald a new stroke or progression of neurologic disease. The speech pathologist should be called early to evaluate the patient, especially if tube feeding is contemplated. Cineradiographic swallowing studies that use liquids and foods of varying consistencies are helpful in determining the presence of aspiration, pooling of ingested liquids and food, and other abnormalities. The results of these studies must be correlated with clinical observations, as there are patients with abnormal findings from evaluations who are able to eat modified diets without clinically significant pulmonary aspirations. Eating-feeding disorders also should be evaluated by the speech pathologist, who may have specific suggestions on feeding techniques.

Respiratory dysfunction, especially breathlessness,

may interfere significantly with eating, and it may necessitate small frequent meals to encourage adequate intake. Nursing staff or other caregivers should be asked to observe patients' breathing during meals for abnormalities or limitations.

Mobility impairment affects eating, in that the ability to maintain an upright posture decreases the risk of aspiration and increases the likelihood of an effective cough in the event of aspiration. Immobility limits the access to food.

Coordination of hand-to-mouth movements is essential for easy handling of common eating utensils. The functional assessment for nutrient intake capacity assumes more importance when the elder has any condition that causes difficulty in handling eating utensils. The occupational therapist can suggest assistive devices, such as partitioned plates, plates with guards that prevent spillage of food, and specially designed forks, spoons, and knives. The patient with poor hand coordination may find it easier to drink soup from a mug, and to eat finger foods, eg, small sandwiches, tomato wedges, hard-boiled eggs, and french fries, which are easy to manipulate. The psychosocial implications of hand incoordination must be acknowledged as well. Patients may be reluctant to eat in public places for fear of appearing messy, or they may limit their participation in social affairs where eating occurs, thus isolating themselves.

The *level of assistance* required at meals can be a serious deterrent to adequate oral intake. Some patients require only that food be cut into appropriate sizes, that meal portions be situated on the table in an accessible place, or that their trays be set up and eating utensils made accessible. Others require hand-feeding with all its potential psychologic implications and difficulties.

The prevalence of eating dependency and the need for hand-feeding have been correlated with immobility, cognitive impairment, upper-extremity dysfunction, modified consistency diets, absence of teeth and dentures, abnormal swallowing, and an increased 6-month mortality rate.[49] There are no studies of the long-term nutritional consequences and clinical outcomes of hand-fed patients, but the amount of time available for hand-feeding should have a significant effect on nutritional status. In the long-term care setting, the time available for hand feeding may be as little as 6 to 10 minutes per patient per meal. In Illinois, the Department of Public Health long-term care standards require that no less than 13 minutes per patient per meal be allocated for hand-feeding. Whether this is an adequate amount of time for feeding, and what the impact is on nutritional status of long-term care patients have not been demonstrated. Also unknown is how often hand-fed patients go on to require enteral tube feeding.[50]

The hand-feeding of patients with cognitive disorders may be difficult. Abnormal eating-feeding behaviors include turning away when food is offered, sucking or biting the spoon, refusing to close the mouth after food has been introduced, holding or "squirreling" food in the cheeks, and spitting the food out. Up to 19% of 400 patients who were studied in one facility exhibited such behaviors during feeding.[51] These behaviors may provoke hostility from the person feeding the patient, setting the stage for elder abuse, either in the home setting or in the long-term care facility. In most facilities, feeding is done by nurses' aides or attendants with little or no medical training and often little understanding of the behavioral abnormalities of demented patients. When caregivers are not properly trained in feeding techniques, hand-feeding can become extremely frustrating, with resultant reductions in the amount of food offered. In-service training for feeders should include techniques for effective hand-feeding, and the psychologic effects of these patients' behaviors on the staff should be addressed.

The *amount of food consumed* throughout a 3-day period can give a good estimate of the adequacy of intake. In the institutional setting, where meals are required to provide the RDA, a patient who consistently consumes less than 70% of meals or does not eat food from all four food groups is at an increased risk of undernutrition.

Laboratory Assessment

Some biochemical, immunologic, and hematologic parameters are altered by aging and may be difficult to interpret in the older individual. However, it is important not to assume that an abnormally low value is due to aging per se.

Serum protein levels are commonly used to assess visceral protein stores. The total serum protein value is less useful than the serum albumin value as a nutritional indicator, because in the presence of elevated globulins levels, the total protein value may be normal if the albumin level is low. The serum albumin level may decline slightly in some elderly persons, leading to a wider range of values, but the reduction is not clinically significant. The albumin value may be affected by an underlying chronic illness, drugs, hydration status, and prolonged bed rest. During periods of acute illness, especially during rapid changes in hydration status, the correlation between serum albumin and visceral protein stores is poor.[8] The 20-day half-life of albumin makes it a poor indicator of early malnutrition. Nevertheless, the serum albumin value, monitored on a periodic basis, remains the most accessible, least expensive, and most widely used biochemical indicator of protein status.

A serum albumin level of 3.0 to 3.5 g/dL is consistent with mild malnutrition; 2.5 to 3.0 g/dL, moderate; and less than 2.5 g/dL, severe.

The *serum transferrin value*, which may be reduced with age, is a useful indicator in acute illness, due to its short (8 to 10 days) half-life. However, transferrin levels are more expensive to obtain than serum albumin levels. Retinol-binding protein and thyroxine-binding prealbumin are sensitive measures of visceral protein status due to their short half-lives, 10 hours and 2 days, respectively, but are expensive and not widely available in clinical settings.

The *serum cholesterol level* has not been routinely used as a nutritional screening parameter. Often, it is low in the presence of protein-calorie malnutrition, which finding has been associated with an increased risk of death within a 1-year period among an elderly, male nursing home population.[52] An elevated serum cholesterol level has implications that will be discussed later in this chapter.

Hemoglobin, hematocrit, serum iron, and iron-binding capacity are commonly used nutritional indicators. A higher proportion of elderly persons have low hemoglobin levels, with anemia present in 12% to 20% of community-living persons.[53] Although most elderly persons have hemoglobin levels in the normal range, some authors have suggested a lower limit of normal of 12 g/dL for both men and women.[53] Among geriatric nursing home patients, anemia is widespread, ranging from 13% to 76%.[26,54] Anemia, lymphopenia, and neutropenia are commonly seen in malnutrition and parallel the depression in bone marrow precursors that accompanies malnutrition.[55] Other nutritional causes of anemia include iron, folic acid, and pyridoxine deficiencies, although a low intake of these nutrients without anemia also has been noted.[26] The incidence of atrophic gastritis increases with age and was found in more than 31% of community-dwelling and institutionalized elderly persons in one study; some persons also had anemia and low serum cobalamin levels.[56] (See also Chapter 26.)

Immunologic changes, including lymphocytopenia and decreased delayed hypersensitivity responses to intradermal antigens, have been observed with advancing age in presumably healthy elderly persons, hyporeactivity to intradermal antigens has been correlated with increased mortality.[57] Similar changes also have been noted in association with a variety of disease states, as well as protein-calorie malnutrition.

Skin testing for delayed hypersensitivity, considered a routine part of nutritional assessment in younger patients, has not been established as valuable for routine screening of nutritional status in elderly individuals. Up to 57% of comunity-living apparently healthy elderly persons in one study had less than two positive reactions to five intradermal antigens.[57] One study of nursing home patients found that 28% of the 227 patients tested had no reaction to any of the seven antigens tested.[54] Skin testing should be performed with at least five antigens before the patient is declared anergic. Nutritional support can improve the lymphopenia, anergy, and decreased bone marrow cell precursors associated with malnutrition.[58] However, anergy may not resolve after nutritional repletion in all elderly patients, perhaps reflecting effects of senescence and not simply malnutrition.[59]

The *total lymphocyte count (TLC)* is a good indicator of protein-calorie malnutrition, and it should be determined routinely as part of nutritional assessment. A TLC ranging from 1,200 to 1,500/mm^3 indicates mild malnutrition; 800 to 1,200/mm^3, moderate; and below 800/mm^3, severe malnutrition.[8]

In summary, nutritional assessment of elderly persons should include the medical and dietary history, physical examination results (including height and weight), functional assessment of capacity for nutrient intake, a complete blood cell count and differential blood cell count, and values for serum albumin, serum electrolytes, calcium, magnesium, and phosphorus.

Routine health maintenance screening for healthy older adults should include nutritional risk factor assessment, with follow-up where needed. Increased surveillance is needed in the perioperative and post–acute illness periods.

Malnutrition

Malnutrition has been documented in 35% to 65% of all hospitalized adults. As the length of hospital stay increases, the likelihood of malnutrition rises from 45% to 75%, due to hypocaloric diets required for diagnostic procedures, underlying illness, and anorexia.[60] Medical care expenditures are demonstrably increased by malnutrition, as are complications of both medical and surgical illness.[61] Among long-term care residents, the prevalence of clinical indicators of malnutrition may be up to 52% and results in increased morbidity, mortality, and medical care expenditures, as well as a lower quality of life.[54]

Malnutrition has been classified according to the primary deficit. When that deficit is one of calories, the result is marasmus, producing depletion of body fat stores; protein stores, including serum albumin, are relatively normal, as are the TLC and skin test reactivity. Kwashiorkor, or protein malnutrition, produces depletion of visceral and somatic (skeletal muscle) proteins, with diminution of serum albumin, the TLC, and skin test reactivity. A mixed picture is often found.

Efforts should be made to identify the sources of nutrient losses and conditions that increase metabolic demands. Marasmus is seen primarily in those situations where there are increased caloric losses, for example, in chronic pancreatitis and steatorrhea. Conditions that impose major metabolic demands increase the risk of protein-calorie malnutrition and include the loss of 10% of usual body weight, a serum albumin level of less than 3 g/dL, draining wounds and abscesses, malabsorption, sepsis, chronic alcoholism, long-term steroid therapy, malignancy, and some antineoplastic drugs.

Nutritional Support

Whenever possible, nutritional support should be initiated early when the patient is at risk of undernutrition, such as after surgical procedures, during exacerbations of chronic medical illness or periods of acute illness, or when drugs with nutrient interactions are started. Although nutritional support often is thought of in terms of enteral tube feeding or parenteral nutrition, nutritional repletion frequently can be accomplished via the oral route, especially when begun early.

Oral supplementation can be achieved inexpensively in the outpatient setting by encouraging the use of protein- and calorie-rich foods, such as peanut butter and cheese. Breakfast consumption should be encouraged in older adults, as many have their highest dietary intakes at this time. Ready-to-eat cereals at breakfast supply most nutrients, including fiber, particularly when milk is used.[62] In persons with milk intolerance, a commercial liquid supplement or a nondairy liquid product may be used. A variety of government-sponsored food programs are available to supplement the diets of low-income elderly persons. The food stamp program allows the purchase of one's choice of foods, but excludes nonfood items; the surplus food distribution program, which has been significantly reduced of late, supplies local food banks with a limited range of foods, including butter, cheese, peanut butter, honey, flour and cornmeal. These can be a significant source of protein and calories for elders on fixed incomes. Congregate meal–dining programs were established as part of the Older Americans Act and provide one hot meal daily to those persons who are able to reach the dining site, usually a senior citizens building, church, or restaurant. Homebound elderly persons may have one hot meal delivered daily to their home through the Meals on Wheels Program.

The addition of oral liquid supplements to a normal diet or a modified consistency diet can improve nutritional status without decreasing appetite. Oral supplements also can be combined with other foods, such as milk shakes or cream soups, to increase their nutrient density. Whenever possible, the patient should

be given the opportunity to taste test the various liquid supplements, to determine the most acceptable product.

Enteral tube feeding is indicated when there is an inability or refusal to eat or to swallow or when there is an inadequate intake in the face of undernutrition. Tube feeding may be performed at home, if the setting is conducive and caregivers are able, or in the institutional setting.

Tube feeding can be used as a supplement to oral intake when undernutrition is present and there are ongoing risk factors for further nutritional depletion. A study of underweight women with hip fractures showed that postoperative supplemental nocturnal tube feeding resulted in an improved nutrient intake, shorter hospital stays, and a decreased time to reach rehabilitation goals.[63]

Nasogastric tube (NGT) feeding takes advantage of normal gastric emptying by delivering a bolus of formula intermittently. Patients who have depressed consciousness, are bedridden, or have a tracheostomy are at the highest risk for pulmonary aspiration, which has been reported in up to 43% of NGT-fed patients.[64] The effects of severe extremity contractures and immobility on aspiration rates have not been defined, but likely are strong as the upright position is difficult to maintain. Complications of the tubes include bacterial sinusitis, parotitis, and otitis media. Most studies of tube feeding come from mixed populations in the acute hospital setting. However, one recent prospective study of 70 elderly tube-fed patients in a long-term care facility reported a 40% 1-year mortality rate in this group of patients.[64]

Nasoenteral (NE) feeding is accomplished by using a smaller bore tube with its tip and feeding ports placed distally, beyond the ligament of Treitz, thus decreasing the risk of aspiration. These tubes can be displaced, and the tubes may migrate back into the stomach, causing aspiration. The NE tube feeding allows continuous infusion of formula into the small intestine by using an enteral infusion pump, at a slow rate so as not to overwhelm the digestive capacity of the small bowel. The continuous delivery of low volumes decreases gastrointestinal symptoms and inhibits obstruction of the tube with clotted formula. However, clotting of formula and tube obstruction are frequent problems that necessitate tube replacement. The small size of these tubes makes accidental tracheal intubation more likely.

Feeding is usually begun at a rate of 50 mL/h, by using a dilute or isotonic formula, and advanced by 25 to 50 mL/12 to 24 h until the appropriate volume is reached. The formula is then adjusted up to full strength as tolerated.

Gastrostomy or jejunostomy feeding is used when tube feedings are expected to be required for more than a month. This route allows for easier nursing care and alleviates the discomfort of the NGT or the NE tube. The percutaneous endoscopic placement of enteral feeding tubes is associated with fewer complications and lower cost than the surgical placement of similar tubes.[65] Although originally begun as a technique for providing enteral feeding in infants, percutaneous endoscopic gastrostomy placement has clearly become an important method of feeding elderly patients with swallowing disabilities.[65] Neurologic and nonobstructive oropharyngeal disorders that compromise swallowing are the most common indications for tube placement. Although it had been hoped that pulmonary aspiration rates would be lower in patients with gastrostomies, studies have shown conflicting results, and it is clear that aspiration still does occur.[65] Another significant complication of long-term gastrostomy tube feeding is stomal leakage of formula and gastric juice. This appears to be more common with surgical gastrostomy and can be managed by using an H_2 blocker to raise the pH of gastric contents that leak onto the surrounding skin and metoclopramide to enhance gastric emptying.[66] The feeding tube must be anchored to the abdominal wall by using tape, a self-retaining outer disk, or another type of tube anchor. Development of granulation tissue at the stoma site is common and can be decreased by anchoring the tube so it does not rotate during manipulation associated with starting feedings and stoma cleansing.

Enteral Formulas

It is unknown if there are age-related differences in the tolerance, absorption, and metabolic responses to enteral formulas. Formula prescriptions are based on nutrient needs, hydration status, underlying illness, and tolerance to formulas once they are in use. Standard formulas provide 1.06 kcal/mL and come in isotonic and hypertonic forms. Isotonic products may be advisable when initiating enteral feeding and in NGT feeding, because gastric emptying is optimal with isotonic solutions. Isotonic formulas also are useful in small-bowel feeding by an infusion pump, as there is less diarrhea than with hypertonic products. When given as the sole nutritional source, in the amounts recommended by the manufacturer, enteral formulas provide 100% of the RDA for protein, calories, and minerals. More concentrated formulas are available that allow provision of nutrients at lower volumes, but close monitoring is required to prevent dehydration. Formulas with higher protein densities are useful in patients with protein-losing states. The use of fiber-containing formulas may improve glucose control in some diabetic patients.

Occasionally, elemental diets are required in patients with Crohn's disease involving the small bowel, short-gut syndrome, enterocutaneous fistulae, and critically ill patients with diarrhea secondary to standard isotonic formulas.

Complications of enteral feeding include nutrient deficiency states, gastrointestinal and metabolic disorders, pulmonary aspiration, and failure to gain weight. Very little information is available on the prevalence of these problems in the long-term care setting; most of the data describe acutely hospitalized patients and do not specifically address the question of age-related differences.

Gastrointestinal problems are commonly reported in tube-fed patients and include diarrhea, vomiting, and constipation.[67] *Diarrhea* may result from a variety of factors, including antibiotics, infectious agents (particularly *Clostridium difficile*), drugs, hypoalbuminemia, and fecal impaction. An elemental diet or albumin infusion may alleviate diarrhea in patients with serum albumin levels below 2.5 g/dL.[68] Rectal examination should be performed to rule out fecal impaction.

Once antibiotic, infectious, and drug-related causes of diarrhea have been eliminated, approaches to management can include switching to an isotonic or fiber-containing formula, slowing the rate, and decreasing the formula volume. However, the latter two actions may result in an inadequate nutrient intake to meet needs. If these measures are unsuccessful, a trial of an antidiarrheal agent should be initiated, by using kaolin-pectin, diphenoxylate, codeine, or tincture of opium.[8]

Vomiting may occur with a rapid intragastric infusion of formula, especially when hypertonic formulas are used. Causes of delayed gastric emptying, such as diabetes or drugs, should be sought and controlled where possible. In addition, some types of gastrostomy tubes may migrate distally, causing a pyloric or small intestinal obstruction. This can be prevented by anchoring the tube to the abdominal wall and by using gastrostomy tubes with an external self-retaining disk.

Constipation may be a problem in some patients, especially those on low-residue formulas. Typically, laxatives or stool softeners are given. However, there is no evidence that stool softeners, such as docusate, are effective in this population, and laxatives can result in significant electrolyte imbalances. Prune juice, given daily or three times per week, can be equally effective in relieving and preventing constipation and is more nutritious and less costly than laxatives or stool softeners.

Metabolic complications of tube feeding include hypernatremia, hyperglycemia, and, most commonly, hyponatremia.[67] Most enteral formulas provide 2 g of sodium or less per day at manufacturers' recommended volumes. It is typical to flush the feeding tube with 100 to 200 mL of water after each feeding and after medications are administered. Excessive amounts of water, especially in those patients with liver, cardiac, or renal disease can lead to hyponatremia, as can simultaneous diuretic therapy. It may be necessary to add sodium chloride to tube feedings or change to a nutrient-dense formula to alleviate hyponatremia. Serum electrolyte values should be monitored periodically.

Aspiration pneumonia poses a major risk to the tube-fed patient, whether an NGT or a gastrostomy tube is being used.[64] Tracheostomy, immobility with inability to maintain an upright position, and delayed gastric emptying all predispose to aspiration. A change in mental status should alert the staff and caregivers to the possibility of pulmonary aspiration.

Failure to gain weight or continued weight loss may result from underlying illness, inadequate tube-feeding prescriptions to meet needs, gastrointestinal or other symptoms that limit the volume and strength of formula used, or malabsorption. Some evidence indicates that older adults have decreased carbohydrate absorptive capacity, although this has not been described in relation to tube feeding.[69] In addition, tube feeding may not evoke maximal pancreatic and biliary secretion.

Total Parenteral Nutrition (TPN)

Elderly persons who are malnourished and require nutritional support are much less likely to receive parenteral nutrition than their younger counterparts.[50] The indications for TPN in elderly patients should depend on the underlying disease, the inability to use the gut for nutrient intake, and the nutrient needs, not the patient's age. The usual clinical situations are infection, postoperative fasting states, and increased protein losses due to bowel disease. Elderly persons with cancer who have a decreased dietary intake and increased fluid and eletrolyte losses due to chemotherapy or radiation therapy should be considered for TPN on the same basis as younger patients. Those with protein-calorie malnutrition who are to receive chemotherapy experience greater bone marrow toxicity and require more intensive nutritional support.

Complications of TPN that may be more likely in elderly persons include hyperglycemia, because of the decline in glucose tolerance with age, and impaired renal function due to high protein concentrations used in the solutions. Careful monitoring of electrolyte and glucose levels, as well as renal function, are imperative. Individualized adjustment of TPN mineral content and trace element supplements is needed, as in young patients.

In the long-term care setting, TPN is seldom used. Most facilities do not have the staffing and cannot provide the monitoring needed for proper management of TPN. Furthermore, inadequate reimbursement for such services has led many facilities to refuse admission to patients receiving TPN.[50]

Stable Healthy Elderly Persons

Healthy ambulatory elderly persons should be advised to eat a variety of foods from the four major food groups, to avoid excessive fat and alcohol, to eat foods high in fiber, and to substitute complex carbohydrates for simple sugars. Breakfast consumption should be encouraged, as should regular exercise. An attempt should be made to provide stable ambulatory or non-ambulatory patients in the institutional, hospital, or homebound setting with the RDA for all nutrients. Meals that are provided in hospitals or long-term care facilities must provide the RDA for all nutrients, as mandated by federal Medicare and Medicaid guidelines and the Joint Commission on the Accreditation of Healthcare Organizations.

The Harris-Benedict equation is used to calculate the basal metabolic rate (BMR) and is based on age, sex, weight, and height. However, it is cumbersome and not used widely by medical practitioners in most clinical situations. Basal energy needs for stable patients who weigh between 60 and 80 kg can be roughly estimated by using the formula: BMR=25 kcal/kg.[8]

About 10% additional kilocalories are added for bedridden patients with minimal activity. It is probably prudent to increase caloric intake somewhat more in agitated bedbound patients or those with hemiballismus, akathisia, and other movement disorders that produce increased activity. Additional energy (10% to 30%) should be allowed for the demands of wheelchair and rehabilitation, physical, and occupational therapy activities. At least 0.8 g/kg/d of protein should be provided, given stable renal function.

Acute Infection

Both energy and protein needs are elevated during acute infection. Fever increases the BMR by 7% per degree Fahrenheit increase over normal. The usual increase in the BMR by 20% to 60% in moderate to severe infection is offset by a decrease in the energy expenditure for activity, which may drop some 25%. Furthermore, malnutrition lowers the BMR by up to 25% after 3 weeks. Thus, even in severe malnutrition with severe sepsis, energy requirements should not exceed 25% of usual needs. An increase in protein allowances should be on the order of 30% during mild infection, and 60% and 100% during moderate and severe illness, respectively.[8] Renal function should be closely monitored during periods of increased protein supplementation.

Decubitus Ulcers

Undernutrition has been recognized as a critical contributor to pressure sores, particularly hypoalbuminemia and decreased zinc and ascorbic acid. Pressure sores also have been associated with hyperglycemia, anemia, and hypocholesterolemia (frequently concomitant with protein-calorie malnutrition).[7,70] Improved healing has been demonstrated following supplementation with protein, zinc, and ascorbic acid, and patients with albumin levels below 3.3 g/dL and total lymphocyte counts under 1,200/mm^3 are candidates for aggressive nutritional intervention.[7,71]

Dementia

Declining dietary intake is common among demented patients, and the ensuing nutritional compromise results in an increased susceptibility to infection, decubitus ulcers, immobility, and other problems. The pathophysiology of a decreased appetite and intake is complex, with memory impairment, disorientation, loss of the significance of food, and impaired judgment all playing a role. In addition, a loss of swallowing reflexes and coordination in some dementing disorders further impair intake. The estimated prevalence of swallowing disorders in various clinical settings has ranged from 25% of patients with stroke in acute care hospitals, to 74% of nursing home patients with feeding disorders.[72] However, it is unknown what proportion of these patients had dementia as a diagnosis, and the studies reported do not focus on the geriatric population. Typical pathologic lesions of the olfactory tract have been identified in Alzheimer's disease, and alterations of taste and smell have been described. A simple strategy for improving food intake may be to liberalize salt and sugar and increase spices in food.

Patients with cognitive impairment may develop swallowing dysfunction during periods of acute medical illness, particularly respiratory disorders. The resulting treatments, including oxygen masks, ventilator support, and frequent use of NGTs or NE-feeding tubes, both mask and aggravate the swallowing dysfunction. Once the patient is stabilized, every effort should be made to restart oral inake, even if supplemental tube feeding is required. The speech pathologist and nursing staff in the acute care hospital setting will be of great value in evaluating the patient, and attempts should be made to restore oral intake, especially if the patient is to be transferred to a nursing home.

There is a growing interest in the increased nutrient needs of patients with Alzheimer's disease who pace or wander. Among patients who walk moderately or constantly, energy expenditures are increased by 600 to 1,600 kcal/d.[73] These patients may lose weight if additional food is not provided, but some are observed to take food from the trays of other patients. Supplemental B-complex vitamins also may be needed, as lower water-soluble vitamin intake has been documented in patients with Alzheimer-type dementia who pace.[73]

Obesity

The most widely used standards for assessment of weights are the 1983 Tables of the Metropolitan Life Insurance Company and the NHANES weight-for-height tables.[74,75] The reliability of these tables, when applied to those persons aged older than 74 years is unclear, as persons above this age were not part of the reference sample. The relationship between mortality and obesity appears to be related to age. While a number of studies have shown an accelerated mortality with increasing weight in younger males, moderately increased weight seems to have a protective effect in elderly persons.[76]

Older obese persons have reduced energy requirements as a function of age, as well as a greater likelihood of reduced physical activity. Their increased fat stores also reduce energy requirements. The problem of obesity in the geriatric patient has not been well studied, and the effects of weight reduction on morbidity, nutritional status, and clinical outcomes are not known. Situations in which weight reduction in those persons greater than 120% over ideal body weight (based on 1983 Metropolitan Life Tables) may be indicated include diabetes mellitus, hypertension, osteoarthritis of the knees and hips, and post–lower extremity amputation. Obese amputees may be hampered in their ability to transfer, and the use of lower-extremity prostheses requires additional energy expenditure, which may be further increased by excessive weight. Caloric restriction below 1,500 kcal/d increases the likelihood of inadequate vitamin and mineral intake, and supplements of water-soluble vitamins should be provided. Use of frequent, small, low-calorie meals may be helpful, especially if coupled with increased exercise.

Atherosclerosis

The risk of atherosclerosis-related mortality and morbidity is clearly increased among younger and middle-aged persons with hyperlipidemia. Most studies of dietary and drug therapy to lower the serum cholesterol level have focused on middle-aged men. The Lipid Research Clinics Coronary Primary Prevention Trial demonstrated the efficacy of cholestyramine in decreasing both the serum cholesterol level and the risk of coronary events. Although one diet trial that involved men aged 54 to 88 years found a reduction in mortality from atherosclerotic disease, total mortality remained unaffected.[77]

The predictive value of the serum cholesterol level in the risk of coronary heart disease declines after the age of 59 years, but still remains significant. In persons aged older than 70 years, the ratio of low-density lipoprotein to high-density lipoprotein cholesterol is of most importance in the risk of coronary disease.

Although the efficacy of drug therapy in lowering the mortality and morbidity associated with hyperlipidemia is unproved in elderly persons, it is not unreasonable to start cholesterol-lowering diets in those persons with elevated levels of total cholesterol and low-density lipoprotein, accompanied by other risk factors for atherosclerosis. A careful balance must be struck between dietary restriction and assuring adequate intake of essential nutrients. Practical dietary measures for lowering the serum cholesterol level are listed in Table 41.4. The desirable level for the serum cholesterol level is under 200 mg/dL and, for low-density lipoprotein, under 130 mg/dL.[10]

Approaches to Dietary Modification in Elderly Persons

Dietary factors that are associated with an increased risk of cardiovascular and cerebrovascular diseases and cancer include excessive consumption of sodium and saturated fat, as well as low consumption of fruits, vegetables, and fiber. While this is generally true, the degree of risk and the potential benefits of risk factor reduction may not be the same for all populations and may be different for the elderly members of various cultural and ethnic groups.

Effective nutrition counseling requires a great deal of skill in communication, patience, general knowledge of dietary practices among different cultural groups, and a willingness to negotiate with the patient to develop a diet that meets nutritional, palatal, and social needs. In no group is this more important than elderly individ-

uals. Food habits are stable behaviors, developed through generations and passed on to individuals. They reflect the manner in which members of a cultural group select, prepare, and consume the available food supply. These behaviors are affected by a wide variety of influences at the societal and individual level, which must be considered whenever attempts are made at starting therapeutic diets. Food preferences in elderly persons take on particular significance during acute illness and at times of loss. Culturally defined food beliefs and values may take precedence over nutrition and health considerations, when elders turn to those food practices that are comfortable and familiar during times of stress. Those persons who would attempt dietary modification in elderly individuals also must have an understanding of the symbolic meaning of food within that culture.[78]

In some situations, the traditional methods of food preparation may be clearly contrary to desired dietary practices. For example, the practice of stewing vegetables with salt pork or pork fat may impede progress toward a low-sodium or low-cholesterol diet. Yet, in the communities in which this practice occurs, the "good cooks" will adhere to these preparation methods, despite nutrition education to the contrary. Strategies for community-wide nutrition life-style change are needed.

Among Asian American, Hispanic, and other ethnic elderly persons, language barriers may pose a major impediment to nutrition education and dietary instruction.[79] Lack of knowledge of traditional foods and preparation methods on the part of nutrition educators, dietitians, and physicians not only impedes appropriate dietary interventions, but compromises the credibility of health professionals' advice. Among immigrants, traditional meal practices, food habits, and beliefs are especially persistent among elderly persons. The prescription of modified diets in elderly persons must be balanced against the adequacy of usual dietary intake and the risk of decreased intake if meals are less palatable. Most dietitians and physicians are trained with and use diet lists of typical American foods and are unfamiliar with how ethnic foods can be exchanged on the list. The role of the dietitian is crucial in instructing patients on dietary modifications that will be compatible with life-style, budget, nutritional goals, and food preferences. It must be borne in mind that food habits become more fixed with time, and dietary modification must be approached with flexibility. Rather than approaching the elderly person with dietary "restrictions," one should attempt to negotiate, by using foods as rewards for compliance with the modified diet. The effects of the increasing level of education and mobility on the food habits of elderly persons also must be investigated to develop rational strategies for dietary

Table 41.4. Dietary approach to hypercholesterolemia.

Approach
Avoid cholesterol-rich foods (egg yolks, organ meats, butter)
Avoid animal fats (remove skin and fat from meat and poultry before cooking)
Substitute soft margarine, skim milk, vegetable oils
Decrease meat intake to less than 8 oz/d
Substitute low-fat cheese (eg, mozzarella)
Eat grains, fruits, vegetables, beans, and cereals
Substitute frozen yogurt for ice cream

intervention in the nation's fastest growing and fastest changing population.

References

1. Harman D. Nutritional implications of the free-radical theory of aging. *J Am Coll Nutr* 1982;1:27–34.
2. Masoro EJ. Food restriction and the aging process. *J Am Geriatr Soc* 1984;32:296-300.
3. Henschen F. Geographic and historical pathology of arteriosclerosis. *J Gerontol* 1953;8:1–5.
4. Food and Nutrition Board. *Recommended Dietary Allowances*. 9th ed. Washington, DC: National Academy of Sciences; 1980.
5. National Institutes of Health, Consensus Development Conference Statement. Osteoporosis. *JAMA* 1984;252:799–802.
6. Clark NGT, Rapaport, JI, DiScala C, et al. Nutritional support of the chronically ill elderly female at risk for elective or urgent surgery. *J Am Coll Nutr* 1988;7:17–26.
7. Constantian MB, ed. *Pressure Ulcers: Principles and Techniques of Management*. Boston, Mass: Little Brown & Co Inc; 1980.
8. Alpers DH, Clouse RE, Stenson WF. *Manual of Nutritional Therapeutics*. Boston, Mass: Little Brown & Co Inc; 1983.
9. Durnin JVGA. Body composition and energy expenditure in elderly people. *Bibl Nutr Dieta* 1983;33:16–30.
10. National Institutes of Health, Consensus Development Conference Statement. Lowering blood cholsterol to prevent heart disease. *JAMA* 1985;253:2080–2086.
11. Willett WC, Stampfer MJ, Colditz GA, et al. Dietary fat and the risk of heart cancer. *N Engl Med* 1987;316:22–28.
12. Hill C, Greco RS, Brooks DL. Alleviation of constipation in the elderly by dietary fiber supplementation. *J Am Geriatr Soc* 1980;28:410–414.
13. Kirby RW, Anderson JW, Sieling B, et al. Oat bran selectively lowers serum low density lipoprotein cholesterol concentrations of hypercholesterolemic men. *Am J Clin Nutr* 1981;34:824–829.
14. Anderson JW, Zettwock H, Feldman T. Cholesterol-lowering effects of psyllium hydrophilic mucilloid for hypercholesterolemic men. *Arch Intern Med* 1988;148:292–297.
15. Kay RM, Grobin W, Track NS. Diets rich in natural fibre improve carbohydrate tolerance in maturity onset non-insulin dependent diabetes. *Diabetologia* 1981;20:18–21.
16. Young VR. Impact of aging on protein metabolism. In: Armbrecht HJ, Prendergast JM, Coe RM, eds. *Nutritional Intervention in the Aging Process*. New York, NY: Springer-Verlag NY/Inc; 1984:27–48.
17. Lindeman RD, Tobin J, Shock NW. Longitudinal study on the rate of decline in renal function with age. *J Am Geriatr Soc* 1985;33:278–285.
18. Tobin J, Spector D. Dietary protein has no effect on future creatinine clearance. *Gerontologist* 1986;26 (suppl):59. Abstract.
19. Barragry JM, France MW, Corless D. Intestinal cholecal-

ciferol absorption in elderly and younger adults. *Clin Sci* 1978;55:2133–2220.
20. Parfitt AM, Gallagher JC, Heaney RP. Vitamin D and bone health in the elderly. *Am J Clin Nutr* 1982;36:1014–1031.
21. Reid JR, Gallagher DJA, Bosworth J. Prophylaxis against vitamin D deficiency in the elderly by regular sunlight exposure. *Age Ageing* 1986;15:35–40.
22. Offerman G, Pinto V, Kruse R. Antiepileptic drugs and vitamin D supplementation. *Epilepsia* 1979;20:3–15.
23. Older MWJ, Dickerson JWT. Thiamine and the elderly orthopaedic patient. *Age Ageing* 1982;11:101–107.
24. Baker H, Frank O Inderjit S, et al. Vitamin profiles in elderly persons living at home or in nursing homes, versus profiles in healthy young subjects. *J Am Geriatr Soc* 1979;27:444–450.
25. Rosenberg IH, Bowman BB, Cooper BA, et al. Folate nutrition in the elderly. *Am J Clin Nutr* 1982;36:1060–1066.
26. Smith JL, Wickiser AA, Korth LL, et al. Nutritional status of an institutionalized aged population. *J Am Coll Nutr* 1984;3:13–25.
27. Carmel R. Pernicious anemia. The expected findings of very low serum cobalamin levels, anemia, and macrocytosis are often lacking. *Arch Intern Med* 1988;148:1712–1714.
28. Garry PJ, Goodwin JS, Hunt WC, et al. Nutritional status in a healthy elderly population: vitamin C. *Am J Clin Nutr* 1982;36:332–339.
29. Newton H, Schorah CJ, Habibzadeh N, et al. The cause and correction of low blood vitamin C concentrations in the elderly. *Am J Clin Nutr* 1985;42:656–659.
30. Jacques PF, Hartz, SC, McGandy RB, et al. Ascorbic acid, HDL, and total plasma cholesterol in the elderly. *J Am Coll Nutr* 1987;6:169–174.
31. Spencer H, Kramer L, Lesniak M, et al. Calcium requirements in humans. *Clin Orthop* 1984;184:270–280.
32. Avioli LV, Calcium and phosphorus. In: Shils ME, Young VR eds. *Modern Nutrition in Health and Disease*. Philadelphia, PA: Lea & Febiger; 1988:142–158.
33. Borchgrevink PC, Jyunge P. Acquired magnesium deficiency and myocardial tolerance to ischemia. *J Am Coll Nutr* 1987;6:355–363.
34. Prasad AS. Zinc in growth and development and spectrum of human zinc deficiency. *J Am Coll Nutr* 1988;7:377–384.
35. Wagner PA, Krista ML, Bailey LB, et al. Zinc status of elderly black Americans from urban low-income households. *Am J Clin Nutr* 1980;33:1771–1777.
36. Bales CW, Steinman LC, Freeland-Graves JH. The effect of age on plasma zinc uptake and taste acuity. *Am J Clin Nutr* 1986;44:664–696.
37. Singer JD, Granahan P, Goodrich N, et al. *Diet and Iron Status: A Study of Relationships: United States, 1971–74*. Hyattsville, Md: US Dept of Health and Human Services, Public Health Service, National Center for Health Statistics.
38. Feller AG, Rudman D, Erve PR. Subnormal concentrations of serum selenium and plasma carnitine in

chronically tube-fed patients. *Am J Clin Nutr* 1987;
45:476–483.

39. Bunker VW, Lawson MS, Delves HT, et al. The uptake
and excretion of chromium by the elderly *Am J Clin Nutr*
1984;39:797–802.

40. Adams CE. *Physician Services in the Long-Term Care
Facility*. Washington, DC: American Health Care Association; 1978.

41. Bowen PE, Mobarhan S, Henderson C, et al. Hypoca-
rotenemia in patients fed enterally with commercial liquid
diets. *JPEN J Parenter Enteral Nutr* 1988;12:485–489.

42. Rodin J. Aging and health: effects of the sense of control.
Science 1986;233:1271–1276.

43. Illinois Dept of Aging. *Elder Abuse and Neglect: The
Illinois Response*. Springfield, Ill: 1987.

44. Henderson CT. Nutrition and malnutrition in the elderly
nursing home patient. *Clin Geriatr Med* 1988;4:527–547.

45. Andres R. Effect of obesity on total mortality. *Int J Obes*
1980;4:381–386.

46. Silver AJ, Morley JE, Strome S, et al. Nutritional status
in an academic nursing home. *J Am Geriatr Soc*
1988;36:487–491.

47. Dwyer JT, Coleman KA, Krall E, et al. Changes in relative weight among institutionalized elderly adults. *J Gerontol* 1987;42:246–250.

48. Friedman PJ, Campbell AG, Caradoc-Davies TH. Prospective trial of a new diagnostic criterion for severe
wasting malnutrition in the elderly. *Age Ageing*
1985;14:149–154.

49. Siebens H, Trupe E, Siebens A. Correlates and consequences of eating dependency in institutionalized elderly.
J Am Geriatr Soc 1986;32:192–198.

50. US Congress Office of Technology Assessment. Nutritional support and hydration. In: *US Congress, Office of
Technology Assessment, Life Sustaining Technologies
and the Elderly, OTA-BA-306*. Washington, DC: US Government Printing Office; 1987:275–329.

51. Michaelsson E, Norberg A, Norberg B. Feeding methods
for demented patients in end stage of life. *Geriatr Nurs
(New York)* 1987;8:69–73.

52. Rudman D, Mattson DE, Nagraj HS, et al. Antecedents
of death in the men of a Veterans Administration nursing
home. *J Am Geriatr Soc* 1987;35:496–502.

53. Centers for Disease Control. *Ten-State Nutrition Survey
in the United States, 1968-1970, IV: Biochemical*. Atlanta, Ga: US Dept of Health, Education, and Welfare
publication HSM 72-8132;1972.

54. Pinchcovsky-Devin GD, Kaminski MV. Incidence of
protein calorie malnutrition in the nursing home population. *J Am Coll Nutr* 1987;6:109–121.

55. Lipschitz DA. Nutrition, aging and the immunohemato-
poietic system. *Clin Geriatr Med* 1987;3:319–328.

56. Krasinski SD, Russell RM, Samloff M, et al. Fundic
atrophic gastritis in an elderly population: effect on hem-
ogobin and several serum nutritional indicators. *J Am
Geriatr Soc* 1986;34:800–806.

57. Roberts-Thomason IC, Whittingham S, Youngchaiyued
U, et al. Ageing, immune response, and mortality. *Lancet*
1974;2:368–370.

58. Lipschitz DA, Mitchell CO. The correctability of the
nutritional, immune and hematopoietic manifestations of
protein calorie malnutrition in the elderly. *J Am Coll Nutr*
1982;1:17–25.

59. Lipschitz DA, Mitchell CO, Steele RW, et al. Nutritional
evaluation and supplementation of elderly subjects participating in a 'Meals on Wheels' program. *JPEN J Parenter Enteral Nutr* 1985;9:343–347.

60. Weinsier RL, Hunker EM, Krumdieck CL, et al. Hospital malnutrition: a prospective evaluation of general medical patients during the course of hospitalization. *Am J
Clin Nutr* 1979;32:418–426.

61. Reilly JJ, Hull SF, Albert N, et al. Economic impact of
malnutrition: a model system for hospitalized patients.
JPEN J Parenter Enteral Nutr 1988;12:371–376.

62. Morgan KJ, Zabik ME, Stampley GL. Breakfast consumption patterns of older Americans. *J Nutr Eld*
1986;5:19–44.

63. Bastow MD, Rawlings J, Allison SP. Benefits of supplementary tube feeding after fractured neck of femur:
a randomized controlled trial. *Br Med J Clin Res*
1983;287:1589–1592.

64. Ciocon JO, Silverstone FA, Graver LM, et al. Tube feedings in elderly patients: indications, benefits and complications. *Arch Intern Med* 1988;148:429–433.

65. Larson DE, Barton DD, Schroeder KW, et al. Percutaneous endoscopic gastrostomy: indications, success, complications, and mortality in 314 consecutive patients.
Gastroenterology 1987;93:48–52.

66. Sriram K, Hammond J. Leakage of feedings and gastric
contents through ostomy sites. *JPEN J Parenter Enteral
Nutr* 1987;10:437.

67. Cataldi-Betcher EL, Seltzer MH, et al. Complications
occurring during enteral nutrition support: a prospective
study. *JPEN J Parenter Enteral Nutr* 1983;7:546–552.

68. Brinson RR, Curtis D, Singh M. Diarrhea in the intensive
care unit: the role of hypoalbuminemia and the response
to a chemically defined diet (case reports and review of
the literature). *J Am Coll Nutr* 1987;6:517–523.

69. Feibusch JM, Holt PR. Impaired absorptive capacity
for carbohydrate in the aging human. *Dig Dis Sci*
1982;27:1095–1100.

70. Verdery RB, Rogers E, Goldberg A. Metabolic profile
and body composition predict decubiti and death in elderly nursing home residents. *J Am Geriatr Soc*
1987;35:89.

71. Pinchcovsky-Devin GD, Kaminski MV. Correlation of
pressure sores and nutritional status. *J Am Geriatr Soc*
1986;34:435–440.

72. Groher ME, Bukatman R. The prevalence of swallowing disorders in two teaching hospitals. *Dysphagia* 1986;
1:3–6.

73. Litchford MD, Wakefield LM. Nutrient intakes and
energy expenditures of residents with senile dementia of
the Alzheimer's type. *J Am Diet Assoc* 1987;87:211–213.

74. 1983 Metropolitan Height and Weight Tables. *Stat Bull
Metrop Insur Co* 1984;64:2–9.

75. National Center for Health Statistics, Carroll AS, Najjar
MF, Fulwood R. Weight by height and age for adults

18–74 years, United States, 1971-74. *Vital Health Stat 11* 1983.

76. Milne JS, Lauder IJ. Factors associated with mortality in older people. *Age Ageing* 1988;7:129–137.

77. Dayton S, Pearce ML, Hashimoto S, et al. A controlled clinical trial of a diet high in unsaturated fat in preventing complications of atherosclerosis. *Circulation* 1969;40 (suppl 2): II-1-II-63.

78. Suitor CJW, Crowley MF. Promoting sound eating habits in different sociocultural situations. In: *Nutrition: Principles and Application in Health Promotion*. Philadelphia, Pa: JB Lippincott; 1984;91–105.

79. Kwan E, Loughrey KA, Brownstein H, et al. Collecting dietary information from non-English speaking elderly. *J Nutr Elder* 1985;5:21–25.

42

Exercise

Eric B. Larson and Robert A. Bruce

Exercise can be considered an important component of overall health promotion. For younger adults, exercise is primarily a recreational activity. Younger adults have considerably more physiologic reserve, in both muscular strength and cardiovascular capacity. Thus, the added strength and capacity provided by the conditioning effect, which results from habitual exercise, is of relatively less benefit for health and well-being. The beneficial effects of exercise for younger persons are most likely to come from cardiovascular risk reduction. Older individuals, by contrast, experience a progressive decline in many physiologic functions, including muscular strength and cardiovascular capacity.[1,2] Habitual exercise, by improving strength and maximum aerobic capacity ($\dot{V}O_2$ max) as a result of conditioning effects, can provide added physiologic reserve as well as enhance well-being by reducing effort and fatigue associated with activities of daily living.[3] Most importantly, habitual exercise in moderation offers the promise of reduced disability and may prolong active life expectancy.[4]

There may be some natural skepticism toward the general topic of health promotion among elderly adults. In particular, shouldn't society concentrate its efforts on the young? Health promotion and risk factor modification unquestionably are important in younger ages, especially efforts to reduce cardiovascular risk factors, early detection of prevalent cancers (breast, cervix, and colon), and correction of behavioral risk factors (especially cigarette smoking and alcohol and substance abuse). The fact that life expectancy at age 65 years averages 14 years for men and 19 years for women is relevant to health promotion in the elderly population.[5] These long periods offer plenty of time for risk reduction and health promotion efforts to provide their beneficial effects. This is particularly important with regard to exercise, where the benefits relate to slowing the rate of declining cardiovascular capacity and muscular strength.[2]

Most older people in advanced countries have grown older during an era when advancing technology at home and in the workplace has promoted a lifestyle characterized by progressively less habitual physical activity. A physically active lifestyle (prior to today's ongoing exercise craze) was usually associated with manual labor, performed by the lower socioeconomic classes, or by the considerable activity provided by raising children. As people aged, they typically became progressively more sedentary. Leisure time was for resting, and heavy physical activity was not viewed as desirable. Thus, it may come as a surprise to many of our older patients when a physician recommends habitual exercise as a "treatment" or means to achieve improved health. Nonetheless, there are compelling reasons to promote exercise and most patients will experience enhanced well-being as a result of the strength and increased fitness associated with habitual exercise.

Exercise and Aging

Dynamic aerobic exercise is commonly defined as the repetitive use of large muscle masses for pleasure or improved fitness and stamina.[3] Aerobic metabolism of muscle increases in proportion to the mass of muscles involved and the intensity of exertion. The functional limits are determined by the body's ability to circulate oxygen and substrates and remove carbon dioxide, metabolites, and heat from the muscles, which is determined by cardiac output and the arterial–mixed venous oxygen (a$-\bar{\text{v}}$ O_2) difference at symptom-limited maximal exercise.[6] Beyond these limits, additional energy for a short interval is achieved by anaerobic metabolism with release of lactate.

A variety of acute changes occur during dynamic aerobic exercise. The circulatory response to dynamic exercise is most prominent in the exercising muscle. Blood flow increases from 4 to 7 mL/100 g/min up to 50 to 70 mL/100 g/min, due to decreased vascular resistance and opening of capillary beds in working muscles.[7] The muscle itself generates adenosine triphosphate (ATP), increases oxygen consumption, and consumes more substrates, especially free fatty acids. Oxygen extraction at the tissue level increases from 5 to 15 mL/100 mL of nutrient flow.[8] Overall, total oxygen uptake increases 10- to 20-fold in well-trained athletes.

Cardiac output increases linearly with oxygen uptake, and heart rate increases linearly with cardiac output.[9] Stroke volume increases to a lesser extent as a result of enhanced systolic emptying. The increase in cardiac output, however, is not sufficient to account for all of the increase in oxygen uptake. Increased extraction of oxygen at the tissue level occurs also.[9]

There is a prominent rise in systolic blood pressure as well as a modest increase in mean arterial pressure. Diastolic blood pressure usually is unchanged or decreases. The vascular beds that are not involved in muscular exercise show increased resistance. In general, venoconstriction occurs in both exercising and nonexercising parts, resulting in increased venous return and thereby contributing to increased cardiac output.[7]

In the working muscle, heat is generated, up to 41°C at maximal effort. A maximum of about 25% of the chemical energy produced is turned into work, 75% is given off as heat and must be dissipated. The most important mechanism for handling excess heat is circulatory; adequate blood flow is required to allow heat to flow from the contracting muscle to the surface for dissipation through the skin. In the lungs, the minute ventilation increases in proportion to the generation of carbon dioxide[8] and aids in heat dissipation.

Most people perform dynamic aerobic exercise repeatedly for a training or conditioning effect. The training effect consists of an increase in the capacity for maximal effort and in circulatory and relative metabolic changes at any given level of submaximal effort. The increase in $\dot{V}O_2$ max that occurs is related to the person's baseline, limitations due to the presence of

any disease, and the intensity and consistency of training.[8] Approximately half the increase is said to occur as a result of peripheral changes, that is, an increase in the capacity of aerobic metabolism and extraction of substrate and oxygen at the tissue level. These peripheral changes include an increased density of mitochondria in the muscle, increased amount of mitochondrial enzymes, and, therefore, an increased capacity to oxidize fat, carbohydrate substrates, and ketones; the amount of myogloblin is increased as is the ability to generate ATP. The net result is an increased capacity for oxygen extraction and a decrease in lactate production during exercise.[10] The other half of the training effect occurs primarily in the cardiovascular system.[8,11] The heart rate and blood pressure are decreased and the stroke volume is increased at any given work level. The increase in maximum aerobic capacity that occurs in conditioning is due to widening the a-$\bar{\text{v}}$ O_2 difference and increasing the stroke volume and cardiac output. Patients with cardiac disease are less likely to experience increased stroke volume with conditioning.

The "therapeutic benefits" of conditioning, however, are probably related not just to increased maximum aerobic capacity; rather, they occur at the submaximal workloads common to everyday activity because of the minor reduction in relative aerobic requirements.[3] With aerobic conditioning, heart rate and blood pressure are proportionately less for any given workload, sympathetic discharge is less, peripheral vascular resistance is less, and the substrate needs of exercising muscle are met to a greater extent by extraction rather than by increased perfusion and perfusion pressure.[8,11] Thus, skeletal muscles are more efficient, and myocardial oxygen requirements are actually less due to the reduction in afterload.

Dynamic exercise may be sustained for hours without fatigue if activity is below 50% of $\dot{V}O_2$ max.[12] To obtain physiologic adaptation, training should begin at lower levels, gradually increasing to 58% to 78% of $\dot{V}O^2$ max or to 70% to 85% of the individual's maximal heart rate.[12,13] Exertion at this level, 20 to 40 minutes three times per week for several weeks, is required for physical conditioning to occur.[12,13] If not maintained, deconditioning occurs. Thus, an active life is necessary to maintain the benefits of such training. When training activities are sustained above 85% of maximal heart rate, the risks of adverse effects are high, especially in persons with coronary heart disease.[14]

Aging alters structures and reduces functions of cells and tissues of all organ systems. The $\dot{V}O_2$ max defines the functional limits of aerobic metabolism and the cardiovascular system which occur with aging.[1,12] (In the absence of bronchopulmonary disease or anemia, neither ventilation nor arterial oxygen content limit $\dot{V}O_2$ max before the cardiovascular limits are obtained.)

Much research has focused on the relationship of $\dot{V}O_2$ max and age. The general results are that $\dot{V}O_2$ max increases with age during growth and in childhood development, reaches a peak with adolescence, and then declines with advancing age.[1,15] The $\dot{V}O_2$ max is higher in men than women, in proportion to differences in amount of skeletal muscle mass. For both men and women, higher values are found in physically active persons compared with sedentary ones. A more appropriate and physiologic measurement involves adjusting $\dot{V}O_2$ max for weight[16] and dividing $\dot{V}O_2$ max in volumes per minute by weight in kilograms. With this correction, the highest value for aerobic capacity is observed during the 1st decade of life, and a roughly linear decline then follows throughout life. The relationship follows the declining maximal heart rate with age.[16]

The rate of decline in $\dot{V}O_2$ max with aging is lower in cross-sectional selective sampling of healthy individuals of different ages than in longitudinal studies of the same persons over time. In cross-sectional studies, the coefficient for this rate of change averages -0.4 mL min^{-1} kg^{-1} y^{-1}, compared with -0.9 mL min^{-1} kg^{-1} y^{-1} in longitudinal studies.[16] When observations were obtained on the same men who remained healthy for several years, this coefficient was about twice that observed for the cross-sectional sample. If the regression line obtained with cross-sectional data is extrapolated to the age at which basal or minimal oxygen uptake is intersected (which represents the minimal aerobic requirement for survival), healthy persons should be living until 110 to 120 years.[12] If the regression line for longitudinal data is similarly extrapolated, it intersects $\dot{V}O_2$ max within 60 to 90 years, which corresponds to the observed survival of healthy persons.[12,16] Actually, the only reliable description of the effects of aging on $\dot{V}O_2$ max is provided by longitudinal measurements in the same persons who remain healthy; such data are difficult to obtain over a period of several decades.[17]

The critical observation with regard to exercise and aging is that the rate of decline in weight-adjusted $\dot{V}O_2$ max with aging is not identical in habitually active men and sedentary men who remain healthy. There are three longitudinal reports of aerobic capacity and aging that provide information on activity status.[16,18–20] Regression lines computed for aerobic capacity and age show a clear separation for active and sedentary men. Moreover, the slopes of the regression lines were remarkably similar for the same categories of men observed in three studies, even though the data were derived from different population samples and with different durations of elapsed time between longitudinal measurements in the same subjects who remained healthy. The slopes of the regression lines calculated from these data were -0.65 ± 1.5 mL min^{-1} kg^{-1} y^{-1}

for physically active men compared with -1.32 ± 0.85 mL min^{-1} kg^{-1} y^{-1} for sedentary men;[16] thus, there is a twofold difference in the rate of decline in $\dot{V}O_2$ max based on habitual activity levels. For men in the 50- to 59-year range, this is equivalent to a 10-year difference in the intersection of the extrapolated regression lines with the $\dot{V}O_2$ max necessary to maintain life (Fig. 42.1).[3,12]

The consequences of a difference in the rate of declining aerobic capacity are obviously important for aging persons. One important consequence is expressed by the concept of functional reserve.[21,22] Functional aerobic reserve can be defined as the amount of reserve between $\dot{V}O_2$ max and the weight-adjusted $\dot{V}O_2$ below which the minimal activity required for survival is no longer possible (3.5 mL/kg/min).[12,21] Figure 42.2 shows that at age 40 years, the difference in rates of $\dot{V}O_2$ max and minimal functional capacity associated with survival (or the functional aerobic reserve) is considerable.[21] Furthermore, the relative difference between conditioned and unconditioned persons is small. As the two curves diverge and one approaches age 60 years, there still is considerable functional aerobic reserve, but the difference between the functional reserves of active and sedentary persons is greater.

By the time a person reaches age 70 years, the functional reserve in the sedentary group becomes much less as aerobic capacity approaches the minimum aerobic requirements for survival, and thus there is more likely to be a clinically significant difference in functional aerobic reserve. The clinical importance of the difference may be manifested as an improved ability to withstand the stress of illness, more rapid recovery from illness or injury, and/or greater likelihood to perform activities of daily living during the course of acute or chronic illnesses.[3,21] These data form the theoretical basis for postulating that aerobic exercise and conditioning may not only prolong life but may also prolong *active* life expectancy[4]—the health benefit most desired by patients.

Exercise Programs for Older Persons

Specific recommendations regarding exercise for older persons should take account of what is presently known. First, habitual exercise in older individuals has been shown to produce a conditioning effect.[23] Second, it has not been shown that exercise in an elderly population prolongs active life expectancy, as suggested earlier in the chapter, or reduces functional impairment.[2,3] The most important concern with regard to the overall health benefits of exercise in older persons is the risk of exercise.[24] That is, except for the risks, exercise is essentially "low cost," should require rela-

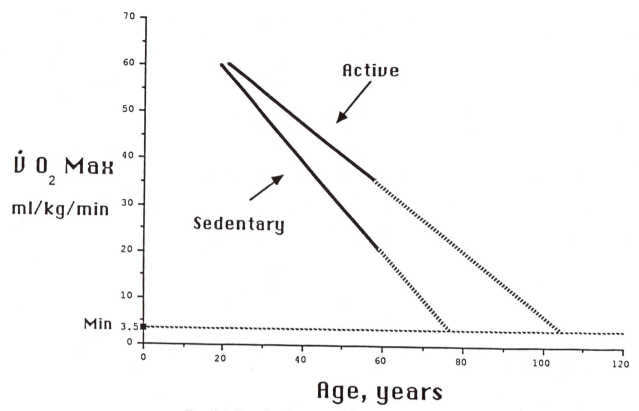

Fig. 42.1. Functional aerobic capacity and age (men).

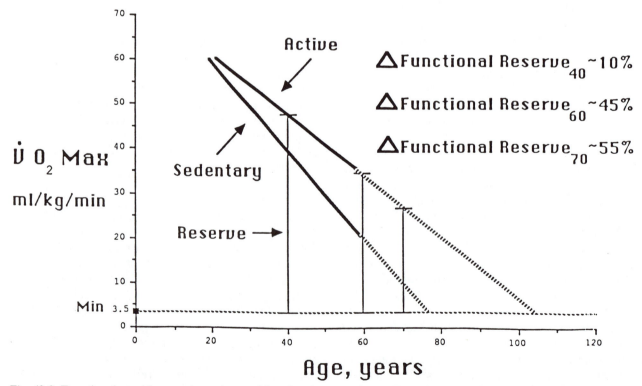

Fig. 42.2. Functional aerobic capacity, aging, and functional reserve (men). From Larson E.B. Health Promotion and Disease Prevention in the Older Adult, *Geriatrics* 1988, 435: 31–38. Reprinted with permission of Edgell Communications.

tively little in the way of health care resources, and, if the individual has time that is not encumbered with other activities (work, raising a family), the marginal cost to the individual of time spent exercising is low. Thus, the key elements to the question of efficacy in older persons are risk and injuries.[24,25]

The hazards of exercise are related to extremes of intensity and duration. When exercise is excessively intense and/or prolonged, extreme fatigue, exhaustion, or delayed recovery is experienced.[26] In addition, more prolonged or intense exercise is associated with increased risk of injury.[27] Other hazards of exercise include hyperthermia, so-called athlete's heart, and, of course, sudden death and nonfatal myocardial infarction.[3] Injuries and sudden death are the most important complications for elderly persons.[3]

The risk of injury has been documented in numerous studies to be directly related to the intensity of training.[3,24,25,27] For example, among participants in the Peach Tree Road Race in Atlanta, there was a nearly linear relationship between miles run per week and the likelihood of suffering an injury in the previous year. At the highest level of training, over 70% of participants had suffered at least one injury the preceding year.[27] On the other hand, studies of a "runners' club" from Stanford demonstrate that habitual exercise need not be associated with increased overall utilization of health services.[28] In this group of patients with a mean age of 58.6 years who ran approximately 27 miles per week, visits to physicians, disability days, and disability levels were more favorable than in a group of community controls. Nonetheless, 35% of the visits to physicians in the runners' club were for running-related injuries.[28]

The risk of sudden death and nonfatal myocardial infarction is quite small, but detectable, during unsupervised activity.[29] Risk factors for sudden death among those participating in exercise programs include attaining a heart rate in excess of 85% of the individual's maximum, marked ST segment depression with exercise despite the absence of chest pain, poor adherence to limiting maximal heart rate, and attainment of above-average $\dot{V}o_2$ max for gender and age due to peripheral mechanisms.[14] Overall, however, Siscovick and colleagues have shown that the risk of primary cardiac arrest in more active individuals is less[29] and that the incidence of primary cardiac arrest attributable to lack of exercise was greatest in older, hypertensive, or obese men.[30]

Thus, any exercise program should be moderate in intensity and duration and should minimize the risks of injury, cardiac arrest, and nonfatal myocardial infarction, as well as excessive fatigue. It is also important to maintain adequate hydration to counteract fluid loss due to sweating.

Four goals should be a part of an exercise program established for older individuals.[21] First, the program should increase conditioning, especially endurance. Second, the intervention should improve muscle strength, especially lower-extremity strength, given the importance of walking to independent functioning. Both of these goals are likely to improve a person's ability to perform activities of daily living, decrease fatigue associated with the day's activity, improve the person's sense of well-being, and perhaps forestall such adverse events as falls by improving muscle strength. The third goal of an exercise program should be to minimize risk, and a fourth goal should be to promote enjoyment without causing excessive fatigue.

The components of the exercise program include two essentials: the first is dynamic aerobic exercise[3,13] in the form of walking, swimming, cycling, jogging, and so forth; the second is a program that promotes lower-extremity strengthening. Also desirable are periods to warm up and cool down and muscle and tendon stretching.[13]

The exercise program should be tailored to the individual. The program should take account of an individual's physical capacities and coexistent disabilities as well as mitigating social, psychological, and economic factors.[13] Among all forms of exercise available to the elderly, brisk walking is perhaps the most ideal and has, in fact, been recommended by a number of groups.[31,32] Brisk walking does produce a training response in older individuals. Physicians and other health professionals should be prepared to give appropriate guidelines for exercise.[13] In particular, habitually sedentary persons may need to be advised of the normal responses to exercise, which include increased heart and respiration rates, mild perspiration, an increased awareness of one's heartbeat, and, at least initially, mild muscle aches. Such responses are normal and do not indicate that a person should stop exercising.[21] The warning signs of *excessive* exercise include severe dyspnea, wheezing, coughing, any form of chest discomfort, excessive perspiration, syncope or near syncope, prolonged fatigue and exhaustion lasting at least half an hour after exercise, and local muscle or joint discomfort. Heart rate guidelines are most appropriate for persons with coexistent cardiac disease. An exercise tolerance test will allow one to calculate the desired heart rate based on the observed or extrapolated maximal heart rate. The desirable heart rate for achieving a conditioning effect is 70% to 80% of maximal heart rate.[12] There also are tables listing average exercise heart rates for various age groups; however, such tables may be less useful given the wide variation in baseline and maximal aerobic capacity seen among elderly persons.

In our own experience, it is perhaps more useful to

teach individual guidelines for pacing. One guideline is the so-called "talk test," in which persons know they are not exercising excessively when they can carry on a normal conversation while exercising. For many elderly persons, a reliable heart rate guide is to aim for an exercise heart rate 15 to 20 beats per minute over their resting heart rate.[33] Most persons who have not exercised excessively will also find that their pulse returns to resting levels or nearly so within 10 minutes after stopping exercise. Finally, it is important to emphasize that exercise for conditioning is not "competition." Many people associate exercise with competition and need to avoid external comparisons. Competitive urges can be focused on the goal of making progress or avoiding decline over time.

Perhaps the most important pacing guide is an emphasis on starting a program slowly and increasing activity by small increments. Many older persons abandon exercise programs because they expect too much too fast, become discouraged, and thereby give up their programs (Table 42.1).

The duration prescribed is driven by the amount of time required to produce the conditioning effect. In general, a minimum of 20 to 30 minutes of aerobic exercise three times per week at 70% to 80% of maximum heart rate is required to achieve a conditioning effect,[3] which will begin approximately 2 weeks after commencing an exercise program. Deconditioning begins as soon as a program is abandoned.

Table 42.1 demonstrates two programs recommended for elderly individuals by advisory groups. Both begin at extremely modest levels (5 minutes of walking three times per week or one quarter mile of walking three times per week) and eventually proceed to a brisk walking pace of 20 to 60 minutes' duration. Programs like this will improve maximum aerobic capacity and may well minimize age-related decline.

Compliance is the major barrier to successful exercise programs for the elderly persons. This is a common issue for many health promotion activities. More research is required to define strategies for improving compliance with habitual exercise recommendations. A related issue is the relative lack of social and community resources for habitual activity. Much of our advancing technology consists of "labor-saving" devices. Especially in our large northern cities, there may be few opportunities and almost no facilities for older persons to get habitual exercise. During the prolonged cold or wet winters, the opportunity for outside activity is particularly restricted. The social issues involved in creating facilities that provide a range of exercises at reasonable costs have yet to be solved. Walking in shopping malls is a solution that works in some communities.

Finally, there is the unsolved issue of whether we should distinguish between the old-old and the young-old in health-promotion activities such as exercise. Little is known or written about exercise in persons over the age of 80 or 85 years—the fastest growing age group in our society. However, as in many other areas of geriatrics, programs should not be guided by simple chronologic age. Functional age and individual abilities are more important determinants of the nature of an exercise health-promotion program.

Table 42.1. Two examples of brisk walking programs.

Week	Program 1,[31] miles of walking	Program 2,[32] minutes of walking
1	¼*	5
2	¼	7
3	½	9
4	¾	11 (approx ½ mile)
5	1	13
6	1	15
7	1 (20 min)	18
8	1½ (30 min)	20 (approx 1 mile)
9	2 (40 min)	23
10	2 (40 min)	26
11	2½ (50 min)	28
12	3 (60 min)	30 (approx 1½ miles)

* Three times weekly. From reference 31. Reprinted with permission.

References

1. Åstrand PO. Physical performance as a function of age. *JAMA* 1968;205:729–733.
2. Larson EB, Bruce RA. Exercise and aging. *Ann Intern Med* 1986;105:783–785.
3. Larson EB, Bruce RA. Health benefits of exercise is an aging society. *Arch Intern Med* 1987;147:353–356.
4. Katz S, Branch LG, Branson MH, et al. Active life expectancy. *N Engl J Med* 1983;309:1218–24.
5. *Aging America, Trends and Projections, 1985–86*. Washington, DC: US Senate Special Committee on Aging, in conjunction with the American Association of Retired Persons, the Federal Council on Aging, and the Administration on Aging; 1986: 498-116-814/42395.
6. Mitchell JN, Sproule BJ, Chapman CV. The physiological meaning of the maximal oxygen intake tests. *J Clin Invest* 1958;37:538–547.
7. Clausen JP. Circulatory adjustments to dynamic exercise and effect of physical training in normal subjects and patients with coronary artery disease. *Prog Cardiovasc Dis* 1976;18:459–495.
8. Wallace AG. Cardiovascular adaptations to exercise. In: Smith LH, Thier SO, eds. *Pathophysiology: The Biological Principles of Disease*. Philadelphia, Pa: WB Saunders Co; 1981:1136–1142.
9. Ekelund LG, Holmgren A. Central hemodynamics during exercise. *Circ Res* 1967;20–21(suppl 1):33–43.
10. Holloszy JO. Adaptations of muscular tissue to training. *Prog Cardiovasc Dis* 1976;18:445–458.

11. Detry JR, Russeau M, Vanderbrouche G, et al. Increased arteriovenous oxygen differences after physical training in coronary heart disease. *Circulation* 1971;44:109–118.

12. Bruce RA. Exercise, functional aerobic capacity and aging: another viewpoint. *Med Sci Sports Exerc* 1984; 16:8–13.

13. Goldberg L, Eliot DL. Prescribing exercise. *West J Med* 1984;141:383–386.

14. Hossack KF, Hartwig R. Cardiac arrest associated with supervised cardiac rehabilitation. *J Cardiac Rehab* 1982;2:402–408.

15. Robinson S. Experimental studies of physical fitness in relationship to age. *Arbeitsphysiologie* 1938;10:251–323.

16. Dehn MM, Bruce RA. Longitudinal variations in maximal oxygen intake with age and activity. *J Appl Physiol* 1972;33:805–807.

17. Bruce RA, DeRouen TA. Longitudinal comparisons of responses to maximal exercise. In: Folinsbee, LA, ed. *Environmental Stress: Individual Adaptations*. New York: Academic Press; 1978:205–224.

18. Dill DB, Robinson S, Ross JC. A longitudinal study of 16 champion runners. *J Sports Med* 1967;7:4–32.

19. Hollman W. *Korperliches Training als Pravention von Herz Kreislauf-Krankheiten*. Stuttgart, West Germany: Hippokrates-Verlag; 1965.

20. Irving JB, Kusumi F, Bruce RA. Longitudinal variations in maximal oxygen consumption in healthy men. *Clin Cardiol* 1980;3:134–136.

21. Larson EB. A general approach to health promotion and disease prevention in the older adult. *Geriatrics*. In press.

22. Williams MA. Clinical implications of aging physiology. *Am J Med* 1984;76:1049–1054.

23. De Vries HA. Physiological effects of an exercise training regimen upon men aged 52 to 88. *J Gerontol* 1970;25:325–336.

24. Koplan JP, Siscovick DS, Goldbaum GM. Risks of exercise: public health view of injuries and hazards. *Public Health Rep* 1985;100:189–194.

25. Siscovick DS, LaBorte RE, Newman JM. The disease-specific benefits and risks of physical activity and exercise. *Public Health Rep* 1985;100:180–188.

26. Bruce RA, Lind AR, Franklin D, et al. The effects of digoxin on fatiguing static and dynamic exercise in man. *Clin Sci* 1968;3:29–42.

27. Koplan JP, Powell KE, Sikes RK, et al. An epidemiologic study of the benefits and risks of running. *JAMA* 1982;248:3118–3121.

28. Lane NE, Bloch DA, Woud PD, et al. Aging, long-distance running and the development of musculoskeletal disability. *Am J Med* 1987;82:772–780.

29. Siscovick DS, Weiss NS, Fletcher RH, et al. The incidence of primary cardiac arrest during vigorous exercise. *N Engl J Med* 1984;311:874–877.

30. Siscovick DS, Weiss NS, Fletcher RH, et al. Habitual vigorous exercise and primary cardiac arrest: effect of other risk factors on the relationship. *J Chronic Dis* 1984;37:625–631.

31. AARP. *Pep Up Your Life: A Fitness Book for Seniors*. Washington, DC, AARP;

32. *Exercise and Your Heart*. Bethesda, Md: National Institutes of Health; 1981. US Dept of Health and Human Services publication.

33. Mielchen SD, Larson EB, Wagner E, et al. *Getting Started: A Guide to Physical Activity for Seniors*. Seattle, Wash: Center for Health Promotion, Group Health Cooperative; 1987.

43

Sleep and Sleep Disorders

Joyce D. Kales, Michael Carvell, and Anthony Kales

Elderly persons frequently complain of problems with their sleep.[1-7] Actually, they often are very concerned about not obtaining enough sleep and/or not feeling refreshed after sleep.[2,4,7] Physicians, however, may feel that some elderly patients are excessively preoccupied with their sleep in a hypochondriacal manner. Thus, not infrequently the elderly's sleep complaints are not given proper attention or are simply dealt with through the hasty prescription of a hypnotic.[2,4] Through such practices, a number of important issues related to the nocturnal as well as daytime life are overlooked, while there is an additional risk of creating certain iatrogenic complications.

The prevalence and intensity of sleep disturbances increases with advancing age.[1,3,4,7] This is due to various factors: physiological, such as age-related changes in sleep patterns; medical, such as more frequent physical ailments and illnesses with symptoms disturbing sleep; psychiatric, including the increased occurrence of affective and organic mental disorders associated with sleep difficulty; pharmacologic, such as use, misuse, and abuse of various drugs directly or indirectly affecting sleep; and social, such as changing rest–activity schedules and consequently sleep–wakefulness patterns.[2-4,8] Thus, there is a need for physicians and particularly those specializing in geriatrics to be aware of the specific characteristics of sleep physiology and pathology in elderly persons, to assess properly the sleep problems of the aged and to effectively treat them. This chapter aims at providing physicians the basic information that will enable them to manage adequately the sleep problems of their elderly patients.

Sleep Patterns and Age

Prior to the modern era of sleep investigations, researchers studying aging focused primarily on the waking individual. Following the discovery of rapid eye movement (REM) sleep[9] and subsequent studies that contributed to our basic understanding of sleep and dream patterns, investigators were provided with a valuable tool for studying an important aspect of the physiology and pathology of aging. Similarly, from a clinical standpoint, physicians have focused much of their attention on a patient's daytime clinical picture and have often neglected complaints of sleeplessness and other forms of nocturnal distress. Much of this neglect relates to a general lack of information about sleep and specifically the misperception that sleep is a fairly uniform, quiescent, stress-free state. We now know that this is not the case. Indeed, research studies have shown that sleep is a complex process. Each night of sleep, which in the sleep laboratory can be demonstrated with objectivity and precision,[10] is characterized by distinct cyclical patterns accompanied by varying degrees of activity in the brain and the body.[11]

Sleep Recording Techniques

The modern sleep laboratory is the ideal setting for the objective assessment of sleep under rigorously controlled conditions.[9,10,12] By having the subjects sleep in sound-attenuated, temperature-controlled rooms, the effects of environmental factors on sleep are minimized. For all sleep laboratory studies electroencephalographic (EEG), electro-oculographic (EOG), and electromyographic (EMG) tracings are recorded (Fig. 43.1). These all-night polygraphic recordings allow for the standardized analysis of sleep and wakefulness patterns on a minute-by-minute basis.

Sleep Stages

In the sleep laboratory, the five sleep stages and wakefulness can be easily identified by characteristic polygraphic patterns. During wakefulness, the EEG pattern is of low amplitude and fast frequency, there are rapid eye movements and eye blinking and a relatively high-amplitude EMG[10] (Fig. 43.2). During the initial transition from wakefulness to sleep, stage 1 sleep usually occurs. It also occurs after any wakefulness during the sleep period. Stage 1 sleep is characterized by slow eye movements; low-amplitude, mixed-frequency EEG activity; and EMG activity which is of lower amplitude than that of relaxed wakefulness. Stages 2, 3, and 4 are characterized by a progressive increase in EEG amplitude and decrease in EEG frequency. During stage 2, sleep spindles (brief bursts of 12–14 cps EEG activity) also occur intermittently. Stages 3 and 4 sleep are often combined and termed slow-wave sleep. During stages 2, 3, and 4, eye movements are absent and EMG activity remains at a lower amplitude than that of wakefulness. Stage 1, 2, 3, and 4 are collectively referred to as non-REM (NREM) sleep.

The overall hypnopolygraphic patterns of REM sleep are distinctly different from the other sleep stages: low-amplitude and mixed-frequency EEG activity resembling that of stage 1; episodic bursts of rapid eye movements; and a markedly reduced level of muscle tonus activity (EMG)[10] (Fig. 43.2).

Sleep Cycles

A young adult's typical night of sleep begins with a brief period of stage 1 followed by stages 2, 3, and 4, respectively[11] (Fig. 43.3). Then the sleep patterns return to stages 3 and 2 and after about 70 to 100 minutes to NREM sleep, the first period of REM sleep occurs. This periodic sequence of sleep stages, ending with a REM period, is defined as a sleep cycle. Averaging about 90 minutes in length, the sleep cycle is repeated four to six times each night, depending on the length of the sleep period which, in turn, changes with age.

While the periodicity of REM sleep is consistent throughout the night, the percentages of sleep stages differ considerably between the first and second halves of the night.[11] As the night progresses, the amount of slow-wave sleep decreases while REM periods increase in length. Thus, slow-wave sleep is more predominant in the first half of the night and REM sleep more predominant late in the second half of the night.[11] For the entire night of sleep, REM sleep constitutes about 20 to 25%; stage 2, 50 to 60%; stages 3 and 4, 10 to

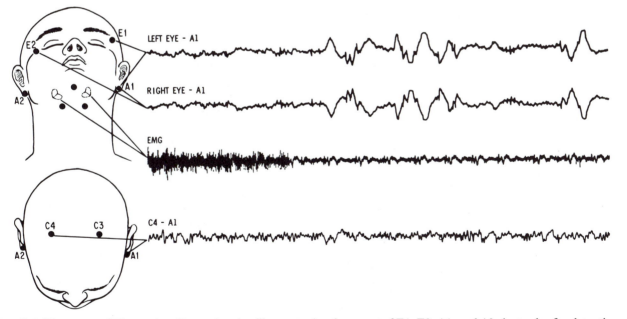

Fig. 43.1. Placement of Electrodes. Upper drawing illustrates the placement of E1, E2, A1, and A2 electrodes for detection of eye movements and also shows two methods for recording tonic EMG from mental and sub-mental muscle areas. Lower drawing illustrates the placement of C3, C4, A1, and A2 electrodes for EEG recording of sleep stages. This epoch illustrates the onset of REM sleep. Note the relatively low voltage, mixed frequency EEG, REMs, and sharp decrease in the tonic EMG. From Bixler & Vela-Bueno, Ref 12

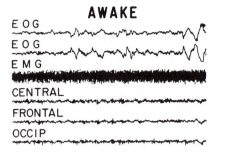

AWAKE

E O G
E O G
E M G
CENTRAL
FRONTAL
OCCIP

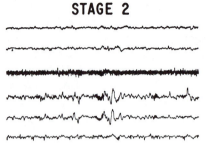

STAGE 2

Fig. 43.2. Stages of Sleep. Notice the high EMG and eye movements during wakefulness, the slow eye movements but absence of EMs during descending stage 1, and REMs with low EMG during stage REM. Stages 2, 3, and 4 are characterized by the slowing of frequency and an increase in amplitude of the EEG. From Bixler & Vela-Bueno, Ref 12

STAGE 1

STAGE 3

REM

STAGE 4

10
$I \mu V$
50
μV

2 sec

20%; and stage 1, 5 to 10% (Fig. 43.3.). In the distribution of wakefulness across an 8-hour nocturnal recording period, the first hour (which includes sleep latency or time to fall asleep) has more wakefulness than any of the remaining seven hours.[13]

Age-Related Sleep Patterns

Age has a number of marked effects on sleep including the length of sleep, its distribution throughout the night, and sleep stage patterns.[13,14] As people grow older they sleep less. The average time spent asleep shortens progressively from 16 hours at birth,[15] to 8 hours in young adults,[13,16] to even less in the elderly.[13,14] However, there is little change in sleep latency across all adult age groups;[13] thus, the increased wakefulness often experienced by the elderly is generally the result of more frequent and prolonged awakenings during the night.[13,14] Sleep distribution throughout the 24-hour period is polyphasic in newborns and infants.[15] From the first year until age 5 or 6, children tend to take one afternoon nap while older children and adults do not regularly nap. With ad-

vanced age, however, napping once again becomes more common.[17]

Even older individuals with no complaint of sleep difficulty have an impaired capacity to maintain sleep. Specifically, in one study,[13] wake time after sleep onset, number of nocturnal awakenings, and both the average duration of these awakenings and final awakenings were all found to be greatest in the oldest age group (50–80 years) when compared with the youngest (19–29 years) and the middle aged (30–49 years) age groups. However, this age-related reduction in sleep efficiency did not appear to involve the individuals' capacity to fall asleep. A number of other studies[14,16,18] have also reported increased sleep disturbance in older age groups in terms of wake time after sleep onset, total sleep time, minutes of total wake time, and number of awakenings.

In regard to sleep stage patterns across the life cycle, REM sleep accounts for about 20 to 25% of total sleep time.[16] In contrast, with age, slow-wave sleep decreases dramatically.[16,19] Children spend about 20 to 25% of total sleep in slow-wave sleep; this percentage begins to decrease in young adulthood and then dimin-

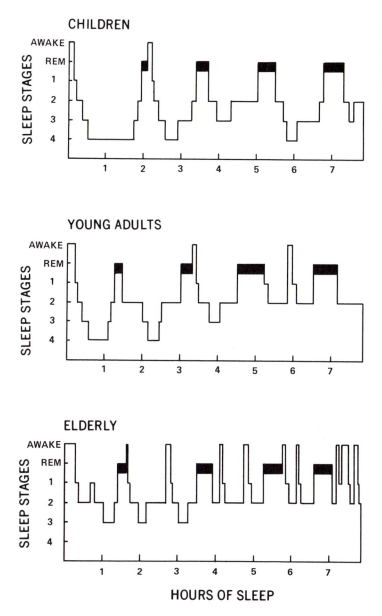

Fig. 43.3. Effects of Age on Sleep. REM sleep (darkened area) occurs cyclically throughout the night at intervals of approximately 90 min in all age groups. REM sleep shows little variation in the different age groups, whereas stage 4 sleep decreases with age. In addition, the elderly have frequent awakenings and a marked increase in total wake time. From Bixler & Vela-Bueno, Ref 12

ishes progressively during middle-age and older years, so that in elderly persons there is little or no slow-wave sleep.

Methods of Assessment

The office assessment of patients with sleep disorders consists of a general medical history and physical examination, a drug history, a thorough psychiatric history, and a comprehensive sleep history.[20] Physicians are well acquainted with these clinical methods except perhaps for the taking of a sleep history. However, provided they have a good knowledge about sleep disorders, they can also be quite effective in assuming this specific task.

Clinical Assessment of Sleep Disorders

The Sleep History

A comprehensive sleep history includes the following components: defining the specific sleep problem, assessing the disorder's clinical course, differentiating between sleep disorders, investigating the family history, evaluating the 24-hour sleep–wakefulness pattern, questioning the bed partner and evaluating the impact of the sleep disorder (Table 43.1).[20] In defining the specific sleep problem for the elderly, it is often important to determine whether a complaint of daytime fatigue, tiredness, or sleepiness is related to poor nocturnal sleep, ie, insomnia, or is a direct manifestation of hypersomnia or excessive sleep. Further, nap taking,

Table 43.1. Guidelines for taking a sleep history.

Define the specific sleep problem
Assess the clinical course of the condition
Distinguish between sleep disorders
Reassess previous diagnoses
Evaluate 24-hour sleep/wakefulness patterns
Question the bed partner
Determine the presence of other sleep disorders
Obtain a family history of sleep disorders
Evaluate the impact of the sleep disorder

From Kales, Ref. 20 & 21.

which is so common in the elderly, should not be confused with hypersomnia.

Assessing the clinical course of sleep disorders can be very helpful in elderly patients.[20] For example, when sleepwalking or night terrors begin suddenly in an elderly person, there should be strong suspicion of some organic factor in the etiology of the disorder. The clinical course of nightmares and night terrors differs considerably; the former are often a chronic or even a life-long problem, whereas the latter may have begun relatively recently.[21] In addition, as will be discussed later, nightmares are relatively easily differentiated from night terrors based on their respective clinical characteristics.

Investigating the family history is helpful in all age groups including the elderly,[20] because patients with certain sleep disorders, such as sleep apnea, narcolepsy, and hypersomnia, as well as night terrors and sleep walking, are likely to have a positive family history of the specific disorders or a closely related sleep disorder.[21,22]

Obtaining a complete 24-hour sleep/wakefulness history rather than simply evaluating only the eight-hour sleep period is of particular importance in the elderly.[20] Often elderly patients complain of severe difficulty with nocturnal sleeplessness; a 24-hour history often reveals that this is related to the practice of taking several naps during the day.[4] In addition, this practice is often associated with low or inconsistent levels of physical activity during the day and irregular schedules including the time for going to bed.

Keeping a sleep diary for 1–2 weeks may be useful in assessing 24-hour sleep–wakefulness patterns.[20] In insomnia, the sleep diary may be helpful in detecting sleep difficulties related to inactivity, daytime napping, and other irregularities in schedules and routines.[4] In disorders of excessive sleep, the diary documents not only symptomatology of the condition but also naps and general activity. The process of keeping a sleep diary can reinforce in some insomniac patients their typical preoccupation with sleeplessness.[4,20] Thus, the use of a sleep diary is generally contraindicated in in-

somniac patients who are obsessive-compulsive or highly hypochondriacal.

Information from the elderly patient's bed partner may provide clinical data that otherwise are unavailable.[20] Whenever a patient presents with a complaint of excessive daytime sleepiness, the bed partner should be questioned to rule out the possibility of sleep apnea.[22] Obstructive sleep apnea is suspected if the bed partner indicates that the patient snores heavily and that there are periodic snorting sounds with intervals of more than 10 to 15 seconds. At times, the frequency and intensity of these snorting sounds may be so disturbing that the bed partner has to move to another room. Because many widowed elderly sleep and even live alone, they can be instructed to ask a relative or friend to observe their sleep on one or two occasions. When such an observer is not available, the patient should utilize a long duration audio recording which is activated just before going to sleep.

While patients with central sleep apnea are less likely to make snorting sounds, other symptoms of sleep apnea may be reported, including choking or gasping during the night, a vague complaint of nocturnal distress, and frequent morning headaches.[22] In these cases, the report of the bed partner or the sleep observer can be most helpful by providing a description of the interruptions of respiration and activity preceding them.[20]

Myoclonus nocturnus[23,24] is another sleep disorder detected most often by the bed partner; or observer who may perceive or complain of jerking movements of the patient's legs during sleep.[20] The jerking movements may distrub the bed partner's sleep to the extent that the partner moves to a separate bed. Finally, because amnesia is characteristically associated with certain episodic nocturnal events[21] such as sleepwalking or night terrors, these disorders are primarily identified by an observer's description.[20]

Medical History

For the elderly patient who complains of sleep difficulty, the medical history is of particular importance. A large proportion of elderly persons have medical problems for which they take medications. These problems or the medications may be a primary cause or a contributing factor to sleep disturbance. Any medical illness associated with discomfort, pain, anxiety, or fear of death may cause insomnia[4] (Table 43.2). In old age, the prevalence of various cardiovascular, respiratory and gastrointestinal disorders, arthritis, cancer and other physical diseases increases dramatically. Therefore, the elderly who present with sleep complaints should be carefully scrutinized for the presence of medical illness.[20] In the case of cardiovascular disorders, sleep may be disrupted by pain, fear, or impaired respiration.

Table 43.2. Medical conditions associated with sleep disturbance.

Cardiovascular Disorders
    Coronary insufficiency
    Left ventricular failure
    Cardiac arrhythmias
Pulmonary Disorders
    Chronic obstructive pulmonary
        disease
    Asthma
    Sleep apnea
Gastrointestinal Disorders
Chronic Renal Insufficiency
Eating Disorders
    Anorexia nervosa
    Obesity
Endocrine Conditions
    Thyroid dysfunction
    Pregnancy
Neurologic Conditions
    Headaches
    Parkinson's disease
    Thalamic lesions

From Kales & Kales, Ref. 4

In chronic obstructive pulmonary disease, sleep is disrupted not only by breathing difficulty but also by the medications used, which can cause anxiety and stimulation.

Because there is always an emotional response to a disease process the physician should assess both physical and emotional factors when a medical condition is associated with a sleep problem. The pain and discomfort of arthritis, neurogenic pain, and various types of headache often contribute to insomnia.[4] The pain experienced during the day in these conditions may be intensified at bedtime, since environmental stimuli diminish and attention is focused internally.

Post-stroke patients as well as those suffering from other neurologic disorders[25] often display a considerable degree of anxiety, which interferes with their sleep; in addition the brain lesion may affect directly the sleep–wakefulness cycle. Elderly patients with malignancies, in addition to dealing with pain, are often overwhelmed with fear and anxiety over the ultimate consequences of their illness.[4] Similarly, patients with angina pectoris or cardiac arrhythmias often fear going to sleep because of a possible attack during the night, when they feel most vulnerable and helpless.[4] Nocturia is a very common cause of sleep disruptions in elderly persons,[26] who have more difficulty getting back to sleep than younger individuals. Secondary enuresis in the elderly often is associated with a condition such as diabetes or a genitourinary tract infection, or it may be due to urinary incontinence, which is common in the

elderly and related to prostatic disorders, cystocele, loss of sphincter control, or regression secondary to dementia.[27] Another common cause of sleep disturbance in elderly persons is musculoskeletal disease, such as fibromyalgia.[28,29]

Obstructive sleep apnea may be caused by oropharyngeal lesions and central sleep apnea is sometimes associated with central nervous system pathology.[30,31] Thus, a careful investigation for a primary condition should be regularly undertaken in the elderly patient with sleep apnea. Further, the medical work-up of patients suspected of having sleep apnea should assess for the presence of cardiovascular problems, because these complications in the sleep apnea patient may be related to increased mortality.[32]

Drug History

A careful drug history[20] is in order whenever evaluating an elderly sleep disorders patient. It is well established that a variety of medications can disturb sleep[4] (Table 43.3). With some of them, such as the stimulants and energizing antidepressants, this effect is expected, particularly when they are taken close to bedtime even in therapeutic doses. With some other drugs, such as the steroids and certain beta adrenergic blockers, the sleep disturbing effect is an unexpected side effect.[4] In the case of beta blockers, those which are highly lipophilic and thus readily cross the blood–brain barrier (eg, propranolol) often cause insomnia and may cause hallucinations and vivid dreams, whereas those which are not lipophilic (eg, nadolol) not only do not disturb sleep but may even have a slightly sleep enhancing effect.[33] Finally, antiparkinsonian medication may cause agitation and hallucinations.

Rebound insomnia may accompany the withdrawal of relatively low doses of short- or intermediate-acting

Table 43.3. Drug-induced insomnia.

Drug Administration
    CNS stimulants
    Steroids
    Bronchodilators
    Beta-blockers
    Methyldopa
    Rauwolfia
    Energizing antidepressants
    Methysergide
    Short half-life benzodiazepines
Drug Withdrawal
    Non-benzodiazepine hypnotics
    Short and intermediate half-life
        benzodiazepines

From Kales & Kales, Ref. 4

benzodiazepine agents,[34] while withdrawal of high doses of non-benzodiazepine hypnotics may cause both insomnia and nightmares.[35] Excessive daytime sleepiness, which can be mistaken for the sleep attacks of narcolepsy, may occur with certain central nervous system depressants, such as hypnotics and sedating antidepressants, especially with inappropriate dosage or scheduling.[20]

Large quantities of coffee or cola taken close to bedtime may also cause difficulty in falling asleep,[36] whereas excessive use of alcohol leads to rapid induction of sleep but, as the drug wears off quickly, to difficulty in staying alseep.[37] Also cigarette smoking is associated with sleep difficulty, while discontinuation of smoking leads to improvement of sleep.[38]

Psychiatric History

In elderly persons, psychologic difficulties are the most frequently associated factor in insomnia. In evaluating for psychologic factors, the physician should be alert to interpersonal difficulties. Marital problems are commonly related to insomnia because poor sleepers are frequently unable to express their feelings and consequently have unsatisfactory interpersonal relationships.[4,39] A person who anticipates problems with sexual performance, as is often the case with the aged, may consciously or unconsciously delay going to bed to avoid sexual relations, and unwittingly create a sleep problem. With advancing age the likelihood of losses of significant others, employment and social status, various sources of narcissistic gratifications, and physical strength and vigor increases. This awareness of loss, along with approaching death, contributes to emerging anxiety and fear, which interfere with sleep quantity and quality and may lead to disturbing dreams.

Determining whether sleep difficulty is associated with psychiatric problems is important.[20] Disturbed sleep, particularly insomnia, is common in many psychiatric conditions, including anxiety states, depression, mania, acute schizophrenia, and organic mental disorders.[40] Of these conditions, depression and organic mental disorders are frequent causes of sleep difficulty in elderly persons.[2] In depressed elderly patients, early morning awakening is the symptom more consistently related to the degree of depression.[41] In contrast, in obsessive-compulsive elderly patients a special problem is difficulty falling asleep. These patients ruminate about their sleep and at bedtime are obsessed with efforts to get to sleep. Actually, by trying to force sleep, performance anxiety occurs and the patient becomes hyperaroused.[4,39]

Elderly patients who have nightmares should be evaluated for underlying psychopathology. They should also be carefully questioned regarding use of medications whose administration (eg, low doses of thioridazine) or withdrawal (eg, from high doses of barbiturates) may lead to increased dreaming and nightmares. Personality patterns of adult nightmare sufferers typically show distrustfulness, alienation, and a chronic schizoid pattern of adjustment.[21] Sleepwalking or night terrors are uncommon in the elderly. When sleepwalking or night terrors have developed recently, the possibility of an organic mental disorder should be carefully scrutinized.[2]

Laboratory Assessment of Sleep Disorders

The sleep laboratory serves as a valuable tool for the study of normal sleep and sleep disorders.[42] Existing clinical information often enables physicians in office practice to recognize specific sleep disorders and to design a treatment approach. When necessary, the physician can recommend diagnostic recordings in the sleep laboratory.

Thorough assessment in the office setting usually suffices for the proper diagnosis and treatment of most sleep disorders by the primary care physician.[20–22] The most notable exception is sleep apnea, a life-threatening nocturnal breathing disorder.[22] Although the physician in the office setting can elicit information strongly suggestive of sleep apnea, sleep laboratory recording is indicated to establish the diagnosis, quantify the severity, and recommend effective treatment. Appropriate use of the sleep laboratory for a number of specific diagnostic purposes is detailed in the following discussion.

Sleep Apnea

The syndrome of sleep apnea is associated with high morbidity because of its pulmonary and cardiovascular sequelae.[22,30,31] Thus, there is a need for prompt and effective evaluation and treatment. When the patient presents with excessive daytime sleepiness, sleep attacks, or unusual snorting or gasping sounds during sleep, the diagnosis of sleep apnea should be suspected. The bedpartner or an observer of the patient's sleep is usually able to confirm the presence of interrupted nocturnal breathing with or without associated snoring, gasping, or gurgling sounds, and morning headache.[20,22] The type of snoring associated with sleep apnea is characteristic: there are periods of breath cessation greater than 10 seconds in duration followed by very loud snorting sounds of about two to four seconds' duration each. Common snoring typically is softer, fluctuates in intensity, and is continuous.[31]

A report of loud snoring especially in patients who are obese or hypertensive also should cause the physician to suspect sleep apnea.[22] Once sleep apnea is suspected clinically, a sleep laboratory recording is in order to determine the type and severity of the condition. There are three types of sleep apnea: central, obstructive, and mixed.[22,30,31] During periods of central apnea, the respiratory center fails to initiate respiratory movements with a cessation of airflow. During periods of obstructive apnea, there is a blockage of airflow in the upper airway despite the presence of respiratory movements.

A thorough sleep laboratory evaluation of a patient suspected of sleep apnea consists of continuous all-night recordings of: standard hypnopolygram (electro-encephalogram, electromyogram, and electrooculogram); the upper airway airflow through nasal and oral thermocouples; and the thoraco-abdominal movements through strain gauges.[42] A sleep apneic event is defined as a complete cessation of airflow lasting at least ten seconds. The diagnosis of sleep apnea is made when there are 30 or more apneic episodes during a night's sleep or an apnea index (the number of events per hour of sleep) of 5 or more.[43] Arterial oxygen saturation (Sao_2) is also measured continuously through an ear oximeter. Finally, an electrocardiogram is routinely recorded throughout the night to detect cardiac abnormalities.

Narcolepsy

The prevalence of narcolepsy is estimated to be one of every thousand persons and is about the same in men and women.[22] The diagnosis is established relatively easily when, as is most often the case, the characteristic irresistible sleep attacks are associated with one or more of three auxiliary symptoms—cataplexy, hypnagogic hallucinations, and sleep paralysis. Studies have shown that the symptom of cataplexy, sudden loss of muscle tone, is pathognomonic or narcolepsy. Thus, for patients with this symptom, diagnostic sleep laboratory recordings are generally of limited usefulness.[22] Because the condition of narcolepsy usually has its onset early in life, the vast majority of elderly narcoleptics have already developed cateplexy and, therefore, are less likely to need a sleep laboratory assessment.

When monitored in the sleep laboratory, narcoleptic patients, particularly those with cataplexy, frequently show the presence of a REM period at sleep onset.[22,42] Thus, in these patients the normal sequence of sleep stages following sleep onset is altered in that the first sleep cycle does not start with a period of 70–100 minutes of non-REM sleep. In addition, narcoleptic patients show a very short sleep latency and an increased amount of wake time after sleep onset. The same abnormalities are seen in daytime naps of narcoleptic patients.

Restless Legs and Nocturnal Myoclonus

Elderly persons are particularly vulnerable to various illnesses, such as diabetes mellitus and renal insufficiency, which may give rise to the syndrome of restless legs.[24] This syndrome not only manifests itself during the day but it is quite disturbing at night, frequently interfering with the patient's getting to sleep. A thorough clinical assessment usually suffices for the detection of the syndrome. However, in certain ambiguous cases a sleep laboratory recording may be needed to confirm the diagnosis.

Nocturnal myoclonic activity and the condition of nocturnal myoclonus[23,24] are observed with about the same prevalence in insomniac patients and non-insomniac subjects.[44] Thus, its etiologic relationship to insomnia is questionable and routine laboratory recordings to rule out nocturnal myoclonus in insomniac patients is not warranted. Actually, it has been proposed that myoclonus is an epiphenomenon of insomnia rather than an etiologic factor.[24] However, whenever the patient or bed partner has a major complaint of nocturnal activity resembling nocturnal myoclonus, the condition should be investigated in the sleep laboratory to establish the diagnosis.

Parasomnias

Among episodic manifestations during sleep, sleep-walking and night terrors in the elderly are of particular clinical significance. If they have been present since childhood or adolescence, they should be considered as evidence of long-lasting psychologic disturbance.[21] If these conditions have developed in older age, especially abruptly, they are most likely related to the presence of an acute brain lesion (eg, ischemia or tumor).[2,25] In such cases, a careful medical workup, including clinical EEG recording and a CAT scan, is necessary. If these tests are inconclusive regarding the nature of the patient's pathology, a sleep laboratory recording using a clinical EEG montage is in order to provide information on brain function during an episode.

Sleep Disturbances And Their Management

Nocturnal Confusional Episodes

Nocturnal confusional episodes are not infrequent in the elderly and often indicate an acute or chronic organic brain dysfunction.[2,45] These episodes are characterized by wandering, disorientation, agitation, or delirium and often are difficult to differentiate from sleepwalking and night terror events. The development of confusion and delirium in the elderly may be facilitated by the presence of medical illness, overmedication, sensory deprivation, immobilization, and sleep loss, all of which are common in the elderly.[2]

Appropriate treatment of nocturnal confusional episodes begins with the identification of underlying organic factors.[2,45] Behavioral and environmental interventions are readily implemented and are effective ways to manage these episodes.[2,4] Reduction of confusing stimuli is best accomplished by maintaining familiar surroundings and minimizing change. Because darkness may facilitate the occurrence of illusions and hallucinations due to impairment of the visual integrative process, use of a nightlight may be helpful.[2]

A thorough drug history begins the pharmacological management of nocturnal confusional episodes in elderly persons and is the most effective means of identifying any excessive or nonessential medication and implementing its gradual reduction and elimination.[2,45] In some cases, psychotic-like behavior may actually be reversed with the discontinuation of some medications. Barbiturate sedatives and hypnotics may further depress the CNS causing mood disorientation and confusion and thus should be avoided.[4] In addition, rapidly eliminated benzodiazepines are contraindicated for this condition, as their rapid removal from the body may lead to rebound phenomena.[34] These drugs may also paradoxically excite an already impaired patient through the mechanism of disinhibition.[46] High-potency antipsychotics (haloperidol and thiothixene) in low doses are the drugs of choice for reducing confusion, agitation, and delirium.[2,4] This in turn promotes sleep through reduction of the patient's anxiety, agitation, perceptual impairment, and wandering behavior. The improved sleep in turn further reduces the symptoms of the confusional state.[2,45]

Medication-Induced Sleep–Wakefulness Disturbances

Certain drugs can cause insomnia either while they are being taken or after their withdrawal while other drugs may cause excessive daytime sleepiness (Table 43.3).[4] Because the prevalence of illnesses is higher in elderly persons, they are more likely to be taking various medications that may cause either insomnia or excessive daytime sleepiness. Additionally, the elderly are generally more vulnerable to the CNS effects and side effects of various medications.[47] Their capacity to metabolize and eliminate drugs is impaired compared to that of younger age groups, which results in protracted and more intense drug action. Also, they more often take multiple drugs which may result in altered pharmacokinetics.

Insomnia may be a consequence of certain drugs' direct effects on the CNS. For example, amphetamines and other CNS stimulants may cause insomnia particularly if they are taken close to bedtime.[4] Other drugs can cause insomnia through their side effects. Drugs used in the treatment of hypertension, such as methyldopa and rauwolfia, frequently produce insomnia.[4] Also, certain beta blockers have been associated with insomnia, vivid dreams, nightmares, and other central nervous system (CNS) side effects.[4] The occurrence of these CNS side effects appears to be related to the drug's capacity to enter the CNS; this, in turn depends on the drug's degree of lipid solubility.[33] It has also been suggested that the occurrence of sleep disturbances with beta blockers might be related to their intrinsic sympathomimetic activity, or partial agonist effect, and to central beta-blockade. Thus, beta blockers with a high degree of lipid solubility and intrinsic sympathomimetic activity, such as propranolol and pinodolol cause insomnia, whereas nadolol, which has low lipid solubility and no intrinsic sympathomimetic activity, does not have a sleep disrupting effect and actually may slightly enhance sleep.[33]

Methysergide, a serotonin-blocking drug that is used to prevent severe migraine, causes side effects of overstimulation and insomnia.[4] Because of their stimulant effects on the CNS, the bronchodilating drugs, which contain ephedrine, theophylline, and norepinephrine, also can lead to sleep difficulties.[4] Other drugs that may cause insomnia are the monoamine oxidase inhibitors used in the treatment of depression, as well as stimulating tricyclic antidepressants (imipramine and protriptyline), and second generation antidepressants, such as nomifensine.[4] In contrast, the sedating tricyclics, such as amitriptyline and doxepine, may cause excessive daytime sleepiness, particularly during the initial period of their administration. Sedating effects of tricyclics may be additive to those of other sedatives, especially alcoholic beverages. Patients taking tricyclic medication should be warned that concomitant use of alcohol may lead to impairment of their ability to drive a car and operate machinery.[4]

The stimulant properties of caffeine in coffee and colas should not be overlooked. Use of caffeine may prolong the time needed to fall asleep and increase wakefulness during the night.[36] Cigarette smoking also disturbs sleep. This is likely a result of increased levels of epinephrine. Thus, people who smoke on a regular basis often sleep poorly and when they stop smoking their sleep can improve considerably.[38]

Depending on their pharmacokinetic profile, benzodiazepine hypnotics may produce either excessive daytime sleepiness (slowly eliminated benzodiazepines) or actually disrupt sleep later in the night (rapidly eliminated benzodiazepines).[4] The more slowly eliminated drugs, such as flurazepam, at higher thera-peutic doses are more likely to accumulate and produce carryover sedation the day following their bedtime ad-ministration, which may result in daytime performance decrements[48] such as disturbances in eye/hand coordi-nation and gait. This is particularly true for elderly persons and thus these drugs should be prescribed at the lowest effective dose and used on an intermittent as-needed basis.

With the rapidly eliminated benzodiazepine drugs, such as triazolam, common side effects are early morn-ing insomnia during drug administration and rebound insomnia following drug withdrawal.[34] Early morning insomnia is a significant increase in wakefulness during the final hours of a nocturnal sleep period that follows the use of a rapidly eliminated hypnotic.[49] This side effect occurs even under the conditions of taking sin-gle, nightly doses for only relatively short periods. Early morning insomnia typically appears after the drug has been taken nightly for relatively short-term periods, when tolerance begins to develop and the drug's effectiveness begins to wear off. As tolerance develops to the hypnotic efficacy of the rapidly elimi-nated drug, sleep generally continues to be improved during the first two-thirds of the night, but it worsens significantly during the last third of the night.[49] Early morning insomnia may not be specific to benzo-diazepines, because it is known that other rapidly elim-inated drugs, such as alcohol, can disrupt sleep.[37] Therefore, special attention should be given to patients who may be using alcohol in addition to hypnotics. Daytime anxiety is a corollary of early morning insom-nia; it consists of an increase in levels of tension and anxiety on days following nights of drug administra-tion.[49]

Rebound insomnia is a specific type of insomnia that follows withdrawal of benzodiazepine drugs with short or intermediate half-lives.[34] When these drugs are withdrawn, nocturnal wakefulness can increase markedly above baseline levels, even under the condi-tions of taking single, nightly doses for only short pe-riods. The frequency and intensity of rebound insom-nia are strongly and inversely related to the half-life of the drug. With short half-life benzodiazepines, rebound insomnia occurs frequently and is severe in intensity.[34] With benzodiazepines of intermediate half-life, rebound insomnia often occurs following withdrawal and is of moderate intensity. Withdrawal of ben-zodiazepines with a long half-life seldom produces withdrawal sleep disturbance. Following withdrawal of benzodiazepines with short elimination half lives and parallel to the development of rebound insomnia, daytime anxiety often rises above baseline levels.[34] This increase in anxiety has been termed rebound anxi-ety. Because benzodiazepine hypnotics with relatively

short half-lives produce frequent and severe rebound phenomena both during administration and especially following withdrawal, these drugs may have a greater potential than intermediate or long half-life ben-zodiazepine hypnotics for reinforcing drug-taking be-havior and eventually leading to hypnotic drug depen-dence.[34]

It should be noted that rebound phenomena have recently been reported to occur with benzodiazepine anxiolytics.[50] Similar to their hypnotic counterparts, benzodiazepine anxiolytics with shorter elimination half-lives, such as lorazepam and alprazolam, are more likely to cause rebound phenomena when compared with the more slowly eliminated drugs, such as di-azepam.

It is important to note that rebound insomnia cannot be avoided simply by using a lower dose of a short elimination half-life benzodiazepine. In one study, the dosage of triazolam was only 0.25 mg hs.[51] While the drug was not clearly effective during its administration, following withdrawal there was a significant degree of rebound insomnia.

Behavioral side effects of benzodiazepines, such as memory impairment, delusions, and confusional states are also more prevalent with relatively low doses of rapidly eliminated anxiolytics (alprazolam and lor-azepam)[50] and hypnotics (triazolam).[51] These side ef-fects are even more frequent in elderly persons, who are generally more sensitive to drug action. For exam-ple, in a recent report, five men, aged 66 to 78 years, without neurologic abnormalities, developed gross confusion with agitation and disinhibition after taking a lower dose of triazolam (0.125 mg or 0.25 mg).[46]

Restless Legs Syndrome and Nocturnal Myoclonus

The restless legs syndrome and nocturnal myoclonus are conditions that appear to overlap and thus may occur together. Typically, the patient is well aware of the symptoms of restless legs, which consist of pares-thesia-like feelings deep within the lower extremities and the unpleasant subjective need to rub or move the limbs.[24] However, it is the bedpartner who usually complains initially of the jerking and kicking move-ments of nocturnal myoclonus. With advancing age, the resltess legs syndrome is more frequent, and the condition occurs more often in those patients who also have diabetes, hypoglycemia, chronic venous insuffi-ciency, uremic neuropathy, prostatitis, vitamin and iron deficiency, or drug withdrawal.[53] Characteris-tically, elderly individuals with the restless legs syn-drome may have difficulty falling alseep. Aside from efforts to treat an identifiable underlying cause, a more general and effective therapy for the restless legs syndrome has yet to be determined.[2]

Nocturnal myoclonus consists of rhythmic and involuntary nonepileptiform periodic jerking or twitching movements of the limbs while falling asleep and during sleep.[23,24] Nocturnal myoclonic activity often is associated with chronic renal insufficiency, sleep apnea, and the use of tricyclic antidepressants.[2,54] Nonetheless, nocturnal myoclonus is also seen in 6% of normal individuals.[44] Although this nocturnal phenomenon has been found to be positively correlated with increasing age, as is insomnia, the clinical relationship between these two conditions is ill defined. Results of a well-controlled study indicate that nocturnal myoclonus occurs at about the same frequency among insomniacs and normal sleepers.[44]

Sleep Disorders And Their Management

Insomnia

The prevalence of complaints of insomnia is high among aged persons.[1,4] Their sleep habits change considerably compared to earlier years (Table 43.4), and most elderly individuals adapt readily to these changes. However, more than any other age group, older persons, especially women, are likely to complain of insomnia.[1,4,6]

Many age-related changes in sleep habits appear to be more a reflection of changes in lifestyle than due to physiologic factors.[2] Specifically, with aging comes retirement or curtailment of work schedules, restructuring of daily routines, and perhaps changes in living arrangements. No longer are sleep habits dictated by the needs of family or employment. With this lessening of daily life structure, the elderly individual may develop a tendency to nap during the day, making nighttime sleep more difficult.[2,4] The problem may be exacerbated by the fact that older individuals are more easily aroused by external stimuli than are the young. Therefore, nighttime may become a particularly anxiety-filled, restless period, especially for elderly individuals living in unsafe neighborhoods or in hospitals and nursing homes, where they experience many sleep disruptions and little privacy.

Regardless of age, insomnia often is associated with pain, discomfort, fear, anxiety or depression.[4,21] In the elderly insomniac, multiple factors (physical, psychological, social) are usually present in cominbation and, therefore, it is often difficult to determine their relative contribution. Among these multiple factors for the development of insomnia in the elderly, special attention should be given to multiple and often serious physical illnesses.[2] Although it is at times difficult to separate

Table 43.4. Insomnia in elderly persons: etiology and treatment.

Age-Related Sleep Cycle Changes
  Educate the patient regarding expected disruptions of sleep-wakefulness patterns with advancing age
  Discourage multiple naps
  Suggest activities, hobbies, and special interests
Situational Stress
  Explain association between stress, arousal, and sleeplessness
  Provide time-limited supportive psychotherapy and behavioral modification measures
Physical Pain/Discomfort
  Treat physical disorders when present
  Provide symptomatic relief for itching, chronic discomfort, or acute pain
Anxiety
  Explore underlying fears
  Encourage appropriate ventilation of conflicts and anger
  Maintain emotional support while providing psychotherapeutic insight
  Recommend relaxation exercises
  Avoid the chronic use of hypnotic medications
Affective Disorders
  Distinguish between dysthymia and major depression
  Identify and explain maladaptive cognitive patterns and negative thinking
  Prescribe sedating antidepressants at bedtime for major depression
Drug-Induced Sleep Disturbance
  Discourage use of caffeine, alcohol, and cigarettes
  Gradually reduce and eliminate nonessential drug intake
  Prescribe hypnotic medication adjunctively and select for efficacy and minimal withdrawal effects
Acute/Chronic Confusional States
  Identify and treat underlying organic illness
  Provide behavioral support and familiar environmental cues
  Judiciously prescribe high-potency, low-dose antipsychotics

From Cadieux, Ref. 2

physical illness from the corollary factors, it is important to give priority to its treatment. Most often, successful treatment of a physical illness leads to dramatic alleviation of the sleep problems.

Because multiple causes usually are present in the elderly, the management of insomnia requires a multidimensional approach to both evaluation and treatment.[4,21] Careful identification of the multiple factors is necessarily based on a careful evaluation. In patients who are more prone to develop hypochondriacal symptoms, a complaint of insomnia may not be given adequate attention. A careful evaluation should be primarily based on a detailed sleep history with special focus on obtaining the 24-hour rest–activity schedule and questioning the bed partner.[20] Also, of great importance for the evaluation of the elderly insomniac are a thorough medical work-up, a detailed drug history, and a psychiatric assessment.

A balanced approach that takes into account the multiple factors usually involved in the development of insomnia in the elderly should be followed in treatment.[2] Education and behavior modification are essential components for all other intervention strategies for insomnia.[4] With the knowledge that sleep patterns change with age, the elderly person may be less concerned that disturbed sleep should be cause for alarm. Practical methods for improving nighttime sleep can be taught such as establishing regular hours for bedtime and arising, eliminating or reducing daytime naps, initiating regular, moderate exercise, and becoming involved in meaningful daily activities.

Optimum sleep in terms of quantity and quality cannot be prescribed by the physician and then carried out in a task-oriented or mechanistic manner by the patient. The physician can, however, clarify misconceptions and refute myths regarding sleep and its functions and can provide elderly patients with the most up-to-date information concerning sleep and rest.[39] In this way, patients can take a realistic look at their own habits, routines, and 24-hour schedules and, with the physician's assistance, can assume responsibility for modifying or removing factors that may have a negative effect on sleep.

The complaint of insomnia often correlates with physical and psychiatric illness.[2,4,21,41] Treatment should be directed towards reversing the disease state, if possible. Particular attention should be given to cardiopulmonary dysfunction, gastrointestinal distress, nocturia, arthritis, and urological dysfunction—all common geriatric ailments that can induce or amplify sleep disturbances.[2,4] Appropriate medical intervention is followed by a lessening of the pain, discomfort, anxiety, and secondary depression associated with these illnesses.

Because of the bias that older patients are more likely to be hypochondriacal and less insightful than younger patients, psychiatrists may avoid treating these patients' underlying emotional problems with psychotherapy.[2] However, a direct psychotherapeutic approach is often helpful in treating elderly patients with insomnia, who tend to have considerable emotional resilience and to become actively involved in the psychotherapy.

Hypnotic medication for elderly insomniac patients should be used only as an adjunct to other approaches.[2,4,21] Prescriptions should be time-limited, and at a dose that is only two-thirds to one-half the usual adult dosage. This dose reduction is necessitated by age-related changes in pharmacokinetics and pharmacodynamics that greatly affect efficacy, safety, and side effects (See Chapter 7).[47]

The benzodiazepines are relatively safe and effective as hypnotic agents. Benzodiazepines differ in their half-lives and rates of absorption; these factors should be considered when a prescription is made.[55] Flurazepam has proven short-term efficacy as well as efficacy with continued use and limited side effects including minimal withdrawal difficulty. As might be expected from flurazepam's slow elimination rate, its primary adverse effect is daytime sedation. A single nightly dose of 15 mg minimizes daytime sedation and has been shown to be effective in elderly insomniac patients.[55] Accumulation and carryover effects may be reduced by using the drug on an occasional, as needed basis. Triazolam, which is a short-acting benzodiazepine (half-life 2–4 hours), has been shown to be efficacious for short-term use.[55] However, its routine use for the elderly is limited by certain disturbing behavioral side effects (amnesia, confusion and delirium)[46,52,55–58] and its undesirable withdrawal profile (rebound insomnia and anxiety).[34,49,55] Temazepam has been shown to be somewhat less efficacious than flurazepam but does not have the severe side effects and withdrawal difficulties associated with triazolam.[55]

Sleep Apnea

The clinical condition of sleep apnea has been rather arbitrarily defined as the cessation of breathing lasting 10 seconds or more that occurs 30 or more times during a 7-hour period of sleep.[22] However, this current diagnostic criterion appears to be inappropriate for older persons, in whom asymptomatic sleep apneic activity appears to be increased. The original cohort used for validation of this criterion did not include elderly persons. Further, the clinical diagnosis of sleep apnea is not determined only by the number of apneic events. Degree of nocturnal oxygen desaturation is a critical measure, and the patient's total clinical picture, including symptom frequency and intensity, must be considered (Table 43.5).[22]

When the above considerations are taken into account, sleep apnea, a condition with potentially life threatening cardiovascular complications, is found to show a peak in the middle-age years.[60] Yet nocturnal apneic activity increases with increasing age, particularly in males, while not infrequently patients found to have the condition of sleep apnea[22] are above 65 years old. Moreover, a number of factors associated with sleep apnea (hypertension, diabetes, obesity, cardiac arrhythmias, etc) are more prevalent in elderly persons. Thus, although the exact prevalence of the condition of sleep apnea has not been well established in the elderly, physicians need to be particularly alert to its identification whenever suspicion of its presence is raised based on clinical evidence.

Treatment recommendations are based on the sever-

Table 43.5. Clinical characteristics of sleep apnea.

Type of apnea	Clinical manifestations
Obstructive apnea	History of snoring and typical intermittant snorting and gasping sounds
	Nocturnal breath cessations observable by bed partner and often perceived by the patient
	Excessive daytime sleepiness and sleep attacks
	Nocturnal body movements, excessive sweating, nocturnal enuresis, loss of libido, morning headaches, obesity, cognitive impairment
	Hypertension and other cardiovascular complications
Central apnea	History of snoring uncharacteristic
	Nocturnal breath cessations often reported
	Usually excessive daytime sleepiness and at times complaints of insomnia

From Kales, Ref. 22

ity of sleep apnea; therefore collection of complete and accurate data is essential.[22,60] If the clinical history and physical examination indicate that the patient may have the sleep apnea syndrome, referral for an 8-hour nocturnal sleep laboratory recording is needed. This evaluation should provide detailed information on the number of apneic events, their duration, the degree of oxygen desaturation and associated ECG abnormalities.[42]

Because the symptoms of sleep apnea are not only debilitating but usually reversible, treatment of this condition is important (Table 43.6).[22] Also, sleep apnea

tends to be more prevalent in elderly patients who are debilitated. Thus, it always is beneficial to correct or reverse, whenever possible, underlying medical illnesses such as congestive heart failure, chronic respiratory disorders, and metabolic abnormalities.[2] Regarding medication, drugs that depress the central ventilatory drive (sedative/hypnotics, barbiturates, narcotics, sedating analgesics, as well as alcohol) should be avoided. Further, for obese elderly patients with apnea, weight loss should be encouraged; however, weight loss dose not guarantee the improvement of sleep apnea.[22] Other non-surgical treatments, such as application of a tongue retaining device at night or of continuous positive airway pressure through the nares, have not been shown to be unequivocally effective, and they require a high degree of compliance.

The main surgical treatment of severe obstructive sleep apnea are uvulopalatopharyngoplasy and tracheostomy.[22] The former is limited to about 50% success rate, while the latter is almost invariably efficacious. Thus, most elderly patients with severe obstructive sleep apnea will require a modified tracheostomy (closed during the day and opened at night) to reverse the disabling daytime symptoms and to prevent or ameliorate the short- and long-term cardiovascular effects of sleep apnea.

The recommendation for tracheostomy is based on the results of the patient's overall clinical and laboratory assessment.[22] Sleep laboratory criteria established for such a recommendation include an apnea index of 20 or greater or a decrease in oxygen saturation of more than 10% below the patient's average presleep value. In addition, major clinical criteria include either daytime symptomatology (eg, excessive daytime sleepiness of an intensity to impair functioning markedly) or cardiovascular complications (eg, hypertension or cardiac arrhythmias). Experience indicates

Table 43.6. Nonpharmacologic treatment of obstructive sleep apnea.

Method	Mechanism of action	Disadvantages
Weight loss	Work of respiration	Difficult to achieve
	Upper airway soft tissue	Inconsistent patient response
		Delay in effect may put patient at increased risk
Nasal continuous positive airway pressure	Prevents upper airway collapse	Administration is complex and uncomfortable making compliance uncertain
		Possible mechanical failure
Nocturnal nasopharyngeal airway	Bypasses obstruction due to nose and tongue	Does not prevent collapse of lateral and posterior pharyngeal walls
		Inconsistent patient response
Uvulopalatopharyngoplasty	Enlarges pharyngeal airspace	Inconsistent patient response
		Possible operative morbidity
Tracheostomy	Bypasses upper airway obstruction	Prosthetic appliance
		Operative morbidity and post-operative complications
		Psychologic adjustments are necessary

From Kales, Ref. 22

that an interdisciplinary team approach that includes the special expertise of a psychiatrist is helpful in reversing the emotional sequelae of sleep apnea syndrome, as well as providing the necessary emotional support if a tracheostomy is indicated.

Narcolepsy

Narcolepsy usually has its onset in adolescence or early adulthood.[22,61,62] It is, however, a life-long disorder and, thus, it is not rare in elderly persons. Narcoleptic patients suffer from excessive daytime sleepiness with irresistible sleep attacks usually occuring in conjunction with one or more of three auxiliary symptoms—cataplexy, sleep paralysis, and hypnagogic hallucinations. Sleep attacks are generally brief, ie, a matter of seconds to a few minutes but may last on occasion up to 30 minutes. They are usually precipitated by sedentary, monotonous activity such as watching television, reading, or driving.

Cataplexy, present in about 70% to 80% of patients with narcolepsy, is a brief (a few seconds to about 2 minutes), sudden loss of muscle control that may cause the person to collapse, while remaining conscious.[22,61,62] This loss of muscle tone frequently occurs in relation to strong emotional experiences such as laughter, surprise, or anger. Sleep paralysis and hypnagogic hallucinations are reported less frequently than is cataplexy. Both symptoms occur during the period of transition between wakefulness and sleep and are of a very short duration. With sleep paralysis there is a temporary loss of muscle tone and a resulting inability to move. Hypnagogic hallucinations are vivid hallucinatory perceptions that occur particularly while falling alseep. Also, about half of narcoleptic patients have disturbed nocturnal sleep.

Auxiliary symptoms are present in 70% to 80% of all narcoleptic patients. Patients without auxiliary symptoms are considered to have so-called independent narcolepsy.[22,61,62] In patients who have cataplexy, REM periods usually occur at or shortly after sleep onset, rather than being preceded by the 70 to 90 minutes of NREM sleep seen in normal persons and many patients with independent narcolepsy.

The elderly narcoleptic has in some respects certain age related advantages: in general, alertness is not as essential as it was before retirement, and often naps may be taken conveniently. However a negative aspect of an elderly narcoleptic is the degree of age-related restrictions superimposed upon the disease-related social and physical restrictions.

The evaluation of narcolepsy begins with a sleep history obtained from the patient and supplemental descriptions of the symptoms from the spouse, roommate, or friends.[20] When cataplexy and the other auxiliary symptoms are present, the diagnosis is established. Diagnostic recordings in the sleep laboratory are indicated for those patients without auxiliary symptoms or in whom sleep apnea is suspected. Sleep laboratory recordings are also indicated for ambiguous cases of narcolepsy, especially those with an onset in old age. Multiple daytime nap recordings may be a useful diagnostic adjunct by detecting sleep-onset REM period or extremely short sleep latencies in narcoleptic patients.[22]

In the psychosocial management of narcolepsy, the physician needs to be aware that this chronic disorder may be misunderstood (Table 43.7).[22,62] Therapeutic naps may be helpful in enhancing daytime alertness. This is relatively easy to accomplish for the elderly narcoleptic who has no job pressure or other conflicting activities. Also, patients should be warned about the potential risk of driving or undertaking activities in situations that would expose them and others to danger in the event of a sleep attack or cataplectic episode.

Table 43.7. Psychosocial consequences of narcolepsy/cataplexy.

Life area	Effects
Interpersonal Relations	Significant others may feel symptoms are under patient's volitional control
	Fear of precipitating symptoms leads to restriction of emotions
	Social interaction decreases to avoid negative experiences
Vocational	Symptoms cause impaired performance and decreased productivity
	Potential for accidents and injury is high
	Supervisors may misinterpret symptomatology of disorder
Educational	Teachers interpret symptoms as indicating dullness or laziness
	Decreased achievement may occur
	Interaction with peers may be impaired
Marital or Family	General increase in tension may occur
	Symptoms may be misunderstood
	Household and driving accidents may be more frequent

From Kales, Ref. 22

The pharmacologic treatment of narcolepsy involves separate treatment for the sleep attacks and for the auxiliary symptoms of cataplexy.[22,61,62] Methylphenidate is the preferred drug for treating the sleep attacks of narcolepsy, primarily because of its prompt action and few side effects.[22] Each of the divided doses is initiated at the lowest possible level (5 mg) and may be gradually increased (usually not to exceed a total daily dose of 60 mg), depending on the patient's response and on the time of day when drowsiness is worst.

Some investigators feel that amphetamines,[62] are preferable for the treatment of narcoleptic sleep attacks. Infrequently, amphetamine therapy in narcoleptic patients can lead to drug dependency or amphetamine psychosis. There is a higher risk for these side-effects in elderly persons because of increased physical and psychological vulnerability.

Imipramine is the drug of choice in the treatment of cataplexy;[22,62] the drug also alleviates sleep paralysis but has little effect on narcoleptic sleep attacks. Generally, the total daily dose of imipramine needed for controlling the symptoms of cataplexy (10 to 75 mg) is much lower than that used for treating depression. Analeptics and imipramine may be combined when a patient requires treatment for both sleep attacks and auxiliary symptoms. But because this combination may produce serious side effects such as hypertension, careful titration and monitoring are necessary, particularly for the patient who may be already hypertensive.

Parasomnias

Parasomnias are episodic disorders occurring during sleep. They include sleepwalking, night terrors, nightmares and enuresis and may occur at any time during the life cycle, but tend to be more prevalent during childhood and early adolescence.[21,63-67] When they appear initially in young adults, their development and, particularly, their persistence have their roots in psychological factors. Although emotional factors may be involved when parasomnias arise in elderly persons, it should be assumed that in these cases the primary etiology is organic until proven otherwise.[2] Use of multiple psychoactive medications, conditions such as brain tumors or metabolic disturbances, and febrile states all have been implicated in the etiology of these disorders.[21]

Sleepwalking and night terrors have been described as disorders of impaired arousal falling along the same pathophysiologic continuum.[21] Usually, they occur out of deep sleep (stages 3 and 4) when patients are more likely to be confused, exhibit low levels of awareness, reactivity, and motor skill. Upon awakening, patients usually are amnesic for the events.[21,63-67] Although they occur at night, sleepwalking and night terrors differ from nocturnal confusional episodes, which are expressions of an impaired mental status in the awake state rather than during sleep.[2,45] To evaluate thoroughly the elderly patient who may have sleepwalking or night terror activity, both physical and psychiatric assessments are necessary.[21] Treatment usually includes protective measures, management of any underlying physical or psychiatric disorders, and education of the family or caregivers regarding the patient's condition.[21,64,66]

Nightmares are vivid, emotionally charged "bad dreams" that occur during REM sleep.[28,65] They may cause the elderly individual to awaken spontaneously and spend long periods of time awake and anxious.[61] Throughout the life cycle, emotional stress and life events generally play a major role in the occurrence of nightmares. However, in elderly persons, nightmares may also be initiated or facilitated by medications such as antihypertensives, neuroleptics, antidepressants, and hypnotics.[21] To treat elderly patients with troublesome nightmares, causative factors must be eliminated or reduced. Medication that can produce nightmares should be removed and replaced with another (eg, replacing propranolol, which can produce nightmares and insomnia, with nadolol); and for emotional distress, insight-oriented psychotherapy often is beneficial.

Nocturia and Nocturnal Incontinence (Enuresis). Nocturia and nocturnal incontinence are common in elderly persons and usually have disruptive effects on sleep patterns.[26] Medical conditions such as congestive heart failure and diabetes, as well as use of diuretics, may cause or contribute to nocturia. Secondary or acquired enuresis is more prevalent in the elderly. The prevalence may be even higher than reported, because most often its presence is quite embarrassing, and consequently the elderly do not readily acknowledge the condition. In contrast to the occurrence of secondary enuresis in childhood, adolescence, and young adulthood, where the condition is most often psychogenic, the underlying etiology is usually organic in nature when enuresis occurs in elderly persons.[2,22,67] The most common cause of bedwetting in the aged is bladder incontinence (See Chapter 38).

Summary

Sleep changes considerably with advancing age both in terms of quantity and patterns; elderly persons experience many more nightly awakenings and a decreased total amount of sleep, as well as demonstrating a marked reduction to total elimination of stages 3 and 4 (slow wave) sleep. Sleep disorders are frequent in elderly persons, with the most prevalent being in order: insomnia, sleep apnea, and narcolepsy. Insomnia is prevalent in all age groups with the greatest frequency being in elderly persons. Sleep apnea has its peak prevalence in middle age while narcolepsy characteristically begins before age 25 and continues throughout life.

Proper assessment of these disorders includes sleep and drug histories and psychiatric evaluation, as well as physical examination. Insomnia in elderly persons may be caused by either or both physical (medical illnesses and medications) and emotional (losses, loneliness, isolation, fear of death) factors. Because sleep apnea is a life threatening disorder, its assessment and treatment are critical. In the evaluation, information regarding snoring, gasping, breath cessations, etc, need to be obtained from the bedpartner. When sleep apnea is suspected, sleep laboratory evaluation is indicated. Narcolepsy in elderly persons may not generally present the same difficulties as in earlier years, considering reduced vocational activities. Nevertheless, elderly narcoleptics need to maintain strict cautions in not driving whenever sleepy or otherwise impaired. Finally, when nocturnal confusional episodes or sleepwalking or night terror events occur in an elderly individual, organic factors should be suspected and a thorough evaluation undertaken.

References

1. Bixler EO, Kales A, Soldatos CR, et al.: Prevalence of sleep disorders in the Los Angeles metropolitan area. *Am J Psychiatry* 1979;136:1257–1262.

2. Cadieux RJ, Woolley D, Kales JD: Sleep disorders in the elderly, in Berlin RM, Soldatos CR (eds): *Psychiatric Medicine. Sleep Disorders in Psychiatric Practice, 1986.* Longwood, FL, Ryandic Publishing, 1987, pp 165–180.

3. Dement WC, Miles LE, Carskadon MA: "White paper" on sleep and aging. *J Am Geriatr Soc* 1982;30:25–50.

4. Kales A, Kales JD: *Evaluation and Treatment of Insomnia.* New York, Oxford University Press, 1984.

5. Kales JD: Aging and sleep, in Rochstein M, Goldman R (eds.): *Physiology and Pathology of Human Aging.* New York, Academic Press, Inc, 1975, pp 188–202.

6. Reynolds CF, Spiker DG, Hanin I, et al: Electroencephalographic sleep, aging, and psychopathology: New data and state of the art. *Biol Psychiatry* 1983;18:139–155.

7. Tune G: Sleep and wakefulness in 509 normal adults. *Br J Med Psychol* 1969;42:75–80.

8. Prinz PN: Sleep patterns in the healthy aged: Relationship with intellectual function. *J Gerontol* 1977;32:179–186.

9. Aserinsky E, Kleitman N: Regularly occurring periods of eye motility and concomitant phenomena during sleep. *Science* 1953;118:273–274.

10. Rechtschaffen A, Kales A (eds): *A Manual of Standardized Terminology, Techniques, and Scoring System for Sleep Stages of Human Subjects.* NIH no. 204, National Institutes of Health, 1968.

11. William RL, Agnew HW Jr, Webb WB: Sleep patterns in young adults: An EEG study. *Electroencephalogr Clin Neurophysiol* 1964;17:376–381.

12. Bixler EO, Vela-Bueno A: Normal sleep: Physiological, behavioral, and clinical correlates. *Psych Annals* 1987;17:437–445.

13. Bixler EO, Kales A, Jacoby JA, et al: Nocturnal sleep and wakefulness: Effects of age and sex in normal sleepers. *Int J Neurosci* 1984;23:33–42.

14. Webb WB: Sleep in older persons: Sleep structures of 50- to 60-year-old men and women. *J Gerontol* 1982;37:581–586.

15. Parmelee AH Jr, Wenner WH, Schulz HR: Infant sleep patterns: From birth to 16 weeks of age. *J Pediatr* 1964;65:576–582.

16. Williams RL, Karacan I, Hursch CJ. *EEG of Human Sleep: Clinical Applications.* New York, John Wiley & Sons, 1974.

17. Webb WB, Agnew HW Jr: Sleep cycling within twenty-four hour periods. *J Exp Psychol* 1967;74:158–160.

18. Feinberg I, Koresko RL, Heller N: EEG sleep patterns as a function of normal and pathological aging in man. *J Psychiatr Res* 1967;5:107–144.

19. Feinberg I, Carlson V. Sleep variables as a function of age in man. *Arch Gen Psychiatry* 1968;18:239–250.

20. Kales A, Soldatos CR, Kales JD: Taking a sleep history. *Am Fam Physician* 1980;22:101–108.

21. Kales A, Soldatos CR, Kales JD: Sleep disorders: Insomnia, sleep-walking, night terrors, nightmares, and enuresis. *Ann Intern Med* 1987;106:582–592.

22. Kales A, Vela-Bueno A, Kales JD: Sleep disorders: Sleep apnea and narcolepsy. *Ann Intern Med* 1987;106:434–443.

23. Coleman RM, Pollak CP, Weitzman ED: Periodic movements in sleep (nocturnal myoclonus): Relation to sleep disorders. *Ann Neurol* 1979;8:416–421.

24. Laugaresi E, Coccagna G, Ceroni GB, et al.: Restless legs syndrome and nocturnal myoclonus, in Gastaut H, Lugaresi E, Bertini-Ceroni G, et al. (eds): *The Abnormalities of Sleep in Man.* Bologna, Aulo Gaggi, 1967, pp 285–294.

25. Culebras A, Magana R: Neurologic disorders and sleep disturbances. *Seminars in Neurology* 1987;7:277–285.

26. Barker JC: Nocturia in the elderly. *Gerontologist* 1988;28:99–104.

27. Williams ME, Pannill FC: Urinary incontinence in the elderly. *Ann Intern Med* 1982;97:895–907.

28. Modolfsky H, Scarisbrick P, England R, Smythe H: Musculoskeletal symptoms and non-REM sleep disturbance in patients with "fibrositis syndrome" and healthy subjects. *Psychosom Med* 1975;37:341–351.

29. Wolfe F: Fibromyalgia in the elderly: Differential diagnosis and treatment. *Geriatrics* 1988;43:57–68.

30. Guilleminault C, Dement WC (eds): *Sleep Apnea Syndromes.* New York, Alan R. Liss, Inc., 1978.

31. Lugaresi E, Coccagna G, Mantovani M: Hypersomnia with periodic apneas, in, Weitzman ED (series ed): *Advances in Sleep Research, vol 4,* New York, Spectrum Publications, 1978.

32. Bliwise D, Carskadon, Carey E, et al.: Longitudinal development of sleep-related respiratory disturbance in adult humans. *J Gerontol* 1984;39:290–293.

33. Kales A, Bixler EO, Vela-Bueno A, et al.: Effects of

578   Joyce D. Kales, Michael Carvell, and Anthony Kales

nadolol on blood pressure, sleep efficiency, and sleep stages. *Clin Pharmacol Ther* 1988;43:655–662.

34. Kales A, Soldatos CR, Bixler EO, et al: Rebound insomnia and rebound anxiety: A review. *Pharmacology* 1983;26:121–137.

35. Kales A, Bixler EO, Tan TL, et al.: Chronic hypnotic-drug use: Ineffectiveness, drug-withdrawal insomnia, and dependence. *JAMA* 1974;227:513–517.

36. Karacan I, Thornby JI, Anch AM, et al.: Dose-related sleep disturbances induced by coffee and caffeine. *Clin Pharmacol Ther* 1976;20:682–689.

37. Rundell OH, Lester BK, Griffiths WJ, et al.: Alcohol and sleep in young adults. *Psychopharmacologia* 1972;26:201–218.

38. Soldatos CR, Kales JD, Scharf MB, et al.: Cigarette smoking associated with sleep difficulty. *Science* 1980;207:551–553.

39. Kales JD, Kales A: Rest and sleep, in Taylor RB, Ureda JR, Denham JW (eds): *Health Promotion. Principles and Clinical Applications*. New York, Appleton-Century-Crofts, 1982, pp 307–337.

40. Soldatos CR, Vela-Bueno A, Kales A: Sleep in psychiatric disorders, in Berlin RM, Soldatos CR (eds): *Psychiatric Medicine. Sleep Disorders in Psychiatric Practice, 1986.* Longwood, FL, Ryandic Publishing, Inc, 1987, pp 119–132.

41. Rodin J, McAvay G, Timko C: A longitudinal study of depressed mood and sleep disturbances in elderly adults. *J Gerontol* 1988;43:45–53.

42. Bixler EO, Robertson JA, Soldatos CR: Sleep laboratory assessment of normal sleep and sleep disorders, in Berlin RM, Soldatos CR (eds): *Psychiatric Medicine. Sleep Disorders in Psychiatric Practice, 1986.* Longwood, FL, Ryandic Publishing, Inc, 1987, pp 105–118.

43. Guilleminault C, Tilkian A, Dement WC: The sleep apnea syndromes. *Annu Rev Med* 1976;27:465–484.

44. Kales A, Bixler EO, Soldatos CR, et al.: Biopsychobehavioral correlates of insomnia, I: Role of sleep apnea and nocturnal myoclonus. *Psychosomatics* 1982;23:589–600.

45. Lipowski ZJ: *Delirium. Acute Brain Failure in Man.* Springfield, IL, Charles S. Thomas, 1980.

46. Patterson J: Triazolam syndrome in the elderly. *South Med J* 1987;80:1425–1426.

47. Prien RF: Problems and practices in geriatric psychopharmacology. *Geriatric Drug Use* 1980;21:213–223.

48. Johnson LC, Chernik DA: Sedative-hypnotics and human performance. *Psychopharmacology,* 1982;76:101–113.

49. Kales A, Soldatos CR, Bixler EO, et al.: Early morning insomnia with rapidly eliminated benzodiazepines. *Science* 1983;220:95–97.

50. Vela-Bueno A, Soldatos CR, Kales A: Anxiety and disordered sleep, in *Handbook of Anxiety, Volume 2: Classification, Etiological Factors and Associated Dis-*

turbances. Amsterdam, Elsevier, (in press), pp 507–543.

51. Kales A, Bixler EO, Vela-Bueno A, et al.: Comparison of short and long half-life benzodiazepine hypnotics: Triazolam and quazepam. *Clin Pharmacol Ther* 1986;40:378–386.

52. Bixler EO, Kales A, Brubaker BH, et al.: Adverse reactions to benzodiazepine hypnotics: Spontaneous reporting system. *Pharmacology* 1987;35:286–300.

53. Young JR, Humphries AQ, DeWolfe VG: Restless leg syndrome. *Geriatrics* 1969;24:167–171.

54. Guilleminault C, Raynal D, Takahashi S, et al.: Evaluation of short-term and long-term treatment of the narcolepsy syndrome with clomipramine hydrochloride. *Acta Neurol Scand* 1976;54:71–87.

55. Kales A, Soldatos CR, Vela-Bueno A: Clinical comparison of benzodiazepine hynotics with short and long elimination half-lives, in Smith DE, Wesson DR (eds): *The Benzodiazepines. Current Standards for Medical Practice.* Lancaster, England, MTP Press Limited, 1985, pp 121–147.

56. Tan TL, Bixler EO, Kales A, Cadieux RJ, Goodman AL: Early morning insomnia, daytime anxiety, and organic mental disorder associated with triazolam. *J Fam Pract,* 1985;20:592–594.

57. Morris HH, Estes ML: Traveler's amnesia: transient global amnesia secondary to triazolam. *JAMA,* 1987;258:945–946.

58. Van der Koref C: Reactions to triazolam. *Lancet,* 1979;2:256.

59. 0.5 mg Halcion withdrawn in FRG, *Scrip,* 1988;1296:3.

60. Kales A, Cadieux RJ, Bixler EO, et al: Severe obstructive sleep apnea—I: onset, clinical course, and characteristics. *J Chron Dis* 1985;38:419–425.

61. Guilleminault C, Dement WC, Passouant P: Narcolepsy, in Wietzman ED (ed): *Advances in Sleep Research, vol 3.* New York, Spectrum Publications, 1976.

62. Roth B. *Narcolepsy and Hypersomnia.* (Prague, Avicenum-Czechloslovak Medical Press) Revised and edited by R Broughton, Basel, Karger, 1980.

63. Kales A, Jacobson A, Paulson MJ, et al: Somnambulism: Psychophysiological correlates, I. All-night EEG studies. *Arch Gen Psychiatry* 1966;14:586–594.

64. Kales A, Soldatos CR, Caldwell AB, et al.: Somnambulism: Clinical characteristics and personality patterns. *Arch Gen Psychiatry* 1980;37:1406–1410.

65. Kales A, Soldatos CR, Caldwell AB, et al: Nightmares: Clinical characteristics and personality patterns. *Am J Psychiatry* 1980;137:1197–1201.

66. Kales JD, Kales A, Soldatos CR, et al.: Night terrors: Clinical characteristics and personality patterns. *Arch Gen Psychiatry* 1980;37:1413–1417.

67. Starfield B: Enuresis: Its pathogenesis and management. *Clin Pediatr (Phila)* 1972;11:343–350.

44

Hypothermia

James B. Reuler

In the minds of many health care practitioners, the problem of hypothermia is associated either with a dramatic presentation that is related to severe environmental exposure in the wilderness or with alcohol intoxication. Over the past 25 years, however, it has become recognized that elderly persons are at risk for developing this disorder, which may present in a subtle fashion. Much work has been done in Great Britain to characterize the epidemiology of hypothermia in elderly persons. For the United States, with its higher latitudes and larger elderly population, this problem likely represents a public health issue, particularly in times of decreasing economic resources. In this chapter, the problem of hypothermia in elderly persons will be discussed. For more broadly based treatises on accidental hypothermia, the reader is referred to several reviews.[1–5]

Pathophysiology

Defined as a core body temperature lower than 35°C, hypothermia represents the body's inability to maintain a constant temperature despite changes in environmental temperature. Any influence that tends to lower the core temperature is met by the mobilization of a number of forces to prevent heat loss and increase heat production. The physical laws involved with heat loss, which are important in the development and prevention of hypothermia, include (1) conduction, or the transfer of heat by direct contact; (2) convection, the transfer of heat by particles of air or water that

have been heated by contact with the body; (3) radiation, the transfer of energy by nonparticulate means, such as heat loss from an unprotected head; and (4) evaporation of water.

With respect to temperature regulation, the body can be viewed as a core protected by several outer layers that modulate heat loss and gain. The skin and subcutaneous tissue, with their thermal receptors, represent the superficial zone and are the most important aspects of the heat exchange mechanism. Body temperature at this level varies with blood flow, ambient air temperature, humidity, and air velocity, and it may drop to nearly environmental temperatures in an attempt to conserve heat. The intermediate zone is the skeletal muscle mass, which ordinarily contributes little to heat production until the core temperature is in danger of falling, at which time the muscles provide heat by the mechanism of shivering. The preoptic anterior hypothalamus integrates these various components of heat exchange with the neural network and acts both through the autonomic nervous system, to provide a rapid control of heat conservation, and through the neuroendocrine axis, resulting in a more gradual increase in heat production.

There are multiple consequences for various organ functions as the body temperature begins to drop. Most obvious is a decrease in the basal metabolic rate, which falls to about 50% of normal at 28°C. Blood pressure initially may rise, but then it gradually falls, with hypotension being clinically significant below 25°C. Most important are the hemodynamic effects, which include the frequent development of atrial fibrillation with mild temperature reductions and more serious high-grade ventricular dysrhythmias and conduction disturbances at temperatures lower than 28°C.

At lower body temperatures, depression of the respiratory center, level of consciousness, and cough reflex may lead to problems with aspiration and respiratory insufficiency. In profound hypothermia, major alterations in acid-base equilibrium also may be seen, with acidosis resulting from respiratory failure and tissue hypoxia. In addition, urine flow may increase as the temperature decreases, secondary to depressed oxidative tubular activities in the kidney. Occurring together with shifts of fluids to the extracellular spaces, this increased flow may render the patient hypovolemic.

Significant effects are manifested in the central nervous system, where the cerebral blood flow decreases by 6% to 7% per 1°C drop in body temperature. This decrease, along with alterations in the microcirculation that are due to increased viscosity, may cause depressed mentation. These central nervous system alterations, combined with a frequently observed hyporeflexia, impalpable pulse, and unmeasurable blood pressure, may cause a patient to appear dead.

Epidemiology

In 1964, the British Medical Association published a memorandum on accidental hypothermia in elderly persons, which included the following statement:

Hypothermia is a serious though unspectacular condition with a very high mortality rate, and its early recognition in general practice is therefore important. It may arise independently as a spontaneous condition or it may be secondary to organic or endogenous causes.

The term, "accidental hypothermia" is employed as it is in common usage and because it emphasizes the cause of the majority of cases in elderly people in which environmental and endogenous factors play a part either singly or together. A large number of elderly people who are found to be hypothermic die either from the condition itself or from the underlying disease or from complications which supervene.[6]

The same year, Geoffrey Taylor, a general practitioner in Great Britain, studied environmental and body temperatures as he made his rounds.[7] He found that the average minimum temperature of the bedrooms of his patients was only 2° to 3° above the ambient environmental temperature, with a low bedroom temperature of −14°C; also, the average oral temperature of his patients was 34.4°C (with a range of 31.6° to 35.7°C).

In 1966, the Royal College of Physicians surveyed 10 hospitals in England and Scotland during 3 winter months and found that 0.68% of all patients admitted had core temperatures less than 35°C, and that 47 of 126 hypothermic patients died.[8] Elderly patients made up 11.25% of the total admissions, but they accounted for 28.6% of all patients admitted with hypothermia. Extrapolating those numbers to all hospital admissions during that period, it was estimated that 9,000 persons could have been admitted with hypothermia. There seemed to be a clear relationship between the incidence of hypothermia and the environmental temperature, since during that period ambient air temperatures dropped to as low as −16°C. Other surveys in Great Britain have found variable prevalences of hypothermia in elderly persons, which ranged up to 11.4% of persons monitored at home and 3.6% of all hospital admissions.[9-13] The most detailed study, the National Hypothermia Survey, involved over 1,000 elderly residents who were evaluated at home with questionnaires. The ambient air temperatures and the mouth and urine temperatures were recorded. These data indicated that 0.58% of elderly persons were hypothermic and 9.6% were "at risk" (35.0 to 35.5°C). If extrapolated, these figures represented over 700,000 elderly citizens who were "at risk." More recent data from Great Britain, however, casts doubt on the assumption that large numbers of elderly persons suffer from clinical hypothermia.[5,14] Methodologic problems with earlier studies that used sublingual or urine temperatures, both of which may give falsely low readings, were cited as reasons for the discrepancies. This postulation has been corroborated by a recent study in the United States[15] that attempted to validate the British survey.[10] Studying 97 elderly patients and using a urine collection method designed to minimize cooling of the sample, the investigators were unable to detect a single instance of hypothermia (defined as a temperature of <35.5°C).

Risk Factors

The development of accidental hypothermia in elderly persons requires some exposure to decreased ambient air temperatures. It appears that, for several reasons, elderly persons are more likely to be faced with an environment in which the ambient air temperature is decreased, and that once in this situation they have fewer physiologic resources available to deal with this stress.

The epidemiologic studies from Great Britain cited above would suggest that many elderly people are exposed to environmental conditions in their homes that approximate ambient environmental temperatures. In the 1972 national survey, 75% of all elderly people had morning living room temperatures lower than 18.3°C (the minimum level recommended by the Council on Housing) when the mean air temperature was 7°C.[13] Those persons who had bedrooms separate from living rooms seemed to be at a greater risk, since the mean bedroom temperatures were significantly lower than the living room temperatures, dropping as low as 5°C.[16]

The decreased environmental temperatures within the home seemed to be directly related to the economic resources of the individual, in that the receipt of supplemental benefits was the only predictor from the analysis of socioeconomic factors that correlated with the development of hypothermia. A more recent survey of at-risk elderly showed that in homes without central heating, median bedroom temperatures were 10°C below the World Health Organization's recommended temperature (18°C).[17] These surveys indicated that elderly persons were more likely to distribute their meager economic resources to food and shelter; therefore, they have inadequate resources for fuel. It also was shown that persons living within public housing projects with central heating were at much less of a risk of developing hypothermia than those living in individual dwellings, particularly dwellings with a separate bedroom and living room.

Thermal comfort, the condition of the mind that expresses satisfaction with the thermal environment,[18] is influenced by several variables, including the activity level, the thermal resistance of clothing (clo value), air temperature and its components, the mean radiant temperature, the relative air velocity, and the water vapor pressure in the ambient air.[19] Elderly persons differ little from younger persons with regard to thermal comfort requirements.[20,21] However, the ability to discriminate peripheral temperature differences seems to deteriorate with age.[21] In general, elderly persons perceive peripheral temperature changes less well than do younger persons; when given the ability to control the environment by selecting preferred temperatures, elderly persons are less precise.[22,23] Collins et al showed that there was a significant difference between young and elderly subjects in their ability to discriminate mean temperature differences using digital thermal sensation.[24] The young subjects were able to discriminate differences in cold exposure of $0.8° \pm 0.2°C$, as opposed to elderly subjects, whose mean discrimination was $2.3° \pm 0.5°C$.

Horvath et al showed that there were no significant changes in heat production, respiratory quotient, or oxygen consumption when elderly persons were put in an environmental temperature of 10°C, whereas there were large increases in each of these parameters in young persons under similar conditions, and they also found that elderly persons did not complain of being cold during such experiences.[25]

Rectal and mean skin temperatures during exposure to cold decrease with age due to a general decrease in the basal metabolic rate and a reduction in heat conductance.[26] When put into a cold environment, young persons have a rapid increase in their metabolic rate and minimize peripheral heat loss by cutaneous vasoconstriction; elderly persons are not as able to increase their metabolic rate or to maintain body heat stores by cutaneous vasoconstriction. It is suggested that this inability to maintain heat stores by cutaneous vasoconstriction is a reflection of an underlying autonomic insufficiency.

In summary, physiologic alterations in elderly persons may predispose to the development of hypothermia. These include a decreasing body core-shell temperature gradient, decreased resting peripheral blood flow, a nonconstrictor pattern of vasomotor response to cold, a higher incidence of orthostatic hypotension, and decreased precision in attaining a preferred temperature.[5,21,23,24,27] Additional factors that have been incriminated include the use of sedative-hypnotic and other neuroleptic drugs often prescribed for insomnia and agitation, which alter the central and peripheral neuroendocrine aspects of heat generation, inhibit shivering, and increase the prevalence of falls, leading to an increased risk of exposure.

The low ambient air temperatures to which elderly persons are exposed may lead to short-term increases in blood pressure and increased blood viscosity,[14,28] both of which may contribute to increased morbidity and mortality due to heart attacks and strokes in the winter months. In hypothermia in an elderly patient, which is usually seen in association with other serious illness, it is often not clear whether the hypothermia caused or resulted from the acute problem, such as a stroke.

Clinical Evaluation

There are numerous clinical settings in which hypothermia occurs.[2] It is important to reemphasize that extreme environmental conditions are not required to precipitate hypothermia, with factors of wind velocity, moisture, alcohol ingestion, inadequate clothing, and duration of exposure all playing important roles. In addition to the predisposing factors that were already mentioned, hypothermia may be a consequence of underlying disease processes. The most common association is with myxedema, with an insufficient calorigenesis providing the mechanism.[29] Approximately 80% of all patients with myxedema will have low body temperatures. This may explain the increased incidence rate of myxedematous comas in the winter months and the risk of sedative drugs in this setting.[30]

A myxedema coma may present a difficult diagnostic problem, because many of the findings of hypothyroidism are mimicked by hypothermia, including edema, abdominal distress, ileus, and delayed deep-tendon reflexes. Also, hypothermia may be a manifestation of hypoglycemia due to exclusion of glucose from central nervous system sites.[31] This can be a problem especially in diabetic elderly patients, who may have difficulty administering insulin due to a visual or other impairment.

Central nervous system disorders, which include cerebral vascular diseases, may lead to alterations in the hypothalamic temperature regulatory center that predispose to hypothermia. In addition, hypothermia is a common manifestation of Wernicke's encephalopathy due to a thiamine deficiency, which usually is seen in the setting of chronic alcohol ingestion and inadequate nutrition. Hypothermia occurs in this setting because of the involvement of the hypothalamic nuclei.

Drug-induced hypothermia may be caused by an interruption of several steps in the thermoregulatory scheme. Depression of the hypothalamic center, inhibition of shivering by a peripheral curarization, and vasodilatation all play a role. This concept is particularly important with respect to elderly persons, due to the frequency with which many of the implicated drugs are prescribed.[12] The postoperative setting also is one in which elderly persons may be vulnerable to the development of core temperature depression. The predilection for development of hypothermia postoperatively will be met with a shivering response that may increase postoperative oxygen demands by up to 500%.[32-34] This factor alone may increase the risk of postoperative complications in an elderly patient, particularly with respect to acute ischemic cardiac disease and metabolic abnormalities. In addition, the decreasing temperature, combined with age-related changes in drug disposition, will lead to an increase in the half-life of many parenterally administered drugs during the perioperative state, thus heightening the possibility of further complications. The risk of hypothermia can be minimized by using anesthetic agents with minimal vasodilator effects, protecting exposed viscera with warmed saline pads, using warmed irrigation and intravenous solutions, using a heating mattress for prolonged surgical procedures, and monitoring temperatures in the postoperative suite. Because of the major thermoregulatory role played by the skin, patients with exfoliative dermatitis also may be at risk for hypothermia, owing to increases in skin blood flow and transepidermal water loss, which lead to heat loss via radiation, conduction, and evaporation.[35,36] Therefore, an elderly patient with an erythroderma may be at particular risk for the development of thermal instability.

In addition to the above-mentioned specific disease entities or clinical settings, hypothermia may accompany any acute or chronic disease in an elderly person, particularly when host defenses are overwhelmed (eg, in the setting of a severe infection). In fact, in the elderly population, the development of hypothermia frequently is a reflection of a combination of several of the above-mentioned factors.

Increased age, complaints of cold hands, a preference for a warmer environment, and the fact that a patient was receiving supplemental benefits all were characteristics that were associated with hypothermia in British studies. The diagnosis should be considered in any elderly person at risk with findings of a progressing confusion, slurring of speech, ataxia, and involuntary movements. Establishing a diagnosis highlights further problems. Many patients present with hypothermia that is not diagnosed until complications supervene. In part, this is due to the fact that standard thermometers record down to only 34.4°C. If the thermometer is not shaken down to begin with, hypothermia patients may be missed altogether. Low-reading thermometers should be available in all hospital emergency rooms and intensive care unit areas. As recommended in the Royal College of Physicians' report,[6,8] any person found to have an oral temperature of 35°C or less should have the core temperature measured.

Physical examination may disclose a clouding of consciousness, and coma frequently supervenes with temperatures under 27°C. The blood pressure may be unmeasurable, the pulse slow or absent, and respirations shallow and infrequent. When the core temperature is lower than 30°C, shivering will be absent and the patient may appear to be in rigor mortis because of increased muscle tone. The pupils may be dilated and sluggishly reactive, deep-tendon reflexes may be either absent or delayed, and heart sounds may be absent. All these findings may combine to lead to a presumptive diagnosis of death at the time of initial evaluation. The above points emphasize the fact that the usual criteria for reversibility are not valid in determining prognosis in a hypothermic patient. Life may be sustained for long periods after an apparent cardiac arrest because of decreased oxygen requirements. Few conclusions can be drawn regarding the nature or extent of complicating disorders until the patient is warmed.

Treatment

The management of a hypothermic patient must focus on both general supportive measures and specific rewarming techniques. For patients with mild hypothermia (core temperature higher than 33.3°C), hospitalization may not be required and management may consist of external rewarming and assuring adequate heating in the living environment. However, a patient with lower core temperature should be hospitalized and monitored more closely, since the lower the core temperature, the more likely the presence of both supervening complications and underlying precipitating disease. In addition to a history and physical examination focusing on the identification of precipitating events, laboratory screening should include plasma glucose, amylase, and renal function studies, as well as coagulation studies.

In a profoundly hypothermic patient, intensive care unit management and continuous electrocardiographic monitoring are imperative because of the frequency of rhythm disturbances. Atrial flutter and fibrillation will revert once the patient is warmed, and ventricular dysrhythmias generally are abolished with correction of hypoxia and acidosis. A hypothermic heart, however, is relatively unresponsive to atropine, electrical pacing, and countershock. If ventricular fibrillation occurs and electroshock is not successful, cardiopulmonary resuscitation (CPR) should be instituted and continued until the core temperature is raised, because successful recovery has been documented after several hours of continued CPR in this setting. The administration of drugs during the period when the patient is profoundly hypothermic may have little therapeutic effect and may cause serious problems when the patient is rewarmed; this highlights the hazards of overmedication in the setting of slowed metabolism of drugs. In this regard, hyperglycemia should be treated cautiously because of the risk of postwarming hypoglycemia. In the setting of chronic hypothermia, volume depletion may be a particular problem, given the tubular dysfunction often seen, in association with diuretic therapy and underlying renal dysfunction in elderly persons. Intravenous fluids may be warmed by passage through a blood-warming coil that is maintained at 37° to 40°C. Other details of specific problems encountered in a profoundly hypothermic patient may be found in general review articles.[1-4]

In conjunction with general supportive maneuvers, mechanisms for rewarming should be instituted. Rewarming methods fall into three categories: (1) passive rewarming, including removal from environmental exposure and the use of insulating materials (eg, blankets or sleeping bags); (2) active external rewarming techniques, including immersion in heated water and the use of electric blankets or heated objects (eg, hot water bottles); and (3) active core rewarming, including the use of intragastric or colonic irrigation, peritoneal dialysis, extracorporeal blood rewarming, and inhalation rewarming.

The use of particular rewarming methods remains a controversial area within hypothermia management. Concern has been raised about the risks of active external rewarming because of inherent physiologic changes that may aggravate the effect of hypothermia on core tissues, thus leading to what has been termed an "after drop" of core temperature after removal of chronic cold stress. However, most survivors of accidental hypothermia have been treated with either passive or active external measures without evidence of significant harm. Recent information suggests that core rewarming is not required for the majority of patients with hypothermia.[37] But the use of core rewarming techniques should be instituted in patients who have profound hypothermia and who have evidence of cardiovascular instability or refractory dysrhythmias. When discussing the use of more aggressive rewarming techniques, it is important to consider the fact that mortality rates in accidental hypothermia do not relate as closely to the degree of temperature depression as to the presence of underlying disease processes.[37-39]

Prevention

The problem of hypothermia in the elderly population is in reality a public health problem. Although most elderly persons maintain reasonable inner body temperatures, a significant minority fail to do so and are at risk for developing hypothermia. Of those at risk, a small proportion have inner body temperatures below the hypothermic level, a small but significant proportion of elderly patients admitted to the hospital are hypothermic, and an unknown number die of hypothermia in hospitals, in their own homes, and elsewhere. The circumstances that surround hypothermia in elderly persons generally are less dramatic than the more well-known settings that involve outdoor recreationists and the alcoholic population. Hypothermia in elderly persons usually develops in an indoor setting that involves socially isolated individuals and is associated with common problems of old age, including immobility and falls. These facts have importance for the planners of social service programs, as well as for health care providers. Policies must focus attention on the provision of adequate heating in both individual and multiunit dwellings for elderly persons and must assure frequent social contact, particularly for the group of elderly persons who live alone in isolated situations and without family support.[40] Priority must be given to increasing public awareness of the problem. In this regard, the National Institute on Aging has begun to make inroads into heightening public awareness by sponsoring workshops for social service agencies and public policy makers, broadcasting messages on radio and television, and publishing written materials for the general public.

References

1. MacLean D, Emslie-Smith D. *Accidental Hypothermia.* Oxford: Blackwell Scientific Publications; 1977.
2. Reuler JB. Hypothermia: pathophysiology, clinical settings, and management. *Ann Intern Med* 1978;89:519–527.
3. Martyn JW. Diagnosing and treating hypothermia. *Can Med Assoc J* 1981;125:1089–1096.
4. Fitzgerald FT, Jessop C. Accidental hypothermia: a report of 22 cases and review of the literature. *Adv Intern Med* 1982;27:127–150.
5. Collins KJ. Hypothermia: the facts. Oxford: Oxford University Press; 1983.
6. Committee on Medical Science, Education, and Research of the British Medical Association. Accidental hypothermia in the elderly. *Br Med J* 1964;2:1255–1258.
7. Taylor G. The problem of hypothermia in the elderly. *Practitioner* 1964;193:761–767.
8. Royal College of Physicians. *Report of the Committee on Accidental Hypothermia.* London Royal College of Physicians; 1966.
9. Hypothermia Subcommittee of the Welfare Group of the Society of Medical Officers of Health. A pilot survey into the occurrence of hypothermia in elderly people living at home. *Public Health* 1968;82:223–229.
10. Fox RH, MacGibbon R, Davies L, et al. Problem of the old and the cold. *Br Med J* 1973;1:21–24.
11. Fox RH, Woodward PM, Exton-Smith AN, et al. Body temperatures in the elderly: a national study of physiological, social and environmental conditions. *Br Med J* 1973;1:200–206.
12. Goldman A, Exton-Smith AN, Francis G, et al. A pilot study of low body temperatures in old people admitted to hospital. *J R Coll Physicians Lond* 1977;11:291–306.
13. Wicks M. *Old and Cold: Hypothermia and Social Policy.* London: Heinemann Educational Books Ltd; 1978.
14. Keatinge W. Medical problems of cold weather. *J R Coll Physicians Lond* 1986;20:283–287.
15. Keilson L, Lambert D, Fabian D, et al. Screening for hypothermia in the ambulatory elderly. *JAMA* 1985;254:1781–1784.
16. Salvosa CB, Payne PR, Wheeler EF. Environmental conditions and body temperatures of elderly women living alone or in local authority home. *Br Med J* 1971;4:656–659.
17. Otty CJ, Roland MO. Hypothermia in the elderly: scope for prevention. *Br Med J* 1987;295:419–420.
18. Benzinger TH. The physiological basis of thermal comfort. In: Fanger PO, Valbjorn O, eds. *Indoor Climate: Effects on Human Comfort, Performance, and Health in Residential, Commercial, and Light-industry Buildings.* Copenhagen: Danish Building Research Institute; 1979:441–476.
19. Fan PO. *Thermal Comfort: Analysis and Applications in Environmental Engineering.* New York: McGraw-Hill International Book Co; 1970.
20. Rohles FH Jr, Johnson MA. Thermal comfort in the elderly. *Trans Am Soc Heating Refrigeration Air Conditioning Engineers* 1972;78:131–137.
21. Collins KJ. Hypothermia and thermal responsiveness in the elderly. In: Fanger PO, Valbjorn O, eds. *Indoor Climate: Effects on Human Comfort, Performance, and Health in Residential, Commercial, and Light-industry Buildings.* Copenhagen: Danish Building Research Institute; 1979:819–833.
22. Watts AJ. Hypothermia in the aged: a study of the role of cold-sensitivity. *Environ Res* 1971;5:119–126.
23. Collins KJ, Exton-Smith AN, Dore C. Urban hypothermia: preferred temperature and thermal perception in old age. *Br Med J* 1981;282:175–177.
24. Collins KJ, Core C, Exton-Smith AN, et al. Accidental hypothermia and impaired temperature homeostasis in the elderly. *Br Med J* 1977;1:353–356.
25. Horvath SM, Radcliffe CE, Hutt BK, et al. Metabolic responses of old people to a cold environment. *J Appl Physiol* 1955;8:145–148.
26. Wagner JA, Robinson S, Marino RP. Age and temperature regulation of humans in neutral and cold environments. *J Appl Physiol* 1974;37:562–565.
27. Macmillan AL, Corbett JL, Johnson RH, et al. Temperature regulation in survivors of accidental hypothermia of the elderly. *Lancet* 1967;2:165–169.
28. Collins KJ. Low indoor temperatures and morbidity in the elderly. *Age Ageing* 1986;15:212–220.
29. Edelman IS. Thyroid thermogenesis. *N Engl J Med* 1974;290:1303–1308.
30. Angel JH, Sash L. Hypothermic coma in myxoedema. *Br Med J* 1960;1:1855–1859.
31. Freinkel N, Metzger BE, Harris E, et al. The hypothermia of hypoglycemia. *N Engl J Med* 1972;287:841–845.
32. Roe CF, Goldberg MH, Blair CS, et al. The influence of body temperature on early postoperative oxygen consumption. *Surgery* 1966;60:85–92.
33. Vaughan MS, Vaughan RW, Cork RC. Postoperative hyothermia in adults: relationship of age, anesthesia, and shivering to rewarming. *Anesth Analg* 1981;60:746–751.
34. Morley-Forster PK. Unintentional hypothermia in the operating room. *Can Anaesth Soc J* 1986;33:516–527.
35. Grice KA, Bettley FR. Skin water loss and accidental hypothermia in psoriasis, ichthyosis, and erythroderma. *Br Med J* 1967;4:195–198.
36. Krook G. Hypothermia in patients with exfoliative dermatitis. *Acta Derm Venereol* 1960;40:124–160.
37. Ledingham I McA, More JG. Treatment of accidental hypothermia: a prospective clinical study. *Br Med J* 1980;2:1102–1105.
38. Hudson LD, Conn RD. Accidental hypothermia: associated diagnoses and prognosis in a common problem. *JAMA* 1974;227:37–40.
39. Miller JW, Danzl DF, Thomas DM. Urban accidental hypothermia: two hundred thirty-five cases. *Ann Emerg Med* 1980;9:456–461.
40. Dawson JA. A case-control study of accidental hypothermia in the elderly in relation to social support and social circumstances. *Community Med* 1987;9:141–145.

45

Pain and Pain Management

Richard Payne and
Gavril W. Pasternak

The principles of pain management[1] are similar for young and old patients (Table 45.1). However, the geriatric population is more likely to experience a number of specific pain problems. Treatment also must be tailored to the elderly patient due to differences in sensitivities to many analgesic agents. This chapter will review the general concept of pain in elderly persons, starting with current knowledge that concerns the role of the nervous system in the modulation of nociperception and the assessment and treatment of specific pain problems in the elderly patient, emphasizing features that are unique to this population, but stressing the importance of a careful evaluation of the pain complaint and the aggressive but judicious use of all available therapeutic modalities for the prompt relief of pain with the minimum amount of adverse effects. Drug therapy for pain will be emphasized, particularly the issues of altered pharmacokinetic and pharmacodynamic responses to a wide variety of pharmacologic agents in the geriatric population (see also Chapter 7).

Pain may be defined as "an unpleasant sensory and emotional experience associated with actual or potential tissue damage, or described in terms of such damage."[2] *Acute pain* is usually straightforward and easily diagnosed. It generally follows tissue injury and is usually associated with objective physical signs of autonomic nervous system activity similar to those associated with anxiety as follows: tachycardia, hypertension, diaphoresis, mydriasis, and pallor.

Chronic pain presents a different clinical picture. It often cannot be ascribed to a specific injury or persists beyond the expected healing time (chronic benign pain) or may be associated with a persistent tissue injury, such as tumor (chronic malignant pain). It may not have a well-defined temporal onset and may not respond to treatments directed at its cause. Chronic pain can be particularly difficult to evaluate. In contrast to acute pain, autonomic signs (sweating, tachycardia, and/or pupillary dilation) may be absent, even in the presence of readily identifiable structural lesions, prompting the inexperienced observer to conclude that the patient does not "look" like he or she is in pain. The evaluation of patients with chronic pain is further complicated by changes in personality, lifestyle, and functional abilities and by symptoms and signs of depression as follows: hopelessness, helplessness, loss of libido and weight, and sleep disturbance.

Pain is subjective, and its description is highly dependent on the experience of the patient, leaving the physician totally dependent on the report of the pain by the patient. Objective observations of grimacing, limping, and tachycardia may be useful in assessing the patient's condition, but these signs may be absent in patients with chronic pain known to be caused by structural lesions. There is no neurophysiologic or chemical test that can measure pain. The clinician does well in the absence of strong contrary evidence to accept the patient's report of pain.

There are several general principles that are useful in the evaluation of the pain complaint. These principles have been detailed recently with respect to the patient with cancer,[3] but the following principles apply generally to all patients with pain, including those who

Table 45.1. Approach to the patient with pain.*

Approach
Elicit a clear history detailing the pain complaint
Differentiate between acute and chronic pain
Detail the onset of the pain
Establish the type, characteristics, and quality of pain
Determine exacerbating and relieving factors
Evaluate any associated symptoms
Perform a careful physical and neurologic examination
Assess the psychologic aspects of the pain complaint
Document a history of prior painful illnesses
Determine the role of pain in functional incapacity
Look for coexistent signs of anxiety and depression
Assess the degree of suffering and psychologic distress
Use appropriate diagnostic tools to determine the extent of disease
Plain x-ray films (not very useful for base of skull, C-7–T-1, and sacrum)
Tomograms (especially useful for base of skull, C1-2 area, C-7–T1, and sacrum)
CT and MRI (particularly helpful for evaluating paraspinal metastases, base of skull, epidural disease, disk problems, and plexopathies)
Bone scans (may not be accurate in radiated regions and may turn abnormal late)
Tumor markers, such as CEA
Surgical exporation and biopsy
Define the pain syndrome
Treat the pain early with adequate doses of medication

* CT indicates computed tomography; MRI, magnetic resonance imaging; and CEA, carcinoembryonic antigen.

are elderly: identify any tissue damage that may be the cause of the pain; recognize significant associated affective and environmental factors; and use whatever methods may support the patient in maintaining personally meaningful activities. In cases where the cause of acute pain is uncertain, establishing a diagnosis is a priority, but symptomatic treatment of pain should be given while the investigation is proceeding. With occasional exceptions, such as the initial examination of the acute abdomen, it is rarely justified to defer analgesia until a diagnosis is made.

Pain Systems

Recent advances in neuroanatomy, physiology, and pharmacology of the peripheral and central nervous system mechanisms of nociperception have been extensively reviewed.[4,5] However, the pathophysiology of pain remains complex and incompletely understood. Clinical pain can be divided into three broad classes: (1) somatic, (2) visceral, and (3) deafferentation or neuropathic. Somatic pain typically is acute and described as aching, sharp, and well localized. In

contrast, visceral pain is poorly localized, often referred, and difficult to describe for many patients.[6] Common examples include right shoulder pain that results from the diaphragmatic irritation of cholecystitis and neck and left arm pain associated with myocardial ischemia. Somatic and visceral pain both result from intense noxious or "tissue-damaging" stimuli that activate nociceptors. The accompanying inflammatory changes often associated with these stimuli further potentiate the pain by releasing algesic compounds that sensitize the nociceptors.

Deafferentation pain results from injury to the peripheral and central nervous system and may persist long after an injury appears to have healed. This type of pain often is very unpleasant, difficult to describe by the patient, and unfamiliar. The mechanisms associated with deafferentation pain are not clear, but nociceptors are not thought to play a major role. Some evidence suggests a central mechanism[7] and the possible involvement of the sympathetic nervous system.[8] Painful diabetic sensory neuropathies, postherpetic neuralgia, causalgia, and thalamic pain are common examples.

Cutaneous and Visceral Pain

Sensory receptors that are preferentially sensitive to noxious or potentially noxious stimuli have been classified morphologically and physiologically. Although best studied in skin, the physiologic properties of cutaneous nociceptors probably apply to visceral and muscular nociceptive units as well. In humans, activation of myelinated nociceptors, which respond almost exclusively to noxious mechanical stimuli,[9] elicit a sharp, stinging pain,[10] whereas activation of unmyelinated nociceptors produces a dull, burning, or aching pain.[11] Nociceptors can be sensitized, particularly after thermal injury to the skin.[9] Sensitization occurs rapidly, often within minutes of an injury, may persist for hours, and may be a physiologic correlate of hyperpathia or allodynia (ie, pain occurring on nonnoxious stimulation). A number of compounds that are released following tissue injury may be involved with the sensitization of nociceptors, including potassium, adenosine triphosphate, bradykinin, and prostaglandins, especially prostaglandin E_2.[4]

Deep pain that originates from skeletal muscle, bone, thoracic, abdominal, and pelvic viscera is much more common than cutaneous pain. Although much less well studied than their cutaneous counterparts, muscle and visceral nociceptors do exist in all organs with anatomic and physiologic properties that are similar to cutaneous nociceptors.[12] Pain that is elicited by muscle nociceptors is typically felt deeply rather than superficially and is often described as aching in quality. Bone and joint pain also is common, particularly in the elderly patient with arthritis. In patients with cancer, metastatic bone disease is the most common pain syndrome.

Visceral pain is poorly localized and typically deep, aching, and/or colicky. It is often referred to cutaneous points, which may be tender. Manipulation of normal viscera in conscious patients does not elicit pain, even when the viscera are cut, burned, or crushed. However, irritation of the mucosal and serosal surfaces, torsion and traction of the mesentery, distention or contraction of a hollow viscus, and impaction will produce pain. Similar stimuli are necessary to provoke pain in the bladder, ureter, or urethra.

The mechanism of *referred pain* is unclear, but possible mechanisms include[5] dual innervation of somatic and visceral structures by common afferent fibers and release of algesic chemicals in the vicinity of somatic afferent fibers. Some experimental data suggest that visceral nociceptor activity may converge with input from somatic afferents into common pools of spinothalamic tract cells in the dorsal horn of the spinal cord.[13] This suggests that pain is referred to remote cutaneous sites because the brain misinterprets the source of the input as coming from the periphery, which normally bombards the central nervous system with sensory stimuli.

Deafferentation (Neuropathic) Pain

Deafferentation pain, the third major type of pain, results from injury to the peripheral and/or central nervous system. Examples include diabetic neuropathy, acute zoster and postherpetic neuralgia, radicular pain from cervical or lumbar disk herniation, metastatic or radiation-induced brachial or lumbosacral plexopathies, and epidural spinal cord and/or cauda equina compression. Pain that results from neural injury often is severe, and it is of a different quality than nociceptive pain. It may be described in terms of "squeezing," with superimposed paroxyms of "burning" or "electrical shocklike" sensations that likely involve spontaneous and ectopic firing of damaged peripheral nerve structures.[14] Peripheral nerve injury also induces epileptiform activity in the medial thalamus in the area of projection of the paleospinothalamic tract. Conversely, stimulation of the medial thalamus produces burning pain in patients who have preexisting deafferentation pain, but not in patients who do not.[15]

The sympathetic nervous system may be involved in these pain states, particularly acute visceral and deafferentation pain.[16] The improvement of pain with sympathetic blockade by local anesthetic drugs or with administration of systemic adrenergic antagonist drugs, such as prazosin or phenoxybenzamine, in patients with reflex sympathetic dystrophy (RDS) is strong evidence in favor of a role for the sympathetic nervous system in these pain states, as is the increase in pain with sympathetic stimulation in some patients with RSD.

Central Modulation of Pain

Ascending Systems

The major ascending pathway for nociceptive input is the spinothalamic tract, which comprises, to a large extent, cells that receive nociceptive and diverse sensory input. The spinothalamic tract consists of two physiologically distinct systems: (1) the neospinothalamic and (2) the paleospinothalamic tracts.

The neospinothalamic tract subserves the sensory-discriminative aspects of pain perception, stimulus localization, and intensity. The phylogenetically older paleospinothalamic tract subserves the arousal, emotional, and affective/suffering components of pain. The neospinothalamic tract ascends in the anterolateral quadrant of the spinal cord and projects monosynaptically to the ventrobasilar thalamic complex that then projects to the somatosensory cortex in the parietal lobe. The paleospinothalamic tract ascends in continuity with the neospinothalamic tract in the anterolateral quadrant of the spinal cord and projects diffusely to the reticular formation in the brain stem and the posterior and the intralaminar nuclei of the thalamus.[16] The neurophysiologic mechanisms that encode pain in the face are subserved through the spinal trigeminal nucleus and are analgous to those described above.[17]

Melzack and Wall[18] postulated that the balance of activity between myelinated (large-fiber) and unmyelinated (small-fiber) afferents on dorsal horn transmission cells was important to the perceived intensity of pain: the Gate Control Theory.

The Cerebral Cortex and Pain

The role of the cortex in the perception of pain remains controversial. Some studies suggest that pain is not altered by large lesions of the cerebral hemispheres, including the somatosensory cortex, while others report that small lesions of the cortex are associated with the loss of pain perception. Although the exact role of the cortex in pain still is unclear, evidence in humans does suggest that the cortex plays a role in pain: (1) one can identify nociceptive-specific neurons in the SI cortex that contain projections from the VPL nucleus of the thalamus,[19] (2) stimulation of an exposed cortex in humans sometimes produces pain,[19] (3) pain is sometimes experienced in epileptic aurae,[20] and (4) lesions of the cortex can produce a syndrome that mimics thalamic pain.[16] However, it is clear that the involvement of the cortex in pain perception is very different from its involvement in other sensations.

Descending Systems

Descending pathways from the brain stem to the spinal cord are important modulators of nociceptive information. Serotoninergic and catecholaminergic terminals that have been demonstrated on the dendrites of dorsal horn neurons originate from these descending brain-stem projections.[21]

Electrical stimulation of the periaqueductal gray matter or nucleus raphe magnus, or microinjection of morphine at these sites, produces total-body analgesia without concomitant motor, sensory, or autonomic blockade.[22] Analgesia is blocked by prior section of the dorsal longitudinal fasciculus. Both serotonin and the enkephalins have been implicated in this effect, since both the opiate antagonist naloxone and the serotonin synthesis inhibitor p-chlorophenylamine reverse it.[5] The importance of nonopiate transmitters in this system may help to explain the analgesic activity of other drugs, particularly the psychotropic agents. For example, tricyclic antidepressants are useful analgesic agents in a variety of pain syndromes, including cancer, independent of their antidepressant activity.[5,23,24] The ability of physiologic stimuli, such as stress, to activate this system has led to the suggestion that activation of this descending control system may account for the phenomenon of placebo analgesia and the apparent analgesic effects of acupuncture and hypnosis.[5]

Endogenous Opioid Systems

The presence of endogenous systems that are capable of modulating the perception of pain has been inferred for decades, based in large part on the study by Beecher[25] during World War II. In this study, he compared the analgesic requirements for soldiers who were wounded on the beaches of Anzio, Italy, with those of civilians who were undergoing elective surgery here in the United States and found that the soldiers required far less medication despite their more severe wounds. Experimental evidence for this system came much later.[26–28] In these investigations, electrical stimulation of specific brain regions, such as the periaqueductal gray matter, elicited a profound anal-

gesia that could be antagonized by the opiate-selective antagonist naloxone, suggesting the release of endogenous opioid materials. We know now that this system comprises a family of opioid peptides and their receptors, through which opiates act.

The enkephalins were the first opioid peptides that were identified.[29,30] Just five amino acids long and differing only in the last residue, these compounds are potent analgesics and have many of the actions observed with classic opiates. A series of additional opioid peptides has been described (Table 45.2),[31] with

Table 45.2. Structures of selected endogenous and synthetic opioid peptides.

Opioid peptides	Structure
Endogenous	
[Leu⁵]enkephalin	H-TYR-GLY-GLY-PHE-Leu-OH
[Met⁵]enkephalin	H-TYR-GLY-GLY-PHE-Met-OH
β-Endorphin	H-TYR-GLY-GLY-PHE-Met-Thr-Ser-Glu-Lys-Ser-Gln-Thr-Pro-Leu-ValThr-Ley-Phe-Lys-Asn-Ala-Ile-Ile-Lys-Asn-Ala-Tyr-Lys-Lys-Gly-Glu-OH
Dynorphin A	H-TYR-GLY-GLY-PHE-Leu-Arg-Arg-Ile-Arg-Pro-Lys-Leu-Lys-Trp-Asp-Asn-Gln-OH
Dynorphin B	H-TYR-GLY-GLY-PHE-Leu-Arg-Arg-Gln-Phe-Lys-Val-Val-Thr
α-Neo-endorphin	H-TYR-GLY-GLY-PHE-Leu-Arg-Lys-Tyr-Pro-Lys-OH
Synthetic: enkephalin analogues	
[D-Ala²,Met⁵]-enkephalinamide (DAMEA)	H-Tyr-D-Ala-Gly-Phe-Met-CONH₂
[D-Ala²,D-Leu⁵]-enkephalin (DADLE)	H-Tyr-D-Ala-Gly-Phe-D-Leu-OH
[D-Ala²,Met⁵]-enkephalin (DALA)	H-Tyr-D-Ala-Gly-Phe-Met-OH
FK-33824	H-Tyr-D-Ala-Gly-Phe(N-CH₃)-Met(O)ol
Metkephamid	H-Tyr-D-Ala-Gly-Phe(N-CH₃)-Met-CONH₂
[D-Pen²,D-Pen⁵]-enkephalin (DPDPE)	H-Tyr-D-Pen-Gly-Phe-D-Pen
[D-Ser²,Leu⁵,Thr⁶]-enkephalin (DSTLE)	H-Tyr-D-Ser-Gly-Phe-Leu-Thr
[D-Ala²,MePhe⁴,-Gly(ol)⁵]enkephalin (DAMPGO or DAGO)	H-Tyr-D-Ala-Gly-MePhe-Gly(ol)

each peptide containing as its first five amino acids the structure of either methionine-enkephalin or leucine-enkephalin. The genes for these compounds have been isolated and characterized. All the peptides can elicit analgesia, but evidence suggests that they may interact with different receptor classes, as described below. Thus, the opioid peptides represent a whole family of neurotransmitters, similar to the monoamines.

One major problem with these peptides is their rapid degradation within the brain. This can be overcome by substitutions of D–amino acids, as exemplified by [D-Ala^2,D-Leu^5]enkephalin (DADL), [D-Pen^2, D-Pen^5]enkephalin (DPDPE), [D-Ala^2,MePhe^4, Gly(ol)^5]enkephalin (DAGO), metkephamid, and FK33824 (Table 45.2). In addition to improving stability, these substitutions also can alter dramatically the selectivity of the ligands. For example, DPDPE is highly selective for the delta opioid receptors, whereas DAGO is selective for mu receptors. These compounds are potent analgesics in humans. DADL has been given intrathecally and found to be approximately fivefold more potent than morphine on a molar basis.[32] Similarly, metkephamid and FK33824 have been reported to be effective systemically.[31]

Opiate receptors were first postulated many years ago, and the possibility of multiple classes was suggested in 1967.[33] They were first demonstrated biochemically in 1973.[34–36] Since then, the field has expanded enormously. Now a variety of receptor subtypes has been identified (Table 45.3). A full description of these subtypes and their pharmacology are reviewed elsewhere.[37] In brief, general classes were defined by their sensitivity for prototypic ligands: mu (morphine), kappa (ketocyclazocine and, more recently, dynorphin), delta (enkephalins), and epsilon (β-endorphin). Subclasses within both the mu[38] and kappa[39] classes also have been identified and

represent distinct receptor subtypes, much like α- and β-adrenergic receptors.

All the various opiate receptor subtypes have their own distinct pharmacologic profile, but each has been implicated in analgesia. Supraspinal opioid mechanisms are the most sensitive in eliciting analgesia and are responsible for analgesia following systemic administration of a drug. Animal studies indicate that mu$_1$ receptors mediate supraspinal analgesia,[40] and results of microinjection studies confirmed the importance of mu$_1$ receptors in analgesia elicited from the periaqueductal gray matter, locus coeruleus, nucleus raphe magnus, and nucleus reticularis gigantocellularis.[41] On the other hand, mu$_2$, delta, and kappa receptors mediate spinal analgesia; mu$_1$ receptors have no role in spinal analgesia. These localizations are important in view of the increasing use of epidural and intrathecal opiate in the treatment of pain. Most clinically available opiates are active at mu receptors, but some, such as levorphanol, also will interact at kappa and delta receptors as well. Thus, these agents may prove to be more valuable than morphine when working at the spinal level. Opiates also elicit a multitude of other actions, including respiratory depression, inhibition of gastrointestinal transit, hormone release, and feeding, which have been classified by the receptors mediating them (Table 45.3).

In summary, the anatomy, physiology, and pharmacology of nociperception and its modification by analgesic drugs has been studied extensively in the past decade. Although the neural mechanisms of nociperception and the stimuli that activate nociceptive and antinociceptive systems in the nervous system are much better understood, the perception of pain involves complex—and much less well understood—neuropsychologic phenomena.

Table 45.3. Classification of opioid receptors.

Opioid receptor	Prototypic ligand*	Actions
Mu		
Mu$_1$	Morphine enkephalins, β-endorphin	Supraspinal analgesia, prolactin release, catalepsy, acetylcholine turnover, feeding (deprivation-induced and free)
Mu$_2$	Morphine, DAMPGO (or DAGO)	Spinal analgesia, respiratory depression, gastrointestinal transit, dopamine turnover, growth hormone release (?)
Delta	Enkephalins, DPDPE	Spinal analgesia, growth hormone release (?), dopamine turnover
Kappa	Ketocyclazocine, dynorphin, U50,488 NalBzoH	Sedation, spinal analgesia, psychotomimetic effects, supraspinal analgesia (?)
Epsilon	β-Endorphin	Analgesia (?)
Sigma	(+)N-Allylnormetazocine (SKF10,047), phencyclidine (PCP)	Psychotomimetic effects

* See text.

Specific Pain Syndromes in the Elderly Population

Several pain syndromes occur with a higher frequency in the elderly population than in younger patients: (1) musculoskeletal disorders, particularly osteoarthritis, which produces chronic neck and back pain; (2) temporal arteritis; (3) postherpetic neuralgia; and (4) pain related to cancer or its therapy.

Musculoskeletal Pain in Elderly Persons

Neck and back pain may be caused by a variety of disorders (Tables 45.4 and 45.5).[42–44] These conditions may produce local bony or soft-tissue pain, or, by virtue of nerve root or spinal cord compression or referred myofascial pain, they may be associated with pain remote from the site of the primary pathologic condition (See also Chapter 17).

Neck pain secondary to cervical spondylosis is a disease of aging. Radiologic manifestations of cervical spondylosis can be seen in more than 50% of patients aged older than 50 years, and in 75% of patients aged older than 65 years.[45] Most patients are asymptomatic, but degenerative disease of the cervical skeleton, including the supporting ligamentous structures, may produce pain and neurologic dysfunction resulting from vertebral body fusion, the ossification of ligamentous structures, and formation of osteophytic bars that allows compression of adjacent nerve roots and spinal cord.

Table 45.4. Differential diagnosis of neck pain in elderly persons.*

Differential diagnosis of neck pain
Lesions in the cervical spine, spinal cord, and meninges
Spondylosis
Fractures and dislocations
Primary and secondary tumors of spinal vertebrae
Meningeal inflammation, infection, or tumor metastasis
Subluxation of the vertebrae (eg, rheumatoid arthritis)
Infection of the vertebrae (eg, osteomyelitis, Pott's disease)
Herniation of the nucleus pulposus
Lesions of the shoulder and brachial plexus
Cervical ribs and thoracic outlet syndrome
Pancoast's tumor of lung
Idiopathic brachial neuritis
Tumor infiltration or radiation-induced fibrosis of the brachial plexus
Bursitis and fibrositis of the shoulder joint
Referred pain from the mediastinum and pharynx

* Modified from Payne.[42,43]

Table 45.5. Differential diagnosis of back pain in elderly persons.*

Differential diagnosis of back pain
Musculoskeletal and neuropathic disorders
Disk herniation
Spondylosis with nerve entrapment
Lumbar stenosis
Spondylolisthesis
Osteoporosis
Myeloma
Primary and metastatic bone tumors
Osteomyelitis and epidural abscess
Visceral pain referred to the back
Pancreatitis and pancreatic carcinoma
Peptic ulcer disease
Nephrolithiasis
Pyelonephritis
Abdominal aortic aneurysm
Ovarian cysts and tumors
Prostatitis and prostate cancer

* Modified from Payne.[48]

The pain of cervical radiculopathy may be of the deep, aching variety, localized to the base of the neck, shoulder girdle, and, classically, the upper fibers of the trapezius muscle. Lancinating and shooting pain, often with a burning quality, which radiates into the arm, forearm, and hand signals cervical root compression. With C-5 root compression, pain, paresthesia, and weakness of the shoulder girdle musculature occur. Compression of the C-6 root produces pain and paresthesia in the anterolateral aspect of the arm, thumb, and second finger; C-7 root compression produces these symptoms in the posterolateral portion of the arm and the the second and third fingers. Finally, compression of the C-8 and/or T-1 nerve roots produces pain, paresthesia, and weakness of the fourth and fifth fingers, the elbow, and the axilla. Note that cervical nerve roots exist above their respective vertebral bodies; therefore, disk herniation at C4-5 will result in C-5 root compression.

Cervical spondylosis results from a slow degenerative process that begins at about the age of 20 years. During the third decade of life, the nucleus pulposus becomes progressively desiccated and fibrotic. In addition, the normal "ball-bearing" movements of the vertebral bodies become abnormal. For example, in flexion, the anterior and posterior contours of the cervical spine increase by 1.5 and 5.0 cm, respectively, with the C5-6 joint being the most mobile.[46] Similarly, the cervical foramina increase in size during extension of the neck. With fibrosis of the facet joints and the progressive dehydration of the nucleus pulposus with aging, this normal movement of the cervical spine is lost, further leading to abnormal biomechanical stresses on the anterior and posterior longitudinal ligaments. The net effect is fibrotic, stiff ligaments and bony osteophytic overgrowths that may produce recurrent trauma to the cord and nerve roots during the constant flexion, extension, and rotation of the cervical spine that occurs with normal head, neck, and body movement. Spondylotic myelopathy is much more likely to occur once the diameter of the spinal canal has been decreased below the normal 9 to 10 mm. The condition of not every patient with symptomatic cervical spondylotic radiculopathy is improved with a foraminotomy, and some patients with this syndrome have apparently normal neural foramina on plain x-ray films.[47] Therefore, nerve root–sleeve fibrosis and root-sleeve stretching without compression also are thought to be important mechanisms of nerve root damage in cervical spondylotic radiculopathy.[46]

Plain films of the cervical spine (with anterior-posterior, lateral, and oblique projections) may be complemented by myelography, computed tomography (CT), or magnetic resonance imaging (MRI). These studies allow visualization and calculation of the diameter of the spinal canal and will demonstrate the site of root and/or spinal cord compression. In addition, they exclude other causes of neck pain associated with upper-extremity neurologic symptoms and signs, including neurofibroma, syringomyelia, and spinal cord tumors (Table 45.4).

Conservative treatment of patients with myelopathy includes the use of a soft cervical collar, physical therapy to preserve function in weakened and spastic arms and legs, and analgesics (typically nonnarcotic, nonsteroidal anti-inflammatory analgesics) for pain. Chiropractic manipulation of the neck is controversial.[46] In some patients, symptoms of cervical root compression diminish with further aging as the spine becomes less mobile due to the accumulated degenerative changes. Surgery is not indicated for pain alone, but to prevent progression of myelopathy, especially weakness and spasticity in the hands and lower extremities. Two basic surgical approaches may be used: (1) anterior exposure of the vertebral body with removal of the osteophyte and/or protruding disk (ie, the Cloward procedure) combined with vertebral body fusion, or (2) posterior exposure of the lamina with laminectomy and nerve root decompression. Improvement in neurologic function, and usually pain, has been reported in up to 74% of patients after laminectomy and in 60% with either fusion or laminectomy for treatment of spondylotic myelopathy.[46] The major indication for surgery in spondylotic myelopathy is severe, persistent pain with progressive radiculopathy. Several studies have reported up to 80% improve-

ment in patients following fusion or foraminotomy, if the nerve root has been adequately decompressed and the cervical spine adequately stabilized.

Back Pain in Elderly Persons

Back pain is common in elderly persons (Table 45.5).[48] The most common causes include (1) disk herniation, (2) lumbar stenosis, (3) osteoporosis with compression fracture, and (4) bone metastasis and epidural spinal cord compression complicating advanced cancer. Diseases of thoracic, abdominal, and pelvic viscera also may produce pain referred to the back but will not be discussed here.

Osteoarthritis associated with age-related "wear-and-tear" trauma to the weight-bearing joints of the spine, knees, and small joints of the hands and feet may produce pain by impingement on nerve roots or nonneural soft tissue. In the lumbar spine, bony overgrowth resulting from these changes may produce narrowing of the neural foramina with resultant pain and loss of function in the innervated muscles and cutaneous distribution. With L-4 radiculopathy, pain may radiate from the lumbar spine to the anterior and medial parts of the thigh, and weakness is present in the quadriceps muscle. The knee jerk may be lost. Compression of the L-5 nerve root produces pain that radiates into the great toe and dorsum of the foot, with weakness of extension of the great toe and foot, as well as weakness of eversion of the entire foot. The ankle jerk may be depressed. Finally, S-1 root dysfunction is manifested by pain that radiates from the back into the buttocks, posterior part of the calf, and lateral aspect of the foot. There may be an overlap with the L-5 root, in that sensory loss and pain may be demonstrated in the great toe, and the ankle jerk also is depressed.

Lumbar spinal stenosis is produced by a combination of degenerative processes that act to ensure the diameter of the spinal canal, thereby promoting compression of the nerve roots and cauda equina in the lower part of the lumbosacral spine. These degenerative changes include osteophyte formation, intervertebral disk bulging, and hypertrophy of the ligamentum flavum.[44] Classically, spinal stenosis presents as "pseudoclaudication," with sharp pain originating in the lower part of the spine, radiating into the buttocks, thigh, or leg that is precipitated by exertion and may be partially relieved by rest. Peripheral vascular disease does not account for these symptoms, which may improve with spinal decompression.

Plain films of the lumbosacral spine and pelvis are helpful in excluding destructive neoplastic processes as the cause of back pain. Oblique views of the lumbar spine may be needed to visualize the neural foramina.

The CT and MRI scanning visualizes neural structures directly and permits the determination of the size of the spinal canal, as well as identifying associated bone destruction or soft-tissue masses.[44,49] Scanning has the additional advantage over myelography of being noninvasive, so it can be performed as an outpatient. The electromyogram (EMG) is useful in confirming the distribution of peripheral nerve and/or root dysfunction.

Management of back pain secondary to osteoarthritis involves bed rest and structured activity. Prolonged bed rest more than 1 week is not advisable, even for an acutely herniated disk and back pain, because it usually does not improve function and may contribute to further bony demineralization or osteoporosis. Traction does not offer any advantages over simple bed rest. Other measures that are frequently helpful in back pain management include the use of transcutaneous nerve stimulation (TENS), treatment of focal muscle pain and spasms with topical ice or heat, and injection of local anesthetics into "trigger points." The use of nonnarcotic analgesics may be helpful for treating acute and chronic pain, and weak narcotic analgesics may be useful for treating acute severe back pain.

Surgery may be indicated for progressive neurologic dysfunction, such as weakness, urinary or fecal incontinence, spasticity, or sensory loss, but it is rarely indicated for pain alone. The risks of surgical intervention, including the use of general anesthetic agents in the geriatric population in which cardiopulmonary diseases are prevalent, must be weighed against the potential benefit. A recent uncontrolled study of 32 patients aged older than 60 years reported the efficacy of a lumbar laminectomy with a diskotomy (and, in one instance, spinal fusion) to be "excellent or good" in 87% of patients who were followed up for an average of 50 months.[50] Intractable pain was the "main indication" for surgery, the complication rate was 18.7%, with no fatalities. However, prospective studies of comparable groups are required to assess the true efficacy of lumbar disk surgery in the geriatric population. Chymopapain offers an alternative to surgery, but this procedure may lead to failure to control symptoms if there is a free disk fragment, and its use has been associated with at least as many complications as surgery.

A detailed discussion of osteoporosis appears in Chapter 15; this obviously is an important age-related cause of back pain when fractures complicate the disorder. The most common fracture sites are the distal part of the forearm (Colles' fracture), the hip, and the vertebral bodies. Therapy for acute bone pain will be discussed below.

Pain syndromes that occur in the patient with cancer will be discussed in the following section, but back pain that complicates malignant neoplasms deserves mention here. Severe neck and back pain are the hallmark of this entity. Pain can be either local over the involved vertebral body or radicular, with the symptoms dependent on the nerve roots involved.

Most instances of spinal cord compression secondary to metastatic cancer can be treated with steroids and radiation therapy. However, surgery is indicated in the following circumstances: (1) the need to establish a histologic diagnosis of cancer, (2) the occurrence of spinal cord compression in an area of a previously irradiated cord or when the tumor is relatively radioresistant, and (3) the occurrence of bony subluxation and spinal instability that complicate vertebral body metastasis. Approximately 80% of patients who are treated while they are still ambulatory will remain so. Only 50% or less who are not ambulatory when treatment is begun will become ambulatory. Hence, early diagnosis and treatment are essential.

Cranial (Temporal) Arteritis

Although patients younger than 40 years of age have been described, temporal arteritis remains predominately a disease in patients aged older than 60 years age (see Chapter 16 for full discussion). The initial clinical manifestations are headache, followed by polymyalgia rheumatica (proximal muscle pain and joint stiffness) and other constitutional symptoms, including fever, malaise, anorexia, and weight loss. Other symptoms include synovitis, scalp tenderness, visual disturbances, including blindness, claudication, and an aortic arch syndrome.

Headache, present in up to 98% of cases, may be quite severe, boring and/or sharp in quality, localized to the regions of the scalp arteries, and often accompanied by scalp tenderness.[51]

Prompt treatment with nonsteroidal antiinflammatory drugs and steroids is strongly indicated. Generally, prednisone is administered until all reversible symptoms are gone, and the results of all laboratory tests return to normal.

Acute Herpetic and Postherpetic Neuralgia

Acute neuralgia that complicates varicella-zoster virus infection can occur at any age, but postherpetic neuralgia, ie, pain that persists beyond 6 months, is much more common in old age.[52,53] In patients older than 80 years of age, the attack rate has been calculated to be 10-fold greater than in children. The pain of postherpetic neuralgia frequently is described as deep, aching, squeezing, sharp, lancinating, and burning. Patients with lancinating or shooting pain may respond to anticonvulsant drugs,[54] such as carbamazepine, whereas those with deep burning and aching pain usually do not respond to carbamazepine, but may improve with tricyclic antidepressants, such as amitriptyline (see also Chapter 25).[55]

Numerous pharmacologic, anesthetic, and surgical therapies have been reported for treatment of acute and postherpetic neuralgia, but the efficacy of only a few, such as amitriptyline, have been proved in well-controlled studies. Most experts recommend the start of therapy with a low dose of amitriptyline, typically 10 to 25 mg/d in a single dose, followed by a gradual increase in dosage to 75 to 100 mg/d, depending on side effects. Keep in mind that many of the side effects associated with amitriptyline can be particularly troublesome in the geriatric population. Occasionally, switching to another tricyclic antidepressant with less anticholinergic potency, such as desipramine, may be useful if the patient experiences the urinary hesitancy, delirium, or dry mouth that frequently accompany amitriptyline therapy. The addition of a neuroleptic, such as fluphenazine, to the antidepressant may be of value.[55] These drugs must be used with caution in the elderly patient due to the risk of tardive dyskinesia. Counterirritation techniques, including the use of TENS also may be efficacious. Recently, topical capsacian, a substance P antagonist, has been used for management of postherpetic neuralgia with mixed results. It is difficult to recommend more invasive therapies, such as somatic or sympathetic nerve blocks, and neuroablative procedures, such as rhizotomy, dorsal root entry zone lesions, or neurolytic blocks, in the absence of controlled studies that demonstrate their efficacy. These procedures should only be considered in truly disabling pain after all other therapies have failed. Also, it is mandatory that aggressive and appropriate psychologic interventions designed to increase the patient's coping abilities and to manage coexisting depression and despair start concomitantly with drug therapy, and certainly before any invasive procedure. Unfortunately, the therapy for intractable postherpetic neuralgia, especially for patients with pain for more than 2 years, is problematic at best.

Cancer Pain in Elderly Persons

The age-specific incidence of cancer for many of the solid tumors that are associated with major pain problems markedly increases over the age of 40 years and progressively increases with each succeeding de-

cade. Pain from invasion of bone and soft tissue by either primary or metastatic tumor is the most common cause of cancer pain. The pain usually is well localized to the lesion, but visceral pain can be referred. Diagnosis of this problem usually is straightforward with the use of CT and MRI scans. Caution must be used with plain x-ray films because they are often falsely negative. Pain management of soft tissue and bone invasion often requires opiate analgesics, described below, and usually is very effective. However, the presence of many of these pain syndromes should alert the physician to underlying problems, such as epidural cord compression associated with spinal metastasis. A full discussion of the syndromes listed in Table 45.6 is beyond the scope of this chapter, but can be found in the review by Foley and Sundarasen.[3] Neuropathic pain syndromes, caused by tumor infiltration or nerve injury from cancer therapy, will be reviewed, since they are particularly difficult to

Table 45.6. Specific pain syndromes associated with cancer.

Pain syndromes
Pain syndromes associated with direct tumor infiltration
Tumor infiltration of bone
Base of skull
Vertebral body
Sacrum
Tumor infiltration of nerve
Peripheral neuropathy
Plexopathies
Brachial plexopathy
Lumbar plexopathy
Sacral plexopathy
Leptomeningeal infiltration of roots
Spinal cord
Epidural spinal cord compression
Intramedullary metastasis
Pain syndromes associated with cancer therapy
Postsurgery syndromes
Postthoracotomy syndrome
Postmastectomy syndrome
Postradical neck syndrome
Phantom-limb syndrome
Postchemotherapy syndromes
Peripheral neuropathy
Aseptic necrosis of the femoral head
Steroid-induced pseudorheumatism
Postherpetic neuralgia
Postradiation syndromes
Radiation-induced fibrosis of brachial and lumbar plexus
Radiation-induced myelopathy
Radiation-induced second primary tumors
Radiation-induced necrosis of bone

manage, especially in the geriatric population, for whom drug toxicity is a greater problem.

In pain syndromes associated with tumor infiltration of nerve, the pain is characterized by constant burning pain with hypesthesias and dysesthesias in an area of sensory loss. The most common causes are tumor compression in the paravertebral or retroperitoneal area or in association with a metastatic tumor in the rib, causing intercostal nerve infiltration. Local and radicular pain are seen with tumor infiltration or compression of nerve peripheral to the paraspinal region, whereas referred pain with or without a radicular component is seen with tumor infiltration of the paraspinal region and more proximal areas. Associated autonomic dysfunction, such as a loss of sweating and a loss of axonal flair response to pin scratch, can help to define the site of the nerve compression or infiltration. The pain is characterized initially as a dull, aching sensation with tenderness to percussion in the distribution of the nerve. Mild paresthesias or dysesthesias can occur as the next sensory symptom, followed by the late appearance of motor symptoms and signs. As the tumor invades the perineurium or compresses the nerve externally, the nature of the pain changes to a burning, dyesthetic sensation. A careful neurologic examination, followed by a CT scan to define the site of nerve compression, are the diagnostic procedures of choice. An EMG can help to define the site of nerve involvement, but it is not diagnostic. Rib erosion and retroperitoneal and paraspinal soft-tissue masses are the most common associated findings.

In patients with a paraspinal tumor, myelography (and/or MRI scanning) often is necessary to exclude epidural extension. Antitumor therapy is the first-line therapy when possible, but interim pain management with analgesics is almost always necessary. Steroids may provide a useful diagnostic test because of both antiinflammatory and antitumor effects, or may act to reduce local swelling, which secondarily relieves pain. However, steroids do not represent a useful long-term management approach due to their role in a number of complications, including peripheral edema, weight gain, hyperglycemia, cataracts, osteoporosis with compression fractures, and an increased risk of infection from immunosuppression.

Brachial Plexopathy

Brachial plexopathy in patients with cancer may be due to tumor invasion of the plexus, trauma during surgery and anesthesia, or secondary to radiation therapy. Radiation can produce nerve damage directly or through radiation-induced tumors, such as malignant schwannoma or fibrosarcoma. Tumor infiltration

and radiation injury are the most common. There are reliable clinical signs and symptoms to distinguish metastatic plexopathy from radiation-induced injury.[56] In patients with tumor-related plexopathies, pain often is quite severe, initially localized to the C-7–T-1 distribution, and, when associated with a Horner's syndrome, suggests impending spinal cord involvement. On the other hand, radiation-induced plexopathy usually presents as C5-6 (or upper trunk involvement), and although lymphedema may be present, pain usually is not as severe as in tumor-related plexopathy.

The CT scan is the diagnostic procedure of choice. Recently, MRI scanning has been advocated and may be a useful means to diagnose metastatic brachial plexopathy. However, comparative studies with CT imaging have not been done, to date. Electrodiagnostic studies (EMGs) are useful in distinguishing tumor infiltration of the brachial plexus from radiation-induced injury. Myokymia, when present, is almost always associated with radiation-induced injury of the plexus. However, radiation-induced fibrosis and tumor can occur simultaneously. Rarely, a biopsy of the brachial plexus may be necessary to distinguish tumor infiltration by recurrent tumor or a new radiation-induced tumor from radiation-induced fibrosis.[1] However, the results of a biopsy are not always definitive.

Brachial plexopathy is a common component of Pancoast's tumors. Pain in a C-8–T-1 distribution, often an early sign, may play an integral role in the diagnosis of the tumor and reliably reflects disease progression. It is the earliest and may be the only sign of epidural cord compression, affecting as many as 50% of patients with Pancoast's tumors. Plain x-ray films and bone scans are not reliable diagnostic tests in assessing this disorder. The initial diagnostic workup should include a CT or MRI scan, tomograms of the vertebral bodies, and myelography to determine the extent of tumor infiltration. Surgery should be directed at removal of all the local tumor and secondary treatment with external radiation therapy and brachytherapy. Pancoast's syndrome is commonly misdiagnosed as cervical disk disease. However, the disk disease appears in a C-8–T-1 distribution in fewer than 5% of patients. The early diagnosis of a tumor is crucial to curative therapy.

Distinguishing between tumor and radiation plexopathies can be difficult, but they often can be diagnosed clinically. Metastasis to the brachial plexus most commonly involves the lower cords, giving rise to neurologic signs and symptoms in the distribution of the C-8 and T-1 roots. In contrast, radiation-induced plexopathy most commonly involves the upper cords of the plexus, predominantly in the distribution of the C-5, C-6, and C-7 roots. Severe pain is most commonly associated with metastatic plexopathy. Horner's syndrome is more commonly associated with metastatic plexopathy than radiation-induced plexopathy and indicates the possibility of an epidural extension of tumor. Finally, neither normal results of a surgical biopsy nor observation for several years for other metastases rule out recurrence of tumor or a new primary tumor.[1]

Lumbosacral Plexus Tumor Infiltration

Involvement of the lumbosacral plexus with tumor commonly is seen in genitourinary, gynecologic, and colonic cancers. Pain often is the earliest symptom, followed later by complaints of paresthesias, numbness, and dysesthesias, leading finally to motor and sensory loss. The distribution of the pain varies with the site of plexus involvement and may be limited to radicular pain. Upper plexus lesions produce pain along the anterior part of the thigh and groin (L-1, L-2, and L-3 distribution), while the pain in lower lesions may radiate into the posterior aspect of the leg to the heel (L-5 and S-1) or into the pelvis.

Jaeckle et al[57] reviewed 85 patients with lumbosacral plexopathy and noted local pain in 72, radicular pain in 72, and referred pain in 37. Local pain in the sacrum or sciatic area was present in 59% of patients, followed by lower back pain in 27% and pain in the groin or lower abdominal quadrant in 21%. Referred pain to the hip or flank occurred in patients with upper plexus lesions, whereas pain in the ankle or the foot occurred in patients with a lower plexopathy. Typically, the pain precedes objective sensory, motor, and autonomic signs for weeks to months (mean, 3 months), and initial CT scans may be normal. Unilateral and bilateral plexopathy with significant motor weakness commonly is associated with an epidural extension, and both CT or MRI scan and myelography are necessary to define the extent of tumor infiltration and/or epidural compression. Plain x-ray films often are not helpful, because the lumbosacral plexus lies within the substance of the psoas muscle and is difficult to visualize. Specific antitumor therapy is dependent on the tumor type, and relief of pain symptoms is directly related to tumor responsiveness. Patients with colorectal and cervical cancers and sarcomas have persistent pain and progressive plexopathy. Pain management in these patients is particularly difficult, because selective analgesia cannot be provided without interfering with motor, sensory, and autonomic functions.

Overall, the management of painful plexopathies is unsatisfactory, but a series of approaches may be effective in treating some patients. All patients should be treated with nonnarcotic and narcotic analgesics. Steroids are helpful in treating patients with significant local swelling. Carbamazepine may be useful for treating acute lancinating pain, and antidepressants may help with dysesthesias. Specific anesthetic and neurosurgical pain management approaches vary with the site of tumor involvement. Epidural local anesthetics can provide local pain relief for lumbosacral plexopathy and can be appropriately titrated to provide only sensory loss, but cannot be maintained for long periods of time because of the development of tolerance to the analgesic effects. Epidural phenol and intrathecal phenol or alcohol are used to produce a chemical neurolysis and can be titrated to produce predominantly sensory changes. However, loss of motor function with the use of these techniques in the management of pain, involving the brachial and lumbosacral plexus, is a significant risk. Subarachnoid administration of phenol and alcohol to block the cauda equina can produce bowel and bladder dysfunction with associated motor loss. No patient should undergo a subarachnoid lumbar block (or spinal opiate administration) with such agents until myelography demonstrates the patency of the subarachnoid space.[58]

A percutaneous or open cordotomy can be very effective with unilateral lumbosacral plexopathy but is less useful in patients with brachial plexopathy where pain radiating to the neck and ears often escapes the cordotomy level. Bilateral pain from a bilateral lumbosacral plexopathy requires a bilateral cordotomy for effective pain control with the consequent risk to bowel and bladder function, as well as motor weakness secondary to bilateral corticospinal tract damage. Epidural and intrathecal morphine infusions can provide analgesia that is selective without interfering with motor, sensory, and autonomic function.[59] Both epidural and intrathecal infusions also are associated with significant systemic uptake of the drug and do not completely obviate the side effects of systemic drug administration. Escalation of dose to offset tolerance can limit the usefulness of this technique.

Dorsal column stimulation and periventricular brain stimulation have been of limited usefulness in this patient population.[22] Behavioral techniques help patients cope with their pain and help to manage the associated symptoms of anxiety and depression that occur with chronic pain and neurologic disability. These syndromes are particularly difficult to manage, and patients are often faced with decisions to undergo novel procedures for only partial relief.[3]

Pain Syndromes Associated With Cancer Therapy

A number of clinical pain syndromes occur in the course of or subsequent to treatment of patients with cancer who undergo surgery, chemotherapy, or radiation therapy. The management of radiation-induced plexopathies is discussed above. Chemotherapy is rarely painful, but associated peripheral neuropathies can be troublesome. Treatment is symptomatic and usually involves antidepressants for treating burning or dysesthesias and carbamazepine for treating lancinating pain. The most difficult syndromes are those of peripheral nerve involvement.

Postthoracotomy Pain

Postthoracotomy pain results from the transection or injury of the intercostal nerve and is most often observed following traction on the ribs with thoracic surgery or rib resection. The immediate postoperative pain occurs in virtually all patients who undergo a thoracotomy and is characterized by an aching sensation in the distribution of the incision with sensory loss with or without autonomic changes. There often is exquisite point tenderness at the most medial and apical points of the scar with a specific trigger point. In most patients, the pain subsides during several months. Recurrence of pain or persistence is most often a result of infection or recurrence of tumor and should be investigated.

We have followed up a small number of patients in whom a traumatic neuroma developed at the site of their previous thoracotomy scar. These patients represent a rare, rather than common, entity, and tumor recurrence, rather than a traumatic neuroma, should be the initial consideration in evaluating such patients with cancer.

Chest x-ray films are insufficient to evaluate recurrent disease, and a CT scan through the chest with bone and soft-tissue windows is the diagnostic procedure of choice before the consideration of intercostal nerve blocks in the management of pain in these syndromes. If the pain management is inadequate or the patient is not actively rehabilitated following surgery, a frozen shoulder and secondary reflex sympathetic dystrophy involving the arm can occur. The nature of the pain in patients with a traumatic neuroma cannot be distinguished from tumor infiltration of the nerve clinically, but the ability to localize a specific trigger point and to provide dramatic pain relief with a local anesthetic blockade strongly suggest a traumatic neuroma.

Postmastectomy Pain

Postmastectomy pain results from injury or interruption of the intercostal brachial nerve and is seen following any surgical procedure on the breast, from lumpectomy to radical mastectomy, or after axillary dissection; the incidence is approximately 5%. The pain may occur immediately following the surgical procedure or as much as 6 months afterward and is characterized as a tight, constricting, burning pain in the posterior aspect of the arm and axilla that radiates across the anterior chest wall. However, the marked anatomic variation in the distribution of the intercostal brachial nerve results in a variable appearance clinically. The nature of the pain and its clinical symptoms should readily distinguish it from a brachial plexopathy secondary to tumor infiltration. The pain is exacerbated by movement of the arm and relieved by immobilization. Patients often posture the arm in a flexed position close to the chest wall and are at risk for the development of a frozen shoulder syndrome if adequate pain relief and postsurgical rehabilitation are not implemented early on. Postoperative complications that lead to fibrosis around the nerve, such as infection or seroma, are particularly likely to cause the syndrome. Typically, a trigger point in the axilla or on the anterior chest wall demonstrates the site of the traumatic neuroma. Breast reconstruction does not alter the tight, constricting sensation in the anterior chest wall that is associated with this syndrome. Pain management in postmastectomy syndrome is similar to the management of any patient with peripheral nerve injury and pain.

Postradical Neck Dissection Pain

Typically, this pain is described as burning in the area of sensory loss and may include dysethesias and intermittent shocklike pain. Like postthoracotomy pain, it is temporally related to the surgical procedure. Recurrence or exacerbation of pain should prompt a full reevaluation to exclude recurrence of tumor. Adenocystic tumors that involve the head and neck typically invade and metastasize locally along the nerve, giving rise to sensory loss, burning dysesthesias, and shocklike shooting and lancinating pain and have a very high incidence of recurrence.

Phantom-Limb Pain

Almost all patients have phantom sensations following amputations, but a number also experience pain distinct from phantom-limb sensation.[60] Phantom-limb pain localized to a portion of the removed limb usually occurs in patients who had pain in the same site before the amputation. Amputation may initially magnify the pain, which slowly fades over time. Stump pain, resulting from a traumatic neuroma, is localized to the site of the surgical scar and appears several months to years following amputation. Stump pain is characterized as a burning, dysesthetic sensation that is exacerbated by movement and blocked by local anesthetic injection. In some patients, the development of a painful phantom-limb several years following surgery represents the earliest sign of tumor recurrence.

Management of peripheral nerve pain in patients with cancer involves a variety of approaches. Following the definition of the nature of the pain and differentiation between tumor infiltration and nerve injury, treatment approaches include the use of systemic narcotic and nonnarcotic analgesics, adjuvant analgesics, TENS, local anesthetic blocks, and (temporary and permanent) surgical procedures. Cryoprobes that are used to freeze the peripheral nerve also have been used in the management of patients with postthoracotomy pain and may be useful in the other syndromes.

Pharmacotherapy for Pain

In the management of pain, the choice of drug therapy is dependent on the cause and type of pain being treated. Analgesics generally are divided into three types: (1) nonsteroidal anti-inflammatory drugs (NSAIDS), (2) opiate analgesics, and (3) the adjuvant analgesics. Acute pain generally is treated with NSAIDS and/or opiates, depending on its severity. Chronic cancer pain usually requires opiates, whereas their use in chronic benign pain remains controversial, particularly in the absence of demonstrable structural lesions.[61] Sharp, achy pain often is well controlled with NSAIDS and opiates, but burning, dysethetic pain is better managed with antidepressants and other adjuvant agents. Lancinating pains usually are treated with carbamazepine. The pharmacologic management of specific pain problems may require specific therapy, such as the headache related to temporal arteritis. Clinicians should not attempt to use all the agents available. Rather, they should be familiar with several drugs in each analgesic class.

Nonopioid Analgesics

Included within this group are the NSAIDS, such as aspirin, fenoprofen, ibuprofen, diflunisal, naproxen, and ketoprofen and acetaminophen (Table 45.7). These "mild" analgesics are widely used for the treatment of acute and chronic pain due to surgery,

Table 45.7. Mild, nonnarcotic analgesics.*

Drug	Usual starting oral dose, mg	Comments	Precautions/ contraindications
Anti-inflamatory agents			
Aspirin	650–1,000	Often used in combination with narcotic-type analgesics	May cause gastric irritation or bleeding, especially with steroids; affects platelet function; avoid in clotting disorders; avoid in liver or renal failure
Ibuprofen	200–400	Greater analgesic potency than aspirin	Like aspirin
Fenoprofen	200	Like ibuprofen	Like ibuprofen
Diflunisal	1,000 (initial dose); 500 every 8 h thereafter	Like ibuprofen, but longer duration of action	Like ibuprofen
Naproxen	500 (initial dose); 250 every 6–8 h thereafter	Like diflunisal	Like ibuprofen
Ketoprofen	25–50	Like ibuprofen	Like ibuprofen
Choline magnesium trisalicylate	1,500	Does not affect platelet function	Like aspirin, except for gastrointestinal and antiplatelet actions
Others			
Acetaminophen	650	Like aspirin, but no anti-inflamatory actions	Overdoses have high liver toxicity

* Modified from the American Pain Society.[79]

trauma, and systemic disease, such as arthritis and cancer. The NSAIDS have analgesic, antipyretic, anti-platelet, and anti-inflammatory actions and differ from opioid analgesics. Foremost, these compounds have a maximal ceiling effect to analgesia. Once the maximal effect has been reached, further increases in drug dosage will not produce additional pain relief, whereas opiates do not demonstrate a ceiling effect clinically. The NSAIDS and acetaminophen do produce tolerance or physical or psychologic dependence and act on pain through peripheral mechanisms, probably by inhibiting prostaglandin E_2 formation by cyclooxygenase. Prostaglandin E_2 sensitizes nociceptors on peripheral nerves to the pain-producing effects of substances, such as bradykinin.

The NSAIDS are used alone for mild-to-moderate pain and in combination with opioids for severe pain. The choice of one drug over another is empiric. Generally, it is best to start with aspirin, acetaminophen, or ibuprofen because of the vast experience with these compounds. Some patients respond to one agent better than others, and patients should be switched to another agent if the first is not adequate. Ibuprofen, fenoprofen, and ketoprofen have short half-lives and the same duration of action as aspirin, whereas diflunisal and naproxen have longer half-lives and longer onset time. Aspirin and NSAIDS may prolong the bleeding time due to inhibition of platelet cyclooxygenase and reduced formation of thromboxane A_2. Acetaminophen is recommended in patients with platelet disorders. Gastric irriation occurs commonly with this class of drugs, and patients should be monitored carefully. The NSAIDS also can cause drug-induced renal insufficiency, particularly in patients with congestive heart failure, chronic renal insufficiency, cirrhosis with ascites, and intravascular volume depletion, as well as in patients being treated with diuretics.

Acetaminophen is equipotent to aspirin in its analgesic and antipyretic effect, but has no anti-inflammatory or antiplatelet action. It also produces less gastric irritation and is the drug of choice in patients who are undergoing surgery or chemotherapy. However, high doses are extremely hepatotoxic, and the dosage should be limited to 4,000 mg/d; even this level may be toxic in patients with preexisting liver damage. Choline magnesium trisalicylate also is an effective analgesic that lacks antiplatelet effects and has fewer gastrointestinal side effects than aspirin.

Opioid Analgesics

Opioid analgesics remain the mainstay in the management of severe acute pain and chronic cancer-related pain.[1,62] Each patient's requirements should be determined, and the choice of drug and its dosage should be individualized. As discussed above, opiates act centrally through binding to opiate receptors. A number of different subtypes of opiate receptors have been identified, including ones selective for morphine (mu), the enkephalins (delta), and dynorphin (kappa). Each receptor class is capable of mediating analgesia independent of the others. Most clinically relevant opiate analgesics are mu (morphinelike), although some, such as levorphanol, also have additional actions at kappa and delta receptors. This is important because tolerance develops at each receptor class indpendently, and patients who are tolerant at one receptor class may still be responsive at another, which explains incomplete cross-tolerance among opiates. Research also indicates that receptor subtypes, responsible for many of the side effects associated with opiate use, such as respiratory depression and inhibition of gastrointestinal transit, are distinct from the subtype that mediates supraspinal analgesia. New, highly selective analgesics with limited side effects and little cross-tolerance may be possible.

Morphine

Morphine is still the standard against which all agents are compared, and all physicians should be familiar with its use. It can be given orally as standard, immediate-release tablets or solutions or as sustained-release preparations, which need only be taken every 8 to 12 hours. The total daily dose of morphine is the same regardless of whether it is given as immediate or sustained release. Morphine also can be employed intramuscularly, intravenously, and intrathecally. Each route of administration has its own advantages and disadvantages. It is also important to remember that the dosage is dependent on the route; oral doses are far higher than parenteral ones due to the first-pass metabolism of an oral drug.

Morphine is metabolized to a variety of compounds, including its 3- and 6-glucuronide. The 3-glucuronide is without activity, but the 6-glucuronide is up to 500-fold more potent than morphine itself when administered directly into the central nervous system.[63] Equally important, morphine and its 6-glucuronide are almost equipotent when given systemically. With long-term dosing, the blood levels of morphine-6-glucuronide are higher than those of morphine. The 6-glucuronide is eliminated by the kidney, perhaps explaining the greater potency of morphine in patients with renal failure and in elderly persons, many of whom have decreased renal function.

General Guidelines for Opiate Use

Choice of Drug

When starting opiate therapy, many physicians prefer to start with a less potent drug, such as codeine, propoxyphene, or oxycodone, and progress to more potent agents. Morphine is the standard strong opioid, and all morphinelike agonists provide similar qualities of analgesia and similar qualities and frequencies of side effects. In practice, however, individual patients respond differently to the various opiates. In general, the drug of choice is morphine. Alternative medications may be chosen for a variety of reasons, including (1) a favorable prior experience with the agent, (2) the availability of a more desirable dosage form (eg, concentrated solutions for injection in emaciated patients or rectal suppositories), (3) the desire for a longer duration of action (eg, methadone, levorphanol, or the sustained-release morphine preparations), and (4) the adverse effects of morphine. A variety of available semisynthetic and synthetic agents are described in Table 45.8.

Mixed agonist/antagonists, such as pentazocine, butorphanol, and buprenorphine, should be used only in opiate-naive patients. In patients who are highly dependent on opiates, these agents may precipitate withdrawal. Even in naive patients, pentazocine has a very high incidence of dysphorias, confusion, and hallucinations and probably should be avoided in elderly persons.

Renal failure also influences the choice of opiates. As noted above, the active morphine metabolite, morphine-6-glucuronide is eliminated by the kidney. In patients with compromised kidney function, the dose of morphine should be lowered. Meperidine use in renal failure also is a problem. Meperidine is a synthetic, short-acting opioid with a poor oral potency. Normeperidine, a metabolite of meperidine, is a central nervous system stimulant that produces anxiety, tremors, myoclonus, and generalized seizures on accumulation with repetitive dosing.[64] This hyperexcitability is not mediated through opiate receptors and cannot be reversed with the opiate antagonist naloxone. Patients with compromised renal function are particularly at risk since normeperidine is eliminated by the kidney. Meperidine should be used cautiously, if at all.

Route of Administration

The first issue to be considered is the route of administration. The oral route is preferred because of its convenience and its ability to provide relatively steady blood levels. A peak drug effect occurs after 1 to 2 hours for most analgesics, which may be a drawback for treating rapidly fluctuating pain. In patients who are unable to take medications orally, rectal administration may prove to be useful.

A parenteral drug is indicated only when the patient is unable to take oral medications. Intramuscular injections have a number of disadvantages, including wide fluctuations in absorption from muscle, a 30- to 60-minute lag to the peak effect, and painful injections. Absorption from deltoid injections may be more rapid than from gluteal, particularly for lipid-soluble opioids, such as methadone.[65] An intravenous bolus provides the most rapid onset of effect, ranging from 1 to 5 minutes for fentanyl to 15 to 30 minutes for morphine. The analgesics also are more potent by this route, and dosages should be adjusted. The major problem with intravenous bolus injections is widely fluctuating blood levels of a drug. In some patients, the peak levels may be associated with undesirable side effects, while pain may break through the low levels. An intravenous infusion provides steady blood levels and the ability to titrate pain relief rapidly.[66] Drugs with shorter half-lives, such as fentanyl, morphine, and hydromorphone, are more easily titrated than long half-life drugs, such as methadone and levorphanol. For stable chronic pain, the oral route is just as effective unless the patient cannot absorb oral medications because of vomiting, dysphagia, or bowel disease. A subcutaneous infusion is another alternative to an intravenous infusion in these cases and will produce equivalent blood levels.[67]

The use of epidural opioids is becoming more common for postoperative pain management, and a number of centers are examining intrathecal administration for chronic cancer-related pain. Most investigators agree that both routes can be very effective, but the question of when they should be chosen instead of a more conventional one remains open. Infusions of epidural bupivacaine alone or in combination with meperidine can provide postoperative pain management, particularly for orthopedic procedures performed below the waist.[68] Patients with cancer who have midline or bilateral pain below the waist who cannot be managed with a systemic opioid may respond to long-term infusion of morphine or other opioids.[59,60] Theoretically, spinal opioids should provide pain relief with fewer side effects, such as sedation, nausea, vomiting, and constipation, because these adverse actions are mediated elsewhere within the neuroaxis. In practice, these side effects, as well as respiratory depression and pruritus, can occur after spinal administration of morphine, which probably reflects the supraspinal redistribution of morphine via

Table 45.8. Moderate-to-strong analgesics.*

	Equianalgesic dose, mg (IM)	Relative potency (PO/IM)	Comments	Precautions and contraindications
Morphinelike agonists Morphine	10	3	Standard of comparison; PO/IM potency is greater with long-term dosing (3) than single dose (6), due to accumulation of the 6-glucuronide	Caution in patients with respiratory disease, increased intracranial pressure, or liver or renal failure
Hydromorphine	1.5	5	Slightly shorter duration of action than morphine	Like morphine
Methadone	10	2	Good oral potency; long plasma half-life (24–36 h)	May accumulate with long-term dosing, causing sedation on days 2–5
Levorphanol	2	2	Long plasma half-life (12–16 h)	May accumulate on days 2–3
Oxymorphone	–	–	Not available orally; 5-mg rectal suppository=to morphine, 5 mg, IM	Like morphine
Heroin	5	6–10	Not available in United States	Like morphine
Meperidine	75	4	Slightly shorter acting than morphine	Normeperidine (toxic metabolite) accumulates with repetitive dosing, causing CNS excitation and seizures, particularly in renal failure; do not use with MAO inhibitors
Codeine	130	1.5	Used orally for less severe pain; inactive, but metabolized to morphine	Like morphine
Oxycodone			Metabolized to oxymorphone; orally, 30-mg equivalent to 60-mg morphine, PO	Like morphine
Mixed agonist-antagonists Pentazocine	60	3	Used orally for less severe pain	May cause psychotomimetic effects; may precipitate withdrawal in dependent patients; contraindicated in myocardial infarction
Nalbuphine	10	NA	Not available orally	Like pentazocine
Butorphanol	2	NA	Not available orally	Like pentazocine
Partial agonists Buprenorphine	0.4	NA	Not available orally	May precipitate withdrawal in dependent patients

* Modified from the American Pain Society.[79] IM indicates intramuscular; PO, by mouth; CNS, central nervous system; MAO, monoamine oxidase; and NA, not available in oral formulation.

blood and cerebrospinal fluid routes.[69] Furthermore, the cross-tolerance between spinal and systemic opiates limits the widespread use of spinal opioids for cancer pain management.

Dose and Frequency

The dose and frequency of administration for a number of commonly used analgesics have recently been reviewed.[80] Requirements among patients can vary tremendously, and each patient needs to be titrated individually. In animal studies, for example, the analgesic potency of morphine among strains of mice can vary by up to 50-fold. Although similar studies have not been performed in humans, major differences in the sensitivity of patients to opiates are likely. Similarly, the pharmacokinetics of these drugs can vary among patients. Thus, each analgesic should be given an adequate trial by gradually increasing the dose until reaching limiting side effects before switching to another drug.

One important issue in pain management is the use of a regular-dosing schedule, as opposed to giving medication as needed. After establishing the optimal dose by titration, analgesics can be administered on an around-the-clock basis with fewer side effects and better pain control. Supplementary "rescue" doses can provide a useful backup. If the pain is allowed to return before giving the next dose of analgesic, the patient is more likely to have periods of undermedication and uncontrolled pain, along with periods of overmedication and drug toxicity. Indeed, patients who take opiates around the clock usually require less medication during a 24-hour period.

Side Effects

Sedation, constipation, nausea, vomiting, and respiratory depression are the most common effects and are seen with virtually all the clinically available opiates. Sedation is best treated by reducing the dose and/or increasing the frequency of administration. Low doses of dextroamphetamine or methylphenidate may be added to increase alertness if the above strategy is unsuccessful.[23] All patients who take opioid analgesics are at risk for constipation and should be given stool softeners and laxatives. Nausea and vomiting should be treated with hydroxyzine or a phenothiazine antiemetic. Opioid-induced ileus has been reversed with metoclopramide.[70]

Respiratory depression rarely is a problem in the treatment of pain with opiates, particularly in patients who are receiving them on a long-term basis, unless the patient has an underlying pulmonary problem. One exception, however, may be the use of opiates in conjunction with general anesthesia. Patients who are receiving long-term opioids develop tolerance to the respiratory depressant actions of opiates in much the same way as to the analgesic actions, and rarely will respiratory problems interfere with dose escalation to compensate for tolerance. In patients who have received a relative overdose of a short half-life opioid drug, physical stimulation may be enough to prevent significant hypoventilation. No patient has died of respiratory depression while he or she was awake. If an opiate antagonist is required to reverse respiratory depression or coma in a patient who has been using opioids on a long-term basis, one should be aware that these patients are exquisitely sensitive to antagonists. A dilute solution of naloxone should be used (0.4 mg in 10 mL of saline solution administered intravenously at the rate of 0.5 mL every 2 minutes). The dose should be titrated to avoid precipitation of profound withdrawal, seizures, and severe pain. Before naloxone administration in a comatose patient, an endotracheal tube should be placed to prevent aspiration. In patients who are receiving meperidine on a long-term basis, naloxone may precipitate seizures by lowering the seizure threshold, allowing the convulsant activity of the active metabolite normeperidine to become evident.

Tolerance

Tolerance, the requirement of a larger dose of a drug to maintain the original effect, is extremely common in opiate use. Tolerance usually occurs in association with physical dependence, but does not imply psychologic dependence. The first sign of the development of tolerance is the decrease in the duration of effective analgesia, followed by a more general loss of pain control. When tolerance develops, the dose of drug should be escalated until pain control is regained. If the increased dosages are not well tolerated by the patient, one should switch to another opiate since cross-tolerance often is incomplete. The following may be done to delay the development of tolerance and to provide effective analgesia in the tolerant patient: (1) combine opioids with nonopioids; (2) switch to an alternate opioid and select one half of the predicted equianalgesic dose as the starting dose, since cross-tolerance among opioids is not complete; or (3) use the oral route in preference to parenteral routes. Since tolerance may be a function of the dose and frequency of administration, intravenous infusions of opioids may produce rapid tolerance.[66]

Physical Dependence

Physical dependence is observed when the opiate is abruptly discontinued or an antagonist is given to patients who are taking opioids on a long-term basis. The abstinence syndrome is characterized by anxiety, irritability, chills alternating with hot flashes, salivation, lacrimation, rhinorrhea, diaphoresis, piloerection, nausea, vomiting, abdominal cramps, insomnia, and, rarely, multifocal myoclonus. The time course of this abstinence syndrome is dependent on the half-life of the opioid. With short half-life drugs, such as morphine or hydromorphone, symptoms may appear in 6 to 12 hours and peak at 24 to 72 hours. With the long half-life drugs methadone and levorphanol, the symptoms may be delayed for several days and are typically less florid. The abstinence syndrome can be avoided by slowly withdrawing chronically used opioids. Withdrawal can be prevented by administering 25% of the previous daily dose. By decreasing the opiate dose by 75% every 2 to 3 days, patients can be easily weaned from the opiate. Of course, pain control may prove to be difficult as the opiate dose is lowered.

Addiction

Psychologic dependence (''addiction'') is defined as a pattern of compulsive drug use that is characterized by a continued craving for an opioid and the need to use the opioid for effects other than pain relief. The patient exhibits drug-seeking behavior and becomes overwhelmingly involved with using and procuring the drug. In the usual medical setting, this behavior may take the form of missed office or clinic appointments with subsequent off-hour calls for prescription renewals; theft or forgery of prescriptions; the solicitation of prescriptions from multiple physicians; theft of drugs from other patients or family members; selling and buying drugs on the street; and the use of prescribed drugs by bizarre means, such as dissolving pills, tablets, and capsules and taking them intravenously. Although most patients who take opioids several times daily for more than 1 month develop some degree of tolerance and physical dependence, the risk of iatrogenic addiction is extremely small, and the fear of opioid addiction should not interfere with treating acute pain and cancer pain. The major factor in the development of psychologic dependence is not drug use alone, but is highly dependent on other medical, social, and economic factors. It is important to emphasize to patients and staff that tolerance or physical dependence is not equivalent to ''addiction.''

Psychologic Issues

Anxiety is common in patients with acute pain. Reassurance and analgesics will often relieve the anxiety without any specific therapy. However, if these measures prove to be inadequate, specific therapy for the anxiety should be considered. Depression also is commonly associated with pain, particularly chronic pain and should be looked for carefully in elderly patients. Antidepressants can prove to be quite helpful by elevating mood, improving sleep and appetite, and possibly providing additional pain relief, particularly in postherpetic neuralgia and diabetic neuropathy.[71,72]

Analgesic Adjuvants

A variety of other drug classes may influence the analgesic actions of opioids or NSAIDS and are important in the management of opioid side effects.

Tricyclic Antidepressants

Controlled trials show that these agents relieve pain that is related to neuropathy and postherpetic neuralgia regardless of whether patients are depressed.[71,72] They are widely used to treat neuropathic pain in patients with cancer secondary to surgery, radiation, chemotherapy, or malignant nerve infiltration and have been reported to be useful, but controlled studies have not yet been done. Amitriptyline has been most extensively studied, but is the least well tolerated due to its potent anticholinergic effects (dry mouth, urinary retention, delirium), sedation, and orthostatic hypotension. Desipramine can be used to avoid sedation or anticholinergic effects, or nortriptyline can be used to minimize orthostatic hypotension. Administration of amitriptyline at bedtime as a single daily dose minimizes daytime side effects and can facilitate sleep. Pain control is usually observed with relatively low amitriptyline doses (25 to 150 mg/kg). The mechanism of action of these agents is not well understood.

Antihistamines

In addition to its antihistaminergic actions, hydroxyzine has analgesic, antiemetic, and mild sedative properties and is a useful adjuvant for anxious or nauseated patients. The usual dose is 25 to 50 mg orally or intramuscularly every 4 to 6 hours, as needed. Hydroxyzine also augments opioid analgesia.

Benzodiazepines

Anxiety and muscle spasm associated with acute pain can be treated with benzodiazepines, such as alprazolam or lorazepam. However, these drugs have no analgesic properties, and their sedative and respiratory depressant effects may decrease the amount of opioid that the patient can tolerate. Therefore, benzodiazepines should be used for anxiety only after adequate doses of analgesics and reassurance have proved to be unsuccessful.

Short-term use of benzodiazepines as hypnotics for sleep problems also may be helpful, but they are not indicated if the sleep disturbance results from inadequate use of analgesics. Many physicians start treatment of insomnia with a short half-life agent, such as triazolam, and use a longer lasting hypnotic, such as temazepam, in the case of repeated awakening (see Chapter 43) Long-term use of benzodiazepines should be avoided when possible owing to their potential to produce physiologic and psychologic dependence.

Caffeine

At doses greater than 65 mg, caffeine potentiates NSAID and opioid analgesia in the treatment of a variety of pain syndromes, including dental pain and headaches. The optimal daily dose of caffeine has not been established, but 100 to 200 mg/d appears to be well tolerated by most patients.[73]

Dextroamphetamine

Like caffeine, amphetamines enhance opiate analgesia.[74] In addition, amphetamines can alleviate some of the sedative effects of opioids, particularly in patients with cancer who have chronic malignant pain. Their use should be restricted to patients in whom no alternative for sedation is available.

Steroids

As noted above, steroids are the drugs of choice for temporal arteritis. They also can be very effective in the management of cancer pain, due to both specific tumor lysis, as in lymphomas, and reduction of edema with the amelioration of painful nerve or spinal cord compression. They are the standard emergency treatment of suspected malignant spinal cord compression and may be useful in the management of pain caused by malignant lesions of the brachial or lumbosacral plexus. In the moribund patient, steroids are usually euphoric and also may increase appetite. Long-term use is associated weight gain, Cushing's syndrome, proximal myopathy, and, rarely, psychosis. Steroids also increase the risk of gastrointestinal bleeding and should be used very cautiously with NSAIDS. Steroid withdrawal deserves special mention due to the high incidence of diffuse arthalgias and exacerbation of pain associated with lowering the dose. This possibility must be considered before concluding that pain exacerbation reflects tumor growth or recurrence.

Phenothiazines

The use of phenothiazines to potentiate opiate analgesia remains controversial, and their use is generally not recommended, because their sedative properties may actually limit the amount of opiate tolerated by the patient. They can be useful in controlling nausea and/or vomiting, particularly when secondary to opiates, but prolonged use risks tardive dyskinesia.

Among the phenothiazines, methotrimeprazine is quite unique. Unlike the others, methotrimeprazine is a potent analgesic equivalent to low-to-moderate doses of morphine. Methotrimeprazine lacks the constipating and respiratory depressant effects of opioids and shows no analgesic cross-tolerance, but sedation and orthostatic hypotension are limiting side effects.

Anticonvulsants

Lancinating pains that arise from peripheral nerve syndromes, such as trigeminal neuralgia, postherpetic neuralgia, glossopharyngeal neuralgia, and posttraumatic neuralgia, can be difficult to manage and may respond poorly to opiates.[54] Similarly, nerve injury caused by cancer or cancer therapy sometimes gives rise to such "ticlike" pains. The drugs of choice for these conditions are the anticonvulsants, particularly carbamazepine.

Special Issues in Pain Management in Elderly Persons

Placebos in pain have been well studied and generally provide relief in up to 30% of subjects, including those with an organic basis for their pain. Thus, a placebo response provides no useful information about the genesis or severity of the pain; it has been suggested that the placebo response may represent the activation of endogenous opioid systems. The age dependence of the placebo response is controversial.[75]

Changes in the pharmacokinetic and pharmacodynamic responses to drugs in elderly persons is reviewed in chapter 7, including differences in absorption, distribution, metabolism, and excretion. Analgesics may be given safely to geriatric patients, but doses usually need adjustment. Morphine is an excellent example. As described earlier, the 6-glucuronide accumulates to levels in the blood greater than morphine with long-term dosing and is eliminated by the kidneys. Renal function may decline with age, so geriatric patients might be expected to have higher and more prolonged levels of morphine-6-glucuronide, resulting in a more pronounced analgesia. Experimentally, intramuscular morphine produces a longer duration of analgesia in older patients. Bellville et al[75] noted a strong correlation between age and pain relief with morphine, with older patients reporting greater relief than younger patients with an equivalent morphine dose. In fact, they noted that age was a more important variable for dose adjustment than height, weight, or other patient characteristics, such as site of pain and type of operation. Similarly, plasma levels of tricyclic compounds usually are higher for a given dose in older than in younger patients.[77] Thus, elderly persons often are more sensitive to many of the analgesics in current use, which serves to emphasize the importance of dose titration as the rule in the pharmacologic management of pain. Typically, physicians undertreat patients with pain.[78] Every effort should be made to avoid the unnecessary suffering that is so common among patients.

References

1. Payne R, Foley KM. Advances in the management of cancer pain. *Cancer Treat Rep* 1984;68:173–183.
2. Merskey H. Classification of chronic pain: description of chronic pain syndromes and definitions of pain terms. *Pain* 1986;3(suppl):S217.
3. Foley KM, Sundaresan N. Management of cancer pain. In: Devita VT, Hellman S, Rosenberg SA, eds. *Principles and Practice of Oncology*. Philadelphia, Pa: JB Lippincott Co; 1985:1940–1941.
4. Raja SN, Meyer RA, Campbell JN. Peripheral mechanisms of somatic pain. *Anesthesiology* 1988;68:571–590.
5. Fields HL. *Pain*. New York, NY: McGraw-Hill International Book Co; 1987.
6. Sinclair DC, Weddel G, Feindel WH. Referred pain and associated phenomena. *Brain* 1948;71:184–211.
7. Albe-Fessard D, Condes-Lara M, Sanderson P, et al. Tentative explaination of the special role played by the areas of paleospinothalamic projection in patients with deafferention pain syndromes. In: Kurger L, Liebeskind JC, eds. *Advances in Pain Research and Therapy*. New York, NY: Raven Press; 1984;6:167–182.
8. Payne R. Neuropathic pain syndromes, with special reference to causalgia and reflex sympathetic dystrophy. *Clin J Pain* 1986;2:59–73.
9. Meyer RA, Campbell JN. Myelinated nociceptive afferent account for the hyperalgesia that follows a burn to the hand. *Science* 1981;213:1527–1529.
10. Wall PD, McMahon SB. Microneurography and its relation to perceived sensation: a critical review. *Pain* 1985;21:209–229.
11. Torebjork HE. Activity in C nociceptors and sensation. In: Kenshalo DR, ed. Sensory Function of the Skin of Humans. New York, NY: Plenum Press; 1979:313–325.
12. Campbell JN, Mayer RA. Primary afferents and hyperalgesia. In: Yaksh TL, ed. *Spinal Afferent Processing*. New York, NY: Plenum Press; 1986:59–81.
13. Milne RJ, Foreman RD, Giesler GJ, Willis WD. Convergence of cutaneous and pelvic visceral nociceptive inputs onto primate spinothalamic neurons. *Pain* 1981; 11:163–181.
14. Culp WJ, Ochoa J. *Abnormal Nerves and Muscles as Impulse Generators*. New York, NY: Oxford University Press Inc; 1982.
15. Tasker RR, Tsuda T, Hawrylyshyn P. Clinical neurophysiological investigation of deafferention pain. In: Bonica JJ, ed. *Advances in Pain Research and Therapy*. New York, NY: Raven Press; 1983;5:718–738.
16. Nathan PW. Pain and the sympathetic nervous system. *J Auton Nerv Syst* 1983;7:363–370.
17. Dubner R, Bennett GJ. Spinal and trigeminal mechanisms of nociception. *Ann Neurol* 1983;6:381–418.
18. Melzack R, Wall PD. Pain mechanism: a new theory. *Science* 1965;150:971–978.
19. Kenshalo DR, Isensee O. Response of primate SI cortical neurons to noxious stimuli. *J Neurophysiol* 1983; 50:1479–1496.
20. Young GB, Blume WT. Painful epileptic seizures. *Brain* 1983;106:537–554.
21. Bausbaum AI. The generation and control of pain. In: Rosenberg, RN, ed. The *Clinical Neurosciences*. New York, NY: Churchill Livingstone Inc; 1983:301–332.
22. Levy RM, Lamb S, Adams JE. Treatment of chronic pain by deep brain stimulation: long term follow-up and review of the literature. *Neurosurgery* 1987;21:885–893.
23. Foley KM. Adjuvant analgesic drugs in cancer pain management. In: Aronoff GM, ed. *Evaluation and Treatment of Chronic Pain*. Baltimore, Md: Urban & Schwartzenberg; 1985b:425–434.
24. Feinmann C. Pain relief by antidepressants: possible mode of action. *Pain* 1985;23:1–8.
25. Beecher HK. Pain in men wounded in battle. *Ann Surg* 1946;123:96–105.
26. Mayer DJ, Liebeskind JC. Pain reduction by focal electrical stimulation of the brain: an anatomical approach. *Brain Res* 1974;68:73–93.
27. Reynolds DV. Surgery in the rat during electrical analgesia induced by focal brain stimulation. *Science* 1969; 164:444–445.
28. Akil H, Mayer DJ, Liebeskind JC. Antagonism of stimulation produced analgesia by naloxone, a narcotic antagonist. *Science* 1974;191:961–962.
29. Hughes J, Smith TH, Kosterlitz JW, et al. Identification of two related pentapeptides from the brain with potent opiate agonist activity. *Nature* 1975;258:577–579.
30. Pasternak GW, Goodman R, Snyder SH. An endogenous morphine like factor in mammalian brain. *Life Sci* 1975;16:1765–1769.
31. Evans CJ, Hammond DL, Frederickson RCA. The opioid peptides. In: Pasternak GW, ed. *The Opiate Receptors*. Clifton, NJ: Humana Press; 1988:23–74.
32. Moulin DE, Max M, Kaiko RF, et al. Efficacy of intrathecal [D-Ala^2,D-Leu^5]enkephalin in cancer patients with chronic pain. *Pain* 1985;23:213–222.
33. Martin WR. Opioid antagonists. *Pharmacol Rev* 1967; 19:463–521.
34. Pert CB, Snyder SH. Opiate receptor: demonstration in nervous tissue. *Science* 1973;179:1011–1014.
35. Terenius L. Characteristics of the 'receptor' for narcotic analgesics in synaptic plasma membrane fractions from rat brain. *Acta Pharmacol Toxicol* 1973;33:377–384.
36. Simon EJ, Hiller JM, Edelman I. Stereo-specific binding of the potent narcotic analgesic ^{3}H-etorphine to rat brain homogenates. *Proc Natl Acad Sci USA* 1973;70:1947–1949.
37. Pasternak GW, ed. *The Opiate Receptors*. Clifton, NJ: Humana Press; 1988.
38. Pasternak GW, Wood PL. Multiple mu opiate receptors. *Life Sci* 1986;38:1889–1898.

39. Zukin RS, Eghbali M, Olive D, et al. Characterization and visualization of rat and guinea pig brain κ opioid receptors: evidence for κ₁ and κ₂ opioid receptors. *Proc Natl Acad Sci USA* 1988;85:4061–4065.

40. Pasternak GW, Childers SR, Snyder SH. Opiate analgesia: evidence for mediation by a subpopulation of opiate receptors. *Science* 1980;208:514–516.

41. Bodnar RJ, Williams CW, Lee SJ, et al. Role of mu₁ opiate receptors in supraspinal opiate analgesia: a microinjection study. *Brain Res* 1988;447:25–37.

42. Payne R. Neck pain in the elderly: a mangement review, I. *Geriatrics* 1987a;42:59–65.

43. Payne R. Neck pain in the elderly: a managment review, II. *Geriatrics* 1987b;42:71–73.

44. Gandy S, Payne R. Back pain in the elderly: updated diagnosis and management. *Geriatrics* 1986;41:59–74.

45. Jefferys RV. The surgical treatment of cervical myelopathy due to spondylosis and disk degeneration. *J Neurol Neurosurg Psychiatry* 1986;49:353.

46. Adams C. Cervical spondylotic radiculopathy and myelopathy. In: Vinken PGJ, Bruyn GW, eds. *Handbook of Clinical Neurology*. Amsterdam, Holland: Elsevier Science Publishers; 1976, vol 26: *Injuries of the Spine and Spinal Cord*, pt 2, p 97.

47. Brooker AE, Barter AW. Cervical spondylosis: clinical study with comparative radiology. *Brain* 1965;88:925.

48. Payne R. Back pain in the elderly. *Geriatrics* 1986;41:59–74.

49. Hall S, Bartleson JD, Onofrio B, et al. Lumbar spinal stenosis: clinical features, diagnostic procedures, and results of surgical treatment in 68 patients. *Ann Intern Med* 1985;103:271–275.

50. Maistrelli GL, Vaughan PA, Evans DC, et al. Lumbar disc herniation in the elderly. *Spine* 1987;12:63–66.

51. Hunder GG, Allen GL. Giant cell arteritis: a review. *Bull Rheum Dis* 1978;29:980–986.

52. Loeser JD. Herpes zoster and postherpetic neuralgia. *Pain* 1986;25:149–164.

53. Portenoy RK, Duma C, Foley KM. Acute herpetic and postherpetic neuralgia: clinical review and current management. Ann Neurol 1986;20:651–664.

54. Swerdlow M. Anticonvulsant drugs and chronic pain. *Clin Neuropharmacol* 1984;7:51–82.

55. Taub A, Collins WF. Observations on the treatment of denervation dysethesia with psychotropic drugs: postherpetic neuralgia, anesthesia dolorosa, peripheral neuropathy. In: Bonica JJ, ed. *Advances in Neurology*. New York, NY: Raven Press; 1974;4:309–315.

56. Kori SH, Krol G, Foley KM. Computed tomographic evaluation of bone and soft tissue metastasis. In: Weiss L, Giklbert HA, eds. *Bone Metastases,* monograph series. 1981;3:245–257.

57. Jaeckle K, Young DF, Foley KM. The natural history of lumbosacral plexopathy in cancer patients. *Neurology* 1984;33:8–14.

58. Cherry DA, Gourlay GK, Cousins MJ. Epidural mass associated with lack of efficacy of epidural morphine and undetectable CSF morphine concentrations. *Pain* 1986; 25:69–73.

59. Coombs DW, Mauer LH, Saunders RL. Outcomes and complications of continuous intraspinal narcotic analgesia for cancer pain control. *J Clin Oncol* 1984;2:1414–1420.

60. Sherman RA, Sherman CJ, Parker L. Chronic phantom and stump pain among American veterans: results of a survey. *Pain* 1984;18:83–95.

61. Portenoy RK, Foley KM. Chronic use of opioid analgesics in nonmalignant pain: report on 38 cases. *Pain* 1986;25:171–186.

62. Inturrisi CE, Foley KM. Narcotic analgesics in the management of pain. In: Kuhar M, Pasternak G, eds. *Analgesics: Neurochemical, Behavioral and Clinical Perspectives*. New York, NY: Raven Press; 1984a;257–288.

63. Pasternak GW, Bodnar RJ, Clark JA, et al. Morphine-6-glucuronide, a potent mu agonist. *Life Sci* 1987;41:2845–2849.

64. Kaiko RF, Wallenstein SL, Rogers AG, et al. Narcotics in the elderly. *Med Clin North Am* 1982;66:1079–1089.

65. Kaiko RF, Wallenstein SL, Rogers AG, et al. Clinical analgesic studies and sources of variation in analgesic responses to morphine. In: Foley KM, Inturrisi, eds. *Advances in Pain Research and Therapy*. New York, NY: Raven Press; 1986;8:13–23.

66. Portenoy RK, Moulin DE, Rogers A, et al. IV infusion of opioids for cancer pain: clinical review and guidelines for use. *Cancer Treat Rep* 1986;70:575–581.

67. Bruera E, Brenneis C, MacDonald RN. Continuous sc infusion of narcotics for the treatment of cancer pain: an update. *Cancer Treat Rep* 1987a;71:953–958.

68. Raj PP, Kannar KD, Vigborth E, et al. Comparison of continuous epidural infusion of local anesthetic and administration of systemic narcotics in the management of pain after total knee replacement surgery. *Anesth Analg* 1987;66:401–406.

69. Payne R. Role of epidural and intrathecal narcotics and peptides in the management of pain. *Med Clin North Am* 1987;71:313–327.

70. MacDonald RN, Bruera E, Brennels C, et al. Management of the narcotic bowel syndrome (NBS) in cancer patients using a continuous subcutaneous infusion of metoclopromide (SCIM). *Pain* 1987;4(suppl):S144.

71. Max MB, Culnane M, Schafer SC, et al. Amitriptyline relieves diabetic neuropathy pain in patients with normal or depressed mood. *Neurology* 1987;37:589–596.

72. Max MB, et al. Amitriptyline, but not lorazapam relieve posttherapeutic neuralgia. Neurology 1988;38:1427–1432.

73. Laska EM, Sunshine A, Mueller F, et al. Caffeine as an analgesic adjuvant. *JAMA* 1984;251:1711–1718.

74. Forrest WH, Brown BW, Brown CR, et al. Dextroamphetamine with morphine for treatment of postoperative pain. *N Engl J Med* 1977;296:712–715.

75. Bellville JW, Forrest WH, Miller E, Brown BW. Influence of age on pain relief from analgesics: a study of postoperative patients. *JAMA* 1971;217:1835–1841.

76. Kaiko RF, Foley KM, Grabinski PY, et al. Central

nervous system excitatory effects of meperidine in cancer patients. *Ann Neurol* 1983;13:180–185.

77. Nies A, Robinson DS, Friedman MJ, et al. Relationship between age and tricyclic antidepressant plasma levels. *Am J Psychiatry* 1977;134:790–793.

78. Marks RM, Sachar EJ. Undertreatment of medical inpatients with narcotic analgesics. *Ann Intern Med* 1973;78:173–181.

79. American Pain Society. *Principles of Analgesic Use in Acute Pain and Chronic Cancer Pain*. In Press.

80. Foley KM. The treatment of cancer pain. *N Engl J Med* 1985;313:84–95.

Care Near the End of Life

Donald J. Murphy and Joanne Lynn

Dying has become both a private and a shared process, one that involves not only family, friends and caregivers but society as a whole. Although caring for a dying patient requires intimacy and compassion, it also demands recognition of such societal considerations as ethics, law, and economics. Less than a century ago, people typically died at home. The patient, family and friends, and the physician met at the deathbed with few, if any, constraints imposed by societal concerns. Today most people die while old, hospitalized, and under the care of multiple health care providers. The constraints imposed by society's concerns are many and pervasive. Foresight and thoughtfulness are essential if the care and compassion that dying elderly persons need are regularly to be given.

This chapter will focus first on the societal concerns that affect the care of the dying patients. The focus will then shift to symptom management and other aspects of caring for individual patients.

Policy Considerations

A consensus is emerging that an ordering of ethical principles[1-4] can help guide decisions by a dying patient and his or her caregivers.

Therapeutic Possibilities

The first endeavor must be to consider all courses of care that might provide a better future for a patient by,

for example, prolonging life or relieving suffering. An intervention that is expected to provide no benefit should not be presented to the dying patient as if it were a real therapeutic option. Doing so might well confuse and frustrate a dying patient and his or her family and might also detract from tasks that many dying people still want to accomplish. On the other hand, physicians often err in failing to consider important options that might be desirable to the patient. Forgoing a feeding tube, allowing a patient to live with a devitalized foot rather than amputating, moving the patient home, and prophylactically fixing a long bone with metastases are common examples.

One should consider all potentially beneficial interventions but offer only those interventions that are actually effective. Cardiopulmonary resuscitation (CPR) can be an exception to this mandate. Most institutional policies require that CPR be discussed with everyone, including dying patients, before a do-not-resuscitate order can be written.[5] However, since CPR is clearly futile for some dying elderly patients, discussing it might not be a moral obligation in such a case.[3,4,6] Do-not-resuscitate policies that require discussion of even predictably futile CPR can nevertheless be justified in two ways. First, adherence helps ensure that other, more germane, issues will be discussed with dying patients and their families. Second, the data substantiating the claim that CPR would be futile are not yet well established and accepted for all but a few patients. The physician who must discuss CPR with a patient for whom it would be predictably futile clearly would do well to focus on other more important aspects of designing the plan of care, deciding resuscitation status in passing.

Patient Self-determination

The second characteristic of good decision making is that it supports patients' authority to control their own lives.[1] This principle has become prominent as many elderly patients with chronic and fatal illnesses have markedly varied views about whether they want their lives prolonged if the chance for meaningful recovery is small.[5] The assumption guiding medical decisions has been that life must be prolonged. Therefore, advance directives have come into use to protect the patient's right to refuse therapy that prolongs life at the expense of pain and decreased consciousness and with little or no chance of benefitting the patient. Most would agree that a patient is best served by establishing formal advance directives (ie, a living will or a durable power of attorney [see Chapter 48]) before death is imminent.[1,7–9] Planning in advance of crisis enables the patient and caregivers to focus on those issues that are especially relevant to the patient and his or her particular options and to ensure that thoughtful plans will be implemented when the time comes. Planning allows caregivers to distinguish, for example, between dying patients who maximally value life extension and those who most fear dependency or pain.

Patient's Best Interests

When what the patient actually wants or would want cannot be known, the decisions must be made so as to promote the patient's best interests.[1] Consider a severely demented 83-year-old woman who has been bedridden for the last 3 years. She has never expressed her preferences and has no family or close friends to speak for her. Treating her for pneumonia may be in her best interests early in her course, when fever and cough are uncomfortable and the pneumonia is likely to cause suffering for a protracted period. But, later in her course, after further deterioration and multiple bouts of pneumonia, another episode might cause death quickly without suffering, while the treatment offers only restraints, fear, and a tenuously prolonged life. At both times the therapy can succeed at correcting an abnormality, the pneumonia. However, the therapy is not necessarily in her best interests at both times. Near the end of life, the burdens of treatment for her may outweigh the potential benefits. In other words, the life to be lived with treatment, though possibly longer, might well be less desirable from the patient's perspective than an earlier death with untreated pneumonia.

Deciding what course serves the dying patient's best interests often is difficult. For example, a feeding tube may cure dehydration for an aphasic 79-year-old stroke victim who can no longer drink. If his preferences are not known and there is no consensus among the health care team about his best interests, a trial with a feeding tube would allow the opportunity to assess the potential benefits and burdens of the treatment. If, after a preset period, the benefits seem to outweigh the burdens, the feedings should continue. If not, the feedings can be withdrawn and the patient allowed to die.[10]

Occasionally the professional health care providers and a patient's family member disagree about the patient's best interest. For example, a son, overwhelmed by guilt for not visiting his demented mother, may insist that his mother receive fully aggressive life-extending care. Alternatively, a physician, stressed with daily visits and the demanding care of a complicated patient, may request that the feeding tube be removed from a patient who still finds pleasure in living. Most of these dilemmas can be resolved with family meetings, consultations, and close attention to the psychological needs of those burdened with the decisions.

Other Considerations

Serving the patient's best interests is the foundation of ethical decision making; when those interests are clear, it is difficult to justify disadvantaging the patient in order to limit the adverse effects upon other people (eg, family stress, cost of care, convenience of caregivers). However, these effects upon others may properly be considered in making decisions. Health care professionals must, of course, recognize external factors that influence decisions about care of dying elderly patients. Some of these factors, such as family strain or finances, might appropriately determine choices that are otherwise uncertain.

Other considerations, such as distributive justice in the health care system,[1] are more appropriately considered in public forums, not at the bedside with an individual patient.[1,11] Many health care providers sense the growing conflict between the need to ration health care[12] and the desire to apply the fruits of medical progress to all patients, including frail elderly patients near the end of life.[13] Advocacy for dying patients will be most effective when health care providers understand the economic and political implications of policies regarding the care of dying elderly patients and become active in shaping a health care system that is fair to all in need. In our current health care system, health care providers will have to be honest, learned, and thoughtful in confronting patient care situations where unjust barriers to optimal treatment are common.

Euthanasia

Euthanasia presents a unique moral conundrum that patients and caregivers will increasingly have to address.[14] Adhering to the ethical principles above does not resolve this issue. Proponents argue that euthanasia is permissable in some situations because it respects patient self determination and may be in the patient's best interests by terminating intractable suffering. Opponents argue that euthanasia is never medically indicated, is not really in the patient's best interests, and is not ever in society's best interests.

The pressure for euthanasia arises mostly from people who fear pain, isolation, loss of self-esteem, and loss of control of day-to-day activities. Physical pain can be successfully relieved with proper use of analgesics (see Chapter 45). Similarly, the control of day-to-day choices can be returned to the patient. Feelings of isolation and abandonment can be alleviated with adequate counseling and regular interaction with various support personnel. Psychological and emotional pain, which can be significant in many dying persons, can be effectively eased in most cases. Since the discomforts of dying, actual or anticipated, can be alleviated for almost all patients, the priority should be to do so.

Some patients have intractable suffering before dying despite the best possible care. However, the number that do not respond to good care is very small. Condoning active euthanasia for the sake of these few patients is ill advised because of the effects the policy would have on medical care for all dying patients. Pressure for high-quality care would decrease, morale of health care providers might decline, and the bereaved might suffer unexpected adverse consequences. Physicians therefore should marshal all resources necessary to provide the best death possible for a dying patient. Although adequate resources are not available for many dying persons, euthanasia is an inappropriate and unjustified solution. Society will be better served by more creative solutions, such as the more widespread application of hospice principles[15-17] (and reimbursement for such services). If the trend in the Netherlands[18] continues to extend to the United States,[14-19] euthanasia may become the major controversy in care near the end of life.

Patient Care Considerations

As people age and approach death, whether slowly or abruptly, they hope that health care providers will be competent, minimize discomfort, communicate with the patient and family (or friends) frequently, and be compassionate.

Competent Evaluation

With the dying patient, a competent physician walks the fine line between insufficient and excessive diagnostic evaluation. Offering palliative care for elderly persons with end-stage disease may be inappropriate when a thorough evaluation has a reasonable chance of uncovering a disease for which treatment could prolong life or maximize comfort. Clinicians must be aware of the protean manifestations of many diseases in frail elderly patients.[20]

On the other hand, physicians must guard against practice habits or diagnostic curiosity that might lead to unwarranted and burdensome diagnostic procedures. If the likelihood of a diagnostic evaluation leading to beneficial therapy (or even to the benefits of a more precise prognosis) is very low, caretakers may serve the patient best by proceeding with palliative therapy. For example, one need not instinctively order multiple tests for the elderly dying patient with anasarca and ascites. If findings of a careful examination and basic laboratory tests strongly point to malignant disease, one must ask what chance the patient has of improving if the exact diagnosis is made. If responsible physicians, aware of the many possibilities, estimate that the chance is very small, they probably should not pursue the diagnosis. Invasive or risky tests and frequent hospitalizations likely will add to the discomfort of a fatal illness. That the same providers would not approach a 35-year old in the same manner (the 35-year-old would almost certainly undergo a complete diagnostic evaluation) is not "ageism." It is a realistic appraisal of benefits and individualization of care. The younger person with the same symptoms is more likely to have fully treatable illnesses than widely metastatic and unresponsive malignancy.

Symptom Control

Relentless symptoms, particularly pain, are what dying persons fear most. Alleviation (if not elimination) of these symptoms is a primary goal for the caregivers.[21] The symptom control regimen usually consists of medications and good nursing care. Occasionally, however, more aggressive means will be necessary to provide symptom relief. A short life expectancy (perhaps even a few days) should not preclude consideration of aggressive means of symptom control, such as surgery, radiation therapy, and nerve blocks.

Pain

Although pain (See also Chapter 45) usually is not severe in dying patients, it can be devastating in some cases. Yet, it also can be treated adequately. Chronic pain in a patient with little hope for a meaningful recovery frequently contributes to anxiety, depression, nausea, weakness, insomnia, and other symptoms. Reassuring the patient that the pain can now and will always be controlled is itself therapeutic.

Pain control should be constant for the dying patient. If an analgesic provides pain relief for 3 hours, a regimen administering it every 4 hours is completely inadequate. Lapses in pain control increase the patient's anxiety and loss of control. Unnecessary tension between the patient and nursing staff may result if the patient has to ask for analgesics frequently. Optimal control obviously requires regular communication between the physician and patient.

The determinants of an individual's pain threshold are multiple and complex.[21] Understanding the patient's willingness to report pain and his or her perception of it requires some knowledge of the patient's psychological, social, and spiritual history. As with many aspects of caring for dying elderly patients, a team approach, utilizing the talents of social workers, clergy, and therapists, is most fruitful. Caregivers must be aware of the many manifestations of pain, especially in the dying elderly who may be too debilitated to articulate the degree of pain clearly. Acute confusion (agitation, hallucinations, etc) may well be the change that signals an increase in pain.

With few exceptions, the dying patient who complains of pain should be treated to relieve the pain unless the cause can be removed. Narcotic addiction is not a concern for the dying patient.[21,22] Physical dependence will occur but is irrelevant, and tolerance can be managed by escalating the dosage.

The analgesic regimen needs to be tailored for each patient. For example, salicylates or nonsteroidal anti-inflammatory agents may suffice for one man dying of metastatic prostate cancer, whereas large doses of morphine may be necessary to control a toothache in another. A stepped-care approach, starting with medications such as acetaminophen, should be considered for all patients. The regimen is then determined by the patient's response and potential side effects. Occasionally, it is best to assure the patient of effectiveness by starting with a powerful analgesic that is certain to work (though it might have more side effects) and then to titrate to lower doses and less potent drugs.

Morphine sulfate is the narcotic of choice for treatment of severe pain in most patients. It can be given orally as an elixir (20 mg/mL), tablet (15 mg) or sustained-release tablet (30 mg). Patients who cannot drink or swallow can be medicated subcutaneously, intravenously, or by suppository. Hydromorphone is similar in effect and ease of administration and can be prepared in high concentrations (100 mg/mL) for high-dose parenteral use. Other opiates may be indicated in special circumstances.[23] For example, methadone, which has a longer half-life than morphine, would be helpful for the patient who needs a longer dosing interval. The dose of any narcotic will need readjusting as the disease progresses, the pain threshold rises or falls, and pharmacodynamics change. Constant monitoring is necessary to treat side effects, including sedation, constipation, and nausea. Respiratory depression is very uncommon. If mild, it simply can be monitored. If substantial, it is readily reversed with dilute naloxone. Table 46.1 outlines the most commonly used narcotics and their approximate dose equivalents.

Psychiatric Symptoms

Psychiatric symptoms are common in dying elderly patients. Agitation, disorientation, hallucinations, anxiety, and depression all are stressful symptoms for the patient, family, and caregivers. Calm reassurance often alleviates some of these symptoms. If emotional support does not resolve the symptoms, psychoactive medications may be indicated. Agitation and anxiety can be alleviated with neuroleptics (eg, haloperidol, 0.5 mg/4–6 hours), benzodiazepines (eg, oxazepam, 10 mg), antihistamines (eg, hydroxyzine hydrochloride, 25 mg), sedating antidepressants (eg, doxepin), or barbiturates. As noted before, physical and psychological dependence are irrelevant for the dying person as long as symptoms are controlled.

Depression in the dying elderly patient can also be ameliorated with medications. Although the patient's mood usually is not elevated significantly, benefits such as improved sleep or mental alertness can significantly affect the patient's sense of well-being. An empiric trial of an antidepressant, preferably one with a low anticholinergic profile, such as desipramine, should be tried. Methylphenidate is occasionally helpful for the medically ill depressed elderly patient.[24] Its relatively rapid onset of action (within a few days) is an advantage over the tricyclic antidepressants (which often require a few weeks).

Gastrointestinal Symptoms

Anorexia, nausea, vomiting, diarrhea, and constipation are among the many gastrointestinal tract symptoms that accompany dying. Anorexia is almost universal during the final stages of most diseases. Nevertheless, patients still can derive pleasure from eating, especially in the company of family and

Table 46.1. Approximate equianalgesic doses of narcotics used for chronic pain.*

Drug	Dose, mg	Usual effective interval, h
Codeine	200 PO, 30 IM or SC†	4–6 PO, 3–4 IM or SC
Morphine sulfate	40 PO,‡ 10 IM or SC	4–6 PO, 3–4 IM or SC
Hydromorphone hydrochloride	7.50 PO, 1.5 IM or SC	4–6 PO, 3–4 IM or SC
Methadone hydrochloride	20 PO, 10 IM or SC	Longer § 4–10 PO, 3–6 IM or SC

*Adapted from reference 2. PO indicates orally; IM, intramuscularly; SC, subcutaneously.
†Patients requiring more than 100 mg of codeine orally or 60 mg parenterally usually are given a more potent narcotic.
‡The correct oral-parenteral ratio for morphine is uncertain. For single doses, the ratio is conventionally given as 6 : 1. However, for chronic use, the ratio is probably lower (perhaps as low as 2 : 1).
§The best dosing interval for methadone is uncertain. Despite a long plasma half-life (15–30 hours), the analgesic effect parenterally may be as short as with morphine (3–5 hours).

friends. Catering to the patient's preferences is important, and serving sizes should correspond with the patient's known intake. Five or six small snacks may be more appetizing than the three large meals that are typically served in the hospital. A flexible meal schedule can be coordinated with the dietary service in an institution or with family members (or friends) at home.

Artificial feeding is infrequently indicated to correct malnutrition resulting from anorexia in a dying patient. For example, if a feeding tube or total parenteral nutrition is used for an elderly man with esophageal cancer, he must understand the expected effects and side effects of therapy as well as his right to continue or discontinue the feeding after it has been started.

Hunger and thirst are symptoms that are much less prevalent among dying persons than the public might think. Dying patients rarely complain of hunger during their final weeks. Similarly, thirst (a craving for water) is unusual for a dying patient who receives good basic nursing care, even though the patient may have hyperosmolarity.[25] On the other hand, a dry mouth, sometimes interpreted as thirst, is common. Medications (especially those with anticholinergic properties), dehydration, and mouth-breathing are the most common causes. Glycerin, candies, and beverages can stimulate saliva production. Regular mouth care, including toothbrushing, rinsing, the use of oral swabs, sipping liquids, and sucking on ice, is a high priority for most dying patients.

Nausea and vomiting are caused by a number of reversible factors, particularly medications. If reversible causes have been excluded, empiric treatment with various antiemetics usually is effective. Phenothiazines and related compounds are the most commonly used antiemetics and can be administered orally, intramuscularly, and rectally. Prochlorperazine, chlorpromazine, thiethylperazine, and perphenazine all have antiemetic properties. Other medications (eg, dexamethasone, metoclopramide, dimenhydrinate) should be considered if nausea is unresponsive to phenothiazines, if phenothiazines

cause excessive sedation, hypotension, or extrapyramidal side effects, or if the other effects of these drugs are likely to be beneficial.

Constipation is caused by many problems commonly found in dying elderly patients, particularly immobility and narcotic use. A stepped-care approach, beginning with stool softeners and dietary bran (if the patient tolerates the taste), often is effective and prevents overmedication with multiple laxatives. Yet, many patients will need lactulose, stimulant cathartics, or enemas. Occasionally, stool becomes impacted despite treatment with various preparations, and digital disimpaction is necessary. Any change in the dying patient's functional status (eg, urinary incontinence, decreased appetite, acute confusion) should alert the clinician to the possibility of a fecal impaction.

Diarrhea that is not caused by infectious agents, medications, or other well-defined problems probably is best controlled with Kaopectate or loperamide, which do not have the anticholinergic effects of diphenoxylate with atropine.

Urinary Incontinence

Urinary incontinence is a frustrating problem for the patient, caretakers, and visitors. Transient causes such as a urinary tract infection should be sought and treated if the incontinence is psychologically or physically burdensome for the patient. Chronic or transient incontinence can be controlled with a catheter, particularly if skin breakdown is a threat.

Pressure Sores

Most dying patients are at risk of developing pressure sores, which can be very painful. Relieving pressure is the cornerstone of prevention and treatment. Although many treatments (eg, dressings, aerosols, powders) have been marketed, data clearly demonstrating their efficacy are scant.[26] It is essential to turn the patient regularly and keep the skin dry and the wound clean. Once a pressure sore has developed, one must consider whether it is better to débride or to leave it alone, as may be the case with the dry eschar of heel sores in dying patients. For lesions needing continued dressing, some clinicians prefer wet-to-dry dressings, and others prefer wet-to-wet. Some use synthetic transpiring dressings (see Chapter 39). Generally, the nurse's preference should be considered, because it may be the care with which dressings are changed, and not the dressing itself, that determines the effectiveness and comfort of the healing process. Surgical débridement may be necessary to promote healing and to debulk foul-smelling tissue. However, a patient who is moribund and expected to die soon probably should not undergo a clean-margin débridement, because the result does not warrant the pain.

Pruritus

Therapy for pruritus often fails when the underlying medical problem cannot be corrected, though an emollient (even in the absence of dry skin) and antihistamine should be tried empirically. Pruritus associated with chronic renal failure or hepatic cholestasis often can be alleviated with cholestyramine.[27]

Respiratory Symptoms

Coughing and dyspnea are the two most frequent respiratory symptoms experienced by dying elderly patients. Coughing usually has an identifiable cause that can be treated. Suppression of the cough itself usually requires a narcotic preparation, though it may be worthwhile to try benzonatate or terpin hydrate initially.

Dyspnea can be terrifying, especially if the air hunger is severe. Although the patient may not be hypoxemic, supplemental oxygen administered via nasal cannula is ordinarily indicated, if only because of the psychological benefit it might provide. If underlying causes of dyspnea have been treated as well as possible (eg, therapeutic thoracentesis for a large pleural effusion) and the patient remains dyspneic, the shortness of breath should be alleviated with morphine or hydromorphone. Low doses can effectively reduce air hunger and anxiety during the last hours of life. If low doses are ineffective, higher doses should be tried despite the risk of sedation and respiratory depression. Sedation may be necessary to prevent awareness of terminal suffocation, even though the sedative may hasten death by minutes or hours.[1,28]

Communication

The multiple needs of the dying patient are best met by frequent communication between the patient, family, and individual caregivers. A physician might not un-

derstand the degree and nature of a patient's pain unless he or she discusses this with the nurse's aide who helps turn the patient every 2 hours. Similarly, the nurse may overlook the patient's desire to visit (or avoid) certain people unless he or she discusses the social history with the social worker. A chaplain may help other caregivers meet the patient's spiritual needs. Regular meetings of the caregiving team help ensure that all needs are being addressed.[32]

Compassion

At times caregivers can do little more than simply be present for the dying patient. Symptoms may persist despite the most conscientious efforts to eliminate them. Empathy with the patient may be all the caregiver can provide, but this may well be what the patient most desperately needs. Health care providers are not trained to sit still, hold the patient's hand, and listen (or simply let time pass). Yet this may be the most effective way of encouraging the patient to share feelings of fear, sadness, and anger or discuss the multiple losses that are part of dying. Unfortunately, our preoccupation with a competent evaluation and symptom control often preclude the compassionate response of listening to the innermost feelings of the patient. Again, a team approach is most likely to provide all elements of care near the end of life.

Compassion requires an empathic response to the patient's family and close friends. Providing an aesthetically pleasing "deathbed" and facilitation of bereavement are essential components of care at the end of life.

Aesthetic Considerations

The final moments of a patient's life often are what family and friends remember about the care provided and can have lasting effects on them and on the caregivers. Keeping the patient peaceful and clean is important. If the patient is not already in a quiet and private environment, he or she should be transferred to one if possible. Occasionally, other considerations may outweigh these. For example, a family may prefer that the patient remain in a less private environment (eg, an intensive care unit) if they feel emotionally secure with the caregivers in that particular area. If death is expected within hours, transferring the patient to a setting where the caregivers are unfamiliar may not be in anyone's best interests.

Regardless of the location, attempts should be made to keep the room quiet and peaceful. Lighting should be adequate but not harsh, and noisy monitoring devices should be silenced. Staff members and uninvolved visitors who may be unaware of the circumstances should not be allowed to engage in inappropriate banter or laughter within earshot of the patient's family and friends.

Both the patient and the bed should be kept clean until the body is removed. Clean linen should keep the patient modestly covered. Attempts to eliminate unpleasant odors should be prompt. Frequent monitoring is necessary to detect and clean up (or, perhaps, cover up) vomitus, urine, and feces. Although these tasks are often performed perfunctorily, the final moments of life provide uniquely well-remembered opportunities for all caregivers to respond compassionately, tenderly, and promptly.

Reassurances that the patient is free of pain are necessary for many families and friends. Agonal breathing patterns and noisy respirations (the "death rattle") are particularly bothersome. If the dying process is prolonged and the family remains distressed by noisy respirations, atropine sulfate (0.4 to 0.6 mg given subcutaneously) can be used to dry the secretions. Caregivers should be sensitive to the perceptions (and misperceptions) of family and friends. For example, oxygen should not be removed if a wife is convinced that it is helping her dying husband.

Many family members and friends need physical contact with the dying patient. They should be encouraged to do whatever suits their needs. Holding hands, wiping the patient's forehead with a cloth, hugging, and even helping maintain cleanliness all help facilitate closure with the dying patient. Some people might not feel comfortable with physical contact in this setting, and they should not feel pressured to respond in a particular manner. Clergy and other support personnel should be available if the patient or family desires.

Bereavement

Facilitation of grief is an extremely important, yet often neglected, aspect of care for dying patients.[30] The severity and duration of grieving are so variable that one cannot assume that a survivor's grief is normal or abnormal. Many survivors feel that the death of their loved one is welcome given all that went before. Their grief may be relatively painless. Others, however, find the loss extremely painful and may need months or years to grieve. The fact that the patient was old and frail (and therefore expected to die) does not necessarily mitigate the pain the survivor feels.

The caregivers must assess the needs of the survivors. Since bereavement starts before the patient dies (in prolonged cases, as in Alzheimer's disease, bereavement starts years before the death), the caregivers usually have some idea of the needs of the survivors. A follow-up visit or telephone call within 2 months after the death further clarifies these needs. The survivors benefit from the assurance that their feelings of sadness, anger, anxiety, depression, and even guilt are expected. Periodic follow-up should be part of the routine care for those survivors who need it.

Professional intervention may be warranted if grief leads to self-damaging behavior (or threats of this), substantial daily dysfunction 3 months later, or inability to develop new relationships after a year has passed. Several grief support networks are available in most urban settings.

Survivors who appear unexpectedly callous at the loss of an elder friend or relative may have good reasons for such a response. For example, an individual who has not adequately grieved the loss of his son will probably be unable to adequately grieve the loss of his father. Permitting the pain of grief to enter his consciousness may simply open wounds that are too deep. Health care providers should encourage, but not force, the expression of grief and should be alert to the adverse effects of inadequately resolved grief.

Decisions regarding autopsy, disposition of the body, and funeral arrangements often are made under pressure and at the most difficult time for the survivors. Addressing these considerations before the patient dies is appropriate in many cases. Regardless of the timing, physicians must try to respond empathically, even though this may be their only encounter with the survivors.

Conclusion

Most elderly persons will die in a health care setting. Competent and responsive management of death is possible to achieve and very worthwhile for patient, survivors, and caregivers. Those who care for dying patients must achieve competence in symptom control, decision making, and management of the patient and of the care system.

References

1. *Guidelines on the Termination of Life-Sustaining Treatment and the Care of the Dying: A Report by the Hasting Center.* New York, NY: The Hastings Center; 1987.
2. President's Commission for the Study of Ethical Problems in Medicine and Biomedical and Behavioral Research. *Deciding to Forego Life-Sustaining Treatment.* 1983. Publication 0-402-884.
3. Schneiderman LJ, Spragg RG. Ethical decisions in discontinuing mechanical ventilation. *N Engl J Med* 1988;318:984–988.
4. Tomlinson T, Brody H. Ethics and communication in do-not-resuscitate orders. *N Engl J Med* 1988;318:43–46.

5. *Life-sustaining Technologies and the Elderly.* Washington, DC: US Congress, Office of Technology Assessment; 1987. Publication OTA-BA-306.

6. Murphy, DJ. Do-not-resuscitate orders: time for reappraisal in long-term-care institutions. *JAMA* 1988; 260:2098–2101.

7. Uhlmann RF, Clark H, Pearlman RA. Medical management decisions in nursing home patients: principles and policy recommendations. *Ann Intern Med* 1987;106:879–885.

8. High DM. Planning for decisional incapacity: a neglected area in ethics and aging. *J Am Geriatr Soc* 1987;35:814–820.

9. Schneiderman JS, Arras JD. Counseling patients to counsel physicians on future care in the event of patient incompetence. *Ann Intern Med* 1985;102:693–698.

10. Lynn J. Elderly residents of long-term care facilities. In: Lynn J, ed. *By No Extraordinary Means.* Indianapolis, Ind: Indiana University Press; 1986:163–179.

11. Daniels N. Why saying no to patients in the United States is so hard. *N Engl J Med* 1986;314:1380–1383.

12. Callahan D. *Setting Limits.* New York, NY: Simon & Schuster, Inc Publishers; 1987.

13. Edmunds LH, Stephenson LW, Edie RN. Open-heart surgery in octogenarians. *N Engl J Med* 1988;319:131–136.

14. Callahan D. Vital distinctions, mortal questions: debating euthanasia and health-care costs. *Commonweal* July 15, 1988:397–404.

15. Volicer L, Rheaume Y, Brown J, et al. Hospice approach to the treatment of patients with advanced dementia of the Alzheimer Type. *JAMA* 1986;256:2210–2213.

16. Lynn J. Dying and dementia. *JAMA* 1986;256:2244–2445.

17. Saunders C. Principles of symptom control in terminal care. In: Reidenberg MM, ed. *The Medical Clinics of North America: Clinical Pharmacology of Symptom Control.* Philadelphia, Pa: WB Saunders Co; 1982:1169–1183.

18. Pence GE. Do not go slowly into that dark night: mercy killing in Holland. *Am J Med* 1988;84:139–141.

19. Vaux KL. Debbie's dying and the good death. *JAMA* 1988;259:2140–2141.

20. Minaker KL, Rowe J. Health and disease among the oldest old: a clinical perspective. *Milbank Mem Fund Q* 1985;63:324–349.

21. Twycross RG, Lack SA. *Symptom Control in Far Advanced Cancer: Pain Relief.* London, England: Pitman Books Ltd; 1983:43–55.

22. American College of Physicians, Health and Public Policy Committee. Drug therapy for severe, chronic pain in terminal illness. *Ann Intern Med* 1983;99:870–873.

23. McGivney WT, Crooks GM. The care of patients with severe chronic pain in terminal illness. *JAMA* 1984;251:1182–1188.

24. Salzman C, van der Kolk B. Treatment of depression. In: Salzman C, ed. *Clinical Geriatric Psychopharmacology.* New York, NY: McGraw-Hill International Book Co; 1984:77–115.

25. Schmitz P, O'Brien M. Observations on nutrition and hydration in dying cancer patients. In: Lynn J, ed. *By No Extraordinary Means.* Indianapolis, Ind: Indiana University Press; 1986:29–38.

26. Reuler JB, Cooney TG. The pressure sore: pathophysiology and principles of management. *Ann Intern Med* 1981;94:661–666.

27. Gilchrest BA. Pruritus: pathogenesis, therapy, and significance in systemic disease states. *Arch Intern Med* 1982;142:101–104.

28. Scheel BJ, Lynn J. Care of dying patients. In: Zweibel NR, Cassel CK, eds. *Clinics in Geriatric Medicine: Clinical and Policy Issues in the Care of the Nursing Home Patient.* Philadelphia, Pa: WB Saunders Co; 1988:639–654.

29. Carlson RW, Devich L, Frank RR. Development of a comprehensive supportive care team for the hopelessly ill on a university hospital medical service. *JAMA* 1988;259:378–383.

30. Osterweis KH, Solomon F, Green KH, eds. Bereavement: reactions, consequences, and care. Washington, DC: *National Academy Press*; 1984.

Justice and the Allocation of Health Care Resources

Christine K. Cassel and
Ruth B. Purtilo

This book thoroughly addresses problems confronting elderly individuals, particularly with respect to their health care problems. In this chapter we draw on such considerations but focus on the additional challenges created by acknowledging that elderly persons as a group are contenders for society's inevitably limited resources. One goal of a good society is to arrive at an approach to the allocation of scarce resources that takes into account the unique values and goals of individuals while supporting fairness overall. But whenever prized resources are in limited supply, groups generally viewed favorably, with sympathy, may become viewed as competitors, or even threats, to other groups. It follows that elderly persons may come to be viewed as an economic threat under current circumstances, with the outcome being less than our society's highest ideals and values would support. To understand why this can happen and how it can be avoided requires a careful evaluation of priorities, values, and trends.

One trend is demographic. There is every indication that the number of elderly persons making claims on scarce health care resources will continue to increase. Those over 75 years of age currently represent about 5% of the US population, and by the year 2040 this figure is expected to grow to 11%, with numbers quadrupling from 3.6 million to 13.8 million. Another trend is toward the use of expensive medical technology in the treatment of acute and chronic disease despite expressing grave concern about the costs of health care. Persons over 75 years of age receive the greatest amount of medical care per capita of any age group. They are most likely to be treated with high-technology interventions such as pacemakers, dialysis, intensive life support systems, and extensive diagnostic modalities. In addition, they are the most likely to be in need of long-term care. While long-term care is not represented heavily in Medicare because of the exclusions of Medicare entitlement, it is represented heavily in the overall expenditures on health care for elderly persons. Concern about these rising costs and about the use of elaborate life-sustaining technology in very frail, ill, and dependent persons at the end of life is beginning to generate vigorous debate about the appropriate type and amount of medical care that should be directed to elderly persons.

When discussing health care for elderly persons, it should be kept in mind that the aging of developed societies is a unique phenomenon in human history, but is not limited to America (see Chapter 2). In fact, it is happening to an even greater extent in Japan, Sweden, Denmark, and other Western European countries. We cannot look back in history for models of how other societies have handled social priorities in the face of increasing numbers and proportions of elderly people in their populations. The unique combination of a lowered fertility rate with increased longevity has led to an ''aging society'' (see Chapter 3). Not only are individuals living longer, but by the midpoint of the next century, one in five persons in our society—perhaps even one in four—may be over the age of 65 years. The factors contributing to this change in percentage of elderly persons—decreased fertility and increased longevity—are both commonly cited as indicators of social progress, which is highly valued.

Because of its historical uniqueness, its link to the value of social progress, and its occurrence in other advanced societies, the aging society should not be assumed to be simply "a burden." Active older persons may make positive contributions to this society that far outweigh the negative aspects of having to care for some dependent elderly persons. The positive aspects of experience and wisdom may enrich the "data bank" of the young, who are living in an increasingly complex and dangerous world. Of course, to limit our framework for thinking about the presence of more elderly persons in society to simply a weighing of positive against negative contributions is an unnecessarily impoverished and narrow approach. We have an opportunity to examine specific questions raised by the necessity of resource allocation, especially with regard to health care. Allocation decisions will always be necessary, and informed persons should have a thorough understanding of the complex issues involved.

With so much change in the United States and worldwide, it is to everyone's benefit to reflect on what should be the basis for determining the appropriate type and amount of health care resources for elderly persons. Considerations of justice, especially distributive justice, help to provide guidelines for clear thinking about this complex issue.

Justice Considerations

The idea of justice is as old as western philosophical thought itself and often is described as "giving to each person what is due him or her." Although few would argue with this definition, it is too general to be of much help as an action or policy guide. Aristotle suggested that it would be helpful to divide justice into "species" concepts, among them *compensatory* justice (dealing with the repayment for harms rendered) and *distributive* justice (dealing with the allocation of resources).[1]

In health care, distributive justice considerations directly affect allocation policies and practices. The goal of distributive justice is to limit arbitrary distinctions among individuals or groups, thereby assuring that each party who has a legitimate claim to a good will receive a proper share, while also bearing a proportionate share of the burden. It forms the basis for determining the proportion of the total services, treatments, and other resources an individual should receive and the price to be exacted for those benefits. Therefore, justice is a key principle upon which to base a humane system of health care.

The goal of justice is to eliminate arbitrary decisions. Policymakers sensitive to the moral demands of justice in a situation should seek allocation decisions that are "fair" or "equitable." Three distinct, commonly accepted criteria for achieving an equitable distribution of a resource are (1) the special merits of some persons, (2) the ability of some to make greater societal contributions than others, and (3) the special needs of some persons.

A *merit* notion supports allocating resources in accord with how hard a person tries, or the kind of results he or she is able to achieve. In health care, giving proportionately more to those who can pay for services or have a greater chance of success of recovery and return to the work force often is justified on the basis that in the end the investment will pay off, thereby benefiting all. Allocating unequal amounts on the basis of *societal contribution* is interpreted to include past contributions as well as promised future ones. "Contributions" may be construed broadly, a factor leading to a curious modern argument with respect to elderly persons, as we discuss below. Allocation based on relative *degrees of need* is quite different from the other two approaches. Here the explicit goal is to help diminish the difference in well-being among persons, and the means of achieving this is to provide a proportionately greater amount to the persons who have the greatest deprivation. In health care, need is logically seen as a medical criterion, that is, resources should be devoted to those who are sick and who stand to benefit from care received. It follows that the allocation deemed appropriate for elderly persons will be guided primarily by one of these lines of reasoning. Each is considered in the section that follows.

Justice Considerations, Allocations, and the Elderly Population

Allocation Based on Merit

The health care system today is driven partially by merit thinking, "merit" being judged primarily according to a potential patient's ability to pay for services rendered, which includes insurance coverage. Persons over age 65 years in the United States vary widely with respect to this type of "merit." Most older people do not live in poverty, but neither are they all well off. There is a tendency to classify the elderly as selfishly well-heeled or poverty stricken, but each of these stereotypes is inaccurate (see Chapter 3) The economic status of elderly people is as variable as their physiologic status or their political beliefs. A generation cannot be accurately viewed as a homogeneous block. People are more like what they were when they were young than they are like other old people. For instance, the myth of the elderly voting block is hard to support with data on voting behavior. Public opinion surveys indicate that given a choice between cutting military spending and cutting Medicare, 65% of people 18 to 29 years old, 73% of those 30 to 49, 73% of those 50 to 64, and 71% of those 65 and older said they would prefer to see military cuts, a remarkably uniform response throughout the generations.[2]

Many debates based on merit consideration of elderly persons also underestimate the complexity of economics. Both public and private funds go to health care. The large public portion represented by Medicare attracts the most concern. An important question today is where society wants health care money to come from—general taxation or private payment for those who can afford to pay. That is a question of ideology. It is assumed by many that public spending on health care and medical care for those who cannot pay is bad for the economy, and that the money disappears into a large black hole, making no positive social contribution. However, one of the main tenets of Keynesian economics is that public dollars spent in any arena will stimulate the economy to a certain extent. Ironically, this belief continues to be one of the main justifications for some other aspects of federal spending, especially in the military sector. In fact, spending in the health care arena creates approximately three to four times as many jobs as military spending, and spending on transportation and education would create even more jobs. The health care sector, in spite of its recent decrease in rate of growth, is still one of the most successfully expanding areas within our economy. Many health care issues have shown growth on the stock market and are considered good areas of investment. If drastic cutbacks were to be made in health care spending, through arbitrary limits on spending for elderly persons, for example, thousands of people would be out of work and a major economic depression might ensue. The dollars that go into the health care industry do not just stop there; they are passed along into the economy in the form of wages, which then can be used to purchase goods and housing, further stimulating the economy.

Another concern that grows out of a merit approach to determe health care allocation in an aging society is that retired persons may be deemed not to "merit" the same treatment for a given disorder as their employed counterparts, even among those retired persons who are able to afford health care insurance. For instance, we have observed a tendency by some practitioners to assume that elderly patients surviving a completed stroke cannot benefit from rehabilitation, because so much rehabilitation is focused on treatment of occupational disability and most patients in this group already are retired.[3] This attitude suggests that it is justifiable to withhold treatment in some cases because basic skills needed for an occupation are not needed by the older, retired person. The problem with this position is that these skills are fundamentally useful for other aspects of daily living as well. The distinction is based on an arbitrary judgment about which skills are needed for the elderly person's well-being, and because it is arbitrary this judgment would not stand up to the requirements of justice.

In short, there is very little within a merit approach to allocation that lends itself to an accurate consideration of an elderly individual's specific economic status or to policies that would take into account the wide variation in economic status within this population. Furthermore, a merit approach may be implicitly tied to assumptions about the merit of gainful employment, so that the status of "retired" may lead to unfair judgments against the claims of elderly persons even for basic health care services. Another criterion of allocation is needed.

Allocation Based on Societal Contribution

A common assumption is that the aged are a financial burden on the young. However, there is considerable evidence that elderly persons contribute financially to younger ones. In one poll, 88% of people over the age of 65 years believed that parents have a responsibility to provide their children with a college education, and 85% believed that parents have a responsibility to provide their children with a place to live if they are unable to afford it themselves. Income transfers from the elderly generation to the younger generation are common and, in fact, exceed the amount of income transferred from the middle-aged generation to the elderly generation until the 8th decade[4] (Fig 47.1). It is within the societal contribution approach to allocation issues that the discussion of "intergenerational equity" has come to the forefront in the debate about health care resource allocation for elderly persons. In this context, the money spent on their health care is seen as taking money *away* from children, the latter being judged more deserving of it, more needy, or both.

Indeed, since 1965, poverty among children has increased, while among elderly persons it has decreased. In 1965, when Medicare was instituted, roughly a quarter of older people were living in poverty, compared with around 12% of children. Today, 25 years later, the percentages are reversed.

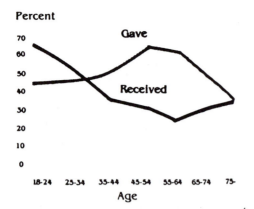

Fig. 47.1. Income transfer by age (from Morgan[4]).

Roughly 15% of older people live below the poverty level, mostly elderly women living alone, but the proportion of children in poverty has risen to 25%. This, however, has been less a direct monetary transfer between the generations than a change in the dynamics of poverty in our society. The children represented in this group are largely urban children living in single-parent families. In spite of these complexities, at a time of growing federal deficits and increasing awareness of government expenditures, these numbers suggest to some that we are overspending on elderly persons, and medical care is an obvious target for spending cuts.

The stakes are high if American society decides to pit one generation against another. The old and the young are not natural adversaries, and the close relationships of grandparents (and now great-grandparents) with the younger generations serves to maintain a network of fidelity and trust in the extended family. Contributions from one generation to another are more than financial; they are made in the form of personal time and effort, or emotional and spiritual support. Therefore, it is wise to consider the shortcomings of the arguments being presented about "intergenerational inequities." A report of the Gerontological Society of America observes that "by framing policy issues in terms of competition and conflict between generations, the inter-generational inequity perspective implies that public benefits to the elderly are a one-way flow from young to old and that there is no exchange between generations."[2] This faulty understanding of the many intergenerational implications of attitudes, life-styles, and changing social policies distracts attention from important social policy questions, such as taxation, value choices about federal spending overall, and policies for the development of new technology, education, housing, and transportation. In a period of a soaring federal deficit, people of all ages have a stake in sound policies that effectively serve to meet the needs of elderly persons as well as

the needs of children and families. In fact, Social Security and Medicare legislation was passed with substantial support from middle-aged individuals who realized that they would be supporting the medical and social expenses for the care of elderly parents and would thus perhaps be unable to buy a home or put their own children through college. It is not only elderly persons who are benefiting from programs to support older people, but all generations. Thus, even at a quick glance the arguments regarding intergenerational equity have serious flaws.

Furthermore, a peculiar and, to us, troubling argument has been imported into the current discussion of intergenerational equity, again distorting clear thinking about allocation. This is the argument that older people have lived a "normal life span" and therefore ought to be willing to step aside in favor of those who have not had such an opportunity.[3] The implication is that older people have already made their societal contribution and that they now should make a societal contribution by *not* accepting health care resources. Taking this reasoning to its logical conclusion, elderly persons would have no further hope of receiving resources because they have already realized or exceeded a reasonable life expectancy. However, the dramatically increasing life expectancy of Americans can be seen as a sign of progress rather than only as an indicator of a problem. Indeed, traditionally, life expectancy has been one of the key health indicators that distinguish the developed from the developing countries. Improvements in social well-being, such as sanitation, nutrition, and control of epidemic and endemic infectious diseases, have provided the basis for dramatic declines in premature death in young adulthood and middle age. In the United States, we still have a good deal of progress to be made in infant mortality compared with other developed countries, but even in this area, we are far ahead of where we were a century ago and where many developing countries are today.

These factors all combine to make it possible for the vast majority of people to live much longer than ever before. The last 2 decades have led us to question our understanding of just what "normal" means when referring to life span. It was expected in the late 1950s and early 1960s that most people would die within a decade after reaching the age of 65 years. Public policy, including Social Security and Medicare, was based on this assumption. In the last 20 years, we have seen that most dramatic increases in life expectancy occur among the oldest people.

While much of the gain in life expectancy early in the century was related to social advances, it is suspected that the advances at very old age are largely due to medical care. With only a few exceptions, most of the new inventions in medical technology developed since the 1950s have had their greatest impact on people over the age of 65 years. The older the patients, the greater the impact has been. Life-sustaining and life-prolonging treatments for coronary artery disease, cardiac valvular disorders, hypertension, thrombotic/embolic disorders, and serious infections—all disorders that are frequently responsible for death in old age—are widely available and widely applied regardless of a patient's age.

If we are thinking about rationing health care and looking at a "normal life span" as a measure of what society owes to a person, this unprecedented, successfully aging society raises difficult questions. If the average life expectancy is between 80 and 90 years and tens of thousands are even living well over 100 years, what then counts as normal? We find that it is the exception rather than the rule for a life pattern to consist only of education, marriage, child rearing, career, retirement, grandchildren, and death. People may be married more than once, have more than one set of children, and have more than one career in a single lifetime. How then are we to judge what is normal? Is it what happened in the good old days? Is it what most people do? Intergenerational inequity as a justification for cutbacks in beneficial medical care for elderly persons (no one is in favor of nonbeneficial medical care) must be examined very carefully. On a very simple level, it is not at all clear that cutting back on Medicare spending would necessarily benefit the poor children of our society. In fact, there is no such guarantee in the current public framework at all. Some experts argue that universal health insurance, which would benefit young and old, is the only morally correct solution.[5] It also may be the most effective cost-containment mechanism, because measures to limit overutilization as well as overpricing can be applied consistently throughout the health care system.

Many of these arguments are based on the concept of the "dependency ratio," a notion that combines aspects of "merit" thinking with "societal contribution" reasoning and that measures the number of persons over the age of 65 years (assumed not to be working) compared with those between the ages of 18 and 64 years (all of whom are assumed to be contributing to the economy). It is in fact children who make up the rest of the dependency ratio, and given that the number of children being born is going down while the number of elderly people is going up, the combined dependency ratio will never at any time during the next 65 years exceed levels it attained in 1964 at the peak of the baby boomers' childhood dependency[6] (Fig 47.2). Further, all of these concepts of the dependency ratio fail to consider such factors as the increasing participation of women in the labor force, the potential for significant portions of the elderly population to work for a longer time, or the effect of economic growth. In short, the issues related to life span and their implications for health care costs and benefits are far more complex than is the thinking usually applied to arguments based on "intergenerational equity" and "normal life span."

Callahan, among others, applies intergenerational equity and the idea of "normal" life span in suggesting an arbitrary age limit for limiting life-sustaining treatment.[7] This may cut off some potentially good years for some individuals, he argues, but has the advantage of being fair: it does not discriminate since all people sooner or later would reach that age. One drawback of such a system is that it does not respond to the wide variability among elderly persons.

To be sure, the issue is a perplexing one deserving of society's most rigorous attention. If an arbitrary uni-

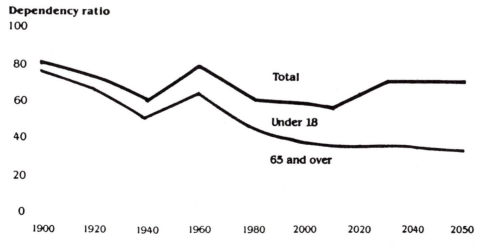

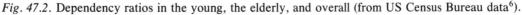

Fig. 47.2. Dependency ratios in the young, the elderly, and overall (from US Census Bureau data[6]).

form cutoff is not to be the answer, the alternative is to figure out a way in which we can make better decisions as to when it is appropriate to allow death to come. In this search, we turn now to a consideration of allocation criteria based primarily on medical need.

Allocation Based on Need

A principle of justice based on need entails the idea that society has an obligation to take care of its own. It is based on an anthropologic assumption that when allocation decisions are made, some persons must be given the advantage of a "handicap" at the outset, in order to make up for certain deprivations they experience. A now classic statement of this approach is found in the *Alva Myrdal Report:*

Equality means that where nature has created great and fundamental differences in abilities, these must not be allowed to determine the individual's chances in life, but rather that society should restore the balance. These differences, in the form of physical or intellectual handicaps, can never be eliminated, but they can be reduced in a generous social climate, and one can work against their leading to social discrimination. Disadvantages inflicted by nature should not be accepted as something we can do nothing about.[8]

In the development of US health policies, attention to need-based reasoning often has been discernible. For example, the idea of "medical indigence" was introduced with the original Medicaid legislation, which asserted that one should not become indigent because of medical expenses. Another competing theme is pervasive in US health policy. Illustrative is the Surgeon General's report identifying the major focus for the 1980s as "disease prevention and health promotion," with one aim being a measurable and achievable "*improvement* in health, function, and independence *for older people.*"[9] Although these goals are laudable, there is little doubt that an emphasis on healthy people can rechannel attention away from chronically ill members of society of all age groups who require extensive health-related services. Overemphasis on preventive measures can even lead to a "blame the victim" attitude toward people suffering from chronic illness or disability.

Clearly an interpretation of justice that begins by considering need creates a favorable environment for assisting sick and chronically ill persons. The governing attitude is the conviction that a person has a claim to realize the highest level of functioning possible, given his or her circumstances. Since independence is an overriding value, persons should be provided with appropriate supports so that they can be as independent as possible. The question is not "does it cost too

much" but rather, "how shall we assume funds for so vital a dimension of societal well-being?" This position does not necessarily include a positive attitude of affection or respect for one's equals; it could as easily be coercive or paternalistic. Nonetheless, since the tension is in favor of helping to assure the basic life and liberty requirements of all persons, promoting independent functioning is a basically positive position. Probably few would argue against the moral soundness of this approach. However, here we run into a snag.

Because needs are almost always greater than resources, depending on how needs are defined, the definition must include logical ways to distinguish levels of need, such as dire, basic, relative or trivial. An approach that rests on allocating according to need requires a social minimum below which no person should fall.[10] Assuming that a more equal life situation for all is an ultimate value to be realized in such allocation decisions, those who are better off will lose liberty to the extent that resources that would permit them more life-style options are redirected to help meet the basic needs of the less well-off.

In the policy arena, then, liberty and justice may be in conflict. At least three approaches to maintaining liberty while realizing justice can be articulated. First, consider the possibility of setting the social minimum high so that everyone can realize a relatively full life (insomuch as physical resources foster it), of allocating sufficient monies for the demands of the situation, and then imposing strict government regulation to help assure that resources are distributed according to need. While the demands of justice are protected, the totalitarian overtones of such an arrangement suggest that liberty is jeopardized. Indeed, to the extent that regulations have been implemented in the United States, such intervention has met sustained resistance. Within the health care system, the value of self-determination or the "liberty" of physicians to market their services according to their professional discretion, patients to choose their providers and to purchase services, and manufacturers to provide a wide range of products so far has created an effective barrier to imposing heavy controls.

A second approach would be to lower the social minimum to subsistence level. This would increase the life-style options of the better-off but decrease it substantially for those requiring services paid for out of public funds. The requirements of responding to need are met, though the underlying ideal of equality is lost. That is, the need may be attended to but there is no guarantee of an impetus to create more equal life choices for all. The motivating concept of "restoring a balance" is dormant. Suspicion that the social minimum would be set unseemly low is a major motive in the political resistance to changing Medicare from a universal to a needs-based entitlement. Clearly, what is desirable, from both the moral and the policy point of view, is a middle way.

With this in mind, and given the ethical trade-offs inherent in the above two approaches, Harvard philosopher John Rawls has introduced the notion that the "maximin" or the "maximum of the minimum liberty" should be available to everyone.[11] He defends equal basic liberties for everyone and provides a fairly expansive notion of what liberty involves. At the very least, he wants each person to be able to work out a life plan that is reasonable for him or her. Each should experience the maximum amount of freedom that everyone else also experiences (thus, the "maximin").

However, he also believes that the exercise of liberty for all means that some persons require more help in obtaining the resources that are prerequisites for exercising life options than do others. He begins by assuming that natural advantages, talents, and strengths do not, in themselves, create a claim for larger shares of basic social and economic goods. The fruits of some natural talents are common assets to be distributed justly. A second assumption is that desirable resources are not necessarily distributed justly by giving equal amounts to everyone. However, unless inequality is shown to be more just, equality is preferred. *The inequalities permitted are those that benefit everyone.*

A key feature of the principle is that it singles out a particular position from which inequalities in resource priorities can be judged. The greater amount of resources given to those who are better off is justified if, and only if, they help create opportunity for equal liberty, and for the attainment of cherished social and economic goods among the less advantaged members of society. That is, more can be given to the better off if there is assurance that those who are deprived will thereby benefit. This is in striking contrast to an approach that pits one generation against another.

Proponents of Rawls defend the approach as a reasonable theoretical framework for developing allocation policies that could meet the heath care needs of the most needy groups while assuring that some incentives for high-quality programs will be built into the overall system of health care. However, others raise doubts regarding the possible degree of difference in resources that would actually exist between the better and less well off in his scheme. At the very least, this should be viewed as one promising approach for working out a golden mean between a totally equalized society and one in which the needs of some are ignored while others reap great benefits.

Even if the Rawlsian approach should provide a workable theoretical model for ascertaining the overall allocations in a society, critical issues remain unanswered concerning health care policy for elderly people.

First, from both theoretical and practical viewpoints, the notion of "need" must be more fully delineated if it is to be an effective starting point for policy deliberation. More attention must be given to distinguishing "needs" from "wants" and "basic" from "felt" needs. The difficult task of trying to categorize various types of need and to measure these effects on the well-being of individuals must be pursued rigorously.

Second, the amount of disability actually experienced by older people who have chronic illness must be ascertained more fully than it has been, in order to gain an accurate picture of the current situation of the elderly population and to project future needs. And, in order to understand need more accurately, a clear account of the benefits of various treatments or interventions must be made. These kinds of data have not been widely sought because of the methodologic difficulties in establishing proper outcome measures in chronic illness.[12] Should we count physical improvement in the same way as psychological improvement? Is maintenance of function in a person with progressive disease as important as improvement of function in a person with the ability to recover? Are assistive interventions that enhance independence or autonomy worth the cost if economic productivity is not at stake?

Third, the criterion of need as a basis for health policy often has led to an emphasis on acute or long-term care for those already affected. Clearly the number of healthy aged persons behooves us to take every opportunity to promote health care policies that also encourage health maintenance and disease prevention as priorities.

In all areas, more research to substantiate claims about the status and needs of older people is required in order for the need criterion of allocation to be applied in a way that would assure fairness to all.

Concluding Thoughts

Decisions about how to allocate society's precious and limited resources will never be easy and should never be automatic. It is not the desire of older people, it would seem, to extend their lives unreasonably and forever. But new technologies as they are developed must be applied in a sensible and appropriate way. The question before us is how to establish what is sensible and what is appropriate. None of the traditional approaches to allocation—including those based on merit, social contribution, or need—is fully adequate for making policies related to older persons' health care. Using an analysis based on justice, we conclude that policies based solely on merit or social contribution criteria have greater ethical failings than those using need as a governing concern.

The aging of society is indeed a sign of progress. The challenge of living in a society that includes many elderly people, some of whom are frail and dependent, requires diligent assessment of how to think about and act on our highest ideals and central values. The challenge of caring for the frail and needy may be seen as another area where social progress can occur. If we can breed compassion and effective systems of health care and social services, as well as breeding silicon chips and new imaging techniques, then we will be a truly advanced society. Indeed, in addition to technical and biologic advances, moral advances will be critically necessary to allow our society to flourish in the 21st century.

References

1. Aristotle; Ross WD, trans. *Nichomachean Ethics Book V*. Vol 9 in *The Works of Aristotle*. New York, NY: Oxford University Press; 1925

2. Kingson ER, Hirshorn Ba, Cornman JM. *The Ties That Bind: The Interdependence of Generations*. Report from the Gerontological Society of America. Washington, DC: Seven Lock Press; 1986.

3. Daniels N. *Just Health Care*. Cambridge, England: Cambridge University Press; 1985.

4. Morgan J.N. The redistribution of income by families and institutions and emergency help patterns. In: Duncan GJ, Morgan JN, eds. *Five Thousand American Families: Patterns of American Progress*. Vol 10: *Analyses of the First Thirteen Years of the Panel Study of Income Dynamics*. Ann Arbor, Mich: Institute for Social Research; 1983.

5. Himmelstein DU, Woolhandler S, Writing Committee of the Working Group on Program Design. A national health program for the United States: a physicians' proposal. *N Engl J Med* 1989;320:102–108.

6. US Bureau of the Census. *Population Projections of the United States by Age, Sex, and Race: 1983 to 2080*. Washington, DC: Government Printing Office; 1984. Current Population Reports, P-25, No. 952.

7. Callahan D. *Setting Limits*. New York, NY: Simon & Shuster Inc Publishers, 1988.

8. *Alva Myrdal Report: Towards Equality*. Stockholm, Sweden Bok Forlaget Prisma; 1971

9. *Healthy People: The Surgeon General's Report on Health Promotion and Diseases Prevention*. Washington DC: US Department of Health, Education, and Welfare; 1979.

10. Brandt RB. *Ethical Theory*. Englewood Cliffs, NJ; 1959.

11. Rawls J. *A Theory of Justice*. Cambridge, Mass: Harvard University Press; 1971.

12. Urban Institute. *Executive Summary of the Comprehensive Needs Study of Individuals with the Most Severe Handicaps*. Contract No. SR-74-54.

48

Medical Treatment and the Physician's Legal Duties

Marshall B. Kapp

In the course of obtaining medical care, the older patient enters into a relationship with one or more physicians, professional staff working under the physician's control, and, frequently, health care entities through which or in which the health care is delivered. These relationships may be described as both contractual (ie, based on a mutual exchange of promises) and fiduciary (ie, based on the necessary trust that accompanies the patient's reliance on the more knowledgeable and powerful health care provider). Under either of these characterizations, the relationships that are formed entail a variety of legal obligations on the part of the physician (as well as ethical obligations; see Chapter 4). These duties are enforceable, and their violation may lead to adverse legal and financial consequences for the physician.

Thus, a working knowledge of treatment-related legal issues is essential to the practicing geriatrician, who needs to understand enforceable requirements and associated potential liabilities. A familiarity with relevant law is also needed because the geriatrician often has the opportunity, and in certain circumstances may be required, to contribute medical expertise to and aid in the resolution of legal issues, as in cases where the physician's affidavit or testimony is the central piece of evidence regarding mental competence in a contested guardianship proceeding.

Many legal issues affecting geriatric practice are basically generic. For instance, physicians must be aware of the legal doctrines of informed consent and confidentiality regardless of the age of their patients. There is nothing inherently distinctive about older

patients from a legal perspective. However, many generic legal issues take on unique twists or special urgency when applied to older patients, owing to considerations of physical or mental decline, impaired sensory perception, a well-developed life history and set of values, the outliving of concerned families or the presence of intermeddling families, and the increased risk of institutionalization. Additionally, there exists a subset of medically related issues that do pertain exclusively to elderly patients, because lawmakers consciously have made age by itself a pertinent criterion; examples include eligibility for Supplemental Security Income and the physical and mental ability of an individual claiming age discrimination to perform a job for which he or she was not hired.

This chapter surveys a few of the more salient legal issues arising in the practice of geriatric medicine, focusing on patient rights and professional obligations. It begins by attempting to deal head-on with the legal topic most prominent in medical minds—professional liability or malpractice—and to put it into some meaningful and realistic perspective in the context of geriatrics. With that as background, the chapter moves to an overview of informed consent, choices in treatment, and research participation, as applied to elderly persons.

What follows naturally from that is an explication of legally sanctioned intervention in medical decision making for older patients, touching on the subjects of advance health care planning for incapacity, guardianship, the family's authority as surrogate decision maker, and particular problems involved in choices concerning life-sustaining treatment. Institutional ethics committees are discussed as one potential mechanism for facilitating decision making in difficult cases. From there, the discussion proceeds to adult protective services. Special dilemmas in confidentiality are then raised. The chapter concludes by exploring the likely relationship between health care cost containment strategies and potential legal liability on the part of the physician.

The Malpractice Cloud[1]

Geriatricians, like practitioners in every other medical specialty, understandably are concerned about the specter of medical malpractice that lurks in the shadow of every clinical decision and action. However, this apprehension often is blown out of proportion and, even and perhaps especially in geriatrics, can result in counterproductive medical decisions and actions that serve both the patient and the physician poorly.[2] Hence, it is important that geriatricians be able to place the malpractice threat in some meaningful perspective so that they are neither lulled into a false sense of complacency nor psychologically paralyzed and prevented from providing clinically effective and respectful care.

At the outset, it should be noted that, although certainly not untouched by the recent malpractice clamor, physicians specializing in treating older patients have in large measure been spared some of the worst aspects of the malpractice problem, at least as compared with their colleagues in other practice areas. Economist Patricia Danzon, in the most important piece of social science research to study this subject to date, found that elderly patients are significantly less likely to file malpractice actions against their physicians than are younger patients, and the claims brought by older patients are likely to result in much lower money damages than would be true for younger plaintiffs.[3] This reluctance of elderly patients to sue health care providers is confirmed by the General Accounting Office's finding that, for malpractice claims that were closed in 1984, less than 14% of the claims filed involved patients over the age of 65 years, and 26% of those claims were filed on behalf of older patients who died during medical treatment.[4] Fourteen percent is a very small figure compared with the much larger proportion of the total health care pie that is consumed by the elderly.[5]

Of the estimated 7,293 malpractice claims brought by Medicare beneficiaries during the General Accounting Office's study period, approximately 3,129 (about 42.9%) were closed with some type of payment. The average indemnity payment for this plaintiff group was $28,352, a figure considerably lower than that awarded to, or settled on for, patient plaintiffs who were not old enough for Medicare.

Several possible reasons have been advanced to explain why older patients tend to bring fewer and less severe malpractice complaints against their physicians and other health care providers than younger patients. These hypothesized explanations speak to characteristics of geriatric practice, elderly patients, and the present legal system through which malpractice claims are processed.

First, there is the argument that the nature of geriatric practice, tending to emphasize conservative management and rehabilitative care, entails fewer and less severe clinical (and hence legal) risks than practice specialties such as surgery, which rely more heavily on dramatic, curative, technologically oriented interventions that are calculated to produce more immediate and definitive results. These results may be either successes or failures, and unsatisfactory results, especially when they come as a surprise to the patient or family, are the genesis of most malpractice claims. For geriatrics, the objectives and expectations of the patient and family ordinarily are more limited and realistic, and hence the probability of serious patient dissatisfaction with unexpectedly bad outcomes is reduced.

Furthermore, even though geriatricians face a tremendous constellation of ethical issues in patient care, ranging from mental competence determinations to confidentiality considerations to decisions about the limitation of life-sustaining treatment, these kinds of issues seldom actually erupt into malpractice claims. The fear of malpractice litigation inspired by these issues is disproportionate to the actual risk.[6]

Second, it has been suggested that older patients as a group are likely to impose less stringent demands and expectations on their physicians than do younger patients, and to be more satisfied with the quality of the medical attention they receive.[7] Elderly people tend to show greater deference to authority figures generally, including those in white coats, than does the population as a whole, whose respect for authority has steadily declined in the last several decades. Older patients, although far from being a homogeneous group in this or any other aspect, for the most part perceive the overall character of their relationships with physicians to be positive. This perception may be accurate, since, despite some data to the contrary,[8] many geriatricians spend more time with the patient and the patient's family than do physicians (particularly specialists) with younger patients, and their posture tends to be supportive and communicative rather than technical.

Finally and perhaps most importantly, the nature of

the American legal system works to keep down the number and severity of legal tort claims brought by or on behalf of older citizens involving allegations of personal injury generally and medical malpractice specifically. This occurs in two ways.

In any personal injury lawsuit, tort doctrine requires that the plaintiff prove by a preponderance of the evidence four basic elements: (1) the nature of the duty owed by the defendant to the plaintiff; (2) the violation or breach of that duty (ie, negligence or fault); (3) some damage or injury suffered by the plaintiff; and (4) a causal relationship between the defendant's breach of duty and the injury incurred by the plaintiff. Proof of the latter two elements frequently presents difficult evidentiary challenges for older individuals contemplating a medical malpractice claim, challenges that are of sufficient magnitude that they often deter the filing of claims that probably would be pursued by younger patients.

Regarding damages, the single most significant element of monetary loss figured into a settlement or jury verdict is the amount of future lost income foregone by the plaintiff as a result of the injury. Older persons, virtually by definition having fewer income-producing years ahead of them, often will be limited in their ability to demonstrate much in the way of this form of financial loss. Thus, the potential economic payout of even a successful malpractice claim prosecuted by an older plaintiff is likely to be modest, deterring its pursuit both by the patient and family and by the attorney who is asked to provide legal representation on the basis of a contingency fee.

Additionally, proving by a preponderance of the evidence the necessary element of causation will be difficult for many older plaintiffs. The allegation that the defendant's negligence was not only the sine qua non ("but for") of the patient's injury but actually the proximate or most direct cause is hard to substantiate when the patient had a preexisting condition of illness and frailty. Since many older patients begin medical treatment already compromised with serious underlying physical or mental infirmities, the requirement of proof that the defendant's negligence was the proximate cause of the injury often is a legally fatal stumbling block, one that is reflected in the low rate of geriatric malpractice claims.

In light of the preceding discussion, why should a geriatrician be very concerned about patient rights or the physician's own legal responsibilities? First, although medical malpractice claims experience in geriatrics has thus far been relatively minimal, some claims indeed are filed. Geriatricians are in a favorable position compared with their colleagues, but they are hardly immune from legal repercussions. Additionally, some have suggested that the growing emphasis on cost containment in health care delivery may impair quality of care and therefore, in the coming months and years, increase the legal liability risks arising in the treatment of older patients (see discussion below).

Second, the physician should be aware that there are many forms of legal regulation of medical practice and its practitioners besides the traditional individual tort lawsuit. For instance, professional licensure and disciplinary provisions, oversight by peer review organizations and other audit agencies of the quality of care provided to Medicare beneficiaries, and new statutory and regulatory requirements for skilled nursing and intermediate care facilities are aspects of legal regulation that exert a direct impact on medical practice (and on the fulfillment of medical administrative roles),[9] quite apart from the patient's ability or inability to pursue litigation seeking money damages. Numerous other examples could be cited.

Finally, legal requirements in most situations represent society's consensus on important ethical issues. While law and ethics are by no means synonymous, in many cases a solid understanding of the permissible legal parameters and the rationale underlying them can assist physicians in defining and carrying out their ethical responsibilities to patients. Hence, the law has an educational as well as a coercive function.

Informed Consent[10]

Competent Patients and the Elements of Consent

As a general legal principle, medical decisions should regularly be made by the person most directly affected by the consequences of each decision, that is, the patient. There are three essential elements that must be present in order for a patient's choice about treatment to be considered legally valid.

First, the patient's participation in the decision-making process and the ultimate decision must be voluntary. The usual definition of voluntariness in the context of consent is that the person giving or withholding consent must be so situated as to be able to exercise free power of choice without the intervention of any element of force, fraud, deceit, duress, overreaching, or other ulterior form of constraint or coercion. It means simply that the person must be free to reject participation in the proposed intervention. The physician must do all possible to minimize any intimidation inherent in the physician-patient relationship, and in the institution-patient relationships when care is provided on an inpatient basis, and to make sure that advice and recommendations are transmitted in as nonpressured and empathetic a manner as possible.

The second fundamental requirement for valid consent is that the patient's agreement be informed. The legal doctrine of informed consent requires that the health care provider, before undertaking an intervention, must disclose certain information to the person who is the subject of the proposed intervention.[11]

The disclosure standard currently enforced in the majority of American jurisdictions is referred to as the "professional," "reasonable physician,"[12] or "community" standard. Under this test, the adequacy of disclosure is judged against the amount and type of information that a reasonable, prudent physician would have disclosed under similar circumstances.

A large minority of jurisdictions have accepted a more expansive standard of information disclosure: the "reasonable patient" or "material risk" standard.[13] This standard dictates that the physician communicate the information that a "reasonable patient" in the same situation would need and want to make a voluntary and knowledgeable decision. Under this test, the patient must be told about all material risks—that is, those factors that might make a difference to a reasonable, average patient under similar circumstances.

The age of a patient may affect what information is material to that person's decision making. For instance, a likely side effect that will not manifest itself for another 20 years may not be very important to an older person. However, the probability that a particular intervention will be accompanied by a great amount of physical pain or discomfort may make quite a difference to an old, frail individual. Physicians always should consider the physical and mental effects of aging, among numerous other factors, when deciding whether information regarding an intervention might be material to the specific person.

Within these standards of disclosure, the particular informational items have usually been enumerated as follows: (1) diagnosis; (2) the nature and purpose of the proposed intervention; (3) the risks, consequences, or perils of the intervention; (4) the probability of success; (5) alternatives; (6) the result anticipated if nothing is done; (7) limitations on the professional or health care facility; and (8) advice (ie, the physician's recommendation).

The third essential element of legally effective consent is that the patient must be mentally competent to think rationally regarding personal care. Where the patient lacks sufficient mental capacity, a substitute or proxy decision maker must be involved (see below). Incapacity and questionable capacity is an especially acute issue for long-term care facilities.

Determinations of Competence

Despite the strong legal presumption toward respect for the individual's autonomous right to make decisions concerning his or her own life, including choices about medical treatment, for a number of older persons the capacity to make and express legally valid decisions has been compromised by biologic factors (eg, dementia, stroke, depression)[14] and, for those who are institutionalized, by the environment in which they find themselves. Particularly when illness occurs in a hospital or a long-term care facility, the ability to make and communicate autonomous choices on important matters may be impaired substantially.

Legal competence refers to a relative, rather than an absolute, degree of ability scale.[15] To say that a person is legally incompetent implies that the individual is below some minimum level of cognitive potential, and not simply that the person has less potential than certain other people.

The great majority of situations where the decision-making capacity of an older patient is called into question are handled on a de facto rather than de jure basis. That is, most such cases quite properly—and without adverse legal consequences—are managed by the physician and health care facility, usually in conjunction with the family, without formal court involvement in determining and acting upon the patient's decision-making impairment.[16]

In most circumstances, competence should be addressed as an ethical matter by those who are closest to the patient, and resort to the courts is neither necessary nor desirable, since it is expensive, time consuming, and emotionally draining. Judicial involvement in determinations of competence should be the exception instead of the rule. The need for such involvement will depend on a variety of factors in any case, including (1) the severity and prognosis of the cognitive impairment; (2) the difficulty and likely consequences of the medical decision to be made; (3) the availability or absence of a suitable surrogate; and (4) the agreement or disagreement among patient, family members, physician, and other relevant actors.

In some situations, such as the patient in a long-term coma or a persistent vegetative state,[17] the determination of incompetence is fairly straightforward. In most circumstances, though, clinical presentations of potential incompetence are more cloudy. These include transient incapacity due to acute illness or medication side effects; mental retardation; mental illness or emotional problems; and physical handicap.[18] Much more is entailed in determining legal status than the simple diagnostic labeling of a clinical condition.[19]

There exists no single, uniform standard of competence. Instead, competence to engage in medical decision making has been only rarely and vaguely defined in statutes and court decisions. In daily practice, it frequently is the attending physician, acting alone and at his or her own discretion, who decides when a person is not capable of making choices and when a substitute should be involved, without using any specific standards for that determination.[20]

In determining competence, the most thoughtful analyses urge that emphasis be placed not on the "objective" nature of the patient's clinical diagnosis or on the specific choice elected by the patient, but rather on the capacity of the patient and the subjective thought process followed in arriving at a "good" or "bad" decision.[21] The proper focus is on functional ability.

In a functional inquiry, the fundamental questions suggested are the following: (1) Can the person make and communicate, by spoken words or otherwise, choices concerning his or her own life? (2) Can the person offer any reasons for the choices made? (3) Are the reasons underlying the choice "rational"? That is, does the patient start with a plausible premise about the facts surrounding the specific medical situation and reason logically from that premise to a conclusion? (4) Is the person able to understand the implications (ie, the likely risks and benefits) of the alternatives presented and the choices that are made, and the fact that those implications apply to that person? (5) Does the person actually understand the implications of those choices?[22]

Under this functional approach, the patient need not understand the scientific theory underlying the physician's recommendations in order to be deemed competent, as long as the patient comprehends the general nature and likely consequences of the choices presented. Also, under this approach, competence must be determined on a decision-specific basis; that is, a patient may be capable of rationally making certain sorts of decisions but not others.[23] The minimally necessary degree of intellectual and emotional capacity may be visualized as falling somewhere on a sliding scale that depends on the nature of the decision being faced.[24] Thus, competence should not be treated as an all-or-nothing affair. Partial competence is not the same thing as incompetence. The patient may be "competent enough" to make the decision in question.

Additionally, competence may improve or deteriorate for a particular patient according to environmental factors, such as the time of day or the day of the week, the physical location, acute, transient medical problems, the presence of other persons supporting or pressuring the patient's decision, and reactions to medications. Health care providers are under an obligation to manipulate environmental barriers to capacity, wherever possible, in an attempt to maximize the decision-making capacity of a patient. Hence, if a decision can be delayed safely until a patient is in a more lucid phase, or if medications can be altered to allow the patient a clearer head to contemplate choices, this is preferable to proceeding unnecessarily on the basis of substituted decision making. Further, many acute physical or mental problems of elderly patients that impair their decision-making capacity can be treated medically successfully, and that course should be pursued vigorously before considering the resident incompetent.[25]

Many older persons are capable of "assisted" consent with a little extra time and effort on the part of health care professionals.[26] For example, an older patient, although unable to process complex information as swiftly and efficiently as a younger person, nevertheless may be able to understand the complexities of a proposed treatment if given enough time to process the information more fully. Physicians should be aware that elderly patients may need more time to work through complex information regarding treatment, and they should not automatically equate the speed with which an older individual processes information with the level of that person's mental competence.

The Research Context

The issue of participation by older persons, particularly those residing within nursing homes, in biomedical and behavioral research protocols is a growing legal concern. The question of legal propriety is especially acute when the topic under study is mental impairment and the proposed subjects are institutionalized as well as cognitively and emotionally compromised. The policy challenge is to protect impaired elderly persons from exploitation and avoidable harm, while facilitating the conduct of important, high-quality research on problems that affect the elderly population disproportionately.[27]

Most biomedical and behavioral research in the United States currently is regulated under federal law that seeks to protect the rights and well-being of potential human subjects.[28] A number of health care practitioners and scholars have suggested that special legal protections should be enacted to safeguard vulnerable older persons from potential abuse, exploitation, coercion, and injury as a result of research participation.[29] These arguments take on particular force when applied to older persons of diminished cognitive capacity who reside in nursing homes.[30] At present, however, there are no particular legal restrictions unique to older research subjects, whether in the community or in institutions; thus, participation by the elderly in research protocols is governed technically by the same law that applies to subjects of all ages.

The older person's competence to consent to research participation therefore is a matter of concern to geriatric researchers and therapists.[31] For incompetent persons, consent for research participation may be obtained legally from those individuals who are empowered to make other decisions on the older person's behalf.[32] Code of Federal Regulation, Title 45, Section 46.102 (d) refers to the use of a "legally authorized representative" for consent to research activities. Other approaches that have been suggested by a National Institute on Aging task force[33] and individual thinkers[34] have included (1) the designation by the older person while still capable of a proxy decision maker to authorize research participation in the event of the subject's subsequent incapacity, (2) special "consent auditors," and (3) increased reliance on institutional review boards to scrutinize and monitor especially carefully research protocols involving older human subjects.

The endeavor of conducting legally and ethically defensible geriatric research, particularly with demented, institutionalized subjects, presents a variety of challenges concerning site and subject selection, competence evaluations, comprehension and retention of relevant information, choice and authority of proxy decision makers, and minimization of coercive influences.[35] Nonetheless, the geriatric research enterprise is an essential one, and the legal challenges must be met appropriately.[36]

Outside Intervention in Medical Decision Making[37]

As just noted, proxy decision making concerning an older person's participation in a research protocol is sometimes necessary when the person lacks the capacity to make decisions rationally. In the same way, physicians involved in the diagnosis and treatment of older patients must frequently deal with substitute decision makers responsible for intervening on behalf of patients whose cognitive deficits are so severe that they prevent the patient from personally making and communicating autonomous choices. The topic of legal intervention by third parties acting for the incompetent patient is a complex and largely unsettled one.

There are several alternative ways to delegate legally what would ordinarily be the patient's authority to make decisions, in order for proxy to exercise that

power on behalf of the incompetent patient. These delegation mechanisms may be categorized as follows: (1) delegation of authority beforehand by the patient, through methods of advance planning; (2) delegation of authority to a substitute by operation of statute, regulation, or broad judicial precedent; (3) informal delegation of authority to a substitute by custom; and (4) delegation of authority to a substitute by a court order in the specific case.

The two most important current devices for advance health care planning are the living will and the durable power of attorney for health care.[38] In addition to allowing a person to give specific advance directions concerning medical treatment in the event of subsequent mental incapacity, in a number of states the living will is a permissible vehicle for designating another individual to act as the proxy or substitute decision maker, to represent one and act on one's behalf in the event of later incompetence and terminal illness. As of mid-1989, 40 states had enacted statutes specifically authorizing the execution of a living will (Table 48.1). In addition, courts in several states (eg, New York) without living will statutes have ruled that the written directive of a competent patient concerning future medical treatment is entitled, as a matter of constitutional and common law, to be given legal effect after the patient becomes incompetent.[39]

Living will statutes vary in detail from state to state and are not without significant problems in interpretation and enforcement.[40] Further, most living will statutes allow the individual to indicate a preference only for limitation of treatment, but not in the other direction.[41] For these and other reasons, many individuals and groups prefer use of the durable power of attorney as an advance planning instrument.[42]

The durable power of attorney is a legal document in which an individual may direct, through the appointment of an agent who is given either general or specific instructions, the making of medical decisions and the management of property in the event of future incapacity.[43] Every state has a durable power of attorney statute, although traditionally they have been used exclusively for asset management purposes. In an attempt at clarification, a few states have enacted statutes in the last few years explicitly creating a durable power of attorney for health care.[44] Even in states without such specific statutes, there appears to be no reason in law or logic to prevent the general durable power of attorney statute from applying to medical decisions.

Personal physicians of older patients have an obligation to initiate frank conversations with patients regarding future treatment preferences and to encourage patients to consider seriously the possible advisability of creating a living will and/or a durable power of

Table 48.1. State living will statutes.

Alabama Natural Death Act, Ala Code §§22-8A-1-10 (1981); Alaska Act Relating to the Rights of the Terminally Ill, Alaska Stat §§18.12.010–.100 (1986); Arizona Medical Treatment Decision, Ariz Rev Stat Ann §§36-3201–3210 (1985); Arkansas Rights of the Terminally Ill or Permanently Unconscious Act, 1987 Ark Acts 713; California Natural Death Act, Cal Health and Safety Code §§7185–7195 (1976); Colorado Medical Treatment Decision Act, Colo Rev Stat §§15-18-101-113, see also Colo. Rev. Stat. §§12-36-117 (1985); Connecticut Removal of Life Support Systems Act, Conn Gen Stat Ann §§190-570–575 (1985); Delaware Death with Dignity Act, Del Code Ann tit 16, §§2501–2509 (1982); District of Columbia Natural Death Act of 1981, DC Code Ann §§6-2421–2430 (1982); Florida Life Prolonging Procedure Act, Fla Stat, chap 84–58, §§765.01–.15 (1984); Georgia Living Wills Act, Ga Code Ann §§31-32-1 to 31-32-12 (1984); Hawaii Medical Treatment Decisions Act, Hawaii Rev Stat §§327D-1 to 327D-27 (1986); Idaho Natural Death Act, Idaho Code §§39-4501–4508 (1977); Illinois Living Will Act, Ill Ann Stat chap 110 1/2 §§701–710 (Smith-Hurd 1984); Indiana Living Wills and Life-Prolonging Procedures Act; Iowa Code chap. 144A.1–114.A11 (1985, amended HF 360 1987 Sess, 72nd Iowa Gen Assembly); Kansas Natural Death Act, Kan Stat Ann §§65–28, 101–109 (1979); Louisiana Declarations Concerning Life-Sustaining Procedures, La Rev Stat 40:1299.58.1–.10 (1984, amend 1985); Maine Living Wills Act, Me Rev Stat Ann title 22, chap 710a (1985); Maryland Life-Sustaining Procedures Act, Md Health General Code Ann §§5-601–614, subtitle 6, Life-Sustaining Procedures (1985); Mississippi Natural Death Act, Miss Code Ann §§41-41-101 to 41-41-121 (1984); Missouri Death-Prolonging Procedures Act, Mo Rev Stat §§459.010–459.055 (1985); Montana Living Will Act, Mont Code Ann §§50-9-101–104, §50-9-111, §§50-9-201–206 (1985); Nevada Withholding of Life-Sustaining Procedures, Nev Rev Stat §§449.540–690 (1977); New Hampshire Living Wills Act, NH Rev Stat Ann chap 137H (1985); New Mexico Right to Die Act, NM Stat Ann §§24-7-1-11 (1977); North Carolina Right to Natural Death Act, NC Gen Stat §§90-320–322 (1977, amend 1979, 1981, 1983); Oklahoma Natural Death Act, Okla Stat title 63, §§3101–3111 (1985); Oregon Rights with Respect to Terminal Illness, Ore Rev Stat §§97.050–.090 (1977, amend 1983); South Carolina Death With Dignity Act, SC Code Ann §44-77-10-160 (1986); Tennessee Right to Natural Death Act, Tenn Code Ann §§32-11-101 to 32-11-111 (1983); Texas Natural Death Act, Tex Stat Ann article 4590h (1977, amend 1979, 1983, 1985); Utah Personal Choice and Living Will Act, Utah Code Ann §§75-2-1101–1118 (1985); Vermont Terminal Care Document Act, Vt Stat Ann title 18, §§5251–5262 and title 13 §1801 (1982); Virginia Natural Death act, Va Code §§54-325.8:1–13 (1983); Washington Natural Death Act, Wash Rev Code Ann §§70.122.010–70.122.905 (1979); West Virginia Natural Death Act, WVa Code

Table 48.1. State living will statutes.

chap 16 article 30 §§1–10 (1984); Wisconsin Natural Death Act, Wis Stat §§154.01 et seq (1984); Wyoming Living Will Act, Wyo Stat §§33-26-144 to 33-26-152 (1984).

attorney while they still retain the mental capacity to do so and the physical health to obviate the need for immediate crisis management.[45,46] Along these lines, this author has advocated use by physicians of a "medical future" device that would enable competent patients of any age to communicate to their physicians values and preferences pertinent to future medical treatment, within a context of normal, noncrisis medical care.[47]

In some circumstances, decision-making authority may devolve or pass from the patient to someone else by operation of a statute, regulation, or judicial precedent. Probably the best known example of this form of substitute decision making is the representative payee concept for regular government benefit payments, including pension and disability checks from the Veterans Administration, Department of Defense, Railroad Retirement Board, and Civil Service; Old Age, Survivors, or Disability Insurance benefit payments under Title 2 of the Social Security Act; and Supplemental Security Income benefit payments to the aged, blind, or disabled under Title 16 of the Social Security Act.

As another example of this type of power delegation, the federal Medicare-Medicaid conditions of participation for skilled nursing and intermediate care facilities provide that the rights of a long-term care resident who is (1) adjudicated incompetent in accordance with state law or (2) found by the physician to be medically incapable of understanding his or her rights devolve to the resident's guardian, next of kin, sponsoring agency(ies), or representative payee. Ironically, in a growing number of jurisdictions, it is in the area of decision making about care of the critically ill patient that statutory, regulatory, and judicial guidance about substitute decision making is clearest.[48]

Living will statutes in several states set forth procedures for decision making on behalf of incompetent persons who have not signed a living will or durable power of attorney.[49] The procedure consists of unanimous agreement between the attending physician, specified relatives (usually in a stated order of preference), and sometimes consultant physicians as well. The trend in enactment and modification of living will legislation in other states also seems to be in this direction. In addition, courts in an increasing number of states are formally recognizing the authority of the family to exercise the incompetent person's decision-making rights on his or her behalf and, just as importantly, most of these judicial decisions explicitly establish legal precedent for families to act in future cases without the need for prior court authorization.

As a general matter, in the absence of a specific statute, regulation, or court order delegating authority to a substitute decision maker, or a court order finding an individual mentally incompetent and appointing another named person to act as guardian or conservator, neither the family as a whole nor any of its individual members (nor any nonrelatives) have any special legal authority to make decisions on behalf of a patient who cannot speak for himself. Nevertheless, it has long been a widely known and implicitly accepted medical custom or convention to rely on families as decision makers for incompetent persons, even in the absence of express legal power. Even where there is no explicit judicial or legislative authorization in one's own state, the legal risk of a physician or health care institution for a good faith treatment decision made in conjunction with an incompetent patient's family is very slight. In fact, with only one exception,[50] every court that has been presented with the question in the context of a concrete case has ratified the family's authority.

In some cases, however, informal substitute decision making—that is, the legal ''muddling through'' process that governs a great deal of medical, and especially geriatric, practice—by the physician and family members may not work. The family members may disagree among themselves. They may make decisions that seem to be at odds with the earlier expressed or implied preferences of the patient or that clearly appear not to be in the patient's best interests (eg, financially or psychologically driven selfish choices). The family may request a course of conduct that seriously contradicts the physician's or facility's own sense of ethical integrity.[51]

When such situations occur, judicial appointment of a guardian or conservator empowered to make decisions on behalf of an incompetent ward may be practically and legally advisable. However, because guardianship often entails an extensive deprivation of the individual's basic rights, may be imposed in the absence of meaningful procedural safeguards,[52] and involves substantial financial, time, and emotional costs, the ''least restrictive alternative'' doctrine dictates that it be pursued only as a last resort when less formal mechanisms of substitute decision making have failed or are unavailable.

Additionally, where guardianship is sought, consideration should be paid to the possibility of strictly limiting it in terms of both time and transferred powers. Since probate courts possess the authority to impose such limitations, under either specific state statutes or their inherent equity powers, physicians who deal with substitute decision makers who purport to be the patient's legal guardian should request to see a copy of the official court order creating the guardianship, in order to verify the existence and extent of the guardian's authority.[53]

Institutional Ethics Committees

One mechanism that may help the physician treating an incompetent patient to avoid the necessity of initiating a formal guardianship procedure is the institutional ethics committee,[54] also referred to by such names as bioethics committee.[55] This entity, which is being established in a growing number of acute care hospitals and long-term care facilities,[56] is essentially an interdisciplinary body within a health care institution that helps the institution and its professional staff to deal with difficult treatment decisions in an ethically, and secondarily in a legally, acceptable manner.

Institutional ethics committees differ among institutions in terms of precise size, composition, structure, procedures, and placement.[57] Functions may include policy drafting, staff education, and/or case consultation on a concurrent or retrospective basis. It has been suggested that consultation with an ethics committee regarding treatment decisions may exert a legal prophylactic effect, in terms of reducing unnecessary guardianship petitions, deterring possible lawsuits against the institution or its staff, and making it easier to defend any malpractice cases filed.[56] As of this writing, only one pending lawsuit has been brought against a health care facility based on the activity of its ethics committee and the projected positive legal effects have yet to be studied systematically.

''Do Not'' Orders

''Do not'' orders from the attending physician to other members of the health care team are predicated on prospectively made decisions to withdraw or withhold certain types of medical interventions from specified patients.[58] Most attention has been devoted, especially in the acute hospital environment, to ''do-not-resuscitate'' (DNR) orders (also known as ''no codes'') or instructions by the physician to refrain from attempts at cardiopulmonary resuscitation (CPR) in the event of a cardiac arrest.[59] However, other kinds of ''do not'' orders also are important, especially in the long-term care environment.[60] Most significant are potential ''do-not-hospitalize'' and ''do-not-treat'' orders.[61]

Legally, deciding about and implementing ''do not''

orders should be handled according to the same substantive principles and procedural guidelines that apply to other treatment decisions.[62] In fact, by allowing and encouraging certain decisions to be made prospectively before a crisis develops, "do not" orders may reduce potential legal risk and certainly should curtail legal anxiety.

The legal status of "do not" orders where the patient is mentally competent is fairly unambiguous. It parallels the situation of medical intervention generally, including intervention that would be life prolonging or even lifesaving. In other words, a competent adult patient has the constitutional, common law, and freedom of religion–based right voluntarily and knowingly to refuse basic (eg, CPR) or advanced cardiac life support or any of its specific components,[63] hospitalization, or any other form of medical intervention and to demand a precisely written "do not" order.

This fundamental right may be overriden by a judicial determination that there exists, under the particular circumstances, a state or societal interest that is compelling enough to justify infringing on the patient's autonomy. Such court rulings are virtually nonexistent, in the absence of minor children who need to be protected from a parent's decision to refuse clearly lifesaving treatment. Put more directly, courts have not ordered competent but critically ill, elderly patients to endure medical interventions over their stated objections, and seldom have physicians requested such rulings, except in relatively rare instances of legal paranoia. The wishes of close family members should be considered by the physician (assuming the competent patient has expressly or by implication authorized family participation in his or her medical care), but should never be permitted to override the decision of a competent patient.

Physicians are advised to assure that every health care setting within which they practice—both acute and long term—has a written policy statement regarding its institutional philosophy and any relevant technologic and staffing limitations concerning various "do not" situations.[64] A copy of this statement should be presented to every competent patient or an incompetent patient's most likely substitute decision maker at or before the time of admission. Extensive and regular professional staff education should be carried out concerning the provider's policies in this area. Physicians should customarily discuss treatment preferences and objectives openly and honestly with patients who are capable of participating in such decisions.[65] As a matter of course, they should document products of these discussions that might provide useful evidence later on of the patient's wishes and the good faith quality of the decision-making process. Some

commentators have even suggested that patients entering a hospital be given a questionnaire or other instrument at the time of admission to survey attitudes toward certain types of medical interventions.[66]

When a competent patient has made a "do not" decision, he or she must be able to reevaluate that decision continually in light of any change in physical or mental condition that materially affects (ie, that might really alter) the possible benefits or burdens of different treatment alternatives. A "do not" decision can be revoked or modified at any time. It is part of the physician's duty to supply the patient at any time with new information pertinent to "do not" decisions.

For the mentally incompetent patient, the situation is a bit less clear-cut legally. Clarification of respective rights and responsibilities may be available from the patient's previously executed advance directive or from the expressions of a legislatively or judicially designated proxy. In the absence of such clarification, "do not" orders are still permissible for incompetent patients according to the same general legal principles governing other kinds of decisions about life-sustaining medical treatment, that is, balancing—from the perspective of the patient—the likely benefits and burdens of the particular intervention. The only pertinent distinction between "do not" orders and other decisions to limit life-prolonging medical interventions lies in the prospective nature of the former.

In an effort to clarify this delicate area further, at least one state legislature has passed recently specific legislation on this subject[67] and one state regulatory agency has issued guidance.[68] The standards of the Joint Commission on the Accreditation of Healthcare Organizations have also been amended to deal with "do not" orders explicitly, with specific provisions on this point effective July 1, 1988, for hospitals and subsequently for nursing homes.

The suggestions offered above concerning the physician's and health care facility's responsibility to adopt, educate about, and communicate concerning a clear policy on "do not" orders applies with full force when incompetent patients are involved. When a patient is not capable of participating fully in decision making, the communication and negotiation about potential "do not" management strategies must encompass available, interested family members. The family has no greater or less legal authority to make "do not" decisions for an incompetent relative than to make other types of medical decisions (see earlier discussion). Even in the absence of specific legal authorization, in this sphere as elsewhere, it is (or should be) the medical custom or convention to involve families in "do not" decisions. From a practical, risk management perspective, extensive interaction with family members concerning such decisions is a prudent, protective practice.

Conversely, whether or not the family possesses the legal authority to veto a physician's proposed "do not" decision has emerged recently as a controversial issue. Proceeding with entry and implementation of a "do not" order in the face of family opposition entails, from a practical standpoint, a certain risk of legal challenge. However, a knowledgeable consensus in the literature appears to be forming that such challenges would be unsuccessful. This opinion assumes that the facts of the case make the "do not" order appropriate in terms of expressed patient wishes, the patient's prognosis, and the imbalance between the likely burdens and benefits of the intervention for the patient.[69]

A communication and negotiation process that is marked by compassion, clarity, and patience should resolve family-physician disagreement peacefully—in either direction—in the vast majority of situations. During such communication with the family, questions should be encouraged and answered candidly. The communication responsibility falls primarily on the attending physician's shoulders, but a vital supporting role in this process should be delegated freely to other trusted members of the health care team, such as nurses, social workers, psychologists, and clergy.

Physicians should explain their reasoning, as well as their diagnoses and prognoses, but they may and generally should present families with the possibility of a "do-not" order by making a recommendation in which the family's concurrence is elicited. This strategy helps to avoid placing families in the position of feeling that they themselves imposed a decision that can afterwards cause them guilt and depression. When the physician explains why mechanical ventilation, artificial feeding, resuscitation, hospitalization, antibiotics, or some other medical interventions would be futile or disproportionately burdensome, family members will seldom dissent if they have placed their trust in the physician. Where serious disagreement does surface and persist, consultation with an institutional ethics committee (discussed above) may be advisable; a judicial declaratory judgment and injunction may be sought as a last resort.

During the communicative process, the family should be informed that the propriety of a "do not" order will be reevaluated regularly and that it can always be rescinded if prognosis or other factors change. As would be true for any clinical action taken on an inaccurate factual basis, a physician or health care institution could be found legally negligent for basing a "do not" order on an incorrect evaluation of the patient's condition and prognosis.

The attending physician should make liberal use of available professional consultations with relevant clinical specialists, while retaining ultimate medical control and responsibility over the case. The judgment of nurses and other team members who are familiar with the patient also should be sought out and considered.

A number of state, local, and national medical societies, as well as ad hoc groups, have addressed the legal and ethical implications of "do not" orders.[70,71] Although such guidelines at this point are voluntary rather than binding, they should carry weight with legislators, courts, medical staffs, and facility-governing boards who struggle with these issues. For this reason, as well as for the ethical direction they may provide, physicians should keep abreast of and involved in the initiatives of their state, local, and national organizations in this sphere, as well as relevant ad hoc groups.

Some uninformed physicians still are fearful that putting nontreatment decisions into writing in the patient's chart may increase the potential exposure to legal liability. This is a serious misperception. Although a degree of sensitivity and discretion must be exercised (eg, do not write the name of DNR patients on a blackboard in a public hallway), nontreatment decisions should be documented thoroughly.[72]

The wishes of the patient (if ascertainable), the family, and significant others should all be recorded. The judgments of involved health care professionals, as well as the reasoning underlying those judgments, should be documented completely and candidly, as well as any attempts to change the minds of patient or family. Honesty and openness in record keeping in this sphere is the best defense for the physician and health care facility against any subsequent allegations of negligence or malevolent intent. Failure to put decisions and orders in writing not only fails to protect the physician but also invites inappropriate responses by other team members based on the mixed and confused signals that are given.

Once a "do not" order has been entered into a medical record, it should remain a permanent part of that record. If it is later modified or rescinded, the modification or rescission also should appear in the record.

Tied to the subject of documentation is the need for communication among appropriate health care team members and institutions once a "do not" order has been written. Going through the agonizing process of decision making serves little purpose if a decision to refrain from certain interventions is not communicated to those responsible for carrying out the "do not" orders, since, in the absence of such orders, the health care team normally is obligated to treat the patient with the full medical arsenal available. Such communication is chiefly an institutional responsibility, and each hospital and nursing home should have a provision in its written policies detailing its procedure for assuring that all members of the health care team involved with a particular patient will be informed accurately and promptly of "do not" orders or other treatment limitations concerning that patient. Regular interdisciplinary case reviews on the various institutional units are one means of communication that should be considered. Special markings on the outside of the medical chart, discreetly but clearly signifying particular treatment instructions, are also a valuable communicative tool.

There will be situations where a resident of a long-term care facility needs to be transferred to an acute care hospital for treatment of a specific remediable problem, such as acute infection, but other treatment limitations may remain appropriate because of the resident's other, underlying, nonremediable deficits. In those circumstances, the nursing home should have a clear, effective, ongoing mechanism in place for communicating "do not" orders directly to health care professionals at the hospital who will be involved in the person's care, as well as to personnel who participate in the transportation of the resident between facilities.[73] Especially since medical staff (and even more particularly the house staff) in acute hospitals may have strong preconceptions about resuscitation and other aggressive therapy for older persons who reside in nursing homes,[74] it is the nursing home's duty to transmit to the receiving hospital, at the time of or before the resident's arrival, as much background as feasible concerning preferences, values, and instructions that should guide treatment for that person. There should be a written provision in the transfer agreement between the nursing home and any other health care institution for the communication of this sort of information.

Finally, decisions to limit specific elements of treatment should not signify total disregard or the "writing off" of an older patient. Neglect of continuing palliative care, as well as medical care that has not been the subject of a "do not" order, could alienate patient and family and expose the physician and health care facility to charges of civil or criminal abandonment, neglect, or even abuse. Alleviating suffering is a basic goal of medical care and a part of the standard of care legally and ethically owed by health care professionals, even where "cure" of underlying disease is no longer possible. Management goals should consist of remaining in physical and emotional contact with the dying person; relieving terminal symptoms (such as pain, confusion, anxiety, or restlessness); providing nourishment and hydration, skin care, bowel and bladder care, and personal grooming; and supporting the family throughout the period of dying, death, and

bereavement.[75] High-dose narcotic agents and sedatives can be used despite the risk of suppressed cerebral function and respiratory depression, because the therapeutic intention is to control the symptoms of human suffering, not to precipitate an earlier death[76] (see Chapter 46).

Adult Protective Services[77]

Until now, this chapter has concentrated exclusively on choices concerning medical decisions facing the older patient. Such considerations, of course, are of paramount importance to the geriatrician. However, there are a multiplicity of other life decisions that need to be made by or on behalf of elderly persons, and the physician with an older patient population regularly is called on to contribute expertise and skills to aid in the making and implementation of these "nonmedical" decisions that frequently carry significant medical consequences. This brings us to the subject of adult protective services.

The concept of adult protective services builds directly both on the legal mechanism of guardianship, discussed earlier, and on the right of a mentally competent adult to give voluntary informed consent to various forms of intervention. It can thus fall at either end of the scale measuring degree of intrusiveness into the life of the older individual concerned. In either event, the physician has an important role to fulfill.

In the past decade and a half, a majority of states have enacted a wide array of programs under the general rubric of adult protective services. The traditional definition of this concept is a system of preventive, supportive, and surrogate services provided to adults living in the community, enabling them to maintain independent living and to avoid abuse and exploitation. Protective services are characterized by two elements that can be mixed in several different ways: the coordinated delivery of services to adults at risk and the actual or potential authority to provide substitute decision making concerning these services.

The services feature consists of an assortment of health, housing, and social services, such as homemaker, house repair, friendly visits, and meals. Ideally, these services are coordinated by a caseworker who is responsible for assessing an older individual's needs and bringing together the available responses. Many state protective services statutes mandate that social service agencies undertake both casework coordination and delivery of services.

The second component of an adult protective services program is authority to intervene on behalf of the client. Ordinarily, the client (if competent), with the encouragement of his physician, will voluntarily delegate this power to the helping party on an informal basis.[78] Where a more formal arrangement is desirable, a power of attorney or durable power of attorney may be appropriate.[79] However, if the client refuses offered assistance but ongoing intervention appears necessary, the legal system may be invoked to authorize appointment of a substitute decision maker over the person's objections.

Some states with adult protective services laws rely, in the case of recalcitrant individuals, on the traditional methods of legal intervention in the lives of elderly persons: involuntary commitment and guardianship. Legislation has been enacted in several jurisdictions, however, that creates special procedures to secure court orders for protective services, for placing the client in an institution, for emergency orders where there is imminent danger to the client's health or safety, or for orders authorizing entry into an uncooperative client's home. These special procedures may be in addition to, or in place of, the existing guardianship apparatus and usually bypass the procedural protections that gradually have been built into extant guardianship laws.

After a court order is obtained, few formal limits are imposed on the agencies that provide services. Protective services are so nebulously defined in many statutes that they may encompass virtually any kind of health or social service, including property management and major medical interventions. Hence, if the court does not expressly limit the services allowed, the agency is free to do virtually as it wishes with the client. A protective services order may, therefore, result in the placement of a person in a hospital, nursing home, boarding home, hospice, or even a mental institution. A physician is well advised, as a matter of standard practice, to ascertain carefully the exact nature and scope of a protective services order before accepting as legally effective the purported informed consent of a public or private social service agency offered on behalf of a patient-client.

Those states that have created new court processes to authorize unsolicited intervention, on either an emergency or a continual basis, also have established standards for identifying candidates for protective services or protective placement. Most of these states follow the same general statutory pattern. First, certain behavioral disabilities are described, such as the inability to care for oneself adequately or to protect oneself from abuse and exploitation by others. Next, a number of causes for this incapacity are listed, most of which involve impairment of mental functioning. "Infirmities of aging," "senility," and "advanced age" are terms commonly used to denote such impairment in elderly persons. In a very few instances, physical impairment alone is considered a sufficient basis for intervention when this condition is likely to lead to self-neglect or victimization by others, even where there is no evidence of mental incompetence; most of these provisions have been invalidated by the courts on constitutional grounds in the last several years.

In the context of adult protective services, geriatricians frequently are called upon to contribute their expertise and skills in (1) identifying candidates for services, (2) providing evidence, (3) exploring voluntary alternatives, and (4) planning and placement. Physicians frequently are in a unique and central position to identify initially those older individuals who meet the eligibility criteria for, and could significantly benefit from, the intervention of an adult protective services program. Notifying a designated social service agency official of the existence and identity of such patients may be incumbent on the physician, depending on that state's mandatory elder abuse and neglect reporting statute.[80]

Just as written reports and live courtroom testimony are vigorously sought from physicians in standard guardianship cases, so too is this form of evidence highly prized in special protective services proceedings. The weight of physician opinion may be even stronger in the latter situation, where less stringent eligibility criteria and procedural formalities empower the presiding probate judge with even broader discretion in making findings and fashioning remedies.

As already mentioned, it is possible (and highly desirable) for adult protection services to be accepted voluntarily by the older person. The physician has a duty to counsel the competent patient about available alternatives and their relative advantages and disadvantages.

Finally, the physician's potential contribution in service planning and placement activities for the nonindependent elderly patient should not be neglected. The ultimate goal is not the obtaining of protective services in and of itself, whether on a voluntary or involuntary basis. Rather, the key is to assure the quality and appropriateness of the services actually provided for the elderly individual involved. Identification, referral, and testimony should not be the end of physician involvement. Social service agencies are not to be used as a convenient dumping ground for unwanted elders, and it is just as possible for an older person without personal resources to be "dumped" harmfully into the community as into a nursing home or public mental institution.

The older individual is entitled to receive reasonable continuity of care from his or her physician. The physician is obligated legally, under the principle of nonabandonment, either to supply that continuity of care directly or to assist in its provision by referral to another competent, willing physician whose services are acceptable to the older person.

Confidentiality

In the course of performing their professional activities, physicians consistently learn very personal, intimate information about their older patients. This knowledge of personal patient information imposes certain duties of confidentiality upon the physician. Fulfilling these duties can, in specific factual situations, raise substantial legal questions.

As a general legal precept, physicians have the duty to hold in confidence all personal patient information entrusted to them, and the patient has the right to expect that this duty will be fulfilled. This obligation has been enforced through numerous civil damage suits based on both statutory (legislative) and common (judge-made) law and embodied in virtually all state professional practice acts and implementing regulations. Regarding civil lawsuits, some states (eg, Texas) have enacted statutes that provide monetary damages for physician breach of confidentiality even if the patient is unable to prove any tangible injury. State practice acts provide that violation of the duty of confidentiality is a potential ground for revoking, denying, or suspending a physician's license to practice medicine.

The patient's reasonable expectation of privacy and the physician's concomitant duty of confidentiality extend to all members of the health care team who are involved in caring for a specific patient. This reflects the fact that the provision of health care is considerably more complex and institutionalized than any single professional-patient relationship would suggest, but it does not cause the traditional legal model of professional and patient contracting with each other to break down. The patient generally makes an agreement with a single physician or facility, and that agreement ordinarily is to have a complex of services performed by a variety of members of a health care team. All professional team members are indirect parties to the agreement and become committed to it by contracting with the employing physician or health care entity (eg, hospital, nursing home, health maintenance organization, Preferred Provider Organization, clinic) to perform certain patient care roles.

A physician's violation of the duty of confidentiality is exacerbated legally when the unauthorized disclosure is both false and injurious to the patient's reputation in the community. In such a case, the patient could bring a civil action against the physician for the tort of defamation (libel if written, slander if spoken). Additionally, repeating to another a false and injurious claim uttered by a patient about a third person also could make the physician legally liable to that third party. Thus, particularly with sensitive and potentially harmful information, extreme discretion is in order.

The difficulty in applying the general legal principles just enumerated to concrete situations involving older patients is that the physician's duty to maintain as confidential the disclosures and medical records of the patient is not an absolute, immutable obligation. The fact that a duty is not absolute does not imply that it fails to occupy an important, even central, place in legal reasoning. However, when a duty is only prima facie, or presumptively applicable, rather than absolute or always applicable, one must consider whether there are relevant factors present that justify or even compel that the prima facie obligation be overridden in a particular case.

The first exception to the usual rule of confidentiality is that a patient may waive, or give up, the right to confidentiality if this is done in a voluntary, competent, and informed manner. This is accomplished daily in the health care area to make information available to third-party payers (such as Medicare and Medicaid), quality-of-care evaluators and auditors (such as inspectors from the Joint Commission on the Accreditation of Healthcare Organizations or reviewers from the state's peer review organization), and other public and private entities, including nursing home ombudsmen and patients' legal representatives. The physician has an affirmative obligation to cooperate fully in the patient-requested release and transfer of medical information. The patient's waiver of the confidentiality right and request for release of information should be honored only once it has been documented thoroughly in writing. Further, the identity and legitimate authority of the record seeker should be verified satisfactorily.

Second, when the rights of innocent third parties are jeopardized, the general requirement of confidentiality may yield. For instance, a physician might be justified or even obligated to inform a municipal transportation department about a serious heart defect or visual dysfunction discovered in one of its bus drivers, which endangers the well-being of unknowing and defenseless passengers and bystanders. More obviously, the expressed threat of a dangerous psychiatric patient to kill a specific victim, coupled with the patient's apparent present ability (not unlikely even for an elderly person in today's climate of easy handgun availability) and intent to make good on the threat, arguably should be reported to the intended victim and to law enforcement officials.[81]

Third, the patient's expectation of confidentiality must yield when the physician is mandated by state law to report to specified public health authorities the existence of certain enumerated conditions reasonably suspected in a patient. The physician should be familiar with the content of such mandatory reporting statutes and regulations in force in his or her own jurisdiction. Such requirements may be based on the state's inherent police power to protect the health, safety, and welfare of society as a whole. This rationale would support, for example, reporting requirements concerning infectious diseases or vital statistics (such as death). Alternatively, reporting of certain conditions may be mandated under the state's *parens patriae* power to protect beneficently those individuals who are unable to care for their own needs. Mandatory reporting of elder abuse or neglect or self-neglect would be justified on this ground (see Chapter 49).[82]

Finally, the physician may be compelled to reveal otherwise confidential patient information by the force of legal process, that is, by a judge's issuance of a court order requiring such release. This is a possibility in any type of lawsuit where the patient's physical or mental condition is in dispute.

The right of privacy may be particularly important to older individuals who, as products of a pre-computer, pre–mass communication age, often assign an even higher value to personal privacy than do members of younger generations. The right of privacy too often is compromised in treating older patients, particularly those with cognitive or emotional deficits.

An older patient who is mentally competent may nonetheless, through appearance or demeanor, leave the impression that his clinical problems and management should be discussed readily with relatives or friends. Every safeguard should be employed to adhere to the ordinary standards of confidentiality unless there is express permission from the patient to do otherwise or the mental condition of the patient is so disabling as to dictate bringing relatives into the decision-making circle. Particularly in situations of marginal or questionable patient competence, the physician should attempt to convince the patient voluntarily to authorize the family's access to information and its active involvement in decision making. When the family or others with appropriate authority are involved, privileged communications about the patient should be carefully handled to avoid unauthorized disclosure beyond those with a right and a need to have access to the information.

Cost Containment and Potential Liability

A dominant theme in current health care policy is an attempt to contain costs by public and private third-party payers. The federal Health Care Financing Administration, which administers Medicare and Medicaid—the primary sources of health care financing for elderly persons in the United States—has taken a leading role in cost control efforts, through such policies as diagnosis-related group reimbursement for hospitals, incentives for physicians to accept Medicare assignment of fees (several states have mandated this as a condition of medical licensure), and encouragement of Medicare beneficiary enrollment in designated health maintenance organizations and competitive medical plans. Other, more far-reaching initiatives are on the horizon as health care costs for the elderly population and everyone else continue to escalate.

An apprehension has been expressed by physicians[83] and attorneys[84] alike that these cost containment efforts may seriously threaten the quality of care received by older patients, causing foreseeable and avoidable injury and thereby expose attending physicians and health care facilities to an increased risk of legal liability. It has been surmised that malpractice claims could be based on such arguments as premature discharge,[85] inadequate testing, inadequate treatment, and denial of access to care.

Many authors have argued that cost constraints would not be accepted under our current jurisprudence as a viable defense to a claim of substandard care, nor should this defense be recognized as valid.[86,87] On the other hand, this author has speculated that cost control values eventually may be incorporated by physicians into standard medical decision making (as they have been in Great Britain) and, thus, may become an implicit part of the standard of medical care to which physicians are held answerable. This would mean that the standard of care would be influenced downward by the need to include considerations of cost containment in the medical decision-making algorithm.[88]

This author also has suggested that, under the current contingency fee system through which plaintiffs are represented by legal counsel in personal injury (including medical malpractice) lawsuits, the type of patient who is most likely to be jeopardized by substandard care driven by cost control strategies— that is, the sick elderly patient—would make a very uninviting potential client for an attorney. This is because the key element of damages in personal injury litigation, lost future wages, ordinarily would be small and the element of a causation link between provider misconduct and any patient injury suffered would be difficult to prove.[89]

Despite a flurry of articles in the professional literature and popular press and a spate of allegations by professional associations and consumer groups versus defensive statements by the government and private insurers, there is still extremely sparse evidence concerning the legal impact on physicians of various cost containment efforts. As of this writing, there has been precisely one reported legal decision in this area, with a few other lawsuits presently working their way through the litigation process. The one decided case, *Wickline v State of California*,[90] has generated an enormous amount of attention.

Mrs Wickline, a (nonelderly) Medicaid-eligible patient, was admitted to the hospital with arterial obstructions in her back and legs. On the date of discharge, her treating physicians requested that the California Medicaid program extend Mrs Wickline's stay for 8 additional days. The Medicaid consulting physician, a general surgeon, approved only a 4-day extension. A few weeks following her discharge, Mrs Wickline reentered the hospital on an emergency basis, at which time the physicians had to amputate her leg to save her life. The specialist who performed the surgery contended that her leg could have been saved had she remained in the hospital for the requested 8 days.

Mrs Wickline brought a negligence action against the state of California, which administered the Medicaid program. The California Court of Appeals ruled against Mrs Wickline. However, the court held that, had Mrs Wickline named the original attending physician as defendant (she did not, presumably because they enjoyed a positive physician-patient relationship), the physician—as the one who actually is responsible for signing discharge documents—could have been held liable for not appealing Medicaid's decision while Mrs Wickline was still hospitalized. Additionally, the court held that, had the attending physician filed an appeal that the Medicaid program then overruled, the state could have been held liable for a negligent discharge decision.

One lesson that most observers have drawn from the *Wickline* case is that a physician has an obligation to advocate[91] for the patient's best medical interests when, in the physician's professional opinion, cost-motivated actions by the third-party payer threaten to imperil quality of care. A related lesson is that fear of potential liability on the part of a third-party payer may be used effectively as a leverage tool by the attending physician to influence third-party payer decisions where the health of the patient is at stake.[92] Fourth-party audit organizations hired by private corporations to review and control utilization of medical services by employees may also be influenced by apprehension of liability.[93]

Conclusion

In some respects, legal liability concerns are less of a factor in geriatrics than in many other branches of medicine. Yet, in many ways, elderly patients offer their physicians a set of unique and complex legal challenges. This chapter has outlined some of the more salient legal considerations confronting and guiding physicians who care for older patients, in the hope of raising consciousness to the benefit of both physicians and the older individuals who depend on them.

References

1. Kapp MB. The malpractice crisis: relevance for geriatrics. *J Am Geriatr Soc*. 1989;37:364–368.
2. Kapp MB, Lo B. Legal perceptions and medical decisionmaking. *Milbank Q* 1986;64(suppl 2):162–202.
3. Danzon PM. New evidence on the frequency and severity of medical malpractice claims. Santa Monica, Calif: Rand Corp Institute for Civil Justice; 1986;18–19.
4. *Medical Malpractice: Characteristics of Claims Closed in 1984*. Washington, DC: United States General Accounting Office. 1987:27–28. Publication GAO/HRD-87-55.
5. American Association of Retired Persons. *A Profile of Older Americans, 1987*. Washington, DC: American Association of Retired Persons; 1987:12–14.
6. Kapp MB. Law, medicine, and the terminally ill: humanizing risk management advice. *Health Care Manage Rev* 1987;12:37–42.
7. *Making Health Care Decisions: The Ethical and Legal Implications of Informed Consent in the Patient-Practitioner Relationship*. Washington, DC: President's Commission for the Study of Ethical Problems in Medicine and Biomedical and Behavioral Research. 1982.
8. Keeler EB, Solomon DH, Beck JC, et al. Effect of patient age on duration of medical encounters on physicians. *Med Care* 1982;20:1101–1108.
9. Levinson SA. *Medical Direction in Long-term Care*. Owings Mills, Md: National Health Publishing; 1988.
10. Kapp MB. Legal perspectives on patients' rights in the nursing home. In: Zweibel NR, Cassel CK, eds. Care of the nursing home patient: clinical and policy concerns. *Clin Geriatr Med* 1988;4:667–679.
11. Marsh FH. Informed consent and the elderly patient. *Clin Geriatr Med* 1986;2:501–510.
12. Rozovsky FA. *Consent to Treatment: a Practical Guide*. Boston, Mass: Little Brown & Co Inc; 1984.
13. Miller L. Informed consent. *JAMA* 1980;244:2100–2103, 2347–2350, 2556–2558, 2661–2662.
14. Larson EB, Lo B, Williams ME. Evaluation and care of elderly patients with dementia. *J Gen Intern Med* 1986;1:116–126.
15. Dubler NN. Coercive placement of elders: protection of choice? *Generations* 1987;11:6–9.
16. Blank K. Depressive illness in the elderly: legal and ethical issues. In: Rosner R, Schwartz HI, eds. *Geriatric Psychiatry and the Law*. New York, NY: Plenum Publishing Corp; 1987:chap 11.
17. Cranford RE. The persistent vegetative state: the medical reality (getting the facts straight). *Hastings Cent Rep* 1988;18:27–323.
18. Munetz M, Lidz C, Meisel A. Informed consent and incompetent medical patients. *J Fam Pract* 1985;20:273–279.

19. Goldstein RL. Non compos mentis: the psychiatrist's role in guardianship and conservatorship proceedings involving the elderly. In: Rosner R, Schwartz HI, eds. *Geriatric Psychiatry and the Law*. New York, NY: Plenum Publishing Corp; 1987:chap 16.

20. Strain JJ, Fulop G. Screening devices for cognitive capacity. *Ann Intern Med* 1987;107:583–585.

21. Meisel A, Roth L, Lidz C. Toward a model of the legal doctrine of informed consent. *Am J Psychiatry* 1977;134:285–289.

22. Roth L, Meisel A, Lidz C. Tests of competency to consent to treatment. *Am J Psychiatry* 1977;134:279–284.

23. Culver C. The clinical determination of competence. In: Kapp MB, Pies H, Doudera AE, eds. *Legal and Ethical Aspects of Health Care for the Elderly*. Ann Arbor, Mich: Health Administration Press, 1985:chap 24.

24. Harris S. Protecting the rights of questionably competent long-term care facility residents. In: Kapp MB, Pies H, Doudera AE, eds. *Legal and Ethical Aspects of Health Care for the Elderly*. Ann Arbor, Mich: Health Administration Press; 1985:chap 17.

25. Heikoff LE. Practical management of the demented elderly. *West J Med* 1986;145:397–399.

26. Caplan A. Let wisdom find a way. *Generations* 1985;10:10–14.

27. Abrams R. Dementia research in the nursing home. *Hosp Community Psychiatry* 1988;39:257–259.

28. Cassel CK. Informed consent for research in geriatrics: history and concepts. *J Am Geriatr Soc* 1987;35:542–544.

29. Ratzan RM. Being old makes you different: the ethics of research with elderly subjects. *Hastings Cent Rep* 1980;10:32–42.

30. Annas GJ, Glantz, LH. Rules for research in nursing homes. *N Engl J Med* 1986;315:1157–1158.

31. Appelbaum PS, Roth LH. Competency to consent to research: a psychiatric overview. *Arch Gen Psychiatry* 1982;39:951–958.

32. Warren JW, Sobal J, Tenney JH, et al. Informed consent by proxy: an issue in research with elderly patients. *N Engl J Med* 1986;315:1124–1128.

33. Melnick VL, Dubler NN, Weisbard A, et al. Clinical research in senile dementia of the Alzheimer's type: suggested guidelines addressing the ethical and legal issues. *J Am Geriatr Soc* 1984;32:531–536.

34. Dubler NN. Legal judgments and informed consent in geriatric research. *J Am Geriatr Soc* 1987;35:545–549.

35. Ratzan RM. Informed consent in clinical geriatrics. *J Am Geriatr Soc* 1984;32:175–176.

36. Hoffman PB, Marron KR, Fillit H, et al. Obtaining informed consent in the teaching nursing home. *J Am Geriatr Soc* 1983;31:565–569.

37. Kapp MB. *Preventing Malpractice in Long-term Care: Strategies for Risk Management*. New York, NY: Springer Publishing Co Inc, 1987:chap 6.

38. Mishkin B. *A Matter of Choice: Planning Ahead for Health Care Decisions: An Information Paper for the United States Senate Special Committee on Aging*. Washington, DC: 1986. Distributed by American Association of Retired Persons.

39. Hirsh HL. Should we enact 'death with dignity' legislation or 'natural death' acts? *Nurs Homes* 1985;34:10–16.

40. Eisendrath SJ, Jonsen AR. The living will: help or hindrance? *JAMA* 1983;249:2054–2058.

41. Kapp MB. Response to the living will furor: directives for maximum care. *Am J Med* 1982;72:855–859.

42. New York State Task Force on Life and the Law. *Life-sustaining Treatment: Making Decisions and Appointing a Health Care Agent*. New York, NY: 1987.

43. Fowler M. Note: appointing an agent to make medical treatment choices. *Columbia Law Rev* 1984;84:985–1031.

44. Steinbrook R, Lo B. Decision making for incompetent patients by designated proxy: California's new law. *N Engl J Med* 1984;310:1598–1601.

45. Angell M. Respecting the autonomy of competent patients. *N Engl J Med* 1984;310:1115–1116.

46. Schneiderman LJ, Arras JD. Counseling patients to counsel physicians on future care in the event of patient incompetence. *Ann Intern Med* 1985;102:693–698.

47. Kapp MB. Advance health care planning: taking a 'medical future.' *South Med J* 1988;81:221–224.

48. Areen J. The legal status of consent obtained from families of adult patients to withhold or withdraw treatment. *JAMA* 1987;258:229–235.

49. *The Physician and the Hopelessly Ill Patient: Legal, Medical and Ethical Guidelines*. New York, NY: Society for the Right to Die. 1985.

50. *In re Storar*, 52 NY2d 363, 420 NE2d 64 (1981).

51. *In the Matter of Jobes*, 108 NJ 394, 529 A2d 419 (1987).

52. US House of Representatives, Subcommittee on Health and Long-term Care of the Select Committee on Aging. *Abuses in Guardianship of the Elderly and Infirm: A National Disgrace*. 100th Congress, 1st Sessions, 1987. Committee Publication 100-641.

53. Appelbaum PS. Limitations on guardianship of the mentally disabled. *Hosp Community Psychiatry* 1982;33:183–184.

54. American Medical Association Judicial Council. Guidelines for ethics committees in health care institutions. *JAMA* 1985;253:2698–2699.

55. Hosford B. *Bioethics Committees: The Health Care Provider's Guide*. Rockville, Md: Aspen Systems Corp; 1986.

56. Brown BA, Miles SH, Aroskar MA. The prevalence and design of ethics committees in nursing homes. *J Am Geriatr Soc* 1987;35:1028–1033.

57. Fost N, Cranford RE. Hospital ethics committees: administrative aspects. *JAMA* 1985;253:2687–2692.

58. Wood JS. Nursing home care. *Clin Geriatr Med* 1986;2:601–615.

59. Kapp MB. Legal and ethical aspects of resuscitation: an annotated bibliography of recent literature. *Resuscitation* 1987;15:289–297.

60. Besdine RW. Decisions to withhold treatment in nursing home residents. *J Am Geriatr Soc* 1983;31:602–606.

61. US Congress, Office of Technology Assessment. *Life-Sustaining Technologies and the Elderly*. Publication OTA-BA-306. 1987; 100th Cong, 1st session.

62. Robertson JA. *The Rights of the Critically Ill*. Cambridge, Mass: Ballinger Publishing Co; 1983.

63. Ross JW, Pugh D. Limited cardiopulmonary resuscitation: the ethics of partial codes. *QRB* 1988;14:4–8.
64. Miles SH, Ryden M. Limited-treatment policies in long-term care facilities. *J Am Geriatr Soc* 1985;33:707–711.
65. Bedell SE, Pelle D, Maher PL, et al. Do-not-resuscitate orders for critically ill patients in the hospital: how are they used and what is their impact? *JAMA* 1986;256:233–237.
66. Stephens R. Do not resuscitate orders: ensuring the patient's participation. *JAMA* 1986;255:240–241.
67. *Do Not Resuscitate Orders*. New York, NY: New York State Task Force on Life and the Law. 1986.
68. *'No Code' Patient Treatment Orders*. Sacramento: California Department of Health Services; 1985. Licensing Procedure Memo 85-10.
69. Blackhall LJ. Must we always use CPR? *N Engl J Med* 1987;317:1281–1285.
70. *Deciding to Forego Life-Sustaining Treatment*. Washington, DC: President's Commission for the Study of Ethical Problems in Medicine and Biomedical and Behavioral Research. 1983.
71. Hastings Center. *Guidelines on the Termination of Life-Sustaining Treatment and the Care of the Dying*. Briarcliff Manor, NY: Hastings Center; 1987.
72. Evans A, Brody B. The do not resuscitate order in teaching hospitals. *JAMA* 1985;253:2236–2239.
73. Miles SH. Advanced directives to limit treatment: the need for portability. *J Am Geriatr Soc* 1987;35:74–76.
74. Farber N, Weiner J, Boyer G, et al. Cardiopulmonary resuscitation: values and decisions—a comparison of health care professionals. *Med Care* 1985;23:1391–1398.
75. Lipton HL. Do-not-resuscitate decisions in a community hospital: implications for quality care. *QRB* 1987;13:226–231.
76. Rango N. The nursing home resident with dementia: clinical care, ethics, and policy implications. *Ann Intern Med* 1985;102:835–841.
77. Kapp MB, Bigot A. *Geriatrics and the Law: Patient Rights and Professional Responsibilities*. New York, NY: Springer Publishing Co Inc; 1985:102–106.
78. Kapp MB. Adult protective services: convincing the patient to consent. *Law Med Health Care* 1983;11:163–167.
79. Kapp MB. Adult protective services: the attorney's role. *Florida Bar J* 1985;59:23–28.
80. American Medical Association Council on Scientific Affairs. Elder abuse and neglect. *JAMA* 1987;257:966–971.
81. Kantor JE. Ethical considerations in geriatric forensic psychiatry. In: Rosner R, Schwartz HI, eds. *Geriatric Psychiatry and the Law*. New York, NY: Plenum Publishing Corp; 1987:chap 19.
82. Quinn MJ, Tomita SK. *Elder Abuse and Neglect: Causes, Diagnosis, and Intervention Strategies*. New York, NY: Springer Publishing Inc; 1986.
83. Johnson DE. Life, death, and the dollar sign: medical ethics and cost containment. *JAMA* 1984;252:223–224.
84. Ludlam JE. Payment systems, cost management, and malpractice. *Hospitals* 1984;58:102–104.
85. American Hospital Association General Counsel's Office. *Discharging Hospital Patients: Legal Implications For Institutional Providers and Health Care Professionals*. Chicago: American Hospital Association; 1987. Legal Memorandum No. 9, Report of the Task Force on Legal Issues in Discharge Planning.
86. Morreim EH. Cost constraints as a malpractice defense. *Hastings Cent Rep* 1988;18:5–10.
87. Lairson AJ. Reexamining the physician's duty of care in response to Medicare's prospective payment system. *Washington Law Rev* 1987;62:791–812.
88. Kapp MB. Health care delivery and the elderly: teaching old patients new tricks. *Cumberland Law Rev* 1986–1987;17:4347–467.
89. Kapp MB. Legal and ethical implications of health care reimbursement by diagnosis related groups. *Law Med Health Care* 1984;12:245–253,278.
90. *Wickline v State of California*, 183 Cal App3d 1175, 228 Cal Rptr 661 (1986).
91. Abrams FA. Patient advocate or secret agent? *JAMA* 1986;256:1784–1785.
92. Smith RP. Insurance carrier liability as a result of preadmission screening and hospital stay guidelines. *Ohio North Law Rev* 1985;12:189–212.
93. Hershey N. Fourth-party audit organizations: practical and legal considerations. *Law Med Health Care* 1986;14:54–65.

Elder Abuse

David O. Staats and Diana Koin

In the 1960s, the syndrome of child abuse was introduced to the medical community.[1] In the 1970s, battered women banded together to counter spouse abuse, and victims of rape and incest also joined forces. Then, in the late 1970s, doctors, social workers, psychologists, sociologists, and lawyers recognized that elderly clients were being maltreated by caregivers. Systematic observations of maltreated elderly persons have partially codified the syndrome of elder abuse and currently are giving rise to improved diagnosis, prevention, and intervention.

The abuse of elderly persons is a syndrome that represents one extreme in the age spectrum of familial violence. Elder abuse has been long noted in literature. Perhaps the best known example is that of Shakespeare's King Lear, the aging monarch who is cruelly victimized by two of his daughters after his judgment and insight fail.

Elder Abuse Defined

Elder abuse is defined as "the infliction of physical pain, injury or debilitating mental anguish, unreasonable confinement, or willful deprivation by a caretaker of services which are necessary to maintain mental and physical health of an elderly person."[2] This definition extends to elderly persons who reside in long-term care facilities (institutional abuse of the elderly) as well as to elderly persons who live with spouses, families, or friends. Besides overt physical assault on an elderly person, this definition encompasses a number of forms of maltreatment. These include unnecessary physical restraint in a bed or chair or an unreasonable confinement to one's home without access to visitors. Also included is the withholding of food, medicines, teeth, eyeglasses, hearing aids, or walking devices that are necessary to sustain the health or activity of an older person. Financial exploitation, a special category of elder abuse that encompasses withholding an elderly person's funds (pension, social security checks, and bank accounts) and willfully mismanaging an older person's money, is also within the scope of the definition, along with sexual abuse.

"Causing debilitating mental anguish" is less readily identified. Abused elderly persons can suffer fear of another person to such an extent that physical or mental functioning is impaired. The fear of being beaten or punished may in some instances be as serious a form of abuse as the actual act. At other times, the threat of institutionalization or abandonment may cause severe mental anguish. In other cases, the neglect of an elderly person's needs by a caregiver constitutes abuse. Failure to provide care to a dependent elderly person, such as giving medications, attending to personal hygiene, and evaluating changes in the elderly person's health status, also constitutes elder abuse.

Contrasting with this definition is self-neglect by elderly persons, such as that due to dementia or psychiatric illness. Other elderly persons have become socially isolated and live in squalor. The aged homeless are also victims of self-neglect.

Elderly persons may be victims of criminals, and although these elderly persons are abused in the process, these events are not classified as elder abuse. Examples of such criminal actions include purse snatching, mugging, and theft in the home. Unscrupulous door-to-door salespersons, con artists who swindle money using scams such as "the bank examiner,"[3] and others who defraud elderly people are not abusers per se under this definition.

Prevalence

No accurate figures can be given for the incidence and prevalence of elder abuse. Available figures suggest that abuse occurs among 2% of the population over 65 years of age; these data are derived from surveys of social welfare agencies correlated with census information on the number of frail and elderly persons in a given area.[4] Recent investigations suggest a prevalence of 32 per 1,000 elderly persons at risk.[5] Where abuse occurs, it tends to be not an isolated incident but rather a pattern of violence in which an older person is repeatedly harmed.

The implementation of mandatory reporting laws (see below) may give more accurate epidemiologic data because of more uniform reporting of elder abuse. Reports of elder abuse seriously understate the actual number of cases. Additionally, the victims in 40% of all cases of documented elder abuse decline any investigation at all.[6] Accurate data from medical records have been difficult to retrieve, because elderly abuse is not included in the International Classification of Disease, ICD-9.

The Setting

Abuse seldom is the presenting complaint of an elderly person in a physician's office. A high index of suspicion is necessary so as not to miss this diagnosis. Repeated bouts of trauma or unexplained deterioration in condition should bring the diagnosis of elder abuse to mind. When abuse occurs, the resultant fractures, burns, malnutrition, dehydration, contusions, decubiti, punctures, and lacerations may be seen in hospital emergency rooms. Because some frail elderly persons are prone to underlying conditions (instability of gait, poor vision, and frequent falls) that give rise to trauma, it may be difficult to differentiate accidental from willful injuries. The simultaneous presence of fresh and healing injuries suggests ongoing episodes of trauma, and elder abuse should be considered in the differential diagnosis. The facts presented may not be congruous with the signs of trauma or neglect that are present. Because intimidation frequently accompanies

elder abuse (but more often because the elderly victim has or has had a close, longstanding, and ongoing relationship with the abusing caregiver), the victim is loathe to report abuse. The abusing caregiver may feel guilt and remorse over the damage that is inflicted, and bringing the abused relative to a hospital emergency room may be a hidden call for help.

As data on elder abuse accumulates, diagnostic strategies evolve. Multple discriminant analysis has yielded screening tools for clients of social service agencies.[7] Others have developed protocols for hospital emergency rooms to assess the likelihood and extent of elder abuse[8,9] Emergency personnel, including ambulance drivers and medical technicians, need to be familiar with common manifestations of elder abuse.

People in an abused elderly person's community with access to that patient's home environment also are likely to detect abuse. These people include neighbors, home health aides, visiting nurses, social service workers, ministers, and the police. When abuse occurs, a physician is less likely to be notified; police or social service agencies are more often contacted.

In a primary care setting or a hospital emergency room, the following observations should raise the index of suspicion that elder abuse has occured. The caregiver may (1) show a loss of control or fear losing control, (2) present a contradictory history or one that does not or cannot explain the injury, (3) project the cause of injury onto a third party, (4) delay bringing in the elderly person for care, (5) overreact or underreact to the seriousness of the situation, (6) complain continuously about problems that are unrelated to the injury, and (7) refuse consent for further diagnostic studies and remove the patient from the facility.

The interactions, including nonverbal communications, of an elderly adult and caregiver also may give clues that abuse is the problem. The anxiety and fearfulness of the elder may be striking. Conversely, he or she may be excessively dependent on the caregiver. If dementia is present, the victim can appear indifferent. An adult child or caregiver may blame the elderly person for what has happened. The caregiver may intentionally refuse to touch, talk, look, or listen to his or her elderly parent or spouse. In some instances, the signs are subtle and observable only by careful attention to clues, such as body language.

Etiologic Factors

A composite rendering of elderly persons most likely to be abused cannot be drawn with precision. Abuse takes place over a wide range of circumstances, and the data that create such a rendering are imperfect.

Nonetheless, there are certain recurrent themes. Dependency is a frequently encountered factor, and it most often arises from multiple medical illnesses and mental impairment. In some elderly persons, dependency is associated with helplessness (ie, a feeling that one is powerless to control life and that no efforts could possibly change the situation). This perceived lack of control, real or not, accelerates the mode of dependency. Alcoholism in elderly persons or their caregivers also may be a factor leading to abuse.

In addition, a victim of abuse is likely to be among the old-old, the mean age being 84 years.[4] Most studies suggest the victim is more often a woman, but men also may be victims of elder abuse. Persons living alone suffer less abuse than those living with a spouse, a child, or others. Elder abuse occurs in all socioeconomic strata, though it is more likely in a low- or middle-class background. Nearly 50% of all victims manifest moderate or severe mental impairment, and only 4% are free from any significant physical ailments.[4,10]

Besides learned dependency on an adult child caregiver, several behavior patterns make an older person particularly at risk for abuse. One of these is having been extremely dependent on a spouse who is now deceased. This dependency is left in a vacuum when a spouse dies, and it may no longer be rewarded with attention and care. It finds fresh expression when the older person comes to live with an adult child, and it creates tensions within the family.

Another behavioral factor that leads to abuse is the elderly person's persistence in an authoritarian role with his or her adult child. By advising, admonishing, and directing the adult child on whom he or she is dependent (in short, by treating the adult as a child), the elderly person creates tension. This attitude is manifested by being intrusive in living arrangements and allowing little privacy for an adult child and his or her family. Insistence on maintaining old patterns of independent functioning, which is at odds with both the new living situation and the present realities of infirmity, often leads to further tensions.

Financial conditions also play a role in placing an older person at risk for abuse. Most commonly, an older person's financial resources and savings are limited, and his or her presence in a caregiver's household imposes a financial burden on the family.[11] This situation can be exacerbated if the older person refuses to apply for financial aid or other services. Other frustrating, tension-provoking scenarios that place an older person at risk for abuse may result from his or her having a lot of money but refusing to spend any of it or using gifts of money in an attempt to control others—usually adult children or more distant relatives. In addition, as economic conditions worsen and Medicaid regulations demand impoverishment for nursing home eligibility, some families attempt to keep an elderly person at home "to preserve the estate."

The Abuser

The portrait of an abuser perhaps emerges even less clearly. Some elder abuse is an extension of spouse abuse into old age. In other cases, adult children, other relatives, or caregivers become abusers. Which factors allow caregivers to care for a debilitated dependent elderly person without being abusive and which predispose them to becoming abusers are not clear. At present, the following characteristics seem to place a caregiver at especially high risk for abusing his or her elderly friend or relative.

Alcoholism and drug dependency in a caregiver enhance the likelihood of abuse, because these persons tend to cope poorly with stresses of any kind. Another factor that enhances the likelihood of elder abuse is mental illness, such as depression or schizophrenia. A limited capacity to express personal needs makes a person psychologically unprepared to meet the dependency needs of an elderly parent, especially when it is coupled with a denial of his or her parent's illness.

Some have suggested cycles of family violence leading to elder abuse. Half of abused elderly men are abused at the hands of their wives[5], and in these cases spouse battering becomes elder abuse. Battered children may perpetrate elder abuse upon formerly abusive parents.[6] Elder abuse may also, of course, occur without a prior history of domestic violence.

The typical abuser has other significant attitudes toward aging. These include negative feelings toward aging in general, a perception that the elderly victim is somehow different from other older persons, and unrealistic expectations of older persons—thinking they are more independent than they actually are or that the caregiver's response to their dependency should be accepted more gracefully. Lifelong unfulfilled expectations may surface and generate anger.

Abusing caregivers frequently insist that the elderly person will never be put in a nursing home. The caregiver underestimates the severity or irreversibility of the elderly person's multiple medical problems and cannot appreciate the magnitude of care that is required to maintain that person as a patient at home.

In terms of living arrangements, social isolation tends to breed abuse by a caregiver, as does a lack of relief in caring for a frail, impaired older person. Outlets for anger and rage are nonexistent. Caregivers sometimes sacrifice their own careers and personal lives to stay at home and care for an older person. Precarious finances are thus further jeopardized.

It would be naive to minimize the stress that is imposed by caring for a frail, dependent parent. Providing care to a person who was once a caregiver reverses both the familial dynamics and the parenting roles. This may lead to conflicting feelings of love and fear toward one's parent. This emotional attachment may pull a caregiver away from his or her spouse and other family members. There often is an unspoken sense of loss and grieving for the person who used to be, for the person whose body now seems inhabited by someone different—sick, peevish, incontinent, and ugly. There are feelings of anger, frustration, and helplessness because of the incontinence, the wandering, and the sleepless nights. A caregiver may be an isolated, fatigued, and careworn person.

Many times, a caregiver is also growing old. The relief and relaxation that was expected after the children have grown and moved away is shattered by a new arrival. This arrival is not a baby, it is one's parent. Rather than the pleasures of watching a child develop, the progress is retrograde. The situation often deteriorates so that an elderly parent becomes increasingly dependent, sick, and messy. Care for an aged parent consumes more and more time, so that there may be few chances for relief or even for going outside; the frustrations and isolation tend to mount. There may be sleep deprivation and fatigue that potentiate abuse. It also may be a caregiver's becoming ill that first brings the problem to medical attention.

Multidisciplinary Scope of Elder Abuse

Elder abuse is an area of geriatric medicine that interfaces broadly with many other disciplines (Fig 49.1). Because of the associated trauma and pain, elder abuse comes within the purview of medicine. Because it involves disturbed family relationships and social interactions, it is also within the purview of social service agencies. Finally, because the abuse of elderly persons may constitute assault and battery, it involves the criminal justice system.

The physician's roles in treating elder abuse are many. In some cases, especially in emergency rooms and geriatric evaluation units, physicians may identify cases of elder abuse. They may refer cases to social service agencies and diagnose and document the illnesses causing incompetency, leading to guardianship and conservatorship. Specific medical interventions can ameliorate symptoms that create stress for the

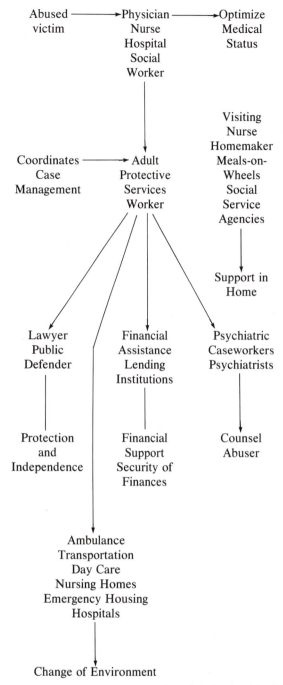

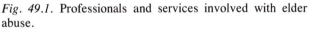

Fig. 49.1. Professionals and services involved with elder abuse.

caregiver. In counseling the family, the physician can set realistic goals on the basis of prognosis and an assessment of needs for care, including home health services, counseling, and respite care.

Legal parameters are an important aspect of elder abuse. In the case of child abuse, most states have the power to make interventions to safeguard the rights and lives of children who are unable to defend themselves. Questions of custody and placement in cases of child abuse then proceed along fairly straightforward lines. For abused elderly persons, however, the situation is different. There is a long tradition in the law that adults have the right of privacy in their own homes and to have information about themselves held as confidential. Also, adults are presumed to be competent to handle personal affairs unless adjudicated to be incompetent. Nonetheless, abused elderly persons who have been maltreated or physically assaulted may be unable to defend themselves.

These tenets may create additional tension and conflict. First, access to a patient may present a problem. A victim of abuse often fails to report that abuse and may decline any further evaluation. The fear of placement in a nursing home may be even greater than the fear of physical abuse. In that case, the right to privacy is brought into conflict with the humane desire to offer help. To enter an abused person's home without his or her permission is considered trespassing. Countering this is the power of the state to regulate activities that bear on the health and safety of its citizens and the doctrine of the law termed *parens patriae,* which gives the state authority to act in a parental capacity on behalf of those who are unable to care for themselves or who are dangerous to others. The laws that deal with these issues vary from state to state. Thus, social service workers may not always be allowed to visit an abused person in his or her home. Tact, gentle persistence, patience, diplomacy, and an attitude of offering to help, rather than passing judgment, generally build a framework of trust between abusing families, their elderly relatives, and social service and health workers, so that visits will be allowed. Nurses, who often are trusted as helpers and bringers of relief, may gain entry more easily, especially when the initial emphasis is on relieving the pain of trauma or other symptoms of illness.

Second, a competent person has the right to refuse medical and social services. Unlike children, whose health must be safeguarded by responsible adults, adults have a right to privacy and self-determination. Thus it is possible that an abused elderly person may wish to remain in a dangerous environment or to be left exploited or neglected, even to the point of starvation or death. The right to refuse services can be limited if a person, in doing so, represents a danger to others, or if a person is legally incompetent. If a person is found to be incompetent, a guardian may be appointed by the court. Without such a declaration of incompetency, social service and medial agencies have little authority to intervene, except in a life-threatening emergency.

Abuse of an elderly person generally is a criminal offense, but the victim must file a complaint against the abuser and be willing to further a prosecution

under the law. Criminal prosecutions are almost always counterproductive maneuvers in dealing with elder abuse, since the goals of interventions are to treat the abused, to stop the abuse, to ameliorate the conditions leading to abuse, and to change the behavior of the abuser rather than to punish. Civil law, whose goal is relief rather than punishment, may be used more effectively. Some states have enacted civil laws that pertain to domestic violence wherein restraining orders may be issued against the abusing party. Thus, civil law procedures are more effective than criminal prosecutions in separating the abused and the abuser through the use of temporary restraining orders. Often, however, a victim does not wish his or her family members or caregivers to be involved with the law and, as a result, does not call on the law to intervene. The uncompromising nature of the law mandates its careful use, so that the delicate nature of family interactions is not unduly upset.

Police interact with abused elderly persons in the setting of a crisis. In general, police do not act as social workers; they may intervene in an emergency or if a victim calls for help. Without sufficient evidence of criminal action, it may be difficult for police officers to act. Sometimes, however, the presence of a uniformed officer exerts a calming influence. Social service workers may call upon police officers for escort in dangerous situations and to help document a trail of evidence for subsequent proceedings.

Confidentiality must be strictly maintained. Information that is obtained from an abused victim can be released to other agencies only with the permission of the victim. The question of libel in alleging that elder abuse has taken place recently has been addressed through the passage of state mandatory reporting laws. These laws require the reporting of each alleged incident of elder abuse, usually to a central state agency. These mandatory reporting laws vary slightly from state to state; at present there is no federal legislation on elder abuse.

Such state legislation to facilitate the mandatory reporting of elder abuse serves several purposes: (1) social workers and others do not risk libel by alleging that someone has abused an elderly person; (2) uniform record keeping makes case handling more efficient, prevents repititious involvement of multiple agencies, and gives a clearer picture of the incidence and prevalence of elder abuse; and (3) the attention of health professionals, social service agencies, and the public at large is focused on the problem of elder abuse.

State mandatory reporting laws have not proved to be a panacea.[12] They have been viewed by some as legislative responses to a politicized problem. Lacking clear definition of elder abuse itself and scientific analysis of its causes, these laws nonetheless have provided an impetus to give the problem sufficient attention. Some social workers are forced to construe events as elder abuse for fear of *not* reporting an occurrence.[13] There are many false-positive reports of abuse. Because much elder abuse is occult, and because 40% of all suspected victims decline any evaluation at all, mandatory reporting laws have not comprehensively defined the need for services. In other cases, services for the abused and the abuser have not expanded in parallel with the mandatory reporting laws, so that more accurate detection of elder abuse has not led to better treatment. In some cases, mandatory reporting laws have not been extended to others involved with elder abuse. For example, bankers, fiduciaries, and attorneys usually are not required to report elder abuse.

Mandatory reporting laws have sometimes created difficult ethical questions for physicians.[14] Do physicians maintain patient confidentiality, or, to prevent criminal abuse, is elder abuse reported against the patient's wishes? Also, to what extent ought physicians intervene in the lives of their patients to ameliorate suffering, when such actions necessarily lessen the autonomy of the elderly person to some degree.

The problem of differentiating real elder abuse from paranoid ideation should be mentioned. Elderly people who suffer from paranoia may express the feeling that their caregivers are mistreating them and trying to inflict injury. This paranoid thinking can be distinguished by the fact that the elderly person exhibits other paranoid ideas at a psychiatric interview. It may be helpful to visit a patient's home and observe the situation firsthand; also, psychiatric consultation is recommended.

Intervention

Once a case of elder abuse is identified, treatment is best initiated through a team approach. Because the problem is multidimensional, the solution must also be a multidimensional scope of response. The relationships of agencies and personnel expert in elder abuse is shown in Figure 49.1. The adult protective service worker plays a central role in coordinating intervention. This person usually is a social worker, often with training in gerontology, who helps to provide services for people in danger of being injured. These may involve coordinating the delivery of services or providing substitute decision making. Protective service workers usually are employed by the state or local government and usually are the personnel through whom centralized reporting occurs. While each case needs to be assessed individually, some generalizations about the approaches to specific problems can be made.

If the life of an abused elderly person is in danger through physical abuse, it is an emergency situation. In this case, an elderly person must be removed from the hostile environment to either an emergency shelter or (more likely) a hospital. If necessary, the police may be summoned to prevent mayhem. The arrest and prosecution of the abuser may take place. However, these life-threatening cases are a minority of the cases of elder abuse.

In the majority of cases, the focus is on maintaining the independence and functional capabilities of both the abused elderly person and his or her family or support system. Institutionalization may be the solution to the problem in cases where abuse is a reflection of a need for care that outstrips the caregiver's ability to provide it. In others, however, the tensions that potentiate elder abuse may be ameliorated through optimum medical management that includes providing support in a patient's home. In these cases, an adult protective service worker can work in conjunction with other social service agencies to provide such in-home services as visiting nurses, homemaker services, home health aides, or meals-on-wheels. Day hospitals or day care may provide enough relief for a caregiver to lessen the potential for abuse. Respite care, giving a caregiver a vacation from caring for an elderly relative, also may reduce the potential for abuse. Sending services into the home also means that there are trained outsiders watching and able to offer informal counseling and support.

In the wake of mandatory reporting laws, some outcome data are beginning to accumulate. Of the cases of elder abuse brought to diagnosis and intervention, about 50% of the elderly persons are institutionalized. About 25% receive various home supports, and another 25% decline any assistance at all.[6]

An abuser can be counseled and helped to understand better the elderly persons illnesses. For example, self-help groups for Alzheimer's disease promote better care and peace of mind, reducing the potential for elder abuse. Psychiatric counseling, referral, and treatment in centers for alcoholism or drug abuse also may improve the situation. Anonymous telephone hotlines that provide a calm sympathetic listener on the other end of the line may avert further elder abuse.

In cases of financial exploitation, there are many avenues for providing help. First, an adult protective service worker will assess the financial status of the client. A client's assets may be turned into more usable funds. For example, money that is invested in real estate can be made more accessible. A caseworker also may be able to expidite an application for welfare or Social Security. Direct-deposit checking services or restricted two-signature accounts may prevent the manipulation of funds. Power of attorney may be granted for the management of finances. Conservatorships and guardianships may place control of other details of living in the hands of an advocate of the client, thus circumventing the potential for exploitation. In addition, a caregiver may be entitled to funds for taking care of an elderly relative or be eligible for financial aid in some other form.

The options for intervention that are presented here are complicated in real life by the fact that availability of services varies from area to area within the United States, and by an imperfect linkage among the many organizations and services cited. Coordination of these services is one of the prime goals for an adult protective service worker dealing with elder abuse. In particular, providing services in rural areas usually is more difficult, because the resources may be less accessible or nonexistent.

In dealing with elder abuse, protective service workers often use preplanned protocols[15] that provide a uniform approach to the problem. These protocols indicate what services are needed and which linkages need to be activated. First is an emergency protocol, in which an imminent danger to life and limb exists. Second, there is the competent consenting victim, in which help is arranged along straightforward lines. Third, there is the competent nonconsenting victim, who can make rational decisions but persists in remaining in dangerous situations. This, perhaps, is the most challenging situation and requires a great deal of tact to allow assessment and assistance. Fourth, there is the incompetent client. In this case, an elderly person is incapable of making decisions concerning his or her care. Promoting guardianship of conservatorship normally is the chief goal and difficulty. Regardless of presentation and subsequent protocol, the initial challenges are to gain access to an abused elderly person and to develop trust that facilitates casework.

Finally, the problem of institutional abuse deserves mention. In some nursing homes, the residents are subjected to the same sorts of abuse discussed above. Theft of a nursing home resident's possessions must be viewed as serious. Some nursing home residents, demented as well as nondemented, strike each other, and the nursing home staff may be wrongly accused of elder abuse. The nursing staff, especially nurse's aides, may have little training in dealing with the problems of institutionalized elderly persons. Sometimes there are ethnic, cultural, or linguistic barriers to good care. The high turnover rate of nurse's aides reflects the high stress of the job, the low pay, and low morale. Theft of the staff's possessions compounds the problems. Inadequate staffing accelerates fatigue and frustration for nursing home personnel, particularly on the night shift, when some residents sundown and are disruptive. Families may express their guilt regarding placement of a loved one by being difficult with and demanding of the staff. In addition to physical abuse, wrongful use of restraints and injudicious use of medications are possible elements of elder abuse in the long-term care setting. Prevention of staff burnout lessens the likelihood of institutional elder abuse.

The Nursing Home Bill of Rights codifies a nursing home resident's rights to privacy, security, and good care. The presence of resident councils in nursing homes may address some of these issues of abuse; also, the state ombudsman may have independent means of investigating alleged nursing home abuses.

The best way to prevent elder abuse in nursing homes is to let it be known that such abuse is not tolerated and will be investigated. The tone that is set by the nursing home administration is quite important in this regard. Sometimes there is a fine line between protective restraint and abusive or unnecessary restraint. Detecting abusive attitudes among the staff is critical. Providing education for employees and a means for ventilating pent-up frustrations reduces elder abuse and minimizes staff turnover in nursing homes. Being readily accessible to families and other concerned persons facilitates this process. The formulation of care plans must be based on the premise that assuring order and safety in a setting that enhances every patient's self-sufficiency is a demanding task for all nursing home personnel.

References

1. Kempe CH, Silverman FN, Steele BF, et al. The battered-child syndrome. *JAMA* 1962;181:105–112.
2. United States House of Representatives, Select Committee on Aging. *Elder Abuse: The Hidden Problem*. 96th Congress, 1st session, June 23, 1979. Boston, Mass: GPO 96-220; 1980:50.
3. Block MR. Special problems and vulnerability of women. In: Kosberg JI, ed. *Abuse and Maltreatment of the Elderly*. Boston, Mass: John Wright PSG Publishing Co Inc; 1983:225.
4. Block MR, Sinnott JD. *The Battered Elder Syndrome*. College Park, Md: University of Maryland Center on Aging; 1979.
5. Pillemer K, Finkelhor D. The prevalence of elder abuse: a random sample survey. *Gerontologist* 1988;28:51–57.
6. O'Malley TA, Everitt DE, O'Malley EW, et al. Identifying and preventing family-mediated abuse and neglect of elderly persons. *Ann Intern Med* 1983;98:998–1005.
7. Hwalek MA, Sengstock MC. Assessing the probability of abuse of the elderly: toward development of a clinical screening instrument. *J Appl Gerontol* 1986;5:153–173.

8. Fulmer T, Welte T. Elder abuse screening and intervention. *Nurse Pract* 1986;11:33–38.

9. Quinn MJ, Tomita SK. Elder abuse and neglect. New York, NY: Springer Publishing Co Inc; 1986:267.

10. Koin DB. The King Lear syndrome. Presented at the American Geriatrics Society Annual Meeting; 1979; Washington, DC.

11. Mace NL, Rabins RV. *The Thirty-Six Hour Day*. Baltimore, Md: The Johns Hopkins University Press; 1982.

12. American Medical Association Council on Scientific Affairs: Elder abuse and neglect. *JAMA* 1987;257:966–971.

13. Salend E, Kane RA, Satz M, et al. Elder abuse reporting: limitation of statutes. *Gerontologist* 1984;24:61–67.

14. Faulkner LR. Mandating the reporting of suspected cases of elder abuse: an inappropriate, ineffective and ageist reponse to the abuse of older adults. *Family Law Q* 1982;16:69–91.

15. Villmoure EE, Bergman, eds. *Elder Abuse and Neglect: A Guide for Practitioners and Policy Makers*. Salem, Ore: State of Oregon, Office of Elderly Affairs; 1981.

50

Long-Term Care

Robert L. Kane and Rosalie A. Kane

As with many social programs, long-term care (LTC) was not planned; most countries drifted into programmatic responses to an aging society. It is now necessary to rationalize what has evolved in bits and pieces. LTC poses a special problem because it covers so many aspects of life. It is essentially care in response to chronic dependency. It crosses many boundaries: physical and mental health care, health and social care, social services and housing, formal services, and family care.

The structure of the LTC system is the result of jurisdictional decisions. These allocations of responsibility to social or health agencies have determined the professional nuance of the care provided and its underlying value system. In the United States, the major determinant of care has been the funding source. Although LTC was never designed as a residual welfare program, it evolved that way as universal entitlements were directed to acute care and LTC was essentially forgotten.

Definition and Goals

There is no universally accepted definition of LTC. A useful formal, but descriptive, definition is that LTC consists of a set of health, personal care, and social services delivered over a sustained period to persons who have lost or never acquired some degree of functional capacity, the latter usually being reflected in some index of functional ability. In turn, functioning includes the ability to perform basic self-care activities (such as bathing, dressing, feeding, and transferring) and other functions needed to live independently (such as cooking, cleaning, shopping, taking medications, and managing money).

Such a definition leaves much room for variety. As with the World Health Organization (WHO) definition of health, there is a danger of taking on too much. The vague boundaries are threatening as the costs of care escalate. The nature of LTC suggests that it is a diffuse service. It does have a time dimension, but no one seems exactly sure when it begins, and fewer seem to recognize if and when it ends. At the same time, transitions certainly occur, at least to acute care. Much of LTC begins in the hospital, but where does acute care stop and LTC begin? In the United States, the terms "transitional care" and "postacute care" have emerged to describe a set of services that seem to continue the work of the hospital after discharge.

In contrast to acute care, LTC uses little high technology. It relies on the efforts of generally minimally trained personnel, primarily aides. When one attempts to define the quality of this service, it is necessary to talk about measures of both technical quality and a more amorphous variable, which is usually called "quality of life." Part of the definitional quandary stems from the fact that services, especially LTC, are often established by what is paid for under various programs. In the United States, publicly subsidized LTC has evolved largely as a welfare program for the poor, leaving its recipients with a double burden of disability and social stigma. Disabled physically or cognitively, they are left to their own resources until they are financially impoverished as well.

Because LTC is so much a compensation for lost function, its potential claims are diffuse. Unfortunately, more attention has been given to stemming costs and finding financing mechanisms than to deciding what services are really needed and how they can be better organized to achieve the ends sought. In fact, the ends sought are often unspecified and usually ambiguous. Most authorities recognize an inevitable physical decline as part of LTC, but little attention has been devoted to identifying the kinds of outcomes that can be realistically expected when different forms of care are provided to appropriate target groups.

There persists a general distinction between quality of care (a term with strong professional and technical overtones) and quality of life (often taken to mean something about ambience and environment), but the two are really intertwined. If improvement is the exception, then slowing decline is a realistic goal. If the situation is chronic, then the circumstances surrounding the giving and receiving of care become ever more pertinent to assessing the overall quality of that care. Moreover, the population needing LTC is heterogeneous, and the potential of any given LTC user will vary over time. Thus, goals must be specific to the patient and the situation.

This chapter focuses on the elderly population, which is the single largest group requiring LTC. However, other groups need LTC as well, including the chronically mentally ill, the developmentally disabled, and the physically disabled of all ages. Although many would treat these four groups as a single class, their different needs and available resources, as well as the separate funding and service streams already established to deal with them, argue persuasively against such conceptual lumping. Perhaps, in the end, LTC entitlements will be structured with functional impairment as the key to eligibility for benefits, regardless of age or the etiology of the disability. But the services themselves will need to be tailored to the specific target populations.

At the outset, we will examine some basic questions of epidemiology and values. These issues can be best addressed as a series of questions:

• Who among the elderly is at greatest risk of needing LTC?
• What is the best way to organize LTC? Is there an appropriate balance between community-based and institutional care?
• Who can afford LTC? How many can afford how much?
• What is the total cost of LTC?
• Does it matter who pays the bill?
• What is the role of families? How is it affected by funding?

In the United States, there are several other issues that must frame any discussion of LTC:

• Should persons be doubly burdened with misfortunes of chronic dependency and poverty?
• Do old persons have a right to leave an inheritance?
• How do we protect and support families, especially spouses?
• LTC is essentially a women's issue: because women are the major caregivers and also are at greatest risk for admission to nursing homes.
• What should be the role of the private sector in insuring? In caring?

Who is at Risk of Needing LTC?

Age is an excellent predictor of dysfunction for groups but a poor indicator for individuals. Because one of the hallmarks of aging is increasing variance in almost every parameter, looking at group means can be misleading. However, for general planning purposes age is a very useful indicator.

It is useful to follow the WHO[1] distinction between disease, impairment, disability, and handicap. A disease or condition may produce some kind of recognizable impairment. That impairment can become a disability when it interferes with function. A disability that prevents a person from carrying out the desired social task is a handicap. The measurement of function in elderly persons has matured a great deal in the last several years.[2,3]

In general, the prevalence of chronic conditions increases with age, as might be expected. However, the effects of survivorship mean that the prevalence of those conditions associated with fatality is less likely to increase. As noted in Chapter 2, the prevalence of nonfatal conditions, such as arthritis, increases with age, but that of hypertension and heart disease actually declines slightly in the oldest age group.

As shown in Figure 50.1, the cross-sectional prevalence of disability (measured in several different ways) increases with age. The most common measures of disability refer to the ability to carry out simple functions. Activities of daily living (ADLs) refer to basic tasks required for self-care. These include such things as bathing, dressing, grooming, using the toilet, transferring in and out of bed, remaining continent, and feeding oneself. The most commonly used ADL measure was proposed by Katz and his colleagues over 2 decades ago (see Chapter 6).[4]

Another group of functions, often called instrumental activities of daily living (IADLs), includes slightly more complex tasks needed for contemporary survival on one's own. These include cooking, cleaning house, shopping, managing money, and managing medica-

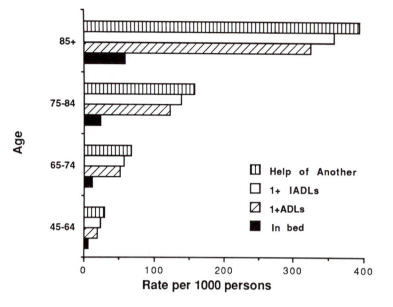

Fig. 50.1. Measures of functional dependency among community elderly, 1979–1980. From BA Fellner, Americans needing home care, Vital and Health Statistics Series 10, No. 153. DHHS Pub. No. (PHS) 86-1581 Public Health Service. Hyattsville, Md: Public Health Service, 1986.

tions. Various investigators have assembled these into scales. A commonly used variant was developed by Lawton et al.[5]

Functional dependency generally indicates a need for human assistance. But for at least one group of dependent elderly, the ADL and IADL measures may not be sufficiently sensitive. Substantial numbers of older persons suffering from dementing disorders, usually Alzheimer's disease, require constant supervision to keep them from harm. Although they do not necessarily need assistance, they may actually need more human effort because they require continuous rather than intermittent oversight.

The degree of risk for LTC is a function of need and available resources. Those in need must have a source of human assistance if they are to survive. Thus, the measurement of need must be carefully addressed. There is an important distinction between residual need and total need. The former refers to the unmet need left by the absence of adequate informal support. Using such an approach immediately penalizes those who do have a possible source of informal care. Indeed, the vast majority of LTC, regardless of funding system, is provided as informal care by unpaid family members and friends. An important question, then, is whether the absence of such care should be required as an eligibility criterion for services. Another issue is whether and how services might be organized to utilize and support informal care.

The central role of informal care in the the provision of LTC has been established repeatedly. A large number of studies show that informal care persists even when organized services are readily accessible; well over 70% of the care given to older persons comes from informal sources. The often-repeated fear that

formal care will drive away informal help seems groundless.

The burden of informal care falls heavily on women, for several demographic as well as social reasons. Because women outlive men by about 5 years and continue to marry older men, they are often both caregivers for their spouses and, later, widows. As a result of these patterns, older women are more likely to live alone (Fig 50.2). After spouses, the

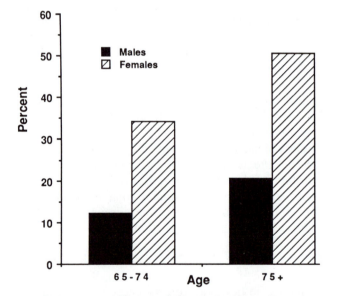

Fig. 50.2. Percent of community elderly living alone, 1984. From MG Kovar, Aging in the eighties, age 65 and over and living alone, contacts with family, friends, and neighbors. Preliminary data from the Supplement on Aging to the National Health Interview Survey: US, January–June 1984. Advance data from Vital and Health Statistics No. 116. DHHS Pub. No. (PHS) 86-1250. Hyattsville, Md: Public Health Service, 1986.

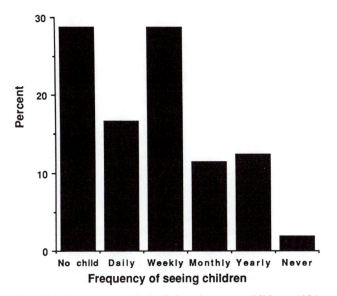

Fig. 50.3. Frequency elderly living alone saw children, 1984. From MG Kovar, Aging in the eighties, age 65 and over and living alone, contacts with family, friends, and neighbors. Preliminary data from the Supplement on Aging to the National Health Interview Survey: US, January–June 1984. Advance data from Vital and Health Statistics No. 116. DHHS Pub. No. (PHS) 86-1250. Hyattsville, Md: Public Health Service, 1986.

next most common group of caregivers is children, again predominantly female children—daughters and daughters-in-law. Even in a mobile society like the United States, older persons maintain frequent contact with their children. As shown in Figure 50.3, the large majority of the 70% of elderly persons with living children see at least one child weekly or more often.

Risk Factors for Admission to Nursing Homes

In general, the lifetime risk of being admitted to a nursing home after age 65 years seems to be about 40%. At the simplest level, persons in nursing homes are more disabled and dependent on others than are those living in the community. There have been several attempts to identify the risk factors associated with admission to nursing homes. These range from simple comparisons of the differences between community-living elderly persons and those dwelling in institutions to complex cross-sectional analyses of multiple variables. Figure 50.4 compares the gross rates for several dependency measures to show the enormous disparity. Some of that difference can be explained by the age, race, and gender distributions of the two groups. Figure 50.5 examines functional parameters among a narrower age band of white women. There still remains considerably more disability in ADLs in the nursing home group, although the rates of vision and hearing impairments are much closer.

Unfortunately there are still very few longitudinal studies on this subject. As can be seen from Figure 50.6, which summarizes the body of work seeking these risk factors, some variables have been frequently tested and others less so.[6] One of the reasons for the variation in findings may be the way the question is posed. Variables such as gender may be very important in univariate analyses, but their contribution is linked to other factors such as available informal care. Other variables are consistently important, but their importance may be circumstantial. For example, social support becomes critical only when

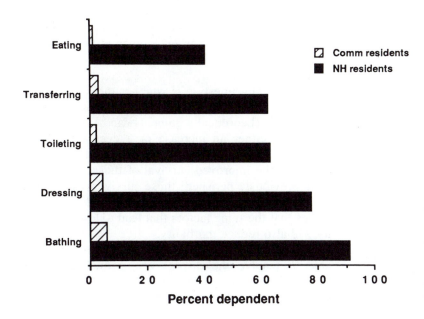

Fig. 50.4. Comparative rates of dependency between elderly persons in the community and in nursing homes. From E. Hing, Use of nursing homes by the elderly: preliminary data from the 1985 National Nursing Home Survey, Advance data from Vital and Health Statistics No. 135. DHHS Pub. No. (PHS) 87-1250. Hyattsville, Md: Public Health Service, 1987.

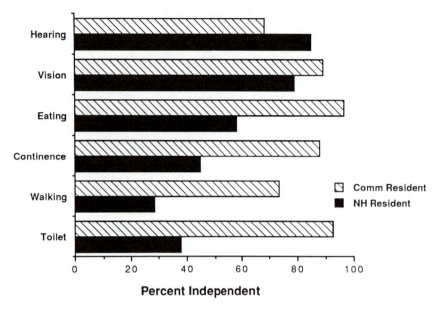

Fig. 50.5. 75–84-year-old white females in nursing home versus in community. From RJ Havlik, MG Liu, MG Kovar et al. (eds.), Health statistics on older persons, US, 1986. Vital and Health Statistics, Series 3, No. 25. DHHS Pub. No. (PHS) 87-1409. Hyattsville, Md: Public Health Service, 1987.

there is disability. Some factors of great importance do not appear in the figure. For example, in anecdotal data, the presence of certain antisocial behaviors, such as wandering (especially at night) and incontinence, are usually credited with a major role in institutionalization.

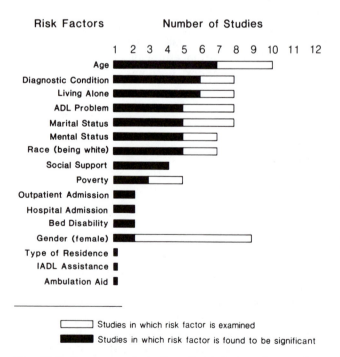

Fig. 50.6. Summary of studies of risk factors for nursing home admission. From RA Kane, RL Kane, *Long Term Care: Principles, Programs, and Policies.* New York, NY: Springer, 1987.

Projecting Risks

By now, the demographic forecast has become a familiar refrain. The disproportionate growth of the elderly part of the population, with even greater growth among the very old, has been combined with contemporary age-specific utilization data to produce frightening glimpses into the future. In the most dire pictures, the bulk of the country's wealth goes to the elderly population, to support a decrepit group.

Planning relies heavily on age and sex as major variables into which to divide the elderly population. Planning based on projections of population age and sex distributions presumes that these age-specific rates are stable. However, the changes in mortality patterns suggest that morbidity rates too may be subject to substantial flux. In truth, there have been remarkable improvements in life expectancy among the elderly population. As noted earlier, women at age 65 years can now expect to live another 20 years, and men another 15.

An important question is whether the current age-specific rates of morbidity will pertain in the next generation. Theoretical arguments can be constructed to predict either an increase or a decrease in age-specific morbidity with time. The projected increase is based on the improved survival of those who would have previously perished; those survivors add to the numbers of the disabled. The projected decrease assumes that the same factors that lead to lower mortality will also reduce morbidity.

As discussed in Chapter 2, the data currently available to resolve the dispute are inconclusive. The general pattern observed from analyses of the annual data from the National Health Interview Survey suggests little improvement in age-specific morbidity rates over the past 10 to 15 years, and perhaps some decline.[7,8] For those 65–74, there is some evidence of increasing morbidity with time, but this is not seen with those age 75 years and older. In truth, both phenomena may be occurring; improved survival may be associated with generally improved health status but may also be adding more disability to the surviving population.[9]

Organization of LTC

Traditionally the benchmark of LTC has been the nursing home. Other modalities of care have been compared with nursing home care in terms of costs and quality. This "alternatives mentality"[10,11] has some unpleasant side effects. It creates a mind-set wherein community care is seen as valuable only to the extent it prevents or reduces nursing home use. Moreover, it tends to deflect attention away from needed improvements in nursing home care on the basis that the real answer is to eliminate the need for nursing homes. The growing body of evidence from both research[12] and practice[13] suggests that efforts to use community services to displace nursing home care are not likely to be successful except in situations where there is a great excess of nursing home beds. The availability of community care facilitates political efforts to limit the supply of nursing home beds. But, community care should be properly viewed as an end itself, not merely a substitute for institutional care. Over and over, older people express strong preferences for remaining in their own homes.

It is increasingly important to distinguish between the site of care and the type of care given at a site. Especially with improvements in technology, it is now possible to provide a vast array of services in the home. The limiting step is no longer feasibility but cost. At some point it is impractical to maintain a person at home either because of the cost of providing paid services or because the social toll on the informal caregivers is too high. It is misleading to think of every admission to a nursing home as a failure.

Many persons are most appropriately cared for in institutions. The real challenge is how to make institutions habitable. This requires attention to creating environments that will not breed dependency and learned helplessness.[14] It means establishing routines and staffing patterns sufficiently flexible to meet the heterogeneous needs and preferences of clients and to permit personal autonomy. In the United States, it means reconsidering the regulations that were designed to promote safety but in practice limit freedom.

It may mean redesigning space to promote privacy and reprogramming with special dementia units.

The nursing home industry experienced great expansion with the passage of Medicaid. The growth of nursing home beds from 1960 to the mid-1970s was exponential, but since then the number of beds has actually declined in proportion to the population. As the regulations tightened and the large real estate–related profits were eliminated, the industry took on a new form. The last decades have seen a growth in chains and networks with more sophisticated management. This shift is prompted by both regulations and economics. The demands of life safety codes require considerable investment in facilities and spelled the end of the "mom and pop" homes that evolved out of boarding houses and the like.

There are almost three times as many nursing homes as acute-care hospitals in the United States. In 1985, there were 16,388 nursing homes, with just over 1.5 million beds, and 5,784 hospitals, with just under 1 million beds.[15] Moreover, while hospitals are running at less than 70% occupancy, nursing homes are over 90% full at all times.

Figure 50.7 contrasts the different levels of LTC facilities. This distinction, which is purportedly based on the intensity of nursing service available and needed, has been widely criticized because of the large variation in definitions of level from one place to another. Thus, one state has a preponderance of skilled facilities and another of intermediate. In the near future, intermediate and skilled care categories will be combined. Nonetheless, some important information is available. Residential care comprises a small proportion of the total beds in the LTC continuum. Residential facilities tend to be smaller; indeed, the more intensive the level of care, the larger the average size of the facility. All types of facilities are heavily occupied. Most would agree that the growth in available beds has not kept pace with the growth in the elderly population. The arguments occur over whether this is a good or bad trend, if we are to increase the proportion of care given in the community. On the one hand, controlling supply is probably the best, if not the only, way to control utilization. At the same time, excess bed capacity may stimulate more competition and hence improve the quality of care, if at the price of more overall use.

Nature of Nursing Home Residents

Nursing home use is very closely tied to age. The general figure of 5% of the elderly population in nursing homes at any time is really an average of widely discrepant numbers. As shown in Figure 50.8,

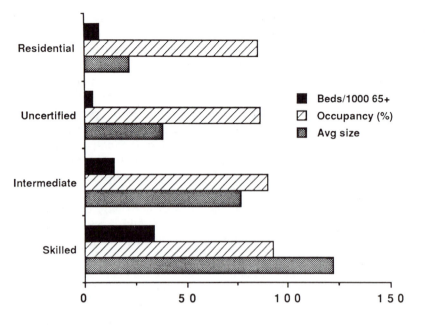

Fig. 50.7. Characteristics of long-term care facilities, 1986. From A. Sirrocco, Nursing and related care homes as reported from the 1986 Inventory of Long-Term Care Places, Advance data from Vital and Health Statistics No. 147. DHHS Pub. No. (PHS) 88-1250. Hyattsville, Md: Public Health Service, 1988.

for those aged 65 to 74 years the rate is closer to 1%, whereas for those aged 85 years and above the rate is over 20%. Figure 50.8 also shows the disproportionate representation of women among nursing home residents. As noted earlier, women are more likely to be living alone. Indeed, widows are especially vulnerable to nursing home admission.

It is important to distinguish between the characteristics of nursing home residents and those of persons entering (or leaving) the nursing home. Data on residents are more like prevalence measures, whereas those for admissions are akin to incidence rates. The prevalence data are more likely to reflect those clients who stay for long periods and thus will contain more

cases of nonfatal chronic problems, such as dementia. Attention to this discrepancy is important in interpreting any data on nursing homes. Similarly, one must be cautious about information on length of stay. Because many nursing home residents are discharged from the nursing home to the hospital, only to return again if they survive the hospitalization, it is misleading to treat each discharge as marking a separate episode of care. In chronic care situations, it is more appropriate to examine continuous patterns of service use. One may refer to these as "LTC careers."

The nature of nursing home residents has changed over time. Figure 50.9 shows how age distribution of persons discharged (alive or dead) has advanced over

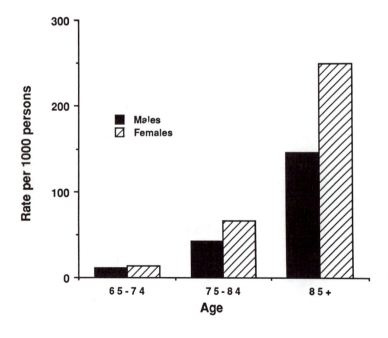

Fig. 50.8. Nursing home use by the elderly, 1985. From E. Hing, Use of nursing homes by the elderly: preliminary data from the 1985 National Nursing Home Survey, Advance data from Vital and Health Statistics No. 135. DHHS Pub. No. (PHS) 87-1250. Hyattsville, Md: Public Health Service, 1987.

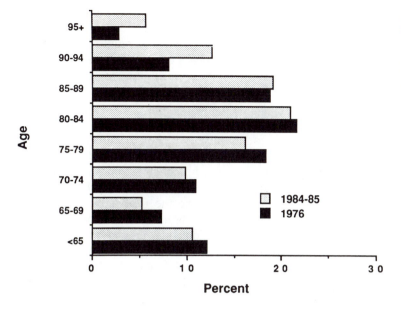

Fig. 50.9. Age of persons discharged from nursing homes, 1976 and 1984–1985. From ES Sek-scenski, Discharges from nursing homes: preliminary data from the 1985 National Nursing Home Survey, Advance data from Vital and Health Statistics No. 142. DHHS Pub. No. (PHS) 87-1250. Hyattsville, Md: Public Health Service, 1987.

the 9-year period between major national surveys. As seen in Figure 50.10, there has been a concomitant increase in disability. In almost every area examined, the proportion of dependent residents has increased. In 1983, hospital reimbursement under Medicare changed to a prospective payment approach, which paid a fixed amount for each of about 470 different types of admissions, based essentially on the patient's primary diagnosis, age, comorbidities, and complications. This approach created an incentive for early

discharge and an expectation that patients going to nursing homes and other forms of postacute care would be sent "quicker and sicker." In fact, the increases in severity of illness among nursing home residents are modest compared to the industry's perceptions about the effects of hospital prospective payment.

Alternatives Mentality

One of the persistent themes in LTC planning has been the expectation that community care will displace nursing home care. Most of the community programs introduced in the last decade have flown under that banner. Indeed, there is currently a waiver program under Medicaid to permit use of funds otherwise targeted for nursing home care to be used for community care, provided there is no overall increase in cost. This fixation on community care as an alternative to nursing home care has several unfortunate consequences.

The most important is the development of false expectations. Study after study has shown that community care will not generally reduce demands for nursing home care. In fact, the projects tended to enroll an impaired population who were not at imminent risk of entering a nursing home. This failure to target, despite active efforts to do so, plus the added costs of extensive case management, designed to encourage community care, made the total cost of adding community care more than that for nursing home care. The recent National Long-term Care Channeling demonstration, a randomized trial of case management with community-based care, showed just

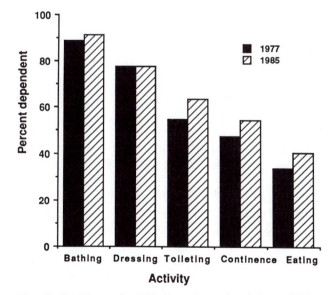

Fig. 50.10. Change in NH dependence level from 1977 to 1985. From E. Hing, Use of nursing homes by the elderly: preliminary data from the 1985 National Nursing Home Survey, Advance data from Vital and Health Statistics No. 135. DHHS Pub. No. (PHS) 87-1250. Hyattsville, Md: Public Health Service, 1987.

this effect[11,12] as has a meta-analysis of the work on this topic.[16]

In Canada, where there are fewer studies but more programs with a balanced set of institutional and community care entitlements, the same phenomenon has been observed.[13,17] Community care will not displace nursing home care unless the supply of nursing home beds is restricted, but community can be a political adjunct in facilitating such a policy of restricted bed supply. In that context, it is a useful step toward the goal.

The emphasis on community care as an alternative fails to recognize that it is an important end in itself. Study after study has shown that older people much prefer to live in the community as long as possible. Indeed, the distaste for nursing home is one reason that the "alternatives" seem to have so little impact. It is essential to recognize the difference between eligibility and use. The argument that persons eligible for nursing home care would have used it had they not received community care greatly overestimates the effect of the latter. Only a small proportion of those eligible for a service actually use it. When the benefit has aversive characteristics and is not highly regarded, the proportion will be even smaller. Thus, even when the population addressed is rather well targeted, it will be hard to show much of an effect in displacement from nursing homes to community care.

The preoccupation with community care and the concomitant belief that nursing home admission represents a community failure may have another pernicious role by distracting attention away from nursing homes at the very time when active reform of the programs is needed. It is therefore important to address the subject of community as a subject in its own right, an important component of LTC.

The Spectrum of Community Care

There is a wide variety of potential services available in the community. Indeed, as mentioned above, the distinction between site and type of care is generally no longer applicable. Almost any form of care can be delivered in the home or under ambulatory auspices. The motivation for community care has varied by time and location. In the United Kingdom, for example, the shortage of chronic-care hospital beds led to an enthusiasm for day hospitals as a means of providing similar services with fewer resources. However, when that concept was exported, it had a different impact in circumstances where the supply of hospital beds was not constrained. In the United States, under the pressure of prospective payment, hospitals have been motivated to discharge patients faster and to avoid many hospitalizations in the first place. There has been

an impressive increase in the use of ambulatory care for many procedures, including extensive surgical procedures that were thought to require hospital admissions only a few years earlier. This new flexibility in care delivery raises opportunities for more innovative ways to approach LTC as well.

An area of confusion has been determining just what institutional care modalities, if any, are actually displaced by community care. For example, home care has at least two separate and presumably distinct components, namely, homemaking and home health. The apparent distinctions are reinforced by the funding mechanisms, because the former is treated as a social service and the latter as a medical one. In practice, the distinctions are less clear, and home health workers often perform homemaking chores. However, home health is more likely actually to substitute for hospital care, whereas homemaking will affect the need for nursing home care. Thus, one may look to the wrong modality of home care for an effect not likely to be produced even under the best circumstances.

Table 50.1 lists a sample of the variety of community resources potentially available to assist LTC recipients. Many planners have expressed great fear that were such resources to become widely available, they would rapidly be inundated. In fact, the opposite seems the case. Figure 50.11 shows how few older persons actually use these services in the course of a year. There is some increase in use with age. The most commonly used services are the senior centers and congregate meals served there. These centers are designed to serve more active elderly persons and provide a gathering place for a variety of social activities.

Links to Acute Care

The interface between is acute care and LTC is poorly articulated, increasing the vulnerability of this already vulnerable clientele. In the United States, this poor

Table 50.1. The spectrum of long-term care.

Site of care	Type of care	Type of service
Nursing home	Postacute	Medical
Home	Respite	Nursing
Day center	Rehabilitative	Homemaking
Day hospital	Chronic	Meal preparation
Residential housing	Hospice	Supervision
Independent living unit		Assistance
Continuing-care retirement community		Case management
		Transportation
Senior center		

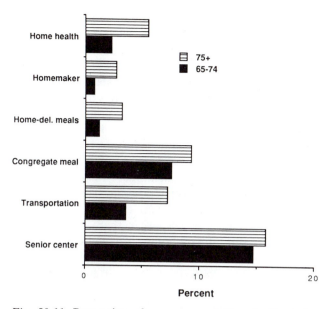

Fig. 50.11. Proportion of persons aged 65 and older using community services, 1984. From R. Stone, Aging in the eighties, age 65 years and over—use of community services: preliminary data from the Supplement on Aging to the National Health Interview Survey: January–June 1984. Advance data from Vital and Health Statistics No. 125. DHHS Pub. No. (PHS) 86-1250. Hyattsville, Md: Public Health Service, 1986.

communication and linkage is exacerbated by the payment system, which covers much of acute care under a federal universal entitlement program but relegates LTC to a residual welfare model for the poor, financed jointly by states and the federal government. This separation is seen in other countries as well, even when both acute care and LTC care are operated under a single agency, and particularly when there is a basic split in responsibility between health and social authorities.

The break is especially inappropriate because of the natural relationship between acute care and LTC for the functionally impaired. People do not cease to need acute care when they enter the LTC system. Moreover, the hospital is the entry point for much of LTC care. Conversely, most patients discharged alive from nursing homes enter the hospital, only to return to the nursing home in a cyclical fashion.[18]

An effective system must bridge this separation to recognize the interdependence of the two. A cost-effective answer to care of chronically dependent elderly persons requires an "investment" philosophy, whereby care given in one sphere is expected to yield benefits in another. Thus, more attention to assessing geriatric patients prior to hospital discharge may readily lead to less inappropriate use of nursing homes.[19] An unresolved issue is how much effort needs to go into assessment to achieve the desired

ends. There is evidence to suggest that interventions of quite different magnitude may all produce positive results.[20] From the opposite perspective, better primary care in nursing homes may help to avoid unnecessary hospitalizations. If physicians are reluctant to care for nursing home residents, other types of practitioners, such as geriatric nurse practitioners, may represent a cost-effective alternative.[21,22]

The interface between acute care and LTC is complicated by the emergence of new forms of care in response to changes in the hospital payment system. Under the pressures of prospective payment systems (PPS), we have begun to talk about postacute, or transitional, care, a reference to a level of treatment that serves as a continuation of hospital care in less expensive settings, including home care, nursing homes, and rehabilitative units. There are, however, striking differences in costs and extent of response to what seem to be similar types of patients at the point of their discharge from hospital. This discrepancy has prompted great interest in learning more about what kinds of patients get what kind of postacute care and what difference it makes.[23,24]

Case Management

One concept that repeatedly surfaces as the answer to a number of divergent problems is case management, ie, the coordination of a group of services on behalf of a defined group of clients. This concept has come to mean quite different things to different groups. At one extreme, the case manager is viewed as an advocate of the client, assisting client and family to obtain a full package of helpful services. At the other end of the continuum, the case manager is viewed as a gatekeeper, preventing the use of unnecessary services and allocating scarce resources where they will do the most good. In a situation of resource constraint, the case manager is expected to distribute the care available in some equitable manner, presumably based on some combination of need and probability of benefit.

The picture is further complicated by the varying levels of empowerment. Case managers sometimes have direct control over resources, authorizing care and payment for it. In other cases, they are brokers and arrangers, whose power is limited to suggesting needed services and making referrals.

Depending on their power and authority, the way case managers are placed in the system of care becomes crucial. A case manager with the authority to purchase care can hardly play an unbiased role as an employee of a provider organization. A provider will have difficulty presenting a disinterested advocacy position for the client. It is unrealistic to expect case managers to act as client advocates and gatekeepers simultaneously. Both they and their clients need to know whom they are working for. If clients are eligible for a variety of services under public funding, case managers are most effectively located in a highly visible organization, from which they can allocate benefits. Depending on local factors, health departments, social service agencies, or area agencies on aging are good contenders for this role.

Financing

A useful aphorism in understanding the organization of care is that "form follows funding." Perhaps nowhere is this observation more true than in the United States, where the very language used to describe care is borrowed directly from the eligibility for coverage under various programs. One of the most visible distinctions can be seen in the way money is channelled to support programs. Table 50.2 compares the sources and distribution of funds for major modalities

Table 50.2. Distribution of LTC spending for fiscal year 1985, by source of payment and type of service* (in billions of dollars).

	Nursing home care	Home care	All LTC
Private sources			
Out of pocket	16.15	3.65	19.80
Insurance	0.30	0.49	0.79
Other	0.28	0.43	0.71
Total private	16.73	4.57	21.30
Federal programs			
Medicare	0.59	2.35	2.94
Medicaid	9.46	0.55	10.01
Veterans administration	0.82	0.01	0.83
Older Americans Act	0.00	0.67	0.67
Title XX	0.00	0.74	0.74
Total federal	10.87	4.32	15.19
State and local programs			
Medicaid	7.74	0.46	8.20
Other	0.42	0.50	0.92
Total state and local	8.16	0.96	9.12
Total public	19.03	5.28	24.31
Total all sources	35.76	9.85	45.61

* Nursing home care expenditures are distributed by levels of facility certification. The levels represented are skilled nursing facilities, intermediate care facilities, combined skilled and intermediate care facilities, intermediate care facilities for the mentally retarded, and uncertified facilities. The home health agency services represented are nursing care, home health aides, speech therapy, physical therapy, occupational therapy, and medical social services. Payments for adult day care, meals, and transportation services are also included in the estimates.
Source: John Holahan and Korbin Liu, "Cost Containment in Long Term Care," Urban Institute Working Paper 1616-01; table based on data supplied by the Congressional Research Service and the Actuarial Research Corporation.

of LTC in fiscal year 1985, the most recent period for data.[25] Of the over $45.5 billion spent on LTC, almost 80% went to nursing homes. About 53% total LTC expenditures came from public sources, mostly Medicaid (a jointly funded federal and state welfare system). This same proportion of public support went for nursing home care and home care, although the latter came from Medicare rather than Medicaid.

In the end, the great concern about LTC is how to pay for it. In the United States, much LTC is not covered by any form of insurance. Instead it comes with the stigma of a poverty program. Hospital care is basically well covered by an entitlement program, Medicare. Patients pay a larger share of the physicians' bills. But nursing home care is essentially paid either out of pocket or under welfare auspices, through Medicaid. Home care, included with drugs and other assorted benefits under the category of "other," is similarly poorly covered by Medicare. There is presently great interest in the potential of private insurance to cover a substantial portion of LTC costs, but analyses suggest that this is unlikely.[26]

Clinicians and policymakers alike have fallen into the habit of accepting the payment coverage as a definition of a service. In the worst scenario, fragmented coverage has led to fragmented care. Even in the best scenario, much effort is devoted to trying to get someone else's budget to cover the costs of care. This budgetary schizophrenia has led to a failure to recognize the natural careers of patients and to make the appropriate investments in care that would enhance future functioning.

Universal coverage is the most desirable situation. Once established, it simplifies many of the problems of organizing and overseeing services. It provides a basis for rational planning and resource distribution with a potential for accountability. The idea of universal covered services is more compatible with countries outside the United States. In the United States, there has been a historical reticence about governmentally organized programs, even when they use private means of delivery. A striking lesson from Canada has been the power of monopsony (a single payer) to control expenditures, with no apparent decrease in quality. This promise of efficiency is all the more attractive at a time when there are pressures to spend more money on health care for the elderly population.

A universal program will not solve all of the problems, however. There still remain the questions of how to control expenditures and how to link acute care and LTC without exploiting either. Some form of gatekeeping, or case management, will be needed to achieve the first objective. The system will likely require some form of capitated budgetary authority with concomitant responsibility. The lessons from the rest of the western world suggest that local control is essential; the larger and more heterogeneous the country, the more appropriate is such local control. The interfacing of acute care and LTC is more uncertain. The health care budget represents the most likely place to find additional resources for LTC programs, but putting the two programs together may lead to health care's simply subsuming LTC rather than to a creative merger. Specific protections, perhaps fostered by careful prenuptial agreements, seem crucial in a successful marriage of the acute care and LTC systems.

References

1. *World Health Organization International Classification of Impairments, Disabilities, and Handicaps: A Manual of Classification Relating to the Consequences of Disease.* Geneva, Switzerland: World Health Organization; 1980.

2. Kane RA, Kane RL. *Assessing the Elderly: A Practical Guide to Measurement.* Lexington, Mass: DC Heath & Co, 1981.

3. McDowell I, Newell C. *Measuring Health: A Guide to Rating Scales and Questionnaires.* New York, NY: Oxford University Press; 1987.

4. Katz S, Ford AB, Moskowitz RW, et al. Studies of illness in the aged: the index of ADL: a standardized measure of biological and psychosocial function. *JAMA* 1963;185:914–919.

5. Lawton MP, Fulcomer M, Kleban, MH. A research and service oriented multilevel assessment instrument. *J Gerontol* 1982;32:91–99.

6. Kane RL, Kane RA. Transitions in Long-term care. In Ory MG, Bond K, eds. *Aging and Health Care.* London: Routledge; 1989;pp 217–243.

7. Verbrugge LM. Longer life but worsening health? trends in health and mortality of middle-aged and older persons. *Milbank Mem Fund Q* 1984;62:475–519.

8. Crimmins EM. Evidence on the compression of morbidity. *Gerontologica Perspecta* 1987;1:45–49.

9. Kane RL, Radosevich D, Vaupel JW. Compression of morbidity: issues and irrelevancies. In: Kane R, Evans JG, Macfadyen DM, eds. *Improving Health in Older People: A World View.* New York, NY: Oxford University Press. In press.

10. Kane RA, Kane RL. *Long-Term Care: Principles, Programs, and Policies.* New York, NY: Springer Publishing Co Inc; 1987.

11. Kane RA. The noblest experiment of them all: learning from the national channeling evaluation. *Health Serv Res* 1988;23:189–198.

12. Carcagno GJ, Kemper P. The evaluation of the National Long-term Care Channeling Demonstration, I: an overview of the channeling demonstration and its evaluation. *Health Serv Res* 1988;23:1–22.

13. Kane RL, Kane RA. *A Will and A Way: What Americans Can Learn About Long-Term Care From Canada.* New York, NY: Columbia University Press; 1985.

14. Rodin J. Aging and health: effects of the sense of control. *Science* 1986;233:1271–1276.

15. US Bureau of the Census. *Statistical Abstract of the United States: 1988.* 108th ed. Washington, DC:, 1987.

16. Berkely Planning Associates. *Evaluation of Coordinated Community Long-term Care Demonstration Projects: Final Report.* Berkeley, Calif: Berkeley Planning Associates; 1985.

17. Kane RA, Kane RL. The feasibility of universal long-term care benefits: ideas from Canada. *New Engl J Med* 1985;12:1357–1363.

18. Lewis MA, Cretin S, Kane RL. The natural history of nursing home patients. *Gerontologist* 1985;25:382–388.

19. Rubenstein LZ, Josephson KR, Wieland GD, et al. Effectiveness of a geriatric evaluation unit: a randomized clinical trial. *New Engl J Med* 1984;311:1664–1670.

20. Kane RL. Beyond caring: the challenge to geriatrics. *J Am Geriatr Soc* 1988;36:467–472.

21. Kane RL, Jorgensen LA, Teteberg B, et al. Is good nursing-home care feasible? *JAMA* 1976;235:516–519.

22. Master RJ, Feltin M, Jainchill J, et al. A continuum of care for the inner city: assessment of its benefits for Boston's elderly and high-risk populations. *N Engl J Med* 1980;302:1434–1440.

23. Gornick M, Hall MJ. Trends in Medicare utilization of SNFs, HHAs, and rehabilitation hospitals. *Health Care Financing Rev.* 1988; annual supplement:27–38.

24. Kane RL, Kane RA. Posthospital care: a mystery and an opportunity. In: Vladeck BC, Alfano GJ, eds. *Medicare and Extended Care: Issues, Problems, and Prospects.* Owings Mills, Md: Rynd Communications; 1987, pp. 37–43.

25. Holahan, J, Liu K. Cost containment in long-term care. Presented at the International Symposium on Controlling Costs While Maintaining Health: The Experience of Canada, the US and the FR of Germany With Alternative Cost-Containment Strategies; June 1988; Bonn, West Germany.

26. Rivlin AM, Wiener JM. *Caring for the Disabled Elderly: Who Will Pay?* Washington, DC: Brookings Institution; 1988.

51

The Physician and the Care of the Nursing Home Resident

Greg A. Sachs and Don Riesenberg

The care of nursing home residents is one of the most challenging and rapidly changing areas in medicine today. Insights from the growing body of knowledge that makes up geriatric medicine have begun to alter radically nursing homes. The nursing home was once seen as a warehouse for the hopeless and helpless aged. Now it is becoming the site of active investigation and treatment of illnesses and iatrogenic conditions, as well as the scene of vigorous efforts to maintain function and dignity. This vitalization of nursing home medicine comes at a most opportune time. The enormous growth of the elderly population who may need hospital and nursing home care is occurring at the same time that reimbursement incentives and regulations are limiting hospital stays. The result is an expanding nursing home population that is more acutely ill than in previous eras. Today's nursing home residents present fascinating and difficult problems in the prevention, diagnosis, and treatment of medical conditions that can be properly addressed only by motivated physicians who accept the challenges of medicine in the nursing home.

Case Presentation

The case of Mrs Jones is one that illustrates many of the exciting elements and challenges in the medical care of nursing home residents:

Mrs Jones is an 82-year old woman with a history of hypertension who was widowed 1 year ago. After her husband's death, Mrs Jones continued to live independently in the community. She did well except for a slight weight loss and recent complaints of difficulty falling asleep. Her local physician prescribed flurazepam hydrochloride (30 mg orally) to be taken at bedtime for the insomnia. One night, about a week after beginning to take the flurazepam, Mrs Jones fell at home, suffering a hip fracture.

After successful replacement of the fractured hip at a nearby hospital, Mrs Jones slowly began to recuperate. After 10 days in the hospital and four sessions in the physical therapy department, this elderly woman was told that she was ready to be discharged from the hospital. However, she still required maximal assistance just to transfer from bed to chair; she was still nearly bedbound. As she had no relatives who could assist in her care at home, Mrs Jones was transferred to a nursing home.

A couple of days after Mrs Jones' admission to the nursing home, a nurse's aide noted that the patient seemed short of breath. Since the original local physician did not continue to care for her after transfer, she was evaluated by one of the nursing home's staff physicians. On examination, Mrs Jones was febrile, somewhat confused, and tachypneic, and she appeared to be volume depleted. Her blood pressure was 140/80 mm Hg supine and 110/60 mm Hg seated. She was tachycardic, but her pulse was regular. The skin over her sacrum was reddened, and on admission a purified protein derivative (PPD) test showed 12 mm of induration. She had decreased breath sounds at the left base and unremarkable cardiac examination findings; specifically, a third heart sound was absent. The neurologic examination findings were nonfocal.

The physician reviewed Mrs Jones' chart and discovered that her medication list included digoxin, hydrochlorothiazide, subcutaneous heparin, docusate sodium, and flurazepam, as well as orders for haloperidol and milk of magnesia as needed. The tests ordered by the physician revealed a serum sodium level of 127 mmol/L and an infiltrate in the left lower lobe.

Many health professionals emphasize the importance of nonphysicians in the care of nursing home residents. For particular residents, the social worker, nurse, or physical therapist is much more important than the physician. However, the case of Mrs Jones clearly is very complicated from the medical standpoint. The physician standing at her bedside is in a unique position to help this patient. This physician is confronted with many interesting and difficult questions in arriving at diagnoses and treatment for Mrs Jones. The potential for a successful outcome, however, goes beyond the resolution of her acute problems. What is at stake is whether or not she gets the kind of care that enables her to be discharged to independent living in the community once again.

Illness Presentation

The first challenge facing the physician at Mrs Jones' bedside is arriving at a diagnosis, or diagnoses, for her acute condition. Making an accurate diagnosis in a nursing home resident tends to be more difficult because of the confounding effects of multiple chronic illnesses, multiple medications and their adverse effects, and the way in which many illnesses have different presentations in elderly patients. Atypical and nonspecific presentations are more common in elderly patients.[1] The changing presentation of illness in older people has been well described for pneumonia[2] and myocardial infarction,[3] where confusion and shortness of breath are common presenting findings. Additionally, pulmonary embolism is a cause of shortness of breath that may be particularly underdiagnosed in nursing home patients. In one recent autopsy study of elderly institutionalized patients, pulmonary embolism was the fourth leading cause of death and caused the greatest antemortem diagnostic confusion (with only 39% of cases correctly diagnosed).[4] Thus, Mrs Jones' confusion and shortness of breath may be a result of pneumonia, myocardial infarction, or pulmonary embolism. This is a diagnostic problem that has crucial implications for treatment and takes rigorous thinking to unravel. Yet, the puzzle of diagnosing acute problems is but a small part of the challenging world of medicine in the nursing home (Table 51.1).

Preventable and Overlooked Illness

One of the most satisfying accomplishments for any physician is to identify and treat reversible problems that were hitherto undiagnosed. While traditionally

Table 51.1. Medical challenges for physicians in the nursing home.

Examples of Prevention
Infection: vaccination (eg, influenza, pneumococcus, tetanus); skin testing (eg, tuberculosis).
Falls: recognition of postprandial hypotension, monitoring of psychotropic medication.
Pressure sores: combating immobility (eg, frequent turning), attention to nutritional status.
Examples of Diagnosis and Treatment
Endocrine disorders: Hypothyroidism, hypoadrenalism, diabetes mellitus
Psychiatric disorders: dementia, depression, paranoia
Cardiopulmonary disorders: acute dyspnea (see case example in text).

seen as a less exciting aspect of medicine, the chance to prevent illness altogether is becoming a fascinating field in its own right. The nursing home is the place where physicians can find ample opportunity to have both of these experiences.

Although the initial challenge to Mrs Jones' new physician is to address her current problems, a subject for later investigation will be the conditions that resulted in nursing home admission in the first place. The former physician had prescribed flurazepam for her insomnia. The possibility of depression must not be overlooked in this elderly woman who was widowed 1 year ago and presents with weight loss and difficulty falling asleep. It has been estimated that as many as 20% of nursing home patients have a primary psychiatric diagnosis and that 70% have psychiatric problems that contribute to their condition.[5] Up to 40% of nursing home residents may have occult depression; many will benefit from treatment.[6] In fact, some patients carrying the diagnosis of dementia may only appear to be demented because of an unrecognized and untreated depression (the pseudodementia of depression).[7] For physicians unfamiliar or uncomfortable with the treatment of psychiatric illness, especially when the patient has complex symptoms, consultation with a psychiatrist will be invaluable. This would go a long way toward changing the estimate that less than 1% of nursing home residents are appropriately evaluated by psychiatrists.[5]

Psychiatric problems are but one example of underdiagnosed and untreated conditions common in the nursing home. Undiagnosed pulmonary embolism has been mentioned as a major cause of death. Malnutrition is widespread in nursing homes, occurring in more than 50% of residents in two studies.[8,9] This is not an irremediable problem; improvement in nutritional status can be achieved.[10] Pressure sores are frequently overlooked until a patient is transferred from a hospital to a nursing home, where the staff is properly sensitized to their critical importance.[11] Although expensive screening tests, such as electrocardiograms, often may be deferred, metabolic and hormonal abnormalities will not be discovered unless physicians periodically order the appropriate laboratory tests.[12] Even infections, a major cause of hospitalization and mortality in nursing home residents,[13] are grossly underdiagnosed.[14]

Because of the magnitude of undiagnosed and untreated illness in the nursing home, tremendous opportunities exist there for the physician who is interested in the prevention of illness. Infectious diseases are of prime concern for a variety of reasons: increased incidence, increased morbidity and mortality, and the potential for rapid spread within the institution. This is the case for influenza,[15] pneumonia,[16] tetanus,[17] and tuberculosis.[18] In fact, nursing home residents figure prominently in controversies over immunizations and chemoprophylaxis.[19–22]

Prevention is not limited to infectious diseases. Opportunities for primary and secondary prevention abound in the areas of malnutrition and pressure sores. The nursing home physician attending to Mrs Jones in our case presentation noted reddening of the skin on her sacrum. Correct diagnosis of this stage 1 pressure sore obviates progression with increased morbidity. Strict adherence to an every-2-hour turning regimen until mobility is achieved will allow this early-stage sore to heal, avoiding the complications of osteomyelitis and sepsis.[23]

Medications

Mrs Jones' medications include hydrochlorothiazide, digoxin, docusate sodium, and flurazepam, as well as orders for haloperidol and milk of magnesia as needed. Her nursing home physician knows several principles of pharmacology in the elderly and the dangers of polymedicine (or polypharmacy) for nursing home residents (also see Chapter 7). Such a physician is able to see sorting through a medication list as a rewarding task. The challenge is to whittle away at the medication list so that each resident is taking only the medicines that are absolutely necessary, with the lowest chance of adverse effects, and in the appropriate geriatric dosages. Mrs Jones' medications certainly deserve scrutiny on many of these accounts.

The first question is to determine just which of these medications, if any, are really necessary. It may be that some of the medications were never indicated or that the indication no longer exists. Mrs Jones' blood pressure is 140/80 mm Hg. Does she really need her diuretic or is her blood pressure lower than usual now because she may be volume depleted or infected? Might it not be more reasonable to attempt to control her blood pressure with nutritional therapy, which can be very effective in a proportion of patients receiving medications?[24] This is especially important to consider in view of the hyponatremia, which may be secondary to the antihypertensive medication. Why is Mrs Jones taking digoxin, and could it be discontinued safely? One study found that 18 of 19 elderly nursing home patients who were in normal sinus rhythm were able to have their digoxin withdrawn without any adverse effects.[25] Docusate sodium and milk of magnesia are medications that are frequently prescribed for elderly nursing home residents with constipation.[26] Often this is done without any thinking about the cause of the constipation or alternative management (diet changes, increased fluid intake, and increased exercise).

Mrs Jones' flurazepam and haloperidol deserve special attention because of the incredible use and misuse of psychotropic agents in nursing homes. Data from the 1984 National Nursing Home Survey Pretest suggest that psychotropics are misused in nursing homes.[27] One third of the residents in this survey were receiving psychotropics. However, two other findings were even more disturbing than the high frequency of use of these drugs: (1) a review panel's determination that less than 50% of the psychotropic medications were fully appropriate in terms of indication, the choice of drug, and proper dosage; and (2) the fact that 21% of residents receiving psychotropics had no mental disorder diagnosis or symptom recorded in their charts. One third of this last group of residents were receiving antipsychotic drugs. This improper use of psychotropic medications must be considered in light of the data mentioned above, suggesting high prevalence of undiagnosed psychiatric conditions in nursing homes. Clearly, the appropriate use of psychotropics is one of the greatest challenges in nursing home medicine.

Mrs Jones' experience with psychotropics actually began as an outpatient when her physician prescribed flurazepam for her insomnia, the etiology of which may well have been depression. Additionally, the particular hypnotic selected is important in elderly patients; flurazepam's prolonged half-life makes it less than ideal for an 82-year-old. Furthermore, the starting dosage of 30 mg/d is excessive in this age group. In fact, Mrs Jones' hip fracture may have been secondary to oversedation with the flurazepam. A case-control study has found that people receiving long-acting hypnotics-anxiolytics have almost double the risk of hip fracture compared with controls not receiving such medications. The same appears to be true for antipsychotic agents and tricyclic antidepressants.[28]

Rehabilitation

Once Mrs Jones' medications and other acute medical difficulties are sorted out, her return to independent living in the community is dependent on effective rehabilitation for her hip fracture. Tragically, many similar patients no longer receive the kind of physical therapy and care that would lead to their regaining function and leaving the nursing home. A study looking at the impact of the prospective payment system (PPS) on hip fracture care in one hospital uncovered some disquieting changes: (1) a decrease in mean length of hospitalization from 16.6 to 10.3 days; (2) a decrease in the mean number of physical therapy sessions from 9.7 to 4.9; (3) an increase in the proportion of patients discharged to a nursing home from 21% to 48%; and (4) an increase in the proportion of patients still in a nursing home 6 months after discharge from 13% to 39%.[29] These findings suggest that the pressures of the PPS led to the earlier discharge of patients with hip fractures, after fewer physical therapy sessions than in the past. This more rapid discharge, in turn, resulted in more patients going to, and remaining in, nursing homes. Further analysis of this study's data demonstrated that the group now at increased risk of nursing home placement is that of elderly women who lack a good home support system. In the pre-PPS era, these women would have been kept in the acute hospital to receive extensive physical therapy until they were able to return home (75% of those with long stays in the pre-PPS era were able to go home).[29]

Mrs Jones, therefore, can be seen as someone caught between the incentives of the PPS and her lack of help at home. She was not allowed to stay in the acute hospital to receive a lengthy rehabilitation course. She is now in the nursing home, where she must be able to obtain adequate physical therapy if she is to make it back to the community. Such patients, who require active rehabilitation efforts, are going to add another challenge to those already faced by physicians in the nursing home: a working knowledge of physical medicine and rehabilitation.

The importance of physiatry in the nursing home cannot be emphasized enough. It is the central element in the care of patients with recent stroke in all sites, including the nursing home. Long-term nursing home residents also can benefit from attention to these kinds of physical needs. Many residents can achieve greater mobility and independence with the appropriate use of physical therapy and assistive devices. The emphasis on physiatry and orthotics on the first certifying examination for added qualification in geriatrics should also serve to highlight the importance of this area for those interested in caring for elderly persons (personal communication, Section of Geriatrics, University of Chicago, May 1988).

Demographic Imperative

The hip fracture data cited above, by Fitzgerald et al[29] is but one study in a growing body of literature on the effects of the PPS, with its emphasis on diagnosis-related groups (DRGs). Because this method of reimbursement has been applied first to Medicare patients, its impact on the cost and quality of health care is being eagerly studied. While it is too early to make final judgments, concern is growing. Many fear that the financial pressures of DRGs result in frail, elderly patients being discharged "sicker and quicker" than in the past. The quality of care for the elderly may be suffering. The price for a shorter average hospital length of stay may be more frequent readmissions, with increased morbidity and mortality for those discharged prematurely the first time around.

Fueling this concern are studies such as that of Fitzgerald et al[29] and one by Sager et al[30] on the impact of Medicare's PPS on Wisconsin nursing homes. Sager et al found remarkable changes in hospitalization and mortality figures only 2 years after the implementation of the system. In Wisconsin's institutionalized elderly Medicaid population, there was a 72% increase in the rate of hospitalization, a 26% decline in the length of stay, a 10.3% decline in hospital deaths, and a 26.2% increase in the rate of deaths in nursing homes. One unifying explanation for these findings is that nursing home residents are being discharged prematurely from the hospital, leading to frequent readmissions and a sicker nursing home population with a higher mortality rate.[30] Obviously, if this is the correct explanation and these findings are replicated, the physicians for nursing home residents will be caring for a much sicker population, with more demanding medical problems.

There are other factors making it more likely that physicians will be caring for a larger and more challenging nursing home population. First, the oft-quoted estimates on the lifetime risk of nursing home residency may be too low. It has been stated that 5% of the elderly are in a nursing home at any given time and that 20% of the elderly population will spend some time in a nursing home.[31] However, investigators recently have used more sophisticated life-table analyses that estimate the lifetime risk of nursing home residency for those reaching 65 years of age at 40%[32] or greater.[33] Thus, medicine in the nursing home is not a practice limited to a small number of frail, elderly patients but is actually a substantial part of caring for this country's aging population.

The aging of our population is the other major factor that is creating a demand for physicians interested in geriatrics in general, and nursing home medicine in particular. This so-called demographic imperative is covered elsewhere in this text (Chapter 2), but it is worth emphasizing a couple of points. The fastest-growing portion of the population is the group over the age of 85 years.[34] The number of elderly people needing to be in a nursing home is expected to expand dramatically, with a projected 278% increase in nursing home residents from 1980 to 2040.[35] There will be far more nursing home beds than hospital beds in this country. Therefore, there are more elderly people, who may have an even greater chance of being in a nursing home than previously thought and who will be subject to financial forces that will place them in nursing homes in a more acutely ill state. This is a challenge for individual physicians (to provide medical care to nursing home residents) and for society.

The Teaching Nursing Home

Robert N. Butler, MD, then the director of the National Institute on Aging, outlined in a 1981 commentary what he thought the response of academic medicine to the challenges of nursing home medicine should be.[36] Butler saw 1981 nursing homes as comparable to "the ancient hospital untouched by science." He called for the establishment of teaching nursing homes that would be the equivalent of the academic-teaching hospital. The teaching nursing home would be affiliated with a major academic medical center having a strong geriatrics section. Research and training would be its goals, in addition to the care of the nursing home residents. Within 3 years, the National Institute on Aging and the Robert Wood Johnson Foundation were supporting a total of 16 teaching nursing home programs.[37] The Veterans Administration system, private organizations, and individual academic medical centers all became involved in the development of academic programs in nursing homes.[38]

By 1987, only 6 years after Dr Butler's call for action, a survey of American medical schools revealed that 90% (109 of 121) had affiliations with at least one nursing home for teaching, research, and/or clinical care (Fig. 51.1).[39] Eight-three percent of medical schools had training programs in nursing homes. The number of schools having teaching programs on the student, house staff, and fellowship levels all in-

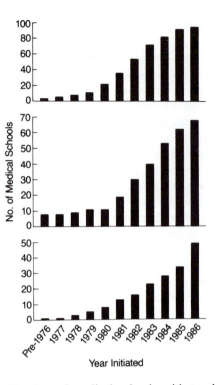

Fig. 51.1. Number of medical schools with teaching programs in nursing homes by year initiated. Top, number with student teaching programs in nursing homes. Center, number with intern/resident training programs in nursing homes. Bottom, number with geriatric fellowship programs in nursing homes. From reference 39.

creased yearly. Though many of these programs are still in their infancy, one academic nursing home already demonstrated significant improvements in residents' functional status, morale, and satisfaction.[40] In this program there was also an increased rate of discharge for patients undergoing long-term rehabilitation, as well a trend toward improved survival (which did not reach statistical significance). All of this, in addition to the initiation of the training aspect of the teaching nursing home, was accomplished with only minimal increases in the cost of running the home.

In addition to clinical care and teaching, 55% of medical schools responding to the 1987 survey by Schneider et al[39] had research programs involving nursing homes. Dementias (including Alzheimer's disease), infections, falls, psychosocial issues, pharmacology, functional assessment and outcomes, urinary incontinence, and pressure sores are just some of the areas of investigation in many of the teaching nursing homes.[39] There is great hope that this academic response to the challenge of nursing home medicine will help create a "thriving intellectual atmosphere"[36] in those institutions.

Ethics in the Nursing Home

While many have eagerly rushed to address research questions in the nursing home, this research has not been without its difficulties. In his call for the teaching nursing home, Butler singled out the patient with Alzheimer's disease as having been ignored as a subject for research up to that point. He believed that the nursing home would be an ideal place for research on dementias of all kinds.[36] However, many ethical issues remain unsettled concerning research in nursing homes, especially when demented residents are involved. Some view nursing home residents, even mentally competent ones, as vulnerable subjects: a captive population by virtue of their living in an institution and at great risk of being coerced into participating in research studies. (Past practices, such as the injection of live malignant cells into residents at the Jewish Chronic Disease Hospital in New York, certainly serve as reminders of the potential for abuse.[41]) There also is concern that protection of nursing home residents has gone too far in the opposite direction. Excessively restrictive regulations may be enacted, and research essential for nursing home residents may be stymied.[42] Many investigators already have found it difficult to recruit subjects for research in nursing homes, even without such restrictions.[43]

The ethical concerns become even more complicated when one is interested in the study of demented residents. The issue of informed consent for research involving demented subjects is especially problematic. One group of investigators who sought proxy consent for a study on the long-term use of urinary catheters was struck by the high rate of refusal (46%) by family members.[44] These investigators went back and interviewed the family members to see if they could understand this refusal rate. The most disturbing finding was that of the 55 proxies who believed that the patient-subject would have refused to participate, 17 (31%) still gave consent, apparently overriding what the patient-subject would have wanted. Obviously, proxy consent is not a panacea for the ethical problems in research on demented residents.

These problems with research in the nursing home are very interesting but represent the concerns of only a minority of physicians actually engaged in research. However, there are ethical dilemmas occurring daily in nursing homes throughout the country that represent yet another challenge for practicing physicians. Difficult decisions involving questions of competency, tube feedings, quality-of-life discussions, care of dying patients, and limitations on treatment and resuscitation efforts are encountered on a regular basis. Physi-

cians working in the nursing home must have a knowledge of ethical principles that will allow them to sort through these difficult issues. The physician caring for nursing home residents also must have the sensitivity and communication skills to discuss such matters with residents and their families. As opposed to the "nursing home of yesteryear as a basically custodial facility,"[45] today's nursing home is a fascinating and challenging place for physicians to practice medicine in all of its richness and diversity, from the purely medical to the psychosocial to the ethical.

Physician Involvement

This chapter has used the case of Mrs Jones to illustrate how interesting and challenging it is to be a physician caring for a nursing home resident. The challenges are plentiful: difficult and subtle differential diagnoses to unravel, new diagnoses to uncover and treat, medications to adjust or discontinue, unanswered questions to research, and ethical problems to confront. The demographic imperative makes the need obvious. Why then do so many physicians avoid taking care of nursing home residents? A nationwide survey of physicians in 15 specialties revealed that only 28% had visited a nursing home in the month prior to the survey.[46] Internists, family practitioners, and cardiologists were the physicians most likely to visit a nursing home. Yet, a subsequent survey directed at these three types of physicians in Michigan still found that almost 60% had not made a nursing home visit in the previous month.[47] The latter study and one other[48] have examined some of the reasons physicians give for not visiting nursing homes: low reimbursement, inconvenience, excessive paperwork, and having too few patients.[47,48] Many of these factors can, and must, be addressed on a policy level in order to encourage physician involvement in the nursing home.

We believe that, especially for younger physicians, much of the reluctance to see nursing home patients is a matter of exposure and education. As one author has put it, "Until recently, clinical research, like clinical training, had almost no contact with the challenging and often fascinating issues inherent in nursing-home medicine."[49] Similarly, a geropsychiatrist has stated that his goal is to make psychiatric services available in the nursing home by educating psychiatrists "to the professional rewards of working with frail older people."[5] We trust that, as more physicians receive training (or continuing education courses) in the nursing home and learn about the unique challenges and rewards involved in practicing medicine there, the "thriving intellectual atmosphere" will draw more and more physicians to the care of this important growing segment of our society.

Conclusion

We now return to the physician standing at Mrs Jones' bedside.

The low-grade fever, dyspnea, confusion, and new infiltrate on the chest x-ray film are suggestive of the diagnosis of pneumonia. Pulmonary embolism is still a possible diagnosis, but the patient was receiving prophylactic therapy for thromboembolic events, and the abnormal chest x-ray film means that ruling out a pulmonary embolism would entail transfer to an acute hospital for a pulmonary angiogram. The physician decides to continue minidose heparin and observe the patient's response to antibiotics for the presumed pneumonia. After appropriate cultures are obtained, the antibiotics chosen are a cephalosporin and an aminoglycoside, because of the patient's toxic appearance.

The hyponatremia may be due to a pulmonary infection or the use of a thiazide diuretic with subsequent volume depletion and continued intake of hypotonic liquids, such as water. It may be difficult to sort out which condition is responsible for the hyponatremia. However, the physician is familiar and comfortable with treating nursing home patients without a single, unifying diagnosis. (Frequently, this physician has had to treat more than one possible diagnosis at a time and see if the results help determine the etiology. After all, even if the etiology is never determined, is that as important as the patient's improvement?)

The thiazide is discontinued and the patient is rehydrated with normal saline. Forty-eight hours later, Mrs Jones is afebrile, no longer confused, and breathing comfortably. Her blood cultures yield Pneumococcus, allowing her physician to change her antibiotic to penicillin alone and rule out pulmonary embolism. Her sodium level is back up to 135 mmol/L, and she remains normotensive without the thiazide.

The physician returns to the patient's medication orders and discontinues the digoxin, flurazepam, haloperidol, docusate sodium, and milk of magnesia. Mrs Jones suffers no adverse effects from the withdrawal of these medications.

As the pneumonia resolves, a trial of an antidepressant is begun. The nursing staff assists Mrs Jones in adhering to an every-2-hours position change regimen until she is more ambulatory. A physical therapist begins working with her. By the end of the antibiotic course, the patient is sleeping well and doing well in her rehabilitation efforts. Her stage I pressure sore has healed.

Records are obtained from the original physician. These reveal that Mrs Jones had a positive PPD reaction in the past. Since her conversion to a positive reaction is not recent, the nursing home physician decides that no treatment is indicated.

After a few more weeks of physical therapy, Mrs Jones is independent in transferring and is able to ambulate with a walker on her own. A team meeting is held to plan her

discharge from the nursing home. All is in order for the discharge, but a home visit by the occupational therapist is done first to see if any adaptations need be made to the home and if there are any obstacles (electrical cords, throw rugs, etc.) that increase the risk of another fall.

Two months later, Mrs Jones goes back to her own home. Her only medication is an antidepressant, which will be discontinued in the future by her new physician—the doctor she met in the nursing home.

References

1. Woodson CE, Sachs GA. Infections in the nursing home: prevention, diagnosis, and management. *Geriatr Clin North Am.* 1988;4:507–525.
2. Marrie TJ, Durrant H, Kwan C. Nursing home-acquired pneumonia: a case-control study. *J Am Gertiatr Soc* 1986;34:697–702.
3. Bayer AJ, Chadha JS, Farag RR, et al. Changing presentation of myocardial infarction with increasing old age. *J Am Geriatr Soc* 1986;34:263–266.
4. Gross JS, Neufeld RR, Libow LS, et al. Autopsy study of the elderly institutional patient: review of 234 autopsies. *Arch Intern Med* 1988;148:173–176.
5. Borson S, Liptzin B, Nininger J, et al. Psychiatry and the nursing home. *Am J Psychiatry* 1987;144:1412–1418.
6. Morley JE. Medical problems in nursing homes. In: *UCLA Board Review Course Syllabus.* 1988:63–68.
7. Bulbena A, Berrios GE. Pseudodementia: facts and Figures. *Br J Psychiatr* 1986;148:87–94.
8. Pinchofsky-Devin GD, Kaminski MV. Correlation of pressure sores and nutritional status. *J Am Geriatr Soc* 1986;34:435–440.
9. Sandman PO, Adolfsson R, Nygren C, et al. Nutritional status and dietary intake in institutionalized patients with Alzheimer's disease and multi-infarct dementia. *J Am Geriatr Soc* 1987;35:31–38.
10. Strome S, Silver A, Morley JE, et al. Increased nutritional status in an academic nursing home. *Fed Proc* 1987;46:900.
11. Shepard MA, Parker D, DeClercque N. The under-reporting of pressure sores in patients transferred between hospital and nursing home. *J Am Geriatr Soc* 1987;35:159–160.
12. Levinstein MR, Ouslander JG, Rubinstein LZ, et al. Yield of routine annual laboratory tests in a skilled nursing home population. *JAMA* 1987;258:1909–1915.
13. Irvine PW, VanBuren N, Crossley K. Causes for hospitalization of nursing home patients: the role of infection. *J Am Geriatr Soc* 1984;32:103–107.
14. Franson TR, Duthie EH, Cooper JE, et al. Prevalence survey of infections and their predisposing factors at a hospital-based nursing home care unit. *J Am Geriatr Soc* 1986;34:95–100.
15. Barker WH. Excess pneumonia and influenza associated hospitalizations during influenza epidemics in the United States, 1970–1978. *Am J Public Health* 1986;76:761–765.
16. Niederman MS, Fein AM: Pneumonia in the elderly. *Geriatr Clin North Am* 1986;2:241–269.

17. LaForce FM, Young LS, Bennet JV. Tetanus in the United States (1965–1966): epidemiologic and clinical features. *N Engl J Med* 1969;280:569–574.

18. Stead WW. Tuberculosis among elderly persons: an outbreak in a nursing home. *Ann Intern Med* 1981; 94:606–610.

19. Patriarca PA, Arden NH, Koplan JP, et al. Prevention and control of type A influenza infections in nursing homes: benefits and costs of four approaches using vaccination and amantadine. *Ann Intern Med* 1987; 107:732–740.

20. Stead WW, To T, Harrison RW, et al. Benefit-risk considerations in preventive treatment for tuberculosis in elderly persons. *Ann Intern Med* 1987;107:843–845.

21. Bentley DW, Iba K, Mamot K, et al. Pneumococcal vaccine in the institutionalized elderly: design of a nonrandomized trial and preliminary results. *Rev Infect Dis* 1981;3(suppl):S71–S81.

22. Sims RV, Steinmann WC, McConville JH, et al. The clinical effectiveness of pneumococcal vaccine in the elderly. *Ann Intern Med* 1988;108:653–657.

23. Reuler JB, Cooney TG. The pressure sore: Pathophysiology and principles of management. *Ann Intern Med* 1981;94:661–666.

24. Stamler R, Stamler J, Grimm R, et al. Nutritional therapy for high blood pressure: Final report of a four-year randomized controlled trial: the Hypertension Control Program. *JAMA* 1987;257:1484–1491.

25. Wilkins CE, Khurana MS. Digitalis withdrawal in elderly nursing home patients. *J Am Geriatr Soc* 1985;33:850–851.

26. Alessi C, Henderson C. Constipation and fecal impaction in the long-term care patient. *Geriatr Clin North Am.* 1988;4:571–588.

27. Burns BJ, Kamerow DB. Psychotropic drug prescriptions for nursing home residents. *J Fam Pract* 1988;26:155–160.

28. Ray WA, Griffin MR, Schaffner W, et al. Psychotropic drug use and the risk of hip fracture. *N Engl J Med* 1987;316:363–369.

29. Fitzgerald JF, Fagan LF, Tierney WM, et al. Changing patterns of hip fracture care before and after implementation of the prospective payment system. *JAMA* 1987;258:218–221.

30. Sager MA, Leventhal EA, Easterling DV. The impact of Medicare's prospective payment system on Wisconsin nursing homes. *JAMA* 1987;257:1762–1766.

31. Kastenbaum RS, Candy SE. The 4% fallacy: methodological and empirical critique of extended care facility program statistics. *Int J Aging Hum Dev* 1973;4:15–21.

32. Cohen MA, Tell EJ, Wallack SS. The lifetime risks and costs of nursing home use among the elderly. *Med Care* 1986;24:1161–1172.

33. McConnel CE. A note on the lifetime risk of nursing home residency. *Gerontologist* 1984;24:193–198.

34. Rosenwaike I. A demographic portrait of the oldest old. *Milbank Mem Fund Q* 1985;63:187–205.

35. Rice DP. The medical care system: past trends and future projections. *NY Med Q* 1986;6:39–70.

36. Butler RN. The teaching nursing home. *JAMA* 1981; 245:1435–1437.

37. Libow LS. The teaching nursing home: past, present, and future. *J Am Geriatr Soc* 1984;32:598–603.

38. Schneider EL. Teaching nursing homes. *N Engl J Med* 1983;308:336–337.

39. Schneider EL, Ory M, Aung ML. Teaching nursing homes revisited: survey of affiliations between American medical schools and long-term-care facilities. *JAMA* 1987;257:2771–2775.

40. Wieland D, Rubinstein LZ, Ouslander JG, et al. Organizing an academic nursing home. *JAMA* 1986;255:2622–2627.

41. Langer E. Human experimentation: cancer studies at Sloan-Kettering stir public debate on medical ethics. *Science* 1964;143:551–553.

42. Cassel CK. Research in nursing homes: ethical issues. *J Am Geriatr Soc* 1985;33:795–799.

43. Ratzan R. Being old makes you different: the ethics of research with elderly subjects. *Hastings Cent Rep* 1980;10(5):32–42.

44. Warren JW, Sobal J, Tenney JH, et al. Informed consent by proxy: an issue with elderly patients. *N Engl J Med* 1986;315:1124–1128.

45. Rossman I. Nursing homes: dim past, bright future. *Geriatr Med Today* 1988;7:23–31.

46. Mitchell JB. Physician visits to nursing homes. *Gerontologist* 1982;22:45–48.

47. Mitchell JB, Hewes HT. Why won't physicians make nursing home visits? *Gerontologist* 1986;26:650–654.

48. Paulson SD. Family physicians' activities in nursing homes: The Minnesota experience. *J Fam Pract* 1987;25:382–385.

49. Avorn J. Nursing-home infections: the context. *N Engl J Med* 1981;305:759–760.

Interdisciplinary Collaboration: Teamwork in Geriatrics

Ruth Ann Tsukuda

Experience has taught us that the complex health care needs of frail elderly patients demand knowledge, skills, and expertise that no single health care discipline alone can provide. It is likely that in addition to physicians and nurses, the skills of social workers, physical therapists, dieticians, pharmacists, and psychologists will be required. Furthermore, these health care professionals also may use the resources of other providers through consultative relationships. From this broad-based collaborative arrangement among health care professionals, the concept of the interdisciplinary geriatric team has developed. These teams bring together health providers from a variety of disciplines to assess, treat, and monitor the health status of elderly patients with multiple, complex, interacting problems.[1-4]

Definitions

The use of a team to address the care needs of elderly patients is an appropriate intervention for delivering health care services to special populations. Teamwork is a special form of interactional interdependence between health care providers, who merge different but complementary skills or viewpoints in the service of patients and in the solution of their health problems. While there have been many definitions of interprofessional teamwork throughout the years, Beckhard's[5] definition may be among the most simple: "A team is a group with a specific task or tasks, the accomplishment of which requires the interdependent

and collaborative efforts of its members." Even this simple definition is based on several important assumptions[6]:

1. The problem is big and/or complex enough to require more than one set of skills or knowledge.
2. The amount of relevant knowledge or skills is so great that one person cannot possess them all.
3. Assembling a group or team of professionals with more than one set of knowledge or skills will enhance the solution of the problem.
4. In the solution of such a problem, the possessors of the relevant skills or knowledge are (at least temporarily) considered to be equal or equally important.
5. All of the involved professionals are working for a common goal for which they are willing to sacrifice some professional security.

Interdisciplinary teamwork, therefore, is a mechanism that formalizes joint action toward mutually defined goals and implies a joint responsibility for actions or decisions to accomplish these goals.

Medical teams are not new. Within the framework of an acute care hospital, they have been widely used to deal with crisis-oriented or life-threatening problems, such as open heart surgery, organ transplantations, burns, and cardiac care, which usually require highly technical and frequently lifesaving interventions and procedures. On such teams, roles are clear, tasks are delegated, and the structure usually is hierarchical. Sometimes, they are monodisciplinary in composition, with teamwork primarily involving different levels of training or skill within a particular specialty area of medicine or surgery.

Other types of teams provide a specific set of services to patients with complex long-term problems (eg, developmental and learning disabilities, speech and hearing problems, stroke rehabilitation). In this setting, effective diagnosis and management usually call for diverse skills and technologies and the collaboration of more than one professional discipline. These teams are now well-accepted mechanisms for delivering care both within and outside of a hospital. In general, they are multidisciplinary in nature, with tasks and services being delivered in sequence or even in different settings according to a predetermined plan. Leadership usually is vested in the discipline with the most training and status, although the management of a patient may fall on other members of a team.

More recently, teamwork has been espoused as a means of better meeting the complex primary health care needs of underserved populations.[7,8] These health care teams are aimed at providing comprehensive primary care to a wide range of individuals or families, usually in an ambulatory setting. In this case, the diversity of the clinical problems that are presented and the broad range of tasks and skills that are required for their solution calls for an interdisciplinary type of approach, which involves interactions among team members, with considerable attention being directed at the negotiation of roles and tasks, as well as the quality of the relationship between team members and between a team and a patient.

In the care of the geriatric patient, the team will often combine the strength of both of these models. Thus, interdisciplinary teams may vary, depending on the nature of the patient problem, the personnel who participate, the setting for practice, the quality of the relationship among members, and the goal to be accomplished.

While the major goal of teamwork, from the viewpoint of a professional, can be simply stated as the achievement of maximum use with minimum redundancy, the following additional advantages have been suggested by the available literature[9]: greater access to other health professions and services; availability of a greater range of knowledge, skills, and services; greater efficiency through coordination and integration of services; increased communication and support among providers; greater opportunity for learning new knowledge and skills; and opportunity to practice at the highest level of skill and training. Advantages to a patient can include availability of a greater range of knowledge, skills, and services; better coordination of care and services; greater convenience; and more opportunity for preventive and educational interventions.

Teamwork in Geriatric Care

The specific issue in geriatrics is how to care better for persons whose problems are chronic and vastly complex. These problems involve multiple systems of the body. They affect multiple dimensions of the life situation, including psychological, emotional, social, and environmental factors, which together may be more debilitating than actual physical impairments. Being able to identify these multiple problems and their potential interactions, to assess the available resources, to define reasonable goals and priorities in treatment, and to develop a plan for continuing care requires a uniquely broad approach. Health among the elderly population consists not so much of the absence of disease, but of learning to lead maximally productive and independent lives through successful adaptation to the normal and abnormal changes of aging, as well as to illness. Even in complex and discouraging situations, a focus on limited but realistic goals may result in noticeable change. If this comprehensive approach to the provision of health care services to elderly patients is to be achieved, it is necessary to involve practitioners of many disciplines in a variety of arrangements and a wide spectrum of patient care facilities and services. Our current mechanisms for delivering health care services in fragmented, uncoordinated, often duplicative practice arrangements may no longer address the challenges faced by an ever-increasing number of frail elderly patients.

The unique challenge in geriatrics, therefore, is the efficient use of a group of providers whose combined and varied inputs can make a significant contribution to the care of these patients. Whether these providers choose to function independently or interdependently in a multidisciplinary or interdisciplinary fashion may be affected by a variety of factors (eg, patient needs and goals, available personnel and resources, physical settings, administrative policies, financial incentives). Also, a commitment to the functional advantages of collaboration and teamwork is required. While these two terms are not necessarily synonymous, they both involve a process of shared planning and action with a joint responsibility for outcomes. The concept of a team formalizes this process, with the additional element of a commitment over time to these goals and responsibilities.

Sites and Settings for Geriatric Teams

The location of services for care to geriatric patients spans the continuum. Care to aging populations is provided in a variety of settings: the patient's own home, foster homes, community-based clinics; senior centers; day-care centers; hospitals and outpatient clinics; and nursing homes and other residential programs. However, it should be noted that the hospital still serves as the major provider of health care services for frail elderly patients. Perhaps in no other environment is the need for teamwork so clear. The hospital that delivers health care in a technologically intensive manner offers health professionals a challenge as they address the multiple and intricate problems of this population. What better environment exists to begin to enhance patient care through improved communication and collaboration among health providers?

The delivery of health care in the hospital is complicated today by the concerns regarding escalating costs of care. As hospital staffs are confronted with the issue of cost containment, the implementation of a well-functioning geriatric team may serve to address some of these issues. For example, a geriatric team that identifies and addresses the needs of a patient soon after his admission, may effect earlier and more appropriate discharge planning, perhaps leading to a decreased length of stay and less chance of readmission.

If patients are discharged earlier, an obvious area for increased services for the geriatric team is in the home setting. The provision of appropriate in-home health care services may help to reduce the cost of care formerly provided in hospitals and nursing homes. Disagreement about actual cost-effectiveness remains, however, and the issue will continue to be debated. Even more important than financial savings, may be the social and psychological benefit people express by being able to remain in a familiar and comfortable home and family setting.

Another traditional site for geriatric care that often professes to use a team approach is the extended-care facility or nursing home. Although representation of various disciplines on the team may vary, it is commonly accepted that a team approach will enhance the well-being of patients in institutional settings.[10]

This discussion does not imply that all elderly patients are receiving care in institutional settings. Most, in fact, receive care through traditional relationships with primary care providers and will not need the vast resources of an interdisciplinary geriatric team. It is important to recognize that when the services of a solo practitioner are sufficient to meet the needs of the patient, it is unrealistic to impose a team approach. The extensive resources of the geriatric team should be used in efficient ways that maximize the potential outcomes of care.

Team Members

Ideally, membership on a health care team is determined by the disciplines and skills that are required to address the problem at hand. In reality, geriatric teams often comprise representatives from disciplines that are available within the organization and may not represent the full spectrum of needed expertise or services. To remedy this problem, new team members may have to be recruited, consultative arrangements may have to be developed, or new training may have to be provided to the available team members.

Among various geriatric teams, the concept of a "core" and "extended" team is common. The core team regularly functions together, ideally on a full-time basis.[11] Minimum membership includes a physician, nurse specialists, and a social worker. It is not at all unusual to see membership expanded to include a dietitian, pharmacist, and psychologist, for these are the disciplines frequently involved in the management of frail elderly patients.[7,12,13] The extended team consists of those members who routinely provide consultation and treatment for these same patients. Often, membership includes physical therapists, speech pathologists, audiologists, and occupational therapists. It is common to observe extended and core team members meeting together in group settings to review, discuss, and plan cooperatively strategies for effective patient management.

In less traditional health care settings, such as a hospice, day-care center, or home, a host of other professionals and nonprofessionals may be required to address the emotional, social, spiritual, and environmental needs of patients and their support systems. These service teams may include the clergy, case managers, home care aides, homemakers, drivers, and volunteers. Once again, the primary concern for team membership is recognizing which resources are necessary to meet the needs of the patient.

Finally, the most important aspect of teamwork is that no matter what the team configuration is, to meet the definition of team, members must work together in a coordinated manner to address the problem(s) at hand. Only through such an approach will teams achieve smooth and effective working relationships.

At a practical level, team members may collaborate or relate to a patient and to each other in a variety of ways. They may be involved in either shared visits, in which a physician and other team members see a patient together, or in alternating or sequential visits, in which each health professional sees a patient independently and meets with other team members at regular intervals to share knowledge and to arrive at appropriate plans. Team members also may "refer" patients to each other for special diagnostic or therapeutic procedures with the expectation that they will be kept informed and reinvolved when necessary. Finally, such visits may be consultative: one member of a team may consult with another member concerning a diagnosis and/or treatment. The particular choice of a collaborative style should be guided mainly by the needs of a patient, the system of care, and by frugality. An ideal team is one that is composed of the smallest number of individuals required to accomplish the task at hand in an efficient and adequate manner.

Much of this discussion presumes that there is a commitment to collaborative practice in the care of geriatric patients. It presumes that geriatric teams know what they are doing, who is doing it, and where it is being done. These decisions may have been reached through an orderly process of needs assessment, program development, and program evaluation, or they may have been determined by administrative mandate or by the availability of funding. In any case, the team must commit itself to the specific programmatic goals to accomplish them. Let us review the geriatric teams in terms of three essential elements necessary for program success: goals, tasks and roles, and leadership and decision making.

Goals and Objectives of Geriatric Teams

The literature on geriatric teams encompasses the breadth of settings where care is provided, including the community, the hospital, and the nursing home. It reflects the findings of programs that are both inpatient and outpatient; yet, not unexpectedly, there are many similarities among stated program goals.

The most commonly reported articles in the literature are those that concern the geriatric assessment or evaluation unit (GEUs). Most frequently, these units are institutionally based in either a hospital or extended hospital setting. However, some GEUs have developed in ambulatory care programs. The GEU programs offer comprehensive interdisciplinary assessment and treatment for frail elderly patients. They focus attention on the provision of comprehensive assessment services, treatment, rehabilitation, and identifying appropriate discharge planning strategies. More specifically, the objectives may include improving diagnosis, improving therapeutic planning, determining optimal placement, enhancing quality of life, improving utilization of scarce health care resources, documenting changes over time, and improving overall functioning.[1,14,15]

Another common approach to improving the care of elderly patients is through the geriatric consultative team. These consultative teams report their major goals as follows: to provide geriatric assessment, to improve discharge planning, to offer preoperative evaluation, and to provide education and research. Often cited are advice to aid in the medical and psychiatric management of frail elderly patients and an increase in rehabilitative services for these patients.[2,3,16–18]

A third approach in providing geriatric team care is the outpatient clinic or ambulatory care model.[19,20] In this setting, a team of health professionals provides services similar to those delivered in inpatient programs, but perhaps to a population that is somewhat less impaired.

Williams et al[4] have stated, "team-oriented outpatient assessment provides a promising way to deliver high quality, satisfying care to older persons without increasing (and possibly decreasing) health care costs." Like their more traditional inpatient counterparts, these geriatric teams address issues that concern functional ability, appropriately identify and use community resources, and provide comprehensive assessment. In summary, the goals of geriatric assessment teams appear to be similar even though the setting in which the programs operate may be different.

The goals of teamwork in a nursing home may be identifying restorative approaches to improving activities of daily living or slowing down the rate of progressive decline. Attention may be directed to bringing team members together with the patient and family members to define appropriate patient treatment goals, which emphasize maintenance or improvement in functional abilities, rather than assessing complex medical problems.

The formulation of programmatic goals is not an easy task, but it remains a cornerstone of team development. Goals serve as the foundation on which future plans of action and performance standards will be implemented.[21,22] Thus, it is essential that the team's goals are clear, specific, and measurable.

Because most teams have multiple, complex, and, sometimes, even competing goals, it may be necessary to set priorities among the established goals and objectives. Finally, it is important to remember that goals are not fixed. In fact, they should be reviewed, evaluated, and redefined as program needs change.

Tasks and Roles

Identification of the disciplines needed to provide necessary services for elderly patients is not sufficient to resolve the important issues of task differentiation and role negotiation on a geriatric team. These are essential elements in team development and need to be accomplished before proceeding further.

A logical outgrowth of defining team goals and objectives is the elaboration of the various tasks and activities by which the goals are to be accomplished. Whenever possible, the differentiation of tasks (things to be done) should precede the negotiations of roles (who is to do them).

In determining what tasks need to be done, it is also necessary to determine *how* things should get done. This involves integrating information, functions, and activities to get the job done efficiently and effectively, with a minimum of confusion and conflict. As the health care system evolves, the work of the team will also change.

These changes in the delivery of health care services involve not only the type of care, but also those who provide care. As the system has evolved, so have different health professionals. The complexity of care has required that professionals acquire new knowledge, skills, and expertise, resulting in a new definition of professional roles and relationships. In geriatrics, as in other areas of health care, there are areas of practice unique to specific disciplines, but there are also considerable areas of overlap with other disciplines. When roles overlap and when expertise is shared, problems may occur.[23] These may include an increased potential for conflict, duplication of efforts, and difficulty in defining professional boundaries. To counteract these potential problems, teams need to spend time defining and communicating expectations of the team and individual members, identifying areas of existing or potential conflict, and clearly assigning roles that are compatible with the skills and experience level of team members. In teams where roles and relationships are ambiguous, it is not at all unusual to observe feelings of misunderstanding, distrust, dissatisfaction, or anger. The definition of who does what is not necessarily easy, but must be addressed if goals are to be accomplished.

In general, services or tasks should be performed by those with the most appropriate training. Complex tasks and decisions should be carried out at the highest level, and simple tasks should be assigned to those with lower levels of skills. By so doing, team members are able to practice at the most appropriate level and are free to perform in areas where their professional expertise is most needed. To accomplish this, team members must have some understanding of the contribution by other team members and the interdependence of team members. The most effective teams will consist of a cohesive group of professionals who have different but complementary skills and who trust and respect the expertise of other team members.

Leadership and Decision Making

Other issues that are related to team practice concern leadership and decision making. These issues are, by definition, partly determined by the nature of the disciplines represented, as well as by the goals and tasks of a team. Conversely, a number of authors have called attention to the traditional power and prestige of the medical profession in defining relationships on teams, as well as in negotiating team issues, such as leadership and decision making.[24] While the team arrangement for delivery of care questions the traditional power dispositions of medicine, it cannot be denied that both historical and medicolegal precedents clearly put power and authority in the hands of a physician in the medical or patient care arena.

At the same time, the emerging norm on many teams appears to be one of equal opportunity for participation and joint responsibility on the part of team members. This involves the concept of "shifting leadership," in which this role is determined less by traditional considerations than by the particular problem to be solved and the particular skills of team members.[7]

Although some teams may choose not to designate a formally appointed leader, it is a misconception that teams can function effectively without leadership. One or more team members must assume responsibility for seeing that plans are developed, tasks are assigned, and work is accomplished.

A major function of a team is to make decisions and solve problems. However, not all decisions need to involve an entire team. While decision making traditionally tends to follow the lines of organizational structure or power and status, the present trend in complex human systems "is to have decisions made as close to the source of the problem as possible, and by those who have the relevant information, regardless of their role or location in the organizational hierarchy."[5] In the clinical area, this means that the team members who best know a patient and the problem should have a major role in reaching and effecting the decision after consulting with, or informing, other members of the team.

In reaching decisions, teams must address what needs to be decided, who should be involved in the decision-making process, who will carry out the decision, and who should be informed about the decision. To facilitate this process, teams need to establish well-functioning systems of communication, involving the opportunity for both formal meetings and informal exchanges of information and well-designed record-keeping systems. The communication system may include problem-oriented medical records, standardized assessment forms familiar to all team members, interdisciplinary case conferences, or bedside rounds that include appropriate team members.

When a heterogeneous group of health professionals is brought together, there will be a diversity of views and differences of opinion about how to address a particular problem. Thus, conflict is inevitable and should be viewed by the team as necessary and desirable if the group is to evolve into an efficient and productive team. Although conflict often is viewed with trepidation, successful confrontation and resolution of differences will have positive results as innovative and creative solutions are determined. Failure to deal with conflict can result in low morale, lack of involvement, anger, lack of trust, and decreased commitment. When this happens, productivity goes down, members become estranged, creativity declines, and, not infrequently, teams fall apart.

Team Development and Maintenance

The technology of team development has derived from several theoretical orientations (eg, general systems, communication sciences, group dynamics, organizational development); various skills and concepts have been identified that can enable a group of health care professionals to work toward achieving more effective teamwork through the collaborative development of rules for governing their work. These rules are needed to cover such areas as goal setting, role definition and negotiation, problem solving, decision making, leadership, and conflict management. The basic assumption is that teams that develop skills in these areas will be better able to perform tasks, whatever their nature.[21]

Major content areas that health teams have experienced as essential to their development include knowledge and skills in management, group process, interpersonal communication, and interdisciplinary or interprofessional interaction. Acquisition of knowledge and skills in these areas will enhance not only the working relationships on a team and with its colleagues, but also will promote a more satisfying environment in which to work.

A frequent mistake of many teams has been to focus on interpersonal needs and issues first, instead of defining the necessary rules and procedures for working together. All too often, when difficulties occur on teams, they are assumed to be the result of basic personality conflicts rather than a lack of procedures for accomplishing tasks together. As a team resolves ambiguities over goals and roles and deals effectively with the issues of leadership, power, and decision making, interpersonal conflict tends to diminish.

Even after a team is well established, the need occasionally arises to go back and rework one or another issue. For example, goals and roles may need to be renegotiated as tasks are successfully accomplished or conditions change. Some reworking of issues may be called for when a new person joins a team. Despite his or her apparent understanding of, and commitment to, the concept of teamwork, each new member must be provided the opportunity to "own" and contribute to the goals of the team. A failure to do this almost always results in problems in other areas, including the interpersonal.

Without outside assistance, it may be extremely difficult for a group of health care professionals to examine their behavior in a fashion that leads to optimal development as a team. The presence of a consultant who calls attention to the process and behavior of a team and defines procedures for working together may enable satisfactory team development.

As with machines, teams need regular and ongoing maintenance. Regular team meetings, plus periodic workshops or retreats for the purpose of processing new or recurring issues with or without outside consultants, are advisable. The essential element is the commitment and legitimation of a regular time and opportunity for team interaction around task and process issues (eg, clinical management, administrative organization, interpersonal communication, ongoing team development). Without this commitment, progress toward teamwork soon dissolves under the pressure of service demands.

Barriers to Teamwork

Much of the foregoing discussion has emphasized the positive aspects of collaboration. However, developing teamwork is not easy. If we examine teamwork in the health professions, we find that from the educational perspective, as well as the practice setting, concepts of teamwork are all too often lacking. The basic structure of our academic institutions offers different theoretical viewpoints, education, and experience for students. Our system of a rigid, standardized, and separate education for health profession students emphasizes unique bodies of expertise, often overshadowing commonalities among disciplines. Is it any wonder that health professionals sometimes have difficulty with developing or working in teams?

Barriers to teamwork in clinical practice occur at

three levels: individual, team, and organizational. At the individual level, barriers may be associated with the acculturation of the individual to the profession, the individual's understanding of his or her role in relation to others, and expectations of teamwork and motivation. It is not uncommon for staff to be assigned to a team because they are the newest persons in the department or because it is a convenient decision. Less frequently do we consider motivation to work in collaborative practice arrangements as a selection criterion for teamwork.

Interactions within the team can inhibit its ability to work effectively. Issues, such as incompatible personalities of team members, struggles for power, leadership, or control, and misunderstandings about roles, may cause problems as the team addresses work to be done. The organizational or environmental setting in which teams operate provide more opportunities for failure. Teams are not free-floating entities; they function within a system that has its own rules, procedures, and expectations. This larger system may be less tolerant of innovative practice arrangements and may, in fact, view the team as a threat to the status quo.

Geriatric Teams and Education

Interdisciplinary geriatric teams offer excellent and innovative teaching resources for students in the health professions. In addition to education in the assessment and management of elderly patients with chronic disease, students are exposed to environments that promote collaboration and cooperation among representatives of many health disciplines.[10,16,25–27] Regardless of the setting, well-functioning geriatric teams allow students to understand the role of their own discipline in the care of elderly patients while gaining understanding of the contribution of other team members. As they acquire new skills, recognition of the interdependent nature of the health care professions, and trust and respect, students gain confidence in the unique aspects of their own discipline as well. Thus, they will appreciate the nature of geriatrics, which builds on an understanding of the individual contributions of team members plus the enhanced perspective of the cooperative team effort.

Evaluating Geriatric Team Programs

Today, the literature in geriatrics is replete with articles concerning geriatric teams and the services provided by them.[1–4,14–20] In general, success has been reported in the areas of improved assessment and diagnosis, better clinical management, improvements in determining discharge plans, and continuing care. However, there are many fundamental issues that have not been adequately addressed. Discussion in this chapter has focused on geriatric teams that care for frail elderly populations. Recognizing the heterogeneity of this population, are we allocating resources in the best ways, or should we be looking at expansion of the geriatric team concept in such areas as prevention? Although research has addressed the outcome of team care, still little is known about the way in which teams organize themselves to provide care. Often, it is difficult to ascertain the unique attributes that allow services performed by a geriatric team to be more effective than those services provided by individual disciplines not using a team approach.

Evaluation research concerning geriatric teams provides a challenging opportunity. It is not enough to study the outcome of care without addressing the process. Studies that link these two elements will contribute to our understanding of how best to use scarce resources as the demand for services increases.

In conclusion, perhaps now is the time to stop debating the usefulness of geriatric teams and focus our attention on improving the effectiveness of this modality that is commonly accepted as relevant and appropriate. T. Franklin Williams,[28] in his 1985 Freeman lecture, best summarized the realities of geriatrics today when he said:

. . . it is clearly impossible for any one professional to address adequately the full range of problems older patients often present, usually at times of crisis—medical or social. The rapid appearance of multidisciplinary geriatric assessment or consultative clinics and services in many settings, staffed with physicians, nurses, and social workers, all of whom are directly involved with the work-up and planning for the care of the patient and family, together with the regular use of other consultants, all speak to the growing recognition of a team approach. To be a "complete geriatrician" means to be a team geriatrician.

References

1. Rubenstein L. Geriatric assessment programs in the US, *Clin Geriatr Med* 1986;2:99–112.
2. Barker W, Williams TF, Zimmer J, et al. Geriatric consultation teams in acute hospitals: impact on back-up of elderly patients. *J Am Geriatr Soc* 1985;33:422–428.
3. Campion E, Jette A, Berkman B. An interdisciplinary consultation service: a controlled trial. *J Am Geriatr Soc* 1983;31:792–796.
4. William ME, Williams TF, Zimmer J, et al. How does the team approach to geriatric evaluation compare with traditional care: a report of a randomized trial. *J Am Geriatr Soc* 1987;35:1071–1078.
5. Beckhard R. Organizational issues in the team delivery

of comprehensive health care. *Milbank Q* 1972;50:287–316.

6. New PK. An analysis of the concept of teamwork. *Community Ment Health J* 1968;4:326–333.

7. Parker AW. *The Team Approach to Primary Health Care*. Berkeley, Calif: University of California; 1972.

8. Beloff JS, Korper M. The health team model and medical care utilization. *JAMA* 1972;219:359–366.

9. Kane RA. *Interprofessional Teamwork, Manpower Monograph 8*. Syracuse, NY: Division of Continuing Education and Manpower Development, Syracuse University School of Social Work; 1975.

10. Thompson RF, Rhyne RL, Stratton MA, et al. Using an interdisciplinary team for geriatric education in a nursing home. *J Med Educ* 1988;63:796–798.

11. Shukla RB. The role of the primary care team in the care of the elderly. *Practitioner* 1981;225:791–797.

12. Andrus LH. The health care team: Concept and reality. In: Kane RI, ed. *New Health Practitioners*. Washington, DC: Fogarty International Series on Teaching of Preventive Medicine; 1975. US Dept of Health, Education, and Welfare publication 75-875.

13. Lamberts H, Riphagen FE. Working together in a team for primary health care: a guide to dangerous country. *J R Coll Gen Pract* 1975;25:745–752.

14. Wisensale SK. An evaluation model for the geriatric assessment team. *Generations* Fall 1987;12:71–73.

15. Robertson D, Christ L, Stalder L. Geriatric assessment unit in a teaching hospital. *Can Med Assoc J* 1986;126:1060–1064.

16. Blumenfield S, Morris J, Sherman F. The geriatric team in the acute care hospital. *J Am Geriatr Soc* 1982;30:660–664.

17. Winograd CH, Gerety M, Brown E, et al. Targeting the hospitalized elderly for geriatric consultation. *J Am Geriatr Soc* 1988;36:1113–1119.

18. Berkman B, Campion E, Swagerty E, et al. Geriatric consultation team: alternate approach to social work discharge planning. *J Gerontol Social Work* Spring 1983;5:77–88.

19. Kerkski D, Drinka T, Carnes M, et al. Post geriatric evaluations unit follow-up: team versus nonteam. *J Gerontol* March 1987;42:191–195.

20. Millman A, Forciea M, Fogel D, et al. A model of interdisciplinary ambulatory geriatric care in a Veterans Administration Medical Center. *Gerontologist* September 1986;26:471–474.

21. Rubin IM, Plovnick, MS, Fry RE. *Improving the Coordination of Care: A Program for Health Team Development*. Cambridge, Mass: Ballinger Publishing Co; 1975.

22. Ducanis AJ, Golin AK. *The Interdisciplinary Health Care Team: Handbook*. Rockville, Md: Aspen Systems Corp; 1979.

23. Rubin IM, Beckard R. Factors influencing the effectiveness of health teams. *Milbank Q* 1972;50:317–335.

24. Friedson E. *Profession of Medicine*. New York, NY: Dodd Mead & Co Inc; 1970.

25. Tsukuda RA, Walsh J. ITTG and GFP: Training physicians for the future. *VA Practitioner* March 1984;1:50–54.

26. Clark P. Participatory health seminars for nursing home residents: a model for multidisciplinary education. *Gerontology Geriatrics Educ* Summer 1984;4:75–84.

27. Clark P, Spence D, Sheehan J. A service learning model for interdisciplinary teamwork in health and aging. *Gerontology Geriatrics Educ* Summer 1986;6:3–16.

28. Williams TF. Geriatrics: the fruition of the clinician reconsidered. *Gerontologist* 1986;26:345–349.

Index